MONOGRAPHS IN CONTACT ALLERGY
Anton C. de Groot

Volume 1: Non-Fragrance Allergens in Cosmetics
Volume 2: Fragrances and Essential Oils

MONOGRAPHS IN CONTACT ALLERGY
VOLUME 2

FRAGRANCES AND ESSENTIAL OILS

MONOGRAPHS IN CONTACT ALLERGY
VOLUME 2

FRAGRANCES AND ESSENTIAL OILS

Anton C. de Groot

With the help of Heleen de Jong in drawing the structural formulas

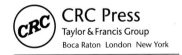

CRC Press
Taylor & Francis Group
Boca Raton London New York

CRC Press is an imprint of the
Taylor & Francis Group, an **informa** business

CRC Press
Taylor & Francis Group
6000 Broken Sound Parkway NW, Suite 300
Boca Raton, FL 33487-2742

© 2019 by Taylor & Francis Group, LLC
CRC Press is an imprint of Taylor & Francis Group, an Informa business

First issued in paperback 2021

No claim to original U.S. Government works

ISBN 13: 978-1-03-207894-6 (pbk)
ISBN 13: 978-0-367-14980-2 (hbk)

Visit the Taylor & Francis Web site at
http://www.taylorandfrancis.com

and the CRC Press Web site at
http://www.crcpress.com

Publisher's Note
The publisher has gone to great lengths to ensure the quality of this reprint but points out that some imperfections in the original copies may be apparent.

Contents

SECTION III   ESSENTIAL OILS

SECTION IV LISTS OF SYNONYMS AND INDEX

PREFACE

Perfumes (fragrances) such as eau de parfum, eau de toilette, deodorant, and aftershave are used by a large portion of the population. In addition, most people have contact with fragrances, often on a daily basis, from their presence in other cosmetics and in household products. Therefore, it can hardly come as a surprise that some consumers will develop contact allergic reactions to one or more fragrance materials. In fact, it has become clear that fragrance allergy is very common. In a 2018 meta-analysis, the pooled prevalence for sensitization to the fragrance mix I (a mixture of 8 fragrance chemicals and an 'indicator' or 'marker' for fragrance contact allergy) in the adult general population was 3.5%. As it is well known that this fragrance mix leaves a considerable number of sensitizations undetected, the author estimates that up to 4.5% of the adult population may be allergic to one or more fragrances. This does not mean that these individuals are all perfume-intolerant, suffer or have suffered from allergic reactions, but they do have the potential to develop allergic contact dermatitis from perfumes or perfumed products.

In the last two decades, much research has been performed in the field of fragrance contact allergy, which has resulted in exciting new discoveries, e.g. that some fragrances which have a low allergenic potential such as linalool and limonene turn into far more potent allergens by oxidation processes, in which strongly allergenic hydroperoxides are formed. The creation and introduction of the fragrance mix II has been another important advancement.

Because of recent developments and the eminent importance of fragrances as causes of contact allergy and allergic contact dermatitis, dermatologists, allergists and other professionals performing patch tests should have (access to) a thorough knowledge of the subject and of individual fragrances, both to provide optimal diagnostic services and to be able to properly counsel patients after the diagnosis of fragrance allergic contact dermatitis has been made. In various recent textbooks on contact dermatitis and in scientific journals, fragrance sensitization has been reviewed. Although these book chapters and articles are useful, they cannot be more than rather superficial (which is of course unavoidable because of limited available space), are always incomplete and the ones published before 2005 lack recent important developments, so that their information is not up-to-date anymore. Not a single individual fragrance has been thoroughly reviewed and relevant information, if searched for, has to be obtained from many different sources.

Therefore, the author, who has been interested in contact allergy to and other side effects of fragrances, essential oils and cosmetics since the early 1980s, decided to create an all-encompassing reference work covering the full spectrum of fragrance chemicals/substances that have caused contact allergy by their presence in fine fragrances, cosmetics, household products or any other materials. Essential oils were included, as they are also used in perfumes and not infrequently cause allergic reactions.

A total of 165 such fragrance chemicals and extracts and 79 essential oils are presented in Monographs. The information provided for each allergen includes a thorough identification with INCI name, chemical/IUPAC name, other names (synonyms), CAS registry number, EC (European Community) number(s), and their molecular and structural formulas (where applicable). Also, a general description/definition of the compounds is provided, the chemical class(es) to which they belong, and whether and where more information can be found in reviews and monographs published by CIR (Cosmetic Ingredient Review), RIFM (Research Institute for Fragrance Materials), IFRA (International Fragrance Association), the Merck Index and European Union SCCS/SCCP/SCCFNP Opinions, and in addition EU and IFRA restrictions on the use of certain fragrances. Advice on patch test concentration and vehicle is given for all fragrances and essential oils discussed.

The information provided also includes – where applicable and available - the results of studies performing patch testing in the general population, in groups of consecutive patients suspected of contact dermatitis (routine testing) and in groups of selected patients, case reports and case series of allergic contact dermatitis, cross-reactions, reports of patch test sensitization, presence in products and chemical analyses, results of ROATs and serial dilution testing, other side effects such as irritant contact dermatitis, photosensitivity, immediate-type reactions, other non-eczematous reactions, systemic side effects from percutaneous absorption and any other information found in literature considered by the author to be relevant to the readers.

This book presents detailed information on contact allergy and allergic reactions to fragrances and essential oils of which a substantial part which will not be found by searching in PubMed and other medical and chemical databases. It gives full coverage of all aspects of fragrance allergens not only for dermatologists and allergists to improve levels of medical knowledge and quality of patient care, but also for the benefit of professionals beyond clinical study and practice, such as chemists working in the fragrance, flavor, cosmetic or essential oils industries, other researchers developing and marketing cosmetic products, and legislators.

This is the second volume in a series of 'Monographs in Contact Allergy', discussing fragrances and essential oils. In the first volume, non-fragrance allergens in cosmetics were presented. In a third volume, contact allergy to topical and systemic drugs is planned to be reviewed in-depth.

Anton de Groot, MD, PhD
Wapserveen, The Netherlands, January 2019

ACKNOWLEDGMENTS

The author is very grateful to the following organizations and individuals:

- to Dr. Matthias Vey, Scientific Director of IFRA (International Fragrance Organization) for giving permission to use data from the IFRA standards for fragrances

- to Joanne Nikitakis, Director, Cosmetic Chemistry, Personal Care Products Council, for permission to use data from the Personal Care Products Council Ingredient Database in the Identification section of each Monograph

- to Dr. Ir. Dirk van Aken, chemist, who gave me much useful chemistry information where my knowledge on the subject was insufficient

- to Heleen de Jong BSc, who spent much time in meticulously drawing the beautiful structural formulas shown in this book

- and to Erich Schmidt, for allowing me to use his analytical data of essential oils previously published in the book `Essential oils: Contact allergy and chemical composition' and for providing analytical data for essential oils newly included in this book

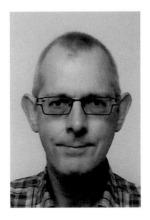
Dr. Ir. Dirk van Aken

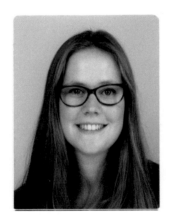
Heleen de Jong BSc

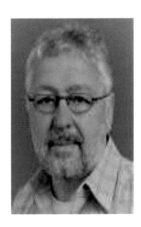
Erich Schmidt

ABOUT THE AUTHOR

Anton C. de Groot, MD, PhD (1951) received his medical and specialist training at the University of Groningen, The Netherlands. In 1980, he started his career as dermatologist in private practice in 's-Hertogenbosch. At that time, he had already become interested in contact allergy and in side effects of drugs by writing the chapter 'Drugs used on the skin' with his mentor prof. Johan Nater, for the famous 'Meyler's Side Effects of Drugs' series. Soon, the subject of this chapter in new Editions and the yearly 'Side Effects of Drugs Annuals' would be expanded to include cosmetics and oral drugs used in dermatology (1980-2000). Contact allergy to cosmetics would become de Groot's main area of interest and expertise and in 1988, he received his PhD degree on his Thesis entitled 'Adverse Reactions to Cosmetics', supervised by prof. Nater.

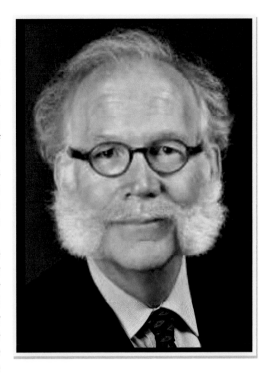

Frustrated by the lack of easily accessible information on the ingredients of cosmetic products, and convinced that compulsory ingredient labeling of cosmetics (which at that time was already implemented in the USA) would benefit both consumers and allergic patients and would lead to only slight and temporary disadvantages to the cosmetics industry, De Groot approached the newly founded European Society of Contact Dermatitis and became Chairman of the Working Party European Community Affairs. The European Commission and its committees, elected legislators, national trade, health departments and the cosmetics industries were extensively lobbied. This resulted in new legislation by the Commission of the European Communities in 1991, making ingredient labeling mandatory for all cosmetic products sold in EC Member States by December 31, 1997.

Anton has been the chairman of the 'Contact Dermatitis Group' of the Dutch Society for Dermatology and Venereology from 1984 to 1998. In 1990, he was one of the founders of the Nederlands Tijdschrift voor Dermatologie en Venereologie (Dutch Journal of Dermatology and Venereology) and was Editor of this scientific journal for 20 years, of which he served 10 years as Editor-in-chief.

De Groot has authored fourteen books, nine of which – all co-authored by Johan Toonstra MD, PhD – are general dermatology books in Dutch for medical students, general practitioners, 'skin therapists' (huidtherapeuten, a paramedical profession largely restricted to The Netherlands) and pedicures and podotherapists. Anton also authored four international books, of which one has had three Editions: 'Unwanted Effects of Cosmetics and Drugs used in Dermatology' (first Edition 1983, second 1985, third 1994). Of his best known book 'Patch Testing' (first Edition 1986, second 1994, third 2008) even a 4th Edition was published, in 2018 (www.patchtesting.info).

His recent international book 'Essential Oils: Contact Allergy and Chemical Composition', that he wrote with Erich Schmidt, appeared in 2016 and was very well received by dermatologists, the essential oils and fragrance industries and other disciplines. Early 2018, the first book in a planned series of 'Monographs in Contact Allergy' was released, discussing 'Non-Fragrance Allergens in Cosmetics'. The current book on 'Fragrances and Essential oils' is the second volume in this series. A third one on 'Topical and Systemic Drugs' is planned to be written in 2019.

In addition to these books, Anton has written over 70 book chapters (mostly in international books), over 125 articles in international journals and some 230 articles in Dutch medical and paramedical journals. He served as board member of several journals including 'Dermatosen' and is currently member of the Editorial Advisory Board of the Journal 'Dermatitis'.

Since 2012, De Groot has been consulting dermatologist and participant in CESES (Consumer Exposure Skin Effects and Surveillance), a Dutch Cosmetovigilance system monitoring side effects of cosmetics in The Netherland, performed by the National Institute for Public Health and the Environment by order of the Netherlands Food and Consumer Product Safety Authority.

Anton de Groot has retired from dermatology practice, but since 2008 regularly teaches general dermatology to junior medical doctors at the University of Groningen. He and his wife Janny have two daughters, both lawyers.

Monographs in Contact Allergy, Volume 2
Fragrances and Essential oils

SECTION 1

RATIONALE AND DATA PROVIDED IN THIS BOOK

CHAPTER 1   INTRODUCTION

1.1 WHY A BOOK WITH MONOGRAPHS ON FRAGRANCES AND ESSENTIAL OILS?

Contact allergy to fragrances is very common, both in patients seen by dermatologists for suspected contact dermatitis and in the general population. In a 2018 meta-analysis of 19 studies covering 19,440 patch tested individuals from the general population, the pooled prevalence for sensitization to the fragrance mix I (a mixture of 8 fragrance chemicals) was 3.5% (2). For Myroxylon pereirae resin, the pooled prevalence of sensitization was 1.8% (2). However, it is well known that these 'markers' (or 'indicators') of fragrance allergy leave a considerable number of fragrance sensitizations undetected, including the majority of reactions to the hydroperoxides of limonene and linalool, which have in recent years become the most prevalent fragrance sensitizers. The author estimates (Chapter 2.6) that up to 4.5% of the adult population may be allergic to one or more fragrances (which does not mean that they are all perfume-intolerant, suffer or have suffered from allergic reactions). Obviously, in patients investigated by dermatologists for suspected contact dermatitis, the prevalence of fragrance sensitization is much higher. In a 2015-2016 study performed in the United Kingdom, for example, of 2084 patients who were tested with the European baseline series and 27 individual fragrances, 359 (17.2%) reacted to at least one fragrance (5). In various other European countries and the USA, fragrance prevalence rates are generally higher than in the U.K., which means that frequencies of fragrance sensitization in the corresponding populations in these countries may well be 20-25% (Chapter 2.6).

In the last two decades, much research has been performed in the field of fragrance contact allergy, notably by European dermatologists. This has resulted in exciting new discoveries, e.g. that fragrances which have a low allergenic potential such as linalool, limonene and geraniol, turn into far stronger haptens by oxidation processes, in which strongly allergenic hydroperoxides are formed. Whereas testing with pure limonene and linalool hardly ever results in positive patch tests, testing with their hydroperoxides has shown that they are in fact very frequent causes of contact allergy and allergic contact dermatitis. One of the reasons for this may be that, both in cosmetics and in household products, these two chemicals belong to the most frequently used perfume ingredients. Another development which has greatly improved reliable testing for fragrance contact allergy was the creation of the fragrance mix II and its addition to the European (and most other) baseline series.

Because of the eminent importance of fragrances as causes of contact allergy and allergic contact dermatitis, it is important that dermatologists, allergists and other professionals performing patch tests should have a thorough knowledge of the subject and individual fragrances, both to provide optimal diagnostic services and to be able to properly counsel patients after the diagnosis of fragrance allergic contact dermatitis has been made. In recent textbooks on contact dermatitis, allergy to fragrances (and sometimes essential oils) are discussed in separate chapters (3,4,6) . Also, in scientific journals, in the period 2000-2017, in some articles the subject of fragrance sensitization has been reviewed (7,8,9,10,11). Although these are useful, they cannot be more than rather superficial (which is of course unavoidable because of limited available space), are always incomplete and the ones published before 2005 lack recent developments such as the experience with the fragrance mix II and the developments with for example limonene and linalool, so that their information is not up-to-date anymore. Not a single individual fragrance allergen has been thoroughly reviewed and relevant information, if searched for, has to be obtained from many different sources.

Therefore, the author, who has been interested in contact allergy to and other side effects of fragrances, essential oils and cosmetics since the early 1980s (17,18,19,20), decided to create an all-encompassing reference work covering the full spectrum of fragrance chemicals/substances that have caused contact allergy. After fully reviewing 'non-fragrance allergens in cosmetics' in *Monographs in Contact Allergy Volume 1* (12), the current work *Monographs in Contact Allergy Volume 2* presents in-depth monographs on all fragrances which have caused contact allergy / allergic contact dermatitis by their presence in fine fragrances, cosmetics, household products or any other materials. Essential oils, which have already been reviewed by the author in a previous work (13) are also included, as they are used in and as fragrances but also in many other applications and not infrequently cause sensitization. Actually, it is conceivable that the frequency of sensitization to essential oils containing high concentrations of limonene such as the Citrus oils and of linalool and linalyl acetate such as lavender oil has greatly been underestimated, because testing was always performed with unoxidized test material.

The author is aware that the terms 'allergen' and 'allergens' are often *sensu stricto* not correct and should read 'hapten' and 'haptens'. However, in scientific journals dedicated to contact dermatitis and contact allergy such as *Contact Dermatitis* and *Dermatitis* the term allergen is still often used and is also familiar to physicians, who are not experts in the field, and to non-physicians. Therefore, the term allergen is used throughout this book.

1.2 DATA PROVIDED IN THIS BOOK

SCOPE AND DATA COLLECTING

This book provides monographs of all fragrance chemicals/substances and essential oils that have caused contact allergy / allergic contact dermatitis from their presence in fine fragrances, other cosmetics, household products, diluted or undiluted essential oils or any other material.

The main sources of information are:
- the journals *Contact Dermatitis* and *Dermatitis*, that were fully screened from their start in 1975 resp. 1990 through December 2018;
- the author's 1988 PhD Thesis *Adverse reactions to cosmetics*, in which all previous literature on cosmetic allergy has been presented (or at least cited) (20);
- the author's books *Unwanted Effects of Cosmetics and Drugs used in Dermatology* (17,18,19) and other reference works: several editions of *Fisher's Contact Dermatitis* (6), Etain Cronin's 1980 book *Contact Dermatitis* (21) and the most recent editions of the books *Contact Dermatitis*, 6th Edition, 2018 (3) and *Kanerva's Occupational Dermatology*, 3rd Edition, 2018 [4]), in both of which the author wrote the chapter 'Fragrances and essential oils';
- the SCCS (Scientific Committee on Consumer Safety) Opinion on Fragrance allergens in cosmetic products, 26-27 June 2012, SCCS/1459/11 (14) and the similar publication in the journal *Contact Dermatitis* (8);
- relevant articles found in literature lists of journal publications used for the book; most of these could be accessed on-line through the Medical Library of the University of Groningen; important articles that were not accessible on-line were requested from the library and obtained digitally;
- all journals available on-line through the Medical Library of the University of Groningen; before finishing and closing a monograph (in the period September 2018-December 2018), the ingredient name was searched for in PubMed and any additional relevant articles and data were added;
- the new journal *Cosmetics* (not currently indexed in MEDLINE) and
- the Monographs on Fragrance materials published by the Research Institute for Fragrance Materials (RIFM).

Sometimes, relevant articles could neither be accessed on-line nor were they requested. If some relevant information was available, e.g. from the Abstract or from being cited in other sources, it was included, in the latter situation mentioning that the information was cited in another article. If data from such articles were missing, this is indicated with 'data missing / specific data unknown / article not read' in the Monograph text.

CRITERIA FOR INCLUSION

To be included in this book, fragrance chemicals/substances and essential oils had to meet one or more of the following criteria:
- they were presented in a case report as cause of allergic contact dermatitis;
- the chemical/substance was mentioned in a list of chemicals that had caused contact allergy / allergic contact dermatitis in groups of patients (1,22,23,24,25,26,27,28,29);
- when a positive patch test to a fragrance or essential oil was specifically stated or implied to be the cause of contact allergy by the author(s);
- the substance caused one or more positive patch test reactions in groups of patients tested with it, either consecutive patients suspected of contact dermatitis (routine testing) or selected patient groups, also when no comments were made on their relevance;
- the fragrances were cited as being causes of pigmented cosmetic dermatitis in the 1970s and 1980s in Japan (15); often, no specific data are available, as the results have been published in Japanese journals only.

Also included are a some chemicals that are not used as fragrances *per se*, but that may be present as allergenic ingredients in botanical products that are themselves used as fragrance materials such as Evernia furfuracea (treemoss) extract (atranol; atranorin; chloroatranol; fumarprotocetraric acid; physodalic acid; physodic acid), Evernia prunastri (oakmoss) extract (atranol; atranorin; chloroatranol; evernic acid; physodic acid (?); usnic acid), Melaleuca alternifolia (tea tree) leaf oil (aromadendrene; ascaridole; ledene; 1,2,4-trihydroxymenthane), and Myroxylon pereirae resin (balsam of Peru) (derivatives) (benzyl isoferulate; coniferyl alcohol; coniferyl benzoate; isoferulic acid).

Not included are fragrances which have shown positive patch tests only in investigations into their sensitizing potential, e.g. in Human Repeat Insult Patch Tests or Maximization tests, e.g. sclareol, phytol and delta-damascone.

DATA PROVIDED IN MONOGRAPHS

The literature search resulted in the identification of 165 fragrance materials (monographed in Chapter 3), 16 non-fragrance allergenic ingredients of botanical fragrance materials (Chapter 4) and 79 essential oils (Chapter 6). For each fragrance chemical/substance or essential oil that was included, the data shown in table 1.1 – when available and applicable - were searched for. For most fragrance chemicals, is has been attempted to provide a full (medical) literature review. However, the data in the essential oils monographs are generally limited to contact allergy / allergic contact dermatitis. Side effects of oral or parenteral administration are largely excluded from discussion.

Table 1.1 Information provided (when available and applicable) in the monographs

IDENTIFICATION	Structural formula
Description/definition	**CONTACT ALLERGY**
Chemical class(es)	Patch testing in the general population
INCI name USA	Patch testing in groups of patients
Chemical/IUPAC name	Case reports and case series
Other names	Cross-reactions, pseudo-cross-reactions and co-
CAS registry number(s)	reactions
EC number(s)	Patch test sensitization
CIR review(s)	Presence in products and chemical analyses
RIFM monograph(s)	Other information
IFRA standard	**OTHER SIDE EFFECTS** [a]
SCCS/SCCP/SCCFNP opinion(s)	Irritant contact dermatitis
ISO standard	Photosensitivity
Merck Index monograph	Immediate-type reactions
Function(s) in cosmetics (EU, USA)	Other non-eczematous contact reactions
EU cosmetic restrictions	Systemic side effects
Patch testing	Miscellaneous side effects
Molecular formula	**OTHER INFORMATION**

[a] For essential oils, other side effects are only presented when encountered 'by chance'; such data were not searched for and on this subject, the essential oils monographs are incomplete and do not provide a full or even broad review

IDENTIFICATION

In the section **IDENTIFICATION** the chemicals are identified by INCI name (EU name; USA name is mentioned only when different from EU name), chemical/IUPAC (International Union of Pure and Applied Chemistry) name, other names (synonyms), CAS (Chemical Abstract Service) registry (www.cas.org) number(s), EC (European Community) (formerly: EINECS [European Inventory of Existing Commercial Chemical Substances]) number(s), and their molecular and structural formulas (where applicable). Also, a general description/definition of the compounds is provided, the chemical class(es) to which they belong, and whether and where more information can be found in reviews and monographs published by CIR (Cosmetic Ingredient Review), the Research Institute for Fragrance Materials (RIFM) and in the Merck Index. Reference is made to any published European Union SCCS (Scientific Committee on Consumer Safety), SCCP (Scientific Committee on Consumer Products) or SCCFNP (Scientific Committee on Cosmetic Products and Non-Food Products Intended for Consumers) Opinions (back to June 1997), EU cosmetic restrictions and, for essential oils, the ISO standard. The functions of the chemicals, both in the EU and the USA are mentioned and an advice on how to patch test the chemical/substance is given in each Monograph. The sources of data provided in the section **IDENTIFICATION** are shown in table 1.2.

Table 1.2 Sources for the information in the section Identification

IDENTIFICATION	Sources (for Legends see below)
Description/definition	1, sometimes 2; for essential oils the descriptions from ref. 13 were used
Chemical class(es)	1
INCI name USA	1
Chemical/IUPAC name	1,2,3,4,5,6,7,13; 4 (IUPAC name)
Other names	1,3,4,5,6,7,13
CAS registry number (s)	1,2,3,4,5,6,7,13; CAS registry numbers have not been validated by the Chemical Abstract Service (www.cas.org) and may therefore be wrong in some cases
EC number(s)	1,2,11
CIR review(s)	8
RIFM monograph(s)	15

Table 1.2 Sources for the information in the section identification (continued)

IDENTIFICATION	Sources (for Legends see below)
IFRA standard	16
SCCS/SCCP/SCCFNP opinion(s)	2,12
ISO standard	14
Merck Index monograph	9
Function(s) in cosmetics (EU, USA)	2 (EU), 1 (USA)
EU cosmetic restrictions	2
Patch testing	10
Molecular formula	1,3,4,5,6,7
Structural formula	1,3,4,5,6,7 (all structural formulas have been drawn by Heleen de Jong BSc)

LEGENDS for Sources

1   The Personal Care Products Council (formerly Cosmetic, Toiletry and Fragrance Association) on-line ingredient database: http://online.personalcarecouncil.org/jsp/Home.jsp (choose Ingredient database) (subscription only); when no description was available (with chemicals not mentioned in the database, ergo no USA INCI name available), the description and chemical classes were assigned by dr. ir. Dirk van Aken, chemist, which was the case in the majority of fragrances

2   The European Commission database with information on cosmetic substances and ingredients CosIng: http://ec.europa.eu/growth/tools-databases/cosing/

3   United States National Library of Medicine ChemIDPlus Advanced database: https://chem.nlm.nih.gov/chemidplus/

4   PubChem: http://pubchem.ncbi.nlm.nih.gov/

5   ChemicalBook Inc.: www.chemicalbook.com

6   Chemspider: www.chemspider.com

7   Miscellaneous databases and websites found through Google search

8   Cosmetic Ingredient Review: http://www.cir-safety.org/

9   The Merck Index online: https://www.rsc.org/merck-index

10 Providers of patch test allergens: Chemotechnique Diagnostics (www.chemotechnique.se), SmartPractice EUROPE (www.smartpracticeeurope.com) and SmartPractice CANADA (www.smartpracticecanada.com). If not available from these suppliers, the test concentration(s) as used in the publication(s) is/are mentioned. If no Patch test concentration/vehicle was given in the article (e.g. the name was mentioned in a list of fragrance allergens with no specifics given), one or more test concentration as mentioned in the author's book 'Patch Testing', 4th Edition, are provided (16)

11 ECHA European Chemicals Agency, EC Inventory: https://echa.europa.eu/information-on-chemicals/ec-inventory

12 European Commission Health and Food Safety Scientific Committees: https://ec.europa.eu/health/scientific_committees/consumer_safety_en

13 The Good Scents Company Information System providing information for the flavor, fragrance, food and cosmetic industries: www.thegoodscentscompany.com

14 International Organization for Standardization: www.iso.org

15 Fragrance monographs published by the Research Institute for Fragrance Materials (RIFM), mostly in the journals *Food and Chemical Toxicology* (1982-2018) and *Food and Cosmetics Toxicology* (<1982)

16 International Fragrance Organization (IFRA): www.ifraorg.org/en-us/standards-library

IFRA standards

In case of restrictions in the use of fragrance materials issued by the International Fragrance Association IFRA, the maximum permitted concentrations in various product categories are shown in each monograph in the following table format. The products belonging to the 11 categories are detailed below.

Table ... 1 IFRA restrictions

Category	Limits	Category	Limits	Category	Limits
1	%	5	%	9	%
2	%	6	%	10	%
3	%	7	%	11	not restricted
4	%	8	%		

IFRA Categories

The following list of the 11 IFRA categories originates from IFRA RIFM QRA Information Booklet Version 7.1, Revised July 9, 2015, reproduced here with written permission of Dr. Matthias Vey, Scientific Director of IFRA, August 2018.

Category 1
Lip products of all types

Children's toys

Category 2
Deodorant and antiperspirant products of all types including any product with intended or reasonably foreseeable use on the axillae or labeled as such (spray, stick, roll-on, under-arm, deocologne and

body spray, etc.)
Nose pore strips
Fragranced bracelets

Category 3
Hydroalcoholic products applied to recently shaved skin (includes aftershave)
Fine fragrance
Eye products of all types (eye shadow, mascara, eyeliner, eye make-up, etc.) including eye care

Men's facial creams and balms
Tampons
Baby creams, lotions, oils
Body paint for children

Category 4
Hydroalcoholic products applied to unshaved skin (includes aqueous based, alcoholic based and hydroalcoholic) like cologne, eau de cologne, eau de parfum or parfum
Hair styling aids sprays of all types (pumps, aerosol sprays, etc.)
Body creams, oils, lotions of all types (except baby creams, lotions and oils)
Fragrancing cream
Body sprays (including body mist) with no intended or

reasonably foreseeable use on the axillae
Solid perfumes
Ingredients of perfume kits
Fragrance compounds for cosmetic kits
Scent pads, foil packs
Scent strips for hydroalcoholic products
Foot care products
Hair deodorant
Body paint (except those for children)

Category 5
Women's facial creams/facial make-up
Hand cream
Hand sanitizers
Facial masks
Baby powder and talc

Hair permanent and other hair chemical treatments (e.g. relaxers) but not hair dyes
Wipes or refreshing tissues for face, neck, hands, body
Dry shampoo or waterless shampoo

Category 6
Mouthwash, including breath sprays

Toothpaste

Category 7
Intimate wipes
Baby wipes

Insect repellent (intended to be applied to the skin)

Category 8
Make-up removers of all types (not including face cleansers)
Hair styling aids non-spray of all types (mousse, gels, leave-in conditioners, etc.)

Nail care
Powders and talcs, all types (except baby powders and talcs)
Hair dyes

Category 9
Conditioner
Liquid soap
Shampoos of all types (including baby shampoos)
Face cleansers of all types (washes, gels, scrubs, etc.)
Shaving creams of all types (stick, gels, foams, etc.)
All depilatories (including waxes for mechanical hair

removal)
Body washes of all types (including baby washes) and shower gels of all types
Bar soap (toilet soap)
Feminine hygiene – pads, liners
Bath gels, foams, mousses, salts, oils and other

products added to bathwater
Facial tissues
Fragranced face masks (not intended to be used as medical device)
Napkins
Paper towels

Toilet paper
Wheat bags
Other aerosols (including air freshener sprays and air freshener pump sprays, but not including deodorants / antiperspirants, hair styling aids sprays)

Category 10

Handwash laundry detergents of all types including concentrates
Fabric softeners of all types including fabric softener sheets
Household cleaning products, other types (fabric cleaners, soft surface cleaners, carpet cleaners, etc.)
Machine wash laundry detergents (liquids, powders, tablets, etc.) including laundry bleach and concentrates

Hand dishwashing detergent including concentrates
Hard surface cleaners of all types (bathroom and kitchen cleansers, furniture polish, etc.)
Diapers
Shampoos for pets
Dry cleaning kits
Scented gloves, socks, tights with moisturizers
Toilet seat wipes

Category 11

All non-skin contact or incidental skin contact including:
Candles
Air fresheners and fragrancing of all types (concentrated aerosol with metered doses (range 0.05-0.5ml/spray), plug-ins, solid substrate, membrane delivery, electrical)
Air delivery systems
Cell phone cases
Potpourri, powders, fragrancing sachets, liquid refills for air fresheners (non-cartridge systems), reed diffusers
Liquid refills for air fresheners (cartridge systems)
Shoe polishes
Deodorizers/maskers not intended for skin contact (e.g. fabric drying machine deodorizers, carpet powders)
Insecticides (mosquito coil, paper, electrical, for clothing etc.) excluding aerosols
Scent delivery system using a dry air technology that

releases a fragrance without sprays, aerosols or heated oils (technology of nebulization)
Air freshening crystals
Toilet blocks
Joss sticks or incense sticks
Machine dishwash detergent and deodorizers
Machine-only laundry detergent (e.g. liquitabs)
Plastic articles (excluding toys)
Fuels
Fragranced lamp ring
Scent pack
Scratch and sniff (sampling technology)
Paints
Cat litter
Animal sprays (all types)
Treatment products for textiles (e.g. starch sprays, fabric treated with fragrances after wash, deodorizers for textiles or fabrics)
Floor wax
Odored distilled water (that can be added to steam irons)

Update of IFRA standards 2019

IFRA Standards addressing sensitizing properties of fragrance ingredients up until the 48th Amendment are based on the so called QRA (Special Issue: Dermal Sensitization Quantitative Risk Assessment for Fragrance Ingredients, Regulatory Toxicology and Pharmacology, Volume 52, number 1, October 2008). With the 49th Amendment, scheduled to be notified in the course of 2019, the revised quantitative risk assessment will be introduced as refined in the IDEA process (www.ideaproject.info), the main refinement of which is the consideration of aggregate exposure (written communication from Dr. Matthias Vey, Scientific Director, IFRA, November 2018).

CONTACT ALLERGY AND ALL OTHER DATA

Patch testing in groups of patients

This section shows the results of studies performing patch testing in groups of consecutive patients suspected of contact dermatitis (routine testing) and in groups of selected patients, e.g. patients suspected of fragrance or cosmetic allergy, patients previously reacting to the fragrance mix I or Myroxylon pereirae resin (balsam of Peru), patients with leg ulcers, nurses with occupational contact dermatitis, or individuals with periocular or lip dermatitis. Data provided include country/countries of the study, period of study, patch test concentration and vehicle used, number of patients tested, number of patients and percentage with positive patch tests, mode of selection, relevance (both percentage and products), other relevant information (in the Comment section) and literature references.

Case reports and case series
Case reports are mostly the description of one, two or three patients with allergic contact dermatitis from the index fragrance. Clinical descriptions are given when only one or a few case reports for a particular chemical/substance have been published. In general, the more case reports were found in literature, the less information is provided (usually limited to number of patients, causative products and sometimes localization of dermatitis). Case series are mostly series of 4 or more patients, but far more often the number of patients in lists of causative ingredients in patients with certain or very probable fragrance allergic contact dermatitis (1,22,23,24,25,26,27,28,29).

General information on cross-reactions, pseudo-cross-reactions and co-reactions
It is often very difficult, if not impossible, to determine whether co-reactions (concomitant positive patch tests) to other fragrances in addition to the index chemical are the result of cross-reactivity (contact allergic reaction to a structurally similar chemical to which the individual has not yet been exposed), of pseudo-cross-reactions (the index chemical and the co-reacting chemical have the same allergenic constituent, contaminant, metabolite or oxidant product) or co-reactions, which are independent of each other. The latter case implies that the patient has been sensitized to the co-reacting chemical at the same time in the culprit allergenic product or at any time previously or later by its presence in this product or one or more other products.

It is well know that patients allergic to fragrances often are polysensitized: they have positive patch test reactions to at least three chemicals or compounds, most often other fragrances or mixtures, including the fragrance mix I, the fragrance mix II, Myroxylon pereirae resin (balsam of Peru), essential oils, and to a far lesser degree colophonium and propolis (both not used as fragrances, but weak 'indicators' or 'markers' of fragrance contact allergy). Although this is often termed 'cross-reactivity', pseudo-cross-reactions and independent sensitization from the presence of a multitude of fragrances in a vast array of products contacting human skin are far more likely scenarios. Even co-reactivity between the related cinnamyl alcohol and cinnamal, for example, are mostly not cross-reactions, as the little allergenic cinnamyl alcohol is converted in the skin into the more potent sensitizer cinnamal.

Examples of pseudo-cross-reactions include co-reactions of fragrance mix I and its 8 ingredients (amyl cinnamal, cinnamal, cinnamyl alcohol, eugenol, Evernia prunastri (oakmoss) extract, geraniol, isoeugenol and hydroxycitro-nellal); fragrance mix II and its 6 ingredients (citral, citronellol, coumarin, farnesol, hexyl cinnamal and hydroxy-isohexyl 3-cyclohexene carboxaldehyde); Myroxylon pereirae resin and some of its ingredients such as coniferyl benzoate, isoeugenol, cinnamic acid, cinnamyl alcohol, benzyl alcohol, benzoic acid and eugenol; Myroxylon pereirae resin and the fragrance mix I, as they share common ingredients (e.g. eugenol, isoeugenol, and cinnamyl alcohol); and Myroxylon pereirae resin and propolis (they share common ingredients such as benzoic acid, benzyl alcohol, benzyl benzoate, benzyl caffeate, benzyl cinnamate, benzyl ferulate, benzyl isoferulate, caffeic acid, cinnamic acid, cinnamyl alcohol, coniferyl benzoate, farnesol, nerolidol and vanillin).

Patients reacting to one essential oil nearly always react to many other essential oils. These often contain the same ingredients, which may partly explain this. Limonene, for example, is present in nearly all essential oils which have caused contact allergy (Chapters 5 and 6). Co-reactivity to individual fragrances and essential oils may be explained by the presence of (high concentrations of) the fragrances in the oil, for example geraniol and palmarosa, citronella, geranium, thyme, rose or melissa oil; linalool and rosewood, coriander fruit, thyme, neroli, lavandin, basil, lavender, spike lavender, petitgrain bigarade, clary sage, ylang-ylang and marjoram essential oils; and limonene and all Citrus essential oils.

In this section in all monographs, chemicals are identified that are certainly or likely able to cross-react or pseudo-cross-react to the monographed chemical/substance, but mostly excluding scenarios as depicted here. In addition, reactions to compounds that are chemically unrelated but appear significantly more often than in patients not allergic to the index chemical are mentioned. Positive patch test reactions to FM I and/or FM II, for example, have a statistically significant association with positive reactions to methylchloroisothiazolinone/methylisothiazo-linone and/or methylisothiazolinone and with positive reactions to formaldehyde. Presumably, fragrances and preservatives are often present in the same consumer products leading to concomitant or successive sensitizations.

Patch test sensitization
Chemicals which have caused late reactions (>7 days) are mentioned in this section. Such late reaction may be a sign of patch test sensitization, but this is only proven when the patients are again tested and then show patch test reactivity at 2-4 days. Retesting has been performed infrequently, and only a for a few fragrances has patch test sensitization been documented beyond doubt, including for alpha-damascone, methyl 2-octynoate, phenylacet-aldehyde and rose ketone-4. This subject is summarized in Chapter 2.8.

Presence in cosmetic products and chemical analyses
Many studies have investigated the (qualitative and/or quantitative) presence of fragrances in cosmetic and other products. Before 2006, most investigators used chemical analysis, usually GC-MS, for qualitative and quantitative determination. Since then, the presence of the target fragrances was usually investigated by screening the product labels for the 26 fragrances that must be labeled since 2005 on cosmetics and detergent products in the EU, if present at > 10 ppm (0.001%) in leave-on products and > 100 ppm (0.01%) in rinse-off products. These are detailed in this section in each monograph.

Other information
This may include results of Repeated Open Application Tests, other provocation tests, serial dilution testing or any other subject related to contact allergy which is not discussed elsewhere.

OTHER SIDE EFFECTS

Irritant contact dermatitis
Irritant contact dermatitis from fragrances has infrequently been reported. Data are discussed in the relevant monographs and summarized in Chapter 2.8.

Photosensitivity
Photosensitivity reactions include photocontact allergy (causing photoallergic contact dermatitis), phototoxicity (causing phototoxic dermatitis) and combined photocontact allergy and contact allergy, causing photoaggravated allergic contact dermatitis, and a few cases of immediate-type photosensitivity reactions. In the past, musk ambrette and 6-coumarin were frequent causes of photoallergic contact dermatitis. They are not used anymore and photosensitivity reactions from fragrance chemicals today are rare.

This section shows the results of studies performing photopatch testing in groups of selected patients, usually individuals suspected of photosensitivity or photocontact allergy. Data provided include country/countries of the study, period of study, photopatch test concentration and vehicle used, number of patients tested, number of patients and percentage with positive patch tests, mode of selection, relevance (both percentage and products), other relevant information (in the Comment section) and literature references. Monographed chemicals that have caused photoallergic contact dermatitis are summarized in Chapter 2.8.

Immediate-type reactions
Cases of immediate-type reactions are presented in this section. Possible symptoms (single or in combination) of such reactions include localized erythema, itching or tingling, localized urticaria, angioedema, generalized urticaria, respiratory symptoms (wheezing, dyspnea, asthma, rhinitis, nasal discharge), cardiac problems (hypotension, bradycardia, ventricular fibrillation or cardiac arrest), gastrointestinal symptoms (abdominal pain, diarrhea, nausea, vomiting) or even anaphylactic shock. Although some fragrance materials are well-known causes of non-immune immediate contact reactions (e.g. cinnamal, cinnamic acid), such reactions from perfumes are hardly ever reported.

Other non-eczematous contact reactions
In this section, other non-eczematous contact reactions from the index fragrances are discussed. A summary of such side effects is presented in Chapter 2.8.

Systemic side effects
In this section, systemic side effects caused by percutaneous resorption of fragrance chemicals are presented. These are rarely caused by the use of fragrances. Benzyl alcohol, benzyl benzoate, benzyl salicylate, camphor, eucalyptol, menthol, methyl salicylate, and thymol have caused or at least have been held responsible for systemic effects, but the causal relationship often was not proven. Also, in the relevant reports, these chemicals were never used as fragrances but rather as ingredient of pharmaceutical preparations and in some cases they were not caused by cutaneous application but by ingestion (camphor) or parenteral administration (benzyl alcohol).

Miscellaneous side effects
This section may provide data on side effects not mentioned in one of the sections above, e.g. respiratory disorders.

OTHER INFORMATION
This section may contain any relevant data on the monographed chemical not related to contact allergy and not discussed elsewhere.

LITERATURE

1   Zaragoza-Ninet V, Blasco Encinas R, Vilata-Corell JJ, Pérez-Ferriols A, Sierra-Talamantes C, Esteve-Martínez A, de la Cuadra-Oyanguren J. Allergic contact dermatitis due to cosmetics: A clinical and epidemiological study in a tertiary hospital. Actas Dermosifiliogr 2016;107:329-336

2   Alinaghi F, Bennike NH, Egeberg A, Thyssen JP, Johansen JD. Prevalence of contact allergy in the general population: A systematic review and meta-analysis. Contact Dermatitis 2018 Oct 29. doi: 10.1111/cod.13119. [Epub ahead of print]

3   Johansen JD, Mahler V, Lepoittevin J-P, Frosch PJ, Eds. Contact Dermatitis, 6th Edition. Berlin Heidelberg: Springer-Verlag, 2018

4   John S, Johansen J, Rustemeyer T, Elsner P, Maibach H, Eds. Kanerva's Occupational Dermatology, 3rd Ed. Cham: Springer, 2018

5   Ung CY, White JML, White IR, Banerjee P, McFadden JP. Patch testing with the European baseline series fragrance markers: a 2016 update. Br J Dermatol 2018;178:776-780

6   Rietschel RL, Fowler JF Jr, Eds. Fisher's Contact Dermatitis, 6th Edition. Hamilton, USA: BC Decker Inc., 2008

7   Johansen JD. Fragrance contact allergy: a clinical review. Am J Clin Dermatol 2003;4:789-798

8   Uter W, Johansen JD, Borje A, Karlberg AT, Lidén C, Rastogi S, et al. Categorization of fragrance contact allergens for prioritization of preventive measures: Clinical and experimental data and consideration of structure–activity relationships. Contact Dermatitis 2013;69;196-230

9   Arribas MP, Soro P, Silvestre JF. Allergic contact dermatitis to fragrances. Part 1. Actas Dermosifiliogr 2012;103:874-879

10 Arribas MP, Soro P, Silvestre JF. Allergic contact dermatitis to fragrances: part 2. Actas Dermosifiliogr 2013;104:29-37

11 Cheng J, Zug KA. Fragrance allergic contact dermatitis. Dermatitis 2014;25:232-245

12 De Groot AC. Monographs in Contact Allergy Volume I. Non-Fragrance Allergens in Cosmetics (Part I and Part 2). Boca Raton, Fl, USA: CRC Press Taylor and Francis Group, 2018 (ISBN 978-1-138-57325-3 and 978-1-138-57338-3)

13 De Groot AC, Schmidt E. Essential oils: contact allergy and chemical composition. Boca Raton, Fl., USA: CRC Press, Taylor and Francis Group, 2016 (ISBN 9781482246407)

14 SCCS (Scientific Committee on Consumer Safety). Opinion on Fragrance allergens in cosmetic products, 26-27 June 2012, SCCS/1459/11. Available at: https://ec.europa.eu/health/sites/health/files/scientific_committees/consumer_safety/docs/sccs_o_102.pdf

15 Nakayama H. Fragrance hypersensitivity and its control. In: Frosch PJ, Johansen JD, White IR, Eds. Fragrances - beneficial and adverse effects. Berlin Heidelberg New York: Springer-Verlag, 1998:83-91

16 De Groot AC. Patch Testing, 4th Edition. Wapserveen, The Netherlands: acdegroot publishing, 2018 (ISBN 978-90-813233-1-4)

17 Nater JP, De Groot AC. Unwanted effects of cosmetics and drugs used in dermatology. Amsterdam: Excerpta Medica, 1983

18 Nater JP, De Groot AC. Unwanted effects of cosmetics and drugs used in dermatology, 2nd Edition. Amsterdam: Elsevier Science Publishers, 1985

19 De Groot AC, Nater JP, Weijland JW. Unwanted effects of cosmetics and drugs used in dermatology, 3rd Edition. Amsterdam: Elsevier Science, 1994

20 De Groot AC. Adverse reactions to cosmetics. PhD Thesis, University of Groningen, The Netherlands, 1988

21 Cronin E. Contact Dermatitis. Edinburgh London New York: Churchill Livingstone, 1980

22 Goossens A. Cosmetic contact allergens. Cosmetics 2016, 3, 5; doi:10.3390/cosmetics3010005

23 Nardelli A, Drieghe J, Claes L, Boey L, Goossens A. Fragrance allergens in 'specific' cosmetic products. Contact Dermatitis 2011;64:212-219

24 De Groot AC, Bruynzeel DP, Bos JD, van der Meeren HL, van Joost T, Jagtman BA, Weyland JW. The allergens in cosmetics. Arch Dermatol 1988;124:1525-1529

25 De Groot AC. Contact allergy to cosmetics: Causative ingredients. Contact Dermatitis 1987;17:26-34

26 Adams RM, Maibach HI, Clendenning WE, Fisher AA, Jordan WJ, Kanof N, et al. A five-year study of cosmetic reactions. J Am Acad Dermatol 1985;13:1062-1069

27 Laguna C, de la Cuadra J, Martín-González B, Zaragoza V, Martínez-Casimiro L, Alegre V. Allergic contact dermatitis to cosmetics. Actas Dermosifiliogr 2009;100:53-60

28 Broeckx W, Blondeel A, Dooms-Goossens A, Achten G. Cosmetic intolerance. Contact Dermatitis 1987;16:189-194

29 Dooms-Goossens, A, Kerre S, Drieghe J, Bossuyt L, DeGreef H. Cosmetic products and their allergens. Eur J Dermatol 1992;2:465-468

Monographs in Contact Allergy, Volume 2
Fragrances and Essential oils

SECTION 2

FRAGRANCES

Chapter 2   Contact allergy to and allergic contact dermatitis from fragrances: a brief review

2.1 INTRODUCTION

Fragrances are an important and frequent cause of contact allergy and allergic contact dermatitis, notably from their presence in fragranced products such as deodorants, fine fragrances and aftershaves, other cosmetics (both leave-on and rinse-off products), household products, topical pharmaceuticals, essential oils, foods, and to a lesser degree industrial products. This chapter gives a brief summary of some important aspects of the subject: 1. The composition of perfumes; 2. How do we come in contact with fragrances; 3. Fragrances that have caused contact allergy / allergic contact dermatitis; 4: Diagnosing fragrance allergy; 5. How frequent is fragrance allergy; 6. Clinical picture of allergic contact dermatitis from fragrances; 7. Products responsible for contact allergy to and allergic contact dermatitis from fragrances; and 8. Occupational contact dermatitis from fragrance allergy.

Individual fragrances, fragrance markers (fragrance mix I, fragrance mix II, Myroxylon pereirae resin [balsam of Peru]) and all essential oils are fully monographed in this book. Other substances that frequently co-react with fragrances such as colophonium (traditionally considered to be a marker for fragrance sensitivity but currently hardly viewed as such) and propolis have been fully reviewed in Volume I of this 'Monographs in Contact Allergy' series (22). A full review of older literature on fragrance allergy was published in 1997 (17). Other useful reviews have been published in 1996 (161), 2003 (23), 2012-2013 (155,156), 2013 (24), 2014 (158) and 2018 (20).

2.2 THE COMPOSITION OF PERFUMES

There are thousands of chemical substances that have an odor, and over 2000, of which 300-400 are of natural origin, are used in the fragrance industry. A perfume consists of a few to several hundred fragrance materials (149). In order to create a modern perfume the perfumer carries out a long series of experiments to determine the optimal balance of the ingredients (149). Since fragrance character evolves over time, the volatility of all raw materials plays a decisive role. The most volatile ingredients are called 'top notes', followed by the bouquet or 'heart note' forming the most essential part of the perfume. The long-lasting materials are known as 'bottom' or 'dry out' (149). In some cases, substances (fixatives) are added to perfumes to prevent the more volatile components from evaporating too easily (47). A fixative may be a fragrance material itself or may be odorless. It is characterized by a low vapor pressure. A perfume is developed for one particular purpose and the composition may have to be changed to retain the same odor if it is incorporated into a different type of product (18).

'Proper' perfumes contain approximately 15-30% of the fragrance compound. They are expensive and too concentrated. The more diluted products such as eau de parfum, eau de toilette, and colognes are therefore much more popular (20). Approximate concentrations of fragrance materials in cosmetics and some household products are shown in Table 2.1.

Table 2.1 Approximate concentrations of perfume in cosmetics and household products (17,18,19,20)

Product	Concentration	Product	Concentration
Aerosol freshener	0.5-2%	Fragranced cream	4%
Bath product	2%	Hair pomade	0.5%
Bathroom cleaner	≤ 5%	Hair spray	0.1-0.5%
Body lotion	0.4%	Laundry powder	0.1-0.3%
Compressed powder	0.5%	Lipstick	1%
Deodorant/antiperspirant	1-3%	Liquid detergent	0.1-1%
Dishwashing liquid	0.1-0.5%	Masking perfume	≤ 0.1%
Eau de cologne	3-5%	Perfume (proper)	15-30%
Eau de parfum	8-15%	Shampoo (undiluted)	0.5%
Eau de toilette	4-8%	Shower gel	1.2%
Face cream	0.3%	Skin care product	0.3-0.5%
Facial make-up	1%	Soap (undiluted)	0.5-2%

Details of the composition of a particular perfume (both in cosmetics used for their scent and in other cosmetic and household products) are usually closely guarded by industry. However, since 2005, in the EU, cosmetic products and detergent products are required to be labeled for the presence of 26 fragrance chemicals (of which 2 are mixtures: Evernia prunastri extract [oakmoss] and Evernia furfuracea extract [treemoss]), if present at >10 parts per million (ppm, 0.001%) in leave-on products and >100 ppm (0.01%) in rinse-off products (table 2.2) (67). Since then, some 15 investigations have studied the presence of these fragrances in certain products by reading the labels (e.g. 60-66). The studies have nearly always been performed in European countries, a few in the USA. The number of products investigated has ranged from 23 to 5588 and the product types varied widely, e.g. 'cosmetic products in hair dye kits', 'fragranced cosmetic products', 'household detergents', 'emollients', 'pediatric cosmetics', 'deodorants', 'liquid household and cleaning products', 'cosmetic products', 'perfumed cosmetics and household products' and 'popular perfumed deodorants'. It can hardly be surprising that the results have varied widely. Indeed, the studies are difficult to compare due to differing parameters such as country, period of investigation, product types, sample sizes, and methods of selection.

Nevertheless, very generally speaking, it appears that – all products taken together - linalool and limonene are used most frequently, followed by citronellol, geraniol, hexyl cinnamal, butylphenyl methylpropional and benzyl salicylate. The least frequently used chemicals appear to be cinnamal, Evernia prunastri extract (oakmoss absolute) Evernia furfuracea extract (treemoss absolute), benzyl cinnamate, anise alcohol, methyl 2-octynoate and amylcinnamyl alcohol. Most products contain at least 3 of the 26 fragrances that need to be labeled. Undoubtedly, they often contain more, but in lower concentrations that need no declaration.

Table 2.2 Fragrances that need to be labeled in the EU in cosmetics and household products [a]

Amyl cinnamal (α-amylcinnamic aldehyde)	Evernia furfuracea (treemoss) extract
Amylcinnamyl alcohol	Evernia prunastri (oakmoss) extract
Anise alcohol (anisyl alcohol)	Farnesol
Benzyl alcohol	Geraniol
Benzyl benzoate	Hexyl cinnamal (α-hexylcinnamic aldehyde)
Benzyl cinnamate	Hydroxycitronellal
Benzyl salicylate	Hydroxyisohexyl 3-cyclohexene carboxaldehyde
Butylphenyl methylpropional (Lilial ®)	(Lyral ®)
Cinnamal (cinnamic aldehyde, cinnamaldehyde)	Isoeugenol
Cinnamyl alcohol	α-Isomethyl ionone (γ-methylionone)
Citral	Limonene
Citronellol	Linalool
Coumarin	Methyl 2-octynoate (methyl heptane carbonate)
Eugenol	

[a] Labeling of the fragrances is only mandatory if present at >10 parts per million (ppm, 0.001%) in leave-on products and >100 ppm (0.01%) in rinse-off products

2.3 HOW DO WE COME IN CONTACT WITH FRAGRANCES?

Cosmetic products that are used primarily for their scent such as perfume, eau de cologne, eau de toilette, deodorant and aftershave, although having the highest concentrations, certainly are not the only source of contact with fragrance materials. In fact, all cosmetics and most household products contain fragrance materials, unless it is stated otherwise. However, even 'unscented' or 'fragrance-free' products may sometime contain a perfume or an essential oil to mask the unpleasant odor of the product or specific ingredients. Examples of products containing fragrances are shown in table 2.3.

Table 2.3 Examples of products containing fragrances (17,20)

Cosmetics including perfumes
Essential oils, e.g. tea tree oil and various oils used in aromatherapy
Fabrics and clothes (after they have been laundered or treated with a fabric softener)
Flavors used in oral hygiene products: toothpaste, mouthwash, dental floss
Household products: detergents, cleaners, softeners, fabric conditioners, deodorising sprays, polishes, solvents, waxes
Industrial products: cutting fluids, electroplating fluids, paints, rubber, plastics, insecticides, herbicides, additives used in air conditioning
Paper and paper products: diapers, facial tissues, moist toilet paper and sanitary napkins
Products used in dentistry (notably eugenol)
Spices including cinnamon, clove, vanilla and cardamom added to foods, soft drinks, lozenges, chewing gum, candies, ice cream and tobacco
Topical drugs (especially essential oils)
Ventilating systems and diffusers

In fact, virtually everyone is in daily contact with fragrance materials. Contact with fragrances may occur from direct product application to the skin or mucous membranes, by occasional contact with an allergen-contaminated product such as towels and pillows, contact with products used by partners, friends or co-workers (consort or connubial contact dermatitis), airborne contact, and systemic exposure by inhalation and ingestion (fragrances, flavors and spices in foods and drinks). Indeed, any part of the body may more or less frequently have contact with fragrances (17,20).

2.4 FRAGRANCES THAT HAVE CAUSED CONTACT ALLERGY / ALLERGIC CONTACT DERMATITIS

The author has found 156 fragrances that have been reported to cause contact allergy / allergic contact dermatitis (from any source) (table 2.5). Most are single chemicals, some are complex mixtures of botanical origin: Evernia furfuracea (treemoss) extract, Evernia prunastri (oakmoss) extract, Ferula galbaniflua gum, methyl ionones (4 chemicals, not botanical), Narcissus poeticus flower extract and Viola odorata leaf extract.

In addition, in another table (table 2.6) patch test results are presented of (a): three compounds that are not used as fragrance materials as such, but are routinely tested as 'indicators' or 'markers' of fragrance contact allergy: fragrance mix I, fragrance mix II and Myroxylon pereirae resin (balsam of Peru), (b): 16 chemicals which are not used as fragrances *per se*, but are potential allergenic ingredients of botanical products which may be applied in perfumery. These botanicals and their respective ingredients are Evernia furfuracea (treemoss) extract (atranol, atranorin, chloroatranol, fumarprotocetraric acid, physodalic acid, physodic acid), Evernia prunastri (oakmoss) extract (atranol, atranorin, chloroatranol, evernic acid, usnic acid), Myroxylon pereirae resin derivatives (benzyl isoferulate, coniferyl alcohol, coniferyl benzoate, isoferulic acid) and Melaleuca alternifolia (tea tree) leaf oil (aromadendrene, ascaridole, ledene, 1,2,4-trihydroxymenthane), and (c): six chemicals, for which contact allergy has not been established with certainty: caprylic alcohol, heptanal, musk, nonanal, nonyl alcohol (1,2) and dehydrodiisoeugenol.

Of these 181 chemicals / mixtures taken together, 17 have been tested in the general population and 71 in routine testing. Patch tests in groups of selected patients (e.g. patients known or suspected to be allergic to fragrances, individuals suspected of cosmetic dermatitis, patients with eyelid / periorbital dermatitis, with allergic contact cheilitis, hairdressers or their clients, patients previously shown to be allergic to Myroxylon pereirae resin or tea tree oil and tested with one or more of their ingredients) have been performed with 140 fragrances. Case reports / series were found for 94 compounds.

It should be realized that for a large number of fragrances (very) little data are available. Thirty-three fragrances have given positive results in a single study only, in which a group of selected patients was tested with a battery of fragrances, leading to a number of positive reactions (ranging from 1-13, mean 3.9, median 2), but where the authors did not comment on their relevance (3-6,21,25-30). With eleven fragrances, patch tests have been performed in the 1970s in Japan, but details are lacking, as the results have been published in Japanese journals only (16).

Generally speaking, in by far most studies performed with fragrances, data on relevance are either completely absent or inadequate. As to case reports and case series, these include the results of retrospective studies in for example groups of patients with cosmetic dermatitis, in which was stated in how many cases specific fragrances were the allergenic ingredient, but without additional supportive data (e.g. 7,9-15). Well-described case reports (clinical picture, patch test results, culprit products, identification of the allergenic ingredients in these products, improvement or healing after avoiding the allergens) constitute a small minority. In total, only 42 fragrances have shown positive results in routine testing *and* in testing in selected groups *and* were reported to be the cause of allergic contact dermatitis in one or more case reports. The data discussed in this section are summarized in table 2.4.

Table 2.4 Key data of fragrances reported as sensitizers

Data	Nr. of fragrances
Fragrances reported to have caused contact allergy / allergic contact dermatitis	156
- single chemicals	150
- mixtures (5 botanical and methyl ionones)	6
Fragrance allergy markers (fragrance mixes I and II, Myroxylon pereirae resin)	3
Chemicals not used as fragrance, but potential allergenic ingredient of botanical fragrances	16
Fragrances, contact allergy not ascertained	6
Tested in general population	17
Tested in consecutive patients suspected of contact dermatitis (routine testing)	71
Tested in groups of selected patients	140
- fragrances positive in a single study in selected patients only, relevance not established	33
Fragrances with Case reports / series	94
Fragrances with positive routine testing *and* testing in selected groups *and* case report(s)	42

In table 2.5, for every of the 156 fragrances that have caused contact allergy / allergic contact dermatitis, the following data – where available – are provided: results of patch testing in the general population (with percentage of positive reactions), of routine testing and testing in groups of selected patients (both with [range of] percentages positive reactions) whether case reports or case series have been documented. Also, for each entry it is indicated whether photosensitivity, immediate-type reactions or patch test sensitization has been reported, and whether they have been identified as causes of pigmented cosmetic dermatitis in Japan in the 1970-1980s only. Similar data are presented for the 25 chemicals (fragrance indicators, allergenic non-fragrance chemicals in botanicals fragrances, fragrances with contact allergy not demonstrated with certainty) shown in table 2.6.

Details for all fragrances and other chemicals can be found in their respective monographs in this book.

Table 2.5 Fragrances that have caused contact allergy / allergic contact dermatitis and nature of investigations

Fragrance	Nature of reports of contact allergy / allergic contact dermatitis			
	General pop.	Routine testing	Selected groups [j]	Case rep.
Acetylcedrene (Vertofix ®)		0.2-1%		+
Acetyl hexamethyl indan (Phantolide ®) [f]			N=1 (5%) (25)	
Acetyl hexamethyl tetralin			N=2 (10%) (25)	
Allylanisole				+
Allyl cyclohexylpropionate			No specific data	+
Ambrettolide			N=6 (3.4%) (5)	
Amyl cinnamal (α-amylcinnamic aldehyde) [g]	0.1%	0.08-1.4%	0.3-15%	+
Amyl cinnamate				+
Amylcinnamyl alcohol [g]		0.1-0.5%	0.5-4%	+
Amyl salicylate		0.2-1%	5%	
Anethole [h]			0.6-33%	+
Anise alcohol [g]		0.03-0.2%	0.1-20%	
Anisylidene acetone			N=2 (1.1%) (3)	
Benzaldehyde [g]			0.2-0.5%	+
Benzyl acetate			0-5.7%	
Benzyl alcohol [g]		0.1-1%	0.2-15%	+
Benzyl benzoate [g,h]		<0.1%-0.3%	0.1-13%	+
Benzyl cinnamate [h]		0.02-0.3%	0.1-19.1%	+
Benzylidene acetone				+
Benzyl isoeugenol		0.09%		
Benzyl propionate [k]			No specific data	
Benzyl salicylate		3.3-8.0%	0.04-22%	+
Butyl acetate				+
Butylphenyl methylpropional (Lilial ®)		0.2-1%	0.4-4%	+
Camphor [g]			5%	+
Camphylcyclohexanol			1.3-2.5%	
3-Carene [f]			18-27%	+
Carvacrol			2.1-19%	
Carvone [g,h]		0.6-2.8%	4.6-40%	+
beta-Caryophyllene		0.5-1.1%		+
Caryophyllene oxide		0.1-0.4%		
Cedrol methyl ether (cedramber)			No specific data	
Cinnamal (cinnamic aldehyde) [f,g,h]	0.8%	0.3-9%	1.4-30%	+
Cinnamic acid [g,h]		1.5%	13-44%	+
Cinnamyl alcohol [f,g,h]	0.3%	0.14-11.2%	1.5-75%	+
Cinnamyl benzoate				+
Cinnamyl cinnamate			20-25%	+
Citral [h]	0.3%	0.3-3.2%	0.4-25%	+
Citral diethyl acetal [k]			No specific data	
Citronellal				+
Citronellol	0.1%	0.07-1%	0.3-35%	+
Coumarin [f,g]	0.1%	0.05-0.7%		
Cuminaldehyde				
5-Cyclohexadecenone [k]			No specific data	

Table 2.5 Fragrances that have caused contact allergy / allergic contact dermatitis and nature of investigations (continued)

Fragrance	Nature of reports of contact allergy / allergic contact dermatitis			
	General pop.	Routine testing	Selected groups [j]	Case rep.
Cyclohexyl acetate			N=1 (0.5%) (6)	
Cyclopentadecanone			N=3 (1.7%) (5)	
p-Cymene			14%	
alpha-Damascone [h]		0.5%		+
beta-Damascone [h]		0.5%		
Diethyl maleate [h]			N=6 (3.3%) (3)	
Dihydrocarveol			N=1 (10%) (26)	
Dihydrocitronellol				+
Dihydrocoumarin [h]			3.7-21%	+
Dihydro pentamethylindanone (Cashmeran ®)			N=1 (0.6%) (4)	
Dimethylbenzyl carbinyl acetate		0.2-0.3%		
Dimethyl citraconate			N=7 (3.8%) (3) [l]	
2,4-Dimethyl-3-cyclohexene carboxaldehyde (Ligustral ®)			N=1 (0.6%) (4)	
Dimethyltetrahydro benzaldehyde			N= 4 (2.3%) (5)	
Ethyl anisate				+
Ethylene dodecanedioate			N=2 (0.9%) (6)	
Ethyl vanillin [g]			N=9 (14%) (83)	
Eucalyptol (1,8-cineole)				+
Eugenol [f,g]	0.2%	0.3-3.4%	1.3-56%	+
Evernia furfuracea (treemoss) extract		1.5-3.3%	2.5-30%	+
Evernia prunastri (oakmoss) extract [f,g]	1.0%	0.7-3.1%	1.9-64%	+
Farnesol	0.4%	0.2-2.5%	0.2-2.5%	+
Ferula galbaniflua gum (galbanum resin)			N=8 (4.8%) (4)	
Geranial		0.4-2.0%		+
Geraniol [g,h]	0.4%	0.2-2.6%	0.6-30%	+
Geranyl acetate				+
Heliotropine (piperonal)		0.4-1.0%	5%	+
Hexadecanolactone (hexadecanolide)			0.6-1.4%	
Hexamethylindanopyran (Galaxolide ®)		0.2%	0.3-3.4%	
cis-3-Hexenyl salicylate			No specific data	+
Hexyl cinnamal (α-hexylcinnamic aldehyde)	0.3%	0.06-0.6%	0.5-7%	+
Hexyl salicylate				+
Hydroxycitronellal [f]	0.5%	0.4-3.8%	1.0-45%	+
Hydroxycitronellol			N=13 (6.0%) (6)	
Hydroxyisohexyl 3-cyclohexene carboxaldehyde (Lyral ®)	1.5%	0.4-4.8%	0.9-40%	+
Ionone (α-irisone)		0.5%	1.1%	+
Isoamyl salicylate		3.7%	0.6%	
Isoeugenol [h]	0.7%	1.0-4.5%	1.3-33%	+
Isoeugenyl acetate		0.8-3.9%		
Isoeugenyl benzoate		0.2%		
Isoeugenyl phenylacetate		0.7%		
Isolongifolanone			N=1 (0.6%) (5)	
alpha-Isomethyl ionone (γ-methyl-ionone)		0.03-0.1%	0.4-2.1%	+
Isopulegol			N=2 (10%) (21)	
Isosafrole			2.3%	
Limonene [g]	see Chapter 3.95 Limonene		0.3-86%	+
Linalool	see Chapter 3.96 Linalool		0.2-20%	+
Linalyl acetate		0.2-2.2%		+

Table 2.5 Fragrances that have caused contact allergy / allergic contact dermatitis and nature of investigations
          (continued)

Fragrance	Nature of reports of contact allergy / allergic contact dermatitis			
	General pop.	Routine testing	Selected groups [j]	Case rep.
Maltol				+
Menthol [g]		0.1%	0.1-40%	+
Menthyl acetate			N=1 (10%) (26)	
Methoxycinnamal				+
Methoxycitronellal [k]			No specific data	
2-Methoxyphenol/2,2-dimethyl-3-me-thylenebicycloheptane hydrogenated (sandela)			N=11 (6.6%) (4) [l]	
Methoxytrimethylheptanol			N=2 (0.9%) (6)	
Methyl p-anisate			0.5%	+
Methyl anthranilate [f]			1-1.9%	
Methyl cinnamate			3-4.2%	
6-Methyl coumarin [f]			0.3-11.9% + (photo)	+ (photo)
Methyldihydrojasmonate (Hedione ®)		0.2%		
Methylenedioxyphenyl methylpropanal (Helional ®)			N=4 (2.4%) (4)	
Methyl eugenol			N=4 (1.8%) (6)	
Methyl ionones				+
5-Methyl-alpha-ionone (α-irone)		0.3%	No specific data	
Methyl isoeugenol		0.3%		
Methyl octine carbonate				+
Methyl 2-octynoate (methyl heptine carbonate) [h]	0.1-0.9%	0.1-0.9%	0.1-5%	
Methyl salicylate [g]		0.1-0.5%	1.3-1.6%	+
3-Methyl-5-(2,2,3-trimethyl-3-cyclo-pentenyl)pent-4-en-2-ol (Ebanol ®)			0.6-2.8%	
Musk ambrette [f]		0.3-0.4% 0.8% (photo)	0.2-10% + (photo)	+ + (photo)
Musk ketone [f]		0.3%	1-2%	+ (& photo)
Musk moskene [f]		1.4%		+
Musk tibetene [f]	Only photocross-reaction to musk ambrette			
Musk xylene		0.7%	2%	+
Myrcene		0.1%	10-35%	+
Narcissus poeticus flower extract		0.5-1.3%	0.5-1.3%	
Neral		0.1-0.9%	2.7%	
Nerol			N=13 (6.0%) (6)	
Nerolidol		3.5%	3-6%	
Nopyl acetate			N=2 (1.1%) (28) [l]	
Pentamethylcyclopent-3-ene-butanol (Sandalore ®)			N=5 (3.0%) (4)	
alpha-Phellandrene			14-63%	+
Phenethyl alcohol			1.1-5%	
Phenylacetaldehyde [g]		1.5%	1.1%	+
Phenylpropanol			0.9%	
alpha-Pinene			50-77%	+
beta-Pinenes		0.2%	9-37%	+
Piperitone			40%	
Propylidene phthalide			N=5 (2.7%) (3)	
D-Pulegone			30%	
Rhodinol			1-5%	
Rose ketone-4 [h,k]			No specific data	
Sabinene			N=2 (10%) (29)	

Table 2.5 Fragrances that have caused contact allergy / allergic contact dermatitis and nature of investigations (continued)

Fragrance	Nature of reports of contact allergy / allergic contact dermatitis			
	General pop.	Routine testing	Selected groups [j]	Case rep.
Safrole [h]			2-7%	
Salicylaldehyde			0.1-2.5%	+
Santalol		No specific data	0.6-1.5%	+
Styryl acetate			N=2 (10%) (30)	
alpha-Terpinene			69-100%	+
4-Terpineol			5-29%	+
alpha-Terpineol		0.1-0.2%	1.3-14%	+
Terpinolene			85-100%	+
Terpinyl acetate [g]			N=1 (5%) (21)	
Tetrahydro-dimethylbenzofuran			N=2 (20%) (26)	
Tetramethyl acetyloctahydronaphthalene (Iso E super ®)		0.2-0.3%	1.7%	
Thymol			1.2-5%	+
Trimethylbenzenepropanol (Majantol ®)		0.2-1.4%	0.8-5.4%	+
5,5,6-Trimethylbicyclohept-2-ylcyclo-hexanol (Isobornyl cyclohexanol) [k]			No specific data	
2,4,6-Trimethyl-4-phenyl-1,3-dioxane (Floropal ®)			N=2 (1.2%) (4)	
Vanillin [g,h]		0.3%	0.1-17%	+
Verdyl acetate (Cyclacet ®)		0.1-0.3%		
Vetiveryl acetate [k]			No specific data	
Viola odorata leaf extract			N=2 (1.2%) (4)	

[a-e] Does not apply; [f] Photosensitivity reported; [g] Immediate-type reactions reported; [h] Patch test sensitization reported; [j] When only one single study is available with one or more positive reactions to the fragrance, the number of positive reactions (N= ..), percentage of positive reactions (in brackets) and the reference (in brackets) is shown. In case of more studies identifying the fragrance as allergen, the *range* of positives is shown. It should be appreciated that the percentages vary considerably for individual fragrances and are strongly dependent on the mode of selecting the patients. Sometimes, data are missing or incomplete, notably from studies which have been published in Japanese journals only; [k] Has only been reported to cause pigmented cosmetic dermatitis in Japan in the 1970s (16); [l] probably includes a number of false-positive reactions. Case rep.: Case reports; General pop.: General population

2.5 DIAGNOSING FRAGRANCE ALLERGY (ADAPTED FROM REF. 20)

Many individuals with contact allergy to fragrance ingredients are aware that they cannot tolerate scented products on their skin and are often able to specifically name product categories that initiated their disease, notably colognes, eaux de toilette, deodorants and lotions (133). However, in a recent study from the UK, 75% of patients that proved to be fragrance-allergic by patch testing, were not aware of this before (49). Indeed, many hypersensitive individuals have never suffered from fragrance allergic contact dermatitis and appear to tolerate perfumes and fragranced products without problems. This may be explained by irritant (false-positive) patch test reactions to fragrances, the absence of relevant allergens in the products used, or their concentration being too low to elicit clinically visible allergic contact reactions. Also, even some that are exposed will not necessarily develop a clinical hypersensitivity reaction (30). Conversely, many more people complain about intolerance to or rashes caused by perfumes or perfumed products than are shown to be allergic by patch testing. This may be attributable to irritant effects of the fragrances or fragranced products or to inadequate diagnostic (patch testing) procedures (24,133).

Full and adequate testing can be complicated, as a perfume may contain over 250 individual ingredients. The European baseline series, which is routinely tested in all patients suspected of contact dermatitis, contains the fragrance hydroxyisohexyl 3-cyclohexene carboxaldehyde (Lyral ®, HICC), and four 'markers' or 'indicators' of fragrance allergy: fragrance mix I (FM I), fragrance mix II (FM II), Myroxylon pereirae resin (balsam of Peru) and colophonium. Colophonium was traditionally considered to be a marker for fragrance allergy, but identifies very few cases not detected by the other markers and is hardly, if at all, viewed as fragrance allergy marker anymore (49).

The FM I has been part of most routine series since the late 1970s and contains 8 fragrance chemicals in a concentration of 1% each: amyl cinnamal, cinnamal, cinnamyl alcohol, eugenol, Evernia prunastri (oakmoss) extract, geraniol, isoeugenol and hydroxycitronellal. The petrolatum vehicle contains 5% sorbitan sesquioleate as emulsifier to ensure even dispersion of the ingredients. The FM I is very useful, but has certain imperfections, which are shown in table 2.7.

Table 2.6 Contact allergy to fragrance indicators, allergenic non-fragrance chemicals in botanicals fragrances, and
fragrances with contact allergy not demonstrated with certainty

Fragrance	Nature of reports of contact allergy / allergic contact dermatitis			
	General pop.	Routine testing	Selected groups	Case rep.
Fragrance indicators				
Fragrance mix I [e,f,g]	3.5% (pooled) (31)	4.5-22.2%	4.5-57%	
Fragrance mix II [f]	1.9%	1.4-8.0%	1.7-19%	
Myroxylon pereirae resin [e,f,g]	1.8% (pooled) (31)	2.4-13.7%	1.7-50%	
Chemicals not used as fragrances per se, but present as possible sensitizers in botanical fragrances				
Aromadendrene [d]			5-71%	
Ascaridole [d]		5.5%	1.5-100%	+
Atranol [a,b]	See Chapter 4.3 Atranol			
Atranorin [a,b,e,g]		1.1%	38%	+
Benzyl isoferulate [c]			2-25%	
Chloroatranol [a,b]	See Chapter 4.6 Chloroatranol			+
Coniferyl alcohol [c]			13%	
Coniferyl benzoate [c,g]			28-81%	
Evernic acid [b,e]			22%	+
Fumarprotocetraric acid [a]	Only cross-reactivity to or from other lichen acids and oakmoss preparations			
Isoferulic acid [c]			1%	
Ledene (viridiflorene)			5-10%	+
Physodalic acid [a]				+
Physodic acid [a]				+
1,2,4-Trihydroxymenthane [d]			25-90%	+
Usnic acid [b,e]			16%	+
Fragrances, contact allergy not demonstrated with certainty				
Caprylic alcohol				+
Dehydrodiisoeugenol			+	
Heptanal				+
Musk				+
Nonanal				+
Nonyl alcohol				+

[a] Potential allergenic ingredient in Evernia furfuracea (treemoss) extract; [b] Potential allergenic ingredient in Evernia prunastri (oakmoss) extract; [c] Potential allergenic ingredient in Myroxylon pereirae resin (derivatives); [d] Potential allergenic ingredient in Melaleuca alternifolia (tea tree) leaf oil; [e] Photosensitivity reported; [f] Immediate-type reactions reported; [g] Patch test sensitization reported; Case rep.: Case reports; General pop.: General population

Table 2.7 Imperfections of the fragrance mix I

May cause irritant reactions
May cause false-negative reactions (negative reaction to the mix, positive reaction to one or more ingredients)
Leaves up to 65% of fragrance sensitivities undetected
Sorbitan sesquioleate may cause an allergic reaction; risk of wrong interpretation as fragrance allergy
Occasional cases of patch test sensitization

When patients allergic to FM I are (concurrently or later) tested with the 8 ingredients ('breakdown testing'), on average 1/3 of the patients does not react to any ingredient. Possible explanations include: 1. false-positive (irritant) reactions to the mix; 2. false-negative reactions to the individual constituents. In most studies, these have been tested at 1% in petrolatum, which is the same as in the mix. That the FM *does* react despite having the same concentration as the constituents that are negative separately may be related to: a. enhancement of elicitation of contact allergic reactions by allergen mixtures (32) or irritants; b. increased skin penetration caused by the (combined) irritancy of other constituents of the mix including sorbitan sesquioleate; or c. the formation of new allergens in the mix (compound allergy). No evidence for this latter scenario is as yet available. As the emulsifier sorbitan sesquioleate (SSO) may cause contact allergic reactions in up to 5-10% of patients tested with the FM I (and can wrongly be interpreted as fragrance allergy), SSO needs always to be tested separately when breakdown testing is performed (33). Addition of SSO to the baseline series would be preferable. Of the ingredients of the FM I, oakmoss absolute is the most frequent sensitizer, followed by isoeugenol, with geraniol and amyl cinnamal by far causing positive reactions the least frequently.

The fragrance mix II was added to the European baseline series in 2008. It consists of 6 ingredients with a total concentration of 14% in petrolatum: citral (1%), citronellol (0.5%), coumarin (2.5%), farnesol (2.5%), hexyl cinnamal (5%) and HICC (2.5%). It has proven its value, as 35-50% of the patients with a positive reaction to FM II do *not* react to the fragrance mix I (34). About one-third of the patients reacting to the FM II have a negative break-down, with no positive reactions to any of its ingredients (34). By far the most frequent sensitizer in the mix is HICC. This fragrance is also part of the baseline series as single chemical in a concentration of 5% and its rate of positive reactions is one of the higher in the baseline series. However, most reactions to HICC are already picked up by the FM II, and the single chemical detects only an additional 0.2%-0.3% positive reactions, which led Swedish researchers to delete it from their national baseline series (35).

The indicators Myroxylon pereirae resin (18) and especially colophonium detect relatively few fragrance sensitivities that are not already identified by reactions to one or both fragrance mixes.

Although extremely useful, the 4 indicators (+ hydroxyisohexyl 3-cyclohexene carboxaldehyde) together leave a considerable number of sensitizations to fragrances (up to 59% [49]) undetected and testing with additional fragrances and/or essential oils may reveal many additional cases of fragrance contact allergy. Nearly 60 fragrance allergens (including indicators and lichen acids, which are themselves not used as fragrances but may be present in treemoss and/or oakmoss extract) are commercially available for patch testing (table 2.8).

When fragrance allergy is suspected on the basis of the patient's history or the clinical presentation, testing a 'fragrance series' is recommended, which should also be performed (in a second session) when fragrance sensitivity is strongly suspected, but the fragrance test substances in the baseline series remain negative (20). In the case of a positive reaction to FM I and/or FM II, subsequently breakdown tests must be done to identify the specific sensitizer(s). In the EU, these must be labeled on cosmetics and detergent products, if present at > 10 ppm (0.001%) in leave-on products and > 100 ppm (0.01%) in rinse-off products, and contact with them can therefore largely be avoided. It is also imperative that all products used by the patients and suspected to cause reactions are patch tested. It has been shown, for example, that relevant allergic reactions to perfumes, deodorants and shaving lotions in about half the cases are *not* identified by any fragrance indicator reacting in the baseline series (36).

In case of dubious (?+) or weak-positive (+) reactions to fragrances, fragrance markers or products used by the patient, repeat testing, use tests or ROATs (Repeated Open Application Tests) are helpful to confirm the allergenic nature of the patch test reaction and aid in establishing the relevance.

Each monograph presents a test concentration and vehicle for patch testing the fragrance discussed; when commercially available, this is indicated. Patch test concentrations and vehicles for other fragrance materials and for all cosmetic products can be found in *Patch Testing*, 4th Edition (2018), written by the author (162).

Table 2.8 Fragrances and fragrance markers commercially available for patch testing

Patch test allergen	Chemotechnique	SmartPractice
Amyl cinnamal (α-amylcinnamic aldehyde)	2%	1%
Amylcinnamyl alcohol	5%	1%
Anethole (*E*-)	5%	
Anise alcohol (anisyl alcohol)	10% Softisan	1%
Atranorin [f]	0.1%	0.1%
Benzaldehyde		5%
Benzyl alcohol	10% Softisan	1% and 5%
Benzyl benzoate	10%	1%
Benzyl cinnamate	10%	5%
Benzyl salicylate	10%	1%
Butylphenyl methylpropional (Lilial®, *p-tert*-butyl-α-methyl-hydrocinnamic aldehyde)	10%	10% [c]
Carvone	5%	5% [b]
Cinnamal (cinnamic aldehyde, cinnamaldehyde)	1%	1%
Cinnamyl alcohol	2%	1%
Citral	2%	2%
Citronellal		2%
Citronellol	1%	1%
Colophonium (colophony, rosin) [a]	20%	20%
Coumarin	5%	5%

Table 2.8 Fragrances and fragrance markers commercially available for patch testing (continued)

Patch test allergen		Chemotechnique	SmartPractice
Dipentene (dl-limonene)			2% [b]
Eugenol		2%	1%
Evernia furfuracea extract (treemoss absolute)		1%	1%
Evernia prunastri extract (oakmoss absolute)		2%	1%
Evernic acid [f]		0.1%	
Farnesol		5%	5%
Fragrance mix I [a]		8%	8%
- amyl cinnamal	1%		
- cinnamal	1%		
- cinnamyl alcohol	1%		
- eugenol	1%		
- geraniol	1%		
- hydroxycitronellal	1%		
- isoeugenol	1%		
- oakmoss absolute	1%		
Fragrance mix A [a] (as Fragrance mix I, oakmoss absolute replaced with sandalwood oil 1%)			8%
Fragrance mix II [a]		14%	14%
- citral	1%		
- citronellol	0.5%		
- coumarin	2.5%		
- farnesol	2.5%		
- hexyl cinnamal	5%		
- hydroxyisohexyl 3-cyclohexene carboxaldehyde (Lyral ®)	2.5%		
Geraniol		2%	1%
Hexyl cinnamal		10%	10%
Hydroxycitronellal		2%	1%
Hydroxyisohexyl 3-cyclohexene carboxaldehyde (Lyral ®)		5%	5%
Isoeugenol		2%	1%
α-Isomethyl ionone (γ-methylionone)		10%	1%
Lichen acid mix [a] (atranorin, evernic acid, usnic acid, each 0.1%)		0.3%	0.3%
d-Limonene [g]		10%	2% and 3% [e]
Limonene hydroperoxides [g]		0.2% and 0.3%	
Linalool [g]		10%	10%
Linalool hydroperoxides [g]		0.5% and 1%	
Menthol		2%	1%
Methyl anthranilate		5%	5% [b]
6-Methylcoumarin		1% and 1% alcohol	
Methyl-2-octynoate (methyl heptine carbonate)		0.2%	
Methyl salicylate			2%
Musk ambrette			5%
Musk ketone		1%	
Musk mix (musk xylene, moskene, ketone, each 1%) [a]		3%	
Musk moskene		1%	
Musk xylene		1%	
Myroxylon pereirae resin (Balsam of Peru) [a]		25%	25%
Narcissus poeticus absolute		2%	2%
Perfume mix [a] (as Fragrance mix I, without amyl cinnamal and oakmoss absolute)		6%	
α-Pinene			15%
Salicylaldehyde			2%
Thymol			1%
Trimethylbenzenepropanol (Majantol ®)		5%	5%

Table 2.8 Fragrances and fragrance markers commercially available for patch testing (continued)

Patch test allergen	Chemotechnique	SmartPractice
Usnic acid [f]	0.1%	0.1%
Vanillin	10%	10%

[a] Not a fragrance ingredient *per se*, but a – weak - indicator of fragrance allergy; [b] Only available at SmartPractice Canada; [c] Only available at SmartPractice Europe; [d] All test substances are in petrolatum unless indicated otherwise; [e] SmartPractice Europe only 2%; [f] Lichen acid; [g] Patch testing should be performed with the hydroperoxides of limonene and linalool
Chemotechnique: Chemotechnique Diagnostics (www.chemotechnique.se); SmartPractice: SmartPractice Europe (www.smartpracticeeurope.com) and SmartPractice Canada (www.smartpracticecanada.com)

2.6 HOW FREQUENT IS FRAGRANCE ALLERGY?

Although fragrances are mostly moderate sensitizers (39), they are among the most frequent causes of contact allergy, presumably from their extremely widespread use. Some fragrances are themselves non-sensitizing or low-sensitizing, but are transformed into a – far stronger sensitizing - hapten outside the skin by chemical transformation from air oxidation or photoactivation (a prehapten) or are transformed into a hapten in the skin (bioactivation), usually via enzymatic catalysis (a prohapten) (37,38). Eugenol and isoeugenol are prohaptens, geranial, limonene, linalool and linalyl acetate are prehaptens, and cinnamyl alcohol, geraniol and alpha-terpinene act both as prohaptens and prehaptens. In recent years it has been shown that autoxidation of linalool, limonene and linalyl acetate forms potently allergenic hydroperoxides. Indeed, linalool and limonene, by patch testing with their hydroperoxides, were identified as very frequent causes of fragrance allergy. When tested with the pure compounds, these chemicals rarely give positive reactions.

Fragrance sensitization is seen more often in female patients and its prevalence increases with age rising above 40 years (153,154)

General population

Fragrance mixes and Myroxylon pereirae resin

In a 2018 meta-analysis of 19 studies covering 19,440 patch tested individuals from the general population, the pooled prevalence for sensitization to the fragrance mix I was 3.5% (women 3.4%, men 2.9%) (31). For Myroxylon pereirae resin (12 studies covering 8002 patch tested individuals) the pooled prevalence of sensitization was 1.8% (women 1.7%, men 1.6%) (31). In the period 2008-2011, in 5 European countries (Sweden, Germany, Netherlands, Portugal, Italy), a random sample of the general population of 3119 individuals aged 18-74 years were patch tested with the FM II. There were 60 reactions (1.9%) to FM II, tested 14% in petrolatum (41,42).

Individual fragrances

In the period 2008-2011, in 5 European countries (Sweden, Germany, Netherlands, Portugal, Italy), a random sample of the general population of 3119 individuals aged 18-74 years were patch tested with the 14 ingredients of the FM I and FM II (42). The percentages positive reactions (in descending order) were as follows: HICC (1.5%), Evernia prunastri (oakmoss) extract (1.0%), cinnamal (0.8%), isoeugenol (0.7%), hydroxycitronellal (0.5%), farnesol (0.4%), geraniol (0.4%), cinnamyl alcohol (0.3%), citral (0.3%), hexyl cinnamal (0.3%), eugenol (0.2%), amyl cinnamal (0.1%), citronellol (0.1%), and coumarin (0.1%) (42). About half of all positive reactions to fragrances and indicators were considered to be relevant based on standardized criteria. Women were affected twice as often (2.5%) as men (1.3%) (42).

From these data it can be concluded that possibly up to 4.5% of the adult general population has contact allergy to one or more fragrances. However, many of them can tolerate perfumes and scented products and do not suffer from, nor have a history of allergic reactions. Even continuous exposure to fragrances to which contact allergy has been established will not necessarily lead to allergic contact dermatitis (30). Indeed, the prevalence of *clinically relevant* fragrance contact allergy has - conservatively - been estimated as 1.9% (42).

Patients patch tested because of suspected contact dermatitis

In a study in 12 European countries performed in the period 2009-2012, 12.7% of a group of over 50,000 consecutive patients patch tested for suspected contact dermatitis (routine testing) had positive reactions to the FM I, the FM II, hydroxyisohexyl 3-cyclohexene carboxaldehyde (HICC), Myroxylon pereirae resin, oil of turpentine (a weak marker for fragrance allergy) or a combination of these (44). In similar 2016 IVDK data, the percentage was nearly 17 (153). However, the actual prevalence of fragrance sensitivity may be considerably higher as these markers fail to detect a large number of fragrance allergic individuals: 58-70% of the many individuals reacting to oxidized limonene or linalool (46,47,48,49) and 40-60% of the reactions to the 26 fragrances that need to be labeled in the EU (49,50). In a 2015-2016 study performed in the UK, of 2084 patients who were tested with the baseline series, the 26 fragrances that need to be labeled including *oxidized* linalool and *oxidized* limonene, and trimethylbenzenepropanol, 359

(17.2%) individuals reacted to at least one fragrance (49). Although the latter would not appear to point at an increased frequency by co-testing additional fragrances including oxidized linalool and limonene, it should be appreciated that fragrance allergy as identified by FM I, FM II and Myroxylon pereirae resin in the United Kingdom has a lower frequency than in several other European countries (49). This means that the actual rate of sensitization in some countries, and notably in the IVDK area (Germany, Switzerland, Austria), may well be above 20% and possibly reach 25%!

In Thailand, 22.1% of a very small group of 312 consecutive patients reacted to the FM I, FM II, Myroxylon pereirae resin or combinations (45). Such combined data are unavailable from the USA, but as the rates of reactions in the NACDG studies for FM I, FM II and Myroxylon pereirae resin are generally higher than in Europe, it may be expected that at least 20% of patients patch tested for suspected allergic contact dermatitis in the USA are allergic to fragrances.

Frequencies of sensitization to individual fragrance markers in routine testing

Generally speaking, in Europe, since 2000, frequencies of sensitization to FM I mostly range from 5% to 9%. This is lower than in the USA, where rates have varied between 9% and 12%. Frequencies of sensitization for Myroxylon pereirae resin in the USA have ranged from 6.6% to 13.7%. Generally speaking, the rates appear to have decreased somewhat in the last decade, ranging in all NACDG studies between 7% and 8%. In multinational multicenter studies performed in Europe,frequencies of sensitization have ranged in a very narrow band of 5.3% to 6.4%. As to the fragrance mix II, most studies scored between 3% and 5.2% positive reactions. In multicenter studies, the rates per center have shown significant variability for all fragrance markers, with a range between 0% and 16% for reactions to fragrance mix I in the 2013-2014 study of the European Surveillance System on Contact Allergies (ESSCA) (27). Colophonium, which is a weaker marker for fragrance sensitization, currently has the lowest prevalence scores, 2.6-2.9% in Europe (44,51) and 1.9-2.5% in the USA (52,53,59). Details and data for other countries (except colophonium) can be found in the respective chapters.

Frequencies of sensitization to individual fragrances in routine testing

Contact allergy to limonene and linalool was long considered to be rare. In recent years, however, limonene hydroperoxides and linalool hydroperoxides (in oxidized limonene and linalool) have gained much attention and have been patch tested in several studies in consecutive patients in European and some other countries. Patch testing with limonene hydroperoxides 0.3% pet. has shown frequencies of sensitization ranging from 2.5% to 9.4%. For linalool hydroperoxides 1% pet. the range was 3.9% to 11.7%. The author thinks it very likely that a number of these reactions have been false-positive. Nevertheless, linalool and limonene, which are both the fragrances most often used in cosmetics and household products, appear to be the most frequent fragrance sensitizers at this moment. Hydroxyisohexyl 3-cyclohexene carboxaldehyde (HICC) probably is the third most frequent fragrance allergen with frequencies of sensitization generally between 1.2-2.5%, but rates up to 4.8% have recently been observed. HICC will be totally banned from cosmetic products in the EU from 23 August 2021 on and the rates are at this moment (2018) already declining.

In six recent studies, the 26 fragrances that need to be labelled in the EU have been patch tested in consecutive patients suspected of contact dermatitis (49,50,54,55,56,58). These include the 8 ingredients of the fragrance mix I (indicated with *) and the six constituents of the fragrance mix II (indicated with **). The results are shown in table 2.9. Evernia furfuracea extract (treemoss absolute) is the most frequently reacting fragrance, with prevalences of 1.5 to 3.3%. It is followed by HICC and 5 components of the FM I: Evernia prunastri extract (oakmoss absolute) (1.2-2.1%), isoeugenol (0.9-2.6%), cinnamyl alcohol (0.6-2.5%), cinnamal (1.2-1.9%), and hydroxycitronellal (0.6-2.2%). All other fragrances score an average frequency of <1%, with the lowest rates for α-isomethyl ionone (0.16%), methyl 2-octynoate (0.16%), amyl cinnamal (0.14%), anise alcohol (0.10%), benzyl cinnamate (0.08%), limonene (not oxidized) (0.06%) and benzyl benzoate (0.04%).

Trimethylbenzenepropanol (Majantol®) was positive in 0.2-1.4% of routinely tested patients and oxidized linalyl acetate scored 2.2% positive reactions in Sweden, with only 0.2% for the unoxidized test material. In the USA, cinnamal appears to be an important fragrance allergen with around 4% positive reactions in the studies of the North American Contact Dermatitis Group (52,53,59).

Frequencies of sensitization in patients with cosmetic dermatitis

In patients suffering from allergic contact dermatitis to cosmetics, 30-45% of the reactions are caused by fragrances (7,8,9).

2.7 CLINICAL PICTURE OF ALLERGIC CONTACT DERMATITIS FROM FRAGRANCES

Contact allergy to fragrances most often causes (aggravation of) dermatitis of the hands, the face (157) and neck (142, 143), and the axillae. Patches of eczema may also be observed in areas where perfumes are dabbed on such as behind the ears, upper chest, elbow flexures and wrists (17). Women are more often affected than men and will typically give a history of a previous rash from a perfume (fine fragrance) or scented deodorant in the axillae (23). Indeed, the fragrances used in deodorants are an important, if not the most important, cause of induction and elicitation of fragrance allergy (23,68,144,148). It is recognised that the axillary skin is a problematic area as it is moist, occluded and is easily irritated. Men are primarily sensitized by deodorants and aftershaves. Micro-traumata from shaving facilitates contact allergy to aftershave fragrances (17,20). Following sensitization by products containing high percentages of fragrances, eczema may appear, or be worsened by, the use of a variety of product types with lower fragrance levels, including other cosmetics, household products, industrial products and flavors.

Table 2.9 Prevalence of sensitization to 26 fragrances labeled in the EU in routine testing (49,50,54,55,56,58)

Fragrance	Range + reactions	Average + reactions [a]	Fragrance	Range + reactions	Average + reactions [a]
Evernia furfuracea extr.	1.5 - 3.3%	2.45%	Coumarin **	0.05 - 0.6%	0.31%
HICC **	1.3 - 4.8%	2.39%	Amycinnamyl alcohol	0.1 - 0.6%	0.30%
Evernia prunastri extr.*	1.2 - 2.1%	1.65%	Citronellol **	0.1 - 0.9%	0.29%
Isoeugenol *	0.9 - 2.6%	1.58%	Linalool (not oxidized) [b]	0.1 - 0.6%	0.28%
Cinnamyl alcohol *	0.6 - 2.5%	1.49%	Benzyl alcohol	0.1 - 0.4%	0.20%
Cinnamal *	1.2 - 1.9%	1.47%	Benzyl salicylate	0.1 - 0.3%	0.19%
Hydroxycitronellal *	0.6 - 2.2%	1.25%	α-Isomethyl ionone	0 - 0.6%	0.16%
Citral **	0.3 - 1.6%	0.84%	Methyl 2-octynoate	0 - 0.3%	0.16%
Eugenol *	0.3 - 1.3%	0.68%	Amyl cinnamal *	0 - 0.2%	0.14%
Farnesol **	0.3 - 0.9%	0.53%	Anise alcohol	0 - 0.2%	0.10%
Hexyl cinnamal **	0.3 - 0.6%	0.48%	Benzyl cinnamate	0 - 0.2%	0.08%
Geraniol *	0 - 1.0%	0.48%	Limonene (unoxidized) [b]	0 - 0.2%	0.06%
Butylphenyl methyl propional	0.3 - 0.7%	0.45%	Benzyl benzoate	0 - 0.1%	0.04%

[a] not adjusted for sample size; [b] tested in 5 studies; + positive; * present in the fragrance mix I; ** present in the fragrance mix II; extr.: Extract; HICC: Hydroxyisohexyl 3-cyclohexene carboxaldehyde

The severity of dermatitis may range from mild to severe with dissemination. Most fragrance allergic reactions are erythematous, more acute lesions with vesicles, oozing and papules may sometimes be observed. Some cases resemble nummular eczema, seborrheic dermatitis, sycosis barbae, or lupus erythematosus. Pustular allergic contact dermatitis has rarely been described (106) as have erythema multiforme-like eruptions (131,132). Lesions in the skin folds may be mistaken for atopic dermatitis. Dermatitis due to perfumes or toilet water tends to be 'streaky'. Hand eczema is common in fragrance-sensitive patients and there is often a possible but not certain association between the dermatitis and fragrance sensitization (145,146,147). Patients may first have irritant dermatitis or atopic dermatitis, which is later complicated by contact allergy to products used for treatment or prevention (hand creams and lotions) of hand dermatitis, or to other perfumed products in the household, hobby, or work environment.

Dyshidrotic eruptions and widespread eruptions are ascribed to ingestion of spices, notably in patients reacting to Myroxylon pereirae resin (systemic contact dermatitis, hematogenic contact dermatitis). Inhalation of high concentrations of fragrance contact allergens may also cause manifest hematogenic contact dermatitis in some individuals (160). Atopic dermatitis located at other body sites, perianal dermatitis and vulvar dermatitis may also be complicated by fragrance allergy. Allergic contact dermatitis in patients with psoriasis may present with a mixed dermatitis – psoriasis picture from the Köbner phenomenon (130). Fragrances present in topical pharmaceutical preparations such as corticosteroids, anti-inflammatory drugs, wound healing, antiseptic-disinfectant, and antihemorrhoidal preparations, can cause iatrogenic allergic contact dermatitis (17,20).

Fragrance sensitization may lead to continuous or periodic dermatitis, sick leave, and impaired quality of life, especially in recently diagnosed young women (69,141).

Pigmented cosmetic dermatitis

In Japan, in the 1960s and 1970s, many female patients developed pigmentation of the face after having facial dermatitis (71). The skin manifestations of this so-called pigmented cosmetic dermatitis consisted of diffuse or patchy brown hyperpigmentation on the cheeks and/or forehead, sometimes the entire face was involved. In severe cases, the pigmentation was black, purple, or blue-black, and in mild cases, it was pale brown. Occasionally, erythematous macules or papules, suggesting a mild contact dermatitis, were observed and itching was also noted at varying times. Pigmented cosmetic dermatitis was shown to be caused by contact allergy to components of cosmetic products, notably essential oils, other fragrance materials, antimicrobials, preservatives and coloring materials (70,71,72). The number of patients with pigmented cosmetic dermatitis decreased strongly after 1978, when major cosmetic companies began to eliminate strong contact sensitizers from their products (70). Since 1980, pigmented cosmetic dermatitis became a rare disease in Japan (73). Fragrances that have been implicated as causes of pigmented cosmetic dermatitis are shown in table 2.10.

Table 2.10 Fragrances that have caused pigmented cosmetic dermatitis (70-73)

Benzaldehyde	Ionone
Benzyl alcohol	alpha-Isomethyl ionone
Benzyl propionate [a]	Isosafrole
Benzyl salicylate	Methoxycitronellal [a]
Cedrol methyl ether	Methyl isoeugenol
Cinnamyl alcohol	Methyl-alpha-ionone
Citral diethyl acetal [a]	Musk moskene
5-Cyclohexadecenone [a]	Rose ketone-4
Eugenol	Tetramethyl acetyloctahydronaphthalene
Evernia prunastri (oakmoss) extract	5,5,6-Trimethylbicyclohept-2-ylcyclohexanol
Geraniol	Vetiveryl acetate [a]
Hydroxycitronellal	

[a] Has only caused pigmented cosmetic dermatitis in Japan in the past; details not available

2.8 OTHER SIDE EFFECTS
Other side effects reported from fragrances include immediate-type reactions (mostly non-immune immediate contact reactions, contact urticaria), photosensitivity, patch test sensitization, respiratory disorders and miscellaneous side effects including irritant contact dermatitis, depigmentation and systemic side effects. None of these currently cause significant clinical problems.

Immediate-type reactions
Several fragrances have been reported to cause immediate-type reactions, mostly non-immune immediate contact reactions (synonym: contact urticaria). Well-known examples are Myroxylon pereirae resin (MP), cinnamal, and cinnamic acid (important ingredient of MP). These substances can, in the proper concentration and vehicle, induce immediate contact reactions in the majority of healthy individuals, mostly with erythema only, sometimes with wheals. Other fragrances that have been reported as causes of contact urticaria are shown in table 2.11. Only a few have caused one or more clinical cases of immediate contact reactions, but rarely from their presence in a perfume (geraniol, terpinyl acetate). All others have been shown to induce such reactions in patch testing with them, where the materials were removed after 20-30 minutes (e.g. 74-78). Usually, however, there was erythema only. Currently, fragrance materials do not cause clinical problems from immediate-type reactions.

Table 2.11 Fragrances that have caused immediate-type reactions

Amyl cinnamal	Ethyl vanillin [a]
Amylcinnamyl alcohol	Eugenol [a]
Anise alcohol	Evernia prunastri (oakmoss) extract
Benzaldehyde [a]	Geraniol [a]
Benzyl alcohol [a]	alpha-Isomethyl ionone [a]
Benzyl benzoate	Limonene
Camphor	Menthol [a]
Carvone [a]	Methyl salicylate
Cinnamal [a]	Myroxylon pereirae resin
Cinnamic acid	Terpinyl acetate [a]
Cinnamyl alcohol	Vanillin
Coumarin	

[a] Clinical manifestations reported

Photosensitivity
At the end of the 1970s up to the mid-1980s, the fragrance material musk ambrette caused many cases of photoallergic contact dermatitis, especially in men, mostly from its presence in aftershave lotions (79). Also in the late 1970s, an epidemic of photocontact dermatitis occurred in people using a popular sunscreen with an increased level of 6-methyl coumarin (80). The reactions occurred primarily in women and developed within several hours after they applied the suntan lotion and went into the sun. The reactions were particularly severe, requiring hospitalization in many cases. Most of the patients' eruptions took weeks to resolve and left (temporary) hyperpigmentation (80). These fragrances were banned by IFRA (International Fragrance Association) and are not

used anymore. Other fragrances that have caused photocontact allergy are shown in table 2.12. Musk ketone, musk moskene, musk tibetene and musk xylene have only photo-cross-reacted to musk ambrette. The other fragrances showed some positive photopatch tests in testing in groups of patients suspected of photosensitivity disorders including photosensitivity dermatitis with actinic reticuloid syndrome (81), but their relevance was never mentioned. Photosensitivity to fragrances currently is not a problem.

Table 2.12 Fragrances that have caused photosensitivity reactions

Acetyl hexamethyl indan	Methyl anthranilate
3-Carene	6-Methyl coumarin [a]
Cinnamal [a]	Musk ambrette [a]
Cinnamyl alcohol	Musk ketone
Coumarin	Musk moskene
Eugenol [a]	Musk tibetene
Evernia prunastri (oakmoss) extract [a]	Musk xylene
Fragrance mix I	Myroxylon pereirae resin [a]
Hydroxycitronellal [a]	

[a] also immediate-type photoreactions reported (mostly interpreted as phototoxicity)

Patch test sensitization

There have been few reports of (definite, probable or possible) patch test sensitization to fragrances (table 2.13). Several patients were sensitized to anethole from a patch test with star anise oil (which contains 84-90% anethole) 0.5%, 1% and 2% in petrolatum (82). Alpha-Damascone, methyl 2-octynoate, phenylacetaldehyde and rose ketone-4 have definitely caused a number of cases of patch test sensitization. Most other fragrances in table 2.13 are constituents of Myroxylon pereirae resin (MP) that were patch tested in patients allergic to this material and that caused one or more positive reactions developing 6 days or later after application. Whether these were simply 'delayed' reactions or indicative of patch test sensitization was not investigated by re-testing (83). In current practice, patch test sensitization is hardly a problem, although the fragrance mix I may probably sensitize occasionally (84,85).

Table 2.13 Fragrances that (may) have caused patch test sensitization

Anethole	Dihydrocoumarin [a]
Benzyl benzoate [c]	Eugenol [c]
Benzyl cinnamate [c]	Fragrance mix I
Carvone [a]	Geraniol
Cinnamal [c]	Isoeugenol [c]
Cinnamic acid [c]	Methyl 2-octynoate [b]
Cinnamyl alcohol [c]	Phenylacetaldehyde [b]
Citral	Rose ketone-4 [b]
alpha- and beta-Damascone [b]	Vanillin [c]
Diethyl maleate	

[a] Probably caused patch test sensitization; [b] Definitely caused patch test sensitization; [c] In patients allergic to Myroxylon pereirae resin and tested with a battery of its ingredients, this fragrance caused one or more positive patch test reactions that developed 6 days or later after application; whether there were simply 'delayed' reactions or indicative of patch test sensitization was not investigated by re-testing (83)

Respiratory disorders

Fragrances are volatile and therefore, in addition to skin exposure, a perfume also exposes the eyes and naso-respiratory tract. Already 35 years ago it was suspected and later confirmed that fragrances can induce or worsen respiratory problems including asthmatic attacks (135,138,139). People may not only experience symptoms from wearing perfume themselves, but also around cosmetic counters, candle shops, and from perfumes worn by other people. Currently, it is estimated that 2-4% of the adult population is affected by respiratory or eye symptoms from such exposures (134). Frequently reported symptoms include dry, itching or watery eyes, nasal irritation, congestion and sneezing, as well as mouth and throat irritation, shortness of breath and cough. Generally, ocular and nasal symptoms are reported more frequently than respiratory symptoms at other locations (140).

A significant association has been found between respiratory complaints related to fragrances and contact allergy to fragrance ingredients, in addition to hand eczema (137). In another study, however, inhalation of high concentrations of fragrance contact allergens in allergic individuals induced some subjective symptoms in a few subjects, but without objective changes (160).

The mechanisms by which fragrance chemicals induce respiratory symptoms in some individuals are unclear. There are no indications that immunological processes are generally involved, but sensory mechanisms may influence the symptoms (136,140).

As to specific fragrance materials, airway irritation has been observed from limonene, and asthma and/or rhinitis has been ascribed to eugenol, limonene, menthol, methyl salicylate and vanillin (table 2.14).

Miscellaneous side effects
Other side effects attributed to fragrances are shown in table 2.14. The causal relationship was not always established beyond doubt. Details can be found in the respective monographs.

Table 2.14 Other side effects attributed to fragrances

Side effect	Implicated fragrances
Airway irritation	Limonene
Alopecia (reversible)	Myroxylon pereirae resin
Asthma and/or rhinitis	Eugenol; limonene; menthol; methyl salicylate; vanillin
Bullous pemphigoid	Benzyl benzoate; cinnamal
Conjunctival cicatrization	Cinnamal
Depigmentation	Benzyl alcohol; cinnamal
Depigmented airborne contact dermatitis	Musk ambrette
Irritant contact dermatitis	Benzyl benzoate; citral; eugenol; isoeugenol; limonene; menthol; methyl salicylate
Irritant contact mucositis	Eucalyptol
Non-trombocytopenic purpura	Menthol
Oral lichen planus	Anethole; cinnamal; eugenol
Orofacial granulomatosis	Carvone; cinnamal; cinnamyl alcohol; menthol; piperitone
Pigmented contact dermatitis	Musk ambrette
Poikiloderma of Civatte [a]	Unspecified
Psoriasis (Köbner reaction)	Linalool
Systemic side effects	Benzyl alcohol; benzyl benzoate; benzyl salicylate; camphor; eucalyptol; menthol; methyl salicylate; thymol
Urticaria	Eugenol; methyl salicylate

[a] Conclusion of the authors: 'Contact sensitization, mostly to perfume ingredients, may develop in poikiloderma of Civatte, possibly playing a pathogenetic part, at least in a subset of patients (150)

2.9 PRODUCTS RESPONSIBLE FOR ALLERGIC CONTACT DERMATITIS FROM FRAGRANCES
Around 80% of the positive patch test reactions to FM I and FM II are clinically relevant (54). Perfumes and deodorants are the most frequent sources of sensitization to and allergic contact dermatitis caused by fragrance ingredients in women, whereas aftershave products and deodorants are most often responsible in men. Thereafter, eczema may appear or be worsened by contact with other fragranced products, such as cosmetics, toiletries, household products, industrial substances, and flavorings (20,24,133).

Products that have caused allergic contact dermatitis from fragrances in (convincing or likely) case reports or case series with the responsible fragrances are shown in table 2.15. Reports of patients allergic to botanical products that may be used as fragrances such as Myroxylon pereirae resin, tea tree oil, oakmoss absolute, tree moss absolute, and essential oils, who were subsequently tested with one or more of their ingredients with positive results are not included, unless the product caused allergic contact dermatitis, the allergen was established and its presence as an ingredient was ascertained or highly likely. The allergenic ingredients in these botanical products can be found in the respective chapters in this book. Essential oils and their allergenic ingredients are fully discussed in Chapters 5 and 6 on Essential oils. Fragrances that have only induced pigmented cosmetic dermatitis in the past (caused by cosmetics, but specific data not available) are shown in table 2.10.

Table 2.15 Products that have caused allergic contact dermatitis from fragrances [a,e]

Product	Causative fragrances [b]
Cosmetics	
Aftershave	Cinnamyl alcohol; eugenol; Evernia prunastri (oakmoss) extract; hydroxycitronellal; isoeugenol; linalool; methyl 2-octynoate
Bath product	Hydroxycitronellal
Deodorant / antiperspirant	Acetylcedrene; benzyl salicylate; butylphenyl methylpropional; coumarin; Evernia prunastri (oakmoss) extract; farnesol; geranial; hexyl cinnamal; hydroxycitronellal; hydroxyisohexyl 3-cyclohexene carboxaldehyde; isoeugenol; usnic acid
Eye cosmetic	Isoeugenol
Eye cream [d]	Allyl cyclohexylpropionate; caprylic alcohol; heliotropine; heptanal; musk; nonanal; nonyl alcohol
Fine fragrance (perfume)	Benzyl salicylate; benzylidene acetone; butylphenyl methylpropional; citral; coumarin; alpha-damascone; eugenol; Evernia prunastri (oakmoss) extract; farnesol; cis-3-hexenyl salicylate; hexyl cinnamal; hydroxycitronellal; hydroxyisohexyl 3-cyclohexene carboxaldehyde; alpha-isomethyl ionone; limonene; linalool; methyl ionones; musk xylene
Foundation lotion / tonic	Hydroxycitronellal; isoeugenol; musk moskene
Hair conditioner	Benzyl salicylate
Hair cream	Eugenol
Hair dye	Benzyl alcohol
Hair lotion	Hydroxycitronellal; linalool; musk ketone
Hair pack	Limonene
Lip cosmetic	Benzyl alcohol; cinnamal; cinnamyl alcohol; citral; geraniol; maltol; methyl 2-octynoate
Make-up, face	Citronellol; geraniol; hydroxycitronellal
Massage cream	Eugenol
Massage oil	Geranial
Moisturizer	Benzyl alcohol; Evernia prunastri (oakmoss) extract; limonene; linalool; musk moskene
Mouthwash	Eugenol; menthol
Nail polish remover	Benzyl salicylate
Permanent waving solution	Evernia prunastri (oakmoss) extract
Rouge	Musk moskene
Shampoo	Benzyl salicylate; limonene; linalool
Shampoo, dry	Cinnamyl alcohol; linalool
Shaving foam	Geraniol
Shower gel	Benzyl salicylate; limonene
Skin care product	Citronellol; dihydrocitronellol; hexyl cinnamal; hydroxycitronellal; alpha-isomethyl Ionone; linalool; methyl 2-octynoate
Soap	Geraniol
Sunscreen	Amyl cinnamal; benzyl alcohol; cinnamyl alcohol; eugenol; Evernia prunastri (oakmoss) extract; geraniol; linalool
Toilet paper / wet wipe / tissue	Cinnamyl alcohol; linalool
Toothpaste	Amyl cinnamal; anethole; carvone; cinnamal; eugenol; menthol; toothpaste
Cosmetics, unspecified	Amyl cinnamal; amylcinnamyl alcohol; anise alcohol; benzyl alcohol; benzyl benzoate; benzyl cinnamate; benzyl salicylate; butyl acetate; butylphenyl methylpropional; cinnamal; cinnamyl alcohol; citral; citronellal; citronellol; coumarin; Evernia furfuracea (treemoss) extract; Evernia prunastri (oakmoss) extract; farnesol; geraniol; hexyl cinnamal; hydroxycitronellal; hydroxyisohexyl 3-cyclohexene carboxaldehyde; isoeugenol; alpha-isomethyl ionone; limonene; linalool; musk ambrette; trimethylbenzenepropanol
Essential oils	Ascaridole; cinnamal; citral; citronellal; eucalyptol; geraniol; geranyl acetate; limonene; linalool; myrcene; alpha-phellandrene; alpha-pinene; beta-pinene; alpha-terpinene; terpinolene; 1,2,5-trihydroxymenthane

Table 2.15 Products that have caused allergic contact dermatitis from fragrances (continued) [a,e]

Product	Causative fragrances [b]
Foods, spices and beverages	Cinnamal; eugenol; limonene
Pharmaceutical products	Amyl cinnamal; amylcinnamyl alcohol; anethole; benzyl alcohol; benzyl benzoate; benzyl salicylate; camphor; cinnamal; cinnamyl alcohol; coumarin; eucalyptol; eugenol; geraniol; heliotropine; hydroxycitronellal; limonene; menthol; methyl salicylate; musk ketone; terpineol; thymol; usnic acid; vanillin
Household products	
Cleanser	Limonene
Fabric softener	Benzyl salicylate
Floor mop	Limonene
Washing detergent	Anethole; eugenol; hydroxycitronellal; limonene; linalool
Washing-up liquid	Geraniol; limonene
Miscellaneous products	
Breath freshener	Cinnamal; cinnamyl alcohol
Cigarette	Menthol
Cod liver oil	Coumarin
Dentistry materials [c]	Eugenol
Exfoliating socks	Linalool
Insect repellent (wipe)	Hydroxycitronellal; linalool
Incense	Musk ambrette; santalol
Lichens	Evernia prunastri (oakmoss) extract
Odor-masking powder	Cinnamal
Ostomy deodorant	Citronellal; Evernia prunastri (oakmoss) extract; limonene
Paint stripper	Limonene
Skin softener plant extract	Cinnamal; cinnamyl alcohol
Throat spray	Menthol
Occupational products	
Baking powder	Anethole
Bark of aspen	Salicylaldehyde
Cleanser	3-Carene; limonene; terpinolene
Coolant	Evernia prunastri (oakmoss) extract
Cosmetics	Citral
Cutting oil	Benzyl alcohol
Degreasing product	Limonene
Dental materials	Eugenol
Essential oils	beta-Caryophyllene; citral; geraniol; limonene
Foods, spices and beverages	Benzyl alcohol; cinnamal; limonene
Fragranced powder (non-cosmetic)	Cinnamal
Glue	Benzyl alcohol
Massage cream / oil	Citral; eugenol
Paint thinner	Limonene
Perfume / fragrance [f]	Benzaldehyde; camphor; cinnamal; citronellol; dipentene; geraniol; linalool; methyl 2-octynoate; phenylacetaldehyde; vanillin
Permanent waving solution	Evernia prunastri (oakmoss) extract
Pinewood sawdust	Limonene
Pressure additive	Limonene
Skin protection cream	Citronellol; geraniol
Solvent	Limonene
Wax polish	Limonene

[a] See individual chapters for details; [b] Includes occupational contacts; [c] Impression materials, filling materials, dental cements, endodontic sealers, periodontal dressing materials and dry socket dressings; [d] All fragrances mentioned in the right column reacted when the components of the perfume in an eye cream was tested in a female patient previously shown to be allergic to the cream; however, they were negative on retesting (1,2); [e] Case reports of photoallergic contact dermatitis are not mentioned

here; see Chapter 3.108 6-Methyl coumarin and Chapter 3.120 Musk ambrette; [f] Includes contacts with the pure fragrance chemical

2.10 OCCUPATIONAL CONTACT DERMATITIS FROM FRAGRANCE ALLERGY

General

It may be expected that fragrances will cause dermatological problems for workers in the cosmetics industry (cosmetic chemists, workers handling the raw materials and the final products, salespeople), beauticians, hairdressers and aromatherapists (the latter group especially from essential oils) (20). Analyses of IVDK data indeed showed an increased risk of fragrance allergy among masseurs/physiotherapists, and also to beauticians, nurses, geriatric nurses, and metal surface workers exposed to metalworking fluids (MWF) (86,151). It was found that that metalworkers added fragrances to the MWF in order to mask their odor (152). Remarkably, hairdressing was not an occupation associated with an increased risk. One can deduce relatively high use of fragrances in the areas mentioned, albeit non-quantifiable (183). Housewives and cleaning personnel may also be endangered by frequent contact with soap, cleansers, dishwashing liquids and other fragranced products (20). In spite of this, surprisingly little information on occupational allergic contact dermatitis from fragrances can be found in literature. This may be because in the majority of people at risk, a definite relationship between dermatitis and fragrances is hard to prove. In many occupations (hairdressers, beauticians, housewives, health personnel [159], cleaning personnel), irritant factors may also be relevant in the etiology of dermatitis and sometimes other allergens are considered of paramount importance. In addition, non-occupational exposure to fragrances occurs in virtually everybody (20).

It appears that fragrances may play a role in some cases of occupational contact dermatitis, but in no single profession are they a major cause of occupational allergic contact dermatitis, and rarely are they the sole etiological factor (20). However, fragrances may play an important role in aggravating hand eczema of other origin (atopic hand eczema, irritant dermatitis, allergic contact dermatitis) by contact with hand cleansers, barrier creams, moisturising preparations, etc. In addition, flavors and spices may be involved in occupational contact dermatitis in bakers, cooks, caterers, and others working in the food industry (43). Only limonene (89), citral (90) and cinnamal have caused a considerable number of occupational sensitizations (20).

Case series

In an early study, all workers in a factory became sensitised to cinnamal (87). In Germany, 26 female workers in a perfume factory were investigated of who six had dermatitis of the hands, forearms and the face. All 26 were tested with four perfumes from the factory and 30 of their ingredients, both individual fragrance compounds and essential oils. The six patients with eczema had many positive reactions. Twelve others were also sensitized to fragrances, but never developed allergic contact dermatitis from working in the factory. The high prevalence of fragrance allergy (18/26, 69%) in this population was the result of poor work hygiene and permanent direct and airborne skin contact. The degree of automation was very low, even the bottle-filling machines had to be operated by hand (30).

Over a period of 2 years, five beauticians working in the same high-end luxury health spa in the United Kingdom developed bilateral hand dermatitis from citral present in massage products and essential oils (90).

In Finland, in the period 2008-2013, occupational limonene allergy was observed in 14 workers who used limonene-containing machine-cleaning detergents and hand cleansers, surface cleaners or dishwashing liquids. In 3 cases, the occupational limonene allergy resulted from work-related use of limonene-containing leave-on cosmetic products (89).

Case reports

Case reports and a few small case series of occupational allergic contact dermatitis from specific fragrances are shown in table 2.16. Cases caused by fragrances where the causative fragrance chemical was not identified (e.g. 88,104,105) are not presented here.

Table 2.16 Case reports of occupational allergic contact dermatitis from specific fragrances

Occupation	Culprit product(s)	Culprit fragrance(s)	Ref.
Aromatherapist(s) (1 or 2)	Essential oils	beta-Caryophyllene; geraniol (n=2); linalool; linalyl acetate; alpha-pinene (n=2)	118
Baker	Cinnamon	Cinnamal	121
Baker	Cinnamon	Cinnamal	122
Bakers (n=2)	Baking cake	Anethole in aniseed oil	112
Bakers (n=2)	Cinnamon	Cinnamal	123
Beauticians (n=5)	Cosmetics and essential oils	Citral	90
Bottle fillers (n=6)	Perfumes	Benzaldehyde (n=3); camphor (n=2); cinnamal (n=2); citronellol (n=1); dipentene (n=3);	30

Table 2.16 Case reports of occupational allergic contact dermatitis from specific fragrances (continued)

Occupation	Culprit product(s)	Culprit fragrance(s)	Ref.
		geraniol (n=6); linalool (n=3)	
Car mechanic	Degreasing agent	D-Limonene	101
Car mechanic	Pinewood sawdust	Limonene	111
Confectioner	Cardamom powder	Limonene	110
Dental assistant	Liquid dental material	Eugenol	125
Dental nurse	Restorative material	Eugenol	96
Dentist	Washing-up liquid	Geraniol	127
Elk researcher	Bark of aspen	Salicylaldehyde	129
Engineer	Coolant	Oakmoss extract	93
Food handler	Beverages	Benzyl alcohol	114
Geriatric nurse	Aftershave	Oakmoss extract	91
Hairdresser	Permanent waving solution	Oakmoss extract	97
Handler of vinyl covers	Odor-masking powder	Cinnamal	95
Histopathology medical worker	Solvent	Limonene	98
Installer of windows	Degreaser	Limonene	108
Joiner in perfume factory	Phenylacetaldehyde	Phenylacetaldehyde	94
Laboratory assistant	Methyl 2-octynoate and methyl octine carbonate	Methyl 2-octynoate and methyl octine carbonate	92
Machine cleaner	Cleanser	3-Carene and terpinolene	117
Masseuse	Massage oil	Geranial	126
Mechanic	Hand cleanser	Limonene	103
Metal grinder	Cutting oil	Benzyl alcohol	113
Metal worker	Protection cream	Geraniol	128
Not specified (n=6)	Cleaning products	D-Limonene	101
Not specified (n=4)	Fruits, flavors, vegetables	D-Limonene	101
Honing machinists	Honing oil	Dipentene (DL-Limonene)	100
Painter / car mechanic	Wax polish	Dipentene (DL-Limonene)	99
Painter / decorator	Hand cleansers	D-Limonene	102
Paint mixer in car factory	Paint thinner	Dipentene (DL-Limonene)	107
Parquet layers (n=2)	2-Part glue catalyst	Benzyl alcohol	116
Physiotherapist	Massage cream	Eugenol	124
Porter	Lemon oil	Limonene	109
Production worker	Vanillin	Vanillin	40
Restaurant worker	Cinnamon	Cinnamal	123
Waiter	Cassia extract	Cinnamal	120
Worker in fragrance plant	Perfume concentrates	Cinnamal	103
Workers in spice factory (n=3)	Cinnamon powder	Cinnamal	119

REFERENCES
1   Larsen WG. Cosmetic dermatitis due to a perfume. Contact Dermatitis 1975;1:142-145
2   Larsen WG. Perfume dermatitis revisited. Contact Dermatitis 1977;3:98
3   Malten KE, van Ketel WG, Nater JP, Liem DH. Reactions in selected patients to 22 fragrance materials. Contact Dermatitis 1984;11:1-10
4   Larsen W, Nakayama H, Lindberg M, Fischer T, Elsner P, Burrows D, et al. Fragrance contact dermatitis: A worldwide multicenter investigation (Part 1). Am J Cont Derm 1996;7:77-83
5   Larsen W, Nakayama H, Fischer, Elsner P, Frosch P, Burrows D, et al. Fragrance contact dermatitis: A worldwide multicenter investigation (Part II). Contact Dermatitis 2001;44:344-346
6   Larsen W, Nakayama H, Fischer T, Elsner P, Frosch P, Burrows D, et al. Fragrance contact dermatitis - a worldwide multicenter investigation (Part III). Contact Dermatitis 2002;46:141-144
7   Adams RM, Maibach HI, for the North American Contact Dermatitis Group. A five-year study of cosmetic reactions. J Am Acad Dermatol 1985;13:1062-1069
8   De Groot AC, Bruynzeel DP, Bos JD, van der Meeren HL, van Joost T, Jagtman BA, Weyland JW. The allergens in cosmetics. Arch Dermatol 1988;124:1525-1529

9   De Groot AC. Adverse reactions to cosmetics. PhD Thesis, University of Groningen, The Netherlands: 1988, chapter 3.4, pp.105-113

10   Zaragoza-Ninet V, Blasco Encinas R, Vilata-Corell JJ, Pérez-Ferriols A, Sierra-Talamantes C, Esteve-Martínez A, de la Cuadra-Oyanguren J. Allergic contact dermatitis due to cosmetics: A clinical and epidemiological study in a tertiary hospital. Actas Dermosifiliogr 2016;107:329-336

11   Laguna C, de la Cuadra J, Martín-González B, Zaragoza V, Martínez-Casimiro L, Alegre V. Allergic contact dermatitis to cosmetics. Actas Dermosifiliogr 2009;100:53-60

12   Goossens A. Cosmetic contact allergens. Cosmetics 2016, 3, 5; doi:10.3390/cosmetics3010005

13   Nardelli A, Drieghe J, Claes L, Boey L, Goossens A. Fragrance allergens in 'specific' cosmetic products. Contact Dermatitis 2011;64:212-219

14   Broeckx W, Blondeel A, Dooms-Goossens A, Achten G. Cosmetic intolerance. Contact Dermatitis 1987;16:189-194

15   Dooms-Goossens, A, Kerre S, Drieghe J, Bossuyt L, DeGreef H. Cosmetic products and their allergens. Eur J Dermatol 1992;2:465-468

16   Nakayama H. Fragrance hypersensitivity and its control. In: Frosch PJ, Johansen JD, White IR, Eds. Fragrances - beneficial and adverse effects. Berlin Heidelberg New York: Springer-Verlag, 1998:83-91

17   De Groot AC, Frosch PJ Adverse reactions to fragrances. A clinical review. Contact Dermatitis 1997;36:57-86

18   Johansen JD. Contact allergy to fragrances: clinical and experimental investigations of the fragrance mix and its ingredients. Contact Dermatitis 2002;46(suppl.3):1-31

19   Cadby PA, Troy WR, Vey MG. Consumer exposure to fragrance ingredients: providing estimates for safety evaluation. Regul Toxicol Pharmacol 2002;36:246-252

20   De Groot AC. Fragrances and essential oils. In: John S, Johansen J, Rustemeyer T, Elsner P, Maibach H (eds). Kanerva's Occupational Dermatology. Cham: Springer, 2018. https://doi.org/10.1007/978-3-319-40221-5_40-2; Online ISBN 978-3-319-40221-5

21   Larsen WG. Perfume dermatitis. A study of 20 patients. Arch Dermatol 1977;113:623-626

22   De Groot AC. Monographs in Contact Allergy Volume I. Non-Fragrance Allergens in Cosmetics (Part I and Part 2). Boca Raton, Fl, USA: CRC Press Taylor and Francis Group, 2018 (ISBN 978-1-138-57325-3 and 978-1-138-57338-3)

23   Johansen JD. Fragrance contact allergy: a clinical review. Am J Clin Dermatol 2003;4:789-798

24   Uter W, Johansen JD, Borje A, Karlberg AT, Lidén C, Rastogi S, et al. Categorization of fragrance contact allergens for prioritization of preventive measures: Clinical and experimental data and consideration of structure–activity relationships. Contact Dermatitis 2013;69;196-230

25   Meynadier JM, Meynadier J, Peyron JL, Peyron L. Formes cliniques des manifestations cutanées d'allergie aux parfums. Ann Dermatol Venereol 1986;113:31-39

26   Saito F, Miyazaki T, Matsuoka Y. Peppermint oil (title incomplete, partly in Japanese). Skin Research 1984;26:636-643 (article in Japanese)

27   Uter W, Amario-Hita JC, Balato A, Ballmer-Weber B, Bauer A, Belloni Fortina A, et al. European Surveillance System on Contact Allergies (ESSCA): results with the European baseline series, 2013/14. J Eur Acad Dermatol Venereol 2017;31:1516-1525

28   De Groot AC, Liem DH, Nater JP, van Ketel WG. Patch tests with fragrance materials and preservatives. Contact Dermatitis 1985;12:87-92

29   Hausen BM. Evaluation of the main contact allergens in oxidized tea tree oil. Dermatitis 2004;15:213-214

30   Schubert HJ. Skin diseases in workers at a perfume factory. Contact Dermatitis 2006;55:81-83

31   Alinaghi F, Bennike NH, Egeberg A, Thyssen JP, Johansen JD. Prevalence of contact allergy in the general population: A systematic review and meta-analysis. Contact Dermatitis 2018 Oct 29. doi: 10.1111/cod.13119. [Epub ahead of print]

32   Bonefeld CM, Geisler C, Gimenéz-Arnau E, Lepoittevin J-P, Uter W, Johansen JD. Immunological, chemical and clinical aspects of exposure to mixtures of contact allergens Contact Dermatitis 2017;77:133-142

33   Geier J, Schnuch A, Lessmann H, Uter W. Reactivity to sorbitan sesquioleate affects reactivity to fragrance mix I. Contact Dermatitis 2015;73:296-304

34   Mowitz M, Svedman C, Zimerson E, Isaksson M, Pontén A, Bruze M. Simultaneous patch testing with fragrance mix I, fragrance mix II and their ingredients in southern Sweden between 2009 and 2015. Contact Dermatitis 2017;77:280-287

35   Engfeldt M, Hagvall L, Isaksson M, Matura M, Mowitz M, Ryberg K, et al. Patch testing with hydroxyisohexyl 3-cyclohexene carboxaldehyde (HICC) – a multicentre study of the Swedish Contact Dermatitis Research Group. Contact Dermatitis 2017;76:34-39

36 Uter W, Geier J, Schnuch A, Frosch PJ. Patch test results with patients' own perfumes, deodorants and shaving lotions: results of the IVDK 1998-2002. J Eur Acad Dermatol Venereol 2007;21:374-379

37 Karlberg A-T, Börje A, Johansen JD, Lidén C, Rastogi S, Roberts D, et al. Activation of non-sensitizing or low-sensitizing fragrance substances into potent sensitizers – prehaptens and prohaptens. Contact Dermatitis 2013;69:323-334

38 Bråred Christensson J, Hagvall L, Karlberg AT. Fragrance allergens, overview with a focus on recent developments and understanding of abiotic and biotic activation. Cosmetics 2017;3:1-19

39 Lidén C, Yazar K, Johansen JD, Karlberg A-T, Uter W, White IR. Comparative sensitizing potencies of fragrances, preservatives, and hair dyes. Contact Dermatitis 2016;75:265-275

40 Wang XS, Xue YS, Jiang Y, Ni HL, Zhu H, Luo BG, Luo SQ. Occupational contact dermatitis in manufacture of vanillin. Chin Med J (Engl) 1987;100:250-254

41 Diepgen TL, Ofenloch RF, Bruze M, Bertuccio P, Cazzaniga S, Coenraads P-J, et al. Prevalence of contact allergy in the general population in different European regions. Br J Dermatol 2016;174:319-329

42 Diepgen TL, Ofenloch R, Bruze M, Cazzaniga S, Coenraads PJ, Elsner P, et al. Prevalence of fragrance contact allergy in the general population of five European countries: a cross-sectional study. Br J Dermatol 2015;173:1411-1419

43 Kanerva L, Estlander T, Jolanki R. Occupational allergic contact dermatitis from spices. Contact Dermatitis 1996;35:157-162

44 Frosch PJ, Johansen JED, Schuttelaar M-LA et al on behalf of the ESSCA network. Patch test results with fragrance markers of the baseline series – analysis of the European Surveillance System on Contact Allergies (ESSCA) network 2009–2012. Contact Dermatitis 2015;73:163-171

45 Vejanurug P, Tresukosol P, Sajjachareonpong P, Puangpet P. Fragrance allergy could be missed without patch testing with 26 individual fragrance allergens. Contact Dermatitis 2016;74:230-235

46 Audrain H, Kenward C, Lovell CR, Green C, Ormerod AD, Sansom J, et al. Allergy to oxidized limonene and linalool is frequent in the UK. Br J Dermatol 2014;171:292-297

47 Bråred Christensson J, Karlberg A-T, Andersen KE, Bruze M, Johansen JD, Garcia-Bravo B, et al. Oxidized limonene and oxidized linalool – concomitant contact allergy to common fragrance terpenes. Contact Dermatitis 2016;74:273-280

48 Deza G, García-Bravo B, Silvestre JF, Pastor-Nieto MA, González-Pérez R, Heras-Mendaza F, et al. Contact sensitization to limonene and linalool hydroperoxides in Spain: a GEIDAC* prospective study. Contact Dermatitis 2017;76:74-80

49 Ung CY, White JML, White IR, Banerjee P, McFadden JP. Patch testing with the European baseline series fragrance markers: a 2016 update. Br J Dermatol 2018;178:776-780

50 Mann J, McFadden JP, White JML, White IR, Banerjee P. Baseline series fragrance markers fail to predict contact allergy. Contact Dermatitis 2014;70:276-281

51 Uter W, Amario-Hita JC, Balato A, Ballmer-Weber B, Bauer A, Belloni Fortina A, et al. European Surveillance System on Contact Allergies (ESSCA): results with the European baseline series, 2013/14. J Eur Acad Dermatol Venereol 2017;31:1516-1525

52 DeKoven JG, Warshaw EM, Belsito DV, Sasseville D, Maibach HI, Taylor JS, et al. North American Contact Dermatitis Group Patch Test Results: 2013-2014. Dermatitis 2017;28:33-46

53 Warshaw EM, Maibach HI, Taylor JS, Sasseville D, DeKoven JG, Zirwas MJ, et al. North American Contact Dermatitis Group patch test results: 2011-2012. Dermatitis 2015;26:49-59

54 Bennike NH, Zachariae C, Johansen JD. Non-mix fragrances are top sensitizers in consecutive dermatitis patients - a cross-sectional study of the 26 EU-labelled fragrance allergens. Contact Dermatitis 2017;77:270-279

55 Heisterberg MV, Menné T, Johansen JD. Contact allergy to the 26 specific fragrance ingredients to be declared on cosmetic products in accordance with the EU cosmetics directive. Contact Dermatitis 2011;65:266-275

56 Van Oosten E, Schuttelaar M-L, Coenraads PJ. Clinical relevance of positive patch test reactions to the 26 EU-labelled fragrances. Contact Dermatitis 2009;61:217-223

57 Bauer K, Garbe D, Surburg H. Common fragrance and flavor materials, 2nd Edn. Wienheim: VCH-Verlagsgesell-schaft, 1990

58 Dittmar D, Schuttelaar MLA. Contact sensitization to hydroperoxides of limonene and linalool: Results of consecutive patch testing and clinical relevance. Contact Dermatitis 2018 Oct 31. doi: 10.1111/cod.13137. [Epub ahead of print]

59 DeKoven JG, Warshaw EM, Zug KA, Maibach HI, Belsito DV, Sasseville D, et al. North American Contact Dermatitis Group patch test results: 2015-2016. Dermatitis 2018;29:297-309

60 Bennike NH, Oturai NB, Müller S, Kirkeby CS, Jørgensen C, Christensen AB, et al. Fragrance contact allergens in 5588 cosmetic products identified through a novel smartphone application. J Eur Acad Dermatol Venereol 2018;32:79-85

61 Buckley DA. Fragrance ingredient labelling in products on sale in the UK. Br J Dermatol 2007;57:295-300

62 Uter W, Yazar K, Kratz E-M, Mildau G, Lidén C. Coupled exposure to ingredients of cosmetic products: I. Fragrances. Contact Dermatitis 2013;69:335-341

63 Yazar K, Johnsson S, Lind M-L, Boman A, Lidén C. Preservatives and fragrances in selected consumer-available cosmetics and detergents. Contact Dermatitis 2011;64:265-272

64 Hamann D, Kishi P, Hamann CR. Consumer hair dye kits frequently contain isothiazolinones, other common preservatives and fragrance allergens. Dermatitis 2018;29:48-49

65 Klaschka U. Contact allergens for armpits - allergenic fragrances specified on deodorants. Int J Hyg Environ Health 2012;215:584-591

66 Wieck S, Olsson O, Kümmerer K, Klaschka U. Fragrance allergens in household detergents. Regul Toxicol Pharmacol 2018;97:163-169

67 EU Directive 2003/15/EC of the European Parliament and of the Council of 27 February 2003 amending Council Directive 76/768/EEC on the approximation of the laws of the Member States relating to cosmetic products. Off J Eur Union 2003;L66:26-35. Available at:
http://eur-lex.europa.eu/LexUriServ/LexUriServ.do?uri=OJ:L:2003:066: 0026:0035:en:PDF

68 Heisterberg MV, Menné T, Andersen KE, Avnstorp C, Kristensen B, Kristensen O, et al. Deodorants are the leading cause of allergic contact dermatitis to fragrance ingredients. Contact Dermatitis 2011;64:258-264

69 Heisterberg MV, Menné T, Johansen JD. Fragrance allergy and quality of life – a case–control study. Contact Dermatitis 2014;70:81-89

70 Nakayama H, Matsuo S, Hayakawa K, Takhashi K, Shigematsu T, Ota S. Pigmented cosmetic dermatitis. Int J Dermatol 1984;23:299-305

71 Nakayama H, Harada R, Toda M. Pigmented cosmetic dermatitis. Int J Dermatol 1976;15:673-675

72 Nakayama H, Hanaoka H, Ohshiro A. Allergen Controlled System. Tokyo: Kanehara Shuppan, 1974

73 Ebihara T, Nakayama H. Pigmented contact dermatitis. Clin Dermatol 1997;15:593-599

74 Becker K, Temesvari E, Nemeth I. Patch testing with fragrance mix and its constituents in a Hungarian population. Contact Dermatitis 1994;30:185-186

75 Emmons WW, Marks JG Jr. Immediate and delayed reactions to cosmetic ingredients. Contact Dermatitis 1985;13:258-265

76 Forsbeck M, Skog E. Immediate reactions to patch tests with balsam of Peru. Contact Dermatitis 1977;3:201-205

77 Temesvári E, Soos G, Podányi B, Kovács I, Nemeth I. Contact urticaria provoked by balsam of Peru. Contact Dermatitis 1978;4:65-68

78 Basketter DA, Wilhelm KP. Studies on non-immune immediate contact reactions in an unselected population. Contact Dermatitis 1996;35:237-240

79 Wojnarowska F, Calnan CD. Contact and photocontact allergy to musk ambrette. Br J Dermatol 1986;114:667-675

80 Jackson RT, Nesbitt LT, DeLeo VA. 6-Methylcoumarin photocontact dermatitis. J Am Acad Dermatol 1980;2:124-127

81 Addo HA, Ferguson J, Johnson BF, Frain-Bell W. The relationship between exposure to fragrance materials and persistent light reaction in photosensitivity dermatitis with actinic reticuloid syndrome. Br J Dermatol 1982;107:261-274

82 Rudzki E, Grzywa Z. Sensitizing and irritating properties of star anise oil. Contact Dermatitis 1976;2:305-308

83 Hjorth N. Eczematous allergy to balsams. Acta Derm Venereol 1961;41(suppl.46):1-216

84 White JML, McFadden JP, White IR. A review of 241 subjects who were patch tested twice: could fragrance mix I cause active sensitization? Br J Dermatol 2008;158:518-521

85 Carlsen BC, Menné T, Johansen JD. 20 years of standard patch testing in an eczema population with focus on patients with multiple contact allergies. Contact Dermatitis 2007;57:76-83

86 Uter W, Schnuch A, Geier J, Pfahlberg A, Gefeller O. Association between occupation and contact allergy to the fragrance mix: a multifactorial analysis of national surveillance data. Occup Environ Med 2001;58:392-398

87 Bonnevie P. Some experiences of war-time industrial dermatoses. Acta Derm Venereol 1948;28:231-237

88 Goodfield MJD, Saihan EM. Fragrance sensitivity in coal miners. Contact Dermatitis 1988;18:81-83

89 Pesonen M, Suomela S, Kuuliala O, Henriks-Eckerman M-L, Aalto-Korte K.Occupational contact dermatitis caused by D-limonene. Contact Dermatitis 2014;71:273-279

90 De Mozzi P, Johnston GA. An outbreak of allergic contact dermatitis caused by citral in beauticians working in a health spa. Contact Dermatitis 2014;70:377-379

91 Dahlquist I, Fregert S. Atranorin and oakmoss contact allergy. Contact Dermatitis 1981;7:168-169

92 English JSC, Rycroft RJG. Allergic contact dermatitis from methyl heptine and methyl octine carbonate. Contact Dermatitis 1988;18:174-175

93 Owen CM, August PJ, Beck MH. Contact allergy to oakmoss resin in a soluble oil. Contact Dermatitis 2000;43:112

94   Sanchez-Politta S, Campanelli A, Pashe-Koo F, Saurat JH, Piletta P. Allergic contact dermatitis to phenylacetal-dehyde: a forgotten allergen? Contact Dermatitis 2007;56:171-172

95   Decapite TJ, Anderson BE. Allergic contact dermatitis from cinnamic aldehyde found in an industrial odour-masking agent. Contact Dermatitis 2004;51:312-313

96   Kanerva L, Estlander T, Jolanki R. Dental nurse's occupational allergic contact dermatitis from eugenol used as a restorative dental material with polymethylmethacrylate. Contact Dermatitis 1998;38:339-340

97   Kanerva L, Jolanki R, Estlander T. Hairdresser's dermatitis caused by oakmoss in permanent waving solution. Contact Dermatitis 1999;41:55

98   Wakelin SH, McFadden JP, Leonard JN, Rycroft RJ. Allergic contact dermatitis from *d*-limonene in a laboratory technician. Contact Dermatitis 1998;38:164-165

99   Martins C, Gonçalo M, Gonçalo S. Allergic contact dermatitis from dipentene in wax polish. Contact Dermatitis 1995;33:126

100 Rycroft RJ. Allergic contact dermatitis from dipentene in honing oil. Contact Dermatitis 1980;6:325-329

101 Karlberg A-T, Dooms-Goossens A. Contact allergy to oxidised *d*-limonene among dermatitis patients. Contact Dermatitis 1997;36:201-206

102 Topham EJ, Wakelin SH. *D*-Limonene contact dermatitis from hand cleansers. Contact Dermatitis 2003;49:108

103 Nethercott JR, Pilger C, O'Blents L, Roy A-M. Contact dermatitis due to cinnamic aldehyde induced in a deodorant manufacturing process. Contact Dermatitis 1983;9:241-242

104 Perper M, Cervantes J, Eber AE, Tosti A. Airborne contact dermatitis caused by fragrance diffusers in Uber cars. Contact Dermatitis 2017;77:116-117

105 Freeman S. Fragrance and nickel: old allergens in new guises. Am J Contact Dermat 1990;1:47-52

106 Verma A, Tancharoen C, Tam MM, Nixon R. Pustular allergic contact dermatitis caused by fragrances. Contact Dermatitis 2015;72:245-248

107 Calnan CD. Allergy to dipentene in paint thinners. Contact Dermatitis 1979;5:123-124

108 Kerre S, Matura M, Goossens A. Allergic contact dermatitis from a degreaser. Contact Dermatitis 2006;55:117-118

109 Keil H. Contact dermatitis due to oil of citronellal. J Invest Dermatol 1947;8:327-334

110 Mobacken H, Fregert S. Allergic contact dermatitis from cardamom. Contact Dermatitis 1975;1:175-176

111 D'Erme AM, Francalanci S, Milanesi N, Ricci L, Gola M. Contact dermatitis due to dipentene and pine oil in an automobile mechanic. Occup Environ Med 2012;69:452

112 Garcia-Bravo B, Pérez Bernal A, Garcia-Hernandez MJ, Camacho F. Occupational contact dermatitis from anethole in food handlers. Contact Dermatitis 1997;37:38

113 Mitchell DM, Beck MH. Contact allergy to benzyl alcohol in a cutting oil reodorant. Contact Dermatitis 1988;18:301-302

114 Schultheiss E. Überempfindlichkeit gegenüber Ionon und Benzylalkohol. Derm Monatsschr 1957;135:629 (article in German). Data cited in ref. 115

115 Fisher AA. Allergic paraben and benzyl alcohol hypersensitivity relationship of the "delayed" and "immediate" varieties. Contact Dermatitis 1975;1:281-284

116 Lodi A, Mancini LL, Pozzi M, Chiarelli G, Crosti C. Occupational airborne allergic contact dermatitis in parquet layers. Contact Dermatitis 1993;29:281-282

117 Castelain PY, Camoin JP, Jouglard J. Contact dermatitis to terpene derivatives in a machine cleaner. Contact Dermatitis 1980;6:358-360

118 Dharmagunawardena B, Takwale A, Sanders KJ, Cannan S, Rodger A, Ilchyshyn A. Gas chromatography: an investigative tool in multiple allergies to essential oils. Contact Dermatitis 2002;47:288-292

119 Meding B. Skin symptoms among workers in a spice factory. Contact Dermatitis 1993;29:202-205

120 De Benito V, Alzaga R. Occupational allergic contact dermatitis from cassia (Chinese cinnamon) as a flavouring agent in coffee. Contact Dermatitis 1999;40:165

121 Guarneri F. Occupational allergy to cinnamal in a baker. Contact Dermatitis 2010;63:294

122 Rastogi SC, Heydorn S, Johansen JD, Basketter DA. Fragrance chemicals in domestic and occupational products. Contact Dermatitis 2001;45:221-225

123 Ackermann L, Aalto-Korte K, Jolanki R, Alanko K. Occupational allergic contact dermatitis from cinnamon including one case from airborne exposure. Contact Dermatitis 2009;60:96-99

124 Sánchez-Pérez J, García-Díez A. Occupational allergic contact dermatitis from eugenol, oil of cinnamon and oil of cloves in a physiotherapist. Contact Dermatitis 1999;41:346-347

125 Ortiz de Frutos FJ, Vergara A, Isarria MJ, del Prado-Sánchez M, Vanaclocha F. Occupational allergic contact eczema in a dental assistant. Actas Dermosifiliogr 2005;96:56-58 (article in Spanish)

126 Hagvall L, Karlberg A-T, Christensson JB. Contact allergy to air-exposed geraniol: clinical observations and report of 14 cases. Contact Dermatitis 2012;67:20-27

127 Murphy LA, White IR. Contact dermatitis from geraniol in washing-up liquid. Contact Dermatitis 2003;49:52

128 Tanko Z, Shab A, Diepgen TL, Weisshaar E. Polyvalent type IV sensitizations to multiple fragrances and a skin protection cream in a metal worker. J Dtsch Dermatol Ges 2009;7:541-543

129 Aalto-Korte K, Valimaa J, Henriks-Eckerman ML, Jolanki R. Allergic contact dermatitis from salicyl alcohol and salicylaldehyde in aspen bark (*Populus tremula*). Contact Dermatitis 2005;52:93-95

130 De Groot AC, Liem DH. Facial psoriasis caused by contact allergy to linalool and hydroxycitronellal in an aftershave. Contact Dermatitis 1983;9:230-232

131 Thompson JA Jr, Wansker BA. A case of contact dermatitis, erythema multiforme, and toxic epidermal necrolysis. J Am Acad Dermatol 1981;5:666-669

132 Seidenari S, Di Nardo A, Motolese A, Pincelli C. Erythema multiforme associated with contact sensitization. Report of 6 cases. G !tal Dermatol Venereal 1990;125:35-40 (article in Italian)

133 SCCS (Scientific Committee on Consumer Safety). Opinion on Fragrance allergens in cosmetic products, 26-27 June 2012, SCCS/1459/11. Available at:
https://ec.europa.eu/health/sites/health/files/scientific_committees/consumer_safety/docs/sccs_o_102.pdf

134 Elberling J, Linneberg A, Dirksen A, Johansen JD, Frolund L, Madsen F, et al. Mucosal symptoms elicited by fragrance products in a population-based sample in relation to atopy and bronchial hyper-reactivity. Clin Exp Allergy 2005;35:75-81

135 Kumar P, Caradonna-Graham VM, Gupta S, Cai X, Rao PN, Thompson J. Inhalation challenge effects of perfume scent strips in patients with asthma. Ann Allergy Asthma Immunol 1995;75:429-433

136 Millqvist E, Bende M, Lowhagen O. Sensory hyperreactivity - a possible mechanism underlying cough and asthma-like symptoms. Allergy 1998;53:1208-1212

137 Elberling J, Linneberg A, Mosbech H, Dirksen A, Frolund L, Madsen F, Nielsen NH, Johansen JD. A link between skin and airways regarding sensitivity to fragrance products? Br J Dermatol 2004;151:1197-1203

138 Guin JD, Berry VK. Perfume sensitivity in adults females. A study of contact sensitivity to a perfume mix in two groups of student nurses. J Am Acad Dermatol 1980;3:299-302

139 De Groot AC, Nater JP, Van der Lende R, Rijcken B. Adverse effects of cosmetics: A retrospective study in the general population. !nt J Cosmetic Science 1987;9:255-259

140 Elberling J. Respiratory symptoms from fragrances and the link with dermatitis. In: Johansen JD, Frosch PJ, Lepoittevin J-D, Eds. Contact Dermatitis, 5th Edition. Heidelberg Dordrecht London New York: Springer, 2011: Chapter 23, 429-436

141 Lysdal SH, Johansen JD. Fragrance contact allergic patients: strategies for use of cosmetic products and perceived impact on life situation. Contact Dermatitis 2009;61:320-324

142 Johansen JD, Andersen TF, Kjoller M, Veien N, Avnstorp C, Andersen KE, et al. Identification of risk products for fragrance contact allergy: a case-referent study based on patients' histories. Am J Contact Dermat 1998;9:80-86

143 Nardelli A, Carbonez A, Ottoy W, Drieghe J, Goossens A. Frequency of and trends in fragrance allergy over a 15-year period. Contact Dermatitis 2008;58:134-141

144 Johansen JD, Andersen TF, Veien N, Avnstorp C, Andersen KE, Menné T. Patch testing with markers of fragrance contact allergy. Do clinical tests correspond to patients' self-reported problems? Acta Derm Venereol 1997;77:149-153

145 Heydorn S, Johansen JD, Andersen KE, Bruze M, Svedman C, White IR, et al. Fragrance allergy in patients with hand eczema - a clinical study. Contact Dermatitis 2003;48:317-323

146 Buckley DA, Rycroft RJ, White IR, McFadden JP. Contact allergy to individual fragrance mix constituents in relation to primary site of dermatitis. Contact Dermatitis 2000;43:304-305

147 Heydorn S, Menné T, Johansen JD. Fragrance allergy and hand eczema – a review. Contact Dermatitis 2003;48:59-66

148 Schnuch A, Uter W, Geier J, Lessmann H, Frosch PJ. Sensitization to 26 fragrances to be labelled according to current European regulation. Results of the IVDK and review of the literature. Contact Dermatitis 2007;57:1-10

149 Harder U. The art of creating a perfume. In: Frosch PJ, Johansen JD, White IR, Eds. Fragrances - beneficial and adverse effects. Berlin: Springer-Verlag, 1998:3-5

150 Katoulis AC, Stavrianeas NG, Katsarou A, Antoniou C, Georgala S, Rigopoulos D, et al. Evaluation of the role of contact sensitization and photosensitivity in the pathogenesis of poikiloderma of Civatte. Br J Dermatol 2002;147:493-497

151 Uter W, Fießler C, Gefeller O, Geier J, Schnuch A. Contact sensitization to fragrance mix I and II, to Myroxylon pereirae resin and oil of turpentine: multifactorial analysis of risk factors based on data of the IVDK network. Flavour Fragr J 2015;30:255-263

152 Geier J, Lessmann H, Schnuch A, Uter W. Contact sensitization in metalworkers with occupational dermatitis exposed to water-based metal working fluids. Results of the research project "FaSt". Int Arch Occup Environ Health 2004;77:543-551

153 Schnuch A, Griem P. Fragrances as allergens. Allergo J Int 2018;27:173-183

154 Buckley DA, Rycroft RJ, White IR, McFadden JP. The frequency of fragrance allergy in patch-tested patients increases with their age. Br J Dermatol 2003;149:986-989

155 Arribas MP, Soro P, Silvestre JF. Allergic contact dermatitis to fragrances. Part 1. Actas Dermosifiliogr 2012;103:874-879

156 Arribas MP, Soro P, Silvestre JF. Allergic contact dermatitis to fragrances: part 2. Actas Dermosifiliogr 2013;104:29-37

157 Katz AS, Sheretz F. Facial dermatitis: patch test results and final diagnosis. Am J Contact Dermat 1999;10:153-156

158 Cheng J, Zug KA. Fragrance allergic contact dermatitis. Dermatitis 2014;25:232-245

159 Buckley DA, Rycroft RJ, White IR, McFadden JP. Fragrance as an occupational allergen. Occup Med (Lond) 2002;52:13-16

160 Schnuch A, Oppel E, Oppel T, Römmelt H, Kramer M, Riu E, et al. Experimental inhalation of fragrance allergens in predisposed subjects: effects on skin and airways. Br J Dermatol 2010;162:598-606

161 Scheinman PL. Allergic contact dermatitis to fragrance: A review. Am J Cont Derm 1996;7:65-76

162 De Groot AC. Patch Testing, 4th Edition. Wapserveen, The Netherlands: acdegroot publishing, 2018 (ISBN 978-90-813233-4-5)

Chapter 3   Monographs of fragrance chemicals and extracts that have caused contact allergy / allergic contact dermatitis

3.0 INTRODUCTION

In this chapter, Monographs of 165 fragrance chemicals and extracts that have caused contact allergy / allergic contact dermatitis are presented. They have a standardized format, which is explained and detailed in Chapter 1.2. The fragrances discussed here are shown in table 3.0.1. A short summary of these data and other general aspects of fragrance allergy (the composition of perfumes; how do we come in contact with fragrances?; fragrances that have caused contact allergy / allergic contact dermatitis; diagnosing fragrance allergy; how frequent is fragrance allergy?; clinical picture of allergic contact dermatitis from fragrances; other side effects; products responsible for allergic contact dermatitis from fragrances; occupational contact dermatitis from fragrance allergy) can be found in Chapter 2. Monographs on chemicals not used as fragrances themselves but present as allergenic ingredients of botanical fragrance materials are presented in Chapter 4 and Monographs on Essential oils in Chapter 6.

Table 3.0.1 Fragrance chemicals and extracts presented in Monographs in Chapter 3

Acetylcedrene	Coumarin
Acetyl hexamethyl indan	Cuminaldehyde
Acetyl hexamethyl tetralin	5-Cyclohexadecenone
Allylanisole	Cyclohexyl acetate
Allyl cyclohexylpropionate	Cyclopentadecanone
Ambrettolide	p-Cymene
Amyl cinnamal	alpha-Damascone
Amyl cinnamate	beta-Damascone
Amylcinnamyl alcohol	Dehydrodiisoeugenol
Amyl salicylate	Diethyl maleate
Anethole	Dihydrocarveol
Anise alcohol	Dihydrocitronellol
Anisylidene acetone	Dihydrocoumarin
Benzaldehyde	Dihydro pentamethylindanone
Benzyl acetate	Dimethylbenzyl carbinyl acetate
Benzyl alcohol	Dimethyl citraconate
Benzyl benzoate	2,4-Dimethyl-3-cyclohexene carboxaldehyde
Benzyl cinnamate	Dimethyltetrahydro benzaldehyde
Benzylidene acetone	Ethyl anisate
Benzyl isoeugenol	Ethylene dodecanedioate
Benzyl propionate	Ethyl vanillin
Benzyl salicylate	Eucalyptol
Butyl acetate	Eugenol
Butylphenyl methylpropional	Evernia furfuracea (treemoss) extract
Camphor	Evernia prunastri (oakmoss) extract
Camphylcyclohexanol	Farnesol
Caprylic alcohol	Ferula galbaniflua gum
3-Carene	Fragrance mix I
Carvacrol	Fragrance mix II
Carvone	Geranial
beta-Caryophyllene	Geraniol
Caryophyllene oxide	Geranyl acetate
Cedrol methyl ether	Heliotropine
Cinnamal	Heptanal
Cinnamic acid	Hexadecanolactone
Cinnamy alcohol	Hexamethylindanopyran
Cinnamyl benzoate	cis-3-Hexenyl salicylate
Cinnamyl cinnamate	Hexyl cinnamal
Citral	Hexyl salicylate
Citral diethyl acetal	Hydroxycitronellal
Citronellal	Hydroxycitronellol
Citronellol	

Table 3.0.1 Fragrance chemicals and extracts presented in Monographs in Chapter 3 (continued)

Hydroxyisohexyl 3-cyclohexene carboxaldehyde	Musk xylene
Ionone	Myrcene
Isoamyl salicylate	Myroxylon pereirae resin
Isoeugenol	Narcissus poeticus flower extract
Isoeugenyl acetate	Neral
Isoeugenyl benzoate	Nerol
Isoeugenyl phenylacetate	Nerolidol
Isolongifolanone	Nonanal
alpha-Isomethyl ionone	Nonyl alcohol
Isopulegol	Nopyl acetate
Isosafrole	Pentamethylcyclopent-3-ene-butanol
Limonene	alpha-Phellandrene
Linalool	Phenethyl alcohol
Linalyl acetate	Phenylacetaldehyde
Maltol	Phenylpropanol
Menthol	alpha-Pinene
Menthyl acetate	beta-Pinenes
Methoxycinnamal	Piperitone
Methoxycitronellal	Propylidene phthalide
2-Methoxyphenol/2,2-dimethyl-3-methyl-enebicycloheptane hydrogenated	D-Pulegone
Methoxytrimethylheptanol	Rhodinol
Methyl p-anisate	Rose ketone-4
Methyl anthranilate	Sabinene
Methyl cinnamate	Safrole
6-Methyl coumarin	Salicylaldehyde
Methyldihydrojasmonate	Santalol
Methylenedioxyphenyl methylpropanal	Styryl acetate
Methyl eugenol	alpha-Terpinene
Methyl ionones	4-Terpineol
5-Methyl-alpha-ionone	alpha-Terpineol
Methyl isoeugenol	Terpinolene
Methyl octine carbonate	Terpinyl acetate
Methyl 2-octynoate	Tetrahydro-dimethylbenzofuran
Methyl salicylate	Tetramethyl acetyloctahydronaphthalene
3-Methyl-5-(2,2,3-trimethyl-3-cyclopentenyl) pent-4-en-2-ol	Thymol
	Trimethylbenzenepropanol
Musk	5,5,6-Trimethylbicyclohept-2-ylcyclohexanol
Musk ambrette	2,4,6-Trimethyl-4-phenyl-1,3-dioxane
Musk ketone	Vanillin
Musk moskene	Verdyl acetate
Musk tibetene	Vetiveryl acetate
	Viola odorata leaf extract

Chapter 3.1 ACETYLCEDRENE

IDENTIFICATION

Description/definition : Acetylcedrene is the polycyclic ketone that conforms to the structural formula shown below

Chemical class(es) : Ketones; polycyclic organic compounds

INCI name USA : Not in the Personal Care Products Council Ingredient Database

Chemical/IUPAC name : (3R-(3α,3αβ,7b,8aα))-1-(2,3,4,7,8,8a-Hexahydro-3,6,8,8-tetramethyl-1H-3a,7-methanoazulen-5-yl)ethan-1-one

Other names : Methyl cedryl ketone; Vertofix ®

CAS registry number(s) : 32388-55-9

EC number(s) : 251-020-3

RIFM monograph(s) : Food Chem Toxicol 2013;62(suppl.1):S152-S166; Food Cosmet Toxicol 1978;16:639 (special issue IV)

SCCS opinion(s) : SCCS/1459/11 (1)

Function(s) in cosmetics : EU: perfuming

Patch testing : 5% pet. (5)

Molecular formula : $C_{17}H_{26}O$

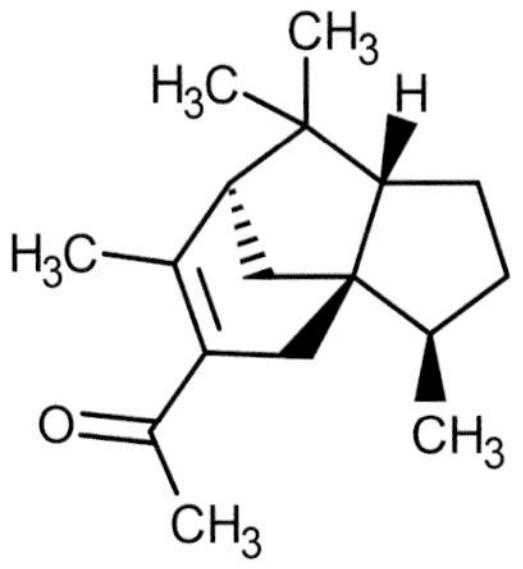

GENERAL

Acetylcedrene is a yellow to brown clear oily liquid; its odor type is woody and its odor at 100% is described as 'woody vetiver amber leather musk cedar' (www.thegoodscentscompany.com). It is a complex mixture obtained from cedar wood oil by the acetylation of terpenes. The principal component of acetylcedrene is methyl cedryl ketone (CAS 32388-55-9) (1).

The INCI name for this fragrance is acetylcedrene, but in most chemical databases it is spelled acetyl cedrene (with blank between acetyl and cedrene).

Presence in essential oils

Acetylcedrene has been identified by chemical analysis in 1 of 91 essential oils, which have caused contact allergy / allergic contact dermatitis: carrot seed oil (8). However, acetylcedrene is not found in nature according to www.thegoodscentscompany.com; therefore, it cannot be excluded that the analytical identification of acetylcedrene has been erroneous.

CONTACT ALLERGY

The SCCS (Scientific Committee on Consumer Safety), in a 2012 Opinion on Fragrance allergens in cosmetic products, has marked acetylcedrene as 'established contact allergen in humans' (1,6). The sensitizing potency of acetylcedrene was classified as 'weak' based on an EC3 value of 13.9% in the LLNA (local lymph node assay) in animal experiments (1,6,7).

Patch testing in groups of patients

Routine testing

In 1997-1998, in 6 European countries, 1855 consecutive patients suspected of contact dermatitis were patch tested with acetylcedrene 5% pet. and there were 3 (0.2%) positive reactions. Their relevance was not specified (5). Before 1995, in Sweden, 100 consecutive patients were tested with acetylcedrene 1% and there was only one positive reaction (1%), which was not relevant (4).

Case reports and case series
A man presented with axillary dermatitis. Upon patch testing, he reacted to 2 deodorants. Ingredient patch testing showed a positive reaction to the perfume in one of the cosmetic products and later to its ingredient acetylcedrene 10.8% in dipropylene glycol. Patch tests to acetylcedrene in dilutions of 0.108%, 0.54% and 1.08% were all negative. Twenty controls had no positive responses to acetylcedrene in the highest concentration (2).

Presence in products and chemical analyses
In 1988, in the USA, 400 perfumes used in fine fragrances, household products and soaps (number of products per category not mentioned) were analyzed for the presence of fragrance chemicals in a concentration of at least 1% and a list of the Top-25 (present in the highest number of products) presented. Acetylcedrene was found to be present in 41% of the fine fragrances (rank number 17), 32% of the household household products (rank number 15) and an unknown percentage of the fragrances used in soaps (3).

LITERATURE

1   SCCS (Scientific Committee on Consumer Safety). Opinion on Fragrance allergens in cosmetic products, 26-27 June 2012, SCCS/1459/11. Available at:
     https://ec.europa.eu/health/sites/health/files/scientific_committees/consumer_safety/docs/sccs_o_102.pdf
2   Handley J, Burrows D. Allergic contact dermatitis from the synthetic fragrances Lyral and acetyl cedrene in separate underarm deodorant preparations. Contact Dermatitis 1994;31:288-290
3   Fenn RS. Aroma chemical usage trends in modern perfumery. Perfumer and Flavorist 1989;14:3-10
4   Frosch PJ, Pilz B, Andersen KE, Burrows D, Camarasa JG, Dooms-Goossens A, et al. Patch testing with fragrances: results of a multicenter study of the European Environmental and Contact Dermatitis Research Group with 48 frequently used constituents of perfumes. Contact Dermatitis 1995;33:333-342
5   Frosch PJ, Johansen JD, Menné T, Pirker C, Rastogi SC, Andersen KE, et al. Further important sensitizers in patients sensitive to fragrances. I. Reactivity to 14 frequently used chemicals. Contact Dermatitis 2002;47:78-85
6   Uter W, Johansen JD, Börje A, Karlberg A-T, Lidén C, Rastogi S, Roberts D, White IR. Categorization of fragrance contact allergens for prioritization of preventive measures: clinical and experimental data and consideration of structure–activity relationships. Contact Dermatitis 2013;69:196-230
7   Scognamiglio J, Letizia CS, Politano VT, Api AM. Fragrance material review on acetyl cedrene. Food Chem Toxicol 2013;62(suppl.1):S152-S166
8   De Groot AC, Schmidt E. Essential oils: contact allergy and chemical composition. Boca Raton, Fl., USA: CRC Press, Taylor and Francis Group, 2016 (ISBN 9781482246407)

Chapter 3.2   ACETYL HEXAMETHYL INDAN

IDENTIFICATION

Description/definition : Acetyl hexamethyl indan is the organic compound that conforms to the structural formula shown below
Chemical class(es) : Ketones
Chemical/IUPAC name : 1-(1,1,2,3,3,6-Hexamethyl-2*H*-inden-5-yl)ethenone
Other names : 5-Acetyl-1,1,2,3,3,6-hexamethylindan; musk indane; Phantolide ®; Fixolide ®; 1,1,2,3,3,6-hexamethylindan-5-yl methyl ketone
CAS registry number(s) : 15323-35-0
EC number(s) : 239-360-0
RIFM monograph(s) : Food Cosmet Toxicol 1979;17:241; Food Cosmet Toxicol 1975;13:693 (special issue II)
IFRA standard : Restricted: leave-on products 2% in finished products, all other products no restrictions (www.ifraorg.org/en-us/standards-library)
SCCS opinion(s) : SCCNFP/0392/00, final (1); SCCNFP/0389/00, final (6)
Function(s) in cosmetics : EU: masking; perfuming. USA: fragrance ingredients
EU cosmetic restrictions : Regulated in Annex III/134 of the Regulation (EC) No. 344/2013
Patch testing : 3% pet. (4)
Molecular formula : $C_{17}H_{24}O$

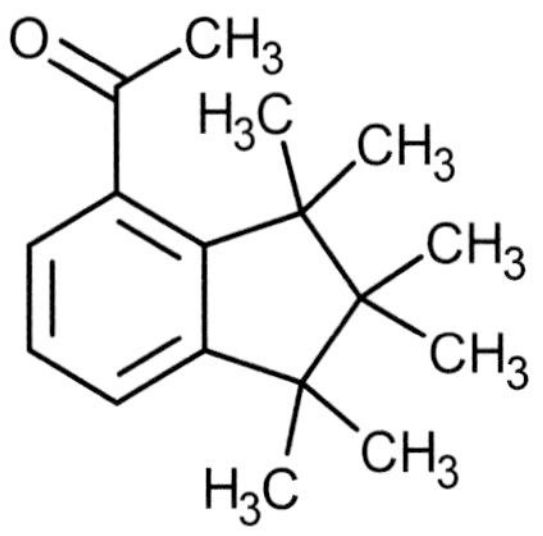

GENERAL

Acetyl hexamethyl indan has the appearance of off-white crystals or solid material; its odor type is musk and its odor at 100% is described as 'strong sweet musk amber powdery dry fruity' (www.thegoodscentscompany.com). It is a synthetic chemical, not found in nature (and consequently not in essential oils).

The name fixolide (not as trade name) is also used as synonym for acetyl hexamethyl tetralin (Chapter 3.3 Acetyl hexamethyl tetralin).

CONTACT ALLERGY

Patch testing in groups of patients
In France, before 1986, 21 patients with dermatitis caused by perfumes were patch tested with a battery of fragrances and essential oils and 1 (5%) reacted to acetyl hexamethyl indan 3% pet. The relevance of this positive patch test reaction was not mentioned (5).

OTHER SIDE EFFECTS

Photosensitivity
Acetyl hexamethyl indan is cited to have caused phototoxic contact dermatitis (2).

LITERATURE

1   SCCNFP (Scientific Committee on Cosmetic Products and Non-Food Products Intended for Consumers). 'An initial list of perfumery materials which must not form part of cosmetic products except subject to the Restrictions and Conditions laid down, 25 September 2001, SCCNFP/0392/00, final. Available at: http://ec.europa.eu/health/archive/ph_risk/committees/sccp/documents/out150_en.pdf
2   Ford R. The toxicology and safety of fragrances. In: Muller PM, Lamparsky D, Eds. Perfumes: art, science, technology. New York: Elsevier, 1991:441-463. Data cited in ref. 3

3   Larsen WG. How do we test for fragrance allergy? In: Frosch PJ, Johansen JD, White IR, Eds. Fragrances - beneficial and adverse effects. Berlin Heidelberg New York: Springer-Verlag, 1998: 76-82

4   De Groot AC. Patch Testing, 4th Edition. Wapserveen, The Netherlands: acdegroot publishing, 2018 (ISBN 978-90-813233-4-5)

5   Meynadier JM, Meynadier J, Peyron JL, Peyron L. Formes cliniques des manifestations cutanées d'allergie aux parfums. Ann Dermatol Venereol 1986;113:31-39

6   Opinion of the Scientific Committee on Cosmetic Products and Non-Food Products Intended for Consumers concerning 'The 1st update of the inventory of ingredients employed in cosmetic products. Section II: Perfume and aromatic raw materials', 24 October 2000, SCCNFP/0389/00, final. Available at: http://ec.europa.eu/health/ph_risk/committees/sccp/documents/out131_en.pdf

Chapter 3.3   ACETYL HEXAMETHYL TETRALIN

IDENTIFICATION

Description/definition   : Acetyl hexamethyl tetralin is the organic compound that conforms to the structural formula shown below
Chemical class(es)   : Ketones
Chemical/IUPAC name   : 1-(3,5,5,6,8,8-Hexamethyl-6,7-dihydronaphthalen-2-yl)ethanone
Other names   : 6-Acetyl-1,1,2,4,4,7-hexamethyltetralin; Tonalide ®; fixolide; musk tetralin; 1-(5,6,7,8-tetrahydro-3,5,5,6,8,8-hexamethyl-2-naphthyl)ethan-1-one
CAS registry number(s)   : 1506-02-1; 21145-77-7
EC number(s)   : 216-133-4; 244-240-6
RIFM monograph(s)   : Food Chem Toxicol 2017;110(suppl.1):S95-S103
SCCS opinion(s)   : SCCNFP/0609/02, final (3)
Function(s) in cosmetics   : EU: masking. USA: fragrance ingredients
EU cosmetic restrictions   : Regulated in Annex III/182 of the Regulation (EC) No. 344/2013
Patch testing   : 4% pet. (2)
Molecular formula   : $C_{18}H_{26}O$

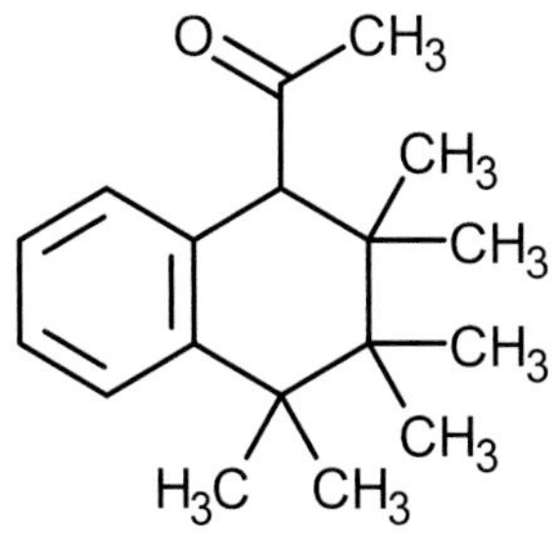

GENERAL

Acetyl hexamethyl tetralin is a white crystalline solid; its odor type is musk and its odor at 100% is described as 'strong sweet amber fruity musk powdery' (www.thegoodscentscompany.com). It is used as a fragrance in cosmetics, detergents, fabric softeners, household cleaning products and air fresheners (U.S. National Library of Medicine). Acetyl hexamethyl tetralin is a synthetic chemical, not found in nature (and consequently not in essential oils).

The name fixolide is also used as trade name for acetyl hexamethyl indan (Chapter 3.2 Acetyl hexamethyl indan).

CONTACT ALLERGY

Patch testing in groups of patients
In France, before 1986, 21 patients with dermatitis caused by perfumes were patch tested with a battery of fragrances and essential oils and 2 (10%) reacted to acetyl hexamethyl tetralin 3% pet. The relevance of these positive patch tests was not mentioned (4).

Presence in products and chemical analyses
In 1988, in the USA, 400 perfumes used in fine fragrances, household products and soaps (number of products per category not mentioned) were analyzed for the presence of fragrance chemicals in a concentration of at least 1% and a list of the Top-25 (present in the highest number of products) presented. Acetyl hexamethyl tetralin was found to be present in an unknown percentage of the fine fragrances, 35% of the household product fragrances and 42% of the fragrances used in soaps (rank number 14 in the latter category) (1).

LITERATURE

1   Fenn RS. Aroma chemical usage trends in modern perfumery. Perfumer and Flavorist 1989;14:3-10
2   De Groot AC. Patch Testing, 4th Edition. Wapserveen, The Netherlands: acdegroot publishing, 2018 (ISBN 978-90-813233-4-5)
3   SCCFNP (Scientific Committee on Cosmetic Products and Non-Food Products Intended for Consumers). Opinion concerning 6-Acetyl-1,1,2,4,4,7-hexamethyltetraline (AHTN), 17 September 2002, SCCNFP/0609/02, final. Available at: http://ec.europa.eu/health/ph_risk/committees/sccp/documents/out176_en.pdf
4   Meynadier JM, Meynadier J, Peyron JL, Peyron L. Formes cliniques des manifestations cutanées d'allergie aux parfums. Ann Dermatol Venereol 1986;113:31-39

Chapter 3.4   ALLYLANISOLE

IDENTIFICATION

Description/definition	: Allylanisole is the benzene derivative that conforms to the structural formula shown below
Chemical class(es)	: Aromatic organic compounds; unsaturated compounds; ethers
INCI name USA	: Not in the Personal Care Products Council Ingredient Database
Chemical/IUPAC name	: 1-Methoxy-4-prop-2-enylbenzene
Other names	: Methyl chavicol; estragole; isoanethole; 1-allyl-4-methoxybenzene
CAS registry number(s)	: 140-67-0
EC number(s)	: 205-427-8
RIFM monograph(s)	: Food Cosmet Toxicol 1976;14:603 (binder, page 540)
IFRA standard	: Restricted (www.ifraorg.org/en-us/standards-library) (table 3.4.1)
Merck Index monograph	: 5030 (Estragole)
Function(s) in cosmetics	: EU: perfuming
Patch testing	: 1% pet. (1)
Molecular formula	: $C_{10}H_{12}O$

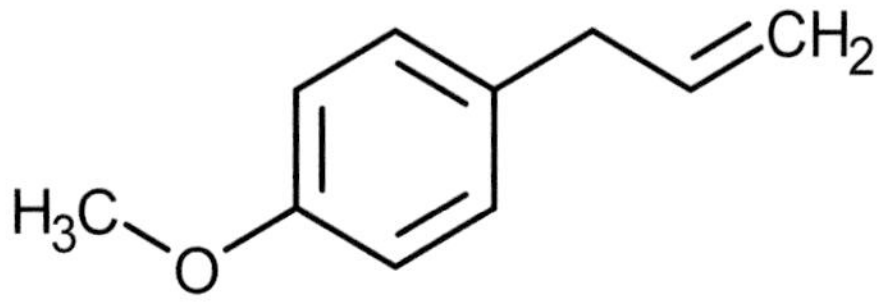

Table 3.4.1 IFRA restrictions for allylanisole

Fine fragrance:	0.2%
Eau de toilette:	0.2%
Other leave-on cosmetic products:	0.01%
Other rinse-off cosmetic products:	0.01%
Non-skin, incidental skin contact products:	0.2%

GENERAL

Allylanisole is a colorless to pale yellow clear liquid; its odor type is anisic and its odor is described as 'sweet, phenolic, anise, harsh, spice, green, herbal, minty' (www.thegoodscentscompany.com).

Presence in essential oils

Allylanisole (methyl chavicol) has been identified by chemical analysis in 38 of 91 (42%) essential oils, which have caused contact allergy / allergic contact dermatitis. In 4 oils, allylanisole belonged to the 'Top-10' of ingredients with the highest concentrations which may be expected in commercial essential oils of this type: basil oil, methyl chavicol type (0.2-87.0%), ravensara oil (0.04-19.9%), star anise oil (0.2-5.9%), and aniseed oil (0.01-3.2%) (2).

CONTACT ALLERGY

Case reports and case series

A patient who was sensitized by patch testing with star anise oil 0.5%, 1% and 2% in petrolatum, was tested with 9 components of star anise oil and reacted to anethole (the main component of star anise oil [2]), methyl chavicol, α-pinene and safrole, all tested 1% in petrolatum (1).

LITERATURE

1   Rudzki E, Grzywa Z. Sensitizing and irritating properties of star anise oil. Contact Dermatitis 1976;2:305-306
2   De Groot AC, Schmidt E. Essential oils: contact allergy and chemical composition. Boca Raton, Fl., USA: CRC Press, Taylor and Francis Group, 2016 (ISBN 9781482246407)

Chapter 3.5   ALLYL CYCLOHEXYLPROPIONATE *

* Not an INCI name, but perfuming name

IDENTIFICATION

Description/definition	: Allyl cyclohexylpropionate is the ester that conforms to the structural formula shown below
Chemical class(es)	: Cyclic organic compounds; unsaturated compounds; esters
INCI name USA	: Not in the Personal Care Products Council Ingredient Database
Chemical/IUPAC name	: Prop-2-enyl 3-cyclohexylpropanoate
Other names	: Allyl cyclohexanepropionate; 2-propenyl 3-cyclohexylpropanoate
CAS registry number(s)	: 2705-87-5
EC number(s)	: 220-292-5
RIFM monograph(s)	: Food Cosmet Toxicol 1973;11:491 and 1081
Function(s) in cosmetics	: EU: perfuming
EU cosmetic restrictions	: Regulated in Annex III/138 of the Regulation (EC) No. 344/2013
Patch testing	: No data available; based on RIFM data, 4% pet. is probably not irritant (2)
Molecular formula	: $C_{12}H_{20}O_2$

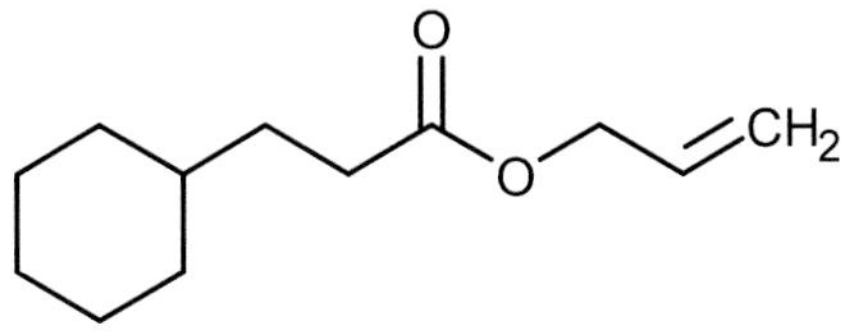

GENERAL

Allyl cyclohexylpropionate is a colorless to pale yellow clear liquid; its odor type is fruity and its odor is described as 'sweet, fruity, pineapple, waxy, apple and green' (www.thegoodscentscompany.com). Allyl cyclohexylpropionate is a synthetic chemical and is not found in nature (and consequently not in essential oils).

CONTACT ALLERGY

Patch testing in groups of patients

While searching for causative ingredients of pigmented cosmetic dermatitis in Japan in the 1970s, both patients with ordinary (nonpigmented) cosmetic dermatitis and women with pigmented cosmetic dermatitis were tested with a large number of fragrance materials. In 1980 the accumulated data enabled the classification of fragrance materials into 4 groups: common sensitizers, rare sensitizers, virtually non-sensitizing fragrances and fragrances considered as non-sensitizers. Allyl cyclohexylpropionate was classified in the group of rare sensitizers, indicating that one or more cases of contact allergy / allergic contact dermatitis to it have been observed (1). More specific data are lacking, the results have largely or solely been published in Japanese journals only.

Case reports and case series

A woman developed allergic contact dermatitis around the eyes from the perfume in an eye cream. When patch tested to its ingredients, there were positive reactions to allyl cyclohexyl propionate and 11 other compounds (4). Two years later, in a Letter to the Editor, the author mentioned that he had retested the patient with the twelve fragrances to which she had previously shown a positive patch test. Only hydroxycitronellal had again given a positive test (3).

LITERATURE

1   Nakayama H. Fragrance hypersensitivity and its control. In: Frosch PJ, Johansen JD, White IR, Eds. Fragrances - beneficial and adverse effects. Berlin Heidelberg New York: Springer-Verlag, 1998:83-91
2   Research Institute for Fragrance Materials (RIFM), cited in De Groot AC. Patch Testing, 4th Edition. Wapserveen, The Netherlands: acdegroot publishing, 2018 (ISBN 978-90-813233-1-4)
3   Larsen WG. Perfume dermatitis revisited. Contact Dermatitis 1977;3:98
4   Larsen WG. Cosmetic dermatitis due to a perfume. Contact Dermatitis 1975;1:142-145

Chapter 3.6   AMBRETTOLIDE

IDENTIFICATION

Description/definition   : Ambrettolide is the cyclic organic compound that conforms to the structural formula
shown below
Chemical class(es)   : Cyclic organic compounds; unsaturated organic compounds; lactones
INCI name USA   : Not in the Personal Care Products Council Ingredient Database
Chemical/IUPAC name   : Oxacycloheptadec-7-en-2-one
Other names   : 6-Hexadecen-16-olide; Ω-6-hexadecenlactone
CAS registry number (s)   : 7779-50-2
EC number(s)   : 231-929-1
RIFM monograph(s)   : Food Chem Toxicol 2011;49(suppl.2):S207-S211; Food Cosmet Toxicol 1975;13:707
(special issue II)
SCCS opinion(s)   : SCCS/1459/11 (1)
Function(s) in cosmetics   : EU: perfuming
Patch testing   : 5% pet. (2)
Molecular formula   : $C_{16}H_{28}O_2$

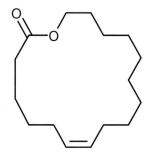

GENERAL

Ambrettolide is a colorless to pale yellow clear liquid; its odor type is soapy and its odor is described as 'sweet, soapy, perfume-like with a heavy fruity undertone' (www.thegoodscentscompany.com). Ambrettolide is a component of Ambrette seed oil (obtained from *Hibiscus abelmoschus* L., Malvaceae) (1).

Presence in essential oils

Ambrettolide has been identified by chemical analysis in 1 of 91 essential oils, which have caused contact allergy / allergic contact dermatitis: chamomile oil German (4).

CONTACT ALLERGY

The SCCS (Scientific Committee on Consumer Safety), in a 2012 Opinion on Fragrance allergens in cosmetic products, has categorized ambrettolide as 'likely fragrance contact allergen by combination of evidence' (1,3).

Testing in groups of patients

In 2000, in Japan, USA and several European countries, 178 patients with known fragrance sensitivity were tested with a series of fragrances and there were 6 (3.4%) positive patch test reactions to ambrettolide 5% pet. The relevance of these reactions was not mentioned (2).

LITERATURE

1   SCCS (Scientific Committee on Consumer Safety). Opinion on fragrance allergens in cosmetic products, 26-27 June 2012, SCCS/1459/11. Available at:
https://ec.europa.eu/health/sites/health/files/scientific_committees/consumer_safety/docs/sccs_o_102.pdf
2   Larsen W, Nakayama H, Fischer T, Elsner P, Frosch P, Burrows D, et al. Fragrance contact dermatitis: A worldwide multicenter investigation (Part II). Contact Dermatitis 2001;44:344-346
3   Uter W, Johansen JD, Börje A, Karlberg A-T, Lidén C, Rastogi S, Roberts D, White IR. Categorization of fragrance contact allergens for prioritization of preventive measures: clinical and experimental data and consideration of structure–activity relationships. Contact Dermatitis 2013;69:196-230
4   De Groot AC, Schmidt E. Essential oils: contact allergy and chemical composition. Boca Raton, Fl., USA: CRC Press, Taylor and Francis Group, 2016 (ISBN 9781482246407)

Chapter 3.7   AMYL CINNAMAL

IDENTIFICATION

Description/definition   : Amyl cinnamal is the organic compound, that conforms to the structural formula shown
                              below
Chemical class(es)   : Aldehydes
Chemical/IUPAC name   : 2-Benzylideneheptanal
Other names   : α-Amylcinnamaldehyde; α-amyl cinnamic aldehyde
CAS registry number(s)   : 122-40-7
EC number(s)   : 204-541-5
CIR review(s)   : Report terminated in 2006 (access: www.cir-safety.org/ingredients)
SCCS opinion(s)   : Various (7); SCCS/1459/11 (8)
RIFM monograph(s)   : Food Chem Toxicol 2015;82(suppl.):S20-S28; Food Cosmet Toxicol 1973;11:855
IFRA standard   : Restricted (www.ifraorg.org/en-us/standards-library) (table 3.7.1)
Function(s) in cosmetics   : EU: perfuming. USA: fragrance ingredients
EU cosmetic restrictions   : Regulated in Annex III/67 of the Regulation (EC) No. 1223/2009, regulated by 2003/15/EC;
                              Must be labeled on cosmetics and detergent products, if present at > 10 ppm (0.001%)
                              in leave-on products and > 100 ppm (0.01%) in rinse-off products
Patch testing   : 1% pet. (SmartPracticeCanada, SmartPractice Europe); 2% pet. (Chemotechnique); also
                              present in the fragrance mix I; TEST ADVICE: 2% pet.
Molecular formula   : $C_{14}H_{18}O$

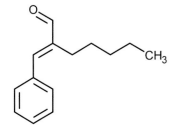

Table 3.7.1 IFRA restrictions for amyl cinnamal

Category [a]	Limits [b]	Category [a]	Limits [b]	Category [a]	Limits [b]
1	0.70%	5	5.60%	9	5.00%
2	0.90%	6	17.10%	10	2.50%
3	3.60%	7	1.80%	11	not restricted
4	10.70%	8	2.00%		

[a] For explanation of categories see pages 6-8
[b] Limits in the finished products

GENERAL

Amyl cinnamal is a pale yellow to yellow clear liquid; its odor type is floral and its odor at 100% is described as 'sweet floral oily fruity herbal jasmin' (www.thegoodscentscompany.com).

Presence in essential oils

Amyl cinnamal has been identified by chemical analysis in none of 91 essential oils, which have caused contact allergy / allergic contact dermatitis (67). It does occur in nature, though (66).

CONTACT ALLERGY

General

The SCCS (Scientific Committee on Consumer Safety), in a 2012 Opinion on Fragrance allergens in cosmetic products, has marked amyl cinnamal as 'established contact allergen in humans' (8,43). The sensitizing potency of amyl cinnamal was classified as 'moderate' based on an EC3 value of 7.6% in the LLNA (local lymph node assay) in animal experiments (8,43).

Amyl cinnamal is a constituent of the fragrance mix I. In groups of patients reacting to the mix and tested with its 8 ingredients, amyl cinnamal scored 0-14.3% positive patch test reactions, median 3.2% and average 3.7%. It has rank number 8 in the list of most frequent reactors in the mix (see Chapter 3.70 Fragrance mix I).

The literature on contact allergy to amyl cinnamal up to 2004 has been reviewed (13).

General population

In the period 2008-2011, in 5 European countries (Sweden, Germany, Netherlands, Portugal, Italy), a random sample of the general population of 3119 individuals aged 18-74 years were patch tested with the FM I, its 8 ingredients, the FM II, its 6 ingredients and Myroxylon pereirae resin. There were 3 reactions (0.1%) to amyl cinnamal (probably erroneously termed amylcinnamyl alcohol, which is not part of the FM I), tested 2% in petrolatum. About half of all positive reactions to fragrances were considered to be relevant based on standardized criteria. Women were affected twice as often as men (60).

Patch testing in groups of patients

Results of studies testing amyl cinnamal in consecutive patients suspected of contact dermatitis (routine testing) back to 1991 are shown in table 3.7.2. Results of testing in groups of *selected* patients (e.g. patients known or suspected to be fragrance-allergic) back to 1975 are shown in table 3.7.3.

Patch testing in consecutive patients suspected of contact dermatitis: routine testing

In 13 studies in which routine testing with amyl cinnamal was performed, rates of sensitization have been low, ranging from 0.08% to 1.4%. Ten had scores of 0.4% or lower (table 3.7.2). In most investigations, no relevance data were provided or specified; in the three that addressed this issue, the relevance rates ranged from 33% to 100%, but the numbers were always very low (one in the study with 100% relevance). Causative products were usually not mentioned or specified, but in one study, of the relevant reactions to any of 26 fragrances tested, 96% were caused by cosmetic products (1).

Table 3.7.2 Patch testing in groups of patients: Routine testing

Years and Country	Test conc. & vehicle	Number of patients tested	positive (%)		Selection of patients (S); Relevance (R); Comments (C)	Ref.
2015-7 Netherlands		821	2	(0.2%)	R: not stated	71
2015-2016 UK	2% pet.	2084	3	(0.1%)	R: not specified for individual fragrances; 25% of patients who reacted to any fragrance or fragrance marker had a positive fragrance history	69
2010-2015 Denmark	1% pet.	6004		(0.14%)	R: present relevance 50%, past relevance 38%	38
2009-2015 Sweden	2% pet.	4483	4	(0.08%)	R: not stated	44
2013-2014 Thailand		312	1	(0.3%)	R: 100%	40
2011-2012 UK	2% pet.	1951	3	(0.15%)	R: not stated	42
2010-2011 China	2% pet.	296		(1.4%)	R: 67% for all fragrances tested together (excluding FM I)	41
2008-2010 Denmark	1% pet.	1503	3	(0.2%)	S: mostly routine testing; R: 33%; C: 100% co-reactivity of FM I, 67% of FM II; of the relevant reactions to any of the 26 fragrances tested, 96% were caused by cosmetic products	1
2005-2008 IVDK	1% pet.	1214		(0.3%)	R: not stated	47
2003-2004 IVDK	1% pet.	2062	4	(0.2%)	R: not stated; C: 75% co-reactivity of FM I	3
<1995 9 European countries + USA	1% pet.	1072	5	(0.5%)	R: not stated	30
1993 EECDRG	1% pet.	709	6	(0.9%)	R: not stated	53
1991 The Netherlands	5% pet.	677	3	(0.4%)	R: not stated	55

EECDRG: European Environmental and Contact Dermatitis Research Group; FM: Fragrance mix; IVDK: Informationsverbund Dermatologischer Kliniken (Germany, Switzerland, Austria)

Patch testing in groups of selected patients

Results of studies patch testing amyl cinnamal in groups of selected patients (mostly patients with known of suspected fragrance sensitivity), rates of positive reactions ranged from 0.3% to 15%. The latter percentage was in a small group of 20 patients with proven fragrance allergy (2). Relevance data are lacking.

Results of testing HICC in groups of patients reacting to the fragrance mix I are shown in Chapter 3.70 Fragrance mix I.

Case reports and case series

Amyl cinnamal was responsible for 2 out of 399 cases of cosmetic allergy where the causal allergen was identified in a study of the NACDG, USA, 1977-1983 (4). In a group of 119 patients with allergic contact dermatitis from cosmetics, investigated in The Netherlands in 1986-1987, one case was caused by amyl cinnamal in a skin care product (27,28).

In a group of 23 patients with (photo)allergic reactions to sunscreens, 4 had positive patch tests to the ingredient amyl cinnamal (29). Amyl cinnamal was stated to be the (or an) allergen in 5 patients in a group of 603 individuals suffering from cosmetic dermatitis, seen in the period 2010-2015 in Leuven, Belgium (37).

Table 3.7.3 Patch testing in groups of patients: Selected patient groups

Years and Country	Test conc. & vehicle	Number of patients tested	positive (%)	Selection of patients (S); Relevance (R); Comments (C)	Ref.
2011-2015 Spain	1% or 2% pet.	1013	22 (2.2%)	S: patients previously reacting to FM I, FM II, Myroxylon pereirae resin or hydroxyisohexyl 3-cyclohexene carboxaldehyde in the baseline series; R: not stated; C: the 2% test substances showed a higher rate of positive reactions than the 1% material	72
2005-10 Netherlands		100	1 (1.0%)	S: patients with known fragrance sensitivity based on a positive patch test to the FM I and/or the FM II; R: not stated	45
2000-2007 USA	2% pet.	254	1 (0.4%)	S: patients who were tested with a supplemental cosmetic screening series; R: 100%; C: weak study: a. high rate of macular erythema and weak reactions; b. relevance figures included 'questionable' and 'past' relevance	11
2000 Japan, Europe, USA	5% pet.	178	4 (2.3%)	S: patients with known fragrance sensitivity; R: not stated	9
1997-2000 Austria	1% pet.	747	2 (0.3%)	S: patients suspected of fragrance allergy; R: not stated	5
<1996 Japan, Europe, USA	5% pet.	167	5 (3.0%)	S: patients known or suspected to be allergic to fragrances; R: not stated	6
1975 USA	2% pet.	20	3 (15%)	S: fragrance-allergic patients; R: not stated	2

Testing in groups of patients reacting to the fragrance mix I
Results of testing amyl cinnamal in groups of patients reacting to the fragrance mix I are shown in Chapter 3.70 Fragrance mix I

FM: Fragrance Mix

In the period 2000-2009, in Leuven, Belgium, an unspecified number of patients had positive patch tests or use tests to a total of 344 cosmetic products *and* positive patch tests to FM I, FM II, and/or to one or more of 28 selected specific fragrance ingredients. In one patient reacting to amyl cinnamal, the presence of this fragrance in the cosmetic product(s) was confirmed by reading the product label (46).

Eight patients had allergic contact dermatitis from a topical pharmaceutical product and all reacted to its ingredient ethylenediamine (a stabilizer) and to the perfume 5% pet. When tested with the 28 individual fragrances of the perfume, there were 5 reactions to amyl cinnamal, 4 to cinnamyl alcohol, 2 to hydroxycitronellal, 2 to benzyl alcohol and one to oakmoss synthetic (36).

In Belgium, in the years before 1986, of 5202 consecutive patients with dermatitis patch tested, 156 were diagnosed with pure cosmetic allergy. Amyl cinnamal was the 'dermatitic ingredient' in 2 (1.3%) patients (frequency in the entire group: 0.1%). It should be realized, however, that only a very limited number of patients was tested with a fragrance series (56).

In a 3-year-period (1979-1981), in one center in the USA, 13 patients reacted to amyl cinnamal (test concentration not mentioned). Most such patients had undergone patch tests with either ingredients of Mycolog ^{TM} cream (the perfume of which contains amyl cinnamal and amylcinnamyl alcohol), a screening tray of perfume ingredients or both. Most reactions were weak (+) and it was suggested that these were not relevant; in 3 patients with very strong reactions, no relevance was found either (62).

One individual had lip dermatitis and stomatitis from contact allergy to amyl cinnamal in toothpaste (59).

Cross-reactions, pseudo-cross-reactions and co-reactions
For general information on cross-/pseudo-cross-/co-reactivity of fragrance chemicals with other fragrances, fragrance markers (fragrance mix I, fragrance mix II, colophonium, Myroxylon pereirae resin [balsam of Peru]) and essential oils see Chapter 1.2 General information on cross-reactions, pseudo-cross-reactions and co-reactions. Co-reactivity with the fragrance mix I can be expected, as the mix contains amyl cinnamal (pseudo-cross-reactions).

There does not appear to be a common hapten for cinnamal and α-amyl cinnamal (65), although some cases of co-reactivity have been observed (63,64). Nevertheless, in a large study performed by the IVDK in the period 2005-2013, twelve out of 296 patients (4.1%) allergic to cinnamal also reacted to amyl cinnamal; conversely, of 43 patients reacting to amyl cinnamal, 12 (28%) co-reacted to cinnamal (70). In the same investigation, of 26 patients reacting to hexyl cinnamal, five (19%) co-reacted to amyl cinnamal. Conversely, of 11 individuals allergic to amyl cinnamal, five (45%) co-reacted to hexyl cinnamal (70).

Of 13 patients reacting to amyl cinnamal, 10 co-reacted to amylcinnamyl alcohol; of 11 patients with positive patch tests to amylcinnamyl alcohol, all co-reacted to amyl cinnamal (62).

In some studies, a significant association between positive reactions to the FM I and to epoxy resin has been found (48,49). Supplementary testing with fragrance mix ingredients showed that the association was related to positive reactions to amyl cinnamal and isoeugenol (49). The clinical implications are not clarified, and the association, which has not been found in several other studies, may be coincidental.

Presence in products and chemical analyses

In various studies, the presence of amyl cinnamal in cosmetic and sometimes other products has been investigated. Before 2006, most investigators used chemical analysis, usually GC-MS, for qualitative and quantitative determination. Since then, the presence of the target fragrances was usually investigated by screening the product labels for the 26 fragrances that must be labeled since 2005 on cosmetics and detergent products in the EU, if present at > 10 ppm (0.001%) in leave-on products and > 100 ppm (0.01%) in rinse-off products. This method, obviously, is less accurate and may result in underestimation of the frequency of the fragrances being present in the product. When they are in fact present, but the concentration is lower than mentioned above, labeling is not required and the fragrances' presence will be missed.

The results of the relevant studies for amyl cinnamal are summarized in table 3.7.4. More detailed information can be found in the corresponding text before and following the table. The percentage of products in which amyl cinnamal was found to be present shows wide variations, which can among other be explained by the selection procedure of the products, the method of investigation (false-negatives with information obtained from labels only) and changes in the use of individual fragrance materials over time (fashion).

In 2017, in the USA, the ingredient labels of 159 hair-dye kits containing 539 cosmetic products (e.g. colorants, conditioners, shampoos, toners) were screened for the most common sensitizers they contain. Amyl cinnamal was found to be present in 32 (6%) of the products (57).

In Denmark, in 2015-2016, 5588 fragranced cosmetic products were examined with a smartphone application for the 26 fragrances that need to be labeled in the EU. Amyl cinnamal was present in 4% of the products (rank number 16) (24).

In Germany, in 2015, fragrance allergens were evaluated based on lists of ingredients in 817 (unique) detergents (all-purpose cleaners, cleaning preparations for special purposes [e.g. bathroom, kitchen, dish-washing] and laundry detergents) present in 131 households. Amyl cinnamal was found to be present in 19 (2%) of the products (68).

Of 179 emollients available in online drugstores in 2014 in Poland, one (0.6%) contained amyl cinnamal, according to information available online (39).

In 2008, 2010 and 2011, 374 deodorants available in German retail shops were randomly selected and their labels checked for the presence of the 26 fragrances that need to be labeled. Amyl cinnamal was found to be present in 34 (9.1%) of the products (61).

In Germany, in the period 2006-2009, 4991 cosmetic products were randomly sampled for an official investigation of conformity of cosmetic products with legal provisions. The labels were inspected for the presence of the 26 fragrances that need to be labeled in the EU. Amyl cinnamal was present in 3% of the products (rank number 16) (23).

In 2008, 66 different fragrance components (including 39 essential oils) were identified in 370 (10% of the total) topical pharmaceutical products marketed in Belgium; one of these (0.3%) contained amyl cinnamal (10).

Amyl cinnamal was present (as indicated by labeling) in 6% of 204 cosmetic products (92 shampoos, 61 hair conditioners, 34 liquid soaps, 17 wet tissues) and in 1% of 97 detergents in Sweden, 2008 (12).

In 2007, in The Netherlands, twenty-three cosmetic products for children were analyzed for the presence of fragrances that need to be labeled. Amyl cinnamal was identified in one of the products (4%) in a concentration of 23 ppm (32).

In January 2006, a study of perfumed cosmetic and household products available on the shelves of U.K. retailers was carried out. Products were included if 'parfum' or 'aroma' was listed among the ingredients. Three hundred products were surveyed and any of 26 mandatory labeling fragrances named on the label were recorded. Amyl cinnamal was present in 22 (7%) of the products (rank number 19) (21).

In 2006, of 88 popular perfume containing deodorants purchased in Denmark, 9 (10%) were labeled to contain amyl cinnamal. Analysis of 24 regulated fragrance substances in 23 selected deodorants (19 spray products, 2 deo-sticks and 2 roll-on deodorants) was performed by GC-MS. Amyl cinnamal was identified in 4 of the products (17%) with a concentration range of 2-165 ppm (26).

In 2006, in The Netherlands, 52 laundry detergents were investigated for the presence of allergenic fragrances by checking their labels and chemical analyses. Amyl cinnamal was found to be present in 5 of the products (10%) in a concentration range of 31- 376 ppm. Amyl cinnamal had rank number 13 in the frequency list (34).

In 2006, the labels of 208 cosmetics for children (especially shampoos, body shampoos and soaps) available in Denmark were checked for the presence of the 26 fragrances that need to be labelled in the EU. Amyl cinnamal was present in 17 products (8.2%), and ranked number 9 in the frequency list. The maximum concentration found for amyl cinnamal was 230 mg/kg (31).

In 2002, in Denmark, 19 air fresheners (6 for cars, 13 for homes) were analyzed for the presence of fragrances that need to be labeled on cosmetics. Amyl cinnamal was found to be present in 5 products (26%) in a concentration range of 640-16,000 ppm and ranked 15 in the frequency list (35).

Table 3.7.4 Presence of amyl cinnamal in products [a]

Year	Country	Product type	Nr. investigated	Nr. of products positive [b]	(%)	Method [c]	Ref.
2017	USA	Cosmetic products in hair-dye kits	539 products in 159 hair-dye kits	32	(6%)	Labeling	52
2015-6	Denmark	Fragranced cosmetic products	5588		(4%)	Labeling	24
2015	Germany	Household detergents	817	19	(2%)	Labeling	68
2014	Poland	Emollients	179	1	(0.6%)	Online info	39
2008-11	Germany	Deodorants	374	34	(9.1%)	Labeling	61
2006-9	Germany	Cosmetic products	4991		(3%)	Labeling	23
2008	Belgium	Fragranced topical pharmaceutical products	370	1	(0.3%)	Labeling	10
2008	Sweden	Cosmetic products	204	12	(6%)	Labeling	12
		Detergents	97	1	(1%)	Labeling	
2007	Netherlands	Cosmetic products for children	23	1	(4%)	Analysis	32
2006	UK	Perfumed cosmetic and household products	300	22	(7%)	Labeling	21
2006	Denmark	Popular perfumed deodorants	88	9	(10%)	Labeling	26
			23	4	(17%)	Analysis	
2006	Netherlands	Laundry detergents	52	5	(10%)	Labeling + analysis	34
2006	Denmark	Rinse-off cosmetics for children	208	17	(8.2%)	Labeling + analysis	31
2002	Denmark	Home and car air fresheners	19	5	(26%)	Analysis	35
2001	Denmark	Women's fine fragrances	10	1	(10%)	Analysis	25
2001	Denmark	Non-cosmetic consumer products	43	2	(5%)	Analysis	33
2000	Denmark, UK, Germany, Italy	Domestic and occupational products	59	5	(8.5%)	Analysis	16
<2000	Sweden	Swedish cosmetic products	42	10	(24%)	Analysis	58
1997-8	Denmark, UK Germany, Sweden	Cosmetics and cosmetic toys for children	25	4	(16%)	Analysis	19
1996-7	Denmark	Deodorants that had caused allergic contact dermatitis	19	5	(26%)	Analysis	50
1996	Five European countries	Fragranced deodorants	70	22	(31%)	Analysis	15
1995-6	Denmark	Perfumes from lower-price range cosmetic products	17	10	(59%)	Analysis	51
1995	Denmark	Cosmetic products based on natural ingredients	42	9	(21%)	Analysis	17
1995	Denmark	The 10 most popular women's perfumes	10	3	(30%)	Analysis	18
1994	Denmark	Cosmetics that had given a positive patch or use test in FM I-allergic patients	23	7	(30%)	Analysis	52
1992	Netherlands	Cosmetic products	300	105	(35%)	Analysis	22
1988	USA	Perfumes used in fine fragrances, household products and soap	400	21-30% (See text for details)		Analysis	20

[a] See the corresponding text below for more details
[b] positive = containing the target fragrance
[c] Labeling: information from the ingredient labels on the product / packaging; Analysis: chemical analysis, most often GC-MS

In January 2001, in Denmark, ten women's fine fragrances were purchased; 5 of these had been launched years ago (1921–1990) and 5 were the latest launches by the same companies, introduced 2 months to 4 years before purchase. They were analyzed for the presence and quantity of the 7 well-identified fragrances present in the FM I (see Chapter 3.70 Fragrance mix I). The analysis revealed that the 5 old perfumes contained a mean of 5 of the 7 target allergens of the FM, while the new perfumes contained a mean of 2.8 of the allergens. The mean concentrations of the target allergens were 2.6 times higher in the old perfumes than in the new perfumes, range 2.2-337 ppm. Amyl cinnamal was present in 1 of the 5 old perfumes, in a concentration of 0.0192% (m/m); in the new perfumes, it was identified in none of the 5 (25).

In 2001, in Denmark, 43 non-cosmetic consumer products (mainly dish-washing products, laundry detergents, and hard and soft surface cleaners) were analyzed for the 26 fragrances that are regulated for labeling in the EU. Amyl cinnamal was present in 2 products (5%) in concentrations of 0.0092 and 0.0284% (m/m) and had rank number 18 in the frequency list (33).

In 2000, fifty-nine domestic and occupational products, purchased in retail outlets in Denmark, England, Germany and Italy were analyzed by GC-MS for the presence of fragrances. The product categories were liquid soap and soap bars (n=13), soft/hard surface cleaners (n=23), fabric conditioners/laundry detergents for hand wash (n=8), dish wash (n=10), furniture polish, car shampoo, stain remover (each n=1) and 2 products used in occupational environments. Amyl cinnamal was present in 5 products (8.5%); quantification was not performed (16).

In Sweden, before 2000, 42 cosmetic products of a Swedish manufacturer were investigated for the presence of the ingredients of the FM I by chemical analysis. Amyl cinnamal was found to be present in 10 of the products (24%) in a concentration range of 9.8-152 ppm with a mean of 68 ppm. Data provided by the manufacturer on the qualitative and quantitative presence of the chemicals was quite different from chemical analyses for some of the fragrances (58).

Twenty-five cosmetics and cosmetic toys for children (5 shampoos and shower gels, 6 perfumes, 1 deodorant (roll-on), 4 baby lotions/creams, 1 baby wipes product, 1 baby oil, 2 lipcare products and 5 toy-cosmetic products: a cosmetic-toy set for blending perfumes and a makeup set) purchased in 1997-1998 in retail outlets in Denmark, Germany, England and Sweden were analyzed in 1998 for the presence of fragrances by GC-MS. Amyl cinnamal was found in 4 products (16%) in a concentration range of ≤0.001-0.388% (w/w). For the analytical data in each product category, the original publication should be consulted (19).

In Denmark, in 1996-1997, nineteen deodorants that had caused axillary allergic contact dermatitis in 14 patients were analyzed for the presence of the 8 constituents of the FM I. Amyl cinnamal was found to be present in 5 (26%) of the products in a concentration range of 0.0008-0.092% (50).

Seventy fragranced deodorants, purchased at retail outlets in 5 European countries in 1996, were analyzed by gas chromatography - mass spectrometry (GC-MS) for the determination of the contents of 21 commonly used fragrance materials. Amyl cinnamal was identified in 22 products (31%) in a concentration range of 1-617 ppm (15).

In Denmark, in 1995-1996, nine perfumes from lower-price cosmetic wash-off products and 8 from stay-on products were analyzed for the presence of the ingredients of the FM I except oakmoss absolute. Amyl cinnamal was present in 5 of the 9 (56%) wash-off product perfumes in a concentration range of 0.0134-1.3477% w/v and in 5 of the 8 (63%) stay-on product perfumes in a concentration range of 0.0050-0.1747% w/v. In one product, amyl cinnamal was detected, but could not be quantified because of interference (51).

In 1995, in Denmark, 42 cosmetic products based on natural ingredients from 12 European and US companies (of which 22 were perfumes and 20 various other cosmetics) were investigated by high-resolution gas chromato-graphy-mass spectrometry (GC-MS) for the presence of 11 fragrances. Amyl cinnamal was present in 8 (36%) of the 22 perfumes in a concentration range of 0.194-3.039 w/w% ; it was also identified in one of the other cosmetics, a body balm, in a concentration of 0.0820% (17).

In Denmark, in 1995, the 10 most popular women's perfumes were analyzed with gas chromatography-mass spectrometry for the presence of 7 ingredients of the Fragrance mix I (all except Evernia prunastri extract). Amyl cinnamal was identified in 3 of the perfumes (30%) with a mean concentration of 0.32% and in a concentration range of 0.03-0.69% (18).

In Denmark, in 1994, 23 cosmetic products, which had either given a positive patch and/or use test in a total of 11 fragrance-mix-positive patients, and which products completely or partly explained present or past episodes of dermatitis, were analyzed for the presence of the constituents of the FM I (with the exception of oakmoss absolute) and a few other fragrances. Amyl cinnamal was found to be present in 7 of the 23 products (30%) in a concentration range of <0.001-0.32% v/v with a mean concentration of 0.066% v/v (52).

In 1992, in The Netherlands, the presence of fragrances was analyzed in 300 cosmetic products. Amyl cinnamal was identified in 35% of the products (rank order 21) (22).

In 1988, in the USA, 400 perfumes used in fine fragrances, household products and soaps (number of products per category not mentioned) were analyzed for the presence of fragrance chemicals in a concentration of at least 1% and a list of the Top-25 (present in the highest number of products) presented. Amyl cinnamal was found to be present in 21% of the fine fragrances (rank number 24), 23% of the household product fragrances (rank number 21) and 30% of the fragrances used in soaps (rank number 22) (20).

OTHER SIDE EFFECTS

Immediate-type reactions
In Hungary, before 1994, in a group of 50 patients reacting to the FM I and tested with its ingredients (test concentrations unknown), there was one immediate contact reaction to amyl cinnamal (54).

LITERATURE

1   Heisterberg MV, Menné T, Johansen JD. Contact allergy to the 26 specific fragrance ingredients to be declared on cosmetic products in accordance with the EU cosmetic directive. Contact Dermatitis 2011;65:266-275
2   Larsen WG. Perfume dermatitis. A study of 20 patients. Arch Dermatol 1977;113:623-626
3   Schnuch A, Uter W, Geier J, Lessmann H, Frosch PJ. Sensitization to 26 fragrances to be labelled according to current European regulation: Results of the IVDK and review of the literature. Contact Dermatitis 2007;57:1-10
4   Adams RM, Maibach HI, for the North American Contact Dermatitis Group. A five-year study of cosmetic reactions. J Am Acad Dermatol 1985;13:1062-1069
5   Wöhrl S, Hemmer W, Focke M, Götz M, Jarisch R. The significance of fragrance mix, balsam of Peru, colophony and propolis as screening tools in the detection of fragrance allergy. Br J Dermatol 2001;145:268-273
6   Larsen W, Nakayama H, Lindberg M, Fischer T, Elsner P, Burrows D, et al. Fragrance contact dermatitis: A worldwide multicenter investigation (Part 1). Am J Cont Derm 1996;7:77-83
7   Various SCCS opinions on amyl cinnamal have been published and are available at: Http://ec.europa.eu/growth/tools-databases/cosing/index.cfm?fuseaction=search.details_v2&id=28325
8   SCCS (Scientific Committee on Consumer Safety). Opinion on Fragrance allergens in cosmetic products, 26-27 June 2012, SCCS/1459/11. Available at: https://ec.europa.eu/health/sites/health/files/scientific_committees/consumer_safety/docs/sccs_o_102.pdf
9   Larsen W, Nakayama H, Fischer T, Elsner P, Frosch P, Burrows D, et al. Fragrance contact dermatitis: A worldwide multicenter investigation (Part II). Contact Dermatitis 2001;44:344-346
10 Nardelli A, D'Hooge E, Drieghe J, Dooms M, Goossens A. Allergic contact dermatitis from fragrance components in specific topical pharmaceutical products in Belgium. Contact Dermatitis 2009;60:303-313
11 Wetter DA, Yiannias JA, Prakash AV, Davis MDP, Farmer SA, el-Azhary RA. Results of patch testing to personal care product allergens in a standard series and a supplemental cosmetic series: an analysis of 945 patients from the Mayo Clinic Contact Dermatitis Group, 2000-2007. J Am Acad Dermatol 2010;63:789-798
12 Yazar K, Johnsson S, Lind M-L, Boman A, Lidén C. Preservatives and fragrances in selected consumer-available cosmetics and detergents. Contact Dermatitis 2011;64:265-272
13 Hostýnek JJ, Maibach HI. Is there evidence that amylcinnamic aldehyde causes allergic contact dermatitis? Exog Dermatol 2004;3:35-46
14 Schnuch A, Lessmann H, Geier J, Frosch PJ, Uter W. Contact allergy to fragrances: frequencies of sensitization from 1996 to 2002. Results of the IVDK. Contact Dermatitis 2004;50:65-76
15 Rastogi SC, Johansen JD, Frosch P, Menné T, Bruze M, Lepoittevin JP, et al. Deodorants on the European market: quantitative chemical analysis of 21 fragrances. Contact Dermatitis 1998;38:29-35
16 Rastogi SC, Heydorn S, Johansen JD, Basketter DA. Fragrance chemicals in domestic and occupational products. Contact Dermatitis 2001;45:221-225
17 Rastogi SC, Johansen JD, Menné T. Natural ingredients based cosmetics. Content of selected fragrance sensitizers. Contact Dermatitis 1996;34:423-426
18 Johansen JD, Rastogi SC, Menné T. Contact allergy to popular perfumes: assessed by patch test, use test and chemical analyses. Br J Dermatol 1996;135:419-422
19 Rastogi SC, Johansen JD, Menné T, Frosch P, Bruze M, Andersen KE, et al. Content of fragrance allergens in children's cosmetics and cosmetic toys. Contact Dermatitis 1999;41:84-88
20 Fenn RS. Aroma chemical usage trends in modern perfumery. Perfumer and Flavorist 1989;14:3-10
21 Buckley DA. Fragrance ingredient labelling in products on sale in the UK. Br J Dermatol 2007;157:295-300
22 Weyland JW. Personal Communication, 1992. Cited in: De Groot AC, Weyland JW, Nater JP. Unwanted effects of cosmetics and drugs used in dermatology, 3rd Ed. Amsterdam: Elsevier, 1994:579
23 Uter W, Yazar K, Kratz E-M, Mildau G, Lidén C. Coupled exposure to ingredients of cosmetic products: I. Fragrances. Contact Dermatitis 2013;69:335-341
24 Bennike NH, Oturai NB, Müller S, Kirkeby CS, Jørgensen C, Christensen AB, et al. Fragrance contact allergens in 5588 cosmetic products identified through a novel smartphone application. J Eur Acad Dermatol Venereol 2018;32:79-85
25 Rastogi SC, Menné T, Johansen JD. The composition of fine fragrances is changing. Contact Dermatitis 2003;48:130-132

26 Rastogi SC, Hellerup Jensen G, Johansen JD. Survey and risk assessment of chemical substances in deodorants. Survey of Chemical Substances in Consumer Products, No. 86 2007. Danish Ministry of the Environment, Environmental Protection Agency. Available at: https://www2.mst.dk/Udgiv/publications/2007/978-87-7052-625-8/pdf/978-87-7052-626-5.pdf

27 De Groot AC, Bruynzeel DP, Bos JD, van der Meeren HL, van Joost T, Jagtman BA, Weyland JW. The allergens in cosmetics. Arch Dermatol 1988;124:1525-1529

28 De Groot AC. Adverse reactions to cosmetics. PhD Thesis, University of Groningen, The Netherlands: 1988, chapter 3.4, pp.105-113

29 Thune P. Contact and photocontact allergy to sunscreens. Photodermatol 1984;1:5-9

30 Frosch PJ, Pilz B, Andersen KE, Burrows D, Camarasa JG, Dooms-Goossens A, et al. Patch testing with fragrances: results of a multicenter study of the European Environmental and Contact Dermatitis Research Group with 48 frequently used constituents of perfumes. Contact Dermatitis 1995;33:333-342

31 Poulsen PB, Schmidt A. A survey and health assessment of cosmetic products for children. Survey of chemical substances in consumer products, No. 88. Copenhagen: Danish Environmental Protection Agency, 2007. Available at: https://www2.mst.dk/udgiv/publications/2007/978-87-7052-638-8/pdf/978-87-7052-639-5.pdf

32 VWA. Dutch Food and Consumer Product Safety Authority. Cosmetische producten voor kinderen: Inventarisatie van de markt en de veiligheidsborging door producenten en importeurs. Report ND04o065/ND05o170, 2007 (Report in Dutch), 2007. Available at: www.nvwa.nl/documenten/communicatie/inspectieresultaten/consument/ 2016m/cosmetische- producten-voor-kinderen

33 Rastogi SC. Survey of chemical compounds in consumer products. Contents of selected fragrance materials in cleaning products and other consumer products. Survey no. 8-2002. Copenhagen, Denmark, Danish Environmental Protection Agency. Available at: http://eng.mst.dk/media/mst/69131/8.pdf

34 Bouma K, Van Peursem AJJ. Marktonderzoek naleving detergenten verordening voor textielwasmiddelen. Dutch Food and Consumer Products Safety Authority (VWA) Report ND06K173, 2006 [in Dutch]. Available at: http://docplayer.nl/41524125-Marktonderzoek-naleving-detergenten-verordening-voor-textielwasmiddelen.html

35 Pors J, Fuhlendorff R. Mapping of chemical substances in air fresheners and other fragrance liberating products. Report Danish Ministry of the Environment, Environmental Protection Agency (EPA). Survey of Chemicals in Consumer Products, No 30, 2003. Available at: http://eng.mst.dk/media/mst/69113/30.pdf

36 Larsen WG. Allergic contact dermatitis to the perfume in Mycolog cream. J Am Acad Dermatol 1979;1:131-133

37 Goossens A. Cosmetic contact allergens. Cosmetics 2016, 3, 5; doi:10.3390/cosmetics3010005

38 Bennike NH, Zachariae C, Johansen JD. Non-mix fragrances are top sensitizers in consecutive dermatitis patients – a cross-sectional study of the 26 EU-labelled fragrance allergens. Contact Dermatitis 2017;77:270-279

39 Osinka K, Karczmarz A, Krauze K, Feleszko W. Contact allergens in cosmetics used in atopic dermatitis: analysis of product composition. Contact Dermatitis 2016;75:241-243

40 Vejanurug P, Tresukosol P, Sajjachareonpong P, Puangpet P. Fragrance allergy could be missed without patch testing with 26 individual fragrance allergens. Contact Dermatitis 2016;74:230-235

41 Liu J, Li L-F. Contact sensitization to fragrances other than fragrance mix I in China. Contact Dermatitis 2015;73:252-253

42 Mann J, McFadden JP, White JML, White IR, Banerjee P. Baseline series fragrance markers fail to predict contact allergy. Contact Dermatitis 2014;70:276-281

43 Uter W, Johansen JD, Börje A, Karlberg A-T, Lidén C, Rastogi S, Roberts D, White IR. Categorization of fragrance contact allergens for prioritization of preventive measures: clinical and experimental data and consideration of structure–activity relationships. Contact Dermatitis 2013;69:196-230

44 Mowitz M, Svedman C, Zimerson E, Isaksson M, Pontén A, Bruze M. Simultaneous patch testing with fragrance mix I, fragrance mix II and their ingredients in southern Sweden between 2009 and 2015. Contact Dermatitis 2017;77:280-287

45 Nagtegaal MJC, Pentinga SE, Kuik J, Kezic S, Rustemeyer T. The role of the skin irritation response in polysensitization to fragrances. Contact Dermatitis 2012;67:28-35

46 Nardelli A, Drieghe J, Claes L, Boey L, Goossens A. Fragrance allergens in 'specific' cosmetic products. Contact Dermatitis 2011;64:212-219

47 Uter W, Geier J, Frosch P, Schnuch A. Contact allergy to fragrances: current patch test results (2005–2008) from the Information Network of Departments of Dermatology. Contact Dermatitis 2010;63:254-261

48 Pontén A, Björk J, Carstensen O, Gruvberger B, Isaksson M, Rasmussen K, Bruze M. Associations between contact allergy to epoxy resin and fragrance mix. Acta Derm Venereol 2004;84:151-152

49 Andersen KE, Porskjær Christensen L, Vølund A, Johansen JD, Paulsen E. Association between positive patch tests to epoxy resin and fragrance mix I ingredients. Contact Dermatitis 2009;60:155-157

50 Johansen JD, Rastogi SC, Bruze M, Andersen KE, Frosch P, Dreier B, et al. Deodorants: a clinical provocation study in fragrance-sensitive individuals. Contact Dermatitis 1998;39:161-165

51 Johansen JD, Rastogi SC, Andersen KE, Menné T. Content and reactivity to product perfumes in fragrance mix positive and negative eczema patients: A study of perfumes used in toiletries and skin-care products. Contact Dermatitis 1997;36:291-296

52 Johansen JD, Rastogi SC, Menné T. Exposure to selected fragrance materials: A case study of fragrance-mix-positive eczema patients. Contact Dermatitis 1996;34:106-110

53 Frosch PJ, Pilz B, Burrows D, Camarasa JG, Lachapelle J-M, Lahti A, et al. Testing with fragrance mix: Is the addition of sorbitan sesquioleate to the constituents useful? Contact Dermatitis 1995;32:266-272

54 Becker K, Temesvari E, Nemeth I. Patch testing with fragrance mix and its constituents in a Hungarian population. Contact Dermatitis 1994;30:185-186

55 De Groot AC, Van der Kley AMJ, Bruynzeel DP, Meinardi MMHM, Smeenk G, van Joost Th, Pavel S. Frequency of false-negative reactions to the fragrance mix. Contact Dermatitis 1993;28:139-140

56 Broeckx W, Blondeel A, Dooms-Goossens A, Achten G. Cosmetic intolerance. Contact Dermatitis 1987;16:189-194

57 Hamann D, Kishi P, Hamann CR. Consumer hair dye kits frequently contain isothiazolinones, other common preservatives and fragrance allergens. Dermatitis 2018;29:48-49

58 Bárány E, Lodén M. Content of fragrance mix ingredients and customer complaints of cosmetic products. Dermatitis 2000;11:74-79

59 Downs AMR, Lear JT, Sansom JE. Contact sensitivity in patients with oral symptoms. Contact Dermatitis 1998;39:258-259

60 Diepgen TL, Ofenloch R, Bruze M, Cazzaniga S, Coenraads PJ, Elsner P, et al. Prevalence of fragrance contact allergy in the general population of five European countries: a cross-sectional study. Br J Dermatol 2015;173:1411-1419

61 Klaschka U. Contact allergens for armpits - allergenic fragrances specified on deodorants. Int J Hyg Environ Health 2012;215:584-591

62 Guin JD, Haffley P. Sensitivity to alpha-amylcinnamic aldehyde and alpha-amylcinnamic alcohol. J Am Acad Dermatol 1983;8:76-80

63 Malten KE. Four bakers showing positive patch tests to a number of fragrance materials, which can also be used as flavors. Acta Derm Venereol 1979;59(suppl.85):117-121

64 Schorr WF. Cinnamic aldehyde allergy. Contact Dermatitis 1975;1:108-111

65 Elahi EN, Wright Z, Hinselwood D, Hotchkiss SA, Basketter DA, Pease CK. Protein binding and metabolism influence the relative skin sensitization potential of cinnamic compounds. Chem Res Toxicol 2004;17:301-310

66 Api AM, Belsito D, Bhatia S, Bruze M, Calow P, Dagli ML, et al. RIFM fragrance ingredient safety assessment, α-amylcinnamaldehyde, CAS registry number 122-40-7. Food Chem Toxicol 2015;82(suppl.):S20-S28

67 De Groot AC, Schmidt E. Essential oils: contact allergy and chemical composition. Boca Raton, Fl., USA: CRC Press, Taylor and Francis Group, 2016 (ISBN 9781482246407)

68 Wieck S, Olsson O, Kümmerer K, Klaschka U. Fragrance allergens in household detergents. Regul Toxicol Pharmacol 2018;97:163-169

69 Ung CY, White JML, White IR, Banerjee P, McFadden JP. Patch testing with the European baseline series fragrance markers: a 2016 update. Br J Dermatol 2018;178:776-780

70 Geier J, Uter W, Lessmann H, Schnuch A. Fragrance mix I and II: results of breakdown tests. Flavour Fragr J 2015;30:264-274

71 Dittmar D, Schuttelaar MLA. Contact sensitization to hydroperoxides of limonene and linalool: Results of consecutive patch testing and clinical relevance. Contact Dermatitis 2018 Oct 31. doi: 10.1111/cod.13137. [Epub ahead of print]

72 Silvestre JF, Mercader P, González-Pérez R, Hervella-Garcés M, Sanz-Sánchez T, Córdoba S, et al. Sensitization to fragrances in Spain: A 5-year multicentre study (2011-2015). Contact Dermatitis. 2018 Nov 14. doi: 10.1111/cod.13152. [Epub ahead of print]

Chapter 3.8   AMYL CINNAMATE

IDENTIFICATION

Description/definition   : Amyl cinnamate is the organic compound that conforms to the structural formula shown
                                       below
Chemical class(es)   : Esters
INCI name USA   : Not in the Personal Care Products Council Ingredient Database
Chemical/IUPAC name   : Pentyl 3-phenyl-2-propenoate
Other names   : Pentyl cinnamate
CAS registry number(s)   : 3487-99-8
EC number(s)   : 222-478-1
RIFM monograph(s)   : Food Chem Toxicol 2007;45(suppl.1):S29-S31; Food Chem Toxicol 2007;45(suppl.1):S1-
                                       S23
Function(s) in cosmetics : EU: perfuming
Patch testing   : 32% pet. (1); based on RIFM data, 8% pet. is probably not irritant (2)
Molecular formula   : $C_{14}H_{18}O_2$

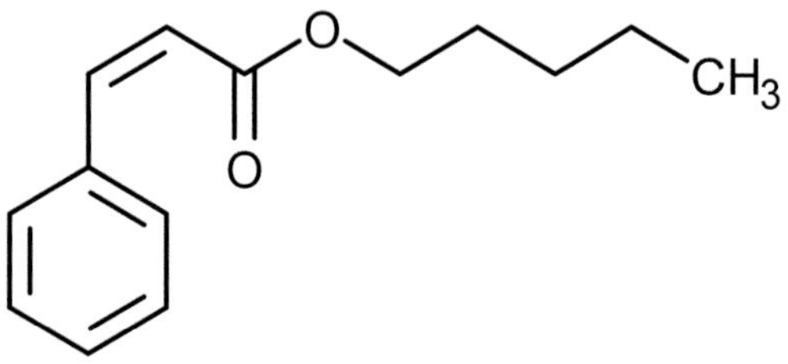

GENERAL

Amyl cinnamate is a colorless to pale yellow clear liquid; its odor type is balsamic and its odor at 100% is described as 'balsam amber cocoa bean orchid labdanum' (www.thegoodscentscompany.com). It is a synthetic chemical, not found in nature (and consequently not in essential oils (3)).

CONTACT ALLERGY

Case reports and case series

A baker was patch tested for hand dermatitis and showed positive reactions to cocoa-powder and 'speculaas-kruiden', a mixture of unknown composition, which he used at work. When subsequently tested with a series of fragrances and flavors, he had positive reactions to amyl cinnamate 32%, hexyl salicylate 12%, citral 0.5%, cinnamal 0.5%, and cinnamyl cinnamate 8%, all in petrolatum. The author was 'inclined' to say that these reactions may have been relevant (1).

Cross-reactions, pseudo-cross-reactions and co-reactions

For general information on cross-/pseudo-cross-/co-reactivity of fragrance chemicals with other fragrances, fragrance markers (fragrance mix I, fragrance mix II, colophonium, Myroxylon pereirae resin [balsam of Peru]) and essential oils see Chapter 1.2 General information on cross-reactions, pseudo-cross-reactions and co-reactions.

   Co-reactions have been observed with cinnamal and cinnamyl cinnamate (1).

LITERATURE

1   Malten KE. Four bakers showing positive patch tests to a number of fragrance materials, which can also be used
      as flavors. Acta Derm Venereol 1979;59(suppl.85):117-121
2   De Groot AC. Patch Testing, 4th Edition. Wapserveen, The Netherlands: acdegroot publishing, 2018, page 49
      (ISBN 978-90-813233-4-5)
3   De Groot AC, Schmidt E. Essential oils: contact allergy and chemical composition. Boca Raton, Fl., USA: CRC Press,
      Taylor and Francis Group, 2016 (ISBN 9781482246407)

Chapter 3.9   AMYLCINNAMYL ALCOHOL

IDENTIFICATION

Description/definition : Amylcinnamyl alcohol is the synthetic fragrance that conforms to the structural formula shown below

Chemical class(es) : Alcohols

Chemical/IUPAC name : 2-Benzylideneheptan-1-ol

Other names : α-Amylcinnamic alcohol; α-amylcinnamyl alcohol; 2-pentylcinnamic alcohol; 2-pentyl-3-phenylprop-2-en-1-ol

CAS registry number(s) : 101-85-9

EC number(s) : 202-982-8

RIFM monograph(s) : Food Chem Toxicol 2007;45(suppl.1):S32-S39; Food Cosmet Toxicol 1974;12:817 (special issue 1)

IFRA standard : Restricted (www.ifraorg.org/en-us/standards-library) (table 3.9.1)

SCCS opinion(s) : Various (5); SCCS/1459/11 (6)

Function(s) in cosmetics : EU: perfuming. USA: fragrance ingredients

EU cosmetic restrictions : Regulated in Annex III/74 of the Regulation (EC) No. 1223/2009, regulated by 2003/15/EC; Must be labeled on cosmetics and detergent products, if present at > 10 ppm (0.001%) in leave-on products and > 100 ppm (0.01%) in rinse-off products

Patch testing : 1% pet. (SmartPracticeEurope, SmartPracticeCanada); 5% pet. (Chemotechnique); recommended test concentration: 5.0% wt./wt. pet. (1)

Molecular formula : $C_{14}H_{20}O$

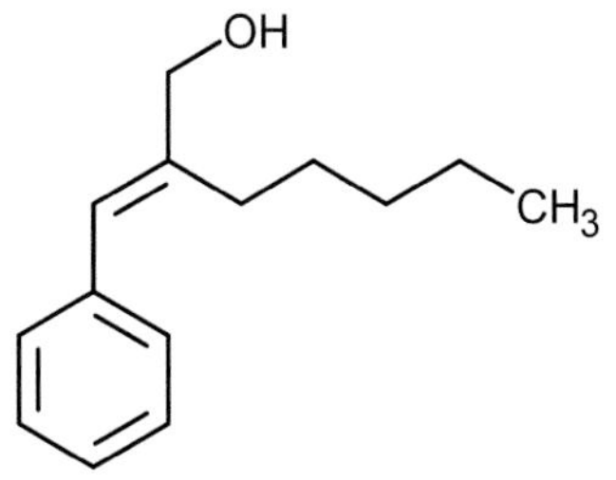

Table 3.9.1 IFRA restrictions for amylcinnamyl alcohol

Category [a]	Limits [b]	Category [a]	Limits [b]	Category [a]	Limits [b]
1	0.10%	5	0.80%	9	5.00%
2	0.10%	6	2.50%	10	2.50%
3	0.50%	7	0.30%	11	not restricted
4	1.60%	8	2.00%		

[a] For explanation of categories see pages 6-8
[b] Limits in the finished products

GENERAL

Amylcinnamyl alcohol is a pale yellow to yellow clear liquid; its odor type is spicy and its odor at 100% is described as 'floral jasmin waxy' (www.thegoodscentscompany.com).

When the fragrance mix I was developed in the late 1970s based on the work of Larsen (29) (see Chapter 3.70 Fragrance mix I), it contained amylcinnamyl alcohol as one of the 8 fragrance ingredients (27,28). It was replaced with amyl cinnamal, but no one seems to know why and when (28). Nevertheless, it is very likely than in later publications (10,11), the name amylcinnamyl alcohol was incorrect and should have read amyl cinnamal (amylcinnamaldehyde).

Presence in essential oils

(E)-Amylcinnamyl alcohol has been identified by chemical analysis in 1 of 91 essential oils, which have caused contact allergy / allergic contact dermatitis: sandalwood oil (at a concentration of 1%) (8). It is, however, a synthetic fragrance, and it is doubtful that it occurs in nature, although, according to the www.goodscentscompany.com, it has also been found in rue oil Cuba at a concentration of 0.61%.

CONTACT ALLERGY

General

The SCCS (Scientific Committee on Consumer Safety), in a 2012 Opinion on Fragrance allergens in cosmetic products, has marked amylcinnamyl alcohol as 'established contact allergen in humans' (6,21). The sensitizing potency of amylcinnamyl alcohol was classified as 'weak' based on an EC3 value of 25% in the LLNA (local lymph node assay) in animal experiments (6,21).

Patch testing in groups of patients

Results of studies testing amylcinnamyl alcohol in consecutive patients suspected of contact dermatitis (routine testing) and those of testing in groups of *selected* patients (e.g. patients with suspected or known fragrance allergy and individuals suspected of cosmetic allergy / intolerance) back to 1984 are shown in table 3.9.2.

In seven studies in which routine testing with amylcinnamyl alcohol was performed, rates of sensitization have invariably been low, ranging from 0.1% to 0.5%. Relevance rates, where mentioned, ranged from 50% to 100%, but the numbers of patients were low (in two studies, 100% relevance related to one patient).

In six studies in which amylcinnamyl alcohol was tested in groups of selected patients, rates of positive reactions ranged from 0.6% to 4%. The highest concentration of 4% was found in 100 patients with known fragrance sensitivity (22). A frequency of sensitization of 3.9% was found in a group of 179 patients suspected of cosmetic allergy, but the concentration used for patch testing (20%) was very high and it is unknown whether this may have resulted in some false-positive, irritant reactions (26). Relevance was not addressed in 5 studies; in the sixth, there was a 61% relevance rate for all positive tested fragrances together (3).

Table 3.9.2 Patch testing in groups of patients

Years and Country	Test conc. & vehicle	Number of patients tested	positive (%)		Selection of patients (S); Relevance (R); Comments (C)	Ref.
Routine testing						
2015-7 Netherlands		821	4	(0.5%)	R: not stated	31
2015-2016 UK	1% pet.	2084	5	(0.2%)	R: not specified for individual fragrances; 25% of patients who reacted to any fragrance or fragrance marker had a positive fragrance history	30
2010-2015 Denmark	1% pet.	6004		(0.14%)	R: present relevance 50%, past relevance 38%	18
2013-2014 Thailand		312	1	(0.3%)	R: 100%	19
2011-2012 UK	1% pet.	1951	6	(0.3%)	R: not stated	20
2008-2010 Denmark	1% pet.	1503	1	(0.1%)	S: mostly routine testing; R: 100%; C: 100% co-reactivity of both FM I and FM II; of the relevant reactions to any of the 26 fragrances tested, 96% were caused by cosmetic products	2
2003-2004 IVDK	1% pet.	1977	7	(0.4%)	R: not stated	4
Testing in groups of selected patients						
2011-2015 Spain	1% or 5% pet.	1013	13	(1.3%)	S: patients previously reacting to FM I, FM II, Myroxylon pereirae resin or hydroxyisohexyl 3-cyclohexene carboxaldehyde in the baseline series and subsequently tested with a fragrance series; R: not stated	32
2006-2011 IVDK	1% pet.	708	5	(0.7%)	S: patients with suspected cosmetic intolerance; R: not stated	17
2005-10 Netherlands		100	4	(4%)	S: patients with known fragrance sensitivity based on a positive patch test to the FM I and/or the FM II; R: not stated	22
2005-2008 IVDK	1% pet.	5650		(0.8%)	S: not specified; R: not stated	23
2005-7 Netherlands	1% pet.	320	2	(0.6%)	S: patients suspected of fragrance or cosmetic allergy; R: 61% relevance for all positive tested fragrances together	3
1984 The Netherlands	20% pet.	179	7	(3.9%)	S: patients suspected of cosmetic allergy; R: not stated	26

FM: Fragrance Mix; IVDK: Informationsverbund Dermatologischer Kliniken (Germany, Switzerland, Austria)

Case reports and case series

A man had perianal allergic contact dermatitis from the perfume in a topical pharmaceutical preparation. When tested with the 28 ingredients of the perfume, there were positive reactions to amylcinnamyl alcohol, cinnamyl alcohol and benzyl alcohol, all tested 5% pet. (7). In a group of 23 patients with (photo)allergic reactions to sunscreens, 2 had positive patch tests to the ingredient amylcinnamyl alcohol (incorrectly termed alpha-amylcinnamic acid (12).

In a 3-year-period (1979-1981), in one center in the USA, 11 patients reacted to amylcinnamyl alcohol (test concentration not mentioned). Most such patients had undergone patch tests for either ingredients of Mycolog cream (the perfume of which contained amyl cinnamal and amylcinnamyl alcohol), a screening tray of perfume ingredients or both. Relevance was not found (25).

Cross-reactions, pseudo-cross-reactions and co-reactions
For general information on cross-/pseudo-cross-/co-reactivity of fragrance chemicals with other fragrances, fragrance markers (fragrance mix I, fragrance mix II, colophonium, Myroxylon pereirae resin [balsam of Peru]) and essential oils see Chapter 1.2 General information on cross-reactions, pseudo-cross-reactions and co-reactions.

Of 11 patients with positive patch tests to amylcinnamyl alcohol, all co-reacted to amyl cinnamal; of 13 patients reacting to amyl cinnamal, 10 co-reacted to amylcinnamyl alcohol (25).

Presence in products and chemical analyses
In various studies, the presence of amylcinnamyl alcohol in cosmetic and sometimes other products has been investigated. Before 2006, most investigators used chemical analysis, usually GC-MS, for qualitative and quantitative determination. Since then, the presence of the target fragrances was usually investigated by screening the product labels for the 26 fragrances that must be labeled since 2005 on cosmetics and detergent products in the EU, if present at > 10 ppm (0.001%) in leave-on products and > 100 ppm (0.01%) in rinse-off products. This method, obviously, is less accurate and may result in underestimation of the frequency of the fragrances being present in the product. When they are in fact present, but the concentration is lower than mentioned above, labeling is not required and the fragrances' presence will be missed.

The results of the relevant studies for amylcinnamyl alcohol are summarized in table 3.9.3. More detailed information can be found in the corresponding text following the table. The percentage of products in which amylcinnamyl alcohol was found to be present was invariably low. In many other studies not mentioned here but discussed in the separate 26 labeled fragrances chapters, the percentage was zero (and therefore not included here).

Table 3.9.3 Presence of amylcinnamyl alcohol in products [a]

Year	Country	Product type	Nr. investigated	Nr. of products positive [b]	(%)	Method [c]	Ref.
2006-9	Germany	Cosmetic products	4991		(0.3%)	Labeling	9
2007	Netherlands	Cosmetic products for children	23	1	(4%)	Analysis	14
2006	Denmark	Rinse-off cosmetics for children	208	6	(2.8%)	Labeling + analysis	13
2002	Denmark	Home and car air fresheners	19	1	(5%)	Analysis	16
2001	Denmark	Non-cosmetic consumer products	43	2	(5%)	Analysis	15

[a] See the corresponding text below for more details
[b] positive = containing the target fragrance
[c] Labeling: information from the ingredient labels on the product / packaging; Analysis: chemical analysis, most often GC-MS

In Germany, in the period 2006-2009, 4991 cosmetic products were randomly sampled for an official investigation of conformity of cosmetic products with legal provisions. The labels were inspected for the presence of the 26 fragrances that need to be labeled in the EU. Amylcinnamyl alcohol was present in 0.3% of the products (rank number 24) (9).

In 2007, in The Netherlands, twenty-three cosmetic products for children were analyzed for the presence of fragrances that need to be labeled. Amylcinnamyl alcohol was identified in one of the products (4%) in a concentration of 30 ppm (14).

In 2006, the labels of 208 cosmetics for children (especially shampoos, body shampoos and soaps) available in Denmark were checked for the presence of the 26 fragrances that need to be labeled in the EU. Amylcinnamyl alcohol was present in 6 products (2.9%), and ranked number 18 in the frequency list (13).

In 2002, in Denmark, 19 air fresheners (6 for cars, 13 for homes) were analyzed for the presence of fragrances that need to be labeled on cosmetics. Amylcinnamyl alcohol was found to be present in one product (5%) in a concentration range of 17-50 ppm (one product?) and ranked 22 in the frequency list (16).

In 2001, in Denmark, 43 non-cosmetic consumer products (mainly dish-washing products, laundry detergents, and hard and soft surface cleaners) were analyzed for the 26 fragrances that are regulated for labeling in the EU. Amylcinnamyl alcohol was present in 2 products (5%); its concentrations were not determined. Its rank number was 19 in the frequency list (15).

OTHER SIDE EFFECTS

Immediate-type reactions

Of 50 individuals who had open tests with amylcinnamyl alcohol 3% pet. on the forearm, 3 (6%) showed local macular erythema after 45 minutes, termed 'contact urticaria' by the authors (24).

LITERATURE

1   Bruze M, Svedman C, Andersen KE, Bruynzeel D, Goossens A, Johansen JD, et al. Patch test concentrations (doses in mg/cm2) for the 12 non-mix fragrance substances regulated by European legislation. Contact Dermatitis 2012;66:131-136

2   Heisterberg MV, Menné T, Johansen JD. Contact allergy to the 26 specificc fragrance ingredients to be declared on cosmetic products in accordance with the EU cosmetic directive. Contact Dermatitis 2011;65:266-275

3   Oosten EJ van, Schuttelaar ML, Coenraads PJ. Clinical relevance of positive patch test reactions to the 26 EU-labelled fragrances. Contact Dermatitis 2009;61:217-223

4   Schnuch A, Uter W, Geier J, Lessmann H, Frosch PJ. Sensitization to 26 fragrances to be labelled according to current European regulation: Results of the IVDK and review of the literature. Contact Dermatitis 2007;57:1-10

5   Various SCCS opinions on amylcinnamyl alcohol have been published and are available at: http://ec.europa.eu/growth/tools-databases/cosing/index.cfm?fuseaction=search.details_v2&id=28325

6   SCCS (Scientific Committee on Consumer Safety). Opinion on Fragrance allergens in cosmetic products, 26-27 June 2012, SCCS/1459/11. Available at: https://ec.europa.eu/health/sites/health/files/scientific_committees/consumer_safety/docs/sccs_o_102.pdf

7   Larsen WG. Perfume dermatitis. A study of 20 patients. Arch Dermatol 1977;113:623-626

8   De Groot AC, Schmidt E. Essential oils: contact allergy and chemical composition. Boca Raton, Fl., USA: CRC Press, Taylor and Francis Group, 2016 (ISBN 9781482246407)

9   Uter W, Yazar K, Kratz E-M, Mildau G, Lidén C. Coupled exposure to ingredients of cosmetic products: I. Fragrances. Contact Dermatitis 2013;69:335-341

10 Enders F, Przybilla B, Ring J. Patch testing with fragrance mix at 16% and 8%, and its individual constituents. Contact Dermatitis 1989;20:237-238

11 Becker K, Temesvari E, Nemeth I. Patch testing with fragrance mix and its constituents in a Hungarian population. Contact Dermatitis 1994;30:185-186

12 Thune P. Contact and photocontact allergy to sunscreens. Photodermatol 1984;1:5-9

13 Poulsen PB, Schmidt A. A survey and health assessment of cosmetic products for children. Survey of chemical substances in consumer products, No. 88. Copenhagen: Danish Environmental Protection Agency, 2007. Available at: https://www2.mst.dk/udgiv/publications/2007/978-87-7052-638-8/pdf/978-87-7052-639-5.pdf

14 VWA. Dutch Food and Consumer Product Safety Authority. Cosmetische producten voor kinderen: Inventarisatie van de markt en de veiligheidsborging door producenten en importeurs. Report ND04o065/ND05o170, 2007 (Report in Dutch), 2007. Available at: www.nvwa.nl/documenten/communicatie/inspectieresultaten/ consument/ 2016m/cosmetische- producten-voor-kinderen

15 Rastogi SC. Survey of chemical compounds in consumer products. Contents of selected fragrance materials in cleaning products and other consumer products. Survey no. 8-2002. Copenhagen, Denmark, Danish Environmental Protection Agency. Available at: http://eng.mst.dk/media/mst/69131/8.pdf

16 Pors J, Fuhlendorff R. Mapping of chemical substances in air fresheners and other fragrance liberating products. Report Danish Ministry of the Environment, Environmental Protection Agency (EPA). Survey of Chemicals in Consumer Products, No 30, 2003. Available at: http://eng.mst.dk/media/mst/69113/30.pdf

17 Dinkloh A, Worm M, Geier J, Schnuch A, Wollenberg A. Contact sensitization in patients with suspected cosmetic intolerance: results of the IVDK 2006-2011. J Eur Acad Dermatol Venereol 2015;29:1071-1081

18 Bennike NH, Zachariae C, Johansen JD. Non-mix fragrances are top sensitizers in consecutive dermatitis patients – a cross-sectional study of the 26 EU-labelled fragrance allergens. Contact Dermatitis 2017;77:270-279

19 Vejanurug P, Tresukosol P, Sajjachareonpong P, Puangpet P. Fragrance allergy could be missed without patch testing with 26 individual fragrance allergens. Contact Dermatitis 2016;74:230-235

20 Mann J, McFadden JP, White JML, White IR, Banerjee P. Baseline series fragrance markers fail to predict contact allergy. Contact Dermatitis 2014;70:276-281

21 Uter W, Johansen JD, Börje A, Karlberg A-T, Lidén C, Rastogi S, Roberts D, White IR. Categorization of fragrance contact allergens for prioritization of preventive measures: clinical and experimental data and consideration of structure–activity relationships. Contact Dermatitis 2013;69:196-230

22 Nagtegaal MJC, Pentinga SE, Kuik J, Kezic S, Rustemeyer T. The role of the skin irritation response in polysensitization to fragrances. Contact Dermatitis 2012;67:28-35

23 Uter W, Geier J, Frosch P, Schnuch A. Contact allergy to fragrances: current patch test results (2005–2008) from the Information Network of Departments of Dermatology. Contact Dermatitis 2010;63:254-261

24 Emmons WW, Marks JG Jr. Immediate and delayed reactions to cosmetic ingredients. Contact Dermatitis 1985;13:258-265

25 Guin JD, Haffley P. Sensitivity to alpha-amylcinnamic aldehyde and alpha-amylcinnamic alcohol. J Am Acad Dermatol 1983;8:76-80

26 De Groot AC, Liem DH, Nater JP, van Ketel WG. Patch tests with fragrance materials and preservatives. Contact Dermatitis 1985;12:87-92

27 Calnan CD, Cronin E, Rycroft RJ. Allergy to perfume ingredients. Contact Dermatitis 1980;6:500-501

28 Storrs FJ. Fragrance. Dermatitis 2007;18:3-7

29 Larsen WG. Perfume dermatitis. A study of 20 patients. Arch Dermatol 1977;113:623-626

30 Ung CY, White JML, White IR, Banerjee P, McFadden JP. Patch testing with the European baseline series fragrance markers: a 2016 update. Br J Dermatol 2018;178:776-780

31 Dittmar D, Schuttelaar MLA. Contact sensitization to hydroperoxides of limonene and linalool: Results of consecutive patch testing and clinical relevance. Contact Dermatitis 2018 Oct 31. doi: 10.1111/cod.13137. [Epub ahead of print]

32 Silvestre JF, Mercader P, González-Pérez R, Hervella-Garcés M, Sanz-Sánchez T, Córdoba S, et al. Sensitization to fragrances in Spain: A 5-year multicentre study (2011-2015). Contact Dermatitis. 2018 Nov 14. doi: 10.1111/cod.13152. [Epub ahead of print]

Chapter 3.10   AMYL SALICYLATE

IDENTIFICATION

Description/definition   : Amyl salicylate is the ester of amyl alcohol and salicylic acid that conforms to the
                                          formula shown below
Chemical class(es)   : Esters
Chemical/IUPAC name   : Pentyl 2-hydroxybenzoate
Other names   : Pentyl salicylate
CAS registry number(s)   : 2050-08-0
EC number(s)   : 218-080-2
RIFM monograph(s)   : Food Chem Toxicol 2007;45(suppl.1):S460-S466; Food Chem Toxicol 2007;45:S318-S361
SCCS opinion(s)   : SCCS/1459/11 (2)
Function(s) in cosmetics   : EU: perfuming; skin conditioning. USA: fragrance ingredients
Patch testing   : 5% pet. (1,6); based on RIFM data, 10% pet. is probably not irritant (8)
Molecular formula   : $C_{12}H_{16}O_3$

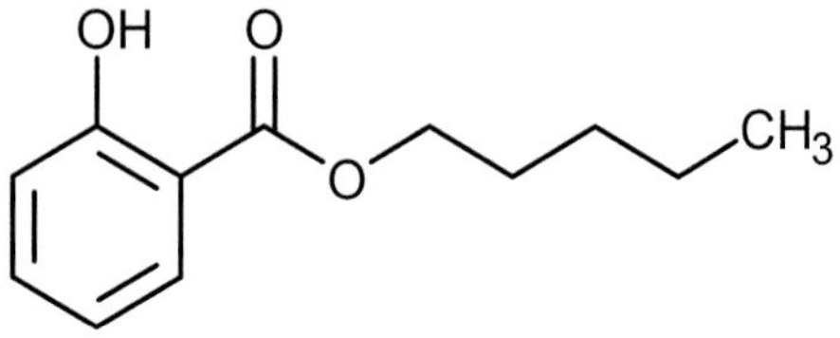

GENERAL

Amyl salicylate is a colorless to pale yellow clear liquid; its odor type is floral and its odor at 100% is described as 'herbal floral clover azalea green sweet chocolate' (www.thegoodscentscompany.com).

Presence in essential oils

Amyl salicylate has been identified by chemical analysis in none of 91 essential oils, which have caused contact allergy / allergic contact dermatitis (9).

CONTACT ALLERGY

General

The SCCS (Scientific Committee on Consumer Safety), in a 2012 Opinion on Fragrance allergens in cosmetic products, has marked amyl salicylate as 'established contact allergen in humans' (2,7).

Testing in groups of patients

Results of studies testing amyl salicylate in consecutive patients suspected of contact dermatitis (routine testing) and those of testing in groups of selected patients are shown in table 3.10.1. In two studies performing routine tests, low frequencies of sensitization of 0.2% and 1% were found (6,10), the latter percentage resulting from one positive patch test in 100 tested patients (10). In one study with selected patients, an early study in a group of 20 fragrance-allergic individuals, there was only one reaction (5%) to amyl salicylate (1). Relevance data were not provided in any of the three investigations.

Table 3.10.1 Patch testing in groups of patients

Years and Country	Test conc. & vehicle	Number of patients tested | positive (%)		Selection of patients (S); Relevance (R); Comments (C)	Ref.
Routine testing					
1997-8 six European countries	5% pet.	1855	3 (0.2%)	R: not stated / specified	6
<1995 Sweden	5% pet.	100	1 (1.0%)	R: not stated	10
	1% pet.	100	0		
Testing in groups of selected patients					
1977 USA	5% pet.	20	1 (5%)	R: not stated	1

Case reports and case series
No case reports of allergic contact dermatitis caused by amyl salicylate have been found.

Presence in products and chemical analyses
In 2000, fifty-nine domestic and occupational products, purchased in retail outlets in Denmark, England, Germany and Italy were analyzed by GC-MS for the presence of fragrances. The product categories were liquid soap and soap bars (n=13), soft/hard surface cleaners (n=23), fabric conditioners/laundry detergents for hand wash (n=8), dish wash (n=10), furniture polish, car shampoo, stain remover (each n=1) and 2 products used in occupational environments. Amyl salicylate was present in 6 products (10%); quantification was not performed (3).

In 1997, 71 deodorants (22 vapo-spray, 22 aerosol spray and 27 roll-on products) were collected in Denmark, England, France, Germany and Sweden and analyzed by gas chromatography – mass spectrometry (GC-MS) for the presence of fragrances and other materials. Amyl / isoamyl salicylate was present in 21 (30%) of the products (4).

In 1988, in the USA, 400 perfumes used in fine fragrances, household products and soaps (number of products per category not mentioned) were analyzed for the presence of fragrance chemicals in a concentration of at least 1% and a list of the Top-25 (present in the highest number of products) presented. Amyl salicylate was found to be present in 32% of the fine fragrances (rank number 20), 24% of the household product fragrances (rank number 19) and 74% of the fragrances used in soaps (rank number 4) (5).

LITERATURE

1   Larsen WG. Perfume dermatitis. A study of 20 patients. Arch Dermatol 1977;113:623-626
2   SCCS (Scientific Committee on Consumer Safety). Opinion on Fragrance allergens in cosmetic products, 26-27 June 2012, SCCS/1459/11. Available at:
    https://ec.europa.eu/health/sites/health/files/scientific_committees/consumer_safety/docs/sccs_o_102.pdf
3   Rastogi SC, Heydorn S, Johansen JD, Basketter DA. Fragrance chemicals in domestic and occupational products. Contact Dermatitis 2001;45:221-225
4   Rastogi SC, Lepoittevin J-P, Johansen JD, Frosch PJ, Menné T, Bruze M, et al. Fragrances and other materials in deodorants: search for potentially sensitizing molecules using combined GC-MS and structure activity relationship (SAR) analysis. Contact Dermatitis 1998;39:293-303
5   Fenn RS. Aroma chemical usage trends in modern perfumery. Perfumer and Flavorist 1989;14:3-10
6   Frosch PJ, Johansen JD, Menné T, Pirker C, Rastogi SC, Andersen KE, et al. Further important sensitizers in patients sensitive to fragrances. I. Reactivity to 14 frequently used chemicals. Contact Dermatitis 2002;47:78-85
7   Uter W, Johansen JD, Börje A, Karlberg A-T, Lidén C, Rastogi S, Roberts D, White IR. Categorization of fragrance contact allergens for prioritization of preventive measures: clinical and experimental data and consideration of structure–activity relationships. Contact Dermatitis 2013;69:196-230
8   De Groot AC. Patch Testing, 4th Edition. Wapserveen, The Netherlands: acdegroot publishing, 2018, page 51 (ISBN 978-90-813233-4-5)
9   De Groot AC, Schmidt E. Essential oils: contact allergy and chemical composition. Boca Raton, Fl., USA: CRC Press, Taylor and Francis Group, 2016 (ISBN 9781482246407)
10 Frosch PJ, Pilz B, Andersen KE, Burrows D, Camarasa JG, Camarasa JG, Dooms-Goossens A, et al. Patch testing with fragrances: results of a multicenter study of the European Environmental and Contact Dermatitis Research Group with 48 frequently used constituents of perfumes. Contact Dermatitis 1995;33:333-342

Chapter 3.11   ANETHOLE

IDENTIFICATION

Description/definition	: Anethole is the substituted aromatic ether that conforms to the structural formula shown below
Chemical class(es)	: Ethers
Chemical/IUPAC name	: 1-Methoxy-4-(1-propenyl)benzene
Other names	: Isoestragole; anise camphor
CAS registry number(s)	: 104-46-1
EC number(s)	: 203-205-5
RIFM monograph(s)	: Food Cosmet Toxicol 1973;11:863 (trans-anethole = E-anethole)
SCCS opinion(s)	: SCCS/1459/11 (2)
Merck Index monograph	: 1906
Function(s) in cosmetics	: EU: denaturant; masking. USA: denaturants; flavoring agents; fragrance ingredients; skin-conditioning agents - miscellaneous
Patch testing	: 5% pet. (Chemotechnique)
Molecular formula	: $C_{10}H_{12}O$

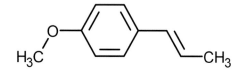

GENERAL

Anethole is a colorless to pale yellow liquid to solid; its odor type is licorice and its odor at 100% is described as 'sweet anise licorice medicinal' (www.thegoodscentscompany.com). Anethole occurs naturally in anise, star anise, and fennel oils, and chickpea seed and is used as a flavor ingredient (U.S. National Library of Medicine). trans-Anethole can be purified from star anise oil (2).

Presence in essential oils

Anethole (any isomer) has been identified by chemical analysis in 35 of 91 essential oils, which have caused contact allergy / allergic contact dermatitis. In two oils, (E)-anethole belonged to the 'Top-10' of ingredients with the highest concentrations which may be expected in commercial essential oils of this type: aniseed oil (91.0-98.6%) and star anise oil (84.3-90.1%) (12).

CONTACT ALLERGY

General

The SCCS (Scientific Committee on Consumer Safety), in a 2012 Opinion on Fragrance allergens in cosmetic products, has marked trans-anethole as 'established contact allergen in humans' (2,9).

Patch testing in groups of patients

Studies in which anethole was patch tested in consecutive patients suspected of contact dermatitis (routine testing) with positive results have not been found. The results of testing anethole in groups of selected patients are shown in table 3.11.1. In four studies, rates of positive reactions were 0.6%, 4.8%, 5% and 33%. The highest frequency was found in a small group of 15 patients who were patch test sensitized by star anise oil, which contains 84-90% anethole (12). Relevance data were generally inadequate.

Case reports and case series

Most reports of allergic contact dermatitis relate to the use of toothpastes containing anethole.

Toothpastes

A woman suffered from an oozing cheilitis for three months with erythema, edema and crusting of the lips and perioral skin. An intra-oral burning sensation, loss of taste and a dry mouth were also present. Patch tests revealed contact allergy to anethole and trans-anethole. The toothpastes' labeling mentioned the presence of 'aroma'; the manufacturers of the toothpastes she used confirmed that nearly all their rinse-off dental products contained (trans-)anethole in concentrations ranging from less than 100 ppm (0.01%) to 1300 ppm (0.13%). The use of an aroma-free compounded toothpaste rapidly led to resolution of the dermatitis, without any recurrence after a follow-up of 2 years (20).

Table 3.11.1 Patch testing in groups of patients: Selected patient groups

Years and Country	Test conc. & vehicle	Number of patients tested	positive (%)	Selection of patients (S); Relevance (R); Comments (C)	Ref.
2000-2007 USA	5% pet.	322	2 (0.6%)	S: patients who were tested with a supplemental cosmetic screening series; R: 100%; C: weak study: a. high rate of macular erythema and weak reactions; b. relevance figures included 'questionable' and 'past' relevance	1
1971-1977 Denmark	5% pet.	41	2 (4.8%)	S: patients who presented with sore mouth, stomatitis and/or dermatitis around the mouth or who were dentist personnel; R: the causative products were supposed to be toothpastes	10
<1976 Poland		15	5 (33%)	S: patients with positive patch tests to star anise oil 1% pet., negative to 0.5% but positive to one or more 'balsams' (Myroxylon pereirae resin, turpentine, wood tars, colophonium); R: not stated; C: star anise oil contains 84-90% anethole (12)	17
1975 USA	1% pet.	20	1 (5%)	S: fragrance-allergic patients; R: not stated	4

Another female patient reported by these authors presented with cheilitis and perioral eczema, dysgeusia and a recalcitrant, dyshidrotic eczema of her right (dominant) hand, related to the use of toothpastes. The regular eating of Dutch licorice ('drop', which contains anethole) also seemed to aggravate the cheilitis. Patch tests revealed sensitization to anethole and trans-anethole. During the patch tests a flare-up of the perioral eczema and of the dyshidrotic hand dermatitis was noted. The patient was prescribed a compounded aroma-free toothpaste, upon which her hand dermatitis disappeared and her perioral eczema significantly improved, although minor flare-ups occasionally still occurred (20).

A woman, using a spearmint-flavored toothpaste, had cheilitis, which healed when the patient stopped using the product. The toothpaste itself was not patch tested, but she reacted to the flavor anethole, which was considered to be the culprit (11). However, its presence in the toothpaste was not ascertained and spearmint oil does not contain anethole (12).

Another female individual was patch tested because of dry mouth, erythema and desquamation of oral mucosa, cheilitis, perioral eczema and loss of taste. She had positive reactions to one of her toothpastes (tested 2% in water) and anethole 5% pet. One of the toothpastes contained anethole, the other fennel, a natural source of anethole. There was a slow resolution of the symptoms after the patient avoided the toothpastes and other sources of anethole (13).

A female patient had sore mouth and cheilitis. She reacted to two toothpastes. In one, the allergens were spearmint oil and its main ingredient carvone, in the other spearmint oil and anethole (which is not an ingredient of spearmint oil (14) .

A girl presented with a 1.5-year history of a pruritic perioral rash without frank lip or intraoral involvement. Patch tests were positive to the toothpaste (open test) and anethole. The manufacturer confirmed that anethole was present in the toothpaste. The patient admitted that she was not particularly tidy when brushing her teeth and her toothpaste would contact much of the perioral area. Her rash improved after discontinuing the use of the product (19).

Early publications from Denmark have described one or more cases of contact allergy to the flavor anethole in toothpastes (5,6).

Other products

Two patients had allergic contact dermatitis from trans-anethole present in the aniseed perfume fraction of a solution to prevent pressure ulcers (16).

One patient from Japan had allergic contact dermatitis of the covered skin areas from anethole added to washing detergents (7).

Two women had occupational allergic contact dermatitis from anise oil and its ingredient anethole from baking cakes containing anise oil. Both also suffered from rhinitis and blepharitis when entering the factory, but whether this was related to their allergy was not mentioned (18).

Patch test sensitization

Of five patients, who were sensitized by patch testing with star anise oil (containing 84-90% anethole [12]), three were tested with anethole 1% in petrolatum, and all reacted. Another of these actively sensitized patients was tested with 9 components of star anise oil and reacted to anethole and three other chemicals: α-pinene, safrole and methylchavicol, all tested 1% in petrolatum (17).

Presence in products and chemical analyses

In 2008, 66 different fragrance components (including 39 essential oils) were identified in 370 (10% of the total) topical pharmaceutical products marketed in Belgium; 9 of these 370 products (2.4%) contained anethole (3).

LITERATURE

1 Wetter DA, Yiannias JA, Prakash AV, Davis MDP, Farmer SA, el-Azhary RA. Results of patch testing to personal care product allergens in a standard series and a supplemental cosmetic series: an analysis of 945 patients from the Mayo Clinic Contact Dermatitis Group, 2000-2007. J Am Acad Dermatol 2010;63:789-798

2 SCCS (Scientific Committee on Consumer Safety). Opinion on Fragrance allergens in cosmetic products, 26-27 June 2012, SCCS/1459/11. Available at: https://ec.europa.eu/health/sites/health/files/scientific_committees/consumer_safety/docs/sccs_o_102.pdf

3 Nardelli A, D'Hooge E, Drieghe J, Dooms M, Goossens A. Allergic contact dermatitis from fragrance components in specific topical pharmaceutical products in Belgium. Contact Dermatitis 2009;60:303-313

4 Larsen WG. Perfume dermatitis. A study of 20 patients. Arch Dermatol 1977;113:623-626

5 Hjorth N, Jervoe P. Allergisk Kontaktstomatitis og Kontaktdermatitis fremkaldt of smagsstoffer i tandpasta. Tandlaegebladet 1967;71:937-942 (article in Danish). Data cited in ref. 15

6 Hjorth N. Toothpaste sensitivity. Contact Dermatitis Newsletter 1967;1:14

7 Nakayama H, Hanaoka H, Ohshiro A. Allergen controlled system (ACS). Tokyo: Kanehara Shuppan, 1974:42. Data cited in ref. 8

8 Mitchell JC. Contact hypersensitivity to some perfume materials. Contact Dermatitis 1975;1:196-199

9 Uter W, Johansen JD, Börje A, Karlberg A-T, Lidén C, Rastogi S, Roberts D, White IR. Categorization of fragrance contact allergens for prioritization of preventive measures: clinical and experimental data and consideration of structure–activity relationships. Contact Dermatitis 2013;69:196-230

10 Andersen KE. Contact allergy to toothpaste flavors. Contact Dermatitis 1978;4:195-198

11 Poon TS, Freeman S. Cheilitis caused by contact allergy to anethole in spearmint flavoured toothpaste. Australas J Dermatol 2006;47:300-301

12 De Groot AC, Schmidt E. Essential oils: contact allergy and chemical composition. Boca Raton, Fl., USA: CRC Press, Taylor and Francis Group, 2016 (ISBN 9781482246407)

13 Franks A. Contact allergy to anethole in toothpaste associated with loss of taste. Contact Dermatitis 1998;38:354-355

14 Grattan CEH, Peachy RD. Contact sensitization to toothpaste flavouring. J Royal Coll Gen Pract 1985;35:498

15 Magnusson B, Wilkinson DS. Cinnamic aldehyde in toothpaste. 1. Clinical aspects and patch tests. Contact Dermatitis 1975;1:70-76

16 Marin-Cabanas I, Bouret AM, Leiva-Salinas M, Frances L, Silvestre JF. Allergic contact dermatitis to anethole in a preventive pressure ulcers solution. J Eur Acad Dermatol Venereol 2014;29:1241

17 Rudzki E, Grzywa Z. Sensitizing and irritating properties of star anise oil. Contact Dermatitis 1976;2:305-308

18 Garcia-Bravo B, Pérez Bernal A, Garcia-Hernandez MJ, Camacho F. Occupational contact dermatitis from anethole in food handlers. Contact Dermatitis 1997;37:38

19 Aschenbeck KA, Hylwa SA. Brushing your way to allergic contact dermatitis: anethole allergy. Dermatitis 2017;28:219-220

20 Horst N, Leysen J, Mellaerts T, Lambert J, Aerts O. Allergic contact cheilitis from anethole-containing toothpastes: a practical solution. J Eur Acad Dermatol Venereol 2017;31:e374-e375

Chapter 3.12   ANISE ALCOHOL

IDENTIFICATION

Description/definition	: Anise alcohol is the organic compound that conforms to the structural formula shown below
Chemical class(es)	: Alcohols; ethers
Chemical/IUPAC name	: (4-Methoxyphenyl)methanol
Other names	: Anisyl alcohol; anisic alcohol
CAS registry number(s)	: 105-13-5
EC number(s)	: 203-273-6
RIFM monograph(s)	: Food Chem Toxicol 2012;50(suppl.2):S134-9; Food Chem Toxicol 2012;50(suppl.2): S117-S119; Food Cosmet Toxicol 1974;12:825 (special issue 1)
IFRA standard	: Restricted (www.ifraorg.org/en-us/standards-library) (table 3.12.1)
SCCS opinion(s)	: Various (6); SCCS/1459/11 (7)
Merck Index monograph	: 1928
Function(s) in cosmetics	: EU: perfuming. USA: fragrance ingredients
EU cosmetic restrictions	: Regulated in Annex III/80 of the Regulation (EC) No. 1223/2009, regulated by 2003/15/EC; Must be labeled on cosmetics and detergent products, if present at > 10 ppm (0.001%) in leave-on products and > 100 ppm (0.01%) in rinse-off products
Patch testing	: 1% pet. (SmartPracticeEurope, SmartPracticeCanada); 10% Softisan (Chemotechnique); recommended test concentration: 10.0% wt./wt. pet. (1)
Molecular formula	: $C_8H_{10}O_2$

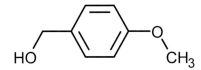

Table 3.12.1 IFRA restrictions for anise alcohol

Category [a]	Limits [b]	Category [a]	Limits [b]	Category [a]	Limits [b]
1	0.04%	5	0.36%	9	5.00%
2	0.06%	6	1.09%	10	2.50%
3	0.23%	7	0.11%	11	not restricted
4	0.68%	8	1.52%		

[a] For explanation of categories see pages 6-8
[b] Limits in the finished products

GENERAL

Anise alcohol is a white to pale yellow liquid to solid; its odor type is powdery and its odor at 100% is described as 'sweet powdery hawthorn lilac rose floral hyacinth' (www.thegoodscentscompany.com).

Presence in essential oils

Anise alcohol has been identified by chemical analysis in 2 of 91 essential oils, which have caused contact allergy / allergic contact dermatitis: aniseed oil and star anise oil (23). In neither of these does it belong to the 'Top-10' ingredients with the highest concentrations.

CONTACT ALLERGY

The SCCS (Scientific Committee on Consumer Safety), in a 2012 Opinion on Fragrance allergens in cosmetic products, has marked anise alcohol as 'established contact allergen in humans' (7,18). The sensitizing potency of anise alcohol was classified as 'moderate' based on an EC3 value of 5.9% in the LLNA (local lymph node assay) in animal experiments (7,18).

The literature on contact allergy to anise alcohol up to 2003 has been reviewed (9).

Patch testing in groups of patients

Results of studies testing anise alcohol in consecutive patients suspected of contact dermatitis (routine testing) and those of testing in groups of *selected* patients (mostly patients suspected or known to be allergic to fragrances) are shown in table 3.12.2.

In five studies in which routine testing with anise alcohol was performed, rates of sensitization have been low, ranging from 0.03% to 0.2%. In four groups of selected patients suspected or known to be allergic to fragrances, between 0.1% and 20% had positive patch tests to anise alcohol. The high percentage of 20 was seen in an early study in a small group of 20 patients with diagnosed fragrance sensitivity (8). In most studies, no relevance data were provided; in the two addressing the issue, 50-100% of the positive patch tests were scored as relevant, but the numbers were always very low. Causative products were usually not mentioned or specified, but in one study, of the relevant reactions to any of 26 fragrances tested, 96% were caused by cosmetic products (2).

Table 3.12.2 Patch testing in groups of patients

Years and Country	Test conc. & vehicle	Number of patients tested	positive (%)		Selection of patients (S); Relevance (R); Comments (C)	Ref.
Routine testing						
2015-2016 UK	1% pet.	2084	3	(0.1%)	R: not specified for individual fragrances; 25% of patients who reacted to any fragrance or fragrance marker had a positive fragrance history	24
2010-2015 Denmark	1% pet.	6004		(0.03%)	R: present relevance 50%, past relevance 50%	16
2011-2012 UK	1% pet.	1951	4	(0.2%)	R: not stated	17
2008-2010 Denmark	1% pet.	1503	1	(0.1%)	S: mostly routine testing; R: 100%; C: 100% co-reactivity of FM I, 0% of FM II; C: of the relevant reactions to any of the 26 fragrances tested, 96% were caused by cosmetic products	2
2003-2004 IVDK	1% pet.	2004	1	(<0.1%)	R: not stated	3
Testing in groups of selected patients						
2011-2015 Spain	1% or 10% pet.	607	14	(2.3%)	S: patients previously reacting to FM I, FM II, Myroxylon pereirae resin or hydroxyisohexyl 3-cyclohexene carboxaldehyde in the baseline series and subsequently tested with a fragrance series; R: not stated	25
2005-2008 IVDK	1% pet.	986		(0.1%)	S: not specified; R: not stated	19
<1996 Japan, Europe, USA	5% pet.	167	3	(1.8%)	S: patients known or suspected to be allergic to fragrances; R: not stated	5
1975 USA		20	4	(20%)	S: fragrance-allergic patients; R: not stated	8

FM: Fragrance Mix; IVDK: Informationsverbund Dermatologischer Kliniken (Germany, Switzerland, Austria)

Case reports and case series
No case reports of allergic contact dermatitis due to sensitization to anise alcohol have been found

Presence in products and chemical analyses
In various studies, the presence of anise alcohol in cosmetic and sometimes other products has been investigated. Before 2006, most investigators used chemical analysis, usually GC-MS, for qualitative and quantitative determination. Since then, the presence of the target fragrances was usually investigated by screening the product labels for the 26 fragrances that must be labeled since 2005 on cosmetics and detergent products in the EU, if present at > 10 ppm (0.001%) in leave-on products and > 100 ppm (0.01%) in rinse-off products. This method, obviously, is less accurate and may result in underestimation of the frequency of the fragrances being present in the product. When they are in fact present, but the concentration is lower than mentioned above, labeling is not required and the fragrances' presence will be missed.

The results of the relevant studies for anise alcohol are summarized in table 3.12.3. More detailed information can be found in the corresponding text before and following the table. The percentage of products in which anise alcohol was found to be present was usually (very) low; anise alcohol appears to be an infrequently used fragrance material.

In 2016, in Sweden, 66 commercially available toothpastes obtained from local pharmacies and supermarkets in Malmö, Sweden were investigated for the presence of flavors by studying the packages and product labels. Anise alcohol was found to be present in 1 (2%) of the products (22).

In Denmark, in 2015-2016, 5588 fragranced cosmetic products were examined with a smartphone application for the 26 fragrances that need to be labeled in the EU. Anise alcohol was present in 0.3% of the products (rank number 22) (12).

In 2008, 2010 and 2011, 374 deodorants available in German retail shops were randomly selected and their labels checked for the presence of the 26 fragrances that need to be labeled. Anise alcohol was found to be present in 9 (2.4%) of the products (21).

Table 3.12.3 Presence of anise alcohol in products [a]

Year	Country	Product type	Nr. investigated	Nr. of products positive [b]	(%)	Method [c]	Ref.
2016	Sweden	Toothpastes	66	1	(2%)	Labeling	22
2015-6	Denmark	Fragranced cosmetic products	5588		(0.3%)	Labeling	12
2008-11	Germany	Deodorants	374	9	(2%)	Labeling	21
2006-9	Germany	Cosmetic products	4991		(0.2%)	Labeling	11
2008	Belgium	Fragranced topical pharmaceutical products	370	1	(0.3%)	Labeling	4
2007	Netherlands	Cosmetic products for children	23	1	(4%)	Analysis	14
2006	UK	Perfumed cosmetic and household products	300	1	(0.3%)	Labeling	10
2006	Denmark	Popular perfumed deodorants	88	2	(2%)	Labeling	13
			23	2	(9%)	Analysis	
2001	Denmark	Non-cosmetic consumer products	43	1	(2%)	Analysis	15

[a] See the corresponding text below for more details

[b] positive = containing the target fragrance

[c] Labeling: information from the ingredient labels on the product / packaging; Analysis: chemical analysis, most often GC-MS

In Germany, in the period 2006-2009, 4991 cosmetic products were randomly sampled for an official investigation of conformity of cosmetic products with legal provisions. The labels were inspected for the presence of the 26 fragrances that need to be labeled in the EU. Anise alcohol was present in 0.2% of the products (rank number 25) (11).

In 2008, 66 different fragrance components (including 39 essential oils) were identified in 370 (10% of the total) topical pharmaceutical products marketed in Belgium; one of these (0.3%) contained anise alcohol (4).

In 2007, in The Netherlands, twenty-three cosmetic products for children were analyzed for the presence of fragrances that need to be labeled. Anise alcohol was identified in one of the products (4%) in a concentration of 22 ppm (14).

In 2006, of 88 popular perfume containing deodorants purchased in Denmark, 2 (2%) were labeled to contain anise alcohol. Analysis of 24 regulated fragrance substances in 23 selected deodorants (19 spray products, 2 deostick and 2 roll-on) was performed by GC-MS. Anise alcohol was identified in 2 of the products (9%) with a concentration range of 1–51 ppm (13).

In January 2006, a study of perfumed cosmetic and household products available on the shelves of U.K. retailers was carried out. Products were included if 'parfum' or 'aroma' was listed among the ingredients. Three hundred products were surveyed and any of 26 mandatory labeling fragrances named on the label were recorded. Anise alcohol was present in one (0.3%) of the products (rank number 24) (10).

In 2001, in Denmark, 43 non-cosmetic consumer products (mainly dish-washing products, laundry detergents, and hard and soft surface cleaners) were analyzed for the 26 fragrances that are regulated for labeling in the EU. Anise alcohol was present in one product (2%) in a concentration of 0.0014% (m/m) and had rank number 21 in the frequency list (15).

OTHER SIDE EFFECTS

Immediate-type reactions

Of 50 individuals who had open tests with anise alcohol 5% pet. on the forearm, 35 (70%) showed local macular erythema after 45 minutes, termed 'contact urticaria' by the authors (20).

LITERATURE

1 Bruze M, Svedman C, Andersen KE, Bruynzeel D, Goossens A, Johansen JD, et al. Patch test concentrations (doses in mg/cm2) for the 12 non-mix fragrance substances regulated by European legislation. Contact Dermatitis 2012;66:131-136

2 Heisterberg MV, Menné T, Johansen JD. Contact allergy to the 26 specific fragrance ingredients to be declared on cosmetic products in accordance with the EU cosmetic directive. Contact Dermatitis 2011;65:266-275

3 Schnuch A, Uter W, Geier J, Lessmann H, Frosch PJ. Sensitization to 26 fragrances to be labelled according to current European regulation: Results of the IVDK and review of the literature. Contact Dermatitis 2007;57:1-10

4 Nardelli A, D'Hooge E, Drieghe J, Dooms M, Goossens A. Allergic contact dermatitis from fragrance components in specific topical pharmaceutical products in Belgium. Contact Dermatitis 2009;60:303-313

5   Larsen W, Nakayama H, Fischer T, Elsner P, Burrows D, Jordan W, et al. Fragrance contact dermatitis: A worldwide multicenter investigation (Part I). Am J Cont Dermat 1996;7:77-83

6   Various SCCS opinions on anise alcohol have been published and are available at: http://ec.europa.eu/growth/tools-databases/cosing/index.cfm?fuseaction=search.details_v2&id=27929&back=1

7   SCCS (Scientific Committee on Consumer Safety). Opinion on Fragrance allergens in cosmetic products, 26-27 June 2012, SCCS/1459/11. Available at: https://ec.europa.eu/health/sites/health/files/scientific_committees/consumer_safety/docs/sccs_o_102.pdf

8   Larsen WG. Perfume dermatitis. A study of 20 patients. Arch Dermatol 1977;113:623-626

9   Hostýnek JJ, Maibach HI. Is there evidence that anisyl alcohol causes allergic contact dermatitis? Exog Dermatol 2003;2:230-233

10 Buckley DA. Fragrance ingredient labelling in products on sale in the UK. Br J Dermatol 2007;157:295-300

11 Uter W, Yazar K, Kratz E-M, Mildau G, Lidén C. Coupled exposure to ingredients of cosmetic products: I. Fragrances. Contact Dermatitis 2013;69:335-341

12 Bennike NH, Oturai NB, Müller S, Kirkeby CS, Jørgensen C, Christensen AB, et al. Fragrance contact allergens in 5588 cosmetic products identified through a novel smartphone application. J Eur Acad Dermatol Venereol 2018;32:79-85

13 Rastogi SC, Hellerup Jensen G, Johansen JD. Survey and risk assessment of chemical substances in deodorants. Survey of Chemical Substances in Consumer Products, No. 86 2007. Danish Ministry of the Environment, Environmental Protection Agency. Available at: https://www2.mst.dk/Udgiv/publications/2007/978-87-7052-625-8/pdf/978-87-7052-626-5.pdf

14 VWA. Dutch Food and Consumer Product Safety Authority. Cosmetische producten voor kinderen: Inventarisatie van de markt en de veiligheidsborging door producenten en importeurs. Report ND04o065/ND05o170, 2007 (Report in Dutch), 2007. Available at: www.nvwa.nl/documenten/communicatie/inspectieresultaten/ consument/2016m/cosmetische- producten-voor-kinderen

15 Rastogi SC. Survey of chemical compounds in consumer products. Contents of selected fragrance materials in cleaning products and other consumer products. Survey no. 8-2002. Copenhagen, Denmark, Danish Environmental Protection Agency. Available at: http://eng.mst.dk/media/mst/69131/8.pdf

16 Bennike NH, Zachariae C, Johansen JD. Non-mix fragrances are top sensitizers in consecutive dermatitis patients – a cross-sectional study of the 26 EU-labelled fragrance allergens. Contact Dermatitis 2017;77:270-279

17 Mann J, McFadden JP, White JML, White IR, Banerjee P. Baseline series fragrance markers fail to predict contact allergy. Contact Dermatitis 2014;70:276-281

18 Uter W, Johansen JD, Börje A, Karlberg A-T, Lidén C, Rastogi S, Roberts D, White IR. Categorization of fragrance contact allergens for prioritization of preventive measures: clinical and experimental data and consideration of structure–activity relationships. Contact Dermatitis 2013;69:196-230

19 Uter W, Geier J, Frosch P, Schnuch A. Contact allergy to fragrances: current patch test results (2005–2008) from the Information Network of Departments of Dermatology. Contact Dermatitis 2010;63:254-261

20 Emmons WW, Marks JG Jr. Immediate and delayed reactions to cosmetic ingredients. Contact Dermatitis 1985;13:258-265

21 Klaschka U. Contact allergens for armpits - allergenic fragrances specified on deodorants. Int J Hyg Environ Health 2012;215:584-591

22 Kroona L, Warfvinge G, Isaksson M, Ahlgren C, Dahlin J, Sörensen Ö, Bruze M. Quantification of L-carvone in toothpastes available on the Swedish market. Contact Dermatitis 2017;77:224-230

23 De Groot AC, Schmidt E. Essential oils: contact allergy and chemical composition. Boca Raton, Fl., USA: CRC Press, Taylor and Francis Group, 2016 (ISBN 9781482246407)

24 Ung CY, White JML, White IR, Banerjee P, McFadden JP. Patch testing with the European baseline series fragrance markers: a 2016 update. Br J Dermatol 2018;178:776-780

25 Silvestre JF, Mercader P, González-Pérez R, Hervella-Garcés M, Sanz-Sánchez T, Córdoba S, et al. Sensitization to fragrances in Spain: A 5-year multicentre study (2011-2015). Contact Dermatitis. 2018 Nov 14. doi: 10.1111/cod.13152. [Epub ahead of print]

Chapter 3.13   ANISYLIDENE ACETONE *
Not an INCI name

IDENTIFICATION

Description/definition	: Anisylidene acetone is the aromatic compound that conforms to the structural formula shown below
Chemical class(es)	: Aromatic compounds; ketones; ethers
INCI name USA	: Not in the Personal Care Products Council Ingredient Database
Chemical/IUPAC name	: 4-(4-Methoxyphenyl)-3-buten-2-one
CAS registry number(s)	: 943-88-4
EC number(s)	: 213-404-9
RIFM monograph(s)	: Food Cosmet Toxicol 1975;13:456
IFRA standard	: Prohibited (www.ifraorg.org/en-us/standards-library)
SCCS opinion(s)	: SCCNFP/0320/00 (1)
EU cosmetic restrictions	: Regulated in Annex II/443 of the Regulation (EC) No. 1223/2009, regulated by 2002/34/EC; Prohibited since 2002
Patch testing	: 2% pet. (3)
Molecular formula	: $C_{11}H_{12}O_2$

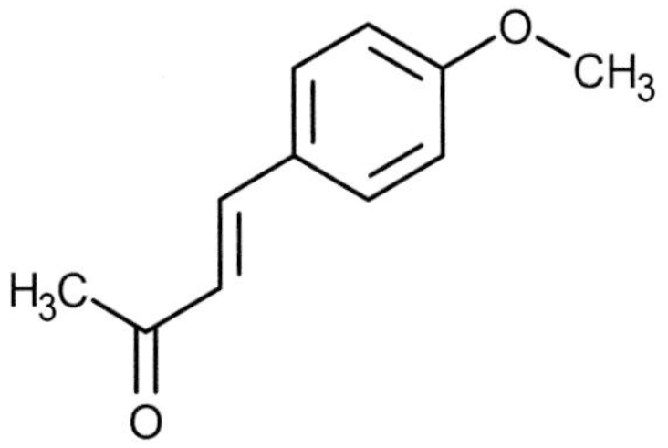

GENERAL

Anisylidene acetone is a white crystalline leaflet. It is a synthetic chemical, not found in nature (and consequently not in essential oils (4)). Anisylidene acetone is prohibited by IFRA (www.ifraorg.org/en-us/standards-library) and the EU because of sensitization and is not used anymore.

CONTACT ALLERGY

Patch testing in groups of patients

Studies in which anisylidene acetone was patch tested in consecutive patients suspected of contact dermatitis (routine testing) with positive results have not been found. In 1983, in The Netherlands, a group of 182 patients suspected of cosmetic allergy was patch tested with anisylidene acetone 2% in petrolatum. There were 2 (1.1%) positive reactions; their relevance was not addressed (2).

Case reports and case series
No cases of allergic contact dermatitis caused by anisylidene acetone have been found.

LITERATURE

1   SCCFNP (Scientific Committee on Cosmetic Products and Non-Food Products Intended for Consumers). Opinion of the Scientific Committee on Cosmetic Products and Non-Food Products Intended for Consumers concerning 'An initial list of perfumery materials which must not form part of fragrances compounds used in cosmetic products', 3 May 2000, SCCNFP/0320/00, final. Available at:
    http://ec.europa.eu/health/archive/ph_risk/committees/sccp/documents/out116_en.pdf
2   Malten KE, van Ketel WG, Nater JP, Liem DH. Reactions in selected patients to 22 fragrance materials. Contact Dermatitis 1984;11:1-10
3   De Groot AC. Patch Testing, 4th Edition. Wapserveen, The Netherlands: acdegroot publishing, 2018 (ISBN 978-90-813233-4-5)
4   De Groot AC, Schmidt E. Essential oils: contact allergy and chemical composition. Boca Raton, Fl., USA: CRC Press, Taylor and Francis Group, 2016 (ISBN 9781482246407)

Chapter 3.14   BENZALDEHYDE

IDENTIFICATION

Description/definition	: Benzaldehyde is the aromatic aldehyde that conforms to the structural formula shown below
Chemical class(es)	: Aldehydes
Chemical/IUPAC name	: Benzaldehyde
Other names	: Benzene carboxaldehyde; benzenecarbaldehyde; artificial almond oil
CAS registry number(s)	: 100-52-7
EC number(s)	: 202-860-4
CIR review(s)	: Int J Toxicol 2006;25(suppl.1):S11-S27 (access: www.cir-safety.org/ingredients)
RIFM monograph(s)	: Food Cosm Toxicol 1976;14:693 (special issue III)
IFRA standard	: Restricted (www.ifraorg.org/en-us/standards-library) (table 3.14.1)
SCCS opinion(s)	: SCCS/1459/11 (3)
Merck Index monograph	: 2330
Function(s) in cosmetics	: EU: denaturant; masking; solvent. USA: denaturants; flavoring agents; fragrance ingredients
Patch testing	: 5% pet. (SmartPracticeEurope, SmartPracticeCanada)
Molecular formula	: C_7H_6O

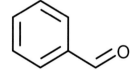

Table 3.14.1 IFRA restrictions for benzaldehyde

Category [a]	Limits [b]	Category [a]	Limits [b]	Category [a]	Limits [b]
1	0.02%	5	0.14%	9	3.00%
2	0.02%	6	0.43%	10	2.50%
3	0.09%	7	0.05%	11	not restricted
4	0.27%	8	0.60%		

[a] For explanation of categories see pages 6-8
[b] Limits in the finished products

GENERAL

Benzaldehyde is a colorless to pale yellow clear liquid; its odor type is fruity and its odor is described as 'almond, fruity, powdery, nutty and benzaldehyde-like' (www.thegoodscentscompany.com). Benzaldehyde occurs naturally in plants. It can be formed in the atmosphere from the reaction of some chemicals with sunlight. Benzaldehyde is an important commercial chemical that is used to make other chemicals, notably benzyl alcohol. Other uses of benzaldehyde include or have included: as a preservative in cosmetics, personal care products, food and select car detailing products, as a solvent for oils, flavoring (it is a key ingredient in natural fruit flavors [10]), in synthetic perfumes and as a tobacco additive (U.S. National Library of Medicine).

Presence in essential oils, Myroxylon pereirae resin (balsam of Peru) and propolis

Benzaldehyde has been identified by chemical analysis in 48 of 92 essential oils, which have caused contact allergy / allergic contact dermatitis. In two oils, benzaldehyde belonged to the 'Top-10' of ingredients with the highest concentrations which may be expected in commercial essential oils of this type: bitter almond oil (60-90%; see Chapter 6.6 Bitter almond oil) and cassia oil (0.9-2.3%) (13). Benzaldehyde may also be present in Myroxylon pereirae resin (balsam of Peru) (12) and in propolis (11).

CONTACT ALLERGY

General

The SCCS (Scientific Committee on Consumer Safety), in a 2012 Opinion on Fragrance allergens in cosmetic products, has marked benzaldehyde as 'established contact allergen in humans' (3,5).

Patch testing in groups of patients

Studies in which benzaldehyde was patch tested in consecutive patients suspected of contact dermatitis (routine testing) with positive results have not been found. Results of testing in groups of *selected* patients (e.g. patients with suspected cosmetic intolerance, individuals suspected of fragrance allergy, patients allergic to Myroxylon pereirae resin (balsam of Peru) are shown in table 3.14.2.

In 3 of 4 studies in groups of selected patients, frequencies of sensitization were low: 0.2%, 0.4% and 0.5%. Relevance was not addressed in any of these investigations (1,4,6). In the 4th study, 100 patients previously shown to be allergic to Myroxylon pereirae resin (balsam of Peru) were patch tested with a number of its constituents, including benzaldehyde 5% in petrolatum, and 10 (10%) had a positive reaction to benzaldehyde (9).

Table 3.14.2 Patch testing in groups of patients: Selected patient groups

Years and Country	Test conc. & vehicle	Number of patients tested	positive (%)	Selection of patients (S); Relevance (R); Comments (C)	Ref.
2006-2011 IVDK	5% pet.	665	3 (0.5%)	S: patients with suspected cosmetic intolerance; R: not stated	4
2005-2008 IVDK	5% pet.	2820	(0.2%)	S: not specified; R: not stated	6
1997-2000 Austria	5% pet.	747	3 (0.4%)	S: patients suspected of fragrance allergy: R: not stated	1
1955-1960 Denmark	5% pet.	100	10 (10.0%)	S: patients allergic to balsam of Peru, of which benzaldehyde may be an ingredient	9

IVDK: Informationsverbund Dermatologischer Kliniken (Germany, Switzerland, Austria)

Case reports and case series

In a perfume factory, three bottle fillers developed occupational allergic contact dermatitis from benzaldehyde. Of twenty people working in the same factory who did *not* have dermatitis, six had positive reactions to this fragrance (2).

Cross-reactions, pseudo-cross-reactions and co-reactions

For general information on cross-/pseudo-cross-/co-reactivity of fragrance chemicals with other fragrances, fragrance markers (fragrance mix I, fragrance mix II, colophonium, Myroxylon pereirae resin [balsam of Peru]) and essential oils see Chapter 1.2 General information on cross-reactions, pseudo-cross-reactions and co-reactions.

Of 12 patients allergic to Myroxylon pereirae resin (balsam of Peru) and tested with oil of bitter almonds (10% in olive oil) and benzaldehyde 5% pet. (an ingredient of both bitter almond oil and balsam of Peru), 6 reacted to both substances (9).

OTHER SIDE EFFECTS

Immediate-type reactions

A male pastry maker presented with recurrent urticaria localized on the dorsa of the hands and forearms. He was indaily contact with various pastry components, including chocolate, caramel, vanilla and cinnamon. There was a clear correlation between his work and the skin lesions, which rapidly disappeared in one to 2 hours on avoiding pastry contact. Patch tests were performed with the European standard series, removed at 20 minutes and read at 20 and 40 minutes. An immediate erythematous and edematous reaction was noted to Myroxylon pereirae resin (balsam of Peru), which persisted for one hour. When tested with several of its components, there were positive immediate reactions to cinnamal and benzaldehyde. After wearing gloves and avoiding skin contact with pastry, lesions did not recur. The authors suggested that the benzaldehyde reaction was a cross-reaction to cinnamal, a well-known cause of non-immunological immediate contact reactions (7).

In a study in the mid-1970's in Sweden, closed patch tests with Myroxylon pereirae resin and 11 of its components were applied to the upper part of the back of five patients for a period of 30 minutes (diagnoses unspecified, some possibly had urticaria). The result was read immediately after removal and every hour thereafter until the reaction disappeared. Benzaldehyde 5% pet. caused one urticarial reaction (8).

A case of urticaria with immediate local and generalized reaction to benzaldehyde and cinnamon oil has been reported from Poland. Details are missing (article not read, in Polish) (14).

LITERATURE

1   Wöhrl S, Hemmer W, Focke M, Götz M, Jarisch R. The significance of fragrance mix, balsam of Peru, colophony and propolis as screening tools in the detection of fragrance allergy. Br J Dermatol 2001;145:268-273

2   Schubert HJ. Skin diseases in workers at a perfume factory. Contact Dermatitis 2006;55:81-83

3   SCCS (Scientific Committee on Consumer Safety). Opinion on Fragrance allergens in cosmetic products, 26-27
     June 2012, SCCS/1459/11. Available at:
     https://ec.europa.eu/health/sites/health/files/scientific_committees/consumer_safety/docs/sccs_o_102.pdf

4   Dinkloh A, Worm M, Geier J, Schnuch A, Wollenberg A. Contact sensitization in patients with suspected cosmetic
     intolerance: results of the IVDK 2006-2011. J Eur Acad Dermatol Venereol 2015;29:1071-1081

5   Uter W, Johansen JD, Börje A, Karlberg A-T, Lidén C, Rastogi S, Roberts D, White IR. Categorization of fragrance
     contact allergens for prioritization of preventive measures: clinical and experimental data and consideration of
     structure–activity relationships. Contact Dermatitis 2013;69:196-230

6   Uter W, Geier J, Frosch P, Schnuch A. Contact allergy to fragrances: current patch test results (2005–2008) from
     the Information Network of Departments of Dermatology. Contact Dermatitis 2010;63:254-261

7   Seite-Beluezza D, El Sayed F, Bazex J. Contact urticaria from cinnamic aldehyde and benzaldehyde in a
     confectioner. Contact Dermatitis 1994;31:272-273

8   Forsbeck M, Skog E. Immediate reactions to patch tests with balsam of Peru. Contact Dermatitis 1977;3:201-205

9   Hjorth N. Eczematous allergy to balsams. Acta Derm Venereol 1961;41(suppl.46):1-216

10   Andersen A. Final report on the safety assessment of benzaldehyde. Int J Toxicol. 2006;25(suppl.1):11-27

11   De Groot AC, Popova MP, Bankova VS. An update on the constituents of poplar-type propolis. Wapserveen, The
     Netherlands: acdegroot publishing, 2014, 11 pages. ISBN/EAN: 978-90-813233-0-7. Available at:
     https://www.researchgate.net/publication/262851225_AN_UPDATE_ON_THE_CONSTITUENTS_OF_POPLAR-
     TYPE_PROPOLIS

12   Mammerler V. Contribution to the analysis and quality control of Peru Balsam. PhD Thesis, University of Vienna,
     Austria, 2007. Available at: http://othes.univie.ac.at/4056/1/2009-03-23_0201578.pdf

13   De Groot AC, Schmidt E. Essential oils: contact allergy and chemical composition. Boca Raton, Fl., USA: CRC Press,
     Taylor and Francis Group, 2016 (ISBN 9781482246407)

14   Ludera-Zimoch G. Case of urticaria with immediate local and generalized reaction to cinnamon oil and
     benzaldehyde. Przegl Dermatol 1981;68:67-70 (article in Polish)

Chapter 3.15   BENZYL ACETATE

IDENTIFICATION

Description/definition : Benzyl acetate is the ester of benzyl alcohol and acetic acid, that conforms to the formula shown below
Chemical class(es) : Esters
Chemical/IUPAC name : Benzyl acetate
Other names : Methyl phenylacetate; methyl α-toluate
CAS registry number(s) : 140-11-4; 101-41-7
EC number(s) : 205-399-7; 202-940-9
RIFM monograph(s) : Food Chem Toxicol 2015;84(suppl.):S15-S24; Food Chem Toxicol 2012;50(suppl.2):S363-S384; Food Cosmet Toxicol 1973;11:875
Merck Index monograph : 1123
Function(s) in cosmetics : EU: masking; perfuming; solvent. USA: fragrance ingredients
Patch testing : 5% pet. (1)
Molecular formula : $C_9H_{10}O_2$

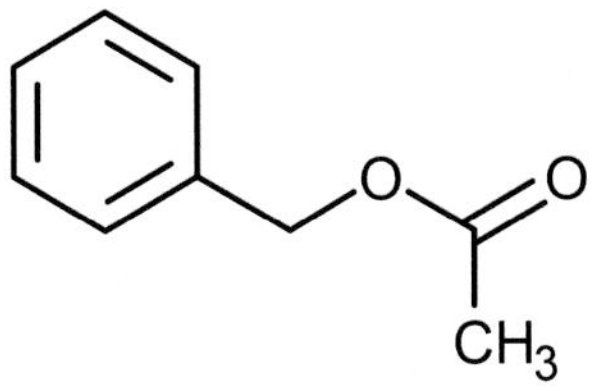

GENERAL

Benzyl acetate is a colorless clear liquid; its odor type is floral and its odor is described as 'sweet, fruity and floral' (www.thegoodscentscompany.com). Uses of benzyl acetate include or have included: in artificial jasmine and other perfumes, soap perfume, for flavoring and as solvent and high boiler for cellulose acetate and nitrate, natural and synthetic resins, oils, lacquers, polishes, printing inks and varnish removers (U.S. National Library of Medicine).

Presence in essential oils and propolis

Benzyl acetate has been identified by chemical analysis in 8 of 91 essential oils, which have caused contact allergy / allergic contact dermatitis. In one oil, benzyl acetate belonged to the 'Top-10' of ingredients with the highest concentrations which may be expected in commercial essential oils of this type: ylang-ylang oil (0.5-17.5%) (10). Benzyl acetate may also be present in propolis (8).

CONTACT ALLERGY

Patch testing in groups of patients

Patch testing in consecutive patients suspected of contact dermatitis: routine testing

Studies in which benzyl acetate was patch tested in consecutive patients suspected of contact dermatitis (routine testing) with positive results have not been found.

Patch testing in groups of selected patients

In the 1970s and 1980s, in Japan, small series of patients with dermatitis, cosmetic dermatitis and facial melanosis were patch tested with benzyl acetate, usually 5% in petrolatum. The frequencies of positive reactions in patients with dermatitis ranged from 0 to 1.9%, in cosmetic dermatitis patients from 1.3-3.8% and in individuals with melanosis of the face from 0 to 5.7%. The results of these studies, which have all been published in Japanese only, have been summarized in a review by the RIFM (9).

In a group of 20 patients allergic to fragrances and tested with a battery of fragrance materials, two reacted to benzyl acetate 5% pet.; relevance was not addressed (1).

Presence in products and chemical analyses

In 2008, 66 different fragrance components (including 39 essential oils) were identified in 370 (10% of the total) topical pharmaceutical products marketed in Belgium; 6 of these 370 products (1.6%) contained benzyl acetate (2).

In 2000, fifty-nine domestic and occupational products, purchased in retail outlets in Denmark, England, Germany and Italy were analyzed by GC-MS for the presence of fragrances. The product categories were liquid soap and soap bars (n=13), soft/hard surface cleaners (n=23), fabric conditioners/laundry detergents for hand wash (n=8), dish wash (n=10), furniture polish, car shampoo, stain remover (each n=1) and 2 products used in occupational environments. Benzyl acetate was present in 8 products; quantification was not performed (4).

Twenty-five cosmetics and cosmetic toys for children (5 shampoos and shower gels, 6 perfumes, 1 deodorant (roll-on), 4 baby lotions/creams, 1 baby wipes product, 1 baby oil, 2 lipcare products and 5 toy-cosmetic products: a cosmetic-toy set for blending perfumes and a makeup set) purchased in 1997-1998 in retail outlets in Denmark, Germany, England and Sweden were analyzed in 1998 for the presence of fragrances by GC-MS. Benzyl acetate was found in 22 products (88%) in a concentration range of ≤0.001-3.359% (w/w). For the analytical data in each product category, the original publication should be consulted (5).

In 1992, in The Netherlands, the presence of fragrances was analyzed in 300 cosmetic products. Benzyl acetate was identified in 78% of the products (rank order 3) (7). In 1988, in the USA, 400 perfumes used in fine fragrances, household products and soaps (number of products per category not mentioned) were analyzed for the presence of fragrance chemicals in a concentration of at least 1% and a list of the Top-25 (present in the highest number of products) presented. Benzyl acetate was found to be present in 74% of the fine fragrances (rank number 4), 63% of the household product fragrances (rank number 4) and 85% of the fragrances used in soaps (rank number 3) (6).

LITERATURE

1   Larsen WG. Perfume dermatitis. A study of 20 patients. Arch Dermatol 1977;113:623-626
2   Nardelli A, D'Hooge E, Drieghe J, Dooms M, Goossens A. Allergic contact dermatitis from fragrance components in specific topical pharmaceutical products in Belgium. Contact Dermatitis 2009;60:303-313
3   Rastogi SC, Johansen JD, Frosch P, Menné T, Bruze M, Lepoittevin JP, et al. Deodorants on the European market: quantitative chemical analysis of 21 fragrances. Contact Dermatitis 1998;38:29-35
4   Rastogi SC, Heydorn S, Johansen JD, Basketter DA. Fragrance chemicals in domestic and occupational products. Contact Dermatitis 2001;45:221-225
5   Rastogi SC, Johansen JD, Menné T, Frosch P, Bruze M, Andersen KE, et al. Content of fragrance allergens in children's cosmetics and cosmetic toys. Contact Dermatitis 1999;41:84-88
6   Fenn RS. Aroma chemical usage trends in modern perfumery. Perfumer and Flavorist 1989;14:3-10
7   Weyland JW. Personal Communication, 1992. Cited in: De Groot AC, Weyland JW, Nater JP. Unwanted effects of cosmetics and drugs used in dermatology, 3rd Ed. Amsterdam: Elsevier, 1994: 579
8   De Groot AC, Popova MP, Bankova VS. An update on the constituents of poplar-type propolis. Wapserveen, The Netherlands: acdegroot publishing, 2014, 11 pages. ISBN/EAN: 978-90-813233-0-7. Available at: https://www.researchgate.net/publication/262851225_AN_UPDATE_ON_THE_CONSTITUENTS_OF_POPLAR-TYPE_PROPOLIS
9   McGinty D, Vitale D, Letizia CS, Api AM. Fragrance material review on benzyl acetate. Food Chem Toxicol 2012;50(suppl.2):S363-S384
10 De Groot AC, Schmidt E. Essential oils: contact allergy and chemical composition. Boca Raton, Fl., USA: CRC Press, Taylor and Francis Group, 2016 (ISBN 9781482246407)

Chapter 3.16 BENZYL ALCOHOL

IDENTIFICATION

Description/definition	: Benzyl alcohol is an aromatic alcohol that conforms to the structural formula shown below
Chemical class(es)	: Alcohols
Chemical/IUPAC name	: Phenylmethanol
CAS registry number(s)	: 100-51-6
EC number(s)	: 202-859-9
CIR review(s)	: Int J Toxicol 2017;36(suppl.3):S5-S30; Int J Toxicol 2001;20(suppl.3):S23-S50 (access: www.cir-safety.org/ingredients)
RIFM monograph(s)	: Food Chem Toxicol 2015;84(suppl.):S1-S14; Food Chem Toxicol 2012;50(suppl.2):S140-S160; Food Cosmet Toxicol 1973;11:1011
IFRA standard	: Restricted (www.ifraorg.org/en-us/standards-library) (table 3.16.1)
SCCS opinion(s)	: SCCS/1459/11 (18); SCCNFP/0389/00, final (100)
Merck Index monograph	: 1124
Function(s) in cosmetics	: EU: perfuming; preservative; solvent; viscosity controlling. USA: external analgesics; fragrance ingredients; oral health care drugs; preservatives; solvents; viscosity decreasing agents
EU cosmetic restrictions	: Regulated in Annexes III/45 and V/34 of the Regulation (EC) No. 344/2013; Must be labeled on cosmetics and detergent products, if present at > 10 ppm (0.001%) in leave-on products and > 100 ppm (0.01%) in rinse-off products
Patch testing	: 1% and 5% pet. (SmartPracticeEurope, SmartPracticeCanada); 10% Softisan (Chemotechnique); recommended test concentration: 10.0% wt./wt. pet. (2)
Molecular formula	: C_7H_8O

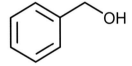

Table 3.16.1 IFRA restrictions for benzyl alcohol

Category [a]	Limits [b]	Category [a]	Limits [b]	Category [a]	Limits [b]
1	0.20%	5	1.40%	9	5.00%
2	0.20%	6	4.30%	10	2.50%
3	0.90%	7	0.40%	11	not restricted
4	2.70%	8	2.00%		

[a] For explanation of categories see pages 6-8
[b] Limits in the finished products

GENERAL

Benzyl alcohol is a colorless clear oily liquid; its odor type is floral and its odor at 100% is described as 'floral rose phenolic balsamic' (www.thegoodscentscompany.com). Benzyl alcohol is used in cosmetics as a fragrance component, preservative, solvent and diluting agent for perfumes and flavors, and viscosity-decreasing agent. It is used as a solvent for surface-coating materials, cellulose esters and ethers, alkyd resins, acrylic resins, fats, dyestuffs, casein (when hot), gelatin, shellac and waxes. It is added in small amounts to surface-coating materials to improve their flow and gloss. In the textile industry, benzyl alcohol is used as an auxiliary in the dyeing of wool, polyamides, and polyesters. In pharmacy it is used as a local anesthetic ingredient in over-the-counter anorectal, oral healthcare and topical analgesic drug products and, because of its antimicrobial effect, as an ingredient of ointments and other preparations (U.S. National Library of Medicine).

Benzyl alcohol is also a starting material for the preparation of numerous benzyl esters that are used as odorants, flavors, stabilizers for volatile perfumes, and plasticizers and is also employed in the extractive distillation of *m*- and *p*-xylenes and *m*- and *p*-cresols. Other uses include or have included heat-sealing of polyethylene films, in color photography as a development accelerator and in microscopy as embedding material (U.S. National Library of Medicine).

Benzyl alcohol may be found, in among other things, adhesives, binders, castings, cleaning agents, construction material, fillings, flooring materials, hardeners, metal coatings, paints/lacquers, photo developers, printings inks, skin care products and injectable solutions (73).

It should be realized that, by far, most adverse reactions to benzyl alcohol reported were from its use as a preservative rather than from its application as a fragrance ingredient. The literature on allergy to benzyl alcohol has been reviewed in 1999 (73) and in 2005 (90).

Presence in essential oils, Myroxylon pereirae resin (balsam of Peru) and propolis

Benzyl alcohol has been identified by chemical analysis in 23 of 91 essential oils, which have caused contact allergy / allergic contact dermatitis. In none of these oils, it belonged to the 'Top-10' of ingredients with the highest concentrations (98). Benzyl alcohol may also be present in propolis (97) and in Myroxylon pereirae resin (Balsam of Peru) (1-2%) (22).

CONTACT ALLERGY

General

The SCCS (Scientific Committee on Consumer Safety), in a 2012 Opinion on Fragrance allergens in cosmetic products, has marked benzyl alcohol as 'established contact allergen in humans' (18,49). The sensitizing potency of benzyl alcohol could not be classified, because no EC3 value was established in the LLNA (local lymph node assay) in animal experiments; higher concentrations should also have been tested (18,49).

Patch testing in groups of patients

Results of patch testing benzyl alcohol in consecutive patients suspected of contact dermatitis (routine testing) are shown in table 3.16.2. Results of testing in groups of *selected* patients (e.g. patients with suspected cosmetic intolerance or fragrance allergy, patients with eyelid dermatitis, individuals with previous reactions to FM I or Myroxylon pereirae resin, patients tested with a preservative series) are shown in table 3.16.3.

Patch testing in consecutive patients suspected of contact dermatitis: routine testing

In ten studies in which benzyl alcohol has been tested in consecutive patients (it is part of the NACDG screening series), low prevalence rates of sensitization have been observed, ranging from 0.1% to 1%; all but one scored 0.4% or lower (table 3.16.2). Relevance scores ranged from 0% to 75%, the latter indicating 'definite + probable relevance' (14). Causative products were usually not mentioned, but in one study, of the relevant reactions to any of 26 fragrances tested, 96% were caused by cosmetic products (3).

Table 3.16.2 Patch testing in groups of patients: Routine testing

Years and Country	Test conc. & vehicle	Number of patients tested	positive (%)		Selection of patients (S); Relevance (R); Comments (C)	Ref.
2015-7 Netherlands		821	3	(0.4%)	R: not stated	105
2015-2016 UK	10% pet.	2084	2	(0.1%)	R: not specified for individual fragrances; 25% of patients who reacted to any fragrance or fragrance marker had a positive fragrance history	104
2010-2015 Denmark	1% pet.	6004		(0.1%)	R: present relevance 40%, past relevance 40%	46
2011-2012 NACDG	1% pet.	4232	18	(0.4%)	R: definite + probable relevance: 72%	42
2011-2012 UK	10% pet.	1951	4	(0.2%)	R: not stated	48
2009-2010 NACDG	1% pet.	4304		(0.2%)	R: definite + probable relevance: 38%	43
2008-2010 Denmark	1% pet.	1508	2	(0.1%)	S: mostly routine testing; R: 0%; C: 50% co-reactivity of both FM I and FM II; of the relevant reactions to any of the 26 fragrances tested, 96% were caused by cosmetic products	3
2001-2010 Australia	5% pet.	4749	49	(1.0%)	R: 14%	44
2007-8200 NACDG	1% pet.	5083		(0.4%)	R: definite + probable relevance: 75%	14
2003-2004 IVDK	1% pet.	2166	7	(0.3%)	R: not stated; C: 29% co-reactivity of FM I	5

FM: Fragrance Mix; IVDK: Informationsverbund Dermatologischer Kliniken (Germany, Switzerland, Austria)
NACDG: North American Contact Dermatitis Group (USA, Canada)

Patch testing in groups of selected patients

Results of testing benzyl alcohol in groups of selected patients (e.g. patients with suspected cosmetic intolerance or fragrance allergy, patients with eyelid dermatitis, individuals with previous reactions to FM I or Myroxylon pereirae resin, patients tested with a preservative series) are shown in table 3.16.3. Frequencies of positive patch test reactions ranged from 0.2 to 15%; generally speaking, however, rates were rather low, in 11/16 studies 1.3% or lower. The high percentage of 15 was observed in an early small study of 20 fragrance-allergic patients (20). Relevance was indicated in two studies: 2/3 (67%) (6) and 29% (101).

Higher rates of reactions to benzyl alcohol were seen in two groups of patients allergic to Myroxylon pereirae resin (8% and 20%), which can possibly be explained by the fact that benzyl alcohol is an ingredient of the resin (22,99).

Table 3.16.3 Patch testing in groups of patients: Selected patient groups

Years and Country	Test conc. & vehicle	Number of patients tested	positive (%)		Selection of patients (S); Relevance (R); Comments (C)	Ref.
2011-2015 Spain	1% or 10% pet.	1013	13	(1.3%)	S: patients previously reacting to FM I, FM II, Myroxylon pereirae resin or hydroxyisohexyl 3-cyclohexene carboxaldehyde in the baseline series and subsequently tested with a fragrance series; R: not stated	106
2006-2011 IVDK	1% pet.	706	2	(0.3%)	S: patients with suspected cosmetic intolerance; R: not stated	45
2006-2010 USA	10% Softisan	100	1	(1.0%)	S: patients with eyelid dermatitis; R: not stated	16
2005-10 Netherlands		100	1	(1.0%)	S: patients with known fragrance sensitivity based on a positive patch test to the FM I and/or the FM II; R: not stated	50
1996-2009 IVDK	1% pet.	79,770	258	(0.3%)	S: not specified; R: not specified; C: decrease in prevalence of sensitization in the period of investigation	9
2005-2008 IVDK	1% pet.	23,257		(0.2%) [a]	S: patients tested with benzyl alcohol as antioxidant in the 'antiseptics in cosmetics and topicals' series; R: not stated	51
2004-2008 Spain	1% pet.	86	2	(2.3%)	S: patients previously reacting to the fragrance mix I or Myroxylon pereirae resin (n=54) or suspected of fragrance contact allergy (n=32); R: not stated	30
2005-7 Netherlands	1% pet.	320	1	(0.3%)	S: patients suspected of fragrance or cosmetic allergy; R: 61% relevance for all positive tested fragrances together	4
2000-2007 USA	1% pet.	869	3	(0.3%)	S: patients who were tested with a supplemental cosmetic screening series; R: 67%; C: weak study: a. high rate of macular erythema and weak reactions; b. relevance figures included 'questionable' and 'past' relevance	6
1993-2006 Australia	1% pet.	4552		(0.4%)	S: not stated; R: 29%	101
1985-1997 Belgium		?	25	?	S: unknown; R: not stated; C: the total number of patients seen was 8521, but is was not specified how many were tested with benzyl alcohol	91
<1996 Japan, Europe, USA	5% pet.	167	2	(1.2%)	S: patients known or suspected to be allergic to fragrances; R: not stated	11
1990-1994 IVDK	1% pet.	11,373	46	(0.4%)	S: patients tested with a preservative series; R: not stated	86
<1985 Netherlands		242	4	(1.7%)	S: randomly selected patients with proven contact allergy of different origins; R: not stated	54
1983 The Netherlands	10% pet.	182	3	(1.6%)	S: patients suspected of cosmetic allergy; R: not stated	19
1975 USA	5% pet.	20	3	(15%)	S: fragrance-allergic patients; R: not stated	20
Testing in patients allergic to Myroxylon pereirae resin (Balsam of Peru)						
1995-1998 Germany	5% pet.	102	8	(8%)	S: patients allergic to balsam of Peru	22
1955-1960 Denmark	5% pet. or 10% alc.	95	19	(20%)	S: patients allergic to balsam of Peru	99

FM: Fragrance mix; IVDK: Informationsverbund Dermatologischer Kliniken (Germany, Switzerland, Austria)

Case reports and case series

Case series
Benzyl alcohol was stated to be the (or an) allergen in one patient in a group of 603 individuals suffering from cosmetic dermatitis, seen in the period 2010-2015 in Leuven, Belgium (40). In the period 1996-2013, in a tertiary referral center in Valencia, Spain, 5419 patients were patch tested. Of these, 628 individuals had allergic contact dermatitis to cosmetics. Benzyl alcohol was the responsible allergen in one case (41). Benzyl alcohol was responsible for 3 out of 399 cases of cosmetic allergy where the causal allergen was identified in a study of the NACDG, USA, 1977-1983 (7).

Thirty patients had allergic contact dermatitis from benzyl alcohol in topical pharmaceutical preparations (17). In Belgium, in the years before 1986, of 5202 consecutive patients with dermatitis patch tested, 156 were diagnosed with pure cosmetic allergy. Benzyl alcohol was the 'dermatitic ingredient' in 2 (1.3%) patients (frequency in the entire group: 0.9%). It should be realized, however, that only a very limited number of patients was tested with a fragrance series (52).

Case reports

Pharmaceutical preparations
Eight patients had allergic contact dermatitis from a topical pharmaceutical product and all reacted to its ingredient ethylenediamine (a stabilizer) and to the perfume 5% pet. When tested with the 28 individual fragrances of the perfume, there were 2 reactions to benzyl alcohol, 5 to amyl cinnamal, 4 to cinnamyl alcohol, 2 to hydroxycitronellal and one to oakmoss synthetic (35). A man had perianal allergic contact dermatitis from benzyl alcohol in the perfume in a topical pharmaceutical preparation (20). A woman, who was allergic to Myroxylon pereirae resin and benzyl alcohol, would develop eczema after application of (cosmetics and) medical preparations containing benzyl alcohol (22).

'Soon' after the injection of a corticosteroid solution in the left wrist for treatment of tendonitis, erythema and pruritus had appeared at the injection site in a female patient. She developed no generalized symptoms. Prick tests with the corticosteroid and a local anesthetic were negative. Patch tests gave positive reactions to benzyl alcohol, the FM I, Myroxylon pereirae resin and several other haptens. The corticosteroid solution proved to contain benzyl alcohol as a preservative. The patient may previously have become sensitized to Myroxylon pereirae resin (in which benzyl alcohol is present) or to a pharmaceutical to treat otitis externa containing benzyl alcohol, from which she would develop 'skin irritation'. Curiously, no tests for immediate-type allergy with benzyl alcohol seem to have been performed (94).

A woman was patch tested because of a 10-year history of dermatitis of the arms and legs. She had many contact allergies including to benzyl alcohol, which was present in several products she used and to which she also reacted: 2 moisturizing lotions, an antibacterial cream, 2 hydrocortisone creams, an antifungal preparation and an immunosuppressive cream to treat dermatitis (90). A male patient reacted to an anti-itch lotion. When tested with the ingredients, he had positive patch tests to benzyl alcohol and the fragrance in the lotion. Gas chromatography showed benzyl alcohol to be present in the perfume (65).

A woman became sensitized to an antifungal topical pharmaceutical. She had positive patch tests and ROATs to the cream and its ingredient benzyl alcohol (72). Another female patient developed dermatitis of the calf with tender, slightly pruritic, bright red dermal swelling from contact allergy to benzyl alcohol in a sclerosing agent used to treat varicose veins at that site (67).

A female individual with facial dermatitis noticed worsening when treating the dermatitis with pimecrolimus cream. She reacted to benzyl alcohol, Myroxylon pereirae resin, FM I and various other fragrances. The pharmaceutical cream contained benzyl alcohol and a provocation test with it (or another 'benzyl alcohol-containing product') caused a flare-up of the dermatitis (96).

Other single case reports also describe allergic contact dermatitis from benzyl alcohol in corticosteroid preparations (61,75,88), antimycotics (62,64,79,88), NSAID-containing pharmaceuticals (66,89) and antibacterial preparations (88).

Cosmetics
One patient had allergic contact dermatitis and contact urticaria from benzyl alcohol in a sunscreen (1). A woman, who was allergic to Myroxylon pereirae resin and benzyl alcohol, noticed lip swelling after usage of a lip balsam containing benzyl alcohol; she would also develop eczema after application of cosmetics and medical preparations containing benzyl alcohol (22).

Another female patient, allergic to Myroxylon pereirae resin and its ingredient benzyl alcohol, would develop eczematous lesions after contact with ointments containing benzyl alcohol and consumption of marzipan, which also contains benzyl alcohol (22). A woman had allergic contact dermatitis from a perfume and a man from an aftershave lotion. There were positive patch test reactions to the product and to benzyl alcohol 1% in pet. in both patients. Although the author ascribed the dermatitis to benzyl alcohol, its presence in these fragranced products was not ascertained (60).

A woman was patch tested because of a 10-year history of dermatitis of the arms and legs. She had many contact allergies including to benzyl alcohol, which was present in several products she used and to which she also reacted: 2 moisturizing lotions and several topical pharmaceutical preparations (90). Another female individual developed allergic contact dermatitis with itching followed by dermatitis and edema on the forehead, periorbital area and behind the auricular folds from benzyl alcohol in a semi-permanent hair dye, which she had used for 2 years without problems. She reacted to both benzyl alcohol 9.5% as provided by the manufacturer of the dye and to benzyl alcohol 1% in the cosmetics series (95).

A positive patch test reaction to benzyl alcohol was ascribed to cosmetic allergy (8).

Other products
An allergic reaction to benzyl alcohol has been reported in a patient working with beverages in an early report. The

patient had been sensitized in childhood to balsam of Peru, which contains benzyl alcohol (59). A metal grinder developed occupational allergic contact dermatitis from a perfume ('reodorant') in a cutting oil. The perfume consisted of 20% vanillin (vanillaldehyde) and 80% benzyl alcohol. The patient had a positive patch test to benzyl alcohol, vanillin was not tested (63).

A man developed severe swelling of his ear canal several hours after earmold impression material containing benzyl alcohol had been placed in the ear canal for several minutes. He had positive patch tests to benzyl alcohol, 2 benzyl alcohol-containing moisturizers and two topical pharmaceuticals containing benzyl alcohol. Tests for immediate-type allergy remained negative (73). Two parquet layers developed occupational allergic airborne contact dermatitis from benzyl alcohol present in the catalyst part of a 2-part glue (78).

Two patients had intractable eyelid dermatitis and recurrent localized delayed-type hypersensitivity reactions (allergic contact dermatitis) after Botox injections containing benzyl alcohol. Patch tests were positive to benzyl alcohol and Myroxylon pereirae resin (102).

Pigmented cosmetic dermatitis

In Japan, in the 1960s and 1970s, many female patients developed pigmentation of the face after having facial dermatitis (37). The skin manifestations of this so-called pigmented cosmetic dermatitis consisted of diffuse or patchy brown hyperpigmentation on the cheeks and/or forehead, sometimes the entire face was involved. In severe cases, the pigmentation was black, purple, or blue-black, and in mild cases, it was pale brown. Occasionally, erythematous macules or papules, suggesting a mild contact dermatitis, were observed and itching was also noted at varying times. Pigmented cosmetic dermatitis was shown to be caused by contact allergy to components of cosmetic products, notably essential oils, other fragrance materials, antimicrobials, preservatives and coloring materials (36,37,38). In a group of 620 Japanese patients with this condition investigated between 1970 and 1980, 1-5% had positive patch test reactions to benzyl alcohol 20% in petrolatum in various time periods versus 0 to 2% in a control group of patients not suffering from pigmented cosmetic dermatitis (36). The number of patients with pigmented cosmetic dermatitis decreased strongly after 1978, when major cosmetic companies began to eliminate strong contact sensitizers from their products (36). Since 1980, pigmented cosmetic dermatitis became a rare disease in Japan (39).

Cross-reactions, pseudo-cross-reactions and co-reactions

For general information on cross-/pseudo-cross-/co-reactivity of fragrance chemicals with other fragrances, fragrance markers (fragrance mix I, fragrance mix II, colophonium, Myroxylon pereirae resin [balsam of Peru]) and essential oils see Chapter 1.2. General information on cross-reactions, pseudo-cross-reactions and co-reactions.

Pseudo-cross-reactivity to Myroxylon pereirae resin, in which benzyl alcohol is present, has been observed very frequently (22,59,63,64,66,73,74,75,76,77,79,88,90,94,96). Indeed, in a series of 25 patients with positive patch test reactions to benzyl alcohol, 19 (76%) co-reacted to Myroxylon pereirae resin (balsam of Peru) and 17 (68%) to the fragrance mix (74). Conversely, only 8% of 102 patients with contact allergy to Myroxylon pereirae reacted to benzyl alcohol (22).

Co-reactions to benzylparaben are sometimes observed (62,63,64,88,95) and have been suggested to be the result of hydrolytic decomposition of benzyl paraben into benzyl alcohol (64).

Presence in products and chemical analyses

In various studies, the presence of benzyl alcohol in cosmetic and sometimes other products has been investigated. Before 2006, most investigators used chemical analysis, usually GC-MS, for qualitative and quantitative determination. Since then, the presence of the target fragrances was usually investigated by screening the product labels for the 26 fragrances that must be labeled since 2005 on cosmetics and detergent products in the EU, if present at > 10 ppm (0.001%) in leave-on products and > 100 ppm (0.01%) in rinse-off products. This method, obviously, is less accurate and may result in underestimation of the frequency of the fragrances being present in the product. When they are in fact present, but the concentration is lower than mentioned above, labeling is not required and the fragrances' presence will be missed.

The results of the relevant studies for benzyl alcohol are summarized in table 3.16.4. More detailed information can be found in the corresponding text following the table. The percentage of products in which benzyl alcohol was found to be present shows wide variations, which can among other be explained by the selection procedure of the products, the method of investigation (false-negatives with information obtained from labels only) and changes in the use of individual fragrance materials over time (fashion).

Table 3.16.4 Presence of benzyl alcohol in products [a]

Year	Country	Product type	Nr. investigated	Nr. of products positive [b]	(%)	Method [c]	Ref.
2017	USA	Cosmetic products in hair-dye kits	539 products in 159 hair-dye kits	77	(14%)	Labeling	55
2016	USA	Facial wipes	178	30	(17%)	Labeling	57
2016	USA	Body washes	50	6	(12%)	Labeling	56
		Bar soaps	50	3	(6%)		
2016	Sweden	Toothpastes	66	3	(5%)	Labeling	93
2015-6	Denmark	Fragranced cosmetic products	5588		(23%)	Labeling	26
2015	Germany	Household detergents	817	50	(6%)	Labeling	103
2015	Sweden	Oxidative hair dyes	26	6	(23%)	Labeling	47
		Non-oxidative hair dyes	35	0		Labeling	
2013	USA	Pediatric cosmetics	187	14	(7%)	Labeling	29
2006-9	Germany	Leave-on cosmetic products	3541	245	(7%)	Labeling	12
2006-9	Germany	Cosmetic products	4991		(9%)	Labeling	25
2008	Belgium	Fragranced topical pharmaceutical products	370	9	(2%)	Labeling	17
2008	Sweden	Cosmetic products	204		(9%)	Labeling	13
		Detergents	97		(1%)	Labeling	
2007	USA	Moisturizers	276	65	(24%)	Labeling	15
2006	UK	Perfumed cosmetic and household products	300	61	(20%)	Labeling	23
2006	Denmark	Popular perfumed deodorants	88	15	(17%)	Labeling	27
			23	6	(26%)	Analysis	
2006	Netherlands	Laundry detergents	52	17	(33%)	Labeling + analysis	33
2006	Denmark	Rinse-off cosmetics for children	208	20	(10%)	Labeling + analysis	31
2002	Denmark	Home and car air fresheners	19	10	(53%)	Analysis	34
2001	Denmark	Non-cosmetic consumer products	43	13	(30%)	Analysis	32
1997-8	Denmark, UK Germany, Sweden	Cosmetics and cosmetic toys for children	25	11	(44%)	Analysis	21
1996	Five European countries	Fragranced deodorants	70	20	(29%)	Analysis	10
1992	Netherlands	Cosmetic products	300		(42%)	Analysis	24

[a] See the corresponding text below for more details
[b] positive = containing the target fragrance
[c] Labeling: information from the ingredient labels on the product / packaging; Analysis: chemical analysis, most often GC-MS

In 2017, in the USA, the ingredient labels 159 hair-dye kits containing 539 cosmetic products (e.g. colorants, conditioners, shampoos, toners) were screened for the most common sensitizers they contain. Benzyl alcohol was found to be present in 77 (14%) of the products (55).

In 2016, in the USA, benzyl alcohol was found to be present in 30 (17%) of 178 facial wipes (57). Of 50 bodywashes available on amazon.com in October 2016 and rated with 4 or 5 starts by customers, 6 (12%) contained benzyl alcohol; of 50 bar soaps, 3 (6%) contained benzyl alcohol (56).

In 2016, in Sweden, 66 commercially available toothpastes obtained from local pharmacies and supermarkets in Malmö, Sweden were investigated for the presence of flavors by studying the packages and product labels. Benzyl alcohol was found to be present in 3 (5%) of the products (93).

In Denmark, in 2015-2016, 5588 fragranced cosmetic products were examined with a smartphone application for the 26 fragrances that need to be labeled in the EU. Benzyl alcohol was present in 23% of the products (rank number 5) (26).

In Germany, in 2015, fragrance allergens were evaluated based on lists of ingredients in 817 (unique) detergents (all-purpose cleaners, cleaning preparations for special purposes [e.g. bathroom, kitchen, dish-washing] and laundry detergents) present in 131 households. Benzyl alcohol was found to be present in 50 (6%) of the products (103).

In Sweden, in 2015, contact allergens were identified on the ingredient labels of 26 oxidative hair dye products (from 4 different product series) and on the labels of 35 non-oxidative hair dye products (from 5 different product series, including so-called herbal hair colors). These products were selected on the basis of being advertised as 'organic', 'natural', or similar, or used in hairdressing salons branded with such attributes. Benzyl alcohol was present in 6 (23%) of the 26 oxidative hair dyes and in zero of the 35 non-oxidative hair dye products (47).

In 2013, in the USA, the allergen content of 187 unique pediatric cosmetics from 6 different retailers marketed in the United States as hypoallergenic was evaluated on the basis of labeling. Inclusion criteria were products marketed as pediatric and 'hypoallergenic', 'dermatologist recommended/tested', 'fragrance free', or 'paraben free'. Benzyl alcohol was found to be present in 14 (7.5%) of the products (29).

In 2008, 2010 and 2011, 374 deodorants available in German retail shops were randomly selected and their labels checked for the presence of the 26 fragrances that need to be labeled. Benzyl alcohol was found to be present in 86 (23.0%) of the products (58).

Benzyl alcohol was present in 245 of 3541 (6.5%) randomly sampled leave-on cosmetic products, Germany, 2006-2009 (12).

In Germany, in the period 2006-2009, 4991 cosmetic products were randomly sampled for an official investigation of conformity of cosmetic products with legal provisions. The labels were inspected for the presence of the 26 fragrances that need to be labeled in the EU. Benzyl alcohol was present in 9% of the products (rank number 11) (25).

In 2008, 66 different fragrance components (including 39 essential oils) were identified in 370 (10% of the total) topical pharmaceutical products marketed in Belgium; 9 of these (2.4%) contained benzyl alcohol (17).

Benzyl alcohol was present (as indicated by labeling) in 9% of 204 cosmetic products (92 shampoos, 61 hair conditioners, 34 liquid soaps, 17 wet tissues) and in 1% of 97 detergents in Sweden, 2008 (13).

Of 276 moisturizers sold in the USA in 2007, 65 (24%) contained benzyl alcohol (15).

In 2006, the labels of 208 cosmetics for children (especially shampoos, body shampoos and soaps) available in Denmark were checked for the presence of the 26 fragrances that need to be labeled in the EU. Benzyl alcohol was present in 20 products (9.6%), and ranked number 7 in the frequency list. Seventeen products were analyzed quantitatively for the fragrances. The maximum concentration found for benzyl alcohol was 790 mg/kg (31).

In 2007, in the USA, under the Voluntary Cosmetic Reporting Program, benzyl alcohol was listed as an ingredient in only 511 cosmetic formulations. Ten years earlier, in 1998, the number had been 322 (92).

In 2006, of 88 popular perfume containing deodorants purchased in Denmark, 15 (17%) were labeled to contain benzyl alcohol. Analysis of 24 regulated fragrance substances in 23 selected deodorants (19 spray products, 2 deostick and 2 roll-on) was performed by GC-MS. Benzyl alcohol was identified in 6 of the products (26%) with a concentration range of 32–166 ppm (27).

In 2006, in The Netherlands, 52 laundry detergents were investigated for the presence of allergenic fragrances by checking their labels and chemical analyses. Benzyl alcohol was found to be present in 17 of the products (33%) in a concentration range of 9-168 ppm. Benzyl alcohol had rank number 7 in the frequency list (33).

In January 2006, a study of perfumed cosmetic and household products available on the shelves of U.K. retailers was carried out. Products were included if 'parfum' or 'aroma' was listed among the ingredients. Three hundred products were surveyed and any of 26 mandatory labeling fragrances named on the label were recorded. Benzyl alcohol was present in 61 (20%) of the products (rank number 14) (23).

In 2002, in Denmark, 19 air fresheners (6 for cars, 13 for homes) were analyzed for the presence of fragrances that need to be labeled on cosmetics. Benzyl alcohol was found to be present in 10 products (53%) in a concentration range of 73-50,000 ppm and ranked 7 in the frequency list (34).

In 2001, in Denmark, 43 non-cosmetic consumer products (mainly dish-washing products, laundry detergents, and hard and soft surface cleaners) were analyzed for the 26 fragrances that are regulated for labeling in the EU. Benzyl alcohol was present in 13 products (30%) in a concentration range of 0.00001-0.2354% (m/m) and had rank number 6 in the frequency list (32).

Twenty-five cosmetics and cosmetic toys for children (5 shampoos and shower gels, 6 perfumes, 1 deodorant (roll-on), 4 baby lotions/creams, 1 baby wipes product, 1 baby oil, 2 lipcare products and 5 toy-cosmetic products: a cosmetic-toy set for blending perfumes and a makeup set) purchased in 1997-1998 in retail outlets in Denmark, Germany, England and Sweden were analyzed in 1998 for the presence of fragrances by GC-MS. Benzyl alcohol was found in 11 products (44%) in a concentration range of ≤0.001-0.652% (w/w). For the analytical data in each product category, the original publication should be consulted (21).

Seventy fragranced deodorants, purchased at retail outlets in 5 European countries in 1996, were analyzed by gas chromatography - mass spectrometry (GC-MS) for the determination of the contents of 21 commonly used fragrance materials. Benzyl alcohol was identified in 20 products in a concentration range of 1-629 ppm. Due to interference by dipropylene glycol, identification of benzyl alcohol was not possible in 36 products (10).

In 1992, in The Netherlands, the presence of fragrances was analyzed in 300 cosmetic products. Benzyl alcohol was identified in 42% of the products (rank order 17) (24).

OTHER SIDE EFFECTS

Immediate-type reactions

One patient had combined contact urticaria and allergic contact dermatitis to benzyl alcohol in a sunscreen (1). A woman who was contact allergic to Myroxylon pereirae resin (Balsam of Peru) and its ingredient benzyl alcohol developed generalized urticaria after injection of a liquid drug containing benzyl alcohol and another one noticed lip swelling after usage of lip balsam containing benzyl alcohol (22). It was not investigated whether these were immediate-type reactions.

Of 50 individuals who had open tests with benzyl alcohol 5% pet. on the forearm, 32 (64%) showed local macular erythema after 45 minutes, termed 'contact urticaria' by the authors (53). One individual developed diffuse angioedema, nausea and fatigue shortly after an intramuscular injection of vitamin B_{12} preserved with benzyl alcohol. Prick tests were negative. Intradermal tests with the commercial solution and with saline with benzyl alcohol were positive, whereas there were no reactions to vitamin B_{12} solution unpreserved or containing parabens (81).

In the evening of the day that a man, who had been exposed to silica for a long time, received an intravenous injection of Gallium 67 preserved with benzyl alcohol for a scintigraphy, he experienced severe itching and joint pains. The following day, he visited the emergency room for a rash over his entire body. The diagnosis of a severe urticarial reaction following the injection of Gallium 67 was entertained. Ten days later, the joint pains increased. They were symmetrical and involved mostly the fingers, hands, elbows, shoulders and knees. The urticarial rash soon disappeared but joint pains would persist for about 5 months. Later, an increase in circulating immune complexes was found and there was a positive prick test to benzyl alcohol 5% in phosphate-buffered saline. The authors postulated that an immune complex-mediated hypersensitivity reaction to the benzyl alcohol found in injectable Gallium 67 may explain the signs and symptoms reported by this patient (82).

One individual treated with benzyl alcohol-preserved parenteral cytarabine, vincristine, and heparin solutions developed a systemic hypersensitivity reaction on three separate occasions. Clinically, the patient presented with fever and a maculopapular rash on the chest and arms, first after 4 hours, and subsequently minutes after injection. None of the reactions were life-threatening or required hospitalization of the patient. Hypersensitivity to benzyl alcohol was confirmed by intradermal skin testing. Treatment with the same drugs using unpreserved diluents caused no reactions (84).

Another patient developed itching, urticaria and arthralgias after an intramuscular injection of vitamin B_{12} solution preserved with benzyl alcohol. No skin tests were performed, but the patient showed a steep drop in platelet count after one hour on 2 occasions, which was not seen in controls. Also, the patient tolerated unpreserved vitamin B_{12} injections without problems (85).

Generalized urticaria in one individual was caused by type-I hypersensitivity to benzyl alcohol in a corticosteroid solution after a periarticular injection for tendonitis of the shoulder (71). A woman had contact urticaria from benzyl alcohol in saline soaks for stasis dermatitis. After one hour, the patch test showed redness and swelling and at D2, there was a wheal with a diameter of 10 cm at the patch test site (87).

A female patient was referred for assessment of possible anaphylactic reactions following vitamin B_{12} injections. When she received an intramuscular injection of vitamin B_{12} (cyanocobalamin 1000 µg), the subject experienced pain at the injection site. Two months later, one hour after her second injection, she reported a sensation of substernal burning and pleuritic pain that resolved over days. Within minutes of her third injection one month later, she felt similar chest discomfort and developed pruritus of the arms and legs, but no rash. The patient was skin tested to three commercial preparations of injectable cyanocobalamin and to the benzyl alcohol (0.9%) preservative found in each. Prick testing was negative but intradermal testing was positive to all 3 preparations and to benzyl alcohol. Pure cyanocobalamin was not tested (28).

Other non-eczematous contact reactions

In one patient, depigmentation of the scalp occurred after use of a benzyl alcohol-containing hair color rinse. There was no clinically evident preceding contact dermatitis. Patch tests were positive to the hair rinse and benzyl alcohol 5% pet. However, neither patch test sites became depigmented. The authors considered this to be benzyl alcohol-induced leukoderma. However, post-inflammatory leukoderma or vitiligo, including Koebner-induced vitiligo, could not be excluded (77).

Systemic side effects

In the 1980s, there have been at least 16 fatalities from benzyl alcohol toxicity in neonates in who sodium chloride for injection, containing 0.9% benzyl alcohol as a preservative, had been used for flushing I.V. catheters (68,69,70). It was also present in many parenteral drug formulations (83). In one study of 10 neonates who died (69), before the onset of symptoms, usually around the second to fourth day, all the infants developed progressive metabolic acidosis, the average anion gap at that time being 29 mmol/l (normal 12-18). Slowly progressive bradycardia, often associated with gasping respiration, soon followed (it was also called the 'gasping syndrome'). Seizures were frequent (eight cases out of ten) and usually developed within 24 hours. The infants became gradually more unresponsive with very depressed EEGs, and eventually they had only reflex movements or occasional gasping respiration. Hypotension leading to cardiovascular collapse was a late finding, usually presaging death. Intracranial hemorrhage was present in six cases. The clinical picture was therefore that of an infant with a severe metabolic acidosis who was unresponsive to treatment and whose symptoms resembled those of a progressive encephalopathy.

The clue to the cause of the acidosis came from examination of the urinary organic acid profile by gas-liquid chromatography. All samples contained huge quantities of benzoic and hippuric acid. Serum benzoic acid values have been measured in five of the infants; values range from 8.4 to 28.7 mmol/l (normal zero). The authors postulated that the benzyl alcohol is metabolized to benzoic acid which is then converted by the liver to hippuric acid. The quantity of the benzoic acid exceeded the capacity of the immature liver for detoxification so that the benzoic acid accumulated in serum, causing the metabolic acidosis (69). When preparations containing benzyl alcohol were removed from nurseries for premature infants, reports of the gasping syndrome and related deaths stopped (83).

LITERATURE

1   Edwards EK Jr. Allergic reactions to benzyl alcohol in a sunscreen. Cutis 1981;28:332-333
2   Bruze M, Svedman C, Andersen KE, Bruynzeel D, Goossens A, Johansen JD, et al. Patch test concentrations (doses in mg/cm2) for the 12 non-mix fragrance substances regulated by European legislation. Contact Dermatitis 2012;66:131-136
3   Heisterberg MV, Menné T, Johansen JD. Contact allergy to the 26 specific fragrance ingredients to be declared on cosmetic products in accordance with the EU cosmetic directive. Contact Dermatitis 2011;65:266-275
4   Oosten EJ van, Schuttelaar ML, Coenraads PJ. Clinical relevance of positive patch test reactions to the 26 EU-labelled fragrances. Contact Dermatitis 2009;61:217-223
5   Schnuch A, Uter W, Geier J, Lessmann H, Frosch PJ. Sensitization to 26 fragrances to be labelled according to current European regulation: Results of the IVDK and review of the literature. Contact Dermatitis 2007;57:1-10
6   Wetter DA, Yiannias JA, Prakash AV, Davis MDP, Farmer SA, el-Azhary RA. Results of patch testing to personal care product allergens in a standard series and a supplemental cosmetic series: an analysis of 945 patients from the Mayo Clinic Contact Dermatitis Group, 2000-2007. J Am Acad Dermatol 2010;63:789-798
7   Adams RM, Maibach HI, for the North American Contact Dermatitis Group. A five-year study of cosmetic reactions. J Am Acad Dermatol 1985;13:1062-1069
8   Kohl L, Blondeel A, Song M. Allergic contact dermatitis from cosmetics: retrospective analysis of 819 patch-tested patients. Dermatology 2002;204:334-337
9   Schnuch A, Lessmann H, Geier J, Uter W. Contact allergy to preservatives. Analysis of IVDK data 1996-2009. Br J Dermatol 2011;164:1316-1325
10 Rastogi SC, Johansen JD, Frosch P, Menné T, Bruze M, Lepoittevin JP, et al. Deodorants on the European market: quantitative chemical analysis of 21 fragrances. Contact Dermatitis 1998;38:29-35
11 Larsen W, Nakayama H, Fischer T, Elsner P, Burrows D, Jordan W, et al. Fragrance contact dermatitis: A worldwide multicenter investigation (Part I). Am J Cont Dermat 1996;7:77-83
12 Schnuch A, Mildau G, Kratz E-M, Uter W. Risk of sensitization to preservatives estimated on the basis of patch test data and exposure, according to a sample of 3541 leave-on products. Contact Dermatitis 2011;65:167-174
13 Yazar K, Johnsson S, Lind M-L, Boman A, Lidén C. Preservatives and fragrances in selected consumer-available cosmetics and detergents. Contact Dermatitis 2011;64:265-272
14 Fransway AF, Zug KA, Belsito DV, Deleo VA, Fowler JF Jr, Maibach HI, et al. North American Contact Dermatitis Group patch test results for 2007-2008. Dermatitis 2013;24:10-21
15 Zirwas MJ, Stechschulte SA. Moisturizer allergy. Diagnosis and management. J Clin Aesthetic Dermatol 2008;1:38-44
16 Wenk KS, Ehrlich AE. Fragrance series testing in eyelid dermatitis. Dermatitis 2012;23:22-26
17 Nardelli A, D'Hooge E, Drieghe J, Dooms M, Goossens A. Allergic contact dermatitis from fragrance components in specific topical pharmaceutical products in Belgium. Contact Dermatitis 2009;60:303-313
18 SCCS (Scientific Committee on Consumer Safety). Opinion on Fragrance allergens in cosmetic products, 26-27 June 2012, SCCS/1459/11. Available at:
    https://ec.europa.eu/health/sites/health/files/scientific_committees/consumer_safety/docs/sccs_o_102.pdf
19 Malten KE, van Ketel WG, Nater JP, Liem DH. Reactions in selected patients to 22 fragrance materials. Contact Dermatitis 1984;11:1-10
20 Larsen WG. Perfume dermatitis. A study of 20 patients. Arch Dermatol 1977;113:623-626
21 Rastogi SC, Johansen JD, Menné T, Frosch P, Bruze M, Andersen KE, et al. Content of fragrance allergens in children's cosmetics and cosmetic toys. Contact Dermatitis 1999;41:84-88
22 Hausen BM. Contact allergy to Balsam of Peru. II. Patch test results in 102 patients with selected balsam of Peru constituents. Am J Cont Derm 2001;12:93-102

23 Buckley DA. Fragrance ingredient labelling in products on sale in the UK. Br J Dermatol 2007;157:295-300

24 Weyland JW. Personal Communication, 1992. Cited in: De Groot AC, Weyland JW, Nater JP. Unwanted effects of cosmetics and drugs used in dermatology, 3rd Ed. Amsterdam: Elsevier, 1994: 579

25 Uter W, Yazar K, Kratz E-M, Mildau G, Lidén C. Coupled exposure to ingredients of cosmetic products: I. Fragrances. Contact Dermatitis 2013;69:335-341

26 Bennike NH, Oturai NB, Müller S, Kirkeby CS, Jørgensen C, Christensen AB, et al. Fragrance contact allergens in 5588 cosmetic products identified through a novel smartphone application. J Eur Acad Dermatol Venereol 2018;32:79-85

27 Rastogi SC, Hellerup Jensen G, Johansen JD. Survey and risk assessment of chemical substances in deodorants. Survey of Chemical Substances in Consumer Products, No. 86 2007. Danish Ministry of the Environment, Environmental Protection Agency. Available at: https://www2.mst.dk/Udgiv/publications/2007/978-87-7052-625-8/pdf/978-87-7052-626-5.pdf

28 Turvey SE, Cronin B, Arnold AD, Twarog FJ, Dioun AF. Adverse reactions to vitamin B12 injections due to benzyl alcohol sensitivity: successful treatment with intranasal cyanocobalamin. Allergy 2004;59:1023-1024

29 Hamann CR, Bernard S, Hamann D, Hansen R, Thyssen JP. Is there a risk using hypoallergenic cosmetic pediatric products in the United States? J Allergy Clin Immunol 2015;135:1070-1071

30 Cuesta L, Silvestre JF, Toledo F, Lucas A, Perez-Crespo M, Ballester I. Fragrance contact allergy: a 4-year retrospective study. Contact Dermatitis 2010;63:77-84

31 Poulsen PB, Schmidt A. A survey and health assessment of cosmetic products for children. Survey of chemical substances in consumer products, No. 88. Copenhagen: Danish Environmental Protection Agency, 2007. Available at: https://www2.mst.dk/udgiv/publications/2007/978-87-7052-638-8/pdf/978-87-7052-639-5.pdf

32 Rastogi SC. Survey of chemical compounds in consumer products. Contents of selected fragrance materials in cleaning products and other consumer products. Survey no. 8-2002. Copenhagen, Denmark, Danish Environmental Protection Agency. Available at: http://eng.mst.dk/media/mst/69131/8.pdf

33 Bouma K, Van Peursem AJJ. Marktonderzoek naleving detergenten verordening voor textielwasmiddelen. Dutch Food and Consumer Products Safety Authority (VWA) Report ND06K173, 2006 [in Dutch]. Available at: http://docplayer.nl/41524125-Marktonderzoek-naleving-detergenten-verordening-voor-textielwasmiddelen.html

34 Pors J, Fuhlendorff R. Mapping of chemical substances in air fresheners and other fragrance liberating products. Report Danish Ministry of the Environment, Environmental Protection Agency (EPA). Survey of Chemicals in Consumer Products, No 30, 2003. Available at: http://eng.mst.dk/media/mst/69113/30.pdf

35 Larsen WG. Allergic contact dermatitis to the perfume in Mycolog cream. J Am Acad Dermatol 1979;1:131-133

36 Nakayama H, Matsuo S, Hayakawa K, Takhashi K, Shigematsu T, Ota S. Pigmented cosmetic dermatitis. Int J Dermatol 1984;23:299-305

37 Nakayama H, Harada R, Toda M. Pigmented cosmetic dermatitis. Int J Dermatol 1976;15:673-675

38 Nakayama H, Hanaoka H, Ohshiro A. Allergen Controlled System. Tokyo: Kanehara Shuppan, 1974

39 Ebihara T, Nakayama H. Pigmented contact dermatitis. Clin Dermatol 1997;15:593-599

40 Goossens A. Cosmetic contact allergens. Cosmetics 2016, 3, 5; doi:10.3390/cosmetics3010005

41 Zaragoza-Ninet V, Blasco Encinas R, Vilata-Corell JJ, Pérez-Ferriols A, Sierra-Talamantes C, Esteve-Martínez A, de la Cuadra-Oyanguren J. Allergic contact dermatitis due to cosmetics: A clinical and epidemiological study in a tertiary hospital. Actas Dermosifiliogr 2016;107:329-336

42 Warshaw EM, Maibach HI, Taylor JS, Sasseville D, DeKoven JG, Zirwas MJ, et al. North American Contact Dermatitis Group patch test results: 2011-2012. Dermatitis 2015;26:49-59

43 Warshaw EM, Belsito DV, Taylor JS, Sasseville D, DeKoven JG, Zirwas MJ, et al. North American Contact Dermatitis Group patch test results: 2009 to 2010. Dermatitis 2013;24:50-59

44 Toholka R, Wang Y-S, Tate B, Tam M, Cahill J, Palmer A, Nixon R. The first Australian Baseline Series: Recommendations for patch testing in suspected contact dermatitis. Australas J Dermatol 2015;56:107-115

45 Dinkloh A, Worm M, Geier J, Schnuch A, Wollenberg A. Contact sensitization in patients with suspected cosmetic intolerance: results of the IVDK 2006-2011. J Eur Acad Dermatol Venereol 2015;29:1071-1081

46 Bennike NH, Zachariae C, Johansen JD. Non-mix fragrances are top sensitizers in consecutive dermatitis patients – a cross-sectional study of the 26 EU-labelled fragrance allergens. Contact Dermatitis 2017;77:270-279

47 Thorén S, Yazar K. Contact allergens in 'natural' hair dyes. Contact Dermatitis 2016;74:302-304

48 Mann J, McFadden JP, White JML, White IR, Banerjee P. Baseline series fragrance markers fail to predict contact allergy. Contact Dermatitis 2014;70:276-281

49 Uter W, Johansen JD, Börje A, Karlberg A-T, Lidén C, Rastogi S, Roberts D, White IR. Categorization of fragrance contact allergens for prioritization of preventive measures: clinical and experimental data and consideration of structure–activity relationships. Contact Dermatitis 2013;69:196-230

50 Nagtegaal MJC, Pentinga SE, Kuik J, Kezic S, Rustemeyer T. The role of the skin irritation response in polysensitization to fragrances. Contact Dermatitis 2012;67:28-35

51 Uter W, Geier J, Frosch P, Schnuch A. Contact allergy to fragrances: current patch test results (2005–2008) from the Information Network of Departments of Dermatology. Contact Dermatitis 2010;63:254-261

52 Broeckx W, Blondeel A, Dooms-Goossens A, Achten G. Cosmetic intolerance. Contact Dermatitis 1987;16:189-194

53 Emmons WW, Marks JG Jr. Immediate and delayed reactions to cosmetic ingredients. Contact Dermatitis 1985;13:258-265

54 Van Joost Th, Stolz E, Van Der Hoek JCS. Simultaneous allergy to perfume ingredients. Contact Dermatitis 1985;12:115-116

55 Hamann D, Kishi P, Hamann CR. Consumer hair dye kits frequently contain isothiazolinones, other common preservatives and fragrance allergens. Dermatitis 2018;29:48-49

56 Siegel JA, Mounessa JS, Dellavalle RP, Dunnick CA. Comparison of contact allergens in bar soaps and liquid body washes. Dermatitis 2018;29:51-53

57 Aschenbeck K. Warshaw EM. Allergenic ingredients in facial wet wipes. Dermatitis 2017;28:353-359

58 Klaschka U. Contact allergens for armpits - allergenic fragrances specified on deodorants. Int J Hyg Environ Health 2012;215:584-591

59 Schultheiss E. Überempfindlichkeit gegenüber Ionon und Benzylalkohol. Derm Monatsschr 1957;135:629 (article in German). Data cited in ref. 60

60 Fisher AA. Allergic paraben and benzyl alcohol hypersensitivity relationship of the "delayed" and "immediate" varieties. Contact Dermatitis 1975;1:281-284

61 Lazzarini S. Contact allergy to benzyl alcohol and isopropyl palmitate, ingredients of topical corticosteroid. Contact Dermatitis 1982;8:349-350

62 Shoji A. Allergic reaction to benzyl alcohol in an antimycotic preparation. Contact Dermatitis 1983;9:510

63 Mitchell DM, Beck MH. Contact allergy to benzyl alcohol in a cutting oil reodorant. Contact Dermatitis 1988;18:301-302

64 Würbach G, Schubert H, Phillipp I. Contact allergy to benzyl alcohol and benzyl paraben. Contact Dermatitis 1993;28:187-188

65 Corazza M, Mantovani L, Maranini C, Virgli A. Allergic contact dermatitis from benzyl alcohol. Contact Dermatitis 1996;34:74-75

66 Aguirre A, Oleaga JM, Zabala R, Izu R, Diaz-Perez JL. Allergic contact dermatitis from Reflex (R) spray. Contact Dermatitis 1994;30:52-53

67 Shmunes E. Allergic dermatitis to benzyl alcohol in an injectable solution. Arch Dermatol 1984;120:1200-1201

68 Food and Drug Administration: Benzyl alcohol may be toxic to newborn. FDA Drug Bull 1982;12:10-11

69 Brown WJ, Buist NRM, Gipson HTC, Huston RK, Kennaway NG. Fatal benzyl alcohol poisoning in a neonatal intensive care unit. Lancet 1982;1(8283):1250

70 Gershanik JJ, Boecler B, Goerge W, et al. The gasping syndrome. Benzyl alcohol (BA) poisoning? Clin Res 1981;29:895A

71 Verecken P, Birringer C, Knitelius A-C, Herbaut D, Germaux M-A. Sensitization to benzyl alcohol: a possible cause of "corticosteroid allergy". Contact Dermatitis 1998;38:106

72 Podda M, Zollner T, Grundmann-Kollmann M, Kaufmann R, Boehncke WH. Allergic contact dermatitis from benzyl alcohol during topical antimycotic treatment. Contact Dermatitis 1999;41:302-303

73 Shaw DW. Allergic contact dermatitis to benzyl alcohol in a hearing aid impression material. Am J Contact Dermat 1999;10:228-232

74 Goossens A. Personal Communication to the author of ref. 73, October 1998 (cited in ref. 73)

75 Jagodzinsky LJ, Taylor JS, Oriba H. Allergic contact dermatitis from topical corticosteroid preparations. Am J Cont Derm 1995;6:67-74

76 Frosch PJ, Raulin C. Contact allergy to bufexamac. Hautarzt 1987;38:331-334 (article in German). Data cited in ref. 73

77 Taylor JS, Maibach HI, Fisher AA, et al. Contact leukoderma associated with the use of hair colors. Cutis 1993;52:273-280

78 Lodi A, Mancini LL, Pozzi M, Chiarelli G, Crosti C. Occupational airborne allergic contact dermatitis in parquet layers. Contact Dermatitis 1993;29:281-282

79 Li M, Gow E. Benzyl alcohol allergy. Australas J Dermatol 1995;36:219-220

80 Hoting E, Kuchmeister B, Hausen BM. Contact allergy to the antifungal agent naftifin. Derm Beruf Umwelt 1987;35:124-127 (article in German). Data cited in ref. 73

81 Grant JA, Bilodeau PA, Guernsey BG, Gardner FH. Unsuspected benzyl alcohol hypersensitivity. N Engl J Med 1982;306:108

82 Commmandeur C, Richard M, Renzi PM. Severe hypersensitivity reaction to injectable Gallium 67 in a worker exposed to silica. Allergy 1992;47:337-339

83 Napke E, Stevens DG. Excipients and additives: hidden hazards in drug products and in product substitution. Can Med Assoc J 1984;131:1449-1452

84 Wilson JP, Solimando DA Jr, Edwards MS. Parenteral benzyl alcohol-induced hypersensitivity reaction. Drug Intell Clin Pharm 1986;20:689-691

85 Lagerholm B, Lodin A, Gentele H. Hypersensitivity to phenylcarbinol preservative in vitamin B$_{12}$ for injection. Acta Allergol 1958;12:295-298

86 Schnuch A, Geier J, Uter W, Frosch PJ. Patch testing with preservatives, antimicrobials and industrial biocides. Results from a multicenter study (IVDK). Br J Dermatol 1998;138:467-476

87 Guin JD, Goodman J. Contact urticaria from benzyl alcohol presenting as intolerance to saline soaks. Contact Dermatitis 2001;45:182-183

88 Sestini S, Mori M, Francalanci S. Allergic contact dermatitis from benzyl alcohol in multiple medicaments. Contact Dermatitis 2004;50:316-317

89 Kleyn CE, Bharati A, King CM. Contact dermatitis from 3 different allergens in Solaraze® gel. Contact Dermatitis 2004;51:215-216

90 Curry EJ, Warshaw EM. Benzyl alcohol allergy: importance of patch testing with personal products. Dermatitis 2005;16:203-208

91 Goossens A, Claes L, Drieghe J, Put E. Antimicrobials: preservatives, antiseptics and disinfectants. Contact Dermatitis 1998;39:133-134

92 Jacob SE, Barron GS. Benzyl alcohol: a covert fragrance. Dermatitis 2007;18:232-233

93 Kroona L, Warfvinge G, Isaksson M, Ahlgren C, Dahlin J, Sörensen Ö, Bruze M. Quantification of L-carvone in toothpastes available on the Swedish market. Contact Dermatitis 2017;77:224-230

94 Kubin ME, Riekki R. Benzyl alcohol allergy mimicking corticosteroid allergy. Contact Dermatitis 2016;75:58-59

95 Carrascosa J-M, Domingo H, Ferrándiz XSC. Allergic contact dermatitis due to benzyl alcohol in a hair dye. Contact Dermatitis 2006;55:124-125

96 Jacob SE, Stechschulte S. Eyelid dermatitis associated with balsam of Peru constituents: benzoic acid and benzyl alcohol. Contact Dermatitis 2008;58:111-112

97 De Groot AC, Popova MP, Bankova VS. An update on the constituents of poplar-type propolis. Wapserveen, The Netherlands: acdegroot publishing, 2014, 11 pages. ISBN/EAN: 978-90-813233-0-7. Available at: https://www.researchgate.net/publication/262851225_AN_UPDATE_ON_THE_CONSTITUENTS_OF_POPLAR-TYPE_PROPOLIS

98 De Groot AC, Schmidt E. Essential oils: contact allergy and chemical composition. Boca Raton, Fl., USA: CRC Press, Taylor and Francis Group, 2016 (ISBN 9781482246407)

99 Hjorth N. Eczematous allergy to balsams. Acta Derm Venereol 1961;41(suppl.46):1-216

100 Opinion of the Scientific Committee on Cosmetic Products and Non-Food Products Intended for Consumers concerning 'The 1st update of the inventory of ingredients employed in cosmetic products. Section II: Perfume and aromatic raw materials', 24 October 2000, SCCNFP/0389/00, final. Available at: http://ec.europa.eu/health/ph_risk/committees/sccp/documents/out131_en.pdf

101 Chow ET, Avolio AM, Lee A, Nixon R. Frequency of positive patch test reactions to preservatives: The Australian experience. Australas J Dermatol 2013;54:31-35

102 Amado A, Jacob SE. Letter: Benzyl alcohol preserved saline used to dilute injectables poses a risk of contact dermatitis in fragrance-sensitive patients. Dermatol Surg 2007;33:1396-1397

103 Wieck S, Olsson O, Kümmerer K, Klaschka U. Fragrance allergens in household detergents. Regul Toxicol Pharmacol 2018;97:163-169

104 Ung CY, White JML, White IR, Banerjee P, McFadden JP. Patch testing with the European baseline series fragrance markers: a 2016 update. Br J Dermatol 2018;178:776-780

105 Dittmar D, Schuttelaar MLA. Contact sensitization to hydroperoxides of limonene and linalool: Results of consecutive patch testing and clinical relevance. Contact Dermatitis 2018 Oct 31. doi: 10.1111/cod.13137. [Epub ahead of print]

106 Silvestre JF, Mercader P, González-Pérez R, Hervella-Garcés M, Sanz-Sánchez T, Córdoba S, et al. Sensitization to fragrances in Spain: A 5-year multicentre study (2011-2015). Contact Dermatitis. 2018 Nov 14. doi: 10.1111/cod.13152. [Epub ahead of print]

Chapter 3.17   BENZYL BENZOATE

IDENTIFICATION

Description/definition   : Benzyl benzoate is the ester of benzyl alcohol and benzoic acid, that conforms to the formula shown below

Chemical class(es)   : Esters

Chemical/IUPAC name   : Benzyl benzoate

CAS registry number(s)   : 120-51-4

EC number(s)   : 204-402-9

CIR review(s)   : Int J Toxicol 2017;36(suppl.3):S5-S30 (access: www.cir-safety.org/ingredients)

RIFM monograph(s)   : Food Cosmet Toxicol 1973;11:1015

IFRA standard   : Restricted (www.ifraorg.org/en-us/standards-library) (table 3.17.1)

SCCS opinion(s)   : SCCS/1459/11 (4); SCCNFP/0389/00, final (39)

Merck Index monograph   : 1127

Function(s) in cosmetics : EU: antimicrobial; perfuming; solvent. USA: fragrance ingredients; pesticides; solvents

EU cosmetic restrictions : Regulated in Annex III/85 of the Regulation (EC) No. 1223/2009, regulated by 2003/15/EC; Must be labeled on cosmetics and detergent products, if present at > 10 ppm (0.001%) in leave-on products and > 100 ppm (0.01%) in rinse-off products

Patch testing   : 1% pet. (SmartPracticeEurope, SmartPracticeCanada); 10% pet. (Chemotechnique); recommended test concentration: 10.0% wt./wt. pet. (1)

Molecular formula   : $C_{14}H_{12}O_2$

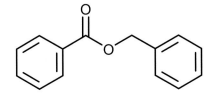

Table 3.17.1 IFRA restrictions for benzyl benzoate

Category [a]	Limits [b]	Category [a]	Limits [b]	Category [a]	Limits [b]
1	1.70%	5	14.0%	9	5.00%
2	2.20%	6	42.80%	10	2.50%
3	8.90%	7	4.50%	11	not restricted
4	26.70%	8	2.00%		

[a] For explanation of categories see pages 6-8
[b] Limits in the finished products

GENERAL

Benzyl benzoate is a colorless to pale yellow clear oily liquid to solid; its odor type is balsamic and its odor is described as 'sweet balsamic floral with fruity nuances' (www.thegoodscentscompany.com). It is one of the main ingredients of Myroxylon pereirae resin (balsam of Peru) and is also present in propolis (6). Benzyl benzoate results from the condensation of benzoic acid and benzyl alcohol (34).

Uses of benzyl benzoate include or have included: pediculicide, acaricide, in synthetic musks, confectionery flavors and chewing gum flavors, fixative, plasticizer for cellulose acetate and nitrocellulose, remedy for scabies, dye carrier, antispasmodic, and repellant for chiggers, mosquitoes and ticks on man (U.S. National Library of Medicine).

Presence in essential oils, Myroxylon pereirae resin (balsam of Peru) and propolis

Benzyl benzoate has been identified by chemical analysis in 28 of 91 essential oils, which have caused contact allergy / allergic contact dermatitis. In four oils, benzyl benzoate belonged to the 'Top-10' of ingredients with the highest concentrations which may be expected in commercial essential oils of this type: ylang-ylang oil (3.5-14.0%), cananga oil (2.6-5.6%), cinnamon leaf oil Sri Lanka (0.6-3.6%), and clove bud/leaf/stem oil (0.03-0.6%) (40). Benzyl benzoate may also be present in Myroxylon pereirae resin (balsam of Peru) (up to 30%) (6) and in propolis (36).

CONTACT ALLERGY

General

The SCCS (Scientific Committee on Consumer Safety), in a 2012 Opinion on Fragrance allergens in cosmetic products, has marked benzyl benzoate as 'established contact allergen in humans' (4,27). The sensitizing potency of benzyl benzoate was classified as 'weak' based on an EC3 value of 17% in the LLNA (local lymph node assay) in animal experiments (4,27).

Patch testing in groups of patients

Results of studies testing benzyl benzoate in consecutive patients suspected of contact dermatitis (routine testing) and those of testing in groups of *selected* patients (e.g. patients with fragrance sensitivity, individuals with suspected cosmetic intolerance) are shown in table 3.17.2.

In 4 studies in which routine testing with benzyl benzoate was performed, very low rates of sensitization of <0.1%-0.3% were observed. Relevance data were inadequate. The rates of sensitization in groups of selected patients ranged from 0.1% to 13%, but were mostly (very) low. The high percentage of 13 was seen in a very small study of 8 patients allergic to propolis (which may contain benzyl benzoate, 36), of who one reacted. In 7 of the 8 studies, no relevance data were provided, in the 8th, it was assumed that nearly all positive reactions were of present or past relevance (7).

In 3 studies in which patients allergic to Myroxylon pereirae resin (balsam of Peru) were patch tested with benzyl benzoate, frequencies of sensitization to this fragrance, which may be an important constituent of balsam of Peru (6), were 3.9%, 7.0% and 12.2% (6,33,37), indicating that benzyl benzoate is not an important allergen in the resin.

Table 3.17.2 Patch testing in groups of patients

Years and Country	Test conc. & vehicle	Number of patients tested	positive (%)		Selection of patients (S); Relevance (R); Comments (C)	Ref.
Routine testing						
2015-2016 UK	1% pet.	2084	3	(0.1%)	R: not specified for individual fragrances; 25% of patients who reacted to any fragrance or fragrance marker had a positive fragrance history	45
2013-2014 Thailand		312	1	(0.3%)	R: 100%	25
2011-2012 UK	1% pet.	1951	2	(0.1%)	R: not stated	26
2003-2004 IVDK	1% pet.	2003	1	(<0.1%)	R: not stated	2
Testing in groups of selected patients						
2006-2011 IVDK	1% pet.	708	1	(0.1%)	S: patients with suspected cosmetic intolerance; R: not stated	24
2005-10 Netherlands		100	2	(2%)	S: patients with known fragrance sensitivity based on a positive patch test to the FM I and/or the FM II; R: not stated	28
2001-2002 Denmark, Sweden	5% pet.	658	1	(0.2%)	S: consecutive patients with hand eczema; R: it was assumed that nearly all positive reactions were of present or past relevance	7
1988-1990 Germany	5% pet.	8	1	(13%)	S: patients allergic to propolis; R: not stated	32
<1986 France	1% pet.	21	1	(5%)	S: patients with dermatitis caused by perfumes; R: not stated	38
1982 France	1% pet.	465	7	(1.5%)	S: patients with suspected allergy to cosmetics, drugs, industrial products or clothes; R: not stated	43
<1982 Italy	5% pet.	73	1	(1%)	S: patients who had been treated for scabies for at least 10 days with either mesulphen, crotamiton or benzyl benzoate; R: not stated; S: it was not specified how many patients had been treated with benzyl benzoate	31
1975 USA	5% pet.	20	1	(5%)	S: fragrance-allergic patients; R: not stated	8
Testing in patients allergic to Myroxylon pereirae resin (balsam of Peru)						
1995-1998 Germany	5% pet.	102	4	(3.9%)	S: patients allergic to balsam of Peru	6
<1976 USA, Canada, Europe		142	10	(7.0%)	S: patients allergic to balsam of Peru	37
1955-1960 Denmark	5% pet.	115	14	(12.2%)	S: patients allergic to balsam of Peru	33

FM: Fragrance mix; IVDK: Informationsverbund Dermatologischer Kliniken (Germany, Switzerland, Austria):

Case reports and case series

Benzyl benzoate was responsible for 1 out of 399 cases of cosmetic allergy where the causal allergen was identified in a study of the NACDG, USA, 1977-1983 (5). Benzyl benzoate was stated to be the (or an) allergen in one patient in a group of 603 individuals suffering from cosmetic dermatitis, seen in the period 2010-2015 in Leuven, Belgium (23).

Five patients had allergic contact dermatitis from benzyl benzoate in topical pharmaceutical preparations (9).

Cross-reactions, pseudo-cross-reactions and co-reactions

For general information on cross-/pseudo-cross-/co-reactivity of fragrance chemicals with other fragrances, fragrance markers (fragrance mix I, fragrance mix II, colophonium, Myroxylon pereirae resin [balsam of Peru]) and essential oils see Chapter 1.2 General information on cross-reactions, pseudo-cross-reactions and co-reactions. Co-reactivity with Myroxylon pereirae resin (MP) may be explained by the presence of benzyl benzoate (up to 30%) in MP (pseudo-cross-reactions).

Patch test sensitization

In 1 patient out of 230 with contact allergy to Myroxylon pereirae resin (balsam of Peru) and tested with benzyl benzoate, there was one positive reaction to 5% pet. that developed 6 days or later after application. Whether this was simply a 'delayed' reaction or indicative of patch test sensitization was not investigated (33).

Presence in products and chemical analyses

In various studies, the presence of benzyl benzoate in cosmetic and sometimes other products has been investigated. Before 2006, most investigators used chemical analysis, usually GC-MS, for qualitative and quantitative determination. Since then, the presence of the target fragrances was usually investigated by screening the product labels for the 26 fragrances that must be labeled since 2005 on cosmetics and detergent products in the EU, if present at > 10 ppm (0.001%) in leave-on products and > 100 ppm (0.01%) in rinse-off products. This method, obviously, is less accurate and may result in underestimation of the frequency of the fragrances being present in the product. When they are in fact present, but the concentration is lower than mentioned above, labeling is not required and the fragrances' presence will be missed.

Table 3.17.3 Presence of benzyl benzoate in products [a]

Year	Country	Product type	Nr. investigated	Nr. of products positive [b]	(%)	Method [c]	Ref.
2015-6	Denmark	Fragranced cosmetic products	5588		(9%)	Labeling	16
2015	Germany	Household detergents	817	17	(2%)	Labeling	44
2008-11	Germany	Deodorants	374	78	(21%)	Labeling	29
2006-9	Germany	Cosmetic products	4991		(9%)	Labeling	15
2008	Belgium	Fragranced topical pharmaceutical products	370	4	(1%)	Labeling	9
2008	Sweden	Cosmetic products	204	8	(4%)	Labeling	3
		Detergents	97	1	(1%)	Labeling	
2007	Netherlands	Cosmetic products for children	23	3	(13%)	Analysis	19
2006	UK	Perfumed cosmetic and household products	300	70	(23%)	Labeling	13
2006	Denmark	Popular perfumed deodorants	88	22	(25%)	Labeling	17
			23	11	(48%)	Analysis	
2006	Netherlands	Laundry detergents	52	6	(12%)	Labeling + analysis	21
2006	Denmark	Rinse-off cosmetics for children	208	19	(9%)	Labeling + analysis	18
2002	Denmark	Home and car air fresheners	19	13	(68%)	Analysis	22
2001	Denmark	Non-cosmetic consumer products	43	11	(26%)	Analysis	20
2000	Denmark, UK, Germany, Italy	Domestic and occupational products	59	6	(10%)	Analysis	11
1997-8	Denmark, UK Germany, Sweden	Cosmetics and cosmetic toys for children	25	17	(68%)	Analysis	12
1996	Five European countries	Fragranced deodorants	70	50	(71%)	Analysis	10
1992	Netherlands	Cosmetic products	300	147	(49%)	Analysis	14

[a] See the corresponding text below for more details
[b] positive = containing the target fragrance
[c] Labeling: information from the ingredient labels on the product / packaging; Analysis: chemical analysis, most often GC-MS

The results of the relevant studies for benzyl benzoate are summarized in table 3.17.3. More detailed information can be found in the corresponding text following the table. The percentage of products in which benzyl benzoate was found to be present shows wide variations, which can among other be explained by the selection procedure of the products, the method of investigation (false-negatives with information obtained from labels only) and changes in the use of individual fragrance materials over time (fashion).

In Denmark, in 2015-2016, 5588 fragranced cosmetic products were examined with a smartphone application for the 26 fragrances that need to be labeled in the EU. Benzyl benzoate was present in 9% of the products (rank number 12) (16).

In Germany, in 2015, fragrance allergens were evaluated based on lists of ingredients in 817 (unique) detergents (all-purpose cleaners, cleaning preparations for special purposes [e.g. bathroom, kitchen, dish-washing] and laundry detergents) present in 131 households. Benzyl benzoate was found to be present in 17 (2%) of the products (44).

In 2008, 2010 and 2011, 374 deodorants available in German retail shops were randomly selected and their labels checked for the presence of the 26 fragrances that need to be labeled. Benzyl benzoate was found to be present in 78 (20.9%) of the products (29).

In Germany, in the period 2006-2009, 4991 cosmetic products were randomly sampled for an official investigation of conformity of cosmetic products with legal provisions. The labels were inspected for the presence of the 26 fragrances that need to be labeled in the EU. Benzyl benzoate was present in 9% of the products (rank number 11) (15).

In 2008, 66 different fragrance components (including 39 essential oils) were identified in 370 (10% of the total) topical pharmaceutical products marketed in Belgium; 4 of these (1.1%) contained benzyl benzoate (9).

Benzyl benzoate was present (as indicated by labeling) in 4% of 204 cosmetic products (92 shampoos, 61 hair conditioners, 34 liquid soaps, 17 wet tissues) and in 1% of 97 detergents in Sweden, 2008 (3).

In 2007, in The Netherlands, twenty-three cosmetic products for children were analyzed for the presence of fragrances that need to be labeled. Benzyl benzoate was identified in 3 of the products (13%) in a concentration range of 50-2654 ppm (19).

In 2006, of 88 popular perfume containing deodorants purchased in Denmark, 22 (25%) were labeled to contain benzyl benzoate. Analysis of 24 regulated fragrance substances in 23 selected deodorants (19 spray products, 2 deostick and 2 roll-on) was performed by GC-MS. Benzyl benzoate was identified in 11 of the products (48%) with a concentration range of 3–4054 ppm (17).

In 2006, in The Netherlands, 52 laundry detergents were investigated for the presence of allergenic fragrances by checking their labels and chemical analyses. Benzyl benzoate was found to be present in 6 of the products (12%) in a concentration range of 4-108 ppm. Benzyl benzoate had rank number 12 in the frequency list (21).

In 2006, the labels of 208 cosmetics for children (especially shampoos, body shampoos and soaps) available in Denmark were checked for the presence of the 26 fragrances that need to be labeled in the EU. Benzyl benzoate was present in 19 products (9.1%), and ranked number 8 in the frequency list. Seventeen products were analyzed quantitatively for the fragrances. The maximum concentration found for benzyl benzoate was 210 mg/kg (18).

In January 2006, a study of perfumed cosmetic and household products available on the shelves of U.K. retailers was carried out. Products were included if 'parfum' or 'aroma' was listed among the ingredients. Three hundred products were surveyed and any of 26 mandatory labeling fragrances named on the label were recorded. Benzyl benzoate was present in 70 (23%) of the products (rank number 13) (13).

In 2002, in Denmark, 19 air fresheners (6 for cars, 13 for homes) were analyzed for the presence of fragrances that need to be labeled on cosmetics. Benzyl benzoate was found to be present in 13 products (68%) in a concentration range of 7.7-10,000 ppm and ranked 4 in the frequency list (22).

In 2001, in Denmark, 43 non-cosmetic consumer products (mainly dish-washing products, laundry detergents, and hard and soft surface cleaners) were analyzed for the 26 fragrances that are regulated for labeling in the EU. Benzyl benzoate was present in 11 products (26%) in a concentration range of 0.0030-0.0152% (m/m) and had rank number 8 in the frequency list (20).

In 2000, fifty-nine domestic and occupational products, purchased in retail outlets in Denmark, England, Germany and Italy were analyzed by GC-MS for the presence of fragrances. The product categories were liquid soap and soap bars (n=13), soft/hard surface cleaners (n=23), fabric conditioners/laundry detergents for hand wash (n=8), dish wash (n=10), furniture polish, car shampoo, stain remover (each n=1) and 2 products used in occupational environments. Benzyl benzoate was present in 6 products (10%) with a mean concentration of 97 ppm and a range of 51-223 ppm (11).

Twenty-five cosmetics and cosmetic toys for children (5 shampoos and shower gels, 6 perfumes, 1 deodorant (roll-on), 4 baby lotions/creams, 1 baby wipes product, 1 baby oil, 2 lipcare products and 5 toy-cosmetic products: a cosmetic-toy set for blending perfumes and a makeup set) purchased in 1997-1998 in retail outlets in Denmark, Germany, England and Sweden were analyzed in 1998 for the presence of fragrances by GC-MS. Benzyl benzoate was found in 17 products (68%) in a concentration range of 0.001-0.134% (w/w). For the analytical data in each product category, the original publication should be consulted (12).

Seventy fragranced deodorants, purchased at retail outlets in 5 European countries in 1996, were analyzed by gas chromatography - mass spectrometry (GC-MS) for the determination of the contents of 21 commonly used fragrance materials. Benzyl benzoate was identified in 50 products (71%) in a concentration range of 1–1075 ppm (10).

In 1992, in The Netherlands, the presence of fragrances was analyzed in 300 cosmetic products. Benzyl benzoate was identified in 49% of the products (rank order 12) (14).

OTHER SIDE EFFECTS

Irritant contact dermatitis
Topical medications containing benzyl benzoate 25% have been used extensively in the past for the treatment of scabies and have caused various 'rashes' within 24 hours, which were probably irritant in nature, presenting on an already inflamed skin of the patient with scabies (34,35).

Immediate-type reactions
Immediate contact reactions (contact urticaria) from benzyl benzoate have been cited in ref. 46.

Other non-eczematous contact reactions
Irritant contact dermatitis from benzyl benzoate may have provoked bullous pemphigoid: A man presented with an acute bullous eruption, which was distributed widely and evenly, following treatment with a 30% benzyl benzoate preparation for scabies. This had been applied to him 2x a day. The patient then developed an erythematous reaction, followed after 2 days by dense bullae. Direct immunofluorescence on perilesional skin showed linear deposits of IgG and complement C3 along the basement membrane zone. Indirect immunofluorescence on normal human skin substance was negative. A patch test with benzyl benzoate 1% pet. was negative (41). The authors cited another case of bullous pemphigoid after therapy of scabies with 30% benzyl benzoate (42).

Systemic side effects
A 2-month-old boy weighing 4.2 kg, who was hospitalized for scabies, was bathed over the body, except for the face, with a solution containing benzyl benzoate (43%), soap (20%), ethyl alcohol (20%), and distilled water (17%). Convulsions appeared 2.5 hours later and were controlled with diazepam. About 1.5 hours later, convulsions recurred requiring even stronger doses of diazepam. There was no hyperthermia, hypocalcemia, or hypoglycemia. The cerebrospinal fluid was normal, as were X-rays of the head. All organic causes and subdural hematoma were eliminated. It was considered highly probable that the condition was iatrogenic and that the etiological agent was the benzyl benzoate. However, this could not be proved, since benzyl benzoate was not found in the urine and since the quantity of urine was too small for analysis of metabolites such as hippuric acid. The boy apparently fully recovered and was in good health when last examined at 6 months of age (30).

LITERATURE

1   Bruze M, Svedman C, Andersen KE, Bruynzeel D, Goossens A, Johansen JD, et al. Patch test concentrations (doses in mg/cm2) for the 12 non-mix fragrance substances regulated by European legislation. Contact Dermatitis 2012;66:131-136

2   Schnuch A, Uter W, Geier J, Lessmann H, Frosch PJ. Sensitization to 26 fragrances to be labelled according to current European regulation: Results of the IVDK and review of the literature. Contact Dermatitis 2007;57:1-10

3   Yazar K, Johnsson S, Lind M-L, Boman A, Lidén C. Preservatives and fragrances in selected consumer-available cosmetics and detergents. Contact Dermatitis 2011;64:265-272

4   SCCS (Scientific Committee on Consumer Safety). Opinion on Fragrance allergens in cosmetic products, 26-27 June 2012, SCCS/1459/11. Available at:
     https://ec.europa.eu/health/sites/health/files/scientific_committees/consumer_safety/docs/sccs_o_102.pdf

5   Adams RM, Maibach HI, for the North American Contact Dermatitis Group. A five-year study of cosmetic reactions. J Am Acad Dermatol 1985;13:1062-1069

6   Hausen BM. Contact allergy to Balsam of Peru. II. Patch test results in 102 patients with selected Balsam of Peru constituents. Am J Contact Derm 2001;12:93-102

7   Heydorn S, Johansen JD, Andersen KE, Bruze M, Svedman C, White IR, et al. Fragrance allergy in patients with hand eczema – a clinical study. Contact Dermatitis 2003;48:317-323

8   Larsen WG. Perfume dermatitis. A study of 20 patients. Arch Dermatol 1977;113:623-626

9   Nardelli A, D'Hooge E, Drieghe J, Dooms M, Goossens A. Allergic contact dermatitis from fragrance components in specific topical pharmaceutical products in Belgium. Contact Dermatitis 2009;60:303-313

10 Rastogi SC, Johansen JD, Frosch P, Menné T, Bruze M, Lepoittevin JP, et al. Deodorants on the European market: quantitative chemical analysis of 21 fragrances. Contact Dermatitis 1998;38:29-35

11 Rastogi SC, Heydorn S, Johansen JD, Basketter DA. Fragrance chemicals in domestic and occupational products. Contact Dermatitis 2001;45:221-225

12 Rastogi SC, Johansen JD, Menné T, Frosch P, Bruze M, Andersen KE, et al. Content of fragrance allergens in children's cosmetics and cosmetic toys. Contact Dermatitis 1999;41:84-88

13 Buckley DA. Fragrance ingredient labelling in products on sale in the UK. Br J Dermatol 2007;157:295-300

14 Weyland JW. Personal Communication, 1992. Cited in: De Groot AC, Weyland JW, Nater JP. Unwanted effects of cosmetics and drugs used in dermatology, 3rd Ed. Amsterdam: Elsevier, 1994: 579

15 Uter W, Yazar K, Kratz E-M, Mildau G, Lidén C. Coupled exposure to ingredients of cosmetic products: I. Fragrances. Contact Dermatitis 2013;69:335-341

16 Bennike NH, Oturai NB, Müller S, Kirkeby CS, Jørgensen C, Christensen AB, et al. Fragrance contact allergens in 5588 cosmetic products identified through a novel smartphone application. J Eur Acad Dermatol Venereol 2018;32:79-85

17 Rastogi SC, Hellerup Jensen G, Johansen JD. Survey and risk assessment of chemical substances in deodorants. Survey of Chemical Substances in Consumer Products, No. 86 2007. Danish Ministry of the Environment, Environmental Protection Agency. Available at: https://www2.mst.dk/Udgiv/publications/2007/978-87-7052-625-8/pdf/978-87-7052-626-5.pdf

18 Poulsen PB, Schmidt A. A survey and health assessment of cosmetic products for children. Survey of chemical substances in consumer products, No. 88. Copenhagen: Danish Environmental Protection Agency, 2007. Available at: https://www2.mst.dk/udgiv/publications/2007/978-87-7052-638-8/pdf/978-87-7052-639-5.pdf

19 VWA. Dutch Food and Consumer Product Safety Authority. Cosmetische producten voor kinderen: Inventarisatie van de markt en de veiligheidsborging door producenten en importeurs. Report ND04o065/ND05o170, 2007 (Report in Dutch), 2007. Available at: www.nvwa.nl/documenten/communicatie/inspectieresultaten/ consument/ 2016m/cosmetische- producten-voor-kinderen

20 Rastogi SC. Survey of chemical compounds in consumer products. Contents of selected fragrance materials in cleaning products and other consumer products. Survey no. 8-2002. Copenhagen, Denmark, Danish Environmental Protection Agency. Available at: http://eng.mst.dk/media/mst/69131/8.pdf

21 Bouma K, Van Peursem AJJ. Marktonderzoek naleving detergenten verordening voor textielwasmiddelen. Dutch Food and Consumer Products Safety Authority (VWA) Report ND06K173, 2006 [in Dutch]. Available at: http://docplayer.nl/41524125-Marktonderzoek-naleving-detergenten-verordening-voor-textielwasmiddelen.html

22 Pors J, Fuhlendorff R. Mapping of chemical substances in air fresheners and other fragrance liberating products. Report Danish Ministry of the Environment, Environmental Protection Agency (EPA). Survey of Chemicals in Consumer Products, No 30, 2003. Available at: http://eng.mst.dk/media/mst/69113/30.pdf

23 Goossens A. Cosmetic contact allergens. Cosmetics 2016, 3, 5; doi:10.3390/cosmetics3010005

24 Dinkloh A, Worm M, Geier J, Schnuch A, Wollenberg A. Contact sensitization in patients with suspected cosmetic intolerance: results of the IVDK 2006-2011. J Eur Acad Dermatol Venereol 2015;29:1071-1081

25 Vejanurug P, Tresukosol P, Sajjachareonpong P, Puangpet P. Fragrance allergy could be missed without patch testing with 26 individual fragrance allergens. Contact Dermatitis 2016;74:230-235

26 Mann J, McFadden JP, White JML, White IR, Banerjee P. Baseline series fragrance markers fail to predict contact allergy. Contact Dermatitis 2014;70:276-281

27 Uter W, Johansen JD, Börje A, Karlberg A-T, Lidén C, Rastogi S, Roberts D, White IR. Categorization of fragrance contact allergens for prioritization of preventive measures: clinical and experimental data and consideration of structure–activity relationships. Contact Dermatitis 2013;69:196-230

28 Nagtegaal MJC, Pentinga SE, Kuik J, Kezic S, Rustemeyer T. The role of the skin irritation response in polysensitization to fragrances. Contact Dermatitis 2012;67:28-35

29 Klaschka U. Contact allergens for armpits - allergenic fragrances specified on deodorants. Int J Hyg Environ Health 2012;215:584-591

30 Hayes WJ Jr, Laws ER Jr, Eds. Handbook of pesticide toxicology. Volume 3. Classes of pesticides. New York, NY: Academic Press, Inc., 1991:1507

31 Meneghini CL, Vena GA, Angelini G. Contact dermatitis to scabicides. Contact Dermatitis 1982;8:285-286

32 Hausen BM, Evers P, Stüwe H-T, König WA, Wollenweber E. Propolis allergy (IV) Studies with further sensitizers from propolis and constituents common to propolis, poplar buds and balsam of Peru. Contact Dermatitis 1992;26:34-44

33 Hjorth N. Eczematous allergy to balsams. Acta Derm Venereol 1961;41(suppl.46):1-216

34 Johnson W, Bergfeld WF, Belsito DV, Hill RA, Klaassen CD, Liebler DC, et al. Safety assessment of benzyl alcohol, benzoic acid and its salts, and benzyl benzoate. Int J Toxicol 2017;36(suppl.3):S5-S30

35 Daughtry DC. Complications following a rapid treatment of scabies. JAMA 1945;127:88-89

36 De Groot AC, Popova MP, Bankova VS. An update on the constituents of poplar-type propolis. Wapserveen, The Netherlands: acdegroot publishing, 2014, 11 pages. ISBN/EAN: 978-90-813233-0-7. Available at: https://www.researchgate.net/publication/262851225_AN_UPDATE_ON_THE_CONSTITUENTS_OF_POPLAR-TYPE_PROPOLIS

37 Mitchell JC, Calnan CD, Clendenning WE, Cronin E, Hjorth N, Magnusson B, et al. Patch testing with some components of balsam of Peru. Contact Dermatitis 1976;2:57-58

38 Meynadier JM, Meynadier J, Peyron JL, Peyron L. Formes cliniques des manifestations cutanées d'allergie aux parfums. Ann Dermatol Venereol 1986;113:31-39

39 Opinion of the Scientific Committee on Cosmetic Products and Non-Food Products Intended for Consumers concerning 'The 1st update of the inventory of ingredients employed in cosmetic products. Section II: Perfume and aromatic raw materials', 24 October 2000, SCCNFP/0389/00, final. Available at: http://ec.europa.eu/health/ph_risk/committees/sccp/documents/out131_en.pdf

40 De Groot AC, Schmidt E. Essential oils: contact allergy and chemical composition. Boca Raton, Fl., USA: CRC Press, Taylor and Francis Group, 2016 (ISBN 9781482246407)

41 Stransky L, Vasileva S, Mateev G. Contact bullous pemphigoid? Contact Dermatitis 1996;35:182

42 Wranicz A, Czernielewski A. TITLE MISSING. Przegl Derm 1974;11:693-696 (cited in ref. 41)

43 Meynadier JM, Meynadier J, Colmas A, Castelain PY, Ducombs G, Chabeau G, et al. Allergy to preservatives. Ann Dermatol Venereol 1982;109:1017-1023

44 Wieck S, Olsson O, Kümmerer K, Klaschka U. Fragrance allergens in household detergents. Regul Toxicol Pharmacol 2018;97:163-169

45 Ung CY, White JML, White IR, Banerjee P, McFadden JP. Patch testing with the European baseline series fragrance markers: a 2016 update. Br J Dermatol 2018;178:776-780

46 De Groot AC. Patch Testing, 4th Edition. Wapserveen, The Netherlands: acdegroot publishing, 2018 (ISBN 978-90-813233-4-5)

Chapter 3.18   BENZYL CINNAMATE

IDENTIFICATION

Description/definition   : Benzyl cinnamate is the ester of benzyl alcohol and cinnamic acid, that conforms to
                             the formula shown below
Chemical class(es)   : Esters
Chemical/IUPAC name   : Benzyl 3-phenylprop-2-enoate
Other names   : Cinnamein
CAS registry number(s)   : 103-41-3
EC number(s)   : 203-109-3
RIFM monograph(s)   : Food Chem Toxicol 2007;45(suppl.1):S40-S48; Food Chem Toxicol 2007;45(suppl.1):S1-
                             S23; Food Cosmet Toxicol 1973;11:1017
IFRA standard   : Restricted (www.ifraorg.org/en-us/standards-library) (table 3.18.1)
SCCS opinion(s)   : Various (7); SCCS/1459/11 (8)
Merck Index monograph   : 1130
Function(s) in cosmetics   : EU: perfuming. USA: fragrance ingredients
EU cosmetic restrictions   : Regulated in Annex III/81 of the Regulation (EC) No. 1223/2009, regulated by 2003/15/EC;
                             Must be labeled on cosmetics and detergent products, if present at > 10 ppm (0.001%)
                             in leave-on products and > 100 ppm (0.01%) in rinse-off products
Patch testing   : 5% pet. (SmartPracticeEurope, SmartPracticeCanada); 10% pet. (Chemotechnique);
                             recommended test concentration: 10.0% wt./wt. pet (1)
Molecular formula   : $C_{16}H_{14}O_2$

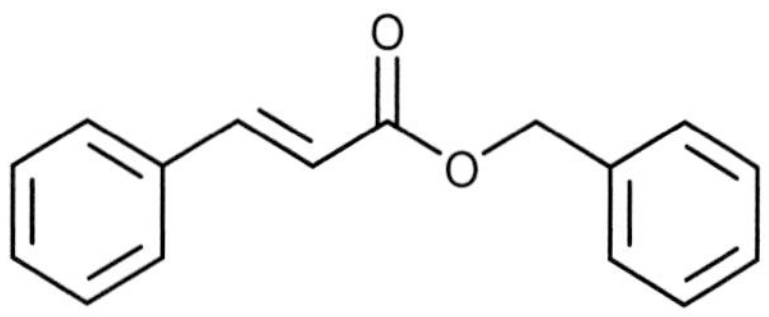

Table 3.18.1 IFRA restrictions for benzyl cinnamate

Category [a]	Limits [b]	Category [a]	Limits [b]	Category [a]	Limits [b]
1	0.10%	5	1.10%	9	5.00%
2	0.20%	6	3.40%	10	2.50%
3	0.70%	7	0.40%	11	not restricted
4	2.10%	8	2.00%		

[a] For explanation of categories see pages 6-8
[b] Limits in the finished products

GENERAL

Benzyl cinnamate is a white to pale yellow solid; its odor type is balsamic and its odor is described as 'sweet, spicy, floral, with a powdery balsamic nuance' (www.thegoodscentscompany.com). It is used in artificial flavors, in perfumes (mainly as a fixative) and as a component of heavy, oriental perfumes (U.S. National Library of Medicine).

Presence in essential oils, Myroxylon pereirae resin (balsam of Peru) and propolis
Benzyl cinnamate has been identified by chemical analysis in two of 91 essential oils, which have caused contact allergy / allergic contact dermatitis: cinnamon bark oil, Sri Lanka and ylang-ylang oil (31). Benzyl cinnamate may also be present in Myroxylon pereirae resin (balsam of Peru) (up to 40%) (5) and in propolis (29).

CONTACT ALLERGY

General
The SCCS (Scientific Committee on Consumer Safety), in a 2012 Opinion on Fragrance allergens in cosmetic products, has marked benzyl cinnamate as 'established contact allergen in humans' (8,21). The sensitizing potency of benzyl cinnamate was classified as 'weak' based on an EC3 value of 18.4% in the LLNA (local lymph node assay) in animal experiments (8,21).

Patch testing in groups of patients

Results of studies testing benzyl cinnamate in consecutive patients suspected of contact dermatitis (routine testing) and those of testing in groups of *selected* patients (e.g. patients with fragrance sensitivity, individuals with suspected cosmetic intolerance, patients allergic to propolis) are shown in table 3.18.2.

In 6 studies in which routine testing with benzyl cinnamate was performed, very low rates of sensitization of 0.02%-0.3% were observed. Relevance ranged from 0 to 100%, but the numbers of allergic patients were very small.

The rates of sensitization to benzyl cinnamate in 7 studies with groups of selected patients ranged from 0.1% to 22%, but 4/7 only scored 1% or lower. The very high percentage of 22 was seen in a small study of 9 patients allergic to propolis (which may contain benzyl cinnamate [29]), of who two reacted to benzyl cinnamate 1% pet. (27). In none of the six studies were relevance data provided. As to the causative products, in one study, of the relevant reactions to any of 26 fragrances tested, 96% were caused by cosmetic products (2).

In 4 investigations in which patients allergic to Myroxylon pereirae resin (balsam of Peru) were patch tested with benzyl cinnamate, frequencies of sensitization to this fragrance, which may be an important constituent of balsam of Peru (up to 40%, ref. 5), ranged from 2.9% to 19.1% (5,26,28,30), indicating that benzyl cinnamate is the allergen or one of the allergens in some 10% of all patients allergic to balsam of Peru (calculated average, adjusted for sample size).

Table 3.18.2 Patch testing in groups of patients

Years and Country	Test conc. & vehicle	Number of patients tested	positive (%)		Selection of patients (S); Relevance (R); Comments (C)	Ref.
Routine testing						
2015-2016 UK	5% pet.	2084	1	(0.05%)	R: not specified for individual fragrances; 25% of patients who reacted to any fragrance or fragrance marker had a positive fragrance history	33
2010-2015 Denmark	5% pet.	6004		(0.02%)	R: present relevance 100%, past relevance 0%	18
2013-2014 Thailand		312	1	(0.3%)	R: 100%	19
2011-2012 UK	5% pet.	1951	3	(0.15%)	R: not stated	20
2008-2010 Denmark	5% pet.	1503	1	(0.1%)	S: mostly routine testing; R: 0%; C: 100% co-reactivity of both FM I and FM II; C: of the relevant reactions to any of the 26 fragrances tested, 96% were caused by cosmetic products	2
2003-2004 IVDK	5% pet.	2042	16	(0.3%)	R: not stated	4
Testing in groups of selected patients						
2011-2015 Spain	5 or 10% pet.	1013	13	(1.3%)	S: patients previously reacting to FM I, FM II, Myroxylon pereirae resin or hydroxyisohexyl 3-cyclohexene carboxaldehyde in the baseline series and subsequently tested with a fragrance series; R: not stated	35
2006-2011 IVDK	5% pet.	708	3	(0.4%)	S: patients with suspected cosmetic intolerance; R: not stated	17
2005-10 Netherlands		100	1	(1%)	S: patients with known fragrance sensitivity based on a positive patch test to the FM I and/or the FM II; R: not stated	22
2005-2008 IVDK	5% pet.	2872		(0.1%)	S: not specified; R: not stated	23
1997-2000 Austria	5% pet.	747	3	(0.4%)	S: patients suspected of fragrance allergy: R: not stated	6
1988-1990 Germany	1% pet.	9	2	(22%)	S: patients allergic to propolis; R: not stated	27
1983 The Netherlands	8% pet.	182	6	(3.3%)	S: patients suspected of cosmetic allergy; R: not stated	25
Testing in patients allergic to Myroxylon pereirae resin (balsam of Peru)						
1995-1998 Germany	5% pet.	102	3	(2.9%)	S: patients allergic to balsam of Peru	5
<1982 Poland	5% pet.	12	1	(9%)	S: patients allergic to Myroxylon pereirae resin and to propolis; C: benzyl cinnamate may be an ingredient of both substances	26
<1976 USA, Canada, Europe		142	11	(7.7%)	S: patients allergic to balsam of Peru	30
1955-1960 Denmark	5% pet.	110	21	(19.1%)	S: patients allergic to balsam of Peru	28

FM: Fragrance Mix; IVDK: Informationsverbund Dermatologischer Kliniken (Germany, Switzerland, Austria)

Case reports and case series

In the period 1996-2013, in a tertiary referral center in Valencia, Spain, 5419 patients were patch tested. Of these, 628 individuals had allergic contact dermatitis to cosmetics. In this group, benzyl cinnamate was the responsible allergen in one case (13).

Patch test sensitization
In 2 patients out of 230 with contact allergy to Myroxylon pereirae resin (balsam of Peru), there was a positive patch test to benzyl cinnamate 5% pet. that developed 6 days or later after application. Whether this was simply a 'delayed' reaction or indicative of patch test sensitization was not well investigated (28).

Cross-reactions, pseudo-cross-reactions and co-reactions
For general information on cross-/pseudo-cross-/co-reactivity of fragrance chemicals with other fragrances, fragrance markers (fragrance mix I, fragrance mix II, colophonium, Myroxylon pereirae resin [balsam of Peru]) and essential oils see Chapter 1.2 General information on cross-reactions, pseudo-cross-reactions and co-reactions. Co-reactivity with Myroxylon pereirae resin (MP) may be explained by the presence of benzyl cinnamate (up to 40%) in MP (pseudo-cross-reactions).

Presence in products and chemical analyses
In various studies, the presence of benzyl cinnamate in cosmetic and sometimes other products has been investigated. Before 2006, most investigators used chemical analysis, usually GC-MS, for qualitative and quantitative determination. Since then, the presence of the target fragrances was usually investigated by screening the product labels for the 26 fragrances that must be labeled since 2005 on cosmetics and detergent products in the EU, if present at > 10 ppm (0.001%) in leave-on products and > 100 ppm (0.01%) in rinse-off products. This method, obviously, is less accurate and may result in underestimation of the frequency of the fragrances being present in the product. When they are in fact present, but the concentration is lower than mentioned above, labeling is not required and the fragrances' presence will be missed.

The results of the relevant studies for benzyl cinnamate are summarized in table 3.18.3. More detailed information can be found in the corresponding text following the table. The percentage of products in which benzyl cinnamate was found to be present ranges from 0.5% to 11%, but the higher frequencies were found in studies with few investigated products only. In general, it may be assumed, that benzyl cinnamate is infrequently used in fragrances.

Table 3.18.3 Presence of benzyl cinnamate in products [a]

Year	Country	Product type	Nr. investigated	Nr. of products positive [b]	(%)	Method [c]	Ref.
2015-6	Denmark	Fragranced cosmetic products	5588		(0.6%)	Labeling	11
2015	Germany	Household detergents	817	1	(0.1%)	Labeling	32
2008-11	Germany	Deodorants	374	7	(2%)	Labeling	24
2006-9	Germany	Cosmetic products	4991		(0.8%)	Labeling	10
2008	Belgium	Fragranced topical pharmaceutical products	370	2	(0.5%)	Labeling	3
2007	Netherlands	Cosmetic products for children	23	1	(4%)	Analysis	15
2006	UK	Perfumed cosmetic and household products	300	10	(3%)	Labeling	9
2006	Denmark	Popular perfumed deodorants	88	3	(3%)	Labeling	12
			23	2	(9%)	Analysis	
2006	Denmark	Rinse-off cosmetics for children	208	6	(3%)	Labeling + analysis	14
2002	Denmark	Home and car air fresheners	19	2	(11%)	Analysis	16

[a] See the corresponding text below for more details
[b] positive = containing the target fragrance
[c] Labeling: information from the ingredient labels on the product / packaging; Analysis: chemical analysis, most often GC-MS

In Denmark, in 2015-2016, 5588 fragranced cosmetic products were examined with a smartphone application for the 26 fragrances that need to be labeled in the EU. Benzyl cinnamate was present in 0.6% of the products (rank number 21) (11).

In Germany, in 2015, fragrance allergens were evaluated based on lists of ingredients in 817 (unique) detergents (all-purpose cleaners, cleaning preparations for special purposes [e.g. bathroom, kitchen, dish-washing] and laundry detergents) present in 131 households. Benzyl cinnamate was found to be present in 1 (0.1%) of the products (32).

In 2008, 2010 and 2011, 374 deodorants available in German retail shops were randomly selected and their labels checked for the presence of the 26 fragrances that need to be labeled. Benzyl cinnamate was found to be present in 7 (1.9%) of the products (24).

In Germany, in the period 2006-2009, 4991 cosmetic products were randomly sampled for an official investigation of conformity of cosmetic products with legal provisions. The labels were inspected for the presence of the 26 fragrances that need to be labeled in the EU. Benzyl cinnamate was present in 0.8% of the products (rank number 23) (10).

In 2008, 66 different fragrance components (including 39 essential oils) were identified in 370 (10% of the total) topical pharmaceutical products marketed in Belgium; 2 of these (0.5%) contained benzyl cinnamate (3).

In 2007, in The Netherlands, twenty-three cosmetic products for children were analyzed for the presence of fragrances that need to be labeled. Benzyl cinnamate was identified in one of the products (4%) in a concentration of 21 ppm (15).

In 2006, the labels of 208 cosmetics for children (especially shampoos, body shampoos and soaps) available in Denmark were checked for the presence of the 26 fragrances that need to be labeled in the EU. Benzyl cinnamate was present in 6 products (2.9%), and ranked number 19 in the frequency list (14).

In 2006, of 88 popular perfume containing deodorants purchased in Denmark, 3 (3%) were labeled to contain benzyl cinnamate. Analysis of 24 regulated fragrance substances in 23 selected deodorants (19 spray products, 2 deostick and 2 roll-on) was performed by GC-MS. Benzyl cinnamate was identified in 2 of the products (9%) with a concentration range of 74–143 ppm (12).

In January 2006, a study of perfumed cosmetic and household products available on the shelves of U.K. retailers was carried out. Products were included if 'parfum' or 'aroma' was listed among the ingredients. Three hundred products were surveyed and any of 26 mandatory labeling fragrances named on the label were recorded. Benzyl cinnamate was present in 10 (3%) of the products (rank number 22) (9).

In 2002, in Denmark, 19 air fresheners (6 for cars, 13 for homes) were analyzed for the presence of fragrances that need to be labeled on cosmetics. Benzyl cinnamate was found to be present in 2 products (11%) in a concentration range of 170-500 ppm and ranked 21 in the frequency list (16).

LITERATURE

1 Bruze M, Svedman C, Andersen KE, Bruynzeel D, Goossens A, Johansen JD, et al. Patch test concentrations (doses in mg/cm2) for the 12 non-mix fragrance substances regulated by European legislation. Contact Dermatitis 2012;66:131-136

2 Heisterberg MV, Menné T, Johansen JD. Contact allergy to the 26 specificc fragrance ingredients to be declared on cosmetic products in accordance with the EU cosmetic directive. Contact Dermatitis 2011;65:266-275

3 Nardelli A, D'Hooge E, Drieghe J, Dooms M, Goossens A. Allergic contact dermatitis from fragrance components in specific topical pharmaceutical products in Belgium. Contact Dermatitis 2009;60:303-313

4 Schnuch A, Uter W, Geier J, Lessmann H, Frosch PJ. Sensitization to 26 fragrances to be labelled according to current European regulation: Results of the IVDK and review of the literature. Contact Dermatitis 2007;57:1-10

5 Hausen BM. Contact allergy to Balsam of Peru. II. Patch test results in 102 patients with selected Balsam of Peru constituents. Am J Contact Derm 2001;12:93-102

6 Wöhrl S, Hemmer W, Focke M, Götz M, Jarisch R. The significance of fragrance mix, balsam of Peru, colophony and propolis as screening tools in the detection of fragrance allergy. Br J Dermatol 2001;145:268-273

7 Various SCCS opinions on benzyl cinnamate have been published and are available at: http://ec.europa.eu/growth/tools-databases/cosing/index.cfm?fuseaction=search.details_v2&id=27930

8 SCCS (Scientific Committee on Consumer Safety). Opinion on Fragrance allergens in cosmetic products, 26-27 June 2012, SCCS/1459/11. Available at: https://ec.europa.eu/health/sites/health/files/scientific_committees/consumer_safety/docs/sccs_o_102.pdf

9 Buckley DA. Fragrance ingredient labelling in products on sale in the UK. Br J Dermatol 2007;157:295-300

10 Uter W, Yazar K, Kratz E-M, Mildau G, Lidén C. Coupled exposure to ingredients of cosmetic products: I. Fragrances. Contact Dermatitis 2013;69:335-341

11 Bennike NH, Oturai NB, Müller S, Kirkeby CS, Jørgensen C, Christensen AB, et al. Fragrance contact allergens in 5588 cosmetic products identified through a novel smartphone application. J Eur Acad Dermatol Venereol 2018;32:79-85

12 Rastogi SC, Hellerup Jensen G, Johansen JD. Survey and risk assessment of chemical substances in deodorants. Survey of Chemical Substances in Consumer Products, No. 86 2007. Danish Ministry of the Environment, Environmental Protection Agency. Available at: https://www2.mst.dk/Udgiv/publications/2007/978-87-7052-625-8/pdf/978-87-7052-626-5.pdf

13 Zaragoza-Ninet V, Blasco Encinas R, Vilata-Corell JJ, Pérez-Ferriols A, Sierra-Talamantes C, Esteve-Martínez A, de la Cuadra-Oyanguren J. Allergic contact dermatitis due to cosmetics: A clinical and epidemiological study in a tertiary hospital. Actas Dermosifiliogr 2016;107:329-336

14 Poulsen PB, Schmidt A. A survey and health assessment of cosmetic products for children. Survey of chemical substances in consumer products, No. 88. Copenhagen: Danish Environmental Protection Agency, 2007.

Available at: https://www2.mst.dk/udgiv/publications/2007/978-87-7052-638-8/pdf/978-87-7052-639-5.pdf

15 VWA. Dutch Food and Consumer Product Safety Authority. Cosmetische producten voor kinderen: Inventarisatie van de markt en de veiligheidsborging door producenten en importeurs. Report ND04o065/ND05o170, 2007 (Report in Dutch), 2007. Available at: www.nvwa.nl/documenten/communicatie/inspectieresultaten/ consument/2016m/cosmetische- producten-voor-kinderen

16 Pors J, Fuhlendorff R. Mapping of chemical substances in air fresheners and other fragrance liberating products. Report Danish Ministry of the Environment, Environmental Protection Agency (EPA). Survey of Chemicals in Consumer Products, No 30, 2003. Available at: http://eng.mst.dk/media/mst/69113/30.pdf

17 Dinkloh A, Worm M, Geier J, Schnuch A, Wollenberg A. Contact sensitization in patients with suspected cosmetic intolerance: results of the IVDK 2006-2011. J Eur Acad Dermatol Venereol 2015;29:1071-1081

18 Bennike NH, Zachariae C, Johansen JD. Non-mix fragrances are top sensitizers in consecutive dermatitis patients – a cross-sectional study of the 26 EU-labelled fragrance allergens. Contact Dermatitis 2017;77:270-279

19 Vejanurug P, Tresukosol P, Sajjachareonpong P, Puangpet P. Fragrance allergy could be missed without patch testing with 26 individual fragrance allergens. Contact Dermatitis 2016;74:230-235

20 Mann J, McFadden JP, White JML, White IR, Banerjee P. Baseline series fragrance markers fail to predict contact allergy. Contact Dermatitis 2014;70:276-281

21 Uter W, Johansen JD, Börje A, Karlberg A-T, Lidén C, Rastogi S, Roberts D, White IR. Categorization of fragrance contact allergens for prioritization of preventive measures: clinical and experimental data and consideration of structure–activity relationships. Contact Dermatitis 2013;69:196-230

22 Nagtegaal MJC, Pentinga SE, Kuik J, Kezic S, Rustemeyer T. The role of the skin irritation response in polysensitization to fragrances. Contact Dermatitis 2012;67:28-35

23 Uter W, Geier J, Frosch P, Schnuch A. Contact allergy to fragrances: current patch test results (2005–2008) from the Information Network of Departments of Dermatology. Contact Dermatitis 2010;63:254-261

24 Klaschka U. Contact allergens for armpits - allergenic fragrances specified on deodorants. Int J Hyg Environ Health 2012;215:584-591

25 Malten KE, van Ketel WG, Nater JP, Liem DH. Reactions in selected patients to 22 fragrance materials. Contact Dermatitis 1984;11:1-10

26 Rudzki E, Grzywa Z. Dermatitis from propolis. Contact Dermatitis 1983;9:40-45

27 Hausen BM, Evers P, Stüwe H-T, König WA, Wollenweber E. Propolis allergy (IV) Studies with further sensitizers from propolis and constituents common to propolis, poplar buds and balsam of Peru. Contact Dermatitis 1992;26:34-44

28 Hjorth N. Eczematous allergy to balsams. Acta Derm Venereol 1961;41(suppl.46):1-216

29 De Groot AC, Popova MP, Bankova VS. An update on the constituents of poplar-type propolis. Wapserveen, The Netherlands: acdegroot publishing, 2014, 11 pages. ISBN/EAN: 978-90-813233-0-7. Available at: https://www.researchgate.net/publication/262851225_AN_UPDATE_ON_THE_CONSTITUENTS_OF_POPLAR-TYPE_PROPOLIS

30 Mitchell JC, Calnan CD, Clendenning WE, Cronin E, Hjorth N, Magnusson B, et al. Patch testing with some components of balsam of Peru. Contact Dermatitis 1976;2:57-58

31 De Groot AC, Schmidt E. Essential oils: contact allergy and chemical composition. Boca Raton, Fl., USA: CRC Press, Taylor and Francis Group, 2016 (ISBN 9781482246407)

32   Wieck S, Olsson O, Kümmerer K, Klaschka U. Fragrance allergens in household detergents. Regul Toxicol Pharmacol 2018;97:163-169

33 Ung CY, White JML, White IR, Banerjee P, McFadden JP. Patch testing with the European baseline series fragrance markers: a 2016 update. Br J Dermatol 2018;178:776-780

34 Oxholm A, Heidenheim M, Larsen E, Batsberg W, Menné T. Extraction and patch testing of methylcinnamate, a newly recognized fraction of balsam of Peru. Dermatitis 1990;1:43-46

35 Silvestre JF, Mercader P, González-Pérez R, Hervella-Garcés M, Sanz-Sánchez T, Córdoba S, et al. Sensitization to fragrances in Spain: A 5-year multicentre study (2011-2015). Contact Dermatitis. 2018 Nov 14. doi: 10.1111/cod.13152. [Epub ahead of print]

Chapter 3.19   BENZYLIDENE ACETONE *
Not an INCI name

IDENTIFICATION

Description/definition : Benzylidene acetone is the aromatic compound that conforms to the structural formula shown below

Chemical class(es) : Aromatic compounds; unsaturated compounds; ketones

INCI name USA : Not in the Personal Care Products Council Ingredient Database

Chemical/IUPAC name : 4-Phenylbut-3-en-2-one

CAS registry number(s) : 122-57-6

EC number(s) : 204-555-1

RIFM monograph(s) : Food Cosmet Toxicol 1973;11:1021

IFRA standard : Prohibited (www.ifraorg.org/en-us/standards-library)

Function(s) in cosmetics : EU: formerly used for perfuming

EU cosmetic restrictions : Regulated in Annex II/356 of the Regulation (EC) No. 1223/2009, regulated by 76/768/EEC; Pohibited since 1976

Patch testing : 0.5% pet. (1)

Molecular formula : $C_{10}H_{10}O$

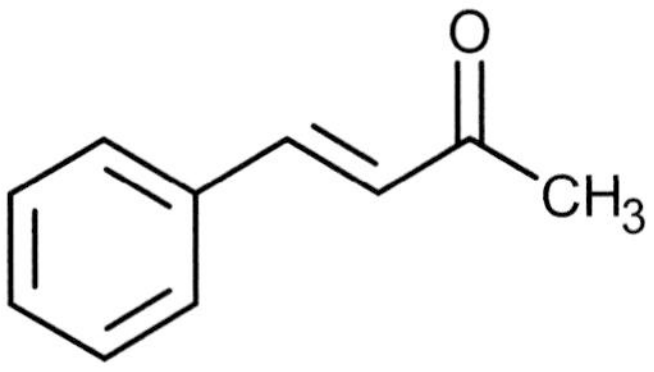

GENERAL

Benzylidene acetone is a white to yellow crystalline solid; its odor type is spicy and its odor at 100% is described as 'sweet, spicy, cinnamon, balsamic, anisyl, powdery and phenolic with jammy, fruity notes' (www.thegoodscents company.com).

Presence in essential oils

Benzylidene acetone has been identified by chemical analysis in none of 91 essential oils, which have caused contact allergy / allergic contact dermatitis (5). It may be present in nature in roasted coffee, soybean and tobacco (www.thegoodscentscompany.com).

CONTACT ALLERGY

General

The sensitizing potency of benzylidene acetone was classified as 'moderate' based on an EC3 value of 3.7% in the LLNA (local lymph node assay) in animal experiments (3,4).

Patch testing in groups of patients

Studies in which benzylidene acetone has been tested in either consecutive patients suspected of contact dermatitis (routine testing) or in groups of selected patients have not been found.

Case reports and case series

A baker had recurrent dyshidrotic eczema of the hands. Routine patch testing was negative, but he reacted to the cinnamon powder he had brought from his work. When tested subsequently with a series of fragrances/flavors, he reacted to benzylidene acetone 0.5%, cinnamyl alcohol 5%, cinnamal 0.5%, cinnamyl benzoate 10% and cinnamyl cinnamate 8%, all in petrolatum. After avoiding skin and mucous membrane contact with cinnamon-containing products and not eating or drinking them, the dermatitis much improved. Another baker with similar symptoms and reacting to cinnamon powder had positive patch tests to the same fragrance materials (including benzylidene acetone) and to methoxycinnamal 4% in petrolatum. The author was 'inclined' to say that these reactions may have been relevant (1).

A man complained of a generalized pruritic eruption of three months' duration. The skin of the trunk and of the extremities was erythematous and excoriated, and that of the axillae, groins, lower part of the abdomen, genitals and hands was particularly involved. The history of the patient revealed that he had been occupied for many years in a cosmetic laboratory preparing creams and the ingredients of these creams were suspected to be the cause of the dermatitis. The patient was advised to avoid contact with the laboratory products. With therapy, the condition gradually improved until a sudden exacerbation of the eruption took place, with severe pruritus, depriving the patient of his sleep. Questioning elicited that the patient did not follow advice strictly. He handled perfume which was incorporated in one of the creams, and it soaked through the cotton gloves which he believed would protect him against contact with the laboratory products. At this time close questioning revealed that the patient had been in the habit, during the past few years, of applying this perfume (jasmine) freely to his skin, particularly in the axillae and groins. Patch tests gave strongly positive reactions to a perfumed cream and (probably) to its jasmine perfume. Later testing revealed that the allergenic culprit was benzylidene acetone, which was added by the manufacturer to the jasmine perfume for the purpose of intensifying its odor (2).

Additional information on contact allergy to benzylidene acetone may be found in ref. 6 (article not read).

LITERATURE

1   Malten KE. Four bakers showing positive patch tests to a number of fragrance materials, which can also be used as flavors. Acta Derm Venereol 1979;59(suppl.85):117-121
2   Bloom D. Eczema venenatum (perfume). Arch Dermatol 1940;42:968-969
3   Uter W, Johansen JD, Börje A, Karlberg A-T, Lidén C, Rastogi S, Roberts D, White IR. Categorization of fragrance contact allergens for prioritization of preventive measures: clinical and experimental data and consideration of structure–activity relationships. Contact Dermatitis 2013;69:196-230
4   SCCS (Scientific Committee on Consumer Safety). Opinion on Fragrance allergens in cosmetic products, 26-27 June 2012, SCCS/1459/11. Available at:
     https://ec.europa.eu/health/sites/health/files/scientific_committees/consumer_safety/docs/sccs_o_102.pdf
5   De Groot AC, Schmidt E. Essential oils: contact allergy and chemical composition. Boca Raton, Fl., USA: CRC Press, Taylor and Francis Group, 2016 (ISBN 9781482246407)
6   Meneghini CL. Cosmetic constituents. Contact Dermatitis Newsletter 1970;8:182

Chapter 3.20   BENZYL ISOEUGENOL

IDENTIFICATION

Description/definition	: Benzyl isoeugenol is the aromatic compound that conforms to the structural formula shown below
Chemical class(es)	: Aromatic compounds; ethers; unsaturated compounds
INCI name USA	: Not in the Personal Care Products Council Ingredient Database
Chemical/IUPAC name	: 2-Methoxy-1-phenylmethoxy-4-prop-1-enylbenzene
Other names	: Isoeugenol benzyl ether
CAS registry number(s)	: 120-11-6
EC number(s)	: 204-370-6
RIFM monograph(s)	: Food Cosmet Toxicol 1973;11:1025
Function(s) in cosmetics	: EU: perfuming
Patch testing	: 1.5% pet. (1); based on RIFM data, 5% pet. is probably not irritant (2)
Molecular formula	: $C_{17}H_{18}O_2$

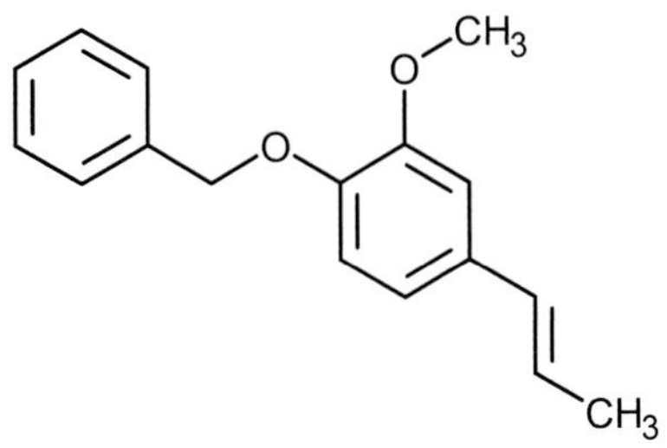

GENERAL

Benzyl isoeugenol is a white to pink crystalline powder; its odor type is spicy and its odor at 100% is described as 'mild spicy balsam carnation' (www.thegoodscentscompany.com). It is a synthetic chemical, not found in nature (and consequently not in essential oils (4)).

CONTACT ALLERGY

Patch testing in groups of patients

In the UK, Denmark, Belgium and Sweden, during 2001-2002, 2261 consecutive patients suspected of contact dermatitis were patch tested with benzyl isoeugenol 1.5% and there were 2 (0.09%) positive reactions. No relevance data were provided. There were no co-reactions to isoeugenol (1).

Case reports and case series
Case reports of allergic contact dermatitis from benzyl isoeugenol have not been found.

Presence in products and chemical analyses
In Denmark, in 2006-2007, 29 hydroalcoholic products of international brands (2 aftershave lotions, 26 eaux de toilette/eaux de parfum [10 for men and 16 for women] and one parfum) were purchased from Danish retail outlets and investigated by GC-MS for the presence of isoeugenol, isoeugenyl acetate, methyl isoeugenol and benzyl isoeugenol. Benzyl isoeugenol was not found in any of the products (3).

LITERATURE

1   Tanaka S, Royds C, Buckley D, Basketter DA, Goossens A, Bruze M, et al. Contact allergy to isoeugenol and its derivatives: problems with allergen substitution. Contact Dermatitis 2004;51:288-291
2   De Groot AC. Patch Testing, 4th Edition. Wapserveen, The Netherlands: acdegroot publishing, 2018 (ISBN 978-90-813233-4-5)
3   Rastogi SC, Johansen JD. Significant exposures to isoeugenol derivates in perfumes. Contact Dermatitis 2008;58:278-281
4   De Groot AC, Schmidt E. Essential oils: contact allergy and chemical composition. Boca Raton, Fl., USA: CRC Press, Taylor and Francis Group, 2016 (ISBN 9781482246407)

Chapter 3.21   BENZYL PROPIONATE

IDENTIFICATION

Description/definition	: Benzyl propionate is the benzyl ester of propanoic acid that conforms to the structural formula shown below
Chemical class(es)	: Aromatic organic compounds; esters
INCI name USA	: Not in the Personal Care Products Council Ingredient Database
Chemical/IUPAC name	: Benzyl propanoate
Other names	: Phenylmethyl propionate; propanoic acid, phenylmethyl ester
CAS registry number(s)	: 122-63-4
EC number(s)	: 204-559-3
RIFM monograph(s)	: Food Chem Toxicol 2016;97(suppl.):S38-S48; Food Chem Toxicol 2012;50(suppl.2):S486-S490; Food Cosmet Toxicol 1975;13:723 (special issue II) (binder, page 140)
Function(s) in cosmetics	: EU: perfuming
Patch testing	: No data available; based on RIFM data, 4% pet. is probably not irritant (2)
Molecular formula	: $C_{10}H_{12}O_2$

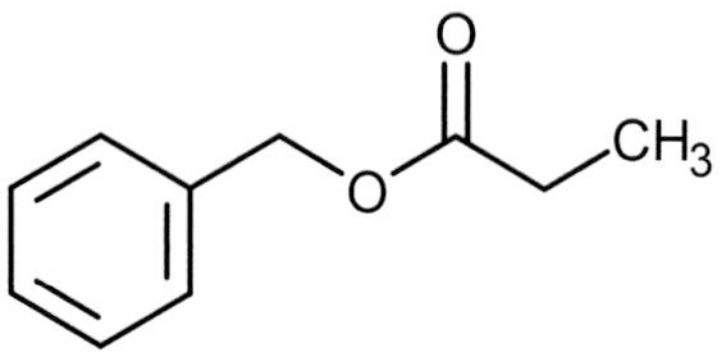

GENERAL

Benzyl propionate is a colorless clear oily liquid; its odor type is fruity and its odor is described as 'sweet, fruity apple and banana, jammy, balsamic, floral with jasmine nuance' (www.thegoodscentscompany.com).

Presence in essential oils

Benzyl propionate has been identified by chemical analysis in 1 of 91 essential oils, which have caused contact allergy / allergic contact dermatitis: rose oil. However, it was found in one old study only, so the question can be raised whether its identification has been correct (1).

CONTACT ALLERGY

Pigmented cosmetic dermatitis

In Japan, in the 1960s and 1970s, many female patients developed pigmentation of the face after having facial dermatitis (5). The skin manifestations of this so-called pigmented cosmetic dermatitis consisted of diffuse or patchy brown hyperpigmentation on the cheeks and/or forehead, sometimes the entire face was involved. In severe cases, the pigmentation was black, purple, or blue-black, and in mild cases, it was pale brown. Occasionally, erythematous macules or papules, suggesting a mild contact dermatitis, were observed and itching was also noted at varying times.

Pigmented cosmetic dermatitis was shown to be caused by contact allergy to components of cosmetic products, notably essential oils, other fragrance materials, antimicrobials, preservatives and coloring materials (4,5,6). In 1973-1974, benzyl propionate was discovered to be one of the causative fragrance materials (3). The number of patients with pigmented cosmetic dermatitis decreased strongly after 1978, when major cosmetic companies began to eliminate strong contact sensitizers from their products (4). Since 1980, pigmented cosmetic dermatitis became a rare disease in Japan (7).

LITERATURE

1   De Groot AC, Schmidt E. Essential oils: contact allergy and chemical composition. Boca Raton, Fl., USA: CRC Press, Taylor and Francis Group, 2016 (ISBN 9781482246407)
2   De Groot AC. Patch Testing, 4th Edition. Wapserveen, The Netherlands: acdegroot publishing, 2018
3   Nakayama H. Fragrance hypersensitivity and its control. In: Frosch PJ, Johansen JD, White IR, Eds. Fragrances - beneficial and adverse effects. Berlin Heidelberg New York: Springer-Verlag, 1998:83-91
4   Nakayama H, Matsuo S, Hayakawa K, Takhashi K, Shigematsu T, Ota S. Pigmented cosmetic dermatitis. Int J Dermatol 1984;23:299-305
5   Nakayama H, Harada R, Toda M. Pigmented cosmetic dermatitis. Int J Dermatol 1976;15:673-675
6   Nakayama H, Hanaoka H, Ohshiro A. Allergen Controlled System. Tokyo: Kanehara Shuppan, 1974
7   Ebihara T, Nakayama H. Pigmented contact dermatitis. Clin Dermatol 1997;15:593-599

Chapter 3.22   BENZYL SALICYLATE

IDENTIFICATION

Description/definition : Benzyl salicylate is the ester of benzyl alcohol and salicylic acid, that conforms to the formula shown below
Chemical class(es) : Esters
Chemical/IUPAC name : Benzyl 2-hydroxybenzoate
CAS registry number(s) : 118-58-1
EC number(s) : 204-262-9
RIFM monograph(s) : Food Chem Toxicol 2007;45(suppl.1):S362-S380 (11); Food Chem Toxicol 2007;45:S318-S361; Food Cosmet Toxicol 1973;11:1029
IFRA standard : Restricted (www.ifraorg.org/en-us/standards-library) (table 3.22.1)
SCCS opinion(s) : Various (39); SCCS/1459/11 (40)
Merck Index monograph : 1144
Function(s) in cosmetics : EU: perfuming; UV-absorber. USA: fragrance ingredients; light stabilizers
EU cosmetic restrictions : Regulated in Annex III/75 of the Regulation (EC) No. 1223/2009, regulated by 2003/15/EC; Must be labeled on cosmetics and detergent products, if present at > 10 ppm (0.001%) in leave-on products and > 100 ppm (0.01%) in rinse-off products
Patch testing : 1% pet. (SmartPracticeEurope, SmartPracticeCanada); 10% pet. (Chemotechnique); recommended test concentration: 10.0% wt./wt. pet. (3)
Molecular formula : $C_{14}H_{12}O_3$

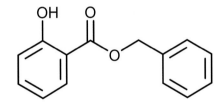

Table 3.22.1 IFRA restrictions for benzyl salicylate

Category [a]	Limits [b]	Category [a]	Limits [b]	Category [a]	Limits [b]
1	0.50%	5	4.20%	9	5.00%
2	0.70%	6	12.80%	10	2.50%
3	2.70%	7	1.30%	11	not restricted
4	8.00%	8	2.00%		

[a] For explanation of categories see pages 6-8
[b] Limits in the finished products

GENERAL

Benzyl salicylate is a colorless to pale yellow clear oily liquid to solid; its odor type is balsamic and its odor at 100% is described as 'balsam clean herbal oily sweet' (www.thegoodscentscompany.com). It is used both as fragrance and as a sunscreen. Benzyl salicylate was the first documented chemical sunscreen to be used in the USA in 1928 (2).

Presence in essential oils and propolis

Benzyl salicylate has been identified by chemical analysis in 7 of 91 essential oils, which have caused contact allergy / allergic contact dermatitis. In one oil, benzyl salicylate belonged to the 'Top-10' of ingredients with the highest concentrations which may be expected in commercial essential oils of this type: ylang-ylang oil (1.2-5.0%) (76). Benzyl salicylate may also be present in propolis (73).

CONTACT ALLERGY

General

The SCCS (Scientific Committee on Consumer Safety), in a 2012 Opinion on Fragrance allergens in cosmetic products, has marked benzyl salicylate as 'established contact allergen in humans' (40,64). The sensitizing potency of benzyl salicylate was classified as 'moderate' based on an EC3 value of 2.9% in the LLNA (local lymph node assay) in animal experiments (40,64).

Patch testing in groups of patients
Results of studies testing benzyl salicylate in consecutive patients suspected of contact dermatitis (routine testing) are shown in table 3.22.2. Results of testing in groups of *selected* patients (e.g. patients with suspected cosmetic intolerance or fragrance sensitivity, individuals with hand eczema) are shown in table 3.22.3.

Patch testing in consecutive patients suspected of contact dermatitis: routine testing
In ten studies in which routine testing with benzyl salicylate was performed, rates of positive reactions have ranged from 0.02% to 2.2%. Seven out of 10 showed frequencies of sensitization of 0.5% or lower. The relevance was not mentioned or specified in 7/10 studies. In the other three investigations, relevance rates ranged from zero to 75%, but the numbers of positive reactions were small. Causative products were usually not mentioned or specified, but in one study, of the relevant reactions to any of 26 fragrances tested, 96% were caused by cosmetic products (4).

Data from Japan
Benzyl salicylate was a frequent cosmetic allergen in Japan in the 1970s and 80s. Prevalences of positive patch test reactions to benzyl salicylate 2% or 5% were observed in 3.3%-8.0% of unselected patients with dermatitis (routine testing): 3.3% (28), 4.0% (17,21), 4.4% (34), 4.8% (16), 5.7% (22), 5.8% (20), 6.5% (14), and 8.0% (25). After efforts to remove benzyl salicylate from cosmetic products in Japan, its prevalence of sensitization dropped in the 1990s in routine testing: 0.8% (31), 1.5% (24), 1.8% (69).

Table 3.22.2 Patch testing in groups of patients: Routine testing

Years and Country	Test conc. & vehicle	Number of patients tested	positive (%)	Selection of patients (S); Relevance (R); Comments (C)	Ref.
2015-7 Netherlands		821	1 (0.1%)	R: not stated	82
2015-2016 UK	1% pet.	2084	3 (0.1%)	R: not specified for individual fragrances; 25% of patients who reacted to any fragrance or fragrance marker had a positive fragrance history	81
2014-2015 USA		600	13 (2.2%)	R: not stated; C: cross-reactions to methyl, phenyl and octyl salicylate	67
2010-2015 Denmark	1% pet.	6004	1 (0.02%)	R: present relevance 0%, past relevance 0%	59
2013-2014 Thailand		312	4 (1.3%)	R: 75%	61
2011-2012 UK	1% pet.	1951	5 (0.3%)	R: not stated	63
2010-2011 China	10% pet.	296	3 (1.0%)	R: 67% for all fragrances tested together (excluding FM I)	62
2008-2010 Denmark	1% pet.	1503	3 (0.2%)	S: mostly routine testing; R: 33%; C: 100% co-reactivity of both FM I and FM II; C: of the relevant reactions to any of the 26 fragrances tested, 96% were caused by cosmetic products	4
2003-2004 IVDK	1% pet.	2041	2 (0.1%)	R: not stated	6
1998-9 Netherlands	2% pet.	1825	10 (0.5%)	R: not stated	13

FM: Fragrance Mix;
IVDK: Informationsverbund Dermatologischer Kliniken (Germany, Switzerland, Austria)

Patch testing in groups of selected patients
Results of studies patch testing benzyl salicylate in groups of selected patients (e.g. patients with suspected cosmetic intolerance or fragrance sensitivity, individuals with hand eczema) are shown in table 3.22.3. In thirteen studies, frequencies of sensitization have ranged from 0.04% to 22%. The highest rate of 22% was seen in a very small group of 9 patients (2 positive reactions) known to be allergic to propolis (which may contain benzyl salicylate) (72). In another small group of 20 patients known to be allergic to fragrances, 2 (10%) reacted to benzyl salicylate (36). Relevance data were mostly absent or inadequate.

Benzyl salicylate has also been tested in patients allergic to Myroxylon pereirae resin (balsam of Peru), which may contain this fragrance (9,75). Frequencies of sensitization were 2.9% (9) and 3.5% (75), indicating that benzyl salicylate is not an important allergen in balsam of Peru,

Data from Japan
Benzyl salicylate was a frequent cosmetic allergen in Japan in the 1970s and 80s. Frequencies in patients suspected of cosmetic dermatitis were 3.2% (15), 3.8% (28), 3.9% (19), 7.7% (34), and 11-25% (32). The highest frequencies of sensitization were observed in women with facial hyperpigmentation (7.8% [18], 13.8% [29], 19.6% [19], 20% [28], 20.8% [37]) termed pigmented cosmetic dermatitis (see the section Pigmented cosmetic dermatitis below). After efforts to remove benzyl salicylate from cosmetic products in Japan, its prevalence of sensitization dropped in the 1990s in patients with cosmetic dermatitis: 0.3% (23), 1.0% (27), 1.9% (26).

Case reports and case series

Benzyl salicylate was stated to be the (or an) allergen in 3 patients in a group of 603 individuals suffering from cosmetic dermatitis, seen in the period 2010-2015 in Leuven, Belgium (57). In the period 1996-2013, in a tertiary referral center in Valencia, Spain, 5419 patients were patch tested. Of these, 628 individuals had allergic contact dermatitis to cosmetics. In this group, benzyl salicylate was the responsible allergen in one case (50).

Table 3.22.3 Patch testing in groups of patients: Selected patient groups

Years and Country	Test conc. & vehicle	Number of patients tested | positive (%)		Selection of patients (S); Relevance (R); Comments (C)	Ref.
2011-2015 Spain	1% or 10% pet.	1013	23 (2.2%)	S: patients previously reacting to FM I, FM II, Myroxylon pereirae resin or hydroxyisohexyl 3-cyclohexene carboxaldehyde in the baseline series and subsequently tested with a fragrance series; R: not stated	84
2011-2015 India	10% pet.	106	6 (5.7%)	S: 74 patient suspected of pigmented cosmetic dermatitis and 32 with suspected allergic cosmetic dermatitis; R: 100%; C: it was not attempted to discriminate 'pigmented cosmetic dermatitis from melasma or other pigmentary disorders	85
2006-2011 IVDK	1% pet.	708	3 (0.4%)	S: patients with suspected cosmetic intolerance; R: not stated	58
2005-10 Netherlands		100	2 (2%)	S: patients with known fragrance sensitivity based on a positive patch test to the FM I and/or the FM II; R: not stated	65
2005-2008 IVDK	1% pet.	3775	(0.04%)	S: not specified; R: not stated	66
2005-7 Netherlands	2% pet.	320	1 (0.3%)	S: patients suspected of fragrance or cosmetic allergy; R: 61% relevance for all positive tested fragrances together	5
2000-2007 USA	2% pet.	870	6 (0.7%)	S: patients who were tested with a supplemental cosmetic screening series; R: 100%; C: weak study: a. high rate of macular erythema and weak reactions; b. relevance figures included 'questionable' and 'past' relevance	7
<2003 Israel		91	2 (2%)	S: patients with a positive or doubtful reaction to the fragrance mix and/or Myroxylon pereirae resin and/or to one or two commercial fine fragrances; R: not stated	51
2001-2 Denmark, Sweden	5% pet.	658	2 (0.3%)	S: consecutive patients with hand eczema; R: it was assumed that nearly all positive reactions were of present or past relevance	35
1997-2000 Austria	1% pet.	747	3 (0.4%)	S: patients suspected of fragrance allergy; R: not stated	12
<1996 Japan, Europe, USA	2% pet.	167	8 (4.8%)	S: patients known or suspected to be allergic to fragrances; R: not stated; C: prevalence in Japan 11.6%, USA 2.8% and Europe 1.1%	33
1988-1990 Germany	2% pet.	9	2 (22%)	S: patients allergic to propolis; R: not stated	72
1975 USA	2% pet.	20	2 (10%)	S: fragrance-allergic patients; R: not stated	36
Testing in patients allergic to Myroxylon pereirae resin (balsam of Peru)					
1995-1998 Germany	2% pet.	102	3 (2.9%)	S: patients allergic to balsam of Peru	9
<1976 USA, Canada, Europe		142	5 (3.5%)	S: patients allergic to balsam of Peru	75

FM: Fragrance mix; IVDK: Informationsverbund Dermatologischer Kliniken (Germany, Switzerland, Austria)

Benzyl salicylate was responsible for 1 out of 399 cases of cosmetic allergy where the causal allergen was identified in a study of the NACDG, USA, 1977-1983 (8). Six of 15 patients using a topical product containing trioxsalen and 5% benzyl salicylate for the treatment of vitiligo became sensitized to benzyl salicylate; it was suggested that the sensitization was caused by phototoxic effects of trioxsalen (2). In an early study on fragrances in Denmark, 31 patients reacted to a perfume from a soap. In twenty-six (84%), benzyl salicylate was the allergenic ingredient (1).

A woman had chronic eyelid erythema and swelling with slight pruritus since 11 months. On examination, weak edema and erythema was observed of the upper and lower eyelids, with a bilateral and symmetrical distribution. Patch tests gave a positive patch test to benzyl salicylate 10% pet. only. Within a month after avoidance of all products containing benzyl salicylate that the patient had contact with (shower gel, deodorant, fabric softener, nail-polish remover, and cologne), the lesions had completely cleared, confirming a diagnosis of allergic contact dermatitis caused by benzyl salicylate (38).

A woman presented with a 2-month history of a rash on her face and around the eyes. Scaly erythematous plaques affecting the upper and lower eyelids and extending to both infraorbital regions were found. Patch test results were positive for benzyl salicylate 10% pet. The patient had come into contact with a hair conditioner and a shampoo that contained this component. After avoidance of these hair products, the lesions disappeared completely (78).

Pigmented cosmetic dermatitis

In Japan, in the 1960s and 1970s, many female patients developed pigmentation of the face after having facial dermatitis (70,71). The skin manifestations of this so-called pigmented cosmetic dermatitis consisted of diffuse or patchy brown hyperpigmentation on the cheeks and/or forehead, sometimes the entire face was involved. In severe cases, the pigmentation was black, purple, or blue-black, and in mild cases, it was pale brown. Occasionally, erythematous macules or papules, suggesting a mild contact dermatitis, were observed and itching was also noted at varying times.

Pigmented cosmetic dermatitis was shown to be caused by contact allergy to components of cosmetic products, notably essential oils, other fragrance materials, antimicrobials, preservatives and coloring materials (32,37,70). In a group of 620 Japanese patients with this condition and non-pigmented recurrent cosmetic dermatitis investigated between 1970 and 1980, 11-25 % had positive patch test reactions to benzyl salicylate 5% in petrolatum in various time periods versus 0-1% in a group of 477 patients with non-cosmetic dermatitis (32). In other studies (possibly some overlap with ref. 32), there were also high frequencies of sensitization to benzyl salicylate in women with facial hyperpigmentation (7.8% [18], 13.8% [29], 19.6% [19], 20% [28], and 20.8% [37]).

The number of patients with pigmented cosmetic dermatitis decreased strongly after 1978, when major cosmetic companies began to eliminate strong contact sensitizers from their products (32,71). Nevertheless, in the mid-1990s, in patients known or suspected to be allergic to fragrances, a rate of 11.6% positive reactions (5/43) to benzyl salicylate was still observed (33).

Recently, in Israel, a male patient was described who had pigmented cosmetic dermatitis from benzyl salicylate in his aftershave (77). In 2013, a woman was reported from Singapore to have developed pigmented cosmetic dermatitis from benzyl salicylate in a facewash. She reacted to both benzyl salicylate and to the facewash containing this fragrance; both patch tests showed pigmentation (80).

Cross-reactions, pseudo-cross-reactions and co-reactions

For general information on cross-/pseudo-cross-/co-reactivity of fragrance chemicals with other fragrances, fragrance markers (fragrance mix I, fragrance mix II, colophonium, Myroxylon pereirae resin [balsam of Peru]) and essential oils see Chapter 1.2 General information on cross-reactions, pseudo-cross-reactions and co-reactions.

Co- or cross-reactions may be observed to methyl salicylate (67), phenyl salicylate (67), octyl salicylate (67) and hexyl salicylate (74).

In Denmark, at the end of the 1960s, an epidemic of contact dermatitis presenting as textile dermatitis occurred in Denmark from contact allergy to Tinopal CH3566 ®, an optical whitener in washing powder. Of 88 allergic individuals who were tested with benzyl salicylate 5% pet. (which was at that time present in the routine series), 16 (18%) showed positive reactions to benzyl salicylate. Although the authors stated that 'the importance of the reactions to benzyl salicylate is uncertain', benzyl salicylate was at that time widely used in toilet soaps (1) and washing powders, so co-exposure and simultaneous or successive sensitization to the optical whitener and the fragrance may be the likely explanation (68).

Presence in products and chemical analyses

In various studies, the presence of benzyl salicylate in cosmetic and sometimes other products has been investigated. Before 2006, most investigators used chemical analysis, usually GC-MS, for qualitative and quantitative determination. Since then, the presence of the target fragrances was usually investigated by screening the product labels for the 26 fragrances that must be labeled since 2005 on cosmetics and detergent products in the EU, if present at > 10 ppm (0.001%) in leave-on products and > 100 ppm (0.01%) in rinse-off products. This method, obviously, is less accurate and may result in underestimation of the frequency of the fragrances being present in the product. When they are in fact present, but the concentration is lower than mentioned above, labeling is not required and the fragrances' presence will be missed.

The results of the relevant studies for benzyl salicylate are summarized in table 3.22.4. More detailed information can be found in the corresponding text following the table. The percentage of products in which benzyl salicylate was found to be present shows wide variations, which can among other be explained by the selection procedure of the products, the method of investigation (false-negatives with information obtained from labels only) and changes in the use of individual fragrance materials over time (fashion).

Table 3.22.4 Presence of benzyl salicylate in products [a]

Year	Country	Product type	Nr. investigated	Nr. of products positive [b]	(%)	Method [c]	Ref.
2015-6	Denmark	Fragranced cosmetic products	5588		(18%)	Labeling	48
2015	Germany	Household detergents	817	86	(11%)	Labeling	79
2015	Sweden	Oxidative hair dye products	26	6	(23%)	Labeling	60
		Non-oxidative	35	4	(11%)	Labeling	
2006-9	Germany	Cosmetic products	4991		(12%)	Labeling	47
2008	Sweden	Cosmetic products	204		(16%)	Labeling	41
		Detergents	97		(2%)	Labeling	
2007	Netherlands	Cosmetic products for children	23	6	(26%)	Analysis	53
2006	UK	Perfumed cosmetic and household products	300	114	(38%)	Labeling	45
2006	Denmark	Popular perfumed deodorants	88	35	(40%)	Labeling	49
			23	11	(48%)	Analysis	
2006	Netherlands	Laundry detergents	52	14	(27%)	Labeling + analysis	55
2006	Denmark	Rinse-off cosmetics for children	208	20	(10%)	Labeling + analysis	52
2002	Denmark	Home and car air fresheners	19	10	(53%)	Analysis	56
2001	Denmark	Non-cosmetic consumer products	43	9	(21%)	Analysis	54
2000	Denmark, UK, Germany, Italy	Domestic and occupational products	59	5	(8%)	Analysis	42
1997-8	Denmark, UK Germany, Sweden	Cosmetics and cosmetic toys for children	25	5	(20%)	Analysis	43
1996	Five European countries	Fragranced deodorants	70	34	(49%)	Analysis	30
1992	Netherlands	Cosmetic products	300		(43%)	Analysis	46
1988	USA	Perfumes used in fine fragrances, household products and soap	400	25-74% (See text)		Analysis	44

[a] See the corresponding text below for more details
[b] positive = containing the target fragrance
[c] Labeling: information from the ingredient labels on the product / packaging; Analysis: chemical analysis, most often GC-MS

In Denmark, in 2015-2016, 5588 fragranced cosmetic products were examined with a smartphone application for the 26 fragrances that need to be labeled in the EU. Benzyl salicylate was present in 18% of the products (rank number 8) (48).

In Sweden, in 2015, contact allergens were identified on the ingredient labels of 26 oxidative hair dye products (from 4 different product series) and on the labels of 35 non-oxidative hair dye products (from 5 different product series, including so-called herbal hair colors). These products were selected on the basis of being advertised as 'organic', 'natural', or similar, or used in hairdressing salons branded with such attributes. Benzyl salicylate was present in 6 (23%) of the 26 oxidative hair dyes and in four (11%) of the 35 non-oxidative hair dye products (60).

In Germany, in 2015, fragrance allergens were evaluated based on lists of ingredients in 817 (unique) detergents (all-purpose cleaners, cleaning preparations for special purposes [e.g. bathroom, kitchen, dish-washing] and laundry detergents) present in 131 households. Benzyl salicylate was found to be present in 86 (11%) of the products (79).

In Germany, in the period 2006-2009, 4991 cosmetic products were randomly sampled for an official investigation of conformity of cosmetic products with legal provisions. The labels were inspected for the presence of the 26 fragrances that need to be labeled in the EU. Benzyl salicylate was present in 12% of the products (rank number 7) (47).

Benzyl salicylate was present (as indicated by labeling) in 16% of 204 cosmetic products (92 shampoos, 61 hair conditioners, 34 liquid soaps, 17 wet tissues) and in 2% of 97 detergents in Sweden, 2008 (41).

In 2007, in The Netherlands, twenty-three cosmetic products for children were analyzed for the presence of fragrances that need to be labeled. Benzyl salicylate was identified in 6 of the products (26%) in a concentration range of 28-2123 ppm (53).

In 2006, the labels of 208 cosmetics for children (especially shampoos, body shampoos and soaps) available in Denmark were checked for the presence of the 26 fragrances that need to be labeled in the EU. Benzyl salicylate was present in 20 products (9.6%), and ranked number 6 in the frequency list (52).

In 2006, of 88 popular perfume containing deodorants purchased in Denmark, 35 (40%) were labeled to contain benzyl salicylate. Analysis of 24 regulated fragrance substances in 23 selected deodorants (19 spray products, 2 deostick and 2 roll-on) was performed by GC-MS. Benzyl salicylate was identified in 11 of the products (48%) with a concentration range of 136-5279 ppm (49).

In 2006, in The Netherlands, 52 laundry detergents were investigated for the presence of allergenic fragrances by checking their labels and chemical analyses. Benzyl salicylate was found to be present in 14 of the products (27%) in a concentration range of 24-448 ppm. Benzyl salicylate had rank number 8 in the frequency list (55).

In January 2006, a study of perfumed cosmetic and household products available on the shelves of U.K. retailers was carried out. Products were included if 'parfum' or 'aroma' was listed among the ingredients. Three hundred products were surveyed and any of 26 mandatory labeling fragrances named on the label were recorded. Benzyl salicylate was present in 114 (38%) of the products (rank number 7) (45).

In 2002, in Denmark, 19 air fresheners (6 for cars, 13 for homes) were analyzed for the presence of fragrances that need to be labeled on cosmetics. Benzyl salicylate was found to be present in 10 products (53%) in a concentration range of 4-13,000 ppm and ranked 8 in the frequency list (56).

In 2001, in Denmark, 43 non-cosmetic consumer products (mainly dish-washing products, laundry detergents, and hard and soft surface cleaners) were analyzed for the 26 fragrances that are regulated for labeling in the EU. Benzyl salicylate was present in 9 products (21%) in a concentration range of 0.0069-0.0587% (m/m) and had rank number 10 in the frequency list (54).

In 2000, fifty-nine domestic and occupational products, purchased in retail outlets in Denmark, England, Germany and Italy were analyzed by GC-MS for the presence of fragrances. The product categories were liquid soap and soap bars (n=13), soft/hard surface cleaners (n=23), fabric conditioners/laundry detergents for hand wash (n=8), dish-wash (n=10), furniture polish, car shampoo, stain remover (each n=1) and 2 products used in occupational environments. Benzyl salicylate was present in 5 products (8%) with a mean concentration of 801 ppm and a range of 293-1614 ppm (42).

Twenty-five cosmetics and cosmetic toys for children (5 shampoos and shower gels, 6 perfumes, 1 deodorant (roll-on), 4 baby lotions/creams, 1 baby wipes product, 1 baby oil, 2 lipcare products and 5 toy-cosmetic products: a cosmetic-toy set for blending perfumes and a makeup set) purchased in 1997-1998 in retail outlets in Denmark, Germany, England and Sweden were analyzed in 1998 for the presence of fragrances by GC-MS. Benzyl salicylate was found in 5 products (20%) in a concentration range of ≤0.001-0.081% (w/w). For the analytical data in each product category, the original publication should be consulted (43).

Seventy fragranced deodorants, purchased at retail outlets in 5 European countries in 1996, were analyzed by gas chromatography - mass spectrometry (GC-MS) for the determination of the contents of 21 commonly used fragrance materials. Benzyl salicylate was identified in 34 products (49%) in a concentration range of 1–18758 ppm (30).

In 1992, in The Netherlands, the presence of fragrances was analyzed in 300 cosmetic products. Benzyl salicylate was identified in 43% of the products (rank order 16) (46).

In 1988, in the USA, 400 perfumes used in fine fragrances, household products and soaps (number of products per category not mentioned) were analyzed for the presence of fragrance chemicals in a concentration of at least 1% and a list of the Top-25 (present in the highest number of products) presented. Benzyl salicylate was found to be present in 74% of the fine fragrances (rank number 5), 25% of the household product fragrances (rank number 18) and 40% of the fragrances used in soaps (rank number 17) (44).

OTHER SIDE EFFECTS

Systemic side effects

Benzyl salicylate has obvious *in vitro* and *in vivo* estrogenic activity; combined with exposure in foods, the dermal exposure of benzyl salicylate in fragrances and other cosmetics may, according to some authors, be a risk for high-volume users (10).

LITERATURE

1 Rothenborg HW, Hjorth N. Allergy to perfumes from toilet soaps and detergents in patients with dermatitis. Arch Dermatol 1968;97:417-421

2 Kahn G. Intensified contact sensitization to benzyl salicylate. Phototoxic effects of topical psoralen therapy. Arch Dermatol 1971;103:497-500

3 Bruze M, Svedman C, Andersen KE, Bruynzeel D, Goossens A, Johansen JD, et al. Patch test concentrations (doses in mg/cm2) for the 12 non-mix fragrance substances regulated by European legislation. Contact Dermatitis 2012;66:131-136

4 Heisterberg MV, Menné T, Johansen JD. Contact allergy to the 26 specific fragrance ingredients to be declared on cosmetic products in accordance with the EU cosmetic directive. Contact Dermatitis 2011;65:266-275

5 Oosten EJ van, Schuttelaar ML, Coenraads PJ. Clinical relevance of positive patch test reactions to the 26 EU-labelled fragrances. Contact Dermatitis 2009;61:217-223

6 Schnuch A, Uter W, Geier J, Lessmann H, Frosch PJ. Sensitization to 26 fragrances to be labelled according to current European regulation: Results of the IVDK and review of the literature. Contact Dermatitis 2007;57:1-10

7 Wetter DA, Yiannias JA, Prakash AV, Davis MDP, Farmer SA, el-Azhary RA. Results of patch testing to personal care product allergens in a standard series and a supplemental cosmetic series: an analysis of 945 patients from the Mayo Clinic Contact Dermatitis Group, 2000-2007. J Am Acad Dermatol 2010;63:789-798

8 Adams RM, Maibach HI, for the North American Contact Dermatitis Group. A five-year study of cosmetic reactions. J Am Acad Dermatol 1985;13:1062-1069

9 Hausen BM. Contact allergy to Balsam of Peru. II. Patch test results in 102 patients with selected Balsam of Peru constituents. Am J Contact Derm 2001;12:93-102

10 Zhang Z, Ja C, Hu Y, et al. The estrogenic potential of salicylate esters and their possible risks in foods and cosmetics. Toxicol Lett 2012;209:146-153

11 Lapczynski A, McGinty D, Jones L, Bhatia S, Letizia CS, Api AM. Fragrance material review on benzyl salicylate. Food Chem Toxicol 2007;45(suppl.1):S362-S380

12 Wöhrl S, Hemmer W, Focke M, Götz M, Jarisch R. The significance of fragrance mix, balsam of Peru, colophony and propolis as screening tools in the detection of fragrance allergy. Br J Dermatol 2001;145:268-273

13 De Groot AC, Coenraads PJ, Bruynzeel DP, Jagtman BA, van Ginkel CJ, Noz K, et al. Routine patch testing with fragrance chemicals in The Netherlands. Contact Dermatitis 2000;42:184-185

14 Asoh S, Sugai T, Yamamoto S, Watanabe K, Okuno F. The incidence of positive reactions to fragrance materials in patch tests and four representative cases with fragrance dermatitis in 1982. Skin Research 1985;25:707-715 (article in Japanese) . Data cited in ref. 11

15 Hayakawa R. Japan Patch Test Research Group. Patch test positive rates of cosmetic ingredients in 1984. Skin Research 1986;28:93-100 (article in Japanese) . Data cited in ref. 11

16 Sugai T. A proposal to the determination of standard test series for patch testing in Japan. Skin Research 1986;28:66-72 (article in Japanese) . Data cited in ref. 11

17 Itoh M, Hosono K, Kantoh H, et al. Patch test results with cosmetic ingredients conducted between 1978 and 1986. J Soc Cosmet Sc 1988;12:27-41. . Data cited in ref. 11

18 Itoh M. Sensitization potency of some phenolic compounds – with special emphasis on the relationship between chemical structure and allergenicity. J Dermatol 1982;9:223-233

19 Ishihara M, Itoh S, Hayashi S, Satake T. Methods of diagnosis in cases of cosmetic dermatitis and facial melanosis in females. Nishinihon Journal of Dermatology 1979;41:426-439 (article in Japanese) . Data cited in ref. 11

20 MJDRG Mid-Japan Contact Dermatitis Research Group, 1984. Determination of suitable concentrations for patch testing of various fragrance materials. A summary of group study conducted over a 6-year period. J Dermatol 1984;11:31-35

21 Itoh M, Ishihara M, Hosono K, et al. Results of patch tests conducted between 1978 and 1985 using cosmetic ingredients. Skin Research 1986;28:110-119 (article in Japanese) . Data cited in ref. 11

22 Hada SC. Standardization of fragrant allergens in patch tests. VI. Studies on the suitable concentration of cinnamic alcohol and cinnamic aldehyde and frequency of sensitivity of benzyl salicylate. Skin Research 1983;25:608-612 (article in Japanese) . Data cited in ref. 11

23 Sugai T. Cosmetic skin diseases in 1994. Environ Dermatol 1996;3:1-7 (article in Japanese) . Data cited in ref. 11

24 Kozuka T, Hayashi H, Hiroyama H, et al. Allergenicity of fragrance materials: Collaborative study of the Second Research Group of the Japanese Society for Cutaneous Health. Environ Dermatol 1996;3:326-335 (article in Japanese) . Data cited in ref. 11

25 Shoji A. Standardization of fragrant allergens in patch tests. V. Studies on the suitable concentration of eugenol and *trans*-isoeugenol, and frequency of sensitivity of benzyl salicylate. Skin Research 1982;24:499-505 (article in Japanese) . Data cited in ref. 11

26   Fujimoto M, Higashi N, Kume, A, et al. Patch test results in 332 patients suspected of cosmetic dermatitis. Environ Dermatol 1997;4:268-276 (article in Japanese) . Data cited in ref. 11

27   Katoh J, Sugai T, Syoji A, Nagareda T, Kuwano A. Multiple sensitizations from fragrance materials during the last one and a half year period at the Osaka Kaisei Hospital. Environ Dermatol 1995;2:178-184 (article in Japanese) . Data cited in ref. 11

28   Nishimura M, Ishihara M, Itoh M, et al. Results of patch tests on cosmetic ingredients conducted between 1979 and 1982. Skin Research 1984;26:945-954 (article in Japanese)

29   Hayakawa R, Ohiwa K, Ukei C, Matsunaga K. Melanosis faciei feminae in 1982. Skin Research 1983;25:690-695 (article in Japanese) . Data cited in ref. 11

30   Rastogi SC, Johansen JD, Frosch P, Menné T, Bruze M, Lepoittevin JP, et al. Deodorants on the European market: quantitative chemical analysis of 21 fragrances. Contact Dermatitis 1998;38:29-35

31   Nagareda T, Sugai T, Shoji A, et al. Incidence of positive reactions to cosmetic products and their ingredients in patch tests and a representative case of cosmetic dermatitis in 1993. Environ Dermatol 1996;3:16-24 (article in Japanese) . Data cited in ref. 11

32   Nakayama H, Matsuo S, Hayakawa K et al. Pigmented cosmetic dermatitis. Int J Dermatol 1984;23:299-305

33   Larsen W, Nakayama H, Lindberg M et al. Fragrance contact dermatitis: A worldwide multicenter investigation (Part 1). Am J Cont Derm 1996;7:77-83

34   Ishihara M, Itoh M, Hosono K, Nishimura M. Some problems with patch tests using fragrance materials. Skin Research 1981;23:808-917 (article in Japanese) (bibliographical data probably incorrect [page numbering]) . Data cited in ref. 11

35   Heydorn S, Johansen JD, Andersen KE, Bruze M, Svedman C, White IR, et al. Fragrance allergy in patients with hand eczema – a clinical study. Contact Dermatitis 2003;48:317-323

36   Larsen WG. Perfume dermatitis. A study of 20 patients. Arch Dermatol 1977;113:623-626

37   Nakayama H, Hanaoka H, Ohshiro A. Allergen Controlled System. Tokyo: Kanehara Shuppan, 1974:42

38   Fernández-Canga P, Ruíz-González I, Varas-Meis E, Valladares-Narganes LM, Rodríguez-Prieto MA. Contact allergy to benzyl salicylate. Contact Dermatitis 2017;76:315-316

39   Various SCCS opinions on benzyl salicylate have been published and are available at: http://ec.europa.eu/growth/tools-databases/cosing/index.cfm?fuseaction=search.details_v2&id=28326

40   SCCS (Scientific Committee on Consumer Safety). Opinion on Fragrance allergens in cosmetic products, 26-27 June 2012, SCCS/1459/11. Available at: https://ec.europa.eu/health/sites/health/files/scientific_committees/consumer_safety/docs/sccs_o_102.pdf

41   Yazar K, Johnsson S, Lind M-L, Boman A, Lidén C. Preservatives and fragrances in selected consumer-available cosmetics and detergents. Contact Dermatitis 2011;64:265-272

42   Rastogi SC, Heydorn S, Johansen JD, Basketter DA. Fragrance chemicals in domestic and occupational products. Contact Dermatitis 2001;45:221-225

43   Rastogi SC, Johansen JD, Menné T, Frosch P, Bruze M, Andersen KE, et al. Content of fragrance allergens in children's cosmetics and cosmetic toys. Contact Dermatitis 1999;41:84-88

44   Fenn RS. Aroma chemical usage trends in modern perfumery. Perfumer and Flavorist 1989;14:3-10

45   Buckley DA. Fragrance ingredient labelling in products on sale in the UK. Br J Dermatol 2007;157:295-300

46   Weyland JW. Personal Communication, 1992. Cited in: De Groot AC, Weyland JW, Nater JP. Unwanted effects of cosmetics and drugs used in dermatology, 3rd Ed. Amsterdam: Elsevier, 1994: 579

47   Uter W, Yazar K, Kratz E-M, Mildau G, Lidén C. Coupled exposure to ingredients of cosmetic products: I. Fragrances. Contact Dermatitis 2013;69:335-341

48   Bennike NH, Oturai NB, Müller S, Kirkeby CS, Jørgensen C, Christensen AB, et al. Fragrance contact allergens in 5588 cosmetic products identified through a novel smartphone application. J Eur Acad Dermatol Venereol 2018;32:79-85

49   Rastogi SC, Hellerup Jensen G, Johansen JD. Survey and risk assessment of chemical substances in deodorants. Survey of Chemical Substances in Consumer Products, No. 86 2007. Danish Ministry of the Environment, Environmental Protection Agency. Available at: https://www2.mst.dk/Udgiv/publications/2007/978-87-7052-625-8/pdf/978-87-7052-626-5.pdf

50   Zaragoza-Ninet V, Blasco Encinas R, Vilata-Corell JJ, Pérez-Ferriols A, Sierra-Talamantes C, Esteve-Martínez A, de la Cuadra-Oyanguren J. Allergic contact dermatitis due to cosmetics: A clinical and epidemiological study in a tertiary hospital. Actas Dermosifiliogr 2016;107:329-336

51   Trattner A, David M. Patch testing with fine fragrances: comparison with fragrance mix, balsam of Peru and a fragrance series. Contact Dermatitis 2003:49:287-289

52 Poulsen PB, Schmidt A. A survey and health assessment of cosmetic products for children. Survey of chemical substances in consumer products, No. 88. Copenhagen: Danish Environmental Protection Agency, 2007. Available at: https://www2.mst.dk/udgiv/publications/2007/978-87-7052-638-8/pdf/978-87-7052-639-5.pdf

53 VWA. Dutch Food and Consumer Product Safety Authority. Cosmetische producten voor kinderen: Inventarisatie van de markt en de veiligheidsborging door producenten en importeurs. Report ND04o065/ND05o170, 2007 (Report in Dutch), 2007. Available at: www.nvwa.nl/documenten/communicatie/inspectieresultaten/consument/2016m/cosmetische- producten-voor-kinderen (in Dutch)

54 Rastogi SC. Survey of chemical compounds in consumer products. Contents of selected fragrance materials in cleaning products and other consumer products. Survey no. 8-2002. Copenhagen, Denmark, Danish Environmental Protection Agency. Available at: http://eng.mst.dk/media/mst/69131/8.pdf

55 Bouma K, Van Peursem AJJ. Marktonderzoek naleving detergenten verordening voor textielwasmiddelen. Dutch Food and Consumer Products Safety Authority (VWA) Report ND06K173, 2006 [in Dutch]. Available at: http://docplayer.nl/41524125-Marktonderzoek-naleving-detergenten-verordening-voor-textielwasmiddelen.html (in Dutch)

56 Pors J, Fuhlendorff R. Mapping of chemical substances in air fresheners and other fragrance liberating products. Report Danish Ministry of the Environment, Environmental Protection Agency (EPA). Survey of Chemicals in Consumer Products, No 30, 2003. Available at: http://eng.mst.dk/media/mst/69113/30.pdf

57 Goossens A. Cosmetic contact allergens. Cosmetics 2016, 3, 5; doi:10.3390/cosmetics3010005

58 Dinkloh A, Worm M, Geier J, Schnuch A, Wollenberg A. Contact sensitization in patients with suspected cosmetic intolerance: results of the IVDK 2006-2011. J Eur Acad Dermatol Venereol 2015;29:1071-1081

59 Bennike NH, Zachariae C, Johansen JD. Non-mix fragrances are top sensitizers in consecutive dermatitis patients – a cross-sectional study of the 26 EU-labelled fragrance allergens. Contact Dermatitis 2017;77:270-279

60 Thorén S, Yazar K. Contact allergens in 'natural' hair dyes. Contact Dermatitis 2016;74:302-304

61 Vejanurug P, Tresukosol P, Sajjachareonpong P, Puangpet P. Fragrance allergy could be missed without patch testing with 26 individual fragrance allergens. Contact Dermatitis 2016;74:230-235

62 Liu J, Li L-F. Contact sensitization to fragrances other than fragrance mix I in China. Contact Dermatitis 2015;73:252-253

63 Mann J, McFadden JP, White JML, White IR, Banerjee P. Baseline series fragrance markers fail to predict contact allergy. Contact Dermatitis 2014;70:276-281

64 Uter W, Johansen JD, Börje A, Karlberg A-T, Lidén C, Rastogi S, Roberts D, White IR. Categorization of fragrance contact allergens for prioritization of preventive measures: clinical and experimental data and consideration of structure–activity relationships. Contact Dermatitis 2013;69:196-230

65 Nagtegaal MJC, Pentinga SE, Kuik J, Kezic S, Rustemeyer T. The role of the skin irritation response in polysensitization to fragrances. Contact Dermatitis 2012;67:28-35

66 Uter W, Geier J, Frosch P, Schnuch A. Contact allergy to fragrances: current patch test results (2005–2008) from the Information Network of Departments of Dermatology. Contact Dermatitis 2010;63:254-261

67 Scheman A, Te R. Contact allergy to salicylates and cross-reactions. Dermatitis 2017;28:291

68 Osmundsen PE, Alani MD. Contact allergy to an optical whitener, 'CPY', in washing powders. Br J Derm 1971;85:61

69 Nagareda T, Sugai T, Shouji A, Katoh J, Mita T, Utsumi M, et al. Incidence of positive reactions to cosmetic products and their ingredients in patch tests and representative cases with cosmetic dermatitis in 1991. Skin Research 1992;34:176-182 (article in Japanese)

70 Nakayama H, Harada R, Toda M. Pigmented cosmetic dermatitis. Int J Dermatol 1976;15:673-675

71 Ebihara T, Nakayama H. Pigmented contact dermatitis. Clin Dermatol 1997;15:593-599

72 Hausen BM, Evers P, Stüwe H-T, König WA, Wollenweber E. Propolis allergy (IV) Studies with further sensitizers from propolis and constituents common to propolis, poplar buds and balsam of Peru. Contact Dermatitis 1992;26:34-44

73 De Groot AC, Popova MP, Bankova VS. An update on the constituents of poplar-type propolis. Wapserveen, The Netherlands: acdegroot publishing, 2014, 11 pages. ISBN/EAN: 978-90-813233-0-7. Available at: https://www.researchgate.net/publication/262851225_AN_UPDATE_ON_THE_CONSTITUENTS_OF_POPLAR-TYPE_PROPOLIS

74 Belsito D, Bickers D, Bruze M, Calow P, Greim H, Hanifin JM, et al. A toxicologic and dermatologic assessment of salicylates when used as fragrance ingredients. Food Chem Toxicol 2007;45:S318-S361

75 Mitchell JC, Calnan CD, Clendenning WE, Cronin E, Hjorth N, Magnusson B, et al. Patch testing with some components of balsam of Peru. Contact Dermatitis 1976;2:57-58

76 De Groot AC, Schmidt E. Essential oils: contact allergy and chemical composition. Boca Raton, Fl., USA: CRC Press, Taylor and Francis Group, 2016 (ISBN 9781482246407)

77 Zaaroura H, Bergman R, Nevet MJ. Pigmented facial contact dermatitis to benzyl salicylate: A comparative histopathological and immunohistochemical study of the involved skin and the positive patch test site. Am J Dermatopathol 2018 Sep 11. doi: 10.1097/DAD.0000000000001258.

78 Tous-Romero F, Prieto-Barrios M, Andrés-Lencina JJ, de Frutos JO. Allergic contact dermatitis caused by benzyl salicylate in hair products. Contact Dermatitis 2018;1–2. https://doi.org/10.1111/cod.13038

79 Wieck S, Olsson O, Kümmerer K, Klaschka U. Fragrance allergens in household detergents. Regul Toxicol Pharmacol 2018;97:163-169

80 Alagappan U, Tay YK, Lim SP. Pigmented contact dermatitis secondary to benzyl salicylate. Acta Derm Venereol 2013;93:590

81 Ung CY, White JML, White IR, Banerjee P, McFadden JP. Patch testing with the European baseline series fragrance markers: a 2016 update. Br J Dermatol 2018;178:776-780

82 Dittmar D, Schuttelaar MLA. Contact sensitization to hydroperoxides of limonene and linalool: Results of consecutive patch testing and clinical relevance. Contact Dermatitis 2018 Oct 31. doi: 10.1111/cod.13137. [Epub ahead of print]

83 Tous-Romero F, Prieto-Barrios M, Andrés-Lencina JJ, de Frutos JO. Allergic contact dermatitis caused by benzyl salicylate in hair products. Contact Dermatitis 2018;79:310-311

84 Silvestre JF, Mercader P, González-Pérez R, Hervella-Garcés M, Sanz-Sánchez T, Córdoba S, et al. Sensitization to fragrances in Spain: A 5-year multicentre study (2011-2015). Contact Dermatitis. 2018 Nov 14. doi: 10.1111/cod.13152. [Epub ahead of print]

85 Sharma VK, Bhatia R, Yadav CP. Clinical profile and allergens in pigmented cosmetic dermatitis and allergic contact dermatitis to cosmetics in India. Dermatitis 2018;29:264-269

Chapter 3.23   BUTYL ACETATE

IDENTIFICATION

Description/definition	: Butyl acetate is the ester of butyl alcohol and acetic acid, that conforms to the formula shown below
Chemical class(es)	: Esters
Chemical/IUPAC name	: Butyl acetate
CAS registry number(s)	: 123-86-4
EC number(s)	: 204-658-1
CIR review(s)	: J Am Coll Toxicol 1989;8:681-705 (access: www.cir-safety.org/ingredients)
RIFM monograph(s)	: Food Cosmet Toxicol 1979;17:515
Merck Index monograph	: 1535
Function(s) in cosmetics	: EU: masking; solvent. USA: fragrance ingredients; solvents
Patch testing	: 25% in olive oil (2); according to data from RIFM, 4% pet. is probably not irritant (3)
Molecular formula	: $C_6H_{12}O_2$

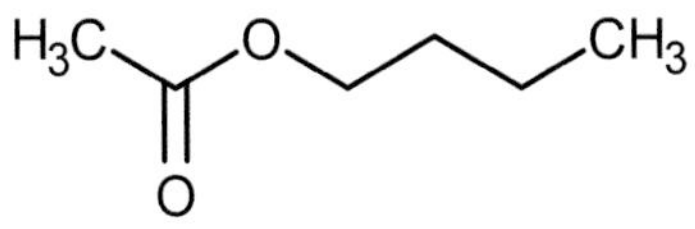

GENERAL

Butyl acetate is a colorless clear liquid; its odor type is ethereal and its odor is described as 'sharp, etherial, diffusive, fruity banana' (www.thegoodscentscompany.com). Butyl acetate is prepared by the slow distillation of butanol and acetic acid in the presence of sulfuric acid (4). Uses of butyl acetate include or have included: in perfumes and as synthetic flavoring ingredient used in producing banana, pear, pineapple and berry flavors; in the manufacture of lacquer, artificial leather, photographic films, plastics and safety glass, in the preservation of foodstuffs; as solvent for gums, resins, lacquer stains, ester-soluble dyes, fats, waxes, cellulose esters, paper coatings and other protective coatings; as dehydrating agent used in processing of oils and pharmaceuticals and as extraction solvent in the manufacture of penicillin (4, U.S. National Library of Medicine).

Presence in essential oils

Butyl acetate has been identified by chemical analysis in seven of 91 essential oils, which have caused contact allergy / allergic contact dermatitis. In none of these, it belonged to the 'Top-10' ingredients (5).

CONTACT ALLERGY

Testing in groups of patients

Studies in which butyl acetate has been tested in either consecutive patients suspected of contact dermatitis (routine testing) or in groups of selected patients have not been found.

Case reports and case series

Butyl acetate was responsible for 1 out of 399 cases of cosmetic allergy where the causal allergen was identified in a study of the NACDG, USA, 1977-1983 (1).

LITERATURE

1   Adams RM, Maibach HI, Clendenning WE, Fisher AA, Jordan WJ, Kanof N, et al. A five-year study of cosmetic reactions. J Am Acad Dermatol 1985;13:1062-1069
2   Fisher's Contact Dermatitis, 6th Edition, 2008; data cited in ref. 3
3   De Groot AC. Patch Testing, 4th Edition. Wapserveen, The Netherlands: acdegroot publishing, 2018 (ISBN 978-90-813233-4-5)
4   Cosmetic Ingredient Review Expert Panel. Final report on the safety assessment of ethyl acetate and butyl acetate. J Am Coll Toxicol 1989;8:681-705
5   De Groot AC, Schmidt E. Essential oils: contact allergy and chemical composition. Boca Raton, Fl., USA: CRC Press, Taylor and Francis Group, 2016 (ISBN 9781482246407)

Chapter 3.24   BUTYLPHENYL METHYLPROPIONAL

IDENTIFICATION

Description/definition	: Butylphenyl methylpropional is the aromatic aldehyde that conforms to the structural formula shown below
Chemical class(es)	: Aldehydes
Chemical/IUPAC name	: 3-(4-*tert*-Butylphenyl)-2-methylpropanal
Other names	: *p-tert*-Butyl-α-methylhydrocinnamic aldehyde; 2-(4-*tert*-butlbenzyl)propionaldehyde; Lilial ®
CAS registry number(s)	: 80-54-6
EC number(s)	: 201-289-8
RIFM monograph(s)	: Food Cosmet Toxicol 1978;16:659 (special issue IV)
IFRA standard	: Restricted (www.ifraorg.org/en-us/standards-library) (table 3.24.1)
SCCS opinion(s)	: SCCS/1591/17, Preliminary version (46); SCCS/1540/14 (7); SCCS/1459/11 (8)
Function(s) in cosmetics	: EU: perfuming. USA: fragrance ingredients
EU cosmetic restrictions	: Regulated in Annex III/83 of the Regulation (EC) No. 1223/2009, regulated by 2003/15/EC; Must be labeled on cosmetics and detergent products, if present at > 10 ppm (0.001%) in leave-on products and > 100 ppm (0.01%) in rinse-off products
Patch testing	: 10% pet. (SmartPracticeEurope, Chemotechnique); recommended test concentration: 10.0% wt./wt. pet. (1)
Molecular formula	: $C_{14}H_{20}O$

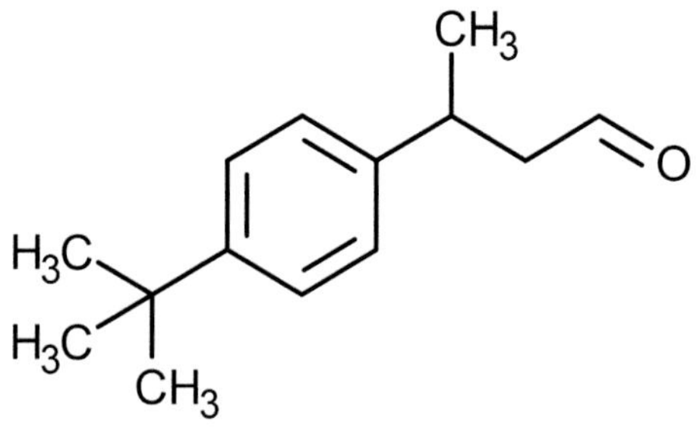

Table 3.24.1 IFRA restrictions for butylphenyl methylpropional

Category [a]	Limits [b]	Category [a]	Limits [b]	Category [a]	Limits [b]
1	0.12%	5	0.98%	9	5.00%
2	0.15%	6	2.97%	10	2.50%
3	0.62%	7	0.31%	11	not restricted
4	1.86%	8	2.00%		

[a] For explanation of categories see pages 6-8
[b] Limits in the finished products

GENERAL

Butylphenyl methylpropional is a colorless to pale yellow clear oily liquid; its odor type is floral and its odor at 100% is described as 'floral muguet watery green powdery cumin' (www.thegoodscentscompany.com). It has repellent activities against the southern house mosquito, *Culex quinquefasciatus*, in laboratory assays (44).

Presence in essential oils

Butylphenyl methylpropional has been identified by chemical analysis in 1 of 91 essential oils, which have caused contact allergy / allergic contact dermatitis: bergamot oil (41). However, butylphenyl methylpropional is a synthetic chemical and is apparently not found in nature (www.thegoodscentscompany.com) and therefore, the analytical identification of this chemical may have been erroneous.

CONTACT ALLERGY

General

The SCCS (Scientific Committee on Consumer Safety), in a 2012 Opinion on Fragrance allergens in cosmetic products, has marked butylphenyl methylpropional as 'established contact allergen in humans' (8,31). The sensitizing potency of butylphenyl methylpropional was classified as 'moderate' based on an EC3 value of 2.9% in the LLNA (local lymph node assay) in animal experiments (8,31). Accordingly, the overall potency classification of butylphenyl methylpropional is a 'moderate sensitizer' (7).

Patch testing in groups of patients

Results of studies testing butylphenyl methylpropional in consecutive patients suspected of contact dermatitis (routine testing) and those of testing in groups of *selected* patients (e.g. patients with suspected or known fragrance sensitivity, individuals with suspected cosmetic intolerance, patients with hand eczema) are shown in table 3.24.2.

In nine studies in which butylphenyl methylpropional was routinely tested, rates of sensitization were always low, ranging from 0.2% to 1% (table 3.24.2). In 6 investigations, no relevance data were provided; in the other 3, relevance ranged from 25% to 100%. In the largest study with 20 patients allergic to butylphenyl methylpropional, the patch test reactions were considered to be presently relevant in 14 patients and of past relevance in two (28).

In 8 studies, in which butylphenyl methylpropional was patch tested in groups of selected patients (e.g. patients with suspected or known fragrance sensitivity, individuals with suspected cosmetic intolerance, patients with hand eczema), frequencies of sensitization were mostly (very) low, ranging from 0.4% to 4%. The latter percentage was found in a group of 100 individuals with known fragrance sensitivity (32). Relevance data were either not provided or inadequate (table 3.24.2).

Table 3.24.2 Patch testing in groups of patients

Years and Country	Test conc. & vehicle	Number of patients tested | positive (%)		Selection of patients (S); Relevance (R); Comments (C)	Ref.
Routine testing					
2015-7 Netherlands		821	6 (0.7%)	R: not stated	45
2015-2016 UK	10% pet.	2084	7 (0.3%)	R: not specified for individual fragrances; 25% of patients who reacted to any fragrance or fragrance marker had a positive fragrance history	43
2010-2015 Denmark	10% pet.	6004	(0.33%)	R: present relevance 70%, past relevance 10%	28
2013-2014 Thailand		312	3 (1.0%)	R: 100%	29
2011-2012 UK	10% pet.	1951	9 (0.5%)	R: not stated	30
2008-2010 Denmark	10% pet.	1503	4 (0.3%)	S: mostly routine testing; R: 25%; C: 100% co-reactivity of FM I, 75% of FM II; C: of the relevant reactions to any of the 26 fragrances tested, 96% were caused by cosmetic products	2
2003-2004 IVDK	10% pet.	2004	8 (0.4%)	R: not stated	4
1998-9 Netherlands	5% pet.	1825	9 (0.5%)	R: not stated	10
1997-8 six European countries	10% pet.	1855	3 (0.2%)	R: not stated / specified	21
Testing in groups of selected patients					
2006-2011 IVDK	10% pet.	707	4 (0.6%)	S: patients with suspected cosmetic intolerance; R: not stated	27
2005-10 Netherlands		100	4 (4%)	S: patients with known fragrance sensitivity based on a positive patch test to the FM I and/or the FM II; R: not stated	32
2005-2008 IVDK	10% pet.	1003	(0.6%)	S: not specified; R: not stated	34
2005-7 Netherlands	1% pet.	320	2 (0.6%)	S: patients suspected of fragrance or cosmetic allergy; R: 61% relevance for all positive tested fragrances together	3
2001-2002 Denmark, Sweden	10% pet.	658	3 (0.5%)	S: consecutive patients with hand eczema; R: it was assumed that nearly all positive reactions were of present or past relevance	5
<1996 Japan, Europe, USA	5% pet.	167	2 (1.2%)	S: patients known or suspected to be allergic to fragrances; R: not stated	6
1977-1985 Japan	10% pet.	685	3 (0.4%)	S: patients suspected of fragrance sensitivity; R: unknown; C: the contents of this article are unknown to the author; some sources (lost during writing) have cited the frequency as 1.1%	39
1984 The Netherlands	20% pet.	179	5 (2.8%)	S: patients suspected of cosmetic allergy; R: not stated; C: false-positive reactions due to excited skin syndrome could not be excluded in some cases	9

FM: Fragrance Mix; IVDK: Informationsverbund Dermatologischer Kliniken (Germany, Switzerland, Austria): RT: Routine Testing

Case reports and case series

In the period 2000-2009, in Leuven, Belgium, an unspecified number of patients had positive patch tests or use tests to a total of 344 cosmetic products *and* positive patch tests to FM I, FM II, and/or to one or more of 28 selected specific fragrance ingredients. In 12 patients reacting to butylphenyl methylpropional, the presence of this fragrance in the cosmetic product(s) was confirmed by reading the product label(s) in 9 individuals (33).

A woman had a history of dermatitis after the use of selected fine fragrances. She reacted to 3 perfumes, and one of these was also positive in a ROAT; however, the fragrance mix was negative. With the help of bioassay-guided chemical fractionation and GC-MS, the ingredients of the allergenic fractions of the fragrance (based on patch testing and ROAT) were identified and tested in the patient. Only butylphenyl methylpropional (Lilial ®) 1% pet. gave a positive reaction (40).

A man developed axillary allergic contact dermatitis from butylphenyl methylpropional ('lilial') in a solid roll-on antiperspirant (38).

Presence in products and chemical analyses

In various studies, the presence of butylphenyl methylpropional in cosmetic and sometimes other products has been investigated. Before 2006, most investigators used chemical analysis, usually GC-MS, for qualitative and quantitative determination. Since then, the presence of the target fragrances was usually investigated by screening the product labels for the 26 fragrances that must be labeled since 2005 on cosmetics and detergent products in the EU, if present at > 10 ppm (0.001%) in leave-on products and > 100 ppm (0.01%) in rinse-off products. This method, obviously, is less accurate and may result in underestimation of the frequency of the fragrances being present in the product. When they are in fact present, but the concentration is lower than mentioned above, labeling is not required and the fragrances' presence will be missed.

Table 3.24.3 Presence of butylphenyl methylpropional in products [a]

Year	Country	Product type	Nr. investigated	Nr. of products positive [b]	(%)	Method [c]	Ref.
2017	USA	Cosmetic products in hair-dye kits	539 products in 159 hair-dye kits	40	(7%)	Labeling	36
2015-6	Denmark	Fragranced cosmetic products	5588		(21%)	Labeling	19
2015	Germany	Household detergents	817	115	(14%)	Labeling	42
2008-11	Germany	Deodorants	374	126	(34%)	Labeling	37
2009	Italy	Liquid household washing and cleaning products	291	93	(32%)	labeling, website info	35
2006-9	Germany	Cosmetic products	4991		(15%)	Labeling	18
2008	Sweden	Cosmetic products	204		(29%)	Labeling	11
		Detergents	97		(9%)	Labeling	
2007	Netherlands	Cosmetic products for children	23	5	(22%)	Analysis	23
2006	UK	Perfumed cosmetic and house-hold products	300	126	(42%)	Labeling	16
2006	Denmark	Popular perfumed deodorants	88	43	(49%)	Labeling	20
			23	16	(70%)	Analysis	
2006	Netherlands	Laundry detergents	52	19	(37%)	Labeling + analysis	25
2006	Denmark	Rinse-off cosmetics for children	208	16	(8%)	Labeling + analysis	22
2002	Denmark	Home and car air fresheners	19	11	(60%)	Analysis	26
2001	Denmark	Non-cosmetic consumer products	43	24	(56%)	Analysis	24
2000	Denmark, UK, Germany, Italy	Domestic and occupational products	59	16	(27%)	Analysis	13
1997-8	Denmark, UK Germany, Sweden	Cosmetics and cosmetic toys for children	25	14	(56%)	Analysis	14
1996	Five European countries	Fragranced deodorants	70	36	(51%)	Analysis	12
1992	Netherlands	Cosmetic products	300		(48%)	Analysis	17
1988	USA	Perfumes used in fine fragrances, household products and soap	400	49-72% (See text)		Analysis	15

[a] See the corresponding text below for more details
[b] positive = containing the target fragrance
[c] Labeling: information from the ingredient labels on the product / packaging; Analysis: chemical analysis, most often GC-MS

The results of the relevant studies for butylphenyl methylpropional are summarized in table 3.24.3. More detailed information can be found in the corresponding text following the table. The percentage of products in which butylphenyl methylpropional was found to be present shows wide variations, which can among other be explained by the selection procedure of the products, the method of investigation (false-negatives with information obtained from labels only) and changes in the use of individual fragrance materials over time (fashion). In general, though, it can be stated that butylphenyl methylpropional is a frequently used fragrance material.

In 2018, butylphenyl methylpropional was found to be present in concentrations of 3 and 8 mg/ml in two eaux de parfum by GC-MS (44).

In 2017, in the USA, the ingredient labels 159 hair-dye kits containing 539 cosmetic products (e.g. colorants, conditioners, shampoos, toners) were screened for the most common sensitizers they contain. Butylphenyl methylpropional was found to be present in 40 (7%) of the products (36).

In Denmark, in 2015-2016, 5588 fragranced cosmetic products were examined with a smartphone application for the 26 fragrances that need to be labeled in the EU. Butylphenyl methylpropional was present in 21% of the products (rank number 7) (19).

In Germany, in 2015, fragrance allergens were evaluated based on lists of ingredients in 817 (unique) detergents (all-purpose cleaners, cleaning preparations for special purposes [e.g. bathroom, kitchen, dish-washing] and laundry detergents) present in 131 households. Butylphenyl methylpropional was found to be present in 115 (14%) of the products (42).

In 2008, 2010 and 2011, 374 deodorants available in German retail shops were randomly selected and their labels checked for the presence of the 26 fragrances that need to be labeled. Butylphenyl methylpropional was found to be present in 126 (33.7%) of the products (37).

In Italy, in 2009, the labels and website product information of 291 liquid household washing and cleaning products were studied for the presence of potential allergens. Butylphenyl methylpropional was found to be present in 93 (32%) of the products (35).

In Germany, in the period 2006-2009, 4991 cosmetic products were randomly sampled for an official investigation of conformity of cosmetic products with legal provisions. The labels were inspected for the presence of the 26 fragrances that need to be labeled in the EU. Butylphenyl methylpropional was present in 15% of the products (rank number 5) (18).

Butylphenyl methylpropional was present (as indicated by labeling) in 29% of 204 cosmetic products (92 shampoos, 61 hair conditioners, 34 liquid soaps, 17 wet tissues) and in 9% of 97 detergents in Sweden, 2008 (11).

In 2007, in The Netherlands, twenty-three cosmetic products for children were analyzed for the presence of fragrances that need to be labeled. Butylphenyl methylpropional was identified in 5 of the products (22%) in a concentration range of 210-5254 ppm (23).

In 2006, of 88 popular perfume containing deodorants purchased in Denmark, 43 (49%) were labeled to contain butylphenyl methylpropional. Analysis of 24 regulated fragrance substances in 23 selected deodorants (19 spray products, 2 deostick and 2 roll-on) was performed by GC-MS. Butylphenyl methylpropional was identified in 16 of the products (70%) with a concentration range of 1–5455 ppm (20).

In January 2006, a study of perfumed cosmetic and household products available on the shelves of U.K. retailers was carried out. Products were included if 'parfum' or 'aroma' was listed among the ingredients. Three hundred products were surveyed and any of 26 mandatory labeling fragrances named on the label were recorded. Butylphenyl methylpropional was present in 126 (42%) of the products (rank number 5) (16).

In 2006, in The Netherlands, 52 laundry detergents were investigated for the presence of allergenic fragrances by checking their labels and chemical analyses. Butylphenyl methyl propional was found to be present in 19 of the products (37%) in a concentration range of 8-795 ppm. Butylphenyl methyl propional had rank number 6 (of 15) in the frequency list (25).

In 2006, the labels of 208 cosmetics for children (especially shampoos, body shampoos and soaps) available in Denmark were checked for the presence of the 26 fragrances that need to be labeled in the EU. Butylphenyl methylpropional was present in 16 products (7.7%), and ranked number 11 in the frequency list. Seventeen products were analyzed quantitatively for the fragrances. The maximum concentration found for butylphenyl methylpropional was 3400 mg/kg (22).

In 2002, in Denmark, 19 air fresheners (6 for cars, 13 for homes) were analyzed for the presence of fragrances that need to be labeled on cosmetics. Butylphenyl methylpropional was found to be present in 11 products (60%) in a concentration range of 450-12,000 ppm and ranked 6 in the frequency list (26).

In 2001, in Denmark, 43 non-cosmetic consumer products (mainly dish-washing products, laundry detergents, and hard and soft surface cleaners) were analyzed for the 26 fragrances that are regulated for labeling in the EU. Butylphenyl methylpropional was present in 24 products (56%) in a concentration range of 0.0009-0.0500% (m/m) and had rank number 2 in the frequency list (24).

In 2000, fifty-nine domestic and occupational products, purchased in retail outlets in Denmark, England, Germany and Italy were analyzed by GC-MS for the presence of fragrances. The product categories were liquid soap and soap bars (n=13), soft/hard surface cleaners (n=23), fabric conditioners/ laundry detergents for hand wash (n=8), dish wash (n=10), furniture polish, car shampoo, stain remover (each n=1) and 2 products used in occupational environments. Butylphenyl methylpropional (Lilial ®) was present in 16 products (27%) with a mean concentration of 99 ppm and a range of 36-214 ppm (13).

Twenty-five cosmetics and cosmetic toys for children (5 shampoos and shower gels, 6 perfumes, 1 deodorant (roll-on), 4 baby lotions/creams, 1 baby wipes product, 1 baby oil, 2 lipcare products and 5 toy-cosmetic products: a cosmetic-toy set for blending perfumes and a makeup set) purchased in 1997-1998 in retail outlets in Denmark, Germany, England and Sweden were analyzed in 1998 for the presence of fragrances by GC-MS. Butylphenyl methylpropional (Lilial ®) was found in 14 products (56%) in a concentration range of 0.003-1.170% (w/w). For the analytical data in each product category, the original publication should be consulted (14).

Seventy fragranced deodorants, purchased at retail outlets in 5 European countries in 1996, were analyzed by gas chromatography - mass spectrometry (GC-MS) for the determination of the contents of 21 commonly used fragrance materials. Butylphenyl methylpropional (Lilial ®) was identified in 36 products (51%) in a concentration range of 1–3732 ppm (12).

In 1992, in The Netherlands, the presence of fragrances was analyzed in 300 cosmetic products. Butylphenyl methylpropional was identified in 48% of the products (rank order 14) (17).

In 1988, in the USA, 400 perfumes used in fine fragrances, household products and soaps (number of products per category not mentioned) were analyzed for the presence of fragrance chemicals in a concentration of at least 1% and a list of the Top-25 (present in the highest number of products) presented. Butylphenyl methylpropional was found to be present in 49% of the fine fragrances (rank number 12), 62% of the household product fragrances (rank number 5) and 72% of the soaps (rank number 5) (15).

LITERATURE

1   Bruze M, Svedman C, Andersen KE, Bruynzeel D, Goossens A, Johansen JD, et al. Patch test concentrations (doses in mg/cm2) for the 12 non-mix fragrance substances regulated by European legislation. Contact Dermatitis 2012;66:131-136
2   Heisterberg MV, Menné T, Johansen JD. Contact allergy to the 26 specificc fragrance ingredients to be declared on cosmetic products in accordance with the EU cosmetic directive. Contact Dermatitis 2011;65:266-75
3   Oosten EJ van, Schuttelaar ML, Coenraads PJ. Clinical relevance of positive patch test reactions to the 26 EU-labelled fragrances. Contact Dermatitis 2009;61:217-223
4   Schnuch A, Uter W, Geier J, Lessmann H, Frosch PJ. Sensitization to 26 fragrances to be labelled according to current European regulation: Results of the IVDK and review of the literature. Contact Dermatitis 2007;57:1-10
5   Heydorn S, Johansen JD, Andersen KE, Bruze M, Svedman C, White IR, et al. Fragrance allergy in patients with hand eczema – a clinical study. Contact Dermatitis 2003;48:317-323
6   Larsen W, Nakayama H, Lindberg M et al. Fragrance contact dermatitis: A worldwide multicenter investigation (Part 1). Am J Cont Derm 1996;7:77–83
7   SCCS (Scientific Committee on Consumer Safety), Opinion on Butylphenyl methylpropional, 12 August 2015, SCCS/1540/14, revision of 16 March 2016 Available at:
    https://ec.europa.eu/health/sites/health/files/scientific_committees/consumer_safety/docs/sccs_o_189.pdf
8   SCCS (Scientific Committee on Consumer Safety). Opinion on Fragrance allergens in cosmetic products, 26-27 June 2012, SCCS/1459/11. Available at:
    https://ec.europa.eu/health/sites/health/files/scientific_committees/consumer_safety/docs/sccs_o_102.pdf
9   De Groot AC, Liem DH, Nater JP, van Ketel WG. Patch tests with fragrance materials and preservatives. Contact Dermatitis 1985;12:87-92
10 De Groot AC, Coenraads PJ, Bruynzeel DP, Jagtman BA, Van Ginkel CJW, Noz K, et al. Routine patch testing with fragrance chemicals in The Netherlands. Contact Dermatitis 2000;42:184-185
11 Yazar K, Johnsson S, Lind M-L, Boman A, Lidén C. Preservatives and fragrances in selected consumer-available cosmetics and detergents. Contact Dermatitis 2011;64:265-272
12 Rastogi SC, Johansen JD, Frosch P, Menné T, Bruze M, Lepoittevin JP, et al. Deodorants on the European market: quantitative chemical analysis of 21 fragrances. Contact Dermatitis 1998;38:29-35
13 Rastogi SC, Heydorn S, Johansen JD, Basketter DA. Fragrance chemicals in domestic and occupational products. Contact Dermatitis 2001;45:221-225
14 Rastogi SC, Johansen JD, Menné T, Frosch P, Bruze M, Andersen KE, et al. Content of fragrance allergens in children's cosmetics and cosmetic toys. Contact Dermatitis 1999;41:84-88
15 Fenn RS. Aroma chemical usage trends in modern perfumery. Perfumer and Flavorist 1989;14:3-10
16 Buckley DA. Fragrance ingredient labelling in products on sale in the UK. Br J Dermatol 2007;157:295-300

17 Weyland JW. Personal Communication, 1992. Cited in: De Groot AC, Weyland JW, Nater JP. Unwanted effects of cosmetics and drugs used in dermatology, 3rd Ed. Amsterdam: Elsevier, 1994:579

18 Uter W, Yazar K, Kratz E-M, Mildau G, Lidén C. Coupled exposure to ingredients of cosmetic products: I. Fragrances. Contact Dermatitis 2013;69:335-341

19 Bennike NH, Oturai NB, Müller S, Kirkeby CS, Jørgensen C, Christensen AB, et al. Fragrance contact allergens in 5588 cosmetic products identified through a novel smartphone application. J Eur Acad Dermatol Venereol 2018;32:79-85

20 Rastogi SC, Hellerup Jensen G, Johansen JD. Survey and risk assessment of chemical substances in deodorants. Survey of Chemical Substances in Consumer Products, No. 86 2007. Danish Ministry of the Environment, Environmental Protection Agency. Available at: https://www2.mst.dk/Udgiv/publications/2007/978-87-7052-625-8/pdf/978-87-7052-626-5.pdf

21 Frosch PJ, Johansen JD, Menné T, Pirker C, Rastogi SC, Andersen KE, et al. Further important sensitizers in patients sensitive to fragrances. I. Reactivity to 14 frequently used chemicals. Contact Dermatitis 2002;47:78-85

22 Poulsen PB, Schmidt A. A survey and health assessment of cosmetic products for children. Survey of chemical substances in consumer products, No. 88. Copenhagen: Danish Environmental Protection Agency, 2007. Available at: https://www2.mst.dk/udgiv/publications/2007/978-87-7052-638-8/pdf/978-87-7052-639-5.pdf

23 VWA. Dutch Food and Consumer Product Safety Authority. Cosmetische producten voor kinderen: Inventarisatie van de markt en de veiligheidsborging door producenten en importeurs. Report ND04o065/ND05o170, 2007 (Report in Dutch), 2007. Available at: www.nvwa.nl/documenten/communicatie/inspectieresultaten/consument/2016m/cosmetische- producten-voor-kinderen

24 Rastogi SC. Survey of chemical compounds in consumer products. Contents of selected fragrance materials in cleaning products and other consumer products. Survey no. 8-2002. Copenhagen, Denmark, Danish Environmental Protection Agency. Available at: http://eng.mst.dk/media/mst/69131/8.pdf

25 Bouma K, Van Peursem AJJ. Marktonderzoek naleving detergenten verordening voor textielwasmiddelen. Dutch Food and Consumer Products Safety Authority (VWA) Report ND06K173, 2006 [in Dutch]. Available at: http://docplayer.nl/41524125-Marktonderzoek-naleving-detergenten-verordening-voor-textielwasmiddelen.html

26 Pors J, Fuhlendorff R. Mapping of chemical substances in air fresheners and other fragrance liberating products. Report Danish Ministry of the Environment, Environmental Protection Agency (EPA). Survey of Chemicals in Consumer Products, No 30, 2003. Available at: http://eng.mst.dk/media/mst/69113/30.pdf

27 Dinkloh A, Worm M, Geier J, Schnuch A, Wollenberg A. Contact sensitization in patients with suspected cosmetic intolerance: results of the IVDK 2006-2011. J Eur Acad Dermatol Venereol 2015;29:1071-1081

28 Bennike NH, Zachariae C, Johansen JD. Non-mix fragrances are top sensitizers in consecutive dermatitis patients – a cross-sectional study of the 26 EU-labelled fragrance allergens. Contact Dermatitis 2017;77:270-279

29 Vejanurug P, Tresukosol P, Sajjachareonpong P, Puangpet P. Fragrance allergy could be missed without patch testing with 26 individual fragrance allergens. Contact Dermatitis 2016;74:230-235

30 Mann J, McFadden JP, White JML, White IR, Banerjee P. Baseline series fragrance markers fail to predict contact allergy. Contact Dermatitis 2014;70:276-281

31 Uter W, Johansen JD, Börje A, Karlberg A-T, Lidén C, Rastogi S, Roberts D, White IR. Categorization of fragrance contact allergens for prioritization of preventive measures: clinical and experimental data and consideration of structure–activity relationships. Contact Dermatitis 2013;69:196-230

32 Nagtegaal MJC, Pentinga SE, Kuik J, Kezic S, Rustemeyer T. The role of the skin irritation response in polysensitization to fragrances. Contact Dermatitis 2012;67:28-35

33 Nardelli A, Drieghe J, Claes L, Boey L, Goossens A. Fragrance allergens in 'specific' cosmetic products. Contact Dermatitis 2011;64:212-219

34 Uter W, Geier J, Frosch P, Schnuch A. Contact allergy to fragrances: current patch test results (2005–2008) from the Information Network of Departments of Dermatology. Contact Dermatitis 2010;63:254-261

35 Magnano M, Silvani S, Vincenzi C, Nino M, Tosti A. Contact allergens and irritants in household washing and cleaning products. Contact Dermatitis 2009;61:337-341

36 Hamann D, Kishi P, Hamann CR. Consumer hair dye kits frequently contain isothiazolinones, other common preservatives and fragrance allergens. Dermatitis 2018;29:48-49

37 Klaschka U. Contact allergens for armpits - allergenic fragrances specified on deodorants. Int J Hyg Environ Health 2012;215:584-591

38 Larsen WG. Allergic contact dermatitis to the fragrance material lilial. Contact Dermatitis 1983;9:158-159

39 Sugai T. Group study IV – farnesol and lily aldehyde. Environ Dermatol 1994;1:213-214 (article in Japanese)

40   Arnau EG, Andersen KE, Bruze M, Frosch PJ, Johansen JD, Menné T, et al. Identification of Lilial ® as a fragrance sensitizer in a perfume by bioassay-guided chemical fractionation and structure-activity relationships. Contact Dermatitis 2000;43:351-358

41   De Groot AC, Schmidt E. Essential oils: contact allergy and chemical composition. Boca Raton, Fl., USA: CRC Press, Taylor and Francis Group, 2016 (ISBN 9781482246407)

42   Wieck S, Olsson O, Kümmerer K, Klaschka U. Fragrance allergens in household detergents. Regul Toxicol Pharmacol 2018;97:163-169

43   Ung CY, White JML, White IR, Banerjee P, McFadden JP. Patch testing with the European baseline series fragrance markers: a 2016 update. Br J Dermatol 2018;178:776-780

44   Zeng F, Xu P, Tan K, Zarbin PHG, Leal WS. Methyl dihydrojasmonate and lilial are the constituents with an "off-label" insect repellence in perfumes. PLoS One 2018;13(6):e0199386

45   Dittmar D, Schuttelaar MLA. Contact sensitization to hydroperoxides of limonene and linalool: Results of consecutive patch testing and clinical relevance. Contact Dermatitis 2018 Oct 31. doi: 10.1111/cod.13137. [Epub ahead of print]

46   SCCS (Scientific Committee on Consumer Safety). Opinion on the safety of Butylphenyl methylpropional (p-BMHCA) in cosmetic products - Submission II -, SCCS/1591/17, Preliminary version, 14 December 2017; available at: ec.europa.eu/health/sites/health/files/scientific_committees/consumer_safety/docs/sccs_o_213.pdf

Chapter 3.25   CAMPHOR

IDENTIFICATION

Description/definition : Camphor is a ketone derived from the wood of the camphor tree, *Cinnamomum camphora* or prepared synthetically; it has two stereoisomers: *D*-camphor and *L*-camphor

Chemical class(es)   : Ketones

SCCS opinion(s)   : SCCS/1459/11 (3)

Merck Index monograph : 3004

Function(s) in cosmetics : EU: denaturant; masking; plasticiser. USA: denaturants; external analgesics; fragrance ingredients; plasticizers

Patch testing   : 1% pet. (SmartPracticeCanada)

Molecular formula   : $C_{10}H_{16}O$

DL-Camphor (mixture of *D*- and *L*-camphor)

Chemical/IUPAC name   : 4,7,7-Trimethylbicyclo[2.2.1]heptan-3-one

CAS registry number(s) : 76-22-2; 464-49-3; 21368-68-3; 8008-51-3

EC number(s)   : 200-945-0; 244-350-4; 207-355-2

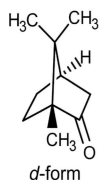

d-form

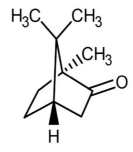

l-form

D-Camphor

Chemical/IUPAC name   : (1*R*,4*R*)-4,7,7-Trimethylbicyclo[2.2.1]heptan-3-one

Other name(s)   : (*R*)-Camphor; (+)-camphor

CAS registry number(s) : 464-49-3; 8022-77-3

EC number(s)   : 207-355-2; 617-014-3; 923-389-7

RIFM monograph(s)   : Food Cosmet Toxicol 1978;16:665 (special issue IV)

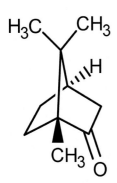

L-Camphor

Chemical/IUPAC name   : (1*S*,4*S*)-4,7,7-Trimethylbicyclo[2.2.1]heptan-3-one
Other name(s)   : (*S*)-Camphor; (-)-camphor
CAS registry number(s) : 464-48-2
EC number(s)   : 207-354-7

GENERAL

Camphor occurs naturally in the fragrant camphor tree *Cinnamomum camphora* and can also be synthetized. Camphor (*D*-) has the appearance of white colorless crystals; its odor type is camphoreous and its odor is described as 'camphoreous, medicinal, mentholic, with a cooling green nuance' (www.thegoodscentscompany.com). Camphor is volatile, reactive and flammable and is irritating to the eyes, skin and mucous membranes. It is used as a plasticizer, moth repellant, in varnish, floor wax, adhesive, as preservative, cosmetic ingredient, and anti-infection agent. Camphor is also used in perfuming industrial products and as flavor for food and beverages. It is common in therapeutic liniments and other pharmaceuticals as a rubefacient/counter-irritant or as a remedy for colds and musculoskeletal pains. In dermatology, when it is applied as lotion (0.1 to 3%), it is an anti-pruritic and surface anesthetic. When applied gently, it creates a feeling of coolness (U.S. National Library of Medicine). Historically, camphor has also been used as an aphrodisiac, abortifacient, antiseptic, and as cardiac and central nervous system stimulant (16).

Presence in essential oils

Camphor (any isomer) has been identified by chemical analysis in 69 of 91 essential oils, which have caused contact allergy / allergic contact dermatitis. In seven oils, camphor belonged to the 'Top-10' of ingredients with the highest concentrations which may be expected in commercial essential oils of this type: sage oil Spanish (11.0-36.0%), spike lavender oil (8.0-35.1%), sage oil Dalmatian (8.5-22.6%), rosemary oil (2.9-24.2%), lavandin oil (5.9-9.9%), coriander fruit oil (2.2-8.0%), and calamus oil (0.02-5.9%) (24).

CONTACT ALLERGY

General

The SCCS (Scientific Committee on Consumer Safety), in a 2012 Opinion on Fragrance allergens in cosmetic products, has marked camphor as 'established contact allergen in humans' (3,8).

Patch testing in groups of patients

Studies in which camphor was patch tested in consecutive patients suspected of contact dermatitis (routine testing) have not been found. In a selected group of 20 patients allergic to fragrances and tested with a battery of fragrance materials, one reacted to camphor 5% pet.; the relevance of this positive reaction was not mentioned (4).

Case reports and case series

Two patients had allergic contact dermatitis from camphor in topical pharmaceutical preparations (1). In a perfume factory, two bottle fillers developed occupational allergic contact dermatitis from camphor. Of twenty people working in the same factory who did *not* have dermatitis, four also had positive reactions to camphor (2).

     A man developed dermatitis from contact allergy to camphor (tested 10% pet.) present in a liquid rubefacient of Asian origin (9). In a clinic in Belgium, in the period 1990-2016, one case of dermatitis caused by contact allergy to camphor from its presence as active principle in a 'topical botanical medicine' has been observed (27).

Presence in products and chemical analyses

In 2008, 66 different fragrance components (including 39 essential oils) were identified in 370 (10% of the total) topical pharmaceutical products marketed in Belgium; 48 of these (13%) contained camphor (1).

In 2000, fifty-nine domestic and occupational products, purchased in retail outlets in Denmark, England, Germany and Italy were analyzed by GC-MS for the presence of fragrances. The product categories were liquid soap and soap bars (n=13), soft/hard surface cleaners (n=23), fabric conditioners/laundry detergents for hand wash (n=8), dish wash (n=10), furniture polish, car shampoo, stain remover (each n=1) and 2 products used in occupational environments. Camphor was present in 7 (12%) products; quantification was not performed (5).

In 1997, 71 deodorants (22 vapo-spray, 22 aerosol spray and 27 roll-on products) were collected in Denmark, England, France, Germany and Sweden and analyzed by gas chromatography – mass spectrometry (GC-MS) for the presence of fragrances and other materials. Camphor was present in 24 (34%) of the products (6).

In 1992, in The Netherlands, the presence of fragrances was analyzed in 300 cosmetic products. Camphor was identified in 31% of the products (rank order 25) (7).

OTHER SIDE EFFECTS

Immediate-type reactions
A woman experienced wheals with marked itching from a perfumed deodorant. Cola, foods flavored with vanilla and vermouth caused digestive symptoms, vomiting and nausea. Epicutaneous tests, read after 30 minutes, showed contact urticaria to Myroxylon pereirae resin, cinnamon oil and camphor. The reactions to Myroxylon pereirae resin and cinnamon oil were certainly relevant, for camphor this was unclear (11).

Systemic side effects
Camphor is often present in over-the-counter remedies, especially for symptomatic relief of 'chest congestion' and muscle aches. When rubbed on the skin, camphor is a rubefacient but, if not vigorously applied, produces a feeling of coolness. However, it is a very toxic chemical and hundreds of cases of poisoning have been reported (13), usually from swallowing by young children (14), but also in adults and from breathing or dermal contact (14) with preparations containing camphor. The progressive severe symptomatology of camphor poisoning has (already 40 years ago) been described as follows (12,13):
1 nausea and vomiting
2 feeling of warmth, headache
3 confusion, vertigo, excitement, restlessness, delirium and hallucinations
4 increased muscular excitability, tremors and jerky movements
5 tremors, progression to seizures, followed by depression
6 coma, central nervous system depression and finally either:
7 death from respiratory failure or from status epilepticus, or
8 slow convalescence
Frequent symptoms are nausea and vomiting and seizures (19).

Even though the risks of camphor are well-known, various case reports of camphor intoxication in young children and sometimes adults from ingestion (17,18,19,20,21,22,23) or dermal application (15,16) have been reported in the previous 20 years (only a few publications are mentioned here). In some countries including Iran, many cases of poisoning are the result of deliberately ingesting camphor by men to decrease libido (19). Most cases obviously are not reported. Indeed, a review of national poison center data from 1990 through 2003 showed approximately 10,000 annual ingestion exposures to camphor-containing products in the USA (16).

In France, two children aged 2 years and 3 months who received a cosmetic baby balm on the skin of their thorax containing eucalyptus, rosemary and lavender essential oils, developed convulsions. As there was no other explanation for this and the 'neurologic toxicity of terpene derivatives is well known' (referring to studies on camphor toxicity), the cosmetic was suspected to be the culprit product. Although no specific terpene ingredient was blamed, the authors discussed the possible role of camphor, menthol and eucalyptol (1,8-cineole). On the basis of these two hardly convincing cases, the product was withdrawn from the market (25).

Camphor in a balm used in 'coin rubbing' may have caused systemic toxicity with vomiting, diarrhea and confusion in a man. After admission to the hospital and supportive treatment, full recovery ensued after 3 days (26).

Only a few publications on camphor poisoning are mentioned here; a full and in-depth discussion is considered to fall outside the scope of this book.

LITERATURE
1   Nardelli A, D'Hooge E, Drieghe J, Dooms M, Goossens A. Allergic contact dermatitis from fragrance components in specific topical pharmaceutical products in Belgium. Contact Dermatitis 2009;60:303-313
2   Schubert HJ. Skin diseases in workers at a perfume factory. Contact Dermatitis 2006;55:81-83
3   SCCS (Scientific Committee on Consumer Safety). Opinion on Fragrance allergens in cosmetic products, 26-27 June 2012, SCCS/1459/11. Available at:

https://ec.europa.eu/health/sites/health/files/scientific_committees/consumer_safety/docs/sccs_o_102.pdf

4   Larsen WG. Perfume dermatitis. A study of 20 patients. Arch Dermatol 1977;113:623-626

5   Rastogi SC, Heydorn S, Johansen JD, Basketter DA. Fragrance chemicals in domestic and occupational products. Contact Dermatitis 2001;45:221-225

6   Rastogi SC, Lepoittevin J-P, Johansen JD, Frosch PJ, Menné T, Bruze M, et al. Fragrances and other materials in deodorants: search for potentially sensitizing molecules using combined GC-MS and structure activity relationship (SAR) analysis. Contact Dermatitis 1998;39:293-303

7   Weyland JW. Personal Communication, 1992. Cited in: De Groot AC, Weyland JW, Nater JP. Unwanted effects of cosmetics and drugs used in dermatology, 3rd Ed. Amsterdam: Elsevier, 1994:579

8   Uter W, Johansen JD, Börje A, Karlberg A-T, Lidén C, Rastogi S, Roberts D, White IR. Categorization of fragrance contact allergens for prioritization of preventive measures: clinical and experimental data and consideration of structure–activity relationships. Contact Dermatitis 2013;69:196-230

9   Vilaplana J, Romaguera C, Campderros L. Contact dermatitis by camphor present in a flushing solution. Actas Dermosifiliogr 2007;98:345-346 (article in Spanish)

10   Stevenson OE, Finch TM. Allergic contact dermatitis from rectified camphor oil in Earex ear drops. Contact Dermatitis 2003;49:51

11   Temesvári E, Soos G, Podányi B, Kovács I, Nemeth I. Contact urticaria provoked by balsam of Peru. Contact Dermatitis 1978;4:65-68

12   De Groot AC, Weyland JW, Nater JP. Unwanted effects of cosmetics and drugs used in dermatology, 3rd Edition. Amsterdam – London – New York – Tokyo: Elsevier, 1994:230-231

13   American Academy of Pediatrics. Committee on Drugs. Camphor: who needs it? Pediatrics 1978;62:404

14   Khine H, Weiss D, Graber N, Hoffman RS, Esteban-Cruciani N, Avner JR. A cluster of children with seizures caused by camphor poisoning. Pediatrics 2009;123:1269-1272

15   Guilbert J, Flamant C, Hallalel F, Doummar D, Frata A, Renolleau S. Anti-flatulence treatment and status epilepticus: a case of camphor intoxication. Emerg Med J 2007;24:859-860

16   Manoguerra AS, Erdman AR, Wax PM, Nelson LS, Caravati EM, Cobaugh DJ, et al. Camphor poisoning: an evidence-based practice guideline for out-of-hospital management. Clin Toxicol (Phila) 2006;44:357-370

17   Uc A, Bishop WP, Sanders KD. Camphor hepatotoxicity. South Med J 2000;93:596-598

18   Cordoba Torres IT, Marino-Nieto J, Barkin HB, Fort AC, Cobas M. Vicks® VapoRub™ intoxication: An unusual presentation of multiorgan failure. J Clin Anesth 2018;48:46-47

19   Rahimi M, Shokri F, Hassanian-Moghaddam H, Zamani N, Pajoumand A, Shadnia S. Severe camphor poisoning, a seven-year observational study. Environ Toxicol Pharmacol 2017;52:8-13

20   Tekin HG, Gökben S, Serdaroğlu G. Seizures due to high dose camphor ingestion. Turk Pediatri Ars 2015;50:248-250

21   Patra C, Sarkar S, Dasgupta MK, Das A. Camphor poisoning: An unusual cause of seizure in children. J Pediatr Neurosci 2015;10:78-79

22   Santos CD, Cabot JC. Persistent effects after camphor ingestion: a case report and literature review. J Emerg Med 2015;48:298-304

23   Love JN, Sammon M, Smereck J. Are one or two dangerous? Camphor exposure in toddlers. J Emerg Med 2004;27:49-54

24   De Groot AC, Schmidt E. Essential oils: contact allergy and chemical composition. Boca Raton, Fl., USA: CRC Press, Taylor and Francis Group, 2016 (ISBN 9781482246407)

25   Laribière A, Miremont-Salamé G, Bertrand S, François C, Haramburu F. Terpènes dans les cosmétiques: 2 cas d'épilepsie. Thérapie 2005;60: 607-609

26   Rampini SK, Schneemann M, Rentsch K, Bachli EB. Camphor intoxication after cao gio (coin rubbing). JAMA 2002;288(1):45

27   Gilissen L, Huygens S, Goossens A. Allergic contact dermatitis caused by topical herbal remedies: importance of patch testing with the patients' own products. Contact Dermatitis 2018;78:177-184

Chapter 3.26 CAMPHYLCYCLOHEXANOL

IDENTIFICATION

Description/definition	: Camphylcyclohexanol is the organic compound that conforms to the formula shown below
Chemical class(es)	: Alcohols
Chemical/IUPAC name	: 1-(1,7,7-Trimethylbicyclo[2.2.1]heptan-2-yl)cyclohexan-1-ol
Other names	: Isobornyl cyclohexanol; santall; Santalex T ®
CAS registry number(s)	: 68877-29-2
EC number(s)	: 272-556-4
Function(s) in cosmetics	: EU: masking; perfuming. USA: fragrance ingredients
Patch testing	: 2% pet. (3); 10% pet. is virtually non-irritant (4)
Molecular formula	: $C_{16}H_{28}O$

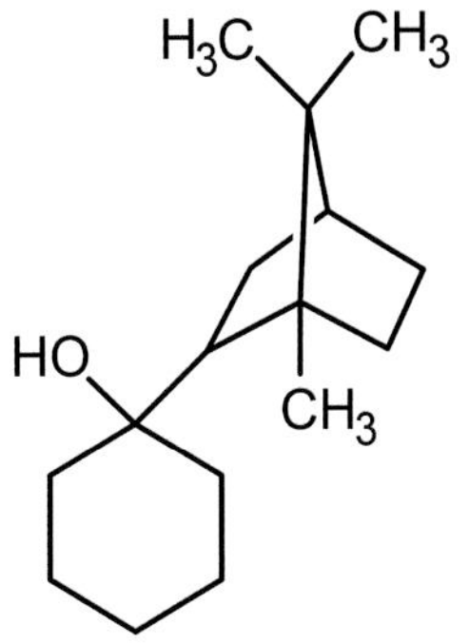

GENERAL

Isobornyl cyclohexanol is a colorless to pale yellow clear very viscous liquid to solid; its odor type is woody and its odor at 100% is described as 'woody clean sandalwood balsam'. It is used in perfumes for fine fragrances, laundry care, and soap as a low cost replacement for sandalwood oil (www.thegoodscentscompany.com). It is a synthetic fragrance not found in nature (and consequently, not in essential oils (5)).

CONTACT ALLERGY

Patch testing in groups of patients

The Mid-Japan Contact Dermatitis Research group (MJDCRG) conducted a 6-year (1976-1981) patch test study with various fragrance chemicals in patients with facial dermatoses. During the year 1979, a total of 327 patients were tested with camphylcyclohexanol (isobornyl cyclohexanol) at concentrations of 10%, 2%, and 1% in white petrolatum. Positive patch test reactions were observed in 2.5%, 1.5% and 0.6% of the patients, respectively. Quite curiously, 2% was chosen as the preferred patch test concentration, although 10% yielded more positive reactions and only one (0.3%) irritant reaction was observed (4).

Also in Japan, 25 of 1949 (1.3%) patients tested with camphylcyclohexanol (isobornyl cyclohexanol, also termed 'synthetic sandalwood oil') between 1979 and 1990 had positive patch test reactions. The patient group was probably selected, but the selection criteria are unknown, as are the test concentration and vehicle and the relevance of the reactions (2).

LITERATURE

1   Bhatia SP, McGinty D, Letizia CS, Api A M. Fragrance material review on alpha-santalol. Food Chem Toxicol 2008;46(suppl.11): S267-S269
2   Utsumi M, Sugai T, Shoji A, Watanabe K, Asoh S, Hashimoto Y. Incidence of positive reactions to sandalwood oil and its related fragrance materials in patch tests and a case of contact allergy to natural and synthetic sandal-wood oil in a museum worker. Skin Res 1992:34(suppl.14):209-213 (article in Japanese). Data cited in ref. 1
3   De Groot AC. Patch Testing, 4th Edition. Wapserveen, The Netherlands: acdegroot publishing, 2018 (ISBN 978-90-813233-4-5)
4   Mid-Japan Contact Dermatitis Research Group. Determination of suitable concentrations for patch testing of various fragrance materials. A summary of group study conducted over a 6-year period. J Dermatol 1984;11:31-35
5   De Groot AC, Schmidt E. Essential oils: contact allergy and chemical composition. Boca Raton, Fl., USA: CRC Press, Taylor and Francis Group, 2016 (ISBN 9781482246407)

Chapter 3.27   CAPRYLIC ALCOHOL

IDENTIFICATION

Description/definition   : Caprylic alcohol is the aliphatic linear alcohol that conforms to the structural formula
                              shown below
Chemical class(es)   : Aliphatic organic compounds; alcohols
INCI name USA   : Not in the Personal Care Products Council Ingredient Database
Chemical/IUPAC name   : Octan-1-ol
Other names   : Alcohol C-8; octanol; 1-octanol; octyl alcohol; capryl alcohol
CAS registry number(s)   : 111-87-5; 67700-96-3; 68603-15-6; 220713-26-8
EC number(s)   : 271-642-9; 606-925-1; 266-920-1; 203-917-6
RIFM monograph(s)   : Food Cosmet Toxicol 1973;11:101; Food Cosmet Toxicol 1973;11:1079 (binder, page 3)
Merck Index monograph   : 8110
Function(s) in cosmetics   : EU: masking; perfuming; viscosity controlling
Patch testing   : 20% pet. (3); according to data from RIFM, 2% pet. is probably not irritant (4);
                              TEST ADVICE: 10% pet.
Molecular formula   : $C_8H_{18}O$

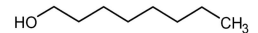

GENERAL

Caprylic alcohol is a colorless clear liquid; its odor type is waxy and its odor is described as 'waxy, green, citrus, aldehydic and floral with a sweet, fatty, coconut nuance' (www.thegoodscentscompany.com).

Presence in essential oils

Caprylic alcohol (1-octanol) has been identified by chemical analysis in 22 of 91 essential oils, which have caused contact allergy / allergic contact dermatitis. In none of these oils, it belonged to the 'Top-10' of ingredients with the highest concentrations (5).

CONTACT ALLERGY

Testing in groups of patients

Studies in which caprylic alcohol has been tested in either consecutive patients suspected of contact dermatitis (routine testing) or in groups of selected patients with positive results have not been found.

Case reports and case series

A woman had allergic contact dermatitis from the perfume in an eye cream. Subsequently, she was tested with 94 individual liquid fragrance materials from this perfume (test concentrations not mentioned). The patient at day 5 had 12 positive patch test reactions, including to caprylic alcohol (alcohol C-8). Three controls were negative. She was not retested, so false-positive reactions due to the excited skin syndrome cannot be excluded (1).

   Indeed, two years later, in a Letter to the Editor, the author mentioned that he had retested the patient with the 12 fragrances to which she had previously shown a positive patch test. Only hydroxycitronellal now had again given a positive reaction (2). This means that, in fact, contact allergy to caprylic alcohol has not been demonstrated thus far beyond doubt.

LITERATURE

1   Larsen WG. Cosmetic dermatitis due to a perfume. Contact Dermatitis 1975;1:142-145
2   Larsen WG. Perfume dermatitis revisited. Contact Dermatitis 1977;3:98
3   Fisher's Contact Dermatitis, 6th Edition, 2008; data cited in ref. 4
4   De Groot AC. Patch Testing, 3rd Edition. Wapserveen, The Netherlands: acdegroot publishing, 2008 (ISBN 978-90-813233-1-4)
5   De Groot AC, Schmidt E. Essential oils: contact allergy and chemical composition. Boca Raton, Fl., USA: CRC Press, Taylor and Francis Group, 2016 (ISBN 9781482246407)

Chapter 3.28   3-CARENE *

* Not officially an INCI name but perfuming name

IDENTIFICATION

Description/definition	: 3-Carene is the cyclohexene derivative that conforms to the structural formula shown below
Chemical class(es)	: Unsaturated organic compounds
INCI name USA	: Not in the Personal Care Products Council Ingredient Database
Chemical/IUPAC name	: 3,7,7-Trimethylbicyclo[4.1.0]hept-3-ene
Other names	: Isodiprene; delta-3-carene; δ-3-carene; S-3-carene
CAS registry number(s)	: 13466-78-9; 74806-04-5
EC number(s)	: 236-719-3
RIFM monograph(s)	: Food Cosmet Toxicol 1973;11:1053 (binder, page 182)
SCCS opinion(s)	: SCCNFP/0389/00 Final (1)
Merck Index monograph	: 3105
Function(s) in cosmetics	: EU: perfuming
EU cosmetic restrictions	: Regulated in Annex III/121 of the Regulation (EC) No. 344/2013
Patch testing	: 10% pet. (1); it may be preferable to test oxidized 3-carene 1% pet. (5)
Molecular formula	: $C_{10}H_{16}$

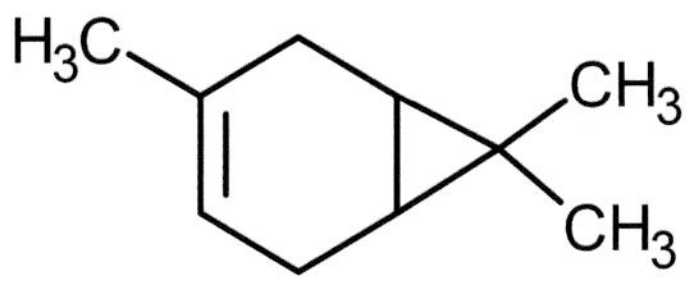

GENERAL

3-Carene is a colorless clear liquid; its odor type is citrus and its odor at 100% is described as 'sweet citrus terpenic fir needle' (www.thegoodscentscompany.com).

Presence in essential oils

3-Carene has been identified by chemical analysis in 69 of 91 essential oils, which have caused contact allergy / allergic contact dermatitis. In 9 oils, 3-carene belonged to the 'Top-10' of ingredients with the highest concentrations which may be expected in commercial essential oils of this type: dwarf pine oil (0.6-34.4%), cypress oil (7.2-25.9%), black pepper oil (4.3-17.6%), angelica root oil (6.4-17.5%), pine needle oil (1.4-13.0%), galbanum resin oil (1.6-9.5%), thuja oil (0.7-8.2%), star anise oil (0.03-0.7%), and turpentine oil (traces-0.3%) (12).

CONTACT ALLERGY

General

3-Carene has not been described as an allergen in perfumes or fragranced products. Contact allergic reactions have developed especially from its presence in oils of turpentine with high concentrations of 3-carene. Turpentine oils with high 3-carene content were those from Scandinavia, the East-European countries, Russia and Indonesia, whereas turpentine oils from the south of France, Spain, Portugal and China contain less of the material and are consequently safer (Chapter 6.75 Turpentine oil).

Indeed, in the 1950s, oil of turpentine was a frequent cause of allergic occupational contact dermatitis, especially in painters. Ceramics workers were also at risk (10,11). 3-Carene itself did not cause sensitization reactions, but the hapten was identified already in the 1950s as an oxidation product of 3-carene: 3-carene hydroperoxide (2,3,4).

The gradual withdrawal of allergenic oil of turpentine from general use, replacement with oil of turpentine with low or zero 3-carene content (e.g. from France and Portugal [6]), replacement with the cheaper and effective petroleum product white spirit, and severe restrictions in some countries of the use of oil of turpentine in paints, solvents and polishes with the specific purpose of reducing occupational dermatitis, led to a sharp decline in the incidence of sensitization in the 1970s. However, there were also other allergens in oil of turpentine including limonene and α-pinene (Chapter 6.75 Turpentine oil).

Patch testing in groups of patients

Results of studies patch testing 3-carene in groups of selected patients, nearly always patients sensitized to oil of turpentine, are shown in table 3.28.1. Frequencies of positive reactions in these patients ranged from 18 to27%, suggesting that it was the allergen or one of the allergens in turpentine oils in every 4 or 5 patients.

Table 3.28.1 Patch testing in groups of patients: Selected patient groups

Years and Country	Test conc. & vehicle	Number of patients tested	positive (%)		Selection of patients (S); Relevance (R); Comments (C)	Ref.
<1996 UK	10% pet.	14	4	(27%)	S: patients with occupational hand dermatitis working in the pottery industry and sensitized to Indonesian turpentine oil with high 3-carene content	11
1985 Spain	15% o.o.	67	16	(24%)	S: patients allergic to oil of turpentine; R: not specified	8
1979-1983 Portugal	15% o.o.	22	4	(18%)	S: patients allergic to oil of turpentine; R: not stated; C: turpentine oil from Portugal was made from *P. pinaster* and *P. pinea*, both of which do not contain 3-carene; the authors suggested that the reactions to 3-carene were caused by imported oil of turpentine	6
1967-1972 France		276	43	(15.6%)	S: patients with plant contact allergy; R: not stated	9

o.o.: Olive oil

Case reports and case series

There are no reports of allergic contact dermatitis caused by 3-carene from its presence in a fragrance or fragranced product. A woman developed occupational allergic contact dermatitis from 3-carene and terpinolene in a cleanser for the machine she worked with. Patch tests were positive to both substances at 5% pet. and 1% in water; 10 controls were negative (7). An unknown number of workers in the ceramics industries in France had occupational allergic contact dermatitis from 3-carene in turpentine oil (10).

OTHER SIDE EFFECTS

Photosensitivity
Photosensitivity to 3-carene has been cited in ref. 5.

LITERATURE

1   SCCFNP (Scientific Committee on Cosmetic Products and Non-Food Products Intended for Consumers). Opinion of the Scientific Committee on Cosmetic Products and Non-Food Products Intended for Consumers concerning 'The 1st update of the inventory of ingredients employed in cosmetic products. Section II: Perfume and aromatic raw materials', 24 October 2000, SCCNFP/0389/00 Final. Available at: http://ec.europa.eu/health/ph_risk/committees/sccp/documents/out131_en.pdf
2   Hellerström S, Thyresson N, Blohm SG, Widmark G. On the nature of the eczematogenic component of oxidized delta 3-carene. J Invest Dermatol 1955;24:217-224
3   Pirilä V, Siltanen E. On the chemical nature of the eczematogenic agent in oil of turpentine. III. Dermatologica 1958;117:1-8
4   Pirilä V, Kilpio O, Olkknen A, Pirilä L, Siltanen E. On the chemical nature of the eczematogens in oil of turpentine. V. Dermatologica 1969;139:183-194
5   De Groot AC. Patch Testing, 4th Edition. Wapserveen, The Netherlands: acdegroot publishing, 2018 (ISBN 978-90-813233-4-5)
6   Cachao P, Menezes Brandao F, Carmo M, Frazao S, Silva M. Allergy to oil of turpentine in Portugal. Contact Dermatitis 1986;14:205-208
7   Castelain PY, Camoin JP, Jouglard J. Contact dermatitis to terpene derivatives in a machine cleaner. Contact Dermatitis 1980;6:358-360
8   Romaguera C, Alomar A, Conde-Salazar L, Camarasa JMG, Grimalt F, Martin Pascual A, et al. Turpentine sensitization. Contact Dermatitis 1986;14:197
9   Fousserau J, Meller JC, Benezra C. Contact allergy to Frullania and Laurus nobilis: cross-sensitization and chemical structure of the allergens. Contact Dermatitis 1975;1:223-230
10   Benezra C, Foussereau J, Maleville J. L'identification chimique des allergènes vegetaux et son interêt dans la prévention de nombreux eczémas allergiques professionels. Maladies Professionnelles de Médecine du Travail et de Securité Sociale 1970;31:539-543 (article in French). Data cited in ref. 11
11   Lear JT, Heagerty AH, Tan BB, Smith AG, English JS. Transient re-emergence of oil of turpentine allergy in the pottery industry. Contact Dermatitis 1996;35:169-172
12   De Groot AC, Schmidt E. Essential oils: contact allergy and chemical composition. Boca Raton, Fl., USA: CRC Press, Taylor and Francis Group, 2016 (ISBN 9781482246407)

Chapter 3.29 CARVACROL

IDENTIFICATION

Description/definition : Carvacrol is the organic compound that conforms to the structural formula shown below
Chemical class(es) : Phenols
Chemical/IUPAC name : 2-Methyl-5-propan-2-ylphenol
Other names : 2-Methyl-5-(1-methylethyl)phenol; 2-hydroxy-*p*-cymene; 5-isopropyl-*o*-cresol; isothymol
CAS registry number(s) : 499-75-2
EC number(s) : 207-889-6
CIR review(s) : Int J Toxicol 2006;25(suppl.1):S29-S127 (access: www.cir-safety.org/ingredients)
RIFM monograph(s) : Food Cosmet Toxicol 1979;17:743 (special issue V)
SCCS opinion(s) : SCCS/1459/11 (1)
Merck Index monograph : 3142
Function(s) in cosmetics : EU: perfuming. USA: fragrance ingredients; skin-conditioning agents - miscellaneous
Patch testing : 5% pet. (2)
Molecular formula : $C_{10}H_{14}O$

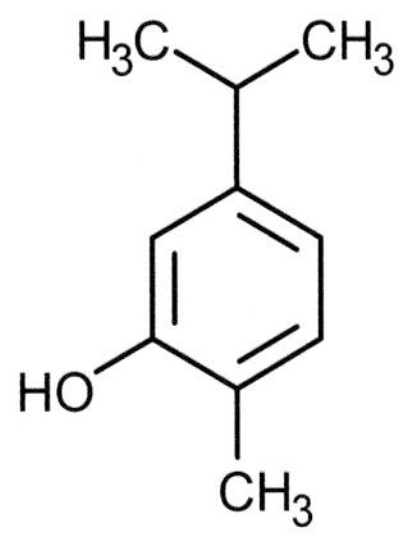

GENERAL

Carvacrol is a colorless to yellow clear viscous liquid; its odor type is spicy and its odor is described as 'spicy, cooling, thymol-like, herbal and camphoreous with smoky nuances' (www.thegoodscentscompany.com). It is not only used in cosmetics as a fragrance, but also as a synthetic flavoring and adjuvant in food, e.g. in alcoholic and non-alcoholic beverages, baked goods, chewing gum, condiment relish, frozen dairy, gelatin pudding and soft candies (5).

Carvacrol is derived from *p*-cymene by sulfonation followed by alkali fusion, but can also be derived from savory, thyme, marjoram, oregano, lovage root, and Spanish thyme oil (1).

Presence in essential oils

Carvacrol has been identified by chemical analysis in 49 of 91 essential oils, which have caused contact allergy / allergic contact dermatitis. In three oils, carvacrol belonged to the 'Top-10' of ingredients with the highest concentrations which may be expected in commercial essential oils of this type: thyme oil (trace-77.8%), black cumin oil (trace-5.8%), and thyme oil Spanish (0.2-5.3%) (6).

CONTACT ALLERGY

General

The SCCS (Scientific Committee on Consumer Safety), in a 2012 Opinion on Fragrance allergens in cosmetic products, has categorized carvacrol as 'likely fragrance contact allergen by combination of evidence' (1,3).

Patch testing in groups of patients

Patch testing in consecutive patients suspected of contact dermatitis: routine testing

Studies in which carvacrol was patch tested in consecutive patients suspected of contact dermatitis (routine testing) with positive results have not been found.

Patch testing in groups of selected patients

Before 1986, in France, 21 patients with dermatitis caused by perfumes were patch tested with a battery of fragrances and essential oils and there were 4 (19%) positive reactions to carvacrol 3% in petrolatum. The authors did not comment on their relevance. Of the 4 positive reactions, 3 were to 'isothymol', which is a synonym of carvacrol, of which the investigators were probably not aware (4).

In 1984, in The Netherlands, 179 patients suspected of cosmetic allergy were tested with a battery of fragrances and preservatives and there were 2 (1.1%) positive reactions to carvacrol 5% pet. Their relevance was not mentioned. It should be appreciated, however, that both patients had multiple positive patch tests reactions, and therefore false-positive reactions due to the excited skin syndrome could not be excluded (2).

Case reports and case series
Case reports of allergic contact dermatitis from carvacrol have not been found.

LITERATURE

1   SCCS (Scientific Committee on Consumer Safety). Opinion on Fragrance allergens in cosmetic products, 26-27 June 2012, SCCS/1459/11. Available at:
     https://ec.europa.eu/health/sites/health/files/scientific_committees/consumer_safety/docs/sccs_o_102.pdf
2   De Groot AC, Liem DH, Nater JP, van Ketel WG. Patch tests with fragrance materials and preservatives. Contact Dermatitis 1985;12:87-92
3   Uter W, Johansen JD, Börje A, Karlberg A-T, Lidén C, Rastogi S, Roberts D, White IR. Categorization of fragrance contact allergens for prioritization of preventive measures: clinical and experimental data and consideration of structure–activity relationships. Contact Dermatitis 2013;69:196-230
4   Meynadier JM, Meynadier J, Peyron JL, Peyron L. Formes cliniques des manifestations cutanées d'allergie aux parfums. Ann Dermatol Venereol 1986;113:31-39 (article in French)
5   Andersen A. Final report on the safety assessment of sodium p-chloro-m-cresol, p-chloro-m-cresol, chlorothymol, mixed cresols, m-cresol, o-cresol, p-cresol, isopropyl cresols, thymol, o-cymen-5-ol, and carvacrol. Int J Toxicol 2006;25(suppl.1):S29-S127
6   De Groot AC, Schmidt E. Essential oils: contact allergy and chemical composition. Boca Raton, Fl., USA: CRC Press, Taylor and Francis Group, 2016 (ISBN 9781482246407)

Chapter 3.30   CARVONE

IDENTIFICATION

Description/definition : Carvone is the terpene that conforms to the structural formula shown below
Chemical class : Ketones
Chemical/IUPAC name : (5R or 5S)-2-Methyl-5-prop-1-en-2-ylcyclohex-2-en-1-one
Other names : L-Carvone; (R)-carvone; D-carvone; (S)-carvone
CAS registry number(s) : 6485-40-1 (L-carvone); 99-49-0 (carvone, natural); 2244-16-8 (D-carvone)
EC number(s) : 229-352-5; 218-827-2; 202-759-5
RIFM monograph(s) : Food Cosmet Toxicol 1978;16:673 (special issue IV) (D-); Food Cosmet Toxicol 1973;11:1057 (L-)
IFRA standard : Restricted (www.ifraorg.org/en-us/standards-library) (table 3.30.1)
SCCS opinion(s) : SCCS/1459/11 (4)
Merck Index monograph : 3144
Function(s) in cosmetics : EU: flavouring; masking; perfuming. USA: flavoring agents; fragrance ingredients
Patch testing : 5% pet. (SmartPracticeCanada, Chemotechnique); 5% pet. from some sources may be marginally irritant (23); the patch test should also be read at D7, otherwise 20% of positive reactions may be missed (25)
Molecular formula : $C_{10}H_{14}O$

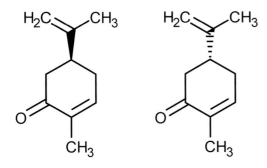

D-carvone   L-carvone

Table 3.30.1 IFRA restrictions for carvone

Category [a]	Limits [b]	Category [a]	Limits [b]	Category [a]	Limits [b]
1	0.08%	5	0.60%	9	5.00%
2	0.10%	6	1.90%	10	2.50%
3	0.40%	7	0.20%	11	not restricted
4	1.20%	8	2.00%		

[a] For explanation of categories see pages 6-8
[b] Limits in the finished products

GENERAL

Carvone is a colorless to pale yellow clear liquid; its odor type is minty and its odor at 100% is described as 'minty licorice' (www.thegoodscentscompany.com). Carvone has different forms: L-carvone, D-carvone and DL-carvone. L-Carvone smells and tastes like spearmint and D-carvone smells like caraway and has a taste like rye bread. It occurs naturally in over 140 plants. L-Carvone is the main ingredient of spearmint oil with concentrations ranging from 60 to 82% (5). D-Carvone occurs naturally in caraway and dill seeds and many essential oils.

Carvone is used as a flavoring for alcoholic beverages and foodstuffs, in personal care products, perfumery and in soaps. L-Carvone is one of several substances found in oxidized D-limonene (26), and there are methods to produce it from D-limonene synthetically (30,31). L-Carvone is produced in larger quantities than D-carvone and is mainly used in oral hygiene products such as toothpaste and mouthwash. Other uses include or have included: as pesticide, plant growth regulator, feed additive for pigs and veterinary use (U.S. National Library of Medicine).

Presence in essential oils

Carvone (any isomer) has been identified by chemical analysis in 51 of 91 essential oils, which have caused contact allergy / allergic contact dermatitis. In one oil, carvone belonged to the 'Top-10' of ingredients with the highest concentrations which may be expected in commercial essential oils of this type: spearmint oil (60.6-82.3%) (5).

CONTACT ALLERGY

General

The SCCS (Scientific Committee on Consumer Safety), in a 2012 Opinion on Fragrance allergens in cosmetic products, has marked carvone as 'established contact allergen in humans' (4,13). The sensitizing potency of carvone was classified as 'moderate' based on an EC3 value of 5.7% in the LLNA (local lymph node assay) in animal experiments (4,13). In other experiments in animals (guinea pigs) both *D*- and *L*-carvone were classified as strong sensitizers (29).

Contact allergy to carvone has infrequently been reported. Most case reports relate to its presence in (spearmint oil in) toothpastes. In Sweden, nearly all toothpastes contain carvone, concentrations ranging from 0.00005 to 0.35% (27). Whether such concentrations may *induce* contact allergy is unknown, but *elicitation* of allergic reactions from carvone in toothpastes has certainly proved possible (7,8,17,18,19,20,21).

There are strong indications that contact allergy to carvone may induce or worsen oral lichen planus / lichenoid lesions (22,25,33); see the section 'Case reports and series / Oral lichen planus and lichenoid lesions' below.

Patch testing in groups of patients

Results of patch testing carvone in consecutive patients suspected of contact dermatitis (routine testing) are shown in table 3.30.2, those of testing in groups of *selected* patients (e.g. patients tested with a dental series, individuals allergic to tea tree oil, patients suspected or oral lichenoid lesions / oral lichen planus, patients who presented with sore mouth, stomatitis and/or dermatitis around the mouth, dentist personnel)) are shown in table 3.30.3.

Patch testing in consecutive patients suspected of contact dermatitis: routine testing

Currently, carvone 5% pet. is part of the screening series of the NACDG. In 6 studies in which routine testing with carvone 5% was performed, frequencies of sensitization ranged from 0.6% to 2.8%. However, in the study with the high frequency of 2.8%, 8 of the 15 carvone-allergic patients were retested and in the second session only 2/8 still reacted, which suggested that irritant reactions may have occurred (23) and give a strong indication that the 2.8% frequency of sensitization is too high. In the 4 studies performed by the NACDG, definite + probable relevance was scored in 12-56% of the carvone-positive subjects (10,11,12,35)

Table 3.30.2 Patch testing in groups of patients: Routine testing

Years and Country	Test conc. & vehicle	Number of patients tested	positive (%)	Selection of patients (S); Relevance (R); Comments (C)	Ref.
2015-2017 NACDG	5% pet.	5594	43 (0.8%)	R: definite + probable relevance: 12%	35
2013-2014 NACDG	5% pet.	4859	34 (0.7%)	R: definite + probable relevance: 27%	10
2011-2012 NACDG	5% pet.	4230	25 (0.6%)	R: definite + probable relevance: 56%	11
2009-2010 NACDG	5% pet.	4302	(1.1%)	R: definite + probable relevance: 29%	12
1997-1998 Sweden	5% pet.	1355	14 (1.0%)	R: not specified, one patient had 'oral lichen'; S: part of a large retrospective study, mostly in selected patients (see below); the test substance was *L*-carvone	25
1991-1992 Denmark	5% pet.	541	15 (2.8%)	R: 2/15 (13%); C: 8 patients were retested, and now only 2 still had positive patch test reactions, suggesting that irritant reactions may have occurred; of the original 15, 9 (60%) co-reacted to the SLS-mix (Compositae)	23

NACDG: North American Contact Dermatitis Group (USA, Canada)

Patch testing in groups of selected patients

Results of studies patch testing carvone in groups of selected patients (e.g. patients tested with a dental series, individuals allergic to tea tree oil, patients suspected or oral lichenoid lesions / oral lichen planus, patients who presented with sore mouth, stomatitis and/or dermatitis around the mouth, dentist personnel) are shown in table 3.30.3. In six studies, frequencies of sensitization ranged from 4.6% to 40%. The two highest rates of positive reactions (13% and 40%) were seen in small groups of patients sensitized to tea tree oil (see the section 'Other information' below for more data). Testing in patients with oral lesions scored between 4.6% and 12% positive reactions. For further information on this subject see the section 'Case reports and series / Oral lichen planus and lichenoid lesions' below.

Table 3.30.3 Patch testing in groups of patients: Selected patient groups

Years and Country	Test conc. & vehicle	Number of patients tested	positive (%)	Selection of patients (S); Relevance (R); Comments (C)	Ref.
1996-2016 Sweden	5% pet.	2866	133 (4.6%)	S: patients tested with a dental series, a cheilitis series or other series containing L-carvone; R: not specified; C: over 75% had oral signs and > 60% had 'oral lichen', which can be explained by referral of the majority of patients by dentists and oral surgeons; nevertheless, in carvone-positive patients, oral lichen was significantly more frequent than in carvone-negative individuals (68% vs. 28%)	25
2001-2010 Australia	5% pet.	178	19 (10.7%)	S: unknown; R: 58%	9
2005-2008 Sweden	5% pet.	83	10 (12%)	S: patients suspected of oral lichen lesions; R: not stated; C: the frequency was considerably higher than in a control group of patients with dermatitis (2.1%)	33
1999-2003 Germany	5% DEP	20	8 (40%)	S: patients with positive patch test reactions to oxidized tea tree oil 5% DEP; 4 reactions to D-carvone and 4 to L-carvone	3
1999 Germany	5% water	8	1 (13%)	S: patients with a positive patch test reaction to oxidized tea tree oil 20% in olive oil; allergy to D-carvone	2
1971-1977 Denmark	5% pet.	41	4 (10%)	S: patients who presented with sore mouth, stomatitis and/or dermatitis around the mouth or who were dentist personnel; R: the causative products were supposed to be toothpastes; C: 2 of the patients also reacted to spearmint oil, in which carvone is the main ingredient	16

DEP: Diethyl phthalate

Case reports and case series

Toothpastes

A woman patch tested for cheilitis reacted to carvone 5% pet. and 2 toothpastes, tested undiluted. The presence of carvone in both products was established by thin layer chromatography and gas chromatography. When the patient stopped using the toothpastes, all symptoms disappeared (17).

A female patient had sore mouth and cheilitis. She reacted to two toothpastes. In one, the allergens were spearmint oil and its main ingredient carvone (19). Another woman had erosive (angular) cheilitis, also from contact allergy to American spearmint oil and its main component carvone in toothpaste (18).

A male patient suffered from cheilitis and erythema and burning of the oral mucosa. He showed a very strong patch test reaction to L-carvone and a weaker (cross)-reaction to D-carvone and also reacted to peppermint oil. L-Carvone constituted 20-30% of the flavor of a toothpaste to which there was also a positive patch test. Later, the patient experienced a recurrence of cheilitis from the use of refreshment lozenges containing carvone (20).

One patient from Germany was allergic to L-carvone (tested 1% pet.) in the spearmint oil flavor in a toothpaste; there was no reaction to D-carvone (21). Early publications from Denmark described one or more cases of contact allergy to carvone in toothpastes (7,8).

Other products

A woman had recurrent desquamative, erythematous, and pruritic dermatitis primarily involving the preauricular cheeks. She reported that the condition had worsened upon subsequent use of a mint-scented hair conditioner. Patch testing revealed a positive reaction to carvone 5% pet. Despite numerous efforts, the authors were unable to definitely confirm with the manufacturers the presence of carvone in the 4 essential oils that were the primary components of the fragrance in the conditioner (tea tree oil, rosemary oil, peppermint oil, lavender oil). However, based on the patient's response to avoidance, they felt it very likely that carvone was present in the product (24).

This conclusion lacks scientific evidence. None of these oils contain appreciable amounts of carvone. However, some patients allergic to tea tree oil have reacted to carvone (2,3,5,6). A possible explanation is that limonene, which was found to be present in commercial tea tree oil (up to 3%) and the other essential oils (lavender up to 1%, peppermint up to 18.5%, rosemary up to 6.7% [5]), were autoxidized to L-carvone (26).

Oral lichen planus and lichenoid lesions

In some studies, an association has been found between allergy to spearmint oil (in which carvone is the main ingredient) or carvone and oral lichen planus / lichenoid lesions (22,25,33).

In the period 1999-2011, in Australia, 1467 selected patients were tested with spearmint oil 2% pet. and 73 (5.0%) had a positive patch test. Of these 73, 19 (26%) reactions were considered to be relevant. Fourteen of these had biopsy-proven oral lichen planus (OLP), of which 7 (50%) co-reacted to carvone. In ten of these patients, the OLP improved >80% after avoidance of spearmint (22).

In 2005-2008, in Sweden, 83 patients referred for suspicion of oral lichen lesions (OLL) and a control group of age- and gender-matched dermatitis patients were patch tested. Ten patients in the OLL group (12.1%) reacted to carvone 5% pet. versus 2 (1.2%) in the dermatitis group; the difference was statistically significant. The authors stated that the clinical relevance of carvone allergy for OLL patients needs to be further elucidated. However, they also mentioned that, at their Department, they had several cases with OLL and/or cheilitis in which the oral lesions or lip lesions disappeared after the patient ceased to use spearmint-containing toothpastes, candy or lozenges (33). There is overlap with the following study.

In Sweden, in the period 1996-2016, 4221 patients were tested with L-carvone 5% pet. in a dental series (n=1938), a cheilitis series (n=500), a dental personnel series (n=460), an oral lichen series (n=259) and/or another series; 1355 were consecutive patients tested in 1997-1998 with carvone in the baseline series (25). There were 147 (3.5%) reactions to carvone. Of these, 73% had oral signs and 57% 'oral lichen' (oral lichen planus or oral lichenoid lesions). The high percentages can easily be explained by the fact that the majority of the patients had been referred by a dentist or oral surgeon. However, when comparing 99 carvone-positive patients to a matched group of carvone-negative patients, the frequency of oral lichen was significantly higher in the group of carvone-positive patients: 67/99 (68%) versus 28/99 (28%) (25). There is overlap with the previous study.

These reports strongly suggest that, for a number of patients, contact allergy to spearmint oil and/or L-carvone may play a role in oral lichen planus / lichenoid lesions, either by causing disease or by aggravating already existing problems (27).

Cross-reactions, pseudo-cross-reactions and co-reactions

For general information on cross-/pseudo-cross-/co-reactivity of fragrance chemicals with other fragrances, fragrance markers (fragrance mix I, fragrance mix II, colophonium, Myroxylon pereirae resin [balsam of Peru]) and essential oils see Chapter 1.2 General information on cross-reactions, pseudo-cross-reactions and co-reactions.

Pseudo-cross-reactions may be observed to spearmint oil (18,19,21,22,25), in which L-carvone is the main ingredient (60-82% [5]). Indeed, of 81 patients allergic to L-carvone, 55 (79%) co-reacted to spearmint oil (25).

L-and D-carvone may (20) or may not (21,29) cross-react. Experimental findings in guinea pigs show no cross-reactivity between both enantiomers (29). Yet, of 6 patients allergic to L-carvone, 3 also had positive patch tests to D-carvone. However, the authors stipulated that these could be considered as simultaneous reactions rather than cross-sensitivity, since the subjects could have been sensitized to both L-and D-carvone (29).

Of 15 patients with a positive patch test to L-carvone 5% pet., 9 (60%) co-reacted to the sesquiterpene lactone-mix. However, when 8 patients were re-tested, only 2 still had positive patch test reactions to L-carvone (23).

Patch test sensitization

Carvone may have caused patch test sensitization in one individual (14). Unfortunately, the test concentration was not mentioned. Of 4221 patients patch tested with L-carvone 5% pet., six had late reactions, from 10 days up to one month after the test application. Two of these patients were re-tested and both showed a reaction on day 3, suggesting patch test sensitization (25). However, the authors stated that they have also observed carvone-positive patients to show positive reactions as late as 21 days upon re-testing, suggesting that a late appearing patch test reaction to carvone may not necessarily need to be a sign of active sensitization (25).

Presence in products and chemical analyses

In 2016, in Sweden, 66 commercially available toothpastes obtained from local pharmacies and supermarkets in Malmö, Sweden were investigated for the presence of L-carvone by studying the packages and product labels and by straight-phase high-performance liquid chromatography for quantitative determination. L-Carvone was found in 64 of 66 toothpastes (97%) in a concentration range of 0.00005 to 0.35%. In 30 of the toothpastes, the concentration was > 0.01%, and in 10 of these the concentration was > 0.1%. Higher concentrations of L-carvone were found if limonene was listed on the label: products with limonene contained 0.059% ±0.074% L-carvone, and products without limonene contained 0.023% ±0.067% L-carvone (27). It is known that limonene may be autoxidized into L-carvone (26), which might explain the higher concentrations of carvone in toothpastes containing limonene. On the other hand, it has previously been shown that only 4% of limonene in petrolatum is transformed into L-carvone by oxidation in 3 months (28). Although it was suggested that the proportion of L-carvone derived from oxidized limonene in toothpaste is therefore most probably very low (27), the behaviour of limonene in toothpaste may well be different from its chemical reactivity in petrolatum.

Other information

Carvone is a minor allergen in tea tree oil. Of 61 patients allergic to tea tree oil and tested with a number of its ingredients in various studies, 5 (8%) reacted to D-carvone and 4 of 54 (7%) tea tree oil-allergic individuals reacted to

L-carvone (6). Commercial batches of tea tree oil (at least fresh ones) do not contain carvone (5). A possible explanation is that in aged samples of this essential oil, carvone is formed from limonene, which is present in concentrations up to 3%, by autoxidation (26). In petrolatum, only 4% of limonene is transformed into *L*-carvone by oxidation in 3 months (28), but this may be different in tea tree oil samples. Low concentrations may yet be sufficient to induce sensitization, as some experimental findings in guinea pigs have suggested *D*- and *L*-carvone both to be strong sensitizers (29).

OTHER SIDE EFFECTS

Immediate-type reactions
A man presented with a 6-month history of swelling of his lips within minutes of contact with toothpaste (1). After a further 5-10 minutes, he would also notice a swelling of his gingiva and shortness of breath. The patient had tried several brands of toothpaste for adults, but experienced the same symptoms with all of them. The only exception was his children's fruit-flavored toothpaste. Open tests were positive to 2 brands of peppermint oil 2% pet. after 15 minutes, to (*R*)- and (*S*)-limonene 1% pet. after 15 minutes (which may be present in peppermint oil in a concentration range of 1-3% and in spearmint oil in a concentration range of 0-22%) and to (*R*)- and (*S*)-carvone 5% pet. after 2 minutes, which is the main ingredient of spearmint oil (57-84%) (5). Quite curiously, the authors did not comment on the composition of the toothpaste(s) the patient had previously used, but they attributed the reaction to carvone, presumably because this was already positive in the open test after 2 minutes. Why menthol, the main ingredient of peppermint oil, was not tested, is unknown (1).

Other non-eczematous contact reactions
A patient with burning mouth syndrome and lupus erythematosus had late patch test reactions to carvone 5%, 2%, 1% pet. and spearmint mix 5% pet. at D19. These were all clinically consistent with SCLE and a biopsy confirmed this diagnosis. Repeat testing gave the same results, so the late reactions were not the result of patch test sensitization. Despite the SCLE aspect of the patch test reactions, the carvone contact allergy was not relevant to either the burning mouth syndrome or the patient's lupus erythematosus (15).

A patient with orofacial granulomatosis had a positive patch test to carvone, which was apparently present in a toothpaste. After stopping the use of this product, partial improvement of the swelling was noted (34).

LITERATURE
1   Hansson C, Bergendorff O, Wallengren J. Contact urticaria caused by carvone in toothpaste. Contact Dermatitis 2011;65:362-364
2   Lippert U, Walter A, Hausen BM, Fuchs Th. Increasing incidence of contact dermatitis to tea tree oil. J Allergy Clin Immunol 2000;105;S43 (abstract 127)
3   Hausen BM. Evaluation of the main contact allergens in oxidized tea tree oil. Dermatitis 2004;15:213-214
4   SCCS (Scientific Committee on Consumer Safety). Opinion on Fragrance allergens in cosmetic products, 26-27 June 2012, SCCS/1459/11. Available at:
    https://ec.europa.eu/health/sites/health/files/scientific_committees/consumer_safety/docs/sccs_o_102.pdf
5   De Groot AC, Schmidt E. Essential oils: contact allergy and chemical composition. Boca Raton, Fl., USA: CRC Press, Taylor and Francis Group, 2016 (ISBN 9781482246407)
6   De Groot AC, Schmidt E. Tea tree oil: contact allergy and chemical composition. Contact Dermatitis 2016;75:129-143
7   Hjorth N, Jervoe P. Allergisk Kontaktstomatitis og Kontaktdermatitis fremkaldt of smagsstoffer i tandpasta. Tandlaegebladet 1967;71:937-942 (article in Danish)
8   Hjorth N. Toothpaste sensitivity. Contact Dermatitis Newsletter 1967;1:14
9   Toholka R, Wang Y-S, Tate B, Tam M, Cahill J, Palmer A, Nixon R. The first Australian Baseline Series: Recommendations for patch testing in suspected contact dermatitis. Australas J Dermatol 2015;56:107-115
10 DeKoven JG, Warshaw EM, Belsito DV, Sasseville D, Maibach HI, Taylor JS, et al. North American Contact Dermatitis Group Patch Test Results: 2013-2014. Dermatitis 2017;28:33-46
11 Warshaw EM, Maibach HI, Taylor JS, Sasseville D, DeKoven JG, Zirwas MJ, et al. North American Contact Dermatitis Group patch test results: 2011-2012. Dermatitis 2015;26:49-59
12 Warshaw EM, Belsito DV, Taylor JS, Sasseville D, DeKoven JG, Zirwas MJ, et al. North American Contact Dermatitis Group patch test results: 2009 to 2010. Dermatitis 2013;24:50-59
13 Uter W, Johansen JD, Börje A, Karlberg A-T, Lidén C, Rastogi S, Roberts D, White IR. Categorization of fragrance contact allergens for prioritization of preventive measures: clinical and experimental data and consideration of structure–activity relationships. Contact Dermatitis 2013;69:196-230

14 Jensen CD, Paulsen E, Andersen KE. Retrospective evaluation of the consequence of alleged patch test sensitization. Contact Dermatitis 2006;55:30-35

15 Deleuran M, Clemmensen O, Andersen KE. Contact lupus erythematosus. Contact Dermatitis 2000;43:169-170

16 Andersen KE. Contact allergy to toothpaste flavors. Contact Dermatitis 1978;4:195-198

17 Corazza M, Levratti A, Virgili A. Allergic contact cheilitis due to carvone in toothpastes. Contact Dermatitis 2002;46:366-367

18 Worm M, Jeep S, Sterry W, Zuberbier T. Perioral contact dermatitis caused by L-carvone in toothpaste. Contact Dermatitis 1998;38:338

19 Grattan CEH, Peachy RD. Contact sensitization to toothpaste flavouring. J Royal Coll Gen Pract 1985;35:498

20 Hausen BM. Toothpaste allergy. Dtsch Med Wochenschr 1984;109:300-302 (article in German)

21 Hausen BM. Zahnpasta-Allergie durch l-carvone. Akt Dermatol 1986;12:23-24 (article in German)

22 Gunatheesan S, Tam MM, Tate B, Tversky J, Nixon R. Retrospective study of oral lichen planus and allergy to spearmint oil. Australas J Dermatol 2012;53:224-228

23 Paulsen E, Andersen KE, Carlsen L, Egsgaard H. Carvone: an overlooked contact allergen cross-reacting with sesquiterpene lactones? Contact Dermatitis 1993;29:138-143

24 Quertermous J, Fowler JF Jr. Allergic contact dermatitis from carvone in hair conditioners. Dermatitis 2010;21:116-117

25 Kroona L, Isaksson M, Ahlgren C, Dahlin J, Bruze M, Warfvinge G. Carvone contact allergy in southern Sweden: A 21-year retrospective study. Acta Derm Venereol 2018 Aug 7. doi: 10.2340/00015555-3009. [Epub ahead of print]

26 Karlberg AT, Magnusson K, Nilsson U. Air oxidation of d-limonene (the citrus solvent) creates potent allergens. Contact Dermatitis 1992;26:332-340

27 Kroona L, Warfvinge G, Isaksson M, Ahlgren C, Dahlin J, Sörensen Ö, Bruze M. Quantification of L-carvone in toothpastes available on the Swedish market. Contact Dermatitis 2017;77:224-230

28 Nilsson U, Magnusson K, Karlberg O, Karlberg AT. Are contact allergens stable in patch test preparations? Investigation of the degradation of d-limonene hydroperoxides in petrolatum. Contact Dermatitis 1999;40:127-132

29 Nilsson AM, Gafvert E, Salvador L, Luthman K, Bruze M, Gruvberger B, Nilsson JL, Karlberg AT. Mechanism of the antigen formation of carvone and related alpha, beta-unsaturated ketones. Contact Dermatitis 2001;44:347-356

30 De Carvalho CCCR, da Fonseca MMR. Carvone: why and how should one bother to produce this terpene. Food Chem 2006;95:413-422

31 Surburg H, Panten J, Eds. Individual fragrance and flavor materials. In: Common Fragrance and Flavor Materials: Preparation, Properties and Uses, 6th Edition. Weinheim, Germany: Wiley-VCH Verlag GmbH & Co, 2016: Chapter 2, 7-192

32 Spiewak R, Samochocki Z, Grubska-Suchanek E, Czarnobilska E, Pasnicki M, Czarnecka-Operacz M, et al. Gallates, as well as hydroperoxides of limonene and linalool, are more frequent and relevant sensitizers than any cosmetic ingredient included in the European Baseline Series. Posters (P075), 13th Congress of the European Society of Contact Dermatitis (ESCD), Manchester, United Kingdom, 14–17 September 2016. Contact Dermatitis 2016;75(suppl.1):87

33 Ahlgren C, Axéll T, Möller H, Isaksson M, Liedholm R, Bruze M. Contact allergies to potential allergens in patients with oral lichen lesions. Clin Oral Investig 2014;18:227-237

34 Patton DW, Ferguson MM, Forsyth A, James J. Oro-facial granulomatosis: a possible allergic basis. Br J Oral Maxillofac Surg 1985;23:235-242

35 DeKoven JG, Warshaw EM, Zug KA, Maibach HI, Belsito DV, Sasseville D, et al. North American Contact Dermatitis Group patch test results: 2015-2016. Dermatitis 2018;29:297-309

Chapter 3.31 BETA-CARYOPHYLLENE

IDENTIFICATION

Description/definition : beta-Caryophyllene is the organic compound that conforms to the structural formula shown below

Chemical class(es) : Hydrocarbons

Chemical/IUPAC name : (1R,4E,9S)-4,11,11-Trimethyl-8-methylidenebicyclo[7.2.0]undec-4-ene

Other names : Caryophyllene; *trans*-caryophyllene

CAS registry number(s) : 87-44-5

EC number(s) : 201-746-1

RIFM monograph(s) : Food Cosmet Toxicol 1973;11:1059

SCCS opinion(s) : SCCS/1459/11 (1)

Merck Index monograph : 3145

Function(s) in cosmetics : EU: masking; perfuming; skin conditioning. USA: fragrance ingredients; skin-conditioning agents - miscellaneous

Patch testing : Oxidation mixture, 3% pet. (7)

Molecular formula : $C_{15}H_{24}$

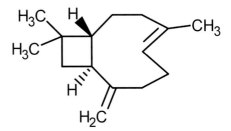

GENERAL

beta-Caryophyllene is a colorless clear oily liquid; its odor type is spicy and its odor at 100% is described as 'sweet woody spice clove dry' (www.thegoodscentscompany.com).

Presence in essential oils, Myroxylon pereirae resin (balsam of Peru) and propolis

beta-Caryophyllene has been identified by chemical analysis in 89 of 91 essential oils, which have caused contact allergy / allergic contact dermatitis. In 35 oils, beta-caryophyllene belonged to the 'Top-10' of ingredients with the highest concentrations. These are shown in table 3.31.1 with the concentration range which may be expected in commercial essential oils of this type (11). β-Caryophyllene may also be present in Myroxylon pereirae resin (balsam of Peru) (12) and in propolis (13).

CONTACT ALLERGY

General

The SCCS (Scientific Committee on Consumer Safety), in a 2012 Opinion on Fragrance allergens in cosmetic products, has marked β-caryophyllene (oxidized) as 'established contact allergen in humans' (1,6).

When beta-caryophyllene is exposed to air at room temperature, it starts to oxidize immediately. After 5 weeks, almost 50% of the original compound is consumed and after 48 weeks only 1% remains (8). Caryophyllene oxide was found to be the major oxidation product. Although hydroperoxides are formed as primary oxidation products in the autoxidation process, they could not be detected in the oxidation mixture; probably, they are quickly decomposed to secondary oxidation products, e.g. alcohols, epoxides, ketones, aldehydes, and polymeric compounds, but mostly to the epoxide caryophyllene oxide, a stable, crystalline compound (8).

Beta-caryophyllene itself is non-sensitizing, but caryophyllene oxide has been shown to be an allergen of moderate strength and beta-caryophyllene air exposed for 10 weeks showed a weak sensitizing capacity in the local lymph node assay (LLNA). Two caryophyllene hydroperoxides, however, were shown to be strongly allergenic in the LLNA (8).

A similar reduction of beta-caryophyllene has been observed in lavender oil exposed to air: only 3.3% of the original amount of beta-caryophyllene (3%) was still present after 45 weeks. In air exposed lavender oil, the same oxidation products of its ingredient beta-caryophyllene are formed as in air oxidized pure beta-caryophyllene (10).

Table 3.31.1 Essential oils containing beta-caryophyllene in the 'Top-10' and concentration range in commercial oil samples (11)

Essential oil	Concentration range (min.-max.)	Essential oil	Concentration range (min.-max.)
Bay oil	0.4 - 1.9%	Lavandin oil	1.0 - 3.7%
Black pepper oil	0.9 - 32.4%	Lavender oil	1.8 - 5.9%
Cajeput oil	0.08 - 5.2%	Lemongrass oil West Indian	0.4 - 3.0%
Cananga oil	32.9 - 38.0%	Melissa oil	0.7 - 29.4%
Carrot seed oil	1.9 - 12.6%	Niaouli oil	0.5 - 4.1%
Cedarwood oil Texas	0.08 - 1.9%	Olibanum oil	1.1 - 4.7%
Cedarwood oil Virginia	0.5 - 1.9%	Palmarosa oil	1.7 - 2.5%
Cinnamon bark oil Sri Lanka	2.7 - 7.5%	Patchouli oil	3.0 - 4.7%
Cinnamon leaf oil Sri Lanka	1.3 - 4.6%	Rosemary oil	0.7 - 6.2%
Clary sage oil	0.6 - 4.0%	Sage oil Dalmatian	1.9 - 7.7%
Clove bud/leaf/stem oil	2.4 - 19.5%	Silver fir oil	0.1 - 4.2%
Costus root oil	1.1 - 3.7%	Spearmint oil	0.09 - 3.0%
Cypress oil	0.2 - 2.1%	Spike lavender oil	0.03 - 1.9%
Dwarf pine oil	0.5 - 5.7%	Star anise oil	0.2 - 0.8%
Eucalyptus citriodora oil	0.5 - 2.6%	Thyme oil Spanish	0.6 - 2.2%
Grapefruit oil	0.1 - 1.2%	Turpentine oil	traces - 3.0%
Hyssop oil	0.8 -3.0%	Ylang-ylang oil	2.5 - 19.0%
Juniper berry oil	2.0 -5.9%		

Patch testing in groups of patients

beta-Caryophyllene has been tested in consecutive patients suspected of contact dermatitis in three studies (table 3.31.2). One of these, an investigation from Denmark (5), was part of an international study (7) and its results were also included in the latter (7). In these investigations, the test substance was an oxidation mixture of beta-caryophyllene, tested 3% in petrolatum (5,7). In an earlier study, 5% pet. was used (4), but it is preferable to use oxidized material, as this contains (one of) the allergenic form(s) of beta-caryophyllene, caryophyllene oxide. Frequencies of sensitization ranged from 0.5% to 1.1%. The relevance of the positive reactions was either not stated (4,5) or not specified for caryophyllene (7).

Table 3.31.2 Patch testing in groups of patients: Routine testing

Years and Country	Test conc. & vehicle	Number of patients tested | positive (%)		Selection of patients (S); Relevance (R); Comments (C)	Ref.
2002-2003 Denmark, Sweden, Belgium, Germany, UK	3% pet., oxidation mixture	1511	8 (0.5%)	R: certain or probable history of fragrance allergy in 58% of all reactions to terpenes (linalool, caryophyllene, caryophyllene oxide and myrcene) tested together; C: two patients co-reacted to caryophyllene oxide	7
2002-2003 Denmark	3% pet., oxidation mixture	262	3 (1.1%)	R: not stated; C: there were also 2 doubtful positive reactions; C: the data of this study are also included in those shown above this entry (ref. 7); all 3 co-reacted to colophonium	5
1998-2000 6 European countries	5% pet.	1606	10 (0.6%)	R: not stated	4

Case reports and case series

Two professional aromatherapists reacted upon patch testing to multiple essential oils. They were also patch tested with caryophyllene (test concentration not stated, probably 5% and 10% pet.), which was found to be present in many of the essential oils by GC-MS, and one of the patients reacted to caryophyllene (2).

Cross-reactions, pseudo-cross-reactions and co-reactions

For general information on cross-/pseudo-cross-/co-reactivity of fragrance chemicals with other fragrances, fragrance markers (fragrance mix I, fragrance mix II, colophonium, Myroxylon pereirae resin [balsam of Peru]) and essential oils see Chapter 1.2 General information on cross-reactions, pseudo-cross-reactions and co-reactions.

Caryophyllene oxide co-reacted in some patients allergic to an oxidation mixture of beta-caryophyllene, which is probably a pseudo-cross-reaction (7). All three patients reacting to the oxidation mixture of beta-caryophyllene in one study co-reacted to colophonium (5).

Presence in products and chemical analyses

In 1997, 71 deodorants (22 vapo-sprays, 22 aerosol sprays and 27 roll-on products) were collected in Denmark, England, France, Germany and Sweden and analyzed by gas chromatography – mass spectrometry (GC-MS) for the presence of fragrances and other materials. Caryophyllene / α-caryophyllene was present in 32 (45%) of the products (9).

In 1992, in The Netherlands, the presence of fragrances was analyzed in 300 cosmetics. Caryophyllene was identified in 33% of the products (rank order 23) (3).

LITERATURE

1   SCCS (Scientific Committee on Consumer Safety). Opinion on Fragrance allergens in cosmetic products, 26-27 June 2012, SCCS/1459/11. Available at:
    https://ec.europa.eu/health/sites/health/files/scientific_committees/consumer_safety/docs/sccs_o_102.pdf

2   Dharmagunawardena B, Takwale A, Sanders KJ, Cannan S, Rodger A, Ilchyshyn A. Gas chromatography: an investigative tool in multiple allergies to essential oils. Contact Dermatitis 2002;47:288-292

3   Weyland JW. Personal Communication, 1992. Cited in: De Groot AC, Weyland JW, Nater JP. Unwanted effects of cosmetics and drugs used in dermatology, 3rd Ed. Amsterdam: Elsevier, 1994:579

4   Frosch PJ, Johansen JD, Menné T, Pirker C, Rastogi SC, Andersen KE, et al. Further important sensitizers in patients sensitive to fragrances. II. Reactivity to essential oils. Contact Dermatitis 2002;47:279-287

5   Paulsen E, Andersen KE. Colophonium and Compositae mix as markers of fragrance allergy: cross-reactivity between fragrance terpenes, colophonium and Compositae plant extracts. Contact Dermatitis 2005;53:285-291

6   Uter W, Johansen JD, Börje A, Karlberg A-T, Lidén C, Rastogi S, Roberts D, White IR. Categorization of fragrance contact allergens for prioritization of preventive measures: clinical and experimental data and consideration of structure–activity relationships. Contact Dermatitis 2013;69:196-230

7   Matura M, Sköld M, Börje A, Andersen KE, Bruze M, Frosch P, et al. Selected oxidized fragrance terpenes are common contact allergens. Contact Dermatitis 2005;52:320-328

8   Sköld M, Karlberg A-T, Matura M, Börje A. The fragrance chemical betacaryophyllene - air oxidation and skin sensitization. Food Chem Toxicol 2006;44:538-545

9   Rastogi SC, Lepoittevin J-P, Johansen JD, Frosch PJ, Menné T, Bruze M, et al. Fragrances and other materials in deodorants: search for potentially sensitizing molecules using combined GC-MS and structure activity relationship (SAR) analysis. Contact Dermatitis 1998;39:293-303

10 Hagvall L, Sköld M, Bråred-Christensson J, Börje A, Karlberg AT. Lavender oil lacks natural protection against autoxidation, forming strong contact allergens on air exposure. Contact Dermatitis 2008;59:143-150

11 De Groot AC, Schmidt E. Essential oils: contact allergy and chemical composition. Boca Raton, Fl., USA: CRC Press, Taylor and Francis Group, 2016 (ISBN 9781482246407)

12 Mammerler V. Contribution to the analysis and quality control of Peru Balsam. PhD Thesis, University of Vienna, Austria, 2007. Available at: http://othes.univie.ac.at/4056/1/2009-03-23_0201578.pdf

13 De Groot AC, Popova MP, Bankova VS. An update on the constituents of poplar-type propolis. Wapserveen, The Netherlands: acdegroot publishing, 2014, 11 pages. ISBN/EAN: 978-90-813233-0-7. Available at:
    https://www.researchgate.net/publication/262851225_AN_UPDATE_ON_THE_CONSTITUENTS_OF_POPLAR-TYPE_PROPOLIS

Chapter 3.32   CARYOPHYLLENE OXIDE

IDENTIFICATION

Description/definition   : Caryophyllene oxide is the bicyclic epoxide that conforms to the structural formula shown
                            below
Chemical class(es)   : Bicyclic organic compounds; epoxides
INCI name USA   : Not in the Personal Care Products Council Ingredient Database
Chemical/IUPAC name   : (1R-(1R*,4R*,6R*,10S*))-4,12,12-Trimethyl-9-methylene-5-oxatricyclo[8.2.0.04,6]do-
                            decane
Other names   : beta-Caryophyllene oxide
CAS registry number(s)   : 1139-30-6
EC number(s)   : 214-519-7
RIFM monograph(s)   : Food Chem Toxicol 1983;21:661-662
Function(s) in cosmetics   : EU: perfuming
Patch testing   : 3.9% pet. (2)
Molecular formula   : $C_{15}H_{24}O$

GENERAL

Caryophyllene oxide is a pale yellow white crystalline solid; its odor type is woody and its odor at 100% is described
as 'sweet fresh dry woody spicy' (www.thegoodscentscompany.com).

Presence in essential oils and propolis

Caryophyllene oxide has been identified by chemical analysis in 79 of 91 essential oils, which have caused contact
allergy / allergic contact dermatitis. In 6 oils, caryophyllene oxide belonged to the 'Top-10' of ingredients with the
highest concentrations which may be expected in commercial essential oils of this type: costus root oil (0.5-4.3%),
hyssop oil (0.2-3.4%), carrot seed oil (0.1-3.1%), spike lavender oil (traces-1.7%), clove oil (0.06-0.6%), and turpentine oil (traces-0.4%) (5). Caryophyllene oxide may also be present in propolis (4).

CONTACT ALLERGY

General

Caryophyllene oxide is the major oxidation product of beta-caryophyllene and is formed when beta-caryophyllene is
exposed to air (autoxidation). After 12 weeks of air exposure of pure beta-caryophyllene at room temperature, the
oxidation mixture contains about 40% caryophyllene oxide. Although hydroperoxides are formed as primary
oxidation products in the autoxidation process, they cannot be detected in the oxidation mixture; probably, they are
quickly decomposed to secondary oxidation products, mostly the epoxide caryophyllene oxide, a stable, crystalline
compound.

Caryophyllene oxide has been shown to be an allergen of moderate strength in the local lymph node assay
(LLNA) (3).

Patch testing in groups of patients

In 2002-2003, in Denmark, Sweden, Belgium, Germany and the United Kingdom, 1511 consecutive patients
suspected of contact dermatitis (routine testing) were patch tested with caryophyllene oxide 3.9% in petrolatum and
there were 2 (0.1%) positive reactions. The relevance of these reactions was not specified, but there was a certain or
probable history of fragrance allergy in 58% of the positive reactions to all terpenes tested (linalool, caryophyllene,
caryophyllene oxide and myrcene) together. Both patients co-reacted to the oxidation mixture of caryophyllene, in
which caryophyllene oxide is the major component (2).

The results of this study from one participating center in Denmark were published separately (1). Of 262 consecutive patients patch tested with caryophyllene oxide 3.9% in petrolatum, one (0.4%) had a positive patch test. Its relevance was not mentioned (1).

Case reports and case series
Case reports of allergic contact dermatitis from caryophyllene oxide have not been found.

Cross-reactions, pseudo-cross-reactions and co-reactions
For general information on cross-/pseudo-cross-/co-reactivity of fragrance chemicals with other fragrances, fragrance markers (fragrance mix I, fragrance mix II, colophonium, Myroxylon pereirae resin [balsam of Peru]) and essential oils see Chapter 1.2 General information on cross-reactions, pseudo-cross-reactions and co-reactions.

Both patients shown to be allergic to caryophyllene oxide 3.9% in petrolatum co-reacted to the oxidation mixture of beta-caryophyllene, in which caryophyllene oxide is the major component (1,2).

LITERATURE

1   Paulsen E, Andersen KE. Colophonium and Compositae mix as markers of fragrance allergy: cross-reactivity between fragrance terpenes, colophonium and Compositae plant extracts. Contact Dermatitis 2005;53:285-291

2   Matura M, Sköld M, Börje A, Andersen KE, Bruze M, Frosch P, et al. Selected oxidized fragrance terpenes are common contact allergens. Contact Dermatitis 2005;52:320-328

3   Sköld M, Karlberg A-T, Matura M, Börje A. The fragrance chemical betacaryophyllene - air oxidation and skin sensitization. Food Chem Toxicol 2006;44:538-545

4   De Groot AC, Popova MP, Bankova VS. An update on the constituents of poplar-type propolis. Wapserveen, The Netherlands: acdegroot publishing, 2014, 11 pages. ISBN/EAN: 978-90-813233-0-7. Available at: https://www.researchgate.net/publication/262851225_AN_UPDATE_ON_THE_CONSTITUENTS_OF_POPLAR-TYPE_PROPOLIS

5   De Groot AC, Schmidt E. Essential oils: contact allergy and chemical composition. Boca Raton, Fl., USA: CRC Press, Taylor and Francis Group, 2016 (ISBN 9781482246407)

Chapter 3.33   CEDROL METHYL ETHER

IDENTIFICATION

Description/definition	: Cedrol methyl ether is the tricyclic organic compound that conforms to the structural formula shown below
Chemical class(es)	: Polycyclic organic compounds; ethers
INCI name USA	: Not in the Personal Care Products Council Ingredient Database
Chemical/IUPAC name	: (3R-(3α,3aβ,6β,7β,8aα))-Octahydro-6-methoxy-3,6,8,8-tetramethyl-1H-3a,7-methanoazulene
Other names	: Cedramber
CAS registry number(s)	: 19870-74-7
EC number(s)	: 243-384-7
RIFM monograph(s)	: Food Chem Toxicol 2008;46(suppl.):S1-S71; Food Cosmet Toxicol 1979;17:747 (special issue V)
Function(s) in cosmetics	: EU: perfuming
Patch testing	: 5% pet. (1)
Molecular formula	: $C_{16}H_{28}O$

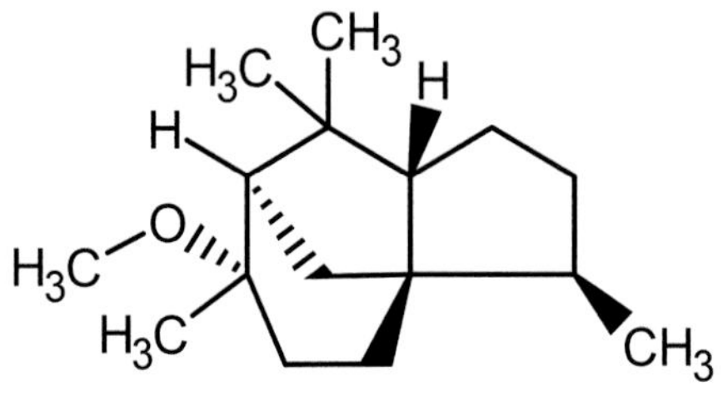

GENERAL

Cedrol methyl ether is a colorless to pale yellow clear liquid; its odor type is woody and its odor at 100% is described as 'woody dry cedar ambergris' (www.thegoodscentscompany.com). It is a synthetic chemical, not found in nature (and consequently not in essential oils (3)).

CONTACT ALLERGY

Patch testing in groups of patients

Before 1996, in Japan, European countries and the USA, 167 patients known or suspected to be allergic to fragrances were patch tested with cedrol methyl ether 5% in petrolatum and there were 3 (1.8%) positive reactions; their relevance was not mentioned (1).

Pigmented cosmetic dermatitis

While searching for causative ingredients of pigmented cosmetic dermatitis in Japan in the 1970s, both patients with ordinary (nonpigmented) cosmetic dermatitis and women with pigmented cosmetic dermatitis were tested with a large number of fragrance materials. In 1980 the accumulated data enabled the classification of fragrance materials into 4 groups: common sensitizers, rare sensitizers, virtually non-sensitizing fragrances and fragrances considered as non-sensitizers. Cedrol methyl ether was classified in the group of rare sensitizers, indicating that one or more cases of contact allergy / allergic contact dermatitis to it have been observed (2). More specific data are lacking, the results have largely or solely been published in Japanese journals only.

Case reports and case series

Case reports of allergic contact dermatitis from cedrol methyl ether have not been found.

LITERATURE

1   Larsen W, Nakayama H, Fischer T, Elsner P, Burrows D, Jordan W, et al. Fragrance contact dermatitis: A worldwide multicenter investigation (Part I). Am J Cont Dermat 1996;7:77-83
2   Nakayama H. Fragrance hypersensitivity and its control. In: Frosch PJ, Johansen JD, White IR, Eds. Fragrances - beneficial and adverse effects. Berlin Heidelberg New York: Springer-Verlag, 1998:83-91
3   De Groot AC, Schmidt E. Essential oils: contact allergy and chemical composition. Boca Raton, Fl., USA: CRC Press, Taylor and Francis Group, 2016 (ISBN 9781482246407)

Chapter 3.34 CINNAMAL

IDENTIFICATION

Description/definition : Cinnamal is the aromatic aldehyde that conforms to the structural formula shown below
Chemical class(es) : Aldehydes
Chemical/IUPAC name : 3-Phenylprop-2-enal
Other names : Cinnamaldehyde; cinnamic aldehyde
CAS registry number(s) : 104-55-2
EC number(s) : 203-213-9
RIFM monograph(s) : Food Chem Toxicol 2005;43:867-923; Food Chem Toxicol 2005;43:799-836; Food Cosm Toxicol 1979;17:253
IFRA standard : Restricted (www.ifraorg.org/en-us/standards-library) (table 3.34.1)
SCCS opinion(s) : SCCNFP/0392/00 (18); SCCS/1459/11 (19); SCCNFP/0389/00, final (52)
Merck Index monograph : 3568
Function(s) in cosmetics : EU: denaturant; flavouring; perfuming. USA: denaturants; flavoring agents; fragrance ingredients
EU cosmetic restrictions : Regulated in Annex III/76 of the Regulation (EC) No. 1223/2009, regulated by 2003/15/EC; Must be labeled on cosmetics and detergent products, if present at > 10 ppm (0.001%) in leave-on products and > 100 ppm (0.01%) in rinse-off products
Patch testing : 1% pet. (SmartPracticeEurope, Chemotechnique, SmartPracticeCanada); also present in the fragrance mix I; 2% pet. is irritant (115,116)
Molecular formula : C_9H_8O

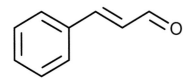

Table 3.34.1 IFRA restrictions for cinnamal

Category [a]	Limits [b]	Category [a]	Limits [b]	Category [a]	Limits [b]
1	0.02%	5	0.05%	9	0.05%
2	0.02%	6	0.40%	10	0.05%
3	0.05%	7	0.04%	11	not restricted
4	0.05%	8	0.05%		

[a] For explanation of categories see pages 6-8
[b] Limits in the finished products

GENERAL

Cinnamal is a pale yellow to dark yellow clear oily liquid; its odor type is spicy and its odor is described as 'cassia, cinnamon, cinnamon bark and red hots' (www.thegoodscentscompany.com). Cinnamal is an important component of cinnamon spice and is used widely in the food and fragrance industry (132). Cinnamal can be found as flavor in beverages and foodstuffs including ice cream, candy, baked goods, chewing gum, condiments, and meats. In electroplating processes, cinnamal is utilized as a brightener. Other applications include or have included its use as a pesticide, as an animal repellent, in compositions to attract insects, for the preparation of corrosion inhibitors, as a polymerization inhibitor for conjugated dienes, and for the coating of metals (U.S. National Library of Medicine).

Cinnamal is one of the eight ingredients of the Fragrance mix I (Chapter 3.70 Fragrance mix I)

Presence in essential oils and propolis

Cinnamal (any isomer) has been identified by chemical analysis in 14 of 91 essential oils, which have caused contact allergy / allergic contact dermatitis. In three oils, (E)-cinnamal belonged to the 'Top-10' of ingredients with the highest concentrations which may be expected in commercial essential oils of this type: cassia oil (75.4-83.1%), cinnamon bark oil Sri Lanka (43.0-72.7%) and cinnamon leaf oil Sri Lanka (0.8-2.8%) (63). Cinnamal may also be present in propolis (149).

CONTACT ALLERGY

General

The SCCS (Scientific Committee on Consumer Safety), in a 2012 Opinion on Fragrance allergens in cosmetic products, has marked cinnamal as 'established contact allergen in humans' (19,59). The sensitizing potency of cinnamal was classified as 'strong' based on an EC3 value of 0.2% in the LLNA (local lymph node assay) in animal experiments (19) and has also in other animal (10,54) and human (11) experiments been shown to be a strong sensitizer.

Cinnamal is a constituent of the fragrance mix I. It is one of the most important sensitizing fragrance substances still in use. In groups of patients reacting to the mix and tested with its 8 ingredients, cinnamal scored 7.0-38.1% positive patch test reactions, median 12.9% and average 16.5%. It has rank number 3 in the list of most frequent reactors in the mix (see Chapter 3.70 Fragrance mix I).

General population

In the period 2008-2011, in 5 European countries (Sweden, Germany, Netherlands, Portugal, Italy), a random sample of the general population of 3119 individuals aged 18-74 years were patch tested with the fragrance mix I, its 8 ingredients, the fragrance mix II, its 6 ingredients and Myroxylon pereirae resin. There were 26 reactions (0.8%) to cinnamal, tested 1% in petrolatum. About half of all positive reactions to fragrances were considered to be relevant based on standardized criteria. Women were affected twice as often as men (95).

Patch testing in groups of patients

Results of patch testing cinnamal in consecutive patients suspected of contact dermatitis (routine testing) are shown in table 3.34.2. Results of testing in groups of selected patients (e.g. patients with suspected cosmetic dermatitis, with known of suspected fragrance allergy, individuals with eyelid dermatitis, with allergic contact cheilitis, patients suffering from anogenital dermatoses, subjects previously reacting to Myroxylon pereirae resin [balsam of Peru]) are shown in table 3.34.3.

Patch testing in consecutive patients suspected of contact dermatitis: routine testing

Cinnamal has been routinely tested in at least 25 studies. Many of these are from the United States, where cinnamal 1% pet. has been part of the screening series of the NACDG (North American Contact Dermatitis Group) for two decades already. Frequencies of sensitization have ranged from 0.3% to 9%. The high 9% prevalence was found in a study from Thailand in a small group of 312 patients, in which other fragrances also scored high rates of sensitization (56). In most investigations, the frequencies of sensitization were generally between 1% and 2.4%. In the USA, a rising trend in percentage of positive reactions to cinnamal can be observed since the 2009-2010 study period of the NACDG. Before that, the frequencies on average were 2.4% (12,13,14,47,81), but in the 2011-2012 period it rose to 3.9% (46), two years later the rate of sensitization to cinnamal had risen to 4.2% (50) and remained stable at that approximate level in 2015-2017 (170). In European countries, recent rates generally range from 1% to 1.5% (2,22,53,58,60,159).

In twelve studies, relevance data were provided for cinnamal. In the NACDG studies, the percentages of definite + probable relevance were generally low, ranging from 22% to 38% (12,13,46,47,50,81,170). In other studies, the percentages of relevant positive patch test reactions – when mentioned - ranged from 45% to 89% (2,7,49,53,56). Culprit products for cinnamal sensitization were never specified, but in one study 96% of the relevant reactions to any of 26 fragrances tested were caused by cosmetic products (2).

Patch testing in groups of selected patients

Results of studies patch testing cinnamal in groups of selected patients (e.g. patients with suspected cosmetic dermatitis, with known of suspected fragrance allergy, individuals with eyelid dermatitis, with allergic contact cheilitis, patients suffering from anogenital dermatoses, subjects previously reacting to Myroxylon pereirae resin [balsam of Peru]) are shown in table 3.34.3.

In 21 investigations, frequencies of sensitization to cinnamal have ranged from 1.4% to 30%. The latter high percentage was seen in a 1975 study from the USA in a small group of 20 patients known to be allergic to fragrances (21). At that time, cinnamal was probably used on a larger scale and at higher concentrations than presently. Other rates of some 10% or more positive reactions have been found, not unexpectedly, in groups of patients known to be allergic to fragrances (9,36,37,38,61,169) (many of who reacted to the fragrance mix I, which contains cinnamal) and also in a group of patients with eyelid dermatitis (15). In two groups of patients allergic to Myroxylon pereirae resin (balsam of Peru), 10% (150) and 21% (92) reacted to cinnamal. Cinnamal is not an ingredient of the balsam, but it does contain cinnamyl alcohol, which is metabolized into the allergenic cinnamal in the skin (130-133). Apart from this, balsam of Peru is of course an indicator for fragrance sensitivity and, in the early study with 21% positive reactions (92), cinnamal was tested at 2% pet., which we now know to cause irritant reactions.

Table 3.34.2 Patch testing in groups of patients: Routine testing

Years and Country	Test conc. & vehicle	Number of patients tested	positive (%)	Selection of patients (S); Relevance (R); Comments (C)	Ref.
2015-2017 NACDG	1% pet.	5594	210 (3.8%)	R: definite + probable relevance: 31%	170
2015-7 Netherlands		821	16 (1.9%)	R: not stated	168
2015-2016 UK	1% pet.	2084	24 (1.2%)	R: not specified for individual fragrances; 25% of patients who reacted to any fragrance or fragrance marker had a positive fragrance history	22
2011-2015 USA	1% pet.	2571	24 (0.9%)	R: not stated	171
2010-2015 Denmark	1% pet.	6004	(1.4%)	R: present relevance 32%, past relevance 68%	53
2009-2015 Sweden	1% pet.	4430	57 (1.3%)	R: not stated	60
2013-2014 NACDG	1% pet.	4858	203 (4.2%)	R: definite + probable relevance: 38%	50
2013-2014 Sweden	1% pet.	616	5 (0.8%)	R: not stated	159
2013-2014 Thailand	1% pet.	312	28 (9.0%)	R: 89%	56
2011-2012 NACDG	1% pet.	4231	164 (3.9%)	R: definite + probable relevance: 34%	46
2011-2012 UK	1% pet.	1951	27 (1.4%)	R: not stated	58
2010-2011 China	1% pet.	296	(0.3%)	R: 67% for all fragrances tested together (excluding FM I)	57
2009-2010 NACDG	1% pet.	4304	(2.3%)	R: definite + probable relevance: 31%	47
2008-2010 Denmark	1% pet.	1503	20 (1.3%)	S: mostly routine testing; R: 45%; C: 90% co-reactivity of FM I, 30% of FM II; C: of the relevant reactions to any of the 26 fragrances tested, 96% were caused by cosmetic products	2
2006-2010 USA	1% pet.	3085	(1.8%)	R: 54%	49
2007-2008 NACDG	1% pet	5079	(2.4%)	R: definite + probable relevance: 38%	13
2005-2008 IVDK	1% pet.	1214	(1.4%)	R: not stated	65
2005-2006 NACDG	1% pet.	4435	(3.1%)	R: definite + probable relevance: 35%	12
2001-2005 USA	1% pet.	3114	(2.0%)	R: 56%	7
2003-2004 NACDG	1% pet.	5138	121 (2.4%)	R: not stated	14
2003-2004 IVDK	1% pet.	2063	21 (1.0%)	R: not stated; C: 70% co-reactivity of FM I	4
2003 NACDG	1% pet.	1603	27 (1.7%)	R: definite + probable relevance: 22%	81
1998-2000 USA	1% pet.	1321	(1.7%)	R: not stated	48
<1995 9 European countries + USA	1% pet.	1072	10 (0.9%)	R: not stated	35
1993 EECDRG	1% pet.	709	6 (0.9%)	R: not stated	73

EECDRG: European Environmental and Contact Dermatitis Research Group; FM: Fragrance mix; IVDK: Informationsverbund Dermatologischer Kliniken (Germany, Switzerland, Austria); NACDG: North American Contact Dermatitis Group (USA, Canada)

The relevance of the positive reactions to cinnamal was hardly ever mentioned or specified. In one study from the USA all 17 positive patch tests were considered to be relevant, but this included 'questionable' and 'past' relevance (5). Culprit products were never mentioned.

Results of testing cinnamal in groups of patients reacting to the fragrance mix I are shown in Chapter 3.70 Fragrance mix I.

Case reports and case series

Case series

Cinnamal was stated to be the (or an) allergen in 23 patients in a group of 603 individuals suffering from cosmetic dermatitis, seen in the period 2010-2015 in Leuven, Belgium (44).

In the period 1996-2013, in a tertiary referral center in Valencia, Spain, 5419 patients were patch tested. Of these, 628 individuals had allergic contact dermatitis to cosmetics. In this group, cinnamal was the responsible allergen in 6 of the cases (32).

In the period 2000-2009, in Leuven, Belgium, an unspecified number of patients had positive patch tests or use tests to a total of 344 cosmetic products *and* positive patch tests to fragrance mix I, fragrance mix II, and/or to one or more of 28 selected specific fragrance ingredients. In one of 5 patients reacting to cinnamal, the presence of this fragrance in the cosmetic product(s) was confirmed by reading the product label(s) (64).

In a group of 146 patients patch tested in the UK between 1982 and 2001 for cheilitis, 22 had relevant positive reactions, of which 3 (14%) were to cinnamal (82).

In 1992, in Sweden, 25 workers in a spice factory who reported some sort of skin reaction (e.g. dry skin, pruritus, skin lesions or hand eczema) were patch tested with cinnamal 2% pet. (a concentration known to cause irritant reactions). Eight had a dubious positive reaction and did not react to the fragrance mix I. Three had positive (+, ++ or +++) reactions and these co-reacted to fragrance mix I. The source was very likely cinnamon powder, with which the workers had regular contact (75).

Table 3.34.3 Patch testing in groups of patients: Selected patient groups

Years and Country	Test conc. & vehicle	Number of patients tested | positive (%)		Selection of patients (S); Relevance (R); Comments (C)	Ref.
2014-2017 USA		502	7 (1.4%)	S: consecutive adult patients with dermatitis; R: not stated; C: the prevalence of sensitization in patients with active atopic dermatitis (3.7%) was significantly higher than in those without (0.8%) which was ascribed to the use of personal care products	162
2011-2015 Spain	1% pet.	1013	96 (9.5%)	S: patients previously reacting to FM I, FM II, Myroxylon pereirae resin or hydroxyisohexyl 3-cyclohexene carboxaldehyde in the baseline series; R: not stated	169
2005-2014 China	1% pet.	6114	340 (5.6%)	S: patients suspected of photodermatoses; R: not stated	80
2007-2011 IVDK	1% pet.	69	4 (5.8%)	S: physical therapists; R: not stated	167
2001-2011 USA	1% pet.	34	2 (6%)	S: patients with allergic contact cheilitis; R: 100%	166
2006-2010 USA	1% pet.	100	11 (11%)	S: patients with eyelid dermatitis; R: not stated	15
2005-10 Netherlands		100	10 (10%)	S: patients with known fragrance sensitivity based on a positive patch test to the FM I and/or the FM II; R: not stated	61
2004-2008 Spain	2% pet.	86	7 (8.1%)	S: patients previously reacting to the fragrance mix I or Myroxylon pereirae (n=54) or suspected of fragrance contact allergy (n=32); R: not stated	37
2005-7 Netherlands	1% pet.	320	5 (1.6%)	S: patients suspected of fragrance or cosmetic allergy; R: 61% relevance for all positive tested fragrances together	3
2000-2007 USA	1% pet.	943	17 (1.8%)	S: patients who were tested with a supplemental cosmetic screening series; R: 100%; C: weak study: a. high rate of macular erythema and weak reactions; b. relevance figures included 'questionable' and 'past' relevance	5
2001-04 NACDG		60	4 (7%)	S: patients with allergic contact cheilitis and relevant contact allergies to allergens in the NACDG series; R: these reactions were probably all relevant, but the causative products were not mentioned	51
1994-2004 USA	1% pet.	265	13 (4.9%)	S: patients with anogenital dermatitis; R: only relevant reactions were mentioned; the rate of sensitization to cinnamal was significantly higher than in a group of routinely tested patients with dermatitis	163
<2003 Israel		91	10 (11%)	S: patients with a positive or doubtful reaction to the fragrance mix and/or Myroxylon pereirae resin and/or to one or two commercial fine fragrances; R: not stated	36
2002-2003 Korea	1% pet.	422	7 (1.7%)	S: patients with suspected cosmetic dermatitis; R: not stated	34
1998-2002 IVDK	1% pet.	29	3 (10%)	S: patients who had a positive reaction to their own deodorant; R: not stated; C: there was a significant difference in percentage positive reactions compared with a control group of dermatitis patients who had *not* reacted to their own deodorant	38
1997-2000 Austria	1% pet.	747	14 (1.9%)	S: patients suspected of fragrance allergy; R: not stated	8
<1996 Japan, Europe, USA	1% pet.	167	24 (14.4%)	S: patients known or suspected to be allergic to fragrances; R: not stated	9
<1985 Netherlands		242	24 (9.1%)	S: randomly selected patients with proven contact allergy of different origins; R: not stated	78
<1976 USA, Canada, Europe		142	14 (9.9%)	S: patients allergic to Myroxylon pereirae resin; R: not stated; cinnamal is not an ingredient of balsam of Peru but probably the sensitizer of cinnamyl alcohol by metabolization of the latter into cinnamal (130-133)	150
1975 USA	1% pet.	20	6 (30%)	S: fragrance-allergic patients; R: not stated	21
1955-1960 Denmark	2% pet.	71	15 (21%)	S: patients allergic to Myroxylon pereirae resin; R: not stated; cinnamal is not an ingredient of balsam of Peru but probably the sensitizer of cinnamyl alcohol by metabolization of the latter into cinnamal 9130-133)	92

Testing in groups of patients reacting to the fragrance mix I
Results of testing cinnamal in groups of patients reacting to the fragrance mix I are shown in Chapter 3.70 Fragrance mix I

FM: Fragrance Mix; IVDK: Informationsverbund Dermatologischer Kliniken (Germany, Switzerland, Austria);
NACDG: North American Contact Dermatitis Group (USA, Canada)

In one center in Belgium, between 1985 and 1990, 3970 patients with dermatitis were patch tested. 462 of these reacted positively to patch tests with cosmetic allergens. The reactions were considered to be relevant in 68%, probably relevant in 25% and doubtfully relevant in 7% of the patients. In the list of 'most common allergens' cinnamal had rank number 9 with 31 reactions. It should be appreciated that not all patients were patch tested with individual fragrances and that the presence of the allergen in cosmetic products causing dermatitis could not always be verified (at that time, ingredient labeling in the EU was not yet mandatory) (151).

In Belgium, in the years before 1986, of 5202 consecutive patients with dermatitis patch tested, 156 were diagnosed with pure cosmetic allergy. Cinnamal was the 'dermatitic ingredient' in 8 (5.1%) patients (frequency in the entire group: 0.8%). It should be realized, however, that only a very limited number of patients was tested with a fragrance series (76).

Cinnamal was responsible for 6 out of 399 cases of cosmetic allergy where the causal allergen was identified in a study of the NACDG, USA, 1977-1983 (6).

In an early study from Denmark, nearly all workers in a factory exposed to high concentrations of cinnamal became sensitized to it (122).

In a perfume factory, two bottle fillers developed occupational allergic contact dermatitis from cinnamal. Of twenty people working in the same factory who did *not* have dermatitis, four also had positive reactions to it (17).

Seven patients had allergic contact dermatitis from a topical medicament containing Chinese cinnamon oil. Five of these co-reacted to the fragrance mix I and to Myroxylon pereirae resin (in one, the baseline series was not tested). Two of the patients also reacted to cinnamyl alcohol and cinnamal. The fragrance mix I contains both of these substances, Chinese cinnamon oil (cassia oil) contains 70-88% cinnamal and 0-1% cinnamyl alcohol (63) and Myroxylon pereirae resin contains a small amount of cinnamyl alcohol (see Chapter 3.126 Myroxylon pereirae resin). The authors concluded that cinnamyl alcohol and cinnamal were 'probably' the sensitizers in the latter two patients (62).

Case reports

Toothpastes

In the period 1985-1998, in a Stomatology Center in the USA, 65 cases were found classified as contact stomatitis caused by cinnamon flavoring agents. In 37 of the 65 cases, causative agents were identified, and the signs and symptoms disappeared after the patients discontinued the use of these agents (foods, toothpastes, and chewing gums). Fifteen of the 37 patients were patch tested with cinnamic acid 5% pet. and cinnamal 2% pet. (which may induce irritant reactions), and 12 reacted positively (not specified to which of the test materials). In 26 patients, toothpastes were considered to be the causative agents or contributory (in combination with foods and/or chewing gum). In nine of these, patch tests had been performed with the cinnamon-derivatives, but it was not specified how many and which ones were positives. The most frequent symptoms and signs of stomatitis were erythema (gingiva, buccal mucosa, tongue) (n=8), epithelial sloughing (n=5) and burning or sore mouth (n=5) (93).

In 1972 a new toothpaste with oil of cassia (containing 70-88% cinnamal) as the main flavoring agent was marketed in the UK and Sweden. Three investigators saw 16 patients with symptoms related to the use of this toothpaste (84,85,86). The symptoms included sore mouth or 'burning' sensation, soreness of the lips, swelling or blistering of the lips, 'burning' or vesiculation of perioral skin, swelling of the tongue and ulceration of the mouth. All but one patient appeared to have been sensitized by the use of the toothpaste. The investigators received all ingredients of the toothpaste from the manufacturer, but concentrated on cassia oil and cinnamal after it was clear that the patients only reacted to these materials. Only 4 patients were tested with the toothpaste itself (all four positive) and cinnamal 1% pet. was positive in 15 of the 16 patients. Most patients tested with cassia oil and cinnamon oil (in both of which cinnamal is the main constituent) had positive reactions to them. The symptoms disappeared 4-10 days after changing the toothpaste in all patients. Several of them later tried the toothpaste again and suffered an immediate return of symptoms (85). The first three patients with contact allergy to this particular toothpaste had been reported in previous publications (87,88). The author of these reports in an addendum stated that, since this article was accepted for publication, 12 other patients had been identified with a similar sensitivity to the toothpaste, all of who had positive patch tests to cinnamal 1% pet. (87). The toothpaste was quickly withdrawn from the market.

A woman suffered from allergic contact cheilitis caused by cinnamal in a toothpaste and a sunscreen lipstick. The toothpaste was not patch tested; the cheilitis completely disappeared after avoiding both products (89).

A man developed cheilitis, stomatitis and eczema of the fingers of the left hand (holding the toothbrush) from contact allergy to cinnamon bark oil, cassia oil and their main ingredient cinnamal (90).

A clear association between the use of cinnamal-containing toothpaste and inflammation of the lips, labial mucosa, and gingivae has been described in a male patient. The sensitivity reaction was verified by a positive patch test with cinnamal. It is uncertain whether the toothpaste itself was tested (91).

In a monograph on contact allergy to balsams (92), one or more cases of contact allergy to cinnamal in toothpastes were apparently described (cited in refs. 93 and 94).

In a clinic in Spain, in a period of 2 years in the 2nd half of the 1970s, of 15 patients suffering from cheilitis, fissures of the lips, and stomatitis, 7 reacted to cinnamal (2% pet., known to be irritant) and to their toothpaste. Five of the 7 also reacted to Myroxylon pereirae resin. Quite surprisingly, the authors did not make any reference to whether the toothpastes contained cinnamal, cassia oil or cinnamon oil (118).

A woman had an erosion of the hard palate surrounded by erythema. When patch tested, she reacted to cinnamal. The cause proved to be a toothpaste she used to clean her new partial maxillary denture with, with a high concentration of cinnamal. This denture was not thoroughly cleaned by the patient before wearing it, holding the allergen in direct contact with her hard palate. The patient discontinued the use of the toothpaste which resulted in a 90% improvement of her symptoms (121).

In a study with several flaws, some patients with oral complaints reacted to cinnamal (or cinnamon), which may have contributed to their complaints by its presence in toothpaste (153).

Spices, foods and flavorings
A woman, who was allergic to cinnamal, developed a widespread and itchy maculopapular skin eruption on the abdomen, arms, chest, legs, and thighs from drinking multiple cups of herbal tea containing 27% cinnamon from *Cinnamomum zeylanicum*, with cinnamal being one of its main components. The patient was diagnosed with systemic allergic dermatitis. Prior skin sensitization had presumably taken place, following the use of scented cosmetics containing cinnamon derivatives (161).

A woman suffered from painful oral erosions which she ascribed to cinnamon-flavored breath mints. Patch tests were positive to cinnamal, crushed cinnamon mints, the fragrance mix I and Myroxylon pereirae resin. The patient challenged herself with the mints on 2 successive days before a clinic visit, and presented with 2 kissing erosions on the mobile and fixed gingival surfaces specifically where the mints had been placed. The patient also ingested mints in the clinic and developed bullous oral lesions that evening, approximately 4 hours later. Discontinuation of exposure to the offending mints led to cessation of lesion development (111).

A male patient had hand eczema for 3 months, which cleared with a 15-day holiday, but relapsed on his return. He had been working for 10 years as a waiter in a coffee house, in which natural cassia extract and synthetic vanillin were added as flavoring agents to the coffee. The patient recovered after he was advised to avoid contact with cassia and is still asymptomatic and working. Patch tests were extremely positive to natural cassia extract and cinnamal (114).

A woman complained of a 2-year history of a burning sensation to her tongue, which was most pronounced at the tip. On physical examination, a very slight erythema was noted at the tip of the tongue, and the papillae on the dorsal aspect of the tongue were slightly atrophic. Patch testing revealed a positive reaction to cinnamal. On further questioning, the patient revealed that every evening, she would eat an apple dipped in cinnamon as a bedtime snack. She often used the tip of her tongue to remove the cinnamon from the surface of the apple. Her symptoms resolved within 3 weeks of discontinuing her bedtime snack (121).

The result of eating cinnamon in one or more individuals allergic to cinnamal have been described in ref. 164 (details missing, article not read)

Occupational allergic contact dermatitis in bakers
In a group of 10 bakers with occupational hand dermatitis, there were two cases of allergic contact dermatitis. One reacted to cinnamon oil, the other to fragrance mix, cinnamal and MP resin. It was not mentioned whether the latter baker had contact with cinnamon, but as it was stated that all positive patch tests were relevant, he probably had (128).

A baker had occupational allergic contact dermatitis of the hands from cinnamal in cinnamon he frequently worked with (127).

Another baker with hand dermatitis had contact with cinnamon regularly. Patch testing revealed positive reactions to cinnamal, cinnamyl alcohol (cross-reaction to cinnamal) and to the fragrance mix I and Myroxylon pereirae resin. Cinnamal is the main ingredient in oil of cinnamon (24).

A baker had recurrent dyshidrotic eczema of the hands. Routine patch testing was negative, but he reacted to the cinnamon powder he had brought from his work. When tested subsequently with a series of fragrances/flavors, he reacted to cinnamal 0.5%, cinnamyl alcohol 5%, cinnamyl benzoate 10% , and cinnamyl cinnamate 8% in petrolatum. After avoiding skin and mucous membrane contact with cinnamon-containing products and not eating or drinking them, the dermatitis much improved. Another baker with similar symptoms and reacting to cinnamon powder had positive patch tests to the same fragrance materials and to o-methoxycinnamal 4% petrolatum. A third baker was patch tested for hand dermatitis and showed positive reactions to cocoa-powder and 'speculaaskruiden', a mixture of unknown composition, which he used at work. When subsequently tested with a series of fragrances and flavors, he had positive reactions to cinnamal 0.5%, amyl cinnamate 32% and cinnamyl cinnamate 8%, all in petrolatum. The author was 'inclined' to say that these reactions may have been relevant (45).

Two bakers and a restaurant worker had occupational allergic contact dermatitis from cinnamon, two on the hands and the third on the face and neck (from airborne contact). They all reacted to cinnamal (the main ingredient of cinnamon), the fragrance mix I (containing cinnamal) and cinnamyl alcohol (which cross-reacts with cinnamal) (106).

Other products

A woman had allergic contact dermatitis from the vulval and anal area from cinnamal and cinnamyl alcohol in sanitary napkins (33).

One or more individuals had an allergic reaction to cinnamal in a topical ophthalmological preparation (details unknown, article not read [102]).

Six patients, seen by one investigator in a period of 10 years, had allergic contact dermatitis from an antiseptic ointment containing oil of cinnamon. Three were tested with cinnamal 1% pet. and they were all positive. Cinnamal was certainly present in the ointment, as the manufacturer had provided cinnamal for patch testing as one of the ingredients of the ointment (119).

A male patient had contact dermatitis of the hands and his left foot from contact allergy to cinnamal in the cinnamon oil with which he treated a wart on his foot (120).

A boy had dermatitis of the face which appeared every time within a few hours after he used scented tissues to wipe his nose. He also had episodes of perianal itching. A patch test to the cardboard center roller, moistened with alcohol, was positive at 48 hours. There were also positive reactions to cinnamal, cinnamyl alcohol, two fragrance mixes and Myroxylon pereirae resin. The facial eruption was clear at the time of testing, but it reappeared approximately 30 minutes to an hour after removal of the patches. Avoidance of perfumed tissues and toilet paper was accompanied by a remission while exposure repeatedly reproduced the condition. Whether the tissues actually contained cinnamyl alcohol or cinnamal was not investigated (99).

A man had allergic contact dermatitis of the right hand and face from cinnamal and cinnamyl alcohol present in an oily mixture of plant extracts used for its skin softening properties (100).

One individual had generalized allergic contact dermatitis from cinnamon oil added to a mud bath in a spa; the patient reacted to cinnamon 'essence', cinnamal, cinnamyl alcohol and eugenol (101). Cinnamal is the main ingredient of cinnamon bark oil (43-73%) and most likely in cinnamon 'essence' (63).

A man handling vinyl covers used for car seat upholstery developed occupational contact dermatitis of the hands and airborne contact dermatitis of the face from contact allergy to cinnamal present in a powder he routinely handled to mask the vinyl odor (112).

A man had a one-week history of vesicular dermatitis on both soles resembling podopompholyx, followed some days later by erysipelas. Two days prior to the onset of the dermatitis, the patient had started to use new commercially available insoles containing cinnamon powder as an odor-neutralizing agent in his shoes. Patch tests were positive to the fragrance mix I, its constituents cinnamal and cinnamyl alcohol and Myroxylon pereirae resin. A strongly positive reaction was also obtained with both the inside and the outside of the cinnamon insole. Whether the cinnamon powder contained cinnamal as main ingredient (as does cinnamon oil) was not investigated (113).

A man working at a plant making room "air fresheners" developed occupational allergic contact of the hands from cinnamal present in 3 perfume concentrates he worked with containing 0.012-0.04% of cinnamal (117).

A young man complained of a sore patch on the hard palate of his mouth. The mucosa in this area was tender and burning. The patient attributed his symptoms to the use of his silicone mouth guard, which he wore when playing hockey. On physical examination, a well-circumscribed patch of pale erythema measuring 2x2 cm was visible on the hard palate. Patch testing revealed contact allergy to cinnamal and cinnamyl alcohol. On further questioning, the patient admitted to using breath fresheners strips, only when wearing his mouth guard, which kept the breath fresheners firmly compressed against his hard palate. The strips proved to contain both cinnamal and cinnamyl alcohol. The patient discontinued the use of the breath freshener strips and the reaction healed and never returned (121).

A woman suffered from allergic contact cheilitis caused by cinnamal in a sunscreen lipstick and a toothpaste. The toothpaste was not patch tested; the cheilitis completely disappeared after avoiding both products (89).

A man presented with follicular pustules and papules and large turgid red plaques in the beard area resembling folliculitis barbae, but mycological and bacterial studies were negative. Because of suspected contact allergy, he was patch tested and reacted to cinnamal, hydroxycitronellal, cinnamyl alcohol, fragrance mix I, Myroxylon pereirae resin, an aftershave and 2 colognes used by his wife. The patient often used a surgeon's mask in his work as dentist and would regularly spray this with perfume (which was patch test-negative). When all perfumes and perfumed products were stopped by him and his wife, the facial eruption subsided completely except for some mild folliculitis barbae. The author stated that 'It is clear that this man had an allergic contact dermatitis of the face due to cinnamyl alcohol, cinnamal and hydroxycitronellal. It was aggravated by his use of a surgeon's mask. The primary source may have been one of his wife's perfumes or one of his own aftershaves'. However, the presence of cinnamal, hydroxycitronellal, and cinnamyl alcohol was not verified in any of the products (146).

A young girl had perioral allergic contact dermatitis from cinnamal in a chap stick and gummy multivitamins (165).

Cross-reactions, pseudo-cross-reactions and co-reactions

For general information on cross-/pseudo-cross-/co-reactivity of fragrance chemicals with other fragrances, fragrance markers (fragrance mix I, fragrance mix II, colophonium, Myroxylon pereirae resin [balsam of Peru]) and essential oils see Chapter 1.2 General information on cross-reactions, pseudo-cross-reactions and co-reactions. Co-reactivity with the fragrance mix I can be expected, as the mix contains cinnamal (pseudo-cross-reactions).

Co-reactivity between cinnamal and cinnamyl alcohol is frequent (24,33,42,45,62,65,70,71,99,100,101,106, 113,121). Indeed, in a large UK study, 63% of patients allergic to cinnamyl alcohol were also allergic to cinnamal, compared with 11% positive patch test reactions to cinnamal in cinnamyl alcohol-negative patients (147). Conversely, among patients with positive reactions to cinnamal, 43 to 53% showed positive reactions to cinnamyl alcohol (4,160). Cinnamyl alcohol is a prohapten, which is transformed in the skin by alcohol dehydrogenase into cinnamal, which acts a hapten, explaining the extensive co-reactivity (130-133) (see Chapter 3.36 Cinnamyl alcohol).

Co-reactions have also been observed with other cinnamon-derivatives: cinnamic acid (92), cinnamyl benzoate, cinnamyl cinnamate, and methoxycinnamal (45). There does not appear to be a common hapten for cinnamal and α-amyl cinnamal (132), although some cases of co-reactivity have been observed (45,120). Nevertheless, in a large study performed by the IVDK in the period 2005-2013, twelve out of 296 patients (4.1%) allergic to cinnamal alsoreacted to amyl cinnamal; conversely, of 43 patients reacting to amyl cinnamal, 12 (28%) co-reacted to cinnamal(160). In the same investigation, 39 patients reacting to cinnamal, 3 (7.7%) had a positive reaction to hexyl cinnamal (160).

No co-reactivity was observed with the cinnamate sunscreens ethylhexyl methoxycinnamate and isoamyl *p*-methoxycinnamate (105). However, two patients with *photo*allergy to isoamyl *p*-methoxycinnamate demonstrated allergic reactions to cinnamal (126).

An association between photocontact allergy to the NSAID ketoprofen and contact allergy to the fragrance mix I has been observed in several studies. Initially, it was though that this co-sensitivity was due to the presence of cinnamal in the fragrance mix I (107,108). Later, however, it was shown that the association is more likely caused by cinnamyl alcohol, which is further discussed in Chapter 3.36 Cinnamyl alcohol.

High concentrations of cinnamal are found in cassia oil (Chapter 6.14 Cassia oil) and in cinnamon bark and cinnamon leaf oil (Chapter 6.17 Cinnamon oil) (63). Co-reactivity of cinnamal and these oils may therefore be expected and has been described many times (62,84,85,86,87,88,90,119).

Patch test sensitization

One patient became sensitized from a patch test with cinnamal 5% pet. (144). In 6 patients out of 230 with contact allergy to Myroxylon pereirae resin (balsam of Peru), there was a positive patch test to cinnamal (5% or 2% pet.) that developed 6 days or later after application. Whether these were simply 'delayed' reactions or indicative of patch test sensitization was not well investigated (92).

Presence in products and chemical analyses

In various studies, the presence of cinnamal in cosmetic and sometimes other products has been investigated. Before 2006, most investigators used chemical analysis, usually GC-MS, for qualitative and quantitative determination. Since then, the presence of the target fragrances was usually investigated by screening the product labels for the 26 fragrances that must be labeled since 2005 on cosmetics and detergent products in the EU, if present at > 10 ppm (0.001%) in leave-on products and > 100 ppm (0.01%) in rinse-off products. This method, obviously, is less accurate and may result in underestimation of the frequency of the fragrances being present in the product. When they are in fact present, but the concentration is lower than mentioned above, labeling is not required and the fragrances' presence will be missed.

The results of the relevant studies for cinnamal are summarized in table 3.34.4. More detailed information can be found in the corresponding text just above and following the table. Generally speaking it can be stated that cinnamal is a little used fragrance material.

In 2016, in Sweden, 66 commercially available toothpastes obtained from local pharmacies and supermarkets in Malmö, Sweden were investigated for the presence of flavors by studying the packages and product labels. Cinnamal was found to be present in 4 (6%) of the products (98).

In Denmark, in 2015-2016, 5588 fragranced cosmetic products were examined with a smartphone application for the 26 fragrances that need to be labeled in the EU. Cinnamal was present in 1% of the products (rank number 20) (1).

In Germany, in 2015, fragrance allergens were evaluated based on lists of ingredients in 817 (unique) detergents (all-purpose cleaners, cleaning preparations for special purposes [e.g. bathroom, kitchen, dish-washing] and laundry detergents) present in 131 households. Cinnamal was found to be present in one (0.1%) of the products (154).

Table 3.34.4 Presence of cinnamal in products [a]

Year	Country	Product type	Nr. investigated	Nr. of products positive [b]	(%)	Method [c]	Ref.
2016	Sweden	Toothpastes	66	4	(6%)	Labeling	98
2015-6	Denmark	Fragranced cosmetic products	5588		(1%)	Labeling	1
2015	Germany	Household detergents	817	1	(0.1%)	Labeling	154
2014	Poland	Emollients	179	1	(0.6%)	Online info	55
2008-11	Germany	Deodorants	374	1	(0.3%)	Labeling	97
2008	Belgium	Fragranced topical pharmaceutical products	370	1	(0.3%)	Labeling	20
2006	UK	Perfumed cosmetic and household products	300	17	(6%)	Labeling	28
2006	Denmark	Popular perfumed deodorants	88	1	(1%)	Labeling	30
			23	1	(4%)	Analysis	
2006	Denmark	Rinse-off cosmetics for children	208	2	(1%)	Labeling + analysis	39
2002	Denmark	Home and car air fresheners	19	3	(16%)	Analysis	41
2001	Denmark	Women's fine fragrances	10	2	(20%)	Analysis	29
2001	Denmark	Non-cosmetic consumer products	43	1	(2%)	Analysis	40
2000	Denmark, UK, Germany, Italy	Domestic and occupational products	59	2	(3%)	Analysis	24
1997-8	Denmark, UK Germany, Sweden	Cosmetics and cosmetic toys for children	25	2	(8%)	Analysis	27
1996-7	Denmark	Deodorants that had caused allergic contact dermatitis	19	1	(5%)	Analysis	72
1996	Five European countries	Fragranced deodorants	70	12	(17%)	Analysis	23
1995	Denmark	Cosmetic products based on natural ingredients	42	1	(2%)	Analysis	25
1995	Denmark	The 10 most popular women's perfumes	10	0	(0%)	Analysis	26

[a] See the corresponding text below for more details
[b] Positive = containing the target fragrance
[c] Labeling: information from the ingredient labels on the product / packaging; Analysis: chemical analysis, most often GC-MS

Of 179 emollients available in online drugstores in 2014 in Poland, one (0.6%) contained cinnamal, according to information available online (55).

In 2008, 2010 and 2011, 374 deodorants available in German retail shops were randomly selected and their labels checked for the presence of the 26 fragrances that need to be labeled. Cinnamal was found to be present in one (0.3%) of the products (97).

In 2008, 66 different fragrance components (including 39 essential oils) were identified in 370 (10% of the total) topical pharmaceutical products marketed in Belgium; one of these (0.3%) contained cinnamal (20).

In 2006, the labels of 208 cosmetics for children (especially shampoos, body shampoos and soaps) available in Denmark were checked for the presence of the 26 fragrances that need to be labeled in the EU. Cinnamal was present in 2 products (1%), and ranked number 21 in the frequency list (39).

In 2006, of 88 popular perfume containing deodorants purchased in Denmark, one (1%) was labeled to contain cinnamal. Analysis of 24 regulated fragrance substances in 23 selected deodorants (19 spray products, 2 deostick and 2 roll-on) was performed by GC-MS. Cinnamal was identified in one of the products (4%) with a concentration of 5 ppm (30).

In January 2006, a study of perfumed cosmetic and household products available on the shelves of U.K. retailers was carried out. Products were included if 'parfum' or 'aroma' was listed among the ingredients. Three hundred products were surveyed and any of 26 mandatory labeling fragrances named on the label were recorded. Cinnamal was present in 17 (6%) of the products (rank number 20) (28).

In 2002, in Denmark, 19 air fresheners (6 for cars, 13 for homes) were analyzed for the presence of fragrances that need to be labeled on cosmetics. Cinnamal was found to be present in 3 products (16%) in a concentration range of 10-63 ppm and ranked 17 in the frequency list (41).

In January 2001, in Denmark, ten women's fine fragrances were purchased; 5 of these had been launched years ago (1921–1990) and 5 were the latest launches by the same companies, introduced 2 months to 4 years before purchase. They were analyzed for the presence and quantity of the 7 well-identified fragrances present in the fragrance mix I (see Chapter 3.70 Fragrance mix I). The analysis revealed that the 5 old perfumes contained a mean of 5 of the 7 target allergens of the fragrance mix, while the new perfumes contained a mean of 2.8 of the allergens. The mean concentrations of the target allergens were 2.6 times higher in the old perfumes than in the new perfumes, range 2.2-337 ppm. Cinnamal was present in 2 of the 5 old perfumes, in a concentration range of 0.02-0.02 % (m/m), mean 0.02%; in the new perfumes, it was identified none of the 5 (29).

In 2001, in Denmark, 43 non-cosmetic consumer products (mainly dish-washing products, laundry detergents, and hard and soft surface cleaners) were analyzed for the 26 fragrances that are regulated for labeling in the EU. Cinnamal was present in one product (2%) in a concentration of 0.0061% (m/m) and had rank number 20 in the frequency list (40).

In 2000, fifty-nine domestic and occupational products, purchased in retail outlets in Denmark, England, Germany and Italy were analyzed by GC-MS for the presence of fragrances. The product categories were liquid soap and soap bars (n=13), soft/hard surface cleaners (n=23), fabric conditioners/laundry detergents for hand wash (n=8), dish- wash (n=10), furniture polish, car shampoo, stain remover (each n=1) and 2 products used in occupational environments. Cinnamal was present in 2 products (3%); quantification was not performed (24).

Seventy fragranced deodorants, purchased at retail outlets in 5 European countries in 1996, were analyzed by gas chromatography - mass spectrometry (GC-MS) for the determination of the contents of 21 commonly used fragrance materials. Cinnamal was identified in 12 products (17%) in a concentration range of 1–424 ppm (23).

Twenty-five cosmetics and cosmetic toys for children (5 shampoos and shower gels, 6 perfumes, 1 deodorant (roll-on), 4 baby lotions/creams, 1 baby wipes product, 1 baby oil, 2 lipcare products and 5 toy-cosmetic products: a cosmetic-toy set for blending perfumes and a makeup set) purchased in 1997-1998 in retail outlets in Denmark, Germany, England and Sweden were analyzed in 1998 for the presence of fragrances by GC-MS. Cinnamal was found in 2 products (8%) in a concentration range of ≤0.001-0.103% (w/w). For the analytical data in each product category, the original publication should be consulted (27).

In Denmark, in 1996-1997, nineteen deodorants that had caused axillary allergic contact dermatitis in 14 patients were analyzed for the presence of the 8 constituents of the fragrance mix I and cinnamal was found to be present in one (5%) of the products in a concentration of 0.0017% (72).

In 1995, in Denmark, 42 cosmetic products based on natural ingredients from 12 European and US companies (of which 22 were perfumes and 20 various other cosmetics) were investigated by high-resolution gaschromatography-mass spectrometry (GC-MS) for the presence of 11 fragrances. Cinnamal was present none of the 22 perfumes and in one of the other cosmetics, a stress buffer gel, in a concentration of 0.0745% (25).

In Denmark, in 1995, the 10 most popular women's perfumes were analyzed with gas chromatography-mass spectrometry for the presence of 7 ingredients of the Fragrance mix I (all except Evernia prunastri extract). Cinnamal was identified in none of the perfumes (26).

Serial dilution testing and Repeated Open Application Tests
Eight patients allergic to cinnamal performed ROATs with a deodorant containing cinnamal in one axilla and with an unscented but otherwise identical deodorant in the other axilla. They started with a deodorant containing 0.032% wt/vol cinnamal; if the ROAT was negative after a week, the concentration of cinnamal was increased to 0.1% and if negative again one week later, to 0.32%. All 8 individuals had a positive ROAT, 2 in the first, 4 in the second and the remaining 2 in the third week of the experiment. There were no reactions to the unscented product (16).

Nine other cinnamal-allergic individuals were patch tested with cinnamal in a dilution series from 2% alc. down to 0.0006%. All nine had positive patch tests, with a lowest concentration that still elicited a response ranging from 2% to 0.002%. Seven also had positive patch tests to cinnamal-containing deodorants, the lowest eliciting concentrations being 0.1% in five and 0.32% in two patients (16). These nine also performed ROATs with cinnamal-containing deodorants and unscented deodorants, beginning with a product containing 0.032% for 2 weeks, continuing with 0.1% for two weeks if the test was negative in the first two weeks and increasing to 0.32% if there was no reaction to 0.1%. One individual reacted to the lowest concentration, 4 to the medium one (0.1%) and three to the highest concentration (0.32%) only. Only one patient had negative ROATs, the individual that had a positive patch test to cinnamal 2% only. No reactions were observed to the unscented deodorants and in 20 controls not allergic to cinnamal, both patch tests and ROATs were negative in all (16).

In serial dilution testing, of 18 patients with a 'clear positive' reaction to cinnamal 2% pet., 15 (83%) also reacted to 1%, 11 (61%) to 0.5%, 5 (27%) to 0.1%, 3 (17%) to 0.05%, 1 (6%) to 0.02% and none to 0.01%, all in petrolatum. These individuals were also patch tested with cinnamal in alcohol with the following results: 13 (72%) reacted to cinnamal 0.8%, three (17%) to 0.1% alc. and 1 (6%) to 0.02% (129).

In the same study, ROATs with alcoholic solutions of cinnamal were performed in 22 patients who previously had shown a positive patch test to the fragrance mix I (8% or 16%) and a positive or dubious reaction upon subsequent testing with cinnamal. The test was done with graded concentrations of cinnamal. For the first 2 weeks, 0.02% was applied, for the next 2 weeks 0.1%, and for the last 2 weeks 0.8% in alcohol. The applications were continued until at least erythema was present or a week had passed from the first symptoms. Subjects with persistent skin reactions at the site of cinnamal application and a negative alcohol control site were classified as positive no matter what the degree of reaction. The results were as follows: 13 patients developed eczema at the site of cinnamal applications. None reacted to the 0.02% alcoholic solution, 8 to 0.1% and 5 only to 0.8% cinnamal solution. No reactions were observed at the alcohol control site. The mean latency period from start of applications to the first visible skin symptoms was 9.6 days for responders to 0.1% cinnamal and 7.4 days for responders to 0.8%, the range being 6-14 and 3-14 days, respectively. Six reacted later than day 7. The outcome of use testing correlated well with the history of the patients regarding adverse reactions to perfumed cosmetics. There was also a good correlation with the patch test results. Thirteen of the 18 (72%) patients with a clearly positive patch test reaction (+ or more) to cinnamal 2% pet. developed a positive use test. Of the 12 with a ++ or +++ reaction, 10 (83%) had a positive use test, of the 6 with a + reaction 3 (50%) were positive in the use test. However, the 4 patients with only a doubtful response (?+) to cinnamal 2% pet. on patch testing were all negative on use testing (129).

Other information

The term 'quenching' was employed to describe the complete abrogation of the sensitizing potential of 3 fragrance chemicals (cinnamal, citral and phenylacetaldehyde) by the presence of certain other fragrance chemicals, notably eugenol and limonene (69). The conclusions were supported by a summary of human predictive test data. Unfortunately, the absence of any details (numbers tested, reproducibility, etc.) have tended to compromise the credibility of the latter report (68). Whilst there is some evidence in man for the occurrence of quenching during the induction of skin sensitization, a much more substantial body of work has failed to find supportive evidence in various animal models, at a chemical level or at elicitation in human subjects with existing allergy (68,143). In a thorough review of the subject in 2000, it was therefore concluded that the existence of quenching of these fragrance allergens by other specific fragrance components should be regarded as a hypothesis still lacking substantive proof (68).

In groups of patients allergic to cinnamal, reduced rates of both 'current' and 'past' atopic dermatitis have been found, which was not the case with fragrances with only cutaneous exposure. It was suggested that such atopic individuals have heightened oral tolerance to dietary haptens (158).

When cinnamal 1% in petrolatum is stored in Finn chambers at room temperature, the concentration of the fragrance decreases by nearly 50% within 8 hours, probably from evaporation. This decrease is lower when the test material is stored in a refrigerator. Therefore, application to the test chamber should be performed as close in time to the patch testing as possible and storage in a refrigerator is recommended (96).

OTHER SIDE EFFECTS

Photosensitivity

Cinnamal has been found to cause immediate and delayed positive photopatch tests, which were considered to be phototoxic in nature (43). Photocontact urticaria has been observed within 20 minutes after photopatch testing with cinnamal in 3 patients (79).

Photopatch testing in groups of patients

The results of 2 studies in which cinnamal was photopatch tested are shown in table 3.34.5. In a study from China, 98 of 6114 patients (1.6%) suspected of photodermatoses had a positive photopatch test to cinnamal, but the relevance of these reactions was not mentioned (80). In a group of 41 patients who were (photo)allergic to UV-absorbers, 2 (5%) had a positive photopatch test to cinnamal 1% pet. (126). Both reactions were relevant, presumably from the presence of cinnamal in sunscreens (but unproven).

Table 3.34.5 Photopatch testing in groups of patients: Selected patient groups

Years and Country	Test conc. & vehicle	Number of patients tested	positive (%)	Selection of patients (S); Relevance (R); Comments (C)	Ref.
2005-2014 China	1% pet.	6114	98 (1.6%)	S: patients suspected of photodermatoses; R: not stated	80
1981-1996 Germany	1% pet.	41	2 (5%)	S: patients (photo)allergic to UV-absorbers; R: both relevant	126

Case reports and case series

One or more individuals had a photoallergic reaction to cinnamal in one or more topical sunscreen preparations (details unknown, article not read [103]).

Immediate-type reactions

It has well been described that cinnamal is capable of causing non-immune immediate contact reactions in the majority of individuals tested, depending on the concentration, vehicle and test location (134).

Cinnamal has also been found to cause immediate positive **photo**patch tests, which were considered to be phototoxic in nature (43). **Photo**contact urticaria has been observed within 20 minutes after photopatch testing with cinnamal in 3 patients (79).

Case reports

A woman experienced swelling of her lips and tongue following use of a cinnamal-containing mouthwash. The patient had noted that lip swelling would occasionally occur after eating cinnamon toast. Testing for contact urticaria was performed by liberally applying the mouthwash, which contained 0.18% cinnamal and had an alcoholic base, with a cotton-tipped applicator to the antecubital fossa of the patient; test sites were left open and read in 15 minutes. The test was positive in both the patient and all 10 controls tested in the same way. When tested with the ingredients of the mouthwash in the same manner, cinnamal in 10% alcohol (test concentration not mentioned, possibly 2%) was positive in the patients and all controls. Sixteen other control subjects complained of intense stinging and burning of the lips, cheeks, and tongue within 30 seconds of rinsing their mouths with the commercial mouthwash. Five complained of numbness or swelling of the lips, cheeks, or tongue within 15 minutes; no symptoms persisted beyond 30 minutes. No subject had any objective evidence of mucosal erythema or edema (134).

Another female patient, who possibly had urticaria, was tested with the ingredients of fragrance mix I, as she had previously shown a positive patch test to fragrance mix I. The materials were applied for just 20 minutes. A strong urticarial reaction was seen to cinnamal and a weak reaction to cinnamyl alcohol. Forty minutes after the test, the patient developed widespread pruritus and erythema, and 5 minutes later, she started to feel faint. A blood pressure reading was unrecordable. She was treated with chlorpheniramine maleate and adrenaline intramuscularly and made a good recovery. Review of the 20 minutes test sites at day 4 identified a positive reaction to cinnamal only. The relevance of the reaction to cinnamal remained unknown, though following identification of this allergy the patient became aware of urticarial reactions and abdominal symptoms following the ingestion of spicy foods (137).

A pastry maker had recurrent urticaria on the dorsa of the hands and forearms, related to his work. He was in daily contact with various pastry components, including chocolate, caramel, vanilla and cinnamon. Skin lesions rapidly disappeared in one or 2 hours on avoiding pastry contact. Patch tests were performed with the European standard series, removed at 20 minutes and read at 20 and 40 minutes. An immediate erythematous and edematous reaction was noted to Myroxylon pereirae resin (balsam of Peru), persistent for 1 hour. An additional series of components of balsam of Peru revealed similar positive reactions to cinnamal (which is in fact not an ingredient of balsam of Peru) and benzaldehyde. After wearing gloves and avoiding skin contact with pastry, lesions did not recur. The authors considered the reaction to benzaldehyde to be a cross-reaction to cinnamal due to the aldehyde function (138).

A woman working in a flower and garden shop complained almost daily of symptoms like generalized pruritus, especially on both hands and forearms without objective clinical signs, dry nose, itching ear and neck, shortness of breath and headache when exposed to 'all odors' since 5 years. Patch testing revealed positive immediate reactions to Myroxylon pereirae resin, cinnamal and benzaldehyde. A bronchial challenge with cinnamal was negative. The relevance of the immediate reactions was unclear and the patient was diagnosed with idiopathic environmental intolerance. One may wonder why this case was published (139).

A boy had urticaria and reacted to cinnamal with both a delayed and immediate patch test. When he stopped eating cinnamon cake, the urticaria disappeared. Eating cinnamon cake again resulted in urticaria within 24 hours (136).

Experimental studies

Of 16 volunteers tested with 0.2% cinnamal in 10% alcohol in the antecubital fossa, all had positive immediate reactions, as manifested by erythema (n=9) or erythema + induration (n=7) . 13/16 also reacted to a 0.1% concentration, but only 2/16 to cinnamal 0.01% in 10% alcohol. When tested on the forearm with cinnamal 0.1% in 10% alcohol, three patients now had negative reactions, 11 erythema only and 2 erythema + induration, indication that the antecubital fossa is the more sensitive location for the test. Only eight of 16 control subjects had positive responses when the vehicle was switched from alcohol to petrolatum. By increasing the concentration tenfold to 2.0% in petrolatum all control subjects again showed positive responses. None of the control subjects reacted to methyl cinnamal or amyl cinnamal, one subject had a weak positive response to cinnamyl alcohol, but five had positive responses to cinnamic acid (all tested 0.2% in alcohol 10%). The responses to cinnamal in the alcoholic vehicle usually appeared within five to 15 minutes; weaker reactions had often completely faded in 30 minutes. Conversely, reactions to cinnamal in petrolatum frequently had a delayed onset of appearance of 45 to 60 minutes. It was concluded that cinnamal can cause non-immunological immediate contact reactions in the majority of all subjects tested, depending on the concentration, vehicle and test location and that a single reading at 30 minutes may result missing positive reactions, both early reactions (that have faded after 30 minutes) and late reactions, appearing only after >30 minutes (134).

In a group of 60 patients with a positive patch test reaction to fragrance mix I and/or MP, 19 (32%) had immediate contact reactions to cinnamal 1% pet. In a control group of 50 non-allergic patients, the percentage of immediate reactions was 28, which was not significantly different. It was concluded that these results underline the non-immunological nature of the immediate contact reactions to cinnamal (66).

In a group of 160 patients with a positive patch test to fragrance mix I, 22 (13.8%) had an immediate contact reaction to cinnamal (67). In Hungary, before 1994, in a group of 50 patients reacting to the fragrance mix I and tested with its ingredients (test concentrations unknown), there were 33 (66%) immediate contact reactions to cinnamal (74). Of 50 individuals who had open tests with cinnamal 1% pet. on the forearm, 38 (76%) showed local macular erythema after 45 minutes, termed 'contact urticaria' by the authors (77).

In 1992, in Sweden, 25 workers in a spice factory who reported some sort of skin reaction (e.g. dry skin, pruritus, skin lesions or hand eczema) were prick tested with cinnamal 5% alc. Four subjects showed local erythema and in 2 there was also wheal formation. Two of the 6 also had positive patch tests to cinnamal 2% pet. (a concentration known to cause irritant reactions). The author did not comment on the significance of these findings (75).

In a study in the mid-1970's in Sweden, closed patch tests with Myroxylon pereirae resin and 11 of its components were applied to the upper part of the back for a period of 30 minutes of 5 patients (diagnoses unspecified, some possibly with urticaria). The result was read immediately after removal and after every hour until the reaction disappeared. Cinnamal (which is not a component of balsam of Peru) 2% pet. caused 4 urticarial reactions (148).

Nine individuals were tested for immediate contact reactions with 0.05 ml cinnamal in alcohol, applied on the skin of the forearm in concentrations of 0.1, 0.3, 1.0, 3 and 10% on a test area of 3.14 cm^2. The site of the tests remained uncovered. There were 6 reactions to cinnamal 10% (3 erythema, 3 whealing + flare), 5 to 3% and one weak reaction to 1%; the lower concentrations all remained negative. Laboratory investigations revealed cinnamal to have a histamine-liberating effect (135).

In a study from the UK, 3 panels of patients and volunteers were tested with cinnamal 2% pet. on the volar aspect of the underarm to investigate non-immune immediate contact reactions (NIICR). In panel A, consisting of 28 patients with (n=10) or without contact allergy to fragrance mix I, in who the material was applied for 40 minutes, 26 (93%) showed some signs of NIICR. In panel B, consisting of 41 consecutive patients of a Contact Clinic tested on the forearm for their immediate contact responses to cinnamal 2% pet. with a covered contact time of 30 minutes, the incidence of NIICR was 56% (n=23). Ten showed contact urticaria and 10 moderate erythema. In panel C, 80 volunteer housewives, in who the contact time was 20 minutes, only two of the 80 subjects (2.5%) failed to produce a more intense reaction to cinnamal than to the petrolatum control alone (140,141).

Of 97 patients with orofacial granulomatosis tested with cinnamal (test concentration and vehicle not mentioned), 9 (9%) showed an immediate-type reaction at 30-60 minutes. These reactions, as were immediate-type reactions to benzoic acid (n=17) and cinnamyl alcohol (n=2), were considered to be type I (immediate) hypersensitivity reactions playing a role in the immunopathology of orofacial granulomatosis. However, no controls were tested, apparently these authors were not aware that benzoic acid and cinnamal are well-known and frequent causes of non-immune immediate contact reactions and no efforts were made to verify a causal role for these chemicals in orofacial granulomatosis (156).

Quenching
The term 'quenching' was employed to describe the complete abrogation of the sensitizing potential of 3 fragrance chemicals (cinnamal, citral and phenylacetaldehyde) by the presence of certain other fragrance chemicals, notably eugenol and limonene (69). However, the same term has also been used to describe the diminution of non-immune immediate contact reactions (NIICR) (140). Eugenol has been reported repeatedly to reduce NIICR induced by cinnamal (140,141,142). The mechanism is unclear, but does not seem to involve a physicochemical interaction between the two fragrance materials (142,145).

Other non-eczematous contact reactions

Lichen planus
A woman had extensive biopsy-proven oral lichen planus. When patch tested, she had a weak positive reaction to cinnamal. The patient stated that she chewed cinnamon-flavored gums and ate cinnamon-flavored candies throughout each day. She discontinued cinnamon gums and candies, and avoided toothpaste containing cinnamal. When seen 1 month later, her oral lichen planus had cleared completely without other treatment (109).

In 3 patients with oral lichen planus and contact allergy to cinnamal, the oral lesions improved after avoidance of flavorings (110).

A female patient presented with a 10-year history of painful ulcerations on her tongue. She reported that she drank large quantities of diet cola and that she used cinnamon-flavored toothpaste and mouthwash nightly. Patch testing elicited positive reactions to balsam of Peru (a fragrance as well as a flavoring agent put in cola drinks) and cinnamal, the main ingredient of cinnamon oil used for flavoring. The patient was put on a restricted diet and a fragrance-free regimen, and her condition resolved (123).

A man had isolated lichen planus of the lips, which was aggravated by spicy foods. Upon patch testing, he reacted to metals, cinnamyl alcohol, cinnamal and benzoic acid. The diagnosis of systemic contact dermatitis from cobalt, nickel, and food fragrances and flavorings was made. Elimination gave improvement, but his 'dermatitis' occasionally flared, always in connection with certain foods (157).

Other non-eczematous contact reactions

A woman developed perioral leukoderma simulating vitiligo, which she attributed to her toothpaste containing cinnamal. A patch test to cinnamal was positive; depigmentation was observed at the patch test site three months after initial application. No changes in pigmentation occurred from a concomitant allergic patch test reaction to neomycin sulfate and *hyper*pigmentation developed at the site of an irritant patch test reaction to nonanoic acid. The perioral hypopigmentation resolved when a toothpaste without cinnamal was substituted. A repeat patch test to cinnamal again showed depigmentation at the patch test site after three months. Neither the clinical history nor physical examination results suggested allergic contact dermatitis. The authors concluded that the depigmenting effect was specific and not simply due to occult post-inflammatory changes from contact allergy, because depigmentation occurred only at the patch test site of cinnamal, but not at the patch test site of the allergic reaction (of equal intensity) to neomycin, *hyper*pigmentation occurred at the patch test sites of the irritant reactions to nonanoic acid, and the perioral leukoderma improved when a toothpaste not containing cinnamal was substituted. However, the mechanism of depigmentation remained unknown. The authors mention a similar case of perioral leukoderma and contact allergy to cinnamal associated with the use of the same commercial brand of toothpaste, which had been observed by other physicians after submitting their manuscript (104).

Two patients with orofacial granulomatosis had positive patch tests to cinnamal, which was (supposed to be) present in toothpaste, vermouth, brandy, gin, and tobacco products. After stopping the use of these products, partial improvement of the swelling was noted in one patient and complete regression in the other (155). One patient had a pemphigoid-like allergic reaction from cinnamal, probably in cinnamon (31). Contact allergy to cinnamal in eyedrops caused conjunctival cicatrization in one individual (125).

LITERATURE

1   Bennike NH, Oturai NB, Müller S, Kirkeby CS, Jørgensen C, Christensen AB, et al. Fragrance contact allergens in 5588 cosmetic products identified through a novel smartphone application. J Eur Acad Dermatol Venereol 2018;32:79-85

2   Heisterberg MV, Menné T, Johansen JD. Contact allergy to the 26 specific fragrance ingredients to be declared on cosmetic products in accordance with the EU cosmetic directive. Contact Dermatitis 2011;65:266-275

3   Oosten EJ van, Schuttelaar ML, Coenraads PJ. Clinical relevance of positive patch test reactions to the 26 EU-labelled fragrances. Contact Dermatitis 2009;61:217-223

4   Schnuch A, Uter W, Geier J, Lessmann H, Frosch PJ. Sensitization to 26 fragrances to be labelled according to current European regulation: Results of the IVDK and review of the literature. Contact Dermatitis 2007;57:1-10

5   Wetter DA, Yiannias JA, Prakash AV, Davis MDP, Farmer SA, el-Azhary RA. Results of patch testing to personal care product allergens in a standard series and a supplemental cosmetic series: an analysis of 945 patients from the Mayo Clinic Contact Dermatitis Group, 2000-2007. J Am Acad Dermatol 2010;63:789-798

6   Adams RM, Maibach HI, for the North American Contact Dermatitis Group. A five-year study of cosmetic reactions. J Am Acad Dermatol 1985;13:1062-1069

7   Davis MDP, Scalf LA, Yiannias JA, Cheng JF, El-Azhary RA, Rohlinger AL, et al. Changing trends and allergens in the patch test standard series. Arch Dermatol 2008;144:67-72

8   Wöhrl S, Hemmer W, Focke M, Götz M, Jarisch R. The significance of fragrance mix, balsam of Peru, colophony and propolis as screening tools in the detection of fragrance allergy. Br J Dermatol 2001;145:268-273

9   Larsen W, Nakayama H, Lindberg M et al. Fragrance contact dermatitis: A worldwide multicenter investigation (Part 1). Am J Cont Derm 1996;7:77–83

10   Andersen KE, Vølund A, Frankild S. The guinea pig maximization test-with a multiple dose design. Acta Derm Venereol 1995;75:463-469

11   Marzulli FN, Maibach HI. Contact allergy: predictive testing of fragrance ingredients in humans by Draize and maximization methods. J Environ Pathol Toxicol 1980;3:235-245

12 Zug KA, Warshaw EM, Fowler JF Jr, Maibach HI, Belsito DL, Pratt MD, et al. Patch-test results of the North American Contact Dermatitis Group 2005-2006. Dermatitis 2009;20:149-160

13 Fransway AF, Zug KA, Belsito DV, DeLeo VA, Fowler JF Jr, Maibach HI, et al. North American Contact Dermatitis Group patch test results for 2007-2008. Dermatitis 2013;24:10-21

14 Warshaw EM, Belsito DV, DeLeo VA, Fowler JF Jr, Maibach HI, Marks JG, et al. North American Contact Dermatitis Group patch-test results, 2003-2004 study period. Dermatitis 2008;19:129-136

15 Wenk KS, Ehrlich AE. Fragrance series testing in eyelid dermatitis. Dermatitis 2012;23:22-26

16 Bruze M, Johansen JD, Andersen KE, Frosch PJ, Lepoittevin JP, Rastogi S, et al. Deodorants: an experimental provocation study with cinnamic aldehyde. J Am Acad Dermatol 2003;48:194-200

17 Schubert HJ. Skin diseases in workers at a perfume factory. Contact Dermatitis 2006;55:81-83

18 SCCNFP (Scientific Committee on Cosmetic Products and Non-Food Products Intended for Consumers). Opinion of the Scientific Committee on Cosmetic Products and Non-Food Products Intended for Consumers concerning 'An initial list of perfumery materials which must not form part of cosmetic products except subject to the Restrictions and Conditions laid down, 25 September 2001, SCCNFP/0392/00, final. Available at: http://ec.europa.eu/health/archive/ph_risk/committees/sccp/documents/out150_en.pdf

19 SCCS (Scientific Committee on Consumer Safety). Opinion on Fragrance allergens in cosmetic products, 26-27 June 2012, SCCS/1459/11. Available at: https://ec.europa.eu/health/sites/health/files/scientific_committees/consumer_safety/docs/sccs_o_102.pdf

20 Nardelli A, D'Hooge E, Drieghe J, Dooms M, Goossens A. Allergic contact dermatitis from fragrance components in specific topical pharmaceutical products in Belgium. Contact Dermatitis 2009;60:303-313

21 Larsen WG. Perfume dermatitis. A study of 20 patients. Arch Dermatol 1977;113:623-626

22 Ung CY, White JML, White IR, Banerjee P, McFadden JP. Patch testing with the European baseline series fragrance markers: a 2016 update. Br J Dermatol 2018;178:776-780

23 Rastogi SC, Johansen JD, Frosch P, Menné T, Bruze M, Lepoittevin JP, et al. Deodorants on the European market: quantitative chemical analysis of 21 fragrances. Contact Dermatitis 1998;38:29-35

24 Rastogi SC, Heydorn S, Johansen JD, Basketter DA. Fragrance chemicals in domestic and occupational products. Contact Dermatitis 2001;45:221-225

25 Rastogi SC, Johansen JD, Menné T. Natural ingredients based cosmetics. Content of selected fragrance sensitizers. Contact Dermatitis 1996;34:423-426

26 Johansen JD, Rastogi SC, Menné T. Contact allergy to popular perfumes: assessed by patch test, use test and chemical analyses. Br J Dermatol 1996;135:419-422

27 Rastogi SC, Johansen JD, Menné T, Frosch P, Bruze M, Andersen KE, et al. Content of fragrance allergens in children's cosmetics and cosmetic toys. Contact Dermatitis 1999;41:84-88

28 Buckley DA. Fragrance ingredient labelling in products on sale in the UK. Br J Dermatol 2007;157:295-300

29 Rastogi SC, Menné T, Johansen JD. The composition of fine fragrances is changing. Contact Dermatitis 2003;48:130-132

30 Rastogi SC, Hellerup Jensen G, Johansen JD. Survey and risk assessment of chemical substances in deodorants. Survey of Chemical Substances in Consumer Products, No. 86 2007. Danish Ministry of the Environment, Environmental Protection Agency. Available at: https://www2.mst.dk/Udgiv/publications/2007/978-87-7052-625-8/pdf/978-87-7052-626-5.pdf

31 Goh CL, Ng SK. Bullous contact allergy from cinnamon. Dermatosen 1988;36:186-187. Cited in: De Groot AC, Weyland JW, Nater JP. Unwanted effects of cosmetics and drugs used in dermatology, 3rd Edition. Amsterdam – London – New York – Tokyo: Elsevier, 1994

32 Zaragoza-Ninet V, Blasco Encinas R, Vilata-Corell JJ, Pérez-Ferriols A, Sierra-Talamantes C, Esteve-Martínez A, de la Cuadra-Oyanguren J. Allergic contact dermatitis due to cosmetics: A clinical and epidemiological study in a tertiary hospital. Actas Dermosifiliogr 2016;107:329-336

33 Larsen WG. Sanitary napkin dermatitis due to the perfume. Arch Dermatol 1979;115:363

34 An S, Lee AY, Lee CH, Kim DW, Hahm JH, Kim KJ, et al. Fragrance contact dermatitis in Korea: a joint study. Contact Dermatitis 2005;53:320-323

35 Frosch PJ, Pilz B, Andersen KE, Burrows D, Camarasa JG, Dooms-Goossens A, et al. Patch testing with fragrances: results of a multicenter study of the European Environmental and Contact Dermatitis Research Group with 48 frequently used constituents of perfumes. Contact Dermatitis 1995;33:333-342

36 Trattner A, David M. Patch testing with fine fragrances: comparison with fragrance mix, balsam of Peru and a fragrance series. Contact Dermatitis 2003:49:287-289

37 Cuesta L, Silvestre JF, Toledo F, Lucas A, Perez-Crespo M, Ballester I. Fragrance contact allergy: a 4-year retrospective study. Contact Dermatitis 2010;63:77-84

38   Uter W, Geier J, Schnuch A, Frosch PJ. Patch test results with patients' own perfumes, deodorants and shaving lotions: results of the IVDK 1998-2002. J Eur Acad Dermatol Venereol 2007;21:374-379

39   Poulsen PB, Schmidt A. A survey and health assessment of cosmetic products for children. Survey of chemical substances in consumer products, No. 88. Copenhagen: Danish Environmental Protection Agency, 2007. Available at: https://www2.mst.dk/udgiv/publications/2007/978-87-7052-638-8/pdf/978-87-7052-639-5.pdf

40   Rastogi SC. Survey of chemical compounds in consumer products. Contents of selected fragrance materials in cleaning products and other consumer products. Survey no. 8-2002. Copenhagen, Denmark, Danish Environmental Protection Agency. Available at: http://eng.mst.dk/media/mst/69131/8.pdf

41   Pors J, Fuhlendorff R. Mapping of chemical substances in air fresheners and other fragrance liberating products. Report Danish Ministry of the Environment, Environmental Protection Agency (EPA). Survey of Chemicals in Consumer Products, No 30, 2003. Available at: http://eng.mst.dk/media/mst/69113/30.pdf

42   Buckley DA, Wakelin SH, Seed PT, Holloway D, Rycroft RJ, White IR, et al. The frequency of fragrance allergy in a patch-test population over a 17-year period. Br J Dermatol 2000;142:279-283

43   Addo HA, Ferguson J, Johnson BF, Frain-Bell W. The relationship between exposure to fragrance materials and persistent light reaction in photosensitivity dermatitis with actinic reticuloid syndrome. Br J Dermatol 1982;107:261-274

44   Goossens A. Cosmetic contact allergens. Cosmetics 2016, 3, 5; doi:10.3390/cosmetics3010005

45   Malten KE. Four bakers showing positive patch tests to a number of fragrance materials, which can also be used as flavors. Acta Derm Venereol 1979;59(suppl.85):117-121

46   Warshaw EM, Maibach HI, Taylor JS, Sasseville D, DeKoven JG, Zirwas MJ, et al. North American Contact Dermatitis Group patch test results: 2011-2012. Dermatitis 2015;26:49-59

47   Warshaw EM, Belsito DV, Taylor JS, Sasseville D, DeKoven JG, Zirwas MJ, et al. North American Contact Dermatitis Group patch test results: 2009 to 2010. Dermatitis 2013;24:50-59

48   Wetter DA, Davis MDP, Yiannias JA, Cheng JF, Connolly SM, el-Azhary RA, et al. Patch test results from the Mayo Contact Dermatitis Group, 1998–2000. J Am Acad Dermatol 2005;53:416-421

49   Wentworth AB, Yiannias JA, Keeling JH, Hall MR, Camilleri MJ, Drage LA, et al. Trends in patch-test results and allergen changes in the standard series: a Mayo Clinic 5-year retrospective review (January 1, 2006, to December 31, 2010). J Am Acad Dermatol 2014;70:269-275

50   DeKoven JG, Warshaw EM, Belsito DV, Sasseville D, Maibach HI, Taylor JS, et al. North American Contact Dermatitis Group Patch Test Results: 2013-2014. Dermatitis 2017;28:33-46

51   Zug KA, Kornik R, Belsito DV, DeLeo VA, Fowler JF Jr, Maibach HI, et al. Patch-testing North American lip dermatitis patients: Data from the North American Contact Dermatitis Group, 2001 to 2004. Dermatitis 2008;19:202-208

52   Dinkloh A, Worm M, Geier J, Schnuch A, Wollenberg A. Contact sensitization in patients with suspected cosmetic intolerance: results of the IVDK 2006-2011. J Eur Acad Dermatol Venereol 2015;29:1071-1081

53   Bennike NH, Zachariae C, Johansen JD. Non-mix fragrances are top sensitizers in consecutive dermatitis patients – a cross-sectional study of the 26 EU-labelled fragrance allergens. Contact Dermatitis 2017;77:270-279

54   Lidén C, Yazar K, Johansen JD, Karlberg A-T, Uter W, White IR. Comparative sensitizing potencies of fragrances, preservatives, and hair dyes. Contact Dermatitis 2016;75:265-275

55   Osinka K, Karczmarz A, Krauze K, Feleszko W. Contact allergens in cosmetics used in atopic dermatitis: analysis of product composition. Contact Dermatitis 2016;75:241-243

56   Vejanurug P, Tresukosol P, Sajjachareonpong P, Puangpet P. Fragrance allergy could be missed without patch testing with 26 individual fragrance allergens. Contact Dermatitis 2016;74:230-235

57   Liu J, Li L-F. Contact sensitization to fragrances other than fragrance mix I in China. Contact Dermatitis 2015;73:252-253

58   Mann J, McFadden JP, White JML, White IR, Banerjee P. Baseline series fragrance markers fail to predict contact allergy. Contact Dermatitis 2014;70:276-281

59   Uter W, Johansen JD, Börje A, Karlberg A-T, Lidén C, Rastogi S, Roberts D, White IR. Categorization of fragrance contact allergens for prioritization of preventive measures: clinical and experimental data and consideration of structure–activity relationships. Contact Dermatitis 2013;69:196-230

60   Mowitz M, Svedman C, Zimerson E, Isaksson M, Pontén A, Bruze M. Simultaneous patch testing with fragrance mix I, fragrance mix II and their ingredients in southern Sweden between 2009 and 2015. Contact Dermatitis 2017;77:280-287

61   Nagtegaal MJC, Pentinga SE, Kuik J, Kezic S, Rustemeyer T. The role of the skin irritation response in polysensitization to fragrances. Contact Dermatitis 2012;67:28-35

62   Schliemann S, Geier J, Elsner P. Fragrances in topical over-the-counter medicaments – a loophole in EU legislation should be closed. Contact Dermatitis 2011;65:367-368

63 De Groot AC, Schmidt E. Essential oils: contact allergy and chemical composition. Boca Raton, Fl., USA: CRC Press, Taylor and Francis Group, 2016 (ISBN 9781482246407)

64 Nardelli A, Drieghe J, Claes L, Boey L, Goossens A. Fragrance allergens in 'specific' cosmetic products. Contact Dermatitis 2011;64:212-219

65 Uter W, Geier J, Frosch P, Schnuch A. Contact allergy to fragrances: current patch test results (2005–2008) from the Information Network of Departments of Dermatology. Contact Dermatitis 2010;63:254-261

66 Tanaka S, Matsumoto Y, Dlova N, Ostlere LS, Goldsmith PC, Rycroft RJG, et al. Immediate contact reactions to fragrance mix constituents and Myroxylon pereirae resin. Contact Dermatitis 2004;51:20-21

67 Temesvári E, Németh I, Baló-Banga MJ, Husz S, Kohánka V, Somos Z, et al. Multicentre study of fragrance allergy in Hungary: Immediate and late type reactions. Contact Dermatitis 2002;46:325-330

68 Basketter D. Quenching: fact or fiction? Contact Dermatitis 2000;43:253-258

69 Opdyke DLJ. Inhibition of sensitization reactions induced by certain aldehydes. Fd Cosmet Toxicol 1976;14:197-198

70 Hendriks SA, van Ginkel CJW. Evaluation of the fragrance mix in the European standard series. Contact Dermatitis 1999;41:161-162

71 Gupta N, Shenoi SD, Balachandran C. Fragrance sensitivity in allergic contact dermatitis. Contact Dermatitis 1999;40:53-54

72 Johansen JD, Rastogi SC, Bruze M, Andersen KE, Frosch P, Dreier B, et al. Deodorants: a clinical provocation study in fragrance-sensitive individuals. Contact Dermatitis 1998;39:161-165

73 Frosch PJ, Pilz B, Burrows D, Camarasa JG, Lachapelle J-M, Lahti A, et al. Testing with fragrance mix: Is the addition of sorbitan sesquioleate to the constituents useful? Contact Dermatitis 1995;32:266-272

74 Becker K, Témesvari E, Nemeth I. Patch testing with fragrance mix and its constituents in a Hungarian population. Contact Dermatitis 1994;30:185-186

75 Meding B. Skin symptoms among workers in a spice factory. Contact Dermatitis 1993;29:202-205

76 Broeckx W, Blondeel A, Dooms-Goossens A, Achten G. Cosmetic intolerance. Contact Dermatitis 1987;16:189-194

77 Emmons WW, Marks JG Jr. Immediate and delayed reactions to cosmetic ingredients. Contact Dermatitis 1985;13:258-265

78 Van Joost Th, Stolz E, Van Der Hoek JCS. Simultaneous allergy to perfume ingredients. Contact Dermatitis 1985;12:115-116

79 Thune P. Photosensitivity and allergy to cosmetics. Contact Dermatitis 1981;7:54-55

80 Hu Y, Wang D, Shen Y, Tanh H. Photopatch testing in Chinese patients over 10 years. Dermatitis 2016;27:137-142

81 Belsito DV, Fowler JF Jr, Sasseville D, Marks JG Jr, DeLeo VA, Storrs FJ. Delayed-type hypersensitivity to fragrance materials in a select North American population. Dermatitis 2006;17:23-28

82 Strauss RM, Orton DI. Allergic contact cheilitis in the United Kingdom: a retrospective study. Dermatitis 2003;14:75-77

83 Endo H, Rees TD. Clinical features of cinnamon-induced contact stomatitis. Compend Contin Educ Dent 2006;27:403-409

84 Magnusson B, Wilkinson DS. Cinnamic aldehyde in toothpaste. 1. Clinical aspects and patch tests. Contact Dermatitis 1975;1:70-76

85 Kirton V, Wilkinson DS. Sensitivity to cinnamic aldehyde in a toothpaste. 2. Further studies. Contact Dermatitis 1975;1:77-80

86 Kirton V, Wilkinson DS. Contact sensitivity to toothpaste. Br Med J 1973;2(5858):115-116

87 Millard L. Acute contact sensitivity to a new toothpaste. J Dent 1973;1:168-170

88 Millard LG. Contact sensitivity to toothpaste. BMJ 1973;1:676

89 Maibach HI. Cheilitis: occult allergy to cinnamic aldehyde. Contact Dermatitis 1986;15:106-107

90 Drake TE, Maibach HI. Allergic contact dermatitis and stomatitis caused by a cinnamic aldehyde-flavored toothpaste. Arch Dermatol 1976;112:202-203

91 Thyne G, Young DW, Ferguson MM. Contact stomatitis caused by toothpaste. NZ Dent J 1989;85(382):124-126

92 Hjorth N. Eczematous allergy to balsams. Acta Derm Venereol 1961;41 (suppl.46):1-216

93 Hausen BM. Toothpaste allergy. Dtsch Med Wochenschr 1984;109:300-302 (article in German)

94 Sainio E-L, Kanerva L. Contact allergens in toothpastes and a review of their hypersensitivity. Contact Dermatitis 1995;33:100-105

95 Diepgen TL, Ofenloch R, Bruze M, Cazzaniga S, Coenraads PJ, Elsner P, et al. Prevalence of fragrance contact allergy in the general population of five European countries: a cross-sectional study. Br J Dermatol 2015;173:1411-1419

96   Mowitz M, Zimerson E, Svedman C, Bruze M. Stability of fragrance patch test preparations applied in test chambers. Br J Dermatol 2012;167:822-827

97   Klaschka U. Contact allergens for armpits - allergenic fragrances specified on deodorants. Int J Hyg Environ Health 2012;215:584-591

98   Kroona L, Warfvinge G, Isaksson M, Ahlgren C, Dahlin J, Sörensen Ö, Bruze M. Quantification of L-carvone in toothpastes available on the Swedish market. Contact Dermatitis 2017;77:224-230

99   Guin JD. Contact dermatitis to perfume in paper products. J Am Acad Dermatol 1981;4:733-734

100 Manzur F, el Sayed F, Bazex J. Contact allergy to cinnamic aldehyde and cinnamic alcohol in Oléophytal®. Contact Dermatitis 1995;32:55

101 Garcia-Abujeta JL, de Larramendi CH, Pomares Berna J, Munoz Palomino E. Mud bath dermatitis due to cinnamon oil. Contact Dermatitis 2005;52:234

102 Frosch PJ, Weickel R, Schmitt T, Krastel H. Nebenwirkungen von ophthalmologischen Externa. Z Hautkr 1988;63:126 (article in German)

103 Fagerlund VL, Kalimo K, Jansén C. Photocontact allergy from sunscreens. Duodecim 1983;99:146 (article in Finnish). Data cited in De Groot AC, Weyland JW, Nater JP. Unwanted effects of cosmetics and drugs used in dermatology, 3rd Edition. Amsterdam – London – New York – Tokyo: Elsevier, 1994

104 Mathias TCG, Maibach HI, Conant MA. Perioral leucoderma simulating vitiligo from use of a toothpaste containing cinnamic aldehyde. Arch Derm 1980;116:1172-1173

105 Pentinga SE, Kuik DJ, Bruynzeel DP, Rustemeyer T. Do 'cinnamon-sensitive' patients react to cinnamate UV filters? Contact Dermatitis 2009;60:210-213

106 Ackermann L, Aalto-Korte K, Jolanki R, Alanko K. Occupational allergic contact dermatitis from cinnamon including one case from airborne exposure. Contact Dermatitis 2009;60:96-99

107 Pigatto P, Bigardi A, Legori A, Valsecchi R, Picardo M. Cross-reactions in patch testing and photopatch testing with ketoprofen, tiaprophenic acid, and cinnamic aldehyde. Am J Contact Dermat 1996;7:220-223

108 Matthieu L, Meuleman L, Van Hecke E, Blondeel A, Dezfoulian B, Constandt L, Goossens A. Contact and photocontact allergy to ketoprofen. The Belgian experience. Contact Dermatitis 2004;50:238-241

109 Hoskyn J, Guin JD. Contact allergy to cinnamal in a patient with oral lichen planus. Contact Dermatitis 2005;52:160-161

110 Yiannias JA, el-Azhary RA, Hand JH, Pakzad SY, Rogers RS III. Relevant contact sensitivities in patients with the diagnosis of oral lichen planus. J Am Acad Dermatol 2000;42:177-182

111 Nadiminti H, Ehrlich A, Udey MC. Oral erosions as a manifestation of allergic contact sensitivity to cinnamon mints. Contact Dermatitis 2005;52:46-47

112 Decapite TJ, Anderson BE. Allergic contact dermatitis from cinnamic aldehyde found in an industrial odour-masking agent. Contact Dermatitis 2004;51:312-313

113 Hartmann K, Hunzelmann N. Allergic contact dermatitis from cinnamon as an odour-neutralizing agent in shoe insoles. Contact Dermatitis 2004;50:253-254

114 De Benito V, Alzaga R. Occupational allergic contact dermatitis from cassia (Chinese cinnamon) as a flavouring agent in coffee. Contact Dermatitis 1999;40:165

115 Speight EL, Lawrence CM. Cinnamic aldehyde 2% pet. is irritant on patch testing. Contact Dermatitis 1990;23:379-380

116 Ferguson J, Sharma S. Cinnamic aldehyde test concentrations. Contact Dermatitis 1984;10:191-192

117 Nethercott JR, Pilger C, O'Blents L, Roy A-M. Contact dermatitis due to cinnamic aldehyde induced in a deodorant manufacturing process. Contact Dermatitis 1983;9:241-242

118 Romaguera C, Grimalt F. Sensitization to cinnamic aldehyde in toothpaste. Contact Dermatitis 1978;4:377-378

119 Calnan CD. Cinnamon dermatitis from an ointment. Contact Dermatitis 1976;2:167-170

120 Schorr WF. Cinnamic aldehyde allergy. Contact Dermatitis 1975;1:108-111

121 Isaac-Renton M, Li MK, Parsons LM. Cinnamon spice and everything not nice: many features of intraoral allergy to cinnamic aldehyde. Dermatitis 2015;26:116-121

122 Bonnevie P. Some experiences of war-time industrial dermatoses. Acta Derm Venereol 1948;28:231-237

123 Jacob SE, Steele T. Tongue erosions and diet cola. Ear Nose Throat J 2007;86:232-233

124 Nixon R. Cinnamon allergy in a baker. Australas J Dermatol 1995;36:41

125 Ostler HB, Okumoto M, Daniels T, Conant MA. Drug-induced cicatrisation of the conjunctiva. Contact Dermatitis 1983;9:155

126 Schauder S, Ippen H. Contact and photocontact sensitivity to sunscreens. Review of a 15-year experience and of the literature. Contact Dermatitis 1997;37:221-232

127 Guarneri F. Occupational allergy to cinnamal in a baker. Contact Dermatitis 2010;63:294

128 Nethercott JR, Holness DL. Occupational dermatitis in food handlers and bakers. J Am Acad Dermatol 1989;21:485-490

129 Johansen JD, Andersen KE, Rastogi SC, Menné T. Threshold responses in cinnamic-aldehyde-sensitive subjects: results and methodological aspects. Contact Dermatitis 1996;34:165-171

130 Basketter DA. Skin sensitization to cinnamic alcohol: The role of skin metabolism. Acta Derm Venereol 1992;72:264-265

131 Smith CK, Moore CA, Elahi EN, Smart AT, Hotchkiss SA. Human skin absorption and metabolism of the contact allergens, cinnamic aldehyde, and cinnamic alcohol. Toxicol Appl Pharmacol 2000;168:189-199

132 Elahi EN, Wright Z, Hinselwood D, Hotchkiss SA, Basketter DA, Pease CK. Protein binding and metabolism influence the relative skin sensitization potential of cinnamic compounds. Chem Res Toxicol 2004;17:301-310

133 Weibel H, Hansen J, Andersen KE. Cross-sensitization patterns in guinea pigs between cinnamaldehyde, cinnamyl alcohol and cinnamic acid. Acta Derm Venereol 1989;69:302-307

134 Mathias CGT, Chappler RR, Maibach HI. Contact urticaria from cinnamic aldehyde. Arch Dermatol 1980;116:74-76

135 Nater JP, De Jong MCJM, Baar AJM, Bleumink E. Contact urticarial skin responses to cinnamaldehyde. Contact Dermatitis 1977;3:151-154

136 Kirton V. Contact urticaria and cinnamic aldehyde. Contact Dermatitis 1978;4:374-375

137 Diba VC, Statham BN. Contact urticaria from cinnamal leading to anaphylaxis. Contact Dermatitis 2003;48:119

138 Seite-Beluezza D, El Sayed F, Bazex J. Contact urticaria from cinnamic aldehyde and benzaldehyde in a confectioner. Contact Dermatitis 1994;31:272-273

139 Harth V, Merget R, Altmann L, Brüning T. Bronchial challenge testing to fragrance component as further diagnostic approach to non-immune immediate contact reactions. Contact Dermatitis 2007;56:175-177

140 Safford RJ, Basketter DA, Allenby CF, Goodwin BF. Immediate contact reactions to chemicals in the fragrance mix and a study of the quenching action of eugenol. Br J Dermatol 1990;123:595-606

141 Allenby CF, Goodwin BFJ, Safford RJ. Diminution of immediate reaction to cinnamic aldehyde by eugenol. Contact Dermatis 1984;11:322-323

142 Guin JD, Meyer BN, Drake RD, Haffley P. The effect of quenching agents on contact urticaria caused by cinnamic aldehyde. J Am Acad Dermatol 1984;10:45-51

143 Basketter DA, Allenby CF. Studies of the quenching phenomenon in delayed contact hypersensitivity reactions. Contact Dermatitis 1991;25:166-171

144 Dooms-Goossens A. Allergic contact dermatitis to ingredients used in topically applied pharmaceutical products and cosmetics. Leuven, Belgium: University Press, 1983. Data cited in ref. 143

145 Susskind R, Majeti VA. Occupational and environmental allergic problems of the skin. J Dermatol 1976;3:3-12

146 Calnan CD. Unusual hydroxycitronellal perfume dermatitis. Contact Dermatitis 1979;5:123

147 Buckley DA, Basketter DA, Smith Pease CK, Rycroft RJG, White IR, McFadden JP. Simultaneous sensitivity to fragrances. Br J Dermatol 2006;154:885-888

148 Forsbeck M, Skog E. Immediate reactions to patch tests with balsam of Peru. Contact Dermatitis 1977;3:201-205

149 De Groot AC, Popova MP, Bankova VS. An update on the constituents of poplar-type propolis. Wapserveen, The Netherlands: acdegroot publishing, 2014, 11 pages. ISBN/EAN: 978-90-813233-0-7. Available at: https://www.researchgate.net/publication/262851225_AN_UPDATE_ON_THE_CONSTITUENTS_OF_POPLAR-TYPE_PROPOLIS

150 Mitchell JC, Calnan CD, Clendenning WE, Cronin E, Hjorth N, Magnusson B, et al. Patch testing with some components of balsam of Peru. Contact Dermatitis 1976;2:57-58

151 Dooms-Goossens, A, Kerre S, Drieghe J, Bossuyt L, DeGreef H. Cosmetic products and their allergens. Eur J Dermatol 1992;2:465-468

152 Opinion of the Scientific Committee on Cosmetic Products and Non-Food Products Intended for Consumers concerning 'The 1st update of the inventory of ingredients employed in cosmetic products. Section II: Perfume and aromatic raw materials', 24 October 2000, SCCNFP/0389/00, final. Available at: http://ec.europa.eu/health/ph_risk/committees/sccp/documents/out131_en.pdf

153 Lamey PJ, Lewis MA, Rees TD, Fowler C, Binnie WH, Forsyth A. Sensitivity reaction to the cinnamonaldehyde component of toothpaste. Br Dent J 1990;168:115-118

154 Wieck S, Olsson O, Kümmerer K, Klaschka U. Fragrance allergens in household detergents. Regul Toxicol Pharmacol 2018;97:163-169

155 Patton DW, Ferguson MM, Forsyth A, James J. Oro-facial granulomatosis: a possible allergic basis. Br J Oral Maxillofac Surg 1985;23:235-242

156 Fitzpatrick L, Healy CM, McCartan BE, Flint SR, McCreary CE, Rogers S. Patch testing for food-associated allergies in orofacial granulomatosis. J Oral Pathol Med 2011;40:10-13

157 Szyfelbein Masterpol K, Gottlieb AB, Scheinman PL. Systemic contact dermatitis presenting as lichen planus of the lip. Dermatitis 2010;21:218-219

158 White JM, White IR, Kimber I, Basketter DA, Buckley DA, McFadden JP. Atopic dermatitis and allergic reactions to individual fragrance chemicals. Allergy 2009;64:312-316

159 Hagvall L, Niklasson IB, Luthman K, Karlberg AT. Can the epoxides of cinnamyl alcohol and cinnamal show new cases of contact allergy? Contact Dermatitis 2018;78:399-405

160 Geier J, Uter W, Lessmann H, Schnuch A. Fragrance mix I and II: results of breakdown tests. Flavour Frag J 2015;30:264-274

161 Mertens M, Gilissen L, Goossens A, Lambert J, Vermander E, Aerts O. Generalized systemic allergic dermatitis caused by *Cinnamomum zeylanicum* in a herbal tea. Contact Dermatitis. 2017 Oct;77(4):259-261.

162 Rastogi S, Patel KR, Singam V, Silverberg JI. Allergic contact dermatitis to personal care products and topical medications in adults with atopic dermatitis. J Am Acad Dermatol. 2018 Jul 25. pii: S0190-9622(18)32316-8. doi: 10.1016/j.jaad.2018.07.017. [Epub ahead of print]

163 Warshaw EM, Furda LM, Maibach HI, Rietschel RL, Fowler JF Jr, Belsito DV, et al. Anogenital dermatitis in patients referred for patch testing: retrospective analysis of cross-sectional data from the North American Contact Dermatitis Group, 1994-2004. Arch Dermatol 2008;144:749-755

164 Hürlimann AF, Wüthrich B. Eating cinnamon in cinnamaldehyde allergy. Hautarzt 1995;46:660-611 (article in German)

165 Matiz C, Jacob SE. Systemic contact dermatitis in children: how an avoidance diet can make a difference. Pediatr Dermatol 2011;28:368-374

166 O'Gorman SM, Torgerson RR. Contact allergy in cheilitis. Int J Dermatol 2016;55:e386-e391

167 Girbig M, Hegewald J, Seidler A, Bauer A, Uter W, Schmitt J. Type IV sensitizations in physical therapists: patch test results of the Information Network of Departments of Dermatology (IVDK) 2007-2011. J Dtsch Dermatol Ges 2013;11:1185-1192

168 Dittmar D, Schuttelaar MLA. Contact sensitization to hydroperoxides of limonene and linalool: Results of consecutive patch testing and clinical relevance. Contact Dermatitis 2018 Oct 31. doi: 10.1111/cod.13137. [Epub ahead of print]

169 Silvestre JF, Mercader P, González-Pérez R, Hervella-Garcés M, Sanz-Sánchez T, Córdoba S, et al. Sensitization to fragrances in Spain: A 5-year multicentre study (2011-2015). Contact Dermatitis. 2018 Nov 14. doi: 10.1111/cod.13152. [Epub ahead of print]

170 DeKoven JG, Warshaw EM, Zug KA, Maibach HI, Belsito DV, Sasseville D, et al. North American Contact Dermatitis Group patch test results: 2015-2016. Dermatitis 2018;29:297-309

171 Veverka KK, Hall MR, Yiannias JA, Drage LA, El-Azhary RA, Killian JM, et al. Trends in patch testing with the Mayo Clinic standard series, 2011-2015. Dermatitis 2018;29:310-315

Chapter 3.35   CINNAMIC ACID

IDENTIFICATION

Description/definition	: Cinnamic acid is the organic compound that conforms to the structural formula shown below
Chemical class(es)	: Carboxylic acids
Chemical/IUPAC name	: 3-Phenylprop-2-enoic acid
Other names	: 3-Phenylacrylic acid
CAS registry number(s)	: 140-10-3; 621-82-9
EC number(s)	: 205-398-1; 210-708-3
RIFM monograph(s)	: Food Chem Toxicol 2005;43:925-943; Food Chem Toxicol 2005;43:799-836; Food Cosmet Toxicol 1978;16:687 (special issue IV)
Merck Index monograph	: 3569
Function(s) in cosmetics	: EU: perfuming; skin conditioning. USA: skin-conditioning agents - miscellaneous
Patch testing	: 5% pet. (1,2)
Molecular formula	: $C_9H_8O_2$

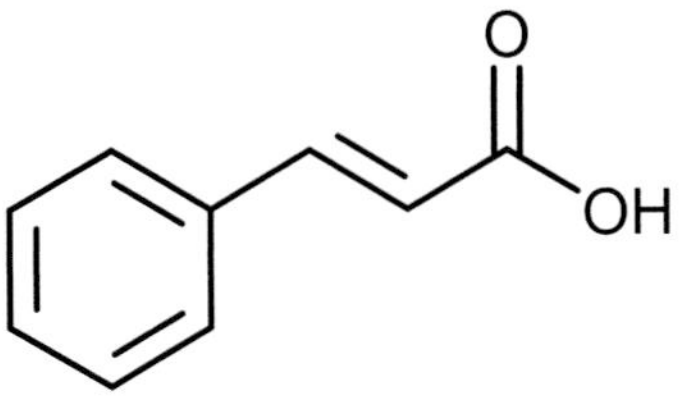

GENERAL

Cinnamic acid is a pale amber powder; its odor type is balsamic and its odor at 100% is described as 'balsam sweet storax' (www.thegoodscentscompany.com).

Presence in essential oils, Myroxylon pereirae resin (balsam of Peru) and propolis

Cinnamic acid (any isomer) has been identified by chemical analysis in 7 of 91 essential oils, which have caused contact allergy / allergic contact dermatitis. In one oil, (E)-cinnamic acid belonged to the 'Top-10' of ingredients with the highest concentrations which may be expected in commercial essential oils of this type: cassia oil (0.2-0.7%) (15). Cinnamic acid may also be present in Myroxylon pereirae resin (balsam of Peru) (3-30%) (2,16) and in propolis (cis- and trans-cinnamic acid) (10).

CONTACT ALLERGY

General

Cinnamic acid is a non- or very weak sensitizer that probably needs to be transformed in the skin into cinnamal, which then acts as a hapten (5). It can be formed in the skin by biotransformation of cinnamal (6).

Patch testing in groups of patients

Results of studies testing cinnamic acid in consecutive patients suspected of contact dermatitis (routine testing) and those of testing in groups of *selected* patients (e.g. patients allergic to propolis, individuals reacting to Myroxylon pereirae resin (in which cinnamic acid may be present in concentrations of 3-30% [2]) are shown in table 3.35.1.

In one early study, cinnamic acid 2% pet. was patch tested in 200 consecutive patients suspected of contact dermatitis (routine testing) and there were 3 (1.5%) positive reactions; their relevance was not mentioned (10).

In a very small study of 9 patients allergic to propolis, 4 (44%) reacted to cinnamic acid (which may be an ingredient of propolis [10]) 5% pet. There have also been 5 studies in which patients allergic to Myroxylon pereirae resin (balsam of Peru) were tested with one or more of its ingredients including cinnamic acid (tested 2% or 5% pet.) (table 3.35.1). Frequencies of sensitization ranged from 13 to 32%, with a mean – adjusted for sample size – of 20%, indicating that cinnamic acid is the allergen or one of the allergens in balsam of Peru in one in every 5 individuals.

Case reports and case series

Convincing case reports of allergic contact dermatitis from cinnamic acid have not been found.

In the period 1985-1998, in a Stomatology Center in the USA, 65 cases were found classified as contact stomatitis caused by cinnamon flavoring agents. In 37 of the 65 cases, causative agents were identified, and the signs and symptoms disappeared after the patients discontinued the use of these agents (foods, toothpastes, and chewing gums). Fifteen of the 37 patients were patch tested with cinnamic acid 5% pet. and cinnamal 2% pet. (which may induce irritant reactions), and 12 reacted positively (not specified to which of the test materials). In 26 patients, toothpastes were considered to be the causative agents or contributory (in combination with foods and/or chewing gum). In nine of these, patch tests had been performed with the cinnamon-derivatives, but, again, it was not specified how many and which ones were positive. The most frequent symptoms and signs of stomatitis were erythema (gingiva, buccal mucosa, tongue) (n=8), epithelial sloughing (n=5) and burning or sore mouth (n=5) (4).

A woman, who suffered repeated exacerbations of dermatitis from cosmetics, had positive reactions to a pharmaceutical ointment, Myroxylon pereirae resin, cinnamic acid 5% pet. and the related cinnamyl alcohol, cinnamal and benzyl cinnamate. The relevance of these findings was uncertain, as the manufacturer of the pharmaceutical denied the presence of fragrances in his product (3).

Table 3.35.1 Patch testing in groups of patients

Years and Country	Test conc. & vehicle	Number of patients tested | positive (%)			Selection of patients (S); Relevance (R); Comments (C)	Ref.
Routine testing						
<1973 Poland	2% pet.	200	3	(1.5%)	R: not stated	17
Testing in groups of selected patients						
1988-1990 Germany	5% pet.	9	4	(44%)	S: patients allergic to propolis; R: not stated	1
Testing in patients allergic to Myroxylon pereirae resin (balsam of Peru)						
1995-1998 Germany	5% pet.	102	33	(32%)	S: patients allergic to balsam of Peru	2
<1990 Denmark	5% pet.	15	2	(13%)	S: patients allergic to balsam of Peru	16
<1976 USA, Canada, Europe		142	26	(18%)	S: patients allergic to balsam of Peru	14
<1973 Poland	2% pet.	16	3	(19%)	S: patients allergic to balsam of Peru	17
1955-1960 Denmark	5% pet.	128	32	(25%)	S: patients allergic to balsam of Peru	9

Cross-reactions, pseudo-cross-reactions and co-reactions

For general information on cross-/pseudo-cross-/co-reactivity of fragrance chemicals with other fragrances, fragrance markers (fragrance mix I, fragrance mix II, colophonium, Myroxylon pereirae resin [balsam of Peru]) and essential oils see Chapter 1.2 General information on cross-reactions, pseudo-cross-reactions and co-reactions. Co-reactivity with Myroxylon pereirae resin (MP) may be explained by the presence of cinnamic acid (3-30%) in MP (pseudo-cross-reactions). In one patient reacting to cinnamic acid, co-reactions have been observed to Myroxylon pereirae resin, cinnamyl alcohol, cinnamal and benzyl cinnamate (3). Co-reactions between cinnamic acid, cinnamal and cinnamyl alcohol (9). In animal experiments, cinnamic acid cross-reacted to cinnamal primary sensitization, but not to cinnamyl alcohol primary sensitization (5).

Patch test sensitization

In 4 patients out of 230 with contact allergy to Myroxylon pereirae resin (balsam of Peru), there was a positive patch test to cinnamic acid 5% pet. that developed 6 days or later after application. Whether these were simply 'delayed' reactions or indicative of patch test sensitization was not well investigated, but one most likely was a case of active sensitization (9).

OTHER SIDE EFFECTS

Immediate-type reactions

Cinnamic acid has long been known to be able to induce non-immune immediate contact reactions (contact urticaria) (12). Of 16 volunteers, who all had positive immediate reactions to cinnamal 0.2% in alcohol 10%, and who were tested with cinnamic acid 0.2% in 10% alcohol in the antecubital fossa, 5 had mild positive immediate reactions, as manifested by erythema (7).

In a study in the mid-1970's in Sweden, closed patch tests with Myroxylon pereirae resin and 11 of its components were applied to the upper part of the back for a period of 30 minutes of 5 patients (diagnoses unspecified, some possibly with urticaria). The result was read immediately after removal and after every hour until the reaction disappeared. Cinnamic acid 5% pet. caused 3 urticarial reactions (8).

Cinnamic acid 5% in petrolatum caused contact urticaria in 85 of 106 (80%) and 87 of 103 (84%) patients in an open test; however, when cinnamic acid was applied in Finn chambers which were removed after 20 minutes, only 29 of 105 test individuals (28%) reacted (11).

Nonimmunologic contact urticaria from cinnamic acid was investigated in 20 male and female volunteers. The subjects were tested with cinnamic acid at dose levels of 50, 100, 250 and 500mM in absolute alcohol. A 10 μl aliquot of cinnamic acid was applied to a 1 cm² area on the upper back and the test sites were observed for erythema and edema every 10-15min over a 2-hour period. No reactions were observed with 50mM cinnamic acid. With the doses of 100,250 and 500mM, the number of patients with erythema rose from 3 to 18 and the number with edema from one with the test dose of 100mM to 9 tested with 500mM cinnamic acid (13).

Two hundred volunteers were tested with *trans*-cinnamic acid 125mM and 500mM in petrolatum for development of immediate contact reactions. Positive reactions were scored on a scale from 1 to 9, where 1 was 'a marginal reaction', 2 'perceptible erythema / perceptible swelling' and 9 'strong 'blister-like' swelling / and 'strong, deep erythema'. (18). With the lower dose of 125 mM, there was no erythema in 113/200 individuals and no edema in 194/200. With 500 mM cinnamic acid, 90/200 had no erythema and 190/200 no edema. *trans*-Cinnamic acid at the doses 500 mM and 125 mM induced lower mean edema (both doses ≤0.06) and erythema (both doses ≤1.2) scores than methyl nicotinate and benzoic acid, but higher mean edema and erythema scores than the negative control, petrolatum (18).

Oral provocation tests

Because of the known capacity of cinnamic acid to produce non-immunologic immediate contact reactions, peroral challenge tests were performed in 106 patients with 200 mg of cinnamic acid in gelatinous capsules, once daily on 4 subsequent days. All objective and subjective symptoms were recorded over a 12 hour period. Erythema was observed in 2 patients and edema was observed in one test individual. Subjective symptoms such as tingling, itching, headache, nausea, diarrhea and sweating were reported by 19 patients (18%) (11).

LITERATURE

1   Hausen BM, Evers P, Stüwe H-T, König WA, Wollenweber E. Propolis allergy (IV) Studies with further sensitizers from propolis and constituents common to propolis, poplar buds and balsam of Peru. Contact Dermatitis 1992;26:34-44

2   Hausen BM. Contact allergy to Balsam of Peru. II. Patch test results in 102 patients with selected Balsam of Peru constituents. Am J Contact Derm 2001;12:93-102

3   Van Ketel WG. Allergy to Nestosyl ointment. Contact Dermatitis 1979;5:193

4   Endo H, Rees TD. Clinical features of cinnamon-induced contact stomatitis. Compend Contin Educ Dent 2006;27:403-409

5   Weibel H, Hansen J, Andersen KE. Cross-sensitization patterns in guinea pigs between cinnamaldehyde, cinnamyl alcohol and cinnamic acid. Acta Derm Venereol 1989;69:302-307

6   Smith CK, Moore CA, Elahi EN, Smart AT, Hotchkiss SA. Human skin absorption and metabolism of the contact allergens, cinnamic aldehyde, and cinnamic alcohol. Toxicol Appl Pharmacol 2000;168:189-199

7   Mathias CGT, Chappler RR, Maibach HI. Contact urticaria from cinnamic aldehyde. Arch Dermatol 1980;116:74-76

8   Forsbeck M, Skog E. Immediate reactions to patch tests with balsam of Peru. Contact Dermatitis 1977;3:201-205

9   Hjorth N. Eczematous allergy to balsams. Acta Derm Venereol 1961;41(suppl.46):1-216

10 De Groot AC, Popova MP, Bankova VS. An update on the constituents of poplar-type propolis. Wapserveen, The Netherlands: acdegroot publishing, 2014, 11 pages. ISBN/EAN: 978-90-813233-0-7. Available at: https://www.researchgate.net/publication/262851225_AN_UPDATE_ON_THE_CONSTITUENTS_OF_POPLAR-TYPE_PROPOLIS

11 Lahti A. Non-immunologic contact urticaria. Acta Derm Venereol 1980;60:3-49

12 Gollhausen R, Kligman AM. Human assay for identifying substances which induce non-allergic contact urticaria: The NICU test. Contact Dermatitis 1985;13:98-106

13 Lahti A, Vaananen A, Kokkonen E, Hannuksela M. Acetylsalicylic acid inhibits nonimmunologic contact urticaria. Contact Dermatitis 1987;16:133-135

14 Mitchell JC, Calnan CD, Clendenning WE, Cronin E, Hjorth N, Magnusson B, et al. Patch testing with some components of balsam of Peru. Contact Dermatitis 1976;2:57-58

15 De Groot AC, Schmidt E. Essential oils: contact allergy and chemical composition. Boca Raton, Fl., USA: CRC Press, Taylor and Francis Group, 2016 (ISBN 9781482246407)

16 Øxholm A, Heidenheim M, Larsen E, Batsberg W, Menné T. Extraction and patch testing of methylcinnamate, a newly recognized fraction of balsam of Peru. Am J Cont Dermat 1990;1:43-46

17 Rudzki E, Kielak D. Sensitivity to some compounds related to Balsam of Peru. Contact Dermatitis Newsletter 1972;nr.13:335-336

18 Basketter DA, Wilhelm KP. Studies on non-immune immediate contact reactions in an unselected population. Contact Dermatitis 1996;35:237-240

Chapter 3.36   CINNAMYL ALCOHOL

IDENTIFICATION

Description/definition	: Cinnamyl alcohol is the organic compound that conforms to the structural formula shown below
Chemical class(es)	: Alcohols
Chemical/IUPAC name	: 3-Phenylprop-2-en-1-ol
Other names	: Cinnamic alcohol
CAS registry number(s)	: 104-54-1
EC number(s)	: 203-212-3
RIFM monograph(s)	: Food Chem Toxicol 2007;45(suppl.1):S1-S23; Food Chem Toxicol 2005;43:799-836; Food Chem Toxicol 2005;43:837-866; Food Cosmet Toxicol 1974;12:855 (special issue I)
IFRA standard	: Restricted (www.ifraorg.org/en-us/standards-library) (table 3.36.1)
SCCS opinion(s)	: SCCNFP/0392/00 (10); SCCS/1459/11 (11); SCCNFP/0389/00, final (111)
Merck Index monograph	: 3573
Function(s) in cosmetics	: EU: flavouring; perfuming. USA: flavoring agents; fragrance ingredients
EU cosmetic restrictions	: Regulated in Annex III/69 of the Regulation (EC) No. 1223/2009, regulated by 2003/15/EC; Must be labeled on cosmetics and detergent products, if present at > 10 ppm (0.001%) in leave-on products and > 100 ppm (0.01%) in rinse-off products
Patch testing	: 1% pet. (SmartPracticeEurope, SmartPracticeCanada); 2% pet. (Chemotechnique); also present in the fragrance mix I; TEST ADVICE: 2% pet.
Molecular formula	: $C_9H_{10}O$

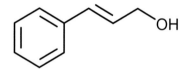

Table 3.36.1 IFRA restrictions for cinnamyl alcohol

Category [a]	Limits [b]	Category [a]	Limits [b]	Category [a]	Limits [b]
1	0.09%	5	0.40%	9	0.40%
2	0.10%	6	2.20%	10	0.40%
3	0.40%	7	0.20%	11	not restricted
4	0.40%	8	0.40%		

[a] For explanation of categories see pages 6-8
[b] Limits in the finished products

GENERAL

Cinnamyl alcohol is a pale yellow solid; its odor type is balsamic and its odor is described as 'cinnamon spice, floral, green and fermented with powdery balsamic nuances' (www.thegoodscentscompany.com). Cinnamyl alcohol is used as fragrance, as fixative for perfume blends, in the flavoring of beverages and foods (it is present in cinnamon spice), as intermediate for the synthesis of cinnamyl esters used in perfumery, and in the manufacturing of photosensitive polymers, lithographic plates and chemical-resistant coatings (U.S. National Library of Medicine).

Presence in essential oils, Myroxylon pereirae resin (balsam of Peru) and propolis
Cinnamyl alcohol (any isomer) has been identified by chemical analysis in 8 of 91 essential oils, which have caused contact allergy / allergic contact dermatitis. In none of these oils, it belonged to the 'Top-10' of ingredients with the highest concentrations (63). Cinnamyl alcohol may also be present in Myroxylon pereirae resin (balsam of Peru) (0.4%) (6) and in propolis (108).

CONTACT ALLERGY

General

The SCCS (Scientific Committee on Consumer Safety), in a 2012 Opinion on Fragrance allergens in cosmetic products, has marked cinnamyl alcohol as 'established contact allergen in humans' (11,59). The sensitizing potency of cinnamyl alcohol was classified as 'weak' based on an EC3 value of 21% in the LLNA (local lymph node assay) in animal experiments (11,59).

Cinnamyl alcohol is a constituent of the fragrance mix I. In groups of patients reacting to the mix and tested with its 8 ingredients, cinnamyl alcohol scored 1.7-42.1% positive patch test reactions, median 11.1% and average 15.2%. It has rank number 4/5/6 (with hydroxycitronellal and eugenol) in the list of most frequent reactors in the mix (see Chapter 3.70 Fragrance mix I).

Cinnamyl alcohol cannot bind to protein (32). This fragrance is thought to be a prohapten, transformed by alcohol dehydrogenase in the skin to cinnamal, which *is* able to bind to protein and act as a hapten (33,34,99). It has also been found that cinnamal adducts can be detected in human and rodent skin treated with both cinnamal and cinnamyl alcohol, indicating these substances could generate a common hapten (35). In addition, epoxycinnamyl alcohol (which is, despite its sensitizing potency, not an important hapten in contact allergy to cinnamon flavor and fragrances [113,115]) and epoxycinnamal have been identified in metabolism studies of cinnamyl alcohol (113).

Indeed, in a large UK study, 63% of patients allergic to cinnamyl alcohol were also allergic to cinnamal, compared with 11% positive patch test reactions to cinnamal in cinnamyl alcohol-negative patients (31). The high rate of simultaneous reactivity to cinnamal and cinnamyl alcohol in humans supports the capacity of human epidermis to interconvert these fragrances (32). However, over 35% of patients allergic to cinnamyl alcohol are *negative* to cinnamal (31,101), which suggests that cinnamyl alcohol may act as an allergen in its own right or via conversion to an allergen other than cinnamal, or via conversion to cinnamal or another sensitizer *outside* the skin (31). Indeed, cinnamyl alcohol readily autoxidizes upon air exposure, and forms cinnamal and epoxycinnamyl alcohol, which are strong sensitizers as determined by the murine local lymph node assay (LLNA) in mice (100) (epoxycinnamyl alcohol is not a clinically important allergen, despite its strong sensitizing capacity [115]). Thus, cinnamyl alcohol is not only a prohapten that is metabolically activated in the skin, but is also readily activated outside the skin by autoxidation, thus acting as a prehapten (100). Conversely, cinnamal can also be biotransformed in the skin into cinnamyl alcohol (32).

In groups of patients allergic to cinnamyl alcohol, reduced rates of both 'current' and 'past' atopic dermatitis have been found, which was not the case with fragrances with only cutaneous exposure. It has been suggested that such atopic individuals have heightened oral tolerance to dietary haptens (118).

The literature on contact allergy to cinnamyl alcohol up to 2004, including older literature and studies from Japan published in Japanese journals only, has been presented in a review from RIFM (102).

See also Chapter 3.70 Fragrance mix I and Chapter 3.126 Myroxylon pereirae resin (balsam of Peru), as some data on cinnamyl alcohol not provided here are presented in those chapters.

General population

In the period 2008-2011, in 5 European countries (Sweden, Germany, Netherlands, Portugal, Italy), a random sample of the general population of 3119 individuals aged 18-74 years were patch tested with the FM I, its 8 ingredients, the FM II, its 6 ingredients and Myroxylon pereirae resin. There were 10 reactions (0.3%) to cinnamyl alcohol, tested 2% in petrolatum. About half of all positive reactions to fragrances were considered to be relevant based on standardized criteria. Women were affected twice as often as men (83).

Patch testing in groups of patients

In the period 1971 to 1986, a series of patch test studies with cinnamyl alcohol were performed in Japan. Frequencies of sensitization ranged from 1-4.0% in patients with dermatitis, from 2.5% to 4.4% in groups of individuals with non-cosmetic dermatitis, it ranged from 1 to 8.1% in patients with pigmented cosmetic dermatitis and from 2.6% to 9.2% in groups of patients with cosmetic dermatitis. Summaries of these studies, which were published in Japanese journals, can be found in a 2005 RIFM review (102).

Results of studies testing cinnamyl alcohol in consecutive patients suspected of contact dermatitis (routine testing) are shown in table 3.36.2. Results of testing in groups of *selected* patients (e.g. patients with known or suspected fragrance or cosmetic dermatitis, individuals with eyelid dermatitis, patients with burning mouth syndrome, individuals suspected of photodermatoses) are shown in table 3.36.3.

Patch testing in consecutive patients suspected of contact dermatitis: routine testing

In fourteen studies in which routine testing with cinnamyl alcohol was performed, frequencies of sensitization have ranged from 0.14% to 11.2% (table 3.36.2). In 8/14 studies, rates were ≤1%. The extremely high percentage of 11.2 was found in a small study from Thailand in which a group of 312 consecutive patients was tested. In this investigation, most other fragrances also had (much) higher scores than in other studies (56).

In 11/14 investigations, no (specific) data on relevance were provided; in the three studies addressing the issue, 60-91% of the positive reactions were scored as relevant (2,54,56). Causative products were usually not mentioned or specified, but in one study, of the relevant reactions to any of 26 fragrances tested, 96% were caused by cosmetic products (2).

Table 3.36.2 Patch testing in groups of patients: Routine testing

Years and Country	Test conc. & vehicle	Number of patients tested | positive (%)			Selection of patients (S); Relevance (R); Comments (C)	Ref.
2015-7 Netherlands		821	8	(1.0%)	R: not stated	122
2015-2016 UK	2% pet.	2084	34	(1.6%)	R: not specified for individual fragrances; 25% of patients who reacted to any fragrance or fragrance marker had a positive fragrance history	119
2010-2015 Denmark	1% pet.	6004		(0.64%)	R: present relevance 60%, past relevance 35%	54
2009-2015 Sweden	2% pet.	4483	35	(0.8%)	R: not stated	60
2013-2014 Thailand		312	35	(11.2%)	R: 91%	56
2013-2014 Sweden	2% pet.	607	7	(1.2%)	R: not stated	115
2011-2012 UK	2% pet.	1951	48	(2.5%)	R: not stated	58
2010-2011 China	2% pet.	296		(5.7%)	R: 67% for all fragrances tested together (excluding FM I)	57
2008-2010 Denmark	1% pet.	1501	10	(0.7%)	S: mostly routine testing; R: 80%; 100% co-reactivity of FM I, 30% of FM II; C: of the relevant reactions to any of the 26 fragrances tested, 96% were caused by cosmetic products	2
2005-2008 IVDK	1% pet.	1214		(0.7%)	R: not stated	65
2003-2004 IVDK	1% pet.	2063	13	(0.6%)	R: not stated; C: 92% co-reactivity of FM I	4
<1995 9 European countries + USA	1% pet.	1072	6	(0.6%)	R: not stated	37
1993 EECDRG	1% pet.	709	1	(0.14%)	R: not stated	73
1991 The Netherlands	5% pet.	677	19	(2.8%)	R: not stated	76

FM: Fragrance mix; IVDK: Informationsverbund Dermatologischer Kliniken (Germany, Switzerland, Austria)

Patch testing in groups of selected patients

Results of studies patch testing cinnamyl alcohol in groups of selected patients (e.g. patients with known or suspected fragrance or cosmetic dermatitis, individuals with eyelid dermatitis, patients with burning mouth syndrome, individuals suspected of photodermatoses) are shown in table 3.36.3. In 13 investigations, frequencies of sensitization to cinnamyl alcohol have ranged from 1.5% to 75%. The extremely high rate of 75% positive reactions was observed in an early small study from the USA in 20 fragrance-allergic patients, when probably high concentrations of cinnamyl alcohol were used in fragrances (13). Other groups with high frequencies of positive reactions (10-15%) were patients with eyelid dermatitis (9) and – not surprisingly – patients with known fragrance sensitivity, (partly) based on a previous reaction to the fragrance mix I, which contains cinnamyl alcohol (39,61,123). In none of the 13 studies were relevance data provided.

Cinnamyl alcohol may be present in Myroxylon pereirae resin (balsam of Peru). In three studies patch testing patients allergic to balsam of Peru with a battery of its ingredients, 20-37% reacted to cinnamyl alcohol (6,107,109). Results of testing cinnamyl alcohol in groups of patients reacting to the fragrance mix I are shown in Chapter 3.71 Fragrance mix II.

Case reports and case series

Case series

Cinnamyl alcohol was stated to be the (or an) allergen in 25 patients in a group of 603 individuals suffering from cosmetic dermatitis, seen in the period 2010-2015 in Leuven, Belgium (50). In the period 1996-2013, in a tertiary referral center in Valencia, Spain, 5419 patients were patch tested. Of these, 628 individuals had allergic contact dermatitis to cosmetics. In this group, cinnamyl alcohol was the responsible allergen in 12 cases (28, overlap with ref. 29).

In the period 2000-2009, in Leuven, Belgium, an unspecified number of patients had positive patch tests or use tests to a total of 344 cosmetic products *and* positive patch tests to FM I, FM II, and/or to one or more of 28 selected specific fragrance ingredients. In 3 of 9 patients reacting to cinnamyl alcohol, the presence of this fragrance in the cosmetic product(s) was confirmed by reading the product label(s) (64). In the period 2000-2007, 202 patients with allergic contact dermatitis caused by cosmetics were seen in Valencia, Spain. In this group, cinnamyl alcohol was the allergen in one individual from its presence in cologne (29, overlap with ref. 28).

In one center in Belgium, between 1985 and 1990, 3970 patients with dermatitis were patch tested. 462 of these reacted positively to patch tests with cosmetic allergens. The reactions were considered to be relevant in 68%, probably relevant in 25% and doubtfully relevant in 7% of the patients. In the list of 'most common allergens' cinnamyl alcohol had rank number 11 with 27 reactions. It should be appreciated that not all patients were patch tested with individual fragrances and that the presence of the allergen in cosmetic products causing dermatitis could not always be verified (at that time, ingredient labeling in the EU was not yet mandatory) (110).

Table 3.36.3 Patch testing in groups of patients: Selected patient groups

Years and Country	Test conc. & vehicle	Number of patients tested	positive (%)	Selection of patients (S); Relevance (R); Comments (C)	Ref.
2011-2015 Spain	1% or 2% pet.	1013	108 (10.7%)	S: patients previously reacting to FM I, FM II, Myroxylon pereirae resin or hydroxyisohexyl 3-cyclohexene carboxaldehyde in the baseline series; R: not stated; C: the 2% test substances showed a higher rate of positive reactions than the 1% material	123
2005-2014 China	1% pet.	6114	342 (5.6%)	S: patients suspected of photodermatoses; R: not stated	81
2008-2012 Canada	1% pet.	132	10 (7.6%)	S: patients with burning mouth syndrome; R: 74% relevance for all allergens together	52
2007-2011 IVDK	1% pet.	69	3 (4.4%)	S: physical therapists; R: not stated	121
2006-2010 USA	2% pet.	100	15 (15%)	S: patients with eyelid dermatitis; R: not stated	9
2005-10 Netherlands		100	13 (13%)	S: patients with known fragrance sensitivity based on a positive patch test to the FM I and/or the FM II; R: not stated	61
2004-2008 Spain	2% pet.	86	12 (14%)	S: patients previously reacting to the fragrance mix I or Myroxylon pereirae (n=54) or suspected of fragrance contact allergy (n=32); R: not stated	39
2005-7 Netherlands	2% pet.	320	8 (2.5%)	S: patients suspected of fragrance or cosmetic allergy; R: 61% relevance for all positive tested fragrances together	3
<2003 Israel		91	5 (5%)	S: patients with a positive or doubtful reaction to the fragrance mix and/or Myroxylon pereirae resin and/or to one or two commercial fine fragrances; R: not stated	38
2002-2003 Korea	2% pet.	422	13 (3.1%)	S: patients with suspected cosmetic dermatitis; R: not stated	36
1997-2000 Austria	1% pet.	747	11 (1.5%)	S: patients suspected of fragrance allergy; R: not stated	7
<1996 Japan, Europe, USA	5% lanolin	167	11 (6.6%)	S: patients known or suspected to be allergic to fragrances; R: not stated	8
1975 USA	4% pet.	20	15 (75%)	S: fragrance-allergic patients; R: not stated	13

Testing in groups of patients reacting to the fragrance mix I
Results of testing cinnamyl alcohol in groups of patients reacting to the fragrance mix I are shown in Chapter 3.70 Fragrance mix I

Testing in patients allergic to Myroxylon pereirae resin (balsam of Peru)

1995-1998 Germany	5% pet.	102	38 (37%)	R: ingredient of Balsam of Peru	6
<1976 USA, Canada, Europe		142	29 (20.4%)	R: ingredient of Balsam of Peru	109
1955-1960 Denmark	5% pet.	93	23 (25%)	R: ingredient of balsam of Peru	107

FM: Fragrance mix

In a group of 119 patients with allergic contact dermatitis from cosmetics, investigated in The Netherlands in 1986-1987, two cases were caused by cinnamyl alcohol in lipstick with UV-filter and in dry shampoo (26,27). In Belgium, in the years before 1986, of 5202 consecutive patients with dermatitis patch tested, 156 were diagnosed with pure cosmetic allergy. Cinnamyl alcohol was the 'dermatitic ingredient' in 6 (3.8%) patients (frequency in the entire group: 0.7%). It should be realized, however, that only a very limited number of patients was tested with a fragrance series (77). Cinnamyl alcohol was responsible for 17 out of 399 cases of cosmetic allergy where the causal allergen was identified in a study of the NACDG, USA, 1977-1983 (5).

Eight patients had allergic contact dermatitis from a topical pharmaceutical product and all reacted to its ingredient ethylenediamine (a stabilizer) and to the perfume 5% pet. When tested with the 28 individual fragrances of the perfume, there were 4 reactions to cinnamyl alcohol, 5 to amyl cinnamal, 2 to benzyl alcohol, 2 to hydroxycitronellal and one to oakmoss synthetic (43).

Seven patients had allergic contact dermatitis from a topical medicament containing Chinese cinnamon oil. Five of these had co-reactions to the fragrance mix I and to Myroxylon pereirae resin (in one, the baseline series was not tested). Two of the patients also reacted to cinnamyl alcohol and cinnamal. The fragrance mix I contains both of these substances, Chinese cinnamon oil (cassia oil) contains 70-88% cinnamal and 0-1% cinnamyl alcohol (63) and Myroxylon pereirae resin contains a small amount of cinnamyl alcohol (see Chapter 3.126 Myroxylon pereirae resin). The authors concluded that cinnamyl alcohol and cinnamal were 'probably' the sensitizers in the latter two patients (62).

In 1992, in Sweden, 25 workers in a spice factory reporting some sort of skin reaction (e.g. dry skin, pruritus, skin lesions or hand eczema) were patch tested with cinnamyl alcohol 2% pet. and there were 3 reactions; all 3 co-reacted to cinnamal and 2 of the 3 to the FM I. The workers had regular contact with cinnamon powder, but this contains little cinnamyl alcohol. Instead, the reactions may have been cross-reactions to cinnamal, the main constituent of cinnamon powder (75).

In a very early study from Russia, workers at a perfumery plant who had developed dermatitis were investigated for allergic reactions to fragrance materials. Ninety-seven of them were skin tested either by a series of 'spot tests' or by tests using a compression method with testing plaster and cells. Reactions to 50% cinnamyl alcohol in olive oil were observed in 13 subjects (85). In a group of 10 patients sensitive to fragrances (in antiphlogistic ointments?), 3 reacted to cinnamyl alcohol. It is unknown whether cinnamyl alcohol was present in the products (article not read, ref. 97).

Case reports

A man had perianal allergic contact dermatitis from the perfume in a topical pharmaceutical preparation. When tested with the 28 ingredients of the perfume, there were positive reactions to cinnamyl alcohol, amylcinnamyl alcohol and benzyl alcohol, all tested 5% pet. (13).One patient had allergic contact dermatitis from cinnamyl alcohol in a 'dry shampoo' (20). A woman developed allergic contact dermatitis from the vulval and anal area from cinnamyl alcohol and cinnamal in sanitary napkins (30).

A baker had recurrent dyshidrotic eczema of the hands. Routine patch testing was negative, but he reacted to the cinnamon powder he had brought from his work and later to cinnamyl alcohol 5%, cinnamal 0.5%, cinnamyl benzoate 10%, cinnamyl cinnamate 8% and benzylidene acetone 0.5%, all in petrolatum. After avoiding skin and mucous membrane contact with cinnamon-containing products and not eating or drinking them, the dermatitis much improved. Another baker with similar symptoms and reacting to cinnamon powder had positive patch tests to the same fragrance materials (including cinnamyl alcohol) and to o-methoxycinnamal 4% in petrolatum. The author was 'inclined' to say that these reactions may have been relevant (51). However, cinnamyl alcohol is – contrary to cinnamal – not an important ingredient of cinnamon powder.

A barber developed contact dermatitis localized to the dorsa of the fingers. He reacted upon patch testing only to his aftershave. Further patch testing with 22 perfume ingredients showed positive reactions to cinnamyl alcohol (5% pet.), hydroxycitronellal (10% pet.), and methyl 2-octynoate (0.5% pet.). By thin layer chromatography, column chromatography and gas chromatography all three fragrance were demonstrated in the aftershave. Whether this was the cause of the dermatitis of his hands was not stated (79).

A woman developed acute allergic contact dermatitis around the anus, which spread to the trunk, legs and face after using moist toilet paper twice. Patch testing revealed allergy to the fragrance-mix, cinnamyl alcohol and isoeugenol. She did not react to the moist toilet paper itself. However, analysis of the perfume in the toilet paper revealed the presence of cinnamyl alcohol (87).

A boy had dermatitis of the face which appeared every time within a few hours after he used scented tissues to wipe his nose. He also had episodes of perianal itching. Patch testing showed positive reactions to cinnamyl alcohol, cinnamal, two fragrance mixes and Myroxylon pereirae resin. The facial eruption was clear at the time of testing, but it reappeared approximately 30 minutes to an hour after removal of the patches. Avoidance of perfumed tissues and toilet paper was accompanied by a remission while exposure repeatedly reproduced the condition. Whether the tissues actually contained cinnamyl alcohol or cinnamal was not investigated (96).

A young man complained of a sore patch on the hard palate of his mouth. The mucosa in this area was tender and burning. The patient attributed his symptoms to the use of his silicone mouth guard, which he wore when playing hockey. On physical examination, a well-circumscribed patch of pale erythema measuring 2x2 cm was visible on the hard palate. Patch testing revealed contact allergy to cinnamyl alcohol and cinnamal. On further questioning, the patient admitted to using breath freshener strips, only when wearing his mouth guard, which kept the breath fresheners firmly compressed against his hard palate. The strips proved to contain both cinnamyl alcohol and cinnamal. The patient discontinued the use of the breath freshener strips and the reaction never returned (103).

A woman with stomatitis upon patch testing reacted to her cinnamon-flavored gum and cinnamyl alcohol, but not to cinnamal or Myroxylon pereirae resin. The authors ascribed her symptoms to contact allergy to cinnamyl alcohol in the chewing gum (104). However, this is most likely incorrect as neither cinnamon oil nor cassia oil (which is often confused with cinnamon oil), which are used in chewing gums, contain appreciable amounts of cinnamyl alcohol (63).

A male patient presented with follicular pustules and papules and large turgid red plaques in the beard area resembling folliculitis barbae, but mycological and bacterial studies were negative. He was patch test positive to cinnamyl alcohol, cinnamal, hydroxycitronellal, FM I, Myroxylon pereirae resin, an aftershave and 2 colognes used by his wife. The patient often used a surgeon's mask in his work as dentist and would regularly spray this with perfume (which was patch test-negative). When all perfumes and perfumed products were stopped by him and his wife, the facial eruption subsided completely except for some mild folliculitis barbae. The author stated that 'It is clear that this man had an allergic contact dermatitis of the face due to cinnamyl alcohol, cinnamal and hydroxycitronellal. It was aggravated by his use of a surgeon's mask. The primary source may have been one of his wife's perfumes or one of his own aftershaves'. However, the presence of cinnamyl alcohol, hydroxycitronellal and cinnamal was not verified in any of the products (106).

A male patient developed allergic contact dermatitis from cinnamyl alcohol present in a sunscreen. He was also photoallergic to ketoprofen (112). The association between cinnamyl alcohol contact allergy and ketoprofen photocontact allergy is well-established (see the section 'Cross-reactions, pseudo-cross-reactions and co-reactions' below). Another man had allergic contact dermatitis of the right hand and face from cinnamyl alcohol and cinnamal present in an oily mixture of plant extracts used for its skin softening properties (98).

Pigmented cosmetic dermatitis

In Japan, in the 1960s and 1970s, many female patients developed pigmentation of the face after having facial dermatitis (45). The skin manifestations of this so-called pigmented cosmetic dermatitis consisted of diffuse or patchy brown hyperpigmentation on the cheeks and/or forehead, sometimes the entire face was involved. In severe cases, the pigmentation was black, purple, or blue-black, and in mild cases, it was pale brown. Occasionally, erythematous macules or papules, suggesting a mild contact dermatitis, were observed and itching was also noted at varying times. Pigmented cosmetic dermatitis was shown to be caused by contact allergy to components of cosmetic products, notably essential oils, other fragrance materials, antimicrobials, preservatives and coloring materials (44,45,46). In a group of 620 Japanese patients with this condition investigated between 1970 and 1980, 1-5% had positive patch test reactions to cinnamyl alcohol 1% in purified lanolin in various time periods versus 1 to 3% in a control group of patients not suffering from pigmented cosmetic dermatitis (44).

Also in Japan, in the period 1971 to 1986, a series of patch test studies with cinnamyl alcohol were performed. Frequencies of sensitization ranged from 1 to 8.1% in patients with pigmented cosmetic dermatitis and from 2.6% to 9.2% in groups of patients with (non-pigmented) cosmetic dermatitis. Summaries of these studies, which were published in Japanese journals, can be found in a 2005 RIFM review (102).

The number of patients with pigmented cosmetic dermatitis decreased strongly after 1978, when major cosmetic companies began to eliminate strong contact sensitizers from their products (44). Since 1980, pigmented cosmetic dermatitis became a rare disease in Japan (47).

Cross-reactions, pseudo-cross-reactions and co-reactions

For general information on cross-/pseudo-cross-/co-reactivity of fragrance chemicals with other fragrances, fragrance markers (fragrance mix I, fragrance mix II, colophonium, Myroxylon pereirae resin [balsam of Peru]) and essential oils see Chapter 1.2 General information on cross-reactions, pseudo-cross-reactions and co-reactions. Co-reactivity with the fragrance mix I can be expected, as the mix contains cinnamyl alcohol (pseudo-cross-reactions). Co-reactivity with Myroxylon pereirae resin (MP) may be explained by the presence of cinnamyl alcohol (0.4%) in MP (pseudo-cross-reactions).

Of 139 patients allergic to cinnamyl alcohol, 87 (63%) were also allergic to cinnamal, compared with 108 (11.1%) of 973 cinnamyl alcohol-negative patients (31). One hundred and twelve of 294 cinnamal-allergic patients (38%) were also allergic to cinnamyl alcohol (48). Co-reactivity between cinnamal and cinnamyl alcohol was also marked in various other studies (65,68,69). In a large study performed by the IVDK in the period 2005-2013, of 296 patients reacting to cinnamal, 158 (53%) also reacted to cinnamyl alcohol; of 235 individuals allergic to cinnamyl alcohol, 158 (67%) co-reacted to cinnamal (120). See 'Contact dermatitis, general' above for more information on the relationship between cinnamyl alcohol and cinnamal.

Co-reactions have also been observed with other cinnamon-derivatives: cinnamyl benzoate, cinnamyl cinnamate, methoxycinnamal, amyl cinnamate (51), and cinnamic acid (107). A patient with photoallergy to isoamyl p-methoxycinnamate demonstrated contact allergic reactions to cinnamyl alcohol and cinnamal (105).

In various studies a significant association between photocontact allergy to the NSAID ketoprofen and contact sensitization to the fragrance mix I (FM I) and Myroxylon pereirae resin (balsam of Peru) (89,94) has been observed (1,89,90,91,92,93,94). In the studies in which the ingredients of the FM I were tested, by far most reactions were observed to cinnamyl alcohol (1,93,94). It has been suggested that this may be due to cross-reactivity, as computerized conformational analysis has shown that there is a strong similarity between the standard structure of cinnamyl alcohol and the UVA–excited ketoprofen structure (1). Indeed, in patients with a reaction to the FM I, who were patch and photopatch tested with ketoprofen and a number of other NSAIDs, there were 23% positive photopatch tests to ketoprofen and 31% to the related NSAID tiaprofenic acid. There was a clear association with contact allergy to cinnamyl alcohol but not with any other ingredient of the FM I. It was concluded that that sensitization to cinnamyl alcohol may be considered a marker of or even a risk factor for photocontact allergy to ketoprofen and tiaprofenic acid (95). Indeed, in the period 1990-2011, in Belgium, 48 of 81 ketoprofen-positive patients were also tested with cinnamyl alcohol, and 37 (77%) reacted positively, whereas only 6 of 45 patients (13%) tested with cinnamal reacted to it; this makes cinnamyl alcohol clearly a potential marker for ketoprofen photosensitization (14).

Patch test sensitization

In three out of 230 patients with contact allergy to Myroxylon pereirae resin (balsam of Peru) and patch tested with cinnamyl alcohol 5% pet. there was a positive patch test to the fragrance that developed 6 days or later after application. Whether these were simply 'delayed' reactions or that they were indicative of patch test sensitization was not well investigated (107).

Of twelve volunteers tested in an irritancy study with *epoxy*cinnamyl alcohol 4%, 2%, 1% and 0.5% pet., three had late strong contact allergic reactions (papules, vesicles, and edema) at all four test sites at D13, D31 and D37, respectively. Of another 207 patients tested with *epoxy*cinnamyl alcohol 0.5%, two had late positive reactions at D18 and D25, resp. (115).

Presence in products and chemical analyses

In various studies, the presence cinnamyl alcohol in cosmetic and sometimes other products has been investigated. Before 2006, most investigators used chemical analysis, usually GC-MS, for qualitative and quantitative determination. Since then, the presence of the target fragrances was usually investigated by screening the product labels for the 26 fragrances that must be labeled since 2005 on cosmetics and detergent products in the EU, if present at > 10 ppm (0.001%) in leave-on products and > 100 ppm (0.01%) in rinse-off products. This method, obviously, is less accurate and may result in underestimation of the frequency of the fragrances being present in the product. When they are in fact present, but the concentration is lower than mentioned above, labeling is not required and the fragrances' presence will be missed.

The results of the relevant studies for cinnamyl alcohol are summarized in table 3.36.4. More detailed information can be found in the corresponding text before and following the table. The percentage of products in which cinnamyl alcohol was found to be present shows wide variations, which can among other be explained by the selection procedure of the products, the method of investigation (false-negatives with information obtained from labels only) and changes in the use of individual fragrance materials over time (fashion). It appears that cinnamyl alcohol is currently far less frequently used in cosmetics and household products, at least in concentrations that need to be labeled (table 3.36.4).

In 2017, in the USA, the ingredient labels 159 hair-dye kits containing 539 cosmetic products (e.g. colorants, conditioners, shampoos, toners) were screened for the most common sensitizers they contain. Cinnamyl alcohol was found to be present in one (0.2%) of the products (80).

In Denmark, in 2015-2016, 5588 fragranced cosmetic products were examined with a smartphone application for the 26 fragrances that need to be labeled in the EU. Cinnamyl alcohol was present in 2% of the products (rank number 18) (23).

In Germany, in 2015, fragrance allergens were evaluated based on lists of ingredients in 817 (unique) detergents (all-purpose cleaners, cleaning preparations for special purposes [e.g. bathroom, kitchen, dish-washing] and laundry detergents) present in 131 households. Cinnnamyl alcohol was found to be present in 5 (0.6%) of the products (114).

Of 179 emollients available in online drugstores in 2014 in Poland, one (0.6%) contained cinnamyl alcohol, according to information available online (55). In 2008, 2010 and 2011, 374 deodorants available in German retail shops were randomly selected and their labels checked for the presence of the 26 fragrances that need to be labeled. Cinnamyl alcohol was found to be present in 6 (1.6%) of the products (88).

In Germany, in the period 2006-2009, 4991 cosmetic products were randomly sampled for an official investigation of conformity of cosmetic products with legal provisions. The labels were inspected for the presence of the 26 fragrances that need to be labeled in the EU. Cinnamyl alcohol was present in 3% of the products (rank number 16) (22).

In 2008, 66 different fragrance components (including 39 essential oils) were identified in 370 (10% of the total) topical pharmaceutical products marketed in Belgium; 5 of these (1.4%) contained cinnamyl alcohol (12).

In 2006, of 88 popular perfume containing deodorants purchased in Denmark, 11 (13%) were labeled to contain cinnamyl alcohol. Analysis of 24 regulated fragrance substances in 23 selected deodorants (19 spray products, 2 deostick and 2 roll-on) was performed by GC-MS. Cinnamyl alcohol was identified in 11 of the products (48%) with a concentration range of 2–503 ppm (25).

In 2006, the labels of 208 cosmetics for children (especially shampoos, body shampoos and soaps) available in Denmark were checked for the presence of the 26 fragrances that need to be labeled in the EU. Cinnamyl alcohol was present in 14 products (6.7%), and ranked number 13 in the frequency list (40).

In January 2006, a study of perfumed cosmetic and household products available on the shelves of U.K. retailers was carried out. Products were included if 'parfum' or 'aroma' was listed among the ingredients. Three hundred products were surveyed and any of 26 mandatory labeling fragrances named on the label were recorded. Cinnamyl alcohol was present in 25 (8%) of the products (rank number 17) (21).

Table 3.36.4 Presence of cinnamyl alcohol in products [a]

Year	Country	Product type	Nr. investigated	Nr. of products positive [b]	(%)	Method [c]	Ref.
2017	USA	Cosmetic products in hair-dye kits	539 products in 159 hair-dye kits		(0.2%)	Labeling	80
2015-6	Denmark	Fragranced cosmetic products	5588		(2%)	Labeling	23
2015	Germany	Household detergents	817	5	(0.6%)	Labeling	114
2014	Poland	Emollients	179	1	(0.6%)	Online info	55
2008-11	Germany	Deodorants	374	6	(2%)	Labeling	88
2006-9	Germany	Cosmetic products	4991		(3%)	Labeling	22
2008	Belgium	Fragranced topical pharmaceutical products	370	5	(1%)	Labeling	12
2006	UK	Perfumed cosmetic and household products	300	25	(8%)	Labeling	21
2006	Denmark	Popular perfumed deodorants	88	11	(13%)	Labeling	25
			23	11	(48%)	Analysis	
2006	Denmark	Rinse-off cosmetics for children	208	14	(7%)	Labeling + analysis	40
2002	Denmark	Home and car air fresheners	19	2	(11%)	Analysis	42
2001	Denmark	Women's fine fragrances	10	4	(40%)	Analysis	24
2001	Denmark	Non-cosmetic consumer products	43	4	(9%)	Analysis	41
2000	Denmark, UK, Germany, Italy	Domestic and occupational products	59	1	(2%)	Analysis	16
<2000	Sweden	Swedish cosmetic products	42	4	(10%)	Analysis	82
1997-8	Denmark, UK Germany, Sweden	Cosmetics and cosmetic toys for children	25	2	(8%)	Analysis	19
1996-7	Denmark	Deodorants that had caused allergic contact dermatitis	19	5	(26%)	Analysis	70
1996	Five European countries	Fragranced deodorants	70	27	(39%)	Analysis	15
1995-6	Denmark	Perfumes from lower-price range cosmetic products	17	8	(47%)	Analysis	71
1995	Denmark	Cosmetic products based on natural ingredients	42	4	(10%)	Analysis	17
1995	Denmark	The 10 most popular women's perfumes	10	6	(60%)	Analysis	18
1994	Denmark	Cosmetics that had given a positive patch or use test in FM I allergic patients	23	12	(53%)	Analysis	72

[a] See the corresponding text below for more details
[b] positive = containing the target fragrance
[c] Labeling: information from the ingredient labels on the product / packaging; Analysis: chemical analysis, most often GC-MS

In January 2001, in Denmark, ten women's fine fragrances were purchased; 5 of these had been launched years ago (1921–1990) and 5 were the latest launches by the same companies, introduced 2 months to 4 years before purchase. They were analyzed for the presence and quantity of the 7 well-identified fragrances present in the FM I (see Chapter 3.70 Fragrance mix I). The analysis revealed that the 5 old perfumes contained a mean of 5 of the 7 target allergens of the FM, while the new perfumes contained a mean of 2.8 of the allergens. The mean concentrations of the target allergens were 2.6 times higher in the old perfumes than in the new perfumes, range 2.2-337. Cinnamyl alcohol was present in 4 of the 5 old perfumes, in a concentration range of 0.068-0.232% (m/m), mean 0.147%; in the new perfumes, it was identified in none of the 5 (24).

In 2002, in Denmark, 19 air fresheners (6 for cars, 13 for homes) were analyzed for the presence of fragrances that need to be labeled on cosmetics. Cinnamyl alcohol was found to be present in 2 products (11%) in a concentration range of 19-320 ppm and ranked 20 in the frequency list (42).

In 2001, in Denmark, 43 non-cosmetic consumer products (mainly dish-washing products, laundry detergents, and hard and soft surface cleaners) were analyzed for the 26 fragrances that are regulated for labeling in the EU.

Cinnamyl alcohol was present in 4 products (9%) in a concentration range of 0.0021-0.0071% (m/m) and had rank number 14 in the frequency list (41).

In 2000, fifty-nine domestic and occupational products, purchased in retail outlets in Denmark, England, Germany and Italy were analyzed by GC-MS for the presence of fragrances. The product categories were liquid soap and soap bars (n=13), soft/hard surface cleaners (n=23), fabric conditioners/laundry detergents for hand wash (n=8), dish wash (n=10), furniture polish, car shampoo, stain remover (each n=1) and 2 products used in occupational environments. Cinnamyl alcohol was present in one product; quantification was not performed (16).

In Sweden, before 2000, 42 cosmetic products of a Swedish manufacturer were investigated for the presence of the ingredients of the FM I by chemical analysis. Cinnamyl alcohol was found to be present in 4 of the products (10%) in a concentration range of 10-35 ppm with a mean of 19 ppm. Data provided by the manufacturer on the qualitative and quantitative presence of the chemicals was quite different from chemical analyses for some of the fragrances (82).

Twenty-five cosmetics and cosmetic toys for children (5 shampoos and shower gels, 6 perfumes, 1 deodorant (roll-on), 4 baby lotions/creams, 1 baby wipes product, 1 baby oil, 2 lipcare products and 5 toy-cosmetic products: a cosmetic-toy set for blending perfumes and a makeup set) purchased in 1997-1998 in retail outlets in Denmark, Germany, England and Sweden were analyzed in 1998 for the presence of fragrances by GC-MS. Cinnamyl alcohol was found in 2 products (8%) in a concentration range of 0.050-3.680% (w/w). For the analytical data in each product category, the original publication should be consulted (19).

In Denmark, in 1996-1997, nineteen deodorants that had caused axillary allergic contact dermatitis in 14 patients were analyzed for the presence of the 8 constituents of the FM I and cinnamyl alcohol was found to be present in 5 (26%) of the products in a concentration range of 0.0001-0.2672% (70).

Seventy fragranced deodorants, purchased at retail outlets in 5 European countries in 1996, were analyzed by gas chromatography - mass spectrometry (GC-MS) for the determination of the contents of 21 commonly used fragrance materials. Cinnamyl alcohol was identified in 27 products (39%) in a concentration range of 6–1169 ppm (15).

In Denmark, in 1995-1996, nine perfumes from lower-price cosmetic wash-off products and 8 from stay-on products were analyzed for the presence of the ingredients of the FM I except oakmoss absolute. Cinnamyl alcohol was present in 4 of the 9 (44%) wash-off product perfumes in a concentration range of 0.0610-0.3288% w/v and in 4 of the 8 (50%) stay-on product perfumes in a concentration range of 0.0119-0.0827% w/v (71).

In 1995, in Denmark, 42 cosmetic products based on natural ingredients from 12 European and US companies (of which 22 were perfumes and 20 various other cosmetics) were investigated by high-resolution gas chromatographymass spectrometry (GC-MS) for the presence of 11 fragrances. Cinnamyl alcohol was present in 3 (14%) of the 22 perfumes in a concentration range of 0.089-2.101 w/w%; it was also identified in one of the other cosmetics (a body balm) in a concentration of 0.0036% (17).

In Denmark, in 1995, the 10 most popular women's perfumes were analyzed with gas chromatography-mass spectrometry for the presence of 7 ingredients of the Fragrance mix I (all except Evernia prunastri extract). Cinnamyl alcohol was identified in 6 of the perfumes (60%) with a mean concentration of 0.27% and in a concentration range of 0.03-0.79% (18).

In Denmark, in 1994, 23 cosmetic products, which had either given a positive patch and/or use test in a total of 11 fragrance-mix-positive patients, and which products completely or partly explained present or past episodes of dermatitis, were analyzed for the presence of the constituents of the FM I (with the exception of oakmoss absolute) and a few other fragrances. Cinnamyl alcohol was found to be present in 12 of the 23 products (52%) in a concentration range of <0.001-0.15% v/v with a mean concentration of 0.003% v/v. It was also present in one other product, but could not be quantified due to interference (72).

OTHER SIDE EFFECTS

Photosensitivity
In China, in the period 2005-2014, 6114 patients suspected of photodermatoses were photopatch tested with cinnamyl alcohol and there were 69 (1.1%) positive photopatch test reactions; their relevance was not mentioned (81).

Immediate-type reactions
In 18 subjects not allergic to fragrances tested for non-immune immediate contact reactions (NIICR), cinnamyl alcohol 2% pet. caused erythema in two individuals (11%) (49). In a group of 60 patients with a positive patch test reaction to FM I and/or Myroxylon pereirae resin, 5 (8%) had immediate contact reactions to cinnamyl alcohol 1% pet. In a control group of 50 non-allergic patients, the percentage of immediate reactions was also 8. It was concluded that these results underline the non-immunological nature of the immediate contact reactions (66).

In a group of 160 patients with a positive patch test to FM I, 13 (8.1%) had an immediate contact reaction to cinnamyl alcohol (67). In Hungary, before 1994, in a group of 50 patients reacting to the FM I and tested with its ingredients (test concentrations unknown), there were 13 (26%) immediate contact reactions to cinnamyl alcohol (74). Of 50 individuals who had open tests with cinnamyl alcohol 5% pet. on the forearm, 39 (78%) showed local macular erythema after 45 minutes, termed 'contact urticaria' by the authors (78).

Of 97 patients with orofacial granulomatosis tested with cinnamyl alcohol (test concentration and vehicle not mentioned), 2 (2%) showed an immediate-type reaction at 30-60 minutes. These reactions, as well as immediate-type reactions to cinnamal (n=9) and benzoic acid (n=17), were considered to be type I (immediate) hypersensitivity reactions playing a role in the immunopathology of orofacial granulomatosis. However, no controls were tested and no efforts were made to verify a causal role for these chemicals in orofacial granulomatosis (116).

Other non-eczematous contact reactions

A man had isolated lichen planus of the lip, which was aggravated by spicy foods. Upon patch testing, he reacted to metals, cinnamyl alcohol, cinnamal and benzoic acid. The diagnosis of systemic contact dermatitis from cobalt, nickel, and food fragrances and flavorings was made. Elimination gave improvement, but his 'dermatitis' occasionally flared, always in connection with certain foods (117).

OTHER INFORMATION

When cinnamyl alcohol 2% in petrolatum is stored in Finn chambers at room temperature, the concentration of the fragrance decreases by 20% or more within 8 hours, probably from evaporation. This decrease is lower when the test material is stored in a refrigerator. Therefore, application to the test chamber should be performed as close in time to the patch testing as possible and storage in a refrigerator is recommended (84).

LITERATURE

1   Foti C, Bonamonte D, Conserva A, Stingeni L, Lisi P, Lionetti N, et al. Allergic and photoallergic contact dermatitis from ketoprofen: evaluation of cross-reactivities by a combination of photopatch testing and computerized conformational analysis. Curr Pharm Des 2008;14:2833-2839

2   Heisterberg MV, Menné T, Johansen JD. Contact allergy to the 26 specific fragrance ingredients to be declared on cosmetic products in accordance with the EU cosmetic directive. Contact Dermatitis 2011;65:266-275

3   Oosten EJ van, Schuttelaar ML, Coenraads PJ. Clinical relevance of positive patch test reactions to the 26 EU-labelled fragrances. Contact Dermatitis 2009;61:217-223

4   Schnuch A, Uter W, Geier J, Lessmann H, Frosch PJ. Sensitization to 26 fragrances to be labelled according to current European regulation: Results of the IVDK and review of the literature. Contact Dermatitis 2007;57:1-10

5   Adams RM, Maibach HI, for the North American Contact Dermatitis Group. A five-year study of cosmetic reactions. J Am Acad Dermatol 1985;13:1062-1069

6   Hausen BM. Contact allergy to Balsam of Peru. II. Patch test results in 102 patients with selected Balsam of Peru constituents. Am J Contact Derm 2001;12:93-102

7   Wöhrl S, Hemmer W, Focke M, Götz M, Jarisch R. The significance of fragrance mix, balsam of Peru, colophony and propolis as screening tools in the detection of fragrance allergy. Br J Dermatol 2001;145:268-273

8   Larsen W, Nakayama H, Fischer T, Elsner P, Burrows D, Jordan W, et al. Fragrance contact dermatitis: A worldwide multicenter investigation (Part I). Am J Cont Dermat 1996;7:77-83

9   Wenk KS, Ehrlich AE. Fragrance series testing in eyelid dermatitis. Dermatitis 2012;23:22-26

10 SCCNFP (Scientific Committee on Cosmetic Products and Non-Food Products Intended for Consumers). Opinion of the Scientific Committee on Cosmetic Products and Non-Food Products Intended for Consumers concerning 'An initial list of perfumery materials which must not form part of cosmetic products except subject to the Restrictions and Conditions laid down, 25 September 2001, SCCNFP/0392/00, final. Available at: http://ec.europa.eu/health/archive/ph_risk/committees/sccp/documents/out150_en.pdf

11 SCCS (Scientific Committee on Consumer Safety). Opinion on Fragrance allergens in cosmetic products, 26-27 June 2012, SCCS/1459/11. Available at: https://ec.europa.eu/health/sites/health/files/scientific_committees/consumer_safety/docs/sccs_o_102.pdf

12 Nardelli A, D'Hooge E, Drieghe J, Dooms M, Goossens A. Allergic contact dermatitis from fragrance components in specific topical pharmaceutical products in Belgium. Contact Dermatitis 2009;60:303-313

13 Larsen WG. Perfume dermatitis. A study of 20 patients. Arch Dermatol 1977;113:623-626

14 Nardelli A, Carbonez A, Drieghe J, Goossens A. Results of patch testing with fragrance mix 1, fragrance mix 2, and their ingredients, and Myroxylon pereirae and colophonium, over a 21-year period. Contact Dermatitis 2013;68:307-313

15 Rastogi SC, Johansen JD, Frosch P, Menné T, Bruze M, Lepoittevin JP, et al. Deodorants on the European market: quantitative chemical analysis of 21 fragrances. Contact Dermatitis 1998;38:29-35

16 Rastogi SC, Heydorn S, Johansen JD, Basketter DA. Fragrance chemicals in domestic and occupational products. Contact Dermatitis 2001;45:221-225

17 Rastogi SC, Johansen JD, Menné T. Natural ingredients based cosmetics. Content of selected fragrance sensitizers. Contact Dermatitis 1996;34:423-426

18 Johansen JD, Rastogi SC, Menné T. Contact allergy to popular perfumes: assessed by patch test, use test and chemical analyses. Br J Dermatol 1996;135:419-422

19 Rastogi SC, Johansen JD, Menné T, Frosch P, Bruze M, Andersen KE, et al. Content of fragrance allergens in children's cosmetics and cosmetic toys. Contact Dermatitis 1999;41:84-88

20 De Groot AC. Contact allergy to cosmetics: causative ingredients. Contact Dermatitis 1987;17:26-34

21 Buckley DA. Fragrance ingredient labelling in products on sale in the UK. Br J Dermatol 2007;157:295-300

22 Uter W, Yazar K, Kratz E-M, Mildau G, Lidén C. Coupled exposure to ingredients of cosmetic products: I. Fragrances. Contact Dermatitis 2013;69:335-341

23 Bennike NH, Oturai NB, Müller S, Kirkeby CS, Jørgensen C, Christensen AB, et al. Fragrance contact allergens in 5588 cosmetic products identified through a novel smartphone application. J Eur Acad Dermatol Venereol 2018;32:79-85

24 Rastogi SC, Menné T, Johansen JD. The composition of fine fragrances is changing. Contact Dermatitis 2003;48:130-132

25 Rastogi SC, Hellerup Jensen G, Johansen JD. Survey and risk assessment of chemical substances in deodorants. Survey of Chemical Substances in Consumer Products, No. 86 2007. Danish Ministry of the Environment, Environmental Protection Agency. Available at: https://www2.mst.dk/Udgiv/publications/2007/978-87-7052-625-8/pdf/978-87-7052-626-5.pdf

26 De Groot AC, Bruynzeel DP, Bos JD, van der Meeren HL, van Joost T, Jagtman BA, Weyland JW. The allergens in cosmetics. Arch Dermatol 1988;124:1525-1529

27 De Groot AC. Adverse reactions to cosmetics. PhD Thesis, University of Groningen, The Netherlands: 1988, chapter 3.4:105-113

28 Zaragoza-Ninet V, Blasco Encinas R, Vilata-Corell JJ, Pérez-Ferriols A, Sierra-Talamantes C, Esteve-Martínez A, de la Cuadra-Oyanguren J. Allergic contact dermatitis due to cosmetics: A clinical and epidemiological study in a tertiary hospital. Actas Dermosifiliogr 2016;107:329-336

29 Laguna C, de la Cuadra J, Martín-González B, Zaragoza V, Martínez-Casimiro L, Alegre V. Allergic contact dermatitis to cosmetics. Actas Dermosifiliogr 2009;100:53-60

30 Larsen WG. Sanitary napkin dermatitis due to the perfume. Arch Dermatol 1979;115:363

31 Buckley DA, Basketter DA, Smith Pease CK, Rycroft RJG, White IR, McFadden JP. Simultaneous sensitivity to fragrances. Br J Dermatol 2006;154:885-888

32 Smith CK, Moore CA, Smart ATS, Hotchkiss SAM. Human skin absorption and metabolism of the contact allergens, cinnamic aldehyde and cinnamic alcohol. Toxicol Appl Pharmacol 2000;168:189-199

33 Weibel H, Hansen J, Andersen KE. Cross-sensitisation patterns in guinea pigs between cinnamaldehyde, cinnamyl alcohol and cinnamic acid. Acta Derm Venereol 1989;69:302-307

34 Basketter DA. Skin sensitisation to cinnamic alcohol: the role of skin metabolism. Acta Derm Venereol 1992;72:264-265

35 Elahi EN, Wright Z, Hinselwood D, Hotchkiss SA, Basketter DA, Pease CK. Protein binding and metabolism influence the relative skin sensitization potential of cinnamic compounds. Chem Res Toxicol 2004;17:301-310

36 An S, Lee AY, Lee CH, Kim DW, Hahm JH, Kim KJ, et al. Fragrance contact dermatitis in Korea: a joint study. Contact Dermatitis 2005;53:320-323

37 Frosch PJ, Pilz B, Andersen KE, Burrows D, Camarasa JG, Dooms-Goossens A, et al. Patch testing with fragrances: results of a multicenter study of the European Environmental and Contact Dermatitis Research Group with 48 frequently used constituents of perfumes. Contact Dermatitis 1995;33:333-342

38 Trattner A, David M. Patch testing with fine fragrances: comparison with fragrance mix, balsam of Peru and a fragrance series. Contact Dermatitis 2003;49:287-289

39 Cuesta L, Silvestre JF, Toledo F, Lucas A, Perez-Crespo M, Ballester I. Fragrance contact allergy: a 4-year retrospective study. Contact Dermatitis 2010;63:77-84

40 Poulsen PB, Schmidt A. A survey and health assessment of cosmetic products for children. Survey of chemical substances in consumer products, No. 88. Copenhagen: Danish Environmental Protection Agency, 2007. Available at: https://www2.mst.dk/udgiv/publications/2007/978-87-7052-638-8/pdf/978-87-7052-639-5.pdf

41 Rastogi SC. Survey of chemical compounds in consumer products. Contents of selected fragrance materials in cleaning products and other consumer products. Survey no. 8-2002. Copenhagen, Denmark, Danish Environmental Protection Agency. Available at: http://eng.mst.dk/media/mst/69131/8.pdf

42 Pors J, Fuhlendorff R. Mapping of chemical substances in air fresheners and other fragrance liberating products. Report Danish Ministry of the Environment, Environmental Protection Agency (EPA). Survey of Chemicals in Consumer Products, No 30, 2003. Available at: http://eng.mst.dk/media/mst/69113/30.pdf

43 Larsen WG. Allergic contact dermatitis to the perfume in Mycolog cream. J Am Acad Dermatol 1979;1:131-133

44 Nakayama H, Matsuo S, Hayakawa K, Takhashi K, Shigematsu T, Ota S. Pigmented cosmetic dermatitis. Int J Dermatol 1984;23:299-305

45 Nakayama H, Harada R, Toda M. Pigmented cosmetic dermatitis. Int J Dermatol 1976;15:673-675

46 Nakayama H, Hanaoka H, Ohshiro A. Allergen Controlled System. Tokyo: Kanehara Shuppan, 1974

47 Ebihara T, Nakayama H. Pigmented contact dermatitis. Clin Dermatol 1997;15:593-599

48 Buckley DA, Wakelin SH, Seed PT, Holloway D, Rycroft RJ, White IR, et al. The frequency of fragrance allergy in a patch-test population over a 17-year period. Br J Dermatol 2000;142:279-283

49 Safford RJ, Basketter DA, Allenby CF, Goodwin BF. Immediate contact reactions to chemicals in the fragrance mix and a study of the quenching action of eugenol. Br J Dermatol 1990;123:595-606

50 Goossens A. Cosmetic contact allergens. Cosmetics 2016, 3, 5; doi:10.3390/cosmetics3010005

51 Malten KE. Four bakers showing positive patch tests to a number of fragrance materials, which can also be used as flavors. Acta Derm Venereol 1979;59(suppl.85):117-121

52 Lynde CB, Grushka M, Walsh SR. Burning mouth syndrome: patch test results from a large case series. J Cutan Med Surg 2014;18:174-179

53 Dinkloh A, Worm M, Geier J, Schnuch A, Wollenberg A. Contact sensitization in patients with suspected cosmetic intolerance: results of the IVDK 2006-2011. J Eur Acad Dermatol Venereol 2015;29:1071-1081

54 Bennike NH, Zachariae C, Johansen JD. Non-mix fragrances are top sensitizers in consecutive dermatitis patients – a cross-sectional study of the 26 EU-labelled fragrance allergens. Contact Dermatitis 2017;77:270-279

55 Osinka K, Karczmarz A, Krauze K, Feleszko W. Contact allergens in cosmetics used in atopic dermatitis: analysis of product composition. Contact Dermatitis 2016;75:241-243

56 Vejanurug P, Tresukosol P, Sajjachareonpong P, Puangpet P. Fragrance allergy could be missed without patch testing with 26 individual fragrance allergens. Contact Dermatitis 2016;74:230-235

57 Liu J, Li L-F. Contact sensitization to fragrances other than fragrance mix I in China. Contact Dermatitis 2015;73:252-253

58 Mann J, McFadden JP, White JML, White IR, Banerjee P. Baseline series fragrance markers fail to predict contact allergy. Contact Dermatitis 2014;70:276-281

59 Uter W, Johansen JD, Börje A, Karlberg A-T, Lidén C, Rastogi S, Roberts D, White IR. Categorization of fragrance contact allergens for prioritization of preventive measures: clinical and experimental data and consideration of structure–activity relationships. Contact Dermatitis 2013;69:196-230

60 Mowitz M, Svedman C, Zimerson E, Isaksson M, Pontén A, Bruze M. Simultaneous patch testing with fragrance mix I, fragrance mix II and their ingredients in southern Sweden between 2009 and 2015. Contact Dermatitis 2017;77:280-287

61 Nagtegaal MJC, Pentinga SE, Kuik J, Kezic S, Rustemeyer T. The role of the skin irritation response in polysensitization to fragrances. Contact Dermatitis 2012;67:28-35

62 Schliemann S, Geier J, Elsner P. Fragrances in topical over-the-counter medicaments – a loophole in EU legislation should be closed. Contact Dermatitis 2011;65:367-368

63 De Groot AC, Schmidt E. Essential oils: contact allergy and chemical composition. Boca Raton, Fl., USA: CRC Press, Taylor and Francis Group, 2016 (ISBN 9781482246407)

64 Nardelli A, Drieghe J, Claes L, Boey L, Goossens A. Fragrance allergens in 'specific' cosmetic products. Contact Dermatitis 2011;64:212-219

65 Uter W, Geier J, Frosch P, Schnuch A. Contact allergy to fragrances: current patch test results (2005–2008) from the Information Network of Departments of Dermatology. Contact Dermatitis 2010;63:254-261

66 Tanaka S, Matsumoto Y, Dlova N, Ostlere LS, Goldsmith PC, Rycroft RJG, et al. Immediate contact reactions to fragrance mix constituents and Myroxylon pereirae resin. Contact Dermatitis 2004;51:20-21

67 Temesvári E, Németh I, Baló-Banga MJ, Husz S, Kohánka V, Somos Z, et al. Multicentre study of fragrance allergy in Hungary: Immediate and late type reactions. Contact Dermatitis 2002;46:325-330

68 Hendriks SA, van Ginkel CJW. Evaluation of the fragrance mix in the European standard series. Contact Dermatitis 1999;41:161-162

69 Gupta N, Shenoi SD, Balachandran C. Fragrance sensitivity in allergic contact dermatitis. Contact Dermatitis 1999;40:53-54

70 Johansen JD, Rastogi SC, Bruze M, Andersen KE, Frosch P, Dreier B, et al. Deodorants: a clinical provocation study in fragrance-sensitive individuals. Contact Dermatitis 1998;39:161-165

71 Johansen JD, Rastogi SC, Andersen KE, Menné T. Content and reactivity to product perfumes in fragrance mix positive and negative eczema patients: A study of perfumes used in toiletries and skin-care products. Contact Dermatitis 1997;36:291-296

72 Johansen JD, Rastogi SC, Menné T. Exposure to selected fragrance materials: A case study of fragrance-mix-positive eczema patients. Contact Dermatitis 1996;34:106-110

73 Frosch PJ, Pilz B, Burrows D, Camarasa JG, Lachapelle J-M, Lahti A, et al. Testing with fragrance mix: Is the addition of sorbitan sesquioleate to the constituents useful? Contact Dermatitis 1995;32:266-272

74 Becker K, Temesvari E, Nemeth I. Patch testing with fragrance mix and its constituents in a Hungarian population. Contact Dermatitis 1994;30:185-186

75 Meding B. Skin symptoms among workers in a spice factory. Contact Dermatitis 1993;29:202-205

76 De Groot AC, Van der Kley AMJ, Bruynzeel DP, Meinardi MMHM, Smeenk G, van Joost Th, Pavel S. Frequency of false-negative reactions to the fragrance mix. Contact Dermatitis 1993;28:139-140

77 Broeckx W, Blondeel A, Dooms-Goossens A, Achten G. Cosmetic intolerance. Contact Dermatitis 1987;16:189-194

78 Emmons WW, Marks JG Jr. Immediate and delayed reactions to cosmetic ingredients. Contact Dermatitis 1985;13:258-265

79 Van Ketel WG. Dermatitis from an aftershave. Contact Dermatitis 1978;4:117

80 Hamann D, Kishi P, Hamann CR. Consumer hair dye kits frequently contain isothiazolinones, other common preservatives and fragrance allergens. Dermatitis 2018;29:48-49

81 Hu Y, Wang D, Shen Y, Tanh H. Photopatch testing in Chinese patients over 10 years. Dermatitis 2016;27:137-142

82 Bárány E, Lodén M. Content of fragrance mix ingredients and customer complaints of cosmetic products. Dermatitis 2000;11:74-79

83 Diepgen TL, Ofenloch R, Bruze M, Cazzaniga S, Coenraads PJ, Elsner P, et al. Prevalence of fragrance contact allergy in the general population of five European countries: a cross-sectional study. Br J Dermatol 2015;173:1411-1419

84 Mowitz M, Zimerson E, Svedman C, Bruze M. Stability of fragrance patch test preparations applied in test chambers. Br J Dermatol 2012;167:822-827

85 Gutman SG, Somov BA. Allergic reactions caused by components of perfumery preparations. Vestn Dermatol Venereol 1968;12:62-66 (article in Russian). Data cited in ref. 102

86 Karlberg A-T, Börje A, Johansen JD, Lidén C, Rastogi S, Roberts D, et al. Activation of non-sensitizing or low-sensitizing fragrance substances into potent sensitizers – prehaptens and prohaptens. Contact Dermatitis 2013;69:323-334

87 De Groot AC, Baar TJM, Terpstra H, Weyland JW. Contact allergy to moist toilet paper. Contact Dermatitis 1991;24:135-136

88 Klaschka U. Contact allergens for armpits - allergenic fragrances specified on deodorants. Int J Hyg Environ Health 2012;215:584-591

89 Matthieu L, Meuleman L, Van Hecke E, Blondeel A, Dezfoulian B, Constandt L, Goossens A. Contact and photocontact allergy to ketoprofen. The Belgian experience. Contact Dermatitis 2004;50:238-241

90 Durieu C, Marguery M-C, Giordano-Labadie F, Journe F, Loche F, Bazex J. Allergies de contact photoaggravées et photoallergies de contact au kétoprofène: 19 Cas. Ann Dermatol Venereol 2001;128:1020-1024

91 Girardin P, Vigan M, Humbert P, Aubin F. Cross-reactions in patch testing with ketoprofen, fragrance mix and cinnamic derivatives. Contact Dermatitis 2006;55:126-128

92 Pigatto P, Bigardi A, Legori A, Valsecchi R, Picardo M. Cross-reactions in patch testing and photopatch testing with ketoprofen, tiaprophenic acid, and cinnamic aldehyde. Am J Contact Dermat 1996;7:220-223

93 Durbize E, Vigan M, Puzenat E, Girardin P, Adessi B, Desprez PH, et al. Spectrum of cross-photosensitization in 18 consecutive patients with contact photoallergy to ketoprofen: associated photoallergies to non-benzophenone-containing molecules. Contact Dermatitis 2003;48:144-149

94 Devleeschouwer V, Roelandts R, Garmyn M, Goossens A. Allergic and photoallergic contact dermatitis from ketoprofen: results of (photo) patch testing and follow-up of 42 patients. Contact Dermatitis 2008;58:159-166

95 Stingeni L, Foti C, Cassano N, Bonamonte D, Vonella M, Vena GA, et al. Photocontact allergy to arylpropionic acid non-steroidal anti-inflammatory drugs in patients sensitized to fragrance mix I. Contact Dermatitis 2010;63:108-110

96 Guin JD. Contact dermatitis to perfume in paper products. J Am Acad Dermatol 1981;4:733-734

97 Novak M. Contact sensitization in perfume composition components in antiphlogistic ointment. Czech Dermatol 1974;49:375-378 (article in Czech). Data cited in: Larsen WG. Perfume dermatitis. A study of 20 patients. Arch Dermatol 1977;113:623-626

98 Manzur F, el Sayed F, Bazex J. Contact allergy to cinnamic aldehyde and cinnamic alcohol in Oléophytal®. Contact Dermatitis 1995;32:55

99 Cheung C, Hotchkiss SAM, Pease CKS. Cinnamic compound metabolism in human skin and the role metabolism may play in determining relative sensitization potency. Int J Dermatol Sci 2003;31:9-19

100 Niklasson IB, Delaine T, Islam MN, Karlsson R, Luthman K, Karlberg A-T. Cinnamyl alcohol oxidizes rapidly upon air exposure. Contact Dermatitis 2013;68:129-138

101 Geier J, Schnuch A. Reaktionen auf Zimtalkohol und Zimtaldehyd. Dermatosen 1997;45:29-33

102 Letizia CS, Cocchiara J, Lalko J, Lapczynski A, Api AM. Fragrance material review on cinnamyl alcohol. Food Chem Toxicol 2005;43:837-866

103 Isaac-Renton M, Li MK, Parsons LM. Cinnamon spice and everything not nice: many features of intraoral allergy to cinnamic aldehyde. Dermatitis 2015;26:116-121

104 Bousquet PJ, Guillot B, Guilhou JJ, Raison-Peyron N. A stomatitis due to artificial cinnamon-flavored chewing gum. Arch Dermatol 2005;141:1466-1467

105 Schauder S, Ippen H. Contact and photocontact sensitivity to sunscreens. Review of a 15-year experience and of the literature. Contact Dermatitis 1997;37:221-232

106 Calnan CD. Unusual hydroxycitronellal perfume dermatitis. Contact Dermatitis 1979;5:123

107 Hjorth N. Eczematous allergy to balsams. Acta Derm Venereol 1961;41(suppl.46):1-216

108 De Groot AC, Popova MP, Bankova VS. An update on the constituents of poplar-type propolis. Wapserveen, The Netherlands: acdegroot publishing, 2014, 11 pages. ISBN/EAN: 978-90-813233-0-7. Available at: https://www.researchgate.net/publication/262851225_AN_UPDATE_ON_THE_CONSTITUENTS_OF_POPLAR-TYPE_PROPOLIS

109 Mitchell JC, Calnan CD, Clendenning WE, Cronin E, Hjorth N, Magnusson B, et al. Patch testing with some components of balsam of Peru. Contact Dermatitis 1976;2:57-58

110 Dooms-Goossens, A, Kerre S, Drieghe J, Bossuyt L, DeGreef H. Cosmetic products and their allergens. Eur J Dermatol 1992;2:465-468

111 Opinion of the Scientific Committee on Cosmetic Products and Non-Food Products Intended for Consumers concerning 'The 1st update of the inventory of ingredients employed in cosmetic products. Section II: Perfume and aromatic raw materials', 24 October 2000, SCCNFP/0389/00, final. Available at: http://ec.europa.eu/health/ph_risk/committees/sccp/documents/out131_en.pdf

112 Foti C, Romita P, Antelmi A. Sunscreen allergy due to cinnamyl alcohol in a ketoprofen-sensitized patient. Eur J Dermatol 2011;21:295

113 Niklasson IB, Ponting DJ, Luthman K, Karlberg A-T. Bioactivation of cinnamic alcohol forms several strong skin sensitizers. Chem Res Toxicol 2014;27:568-575

114 Wieck S, Olsson O, Kümmerer K, Klaschka U. Fragrance allergens in household detergents. Regul Toxicol Pharmacol 2018;97:163-169

115 Hagvall L, Niklasson IB, Luthman K, Karlberg AT. Can the epoxides of cinnamyl alcohol and cinnamal show new cases of contact allergy? Contact Dermatitis 2018;78:399-405

116 Fitzpatrick L, Healy CM, McCartan BE, Flint SR, McCreary CE, Rogers S. Patch testing for food-associated allergies in orofacial granulomatosis. J Oral Pathol Med 2011;40:10-13

117 Szyfelbein Masterpol K, Gottlieb AB, Scheinman PL. Systemic contact dermatitis presenting as lichen planus of the lip. Dermatitis 2010;21:218-219

118 White JM, White IR, Kimber I, Basketter DA, Buckley DA, McFadden JP. Atopic dermatitis and allergic reactions to individual fragrance chemicals. Allergy 2009;64:312-316

119 Ung CY, White JML, White IR, Banerjee P, McFadden JP. Patch testing with the European baseline series fragrance markers: a 2016 update. Br J Dermatol 2018;178:776-780

120 Geier J, Uter W, Lessmann H, Schnuch A. Fragrance mix I and II: results of breakdown tests. Flavour Fragr J 2015;30:264-274

121 Girbig M, Hegewald J, Seidler A, Bauer A, Uter W, Schmitt J. Type IV sensitizations in physical therapists: patch test results of the Information Network of Departments of Dermatology (IVDK) 2007-2011. J Dtsch Dermatol Ges 2013;11:1185-1192

122 Dittmar D, Schuttelaar MLA. Contact sensitization to hydroperoxides of limonene and linalool: Results of consecutive patch testing and clinical relevance. Contact Dermatitis 2018 Oct 31. doi: 10.1111/cod.13137. [Epub ahead of print]

123 Silvestre JF, Mercader P, González-Pérez R, Hervella-Garcés M, Sanz-Sánchez T, Córdoba S, et al. Sensitization to fragrances in Spain: A 5-year multicentre study (2011-2015). Contact Dermatitis. 2018 Nov 14. doi: 10.1111/cod.13152. [Epub ahead of print]

Chapter 3.37   CINNAMYL BENZOATE

IDENTIFICATION

Description/definition   : Cinnamyl benzoate is the benzoic acid ester that conforms to the structural formula
                             shown below
Chemical class(es)   : Aromatic organic compounds; unsaturated compounds; esters
INCI name USA   : Not in the Personal Care Products Council Ingredient Database
Chemical/IUPAC name   : 3-Phenyl-2-propenyl benzoate
Other names   : 3-Phenylallyl benzoate
CAS registry number(s)   : 5320-75-2
EC number(s)   : 226-180-2
RIFM monograph(s)   : Food Chem Toxicol 2007;45(suppl.1):S58-61; Food Chem Toxicol 2007;45(suppl.1):S1-
                             S23; Food Cosmet Toxicol 1976;14:717 (special issue III)
SCCS opinion(s)   : SCCNFP/0389/00, final (5)
Function(s) in cosmetics   : EU: perfuming
Patch testing   : 5%-10% pet. (2)
Molecular formula   : $C_{16}H_{14}O_2$

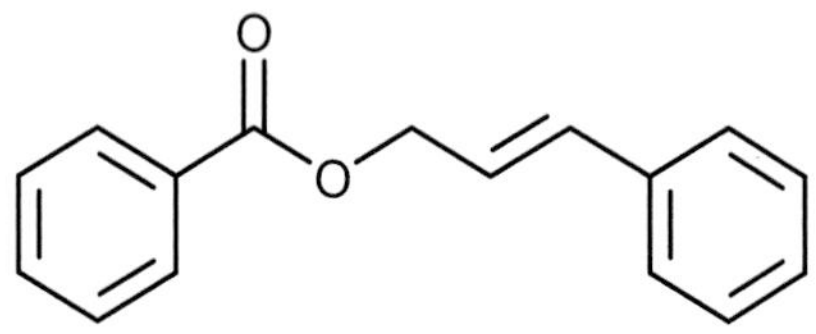

GENERAL

Cinnamyl benzoate is a white crystalline powder; its odor type is balsamic and its odor at 100% is described as 'balsam spicy buttery fruity' (www.thegoodscentscompany.com).

Presence in essential oils and propolis

Cinnamyl benzoate has been identified by chemical analysis in none of 91 essential oils, which have caused contact allergy / allergic contact dermatitis (4). Cinnamyl benzoate may, however, be present in propolis (3).

CONTACT ALLERGY

Testing in groups of patients

Studies in which cinnamyl benzoate has been tested in either consecutive patients suspected of contact dermatitis (routine testing) or in groups of selected patients with positive results have not been found.

Case reports and case series

Convincing case reports of allergic contact dermatitis from cinnamyl benzoate have not been found.

A baker had recurrent dyshidrotic eczema of the hands. Routine patch testing was negative, but he reacted to the cinnamon powder he had brought from his work. When tested subsequently with a series of fragrances/flavors, he reacted to cinnamyl benzoate 10%, cinnamyl alcohol 5%, cinnamal 0.5%, cinnamyl cinnamate 8% and benzylidene acetone 0.5%, all in petrolatum. After avoiding skin and mucous membrane contact with cinnamon-containing products and not eating or drinking them, the dermatitis much improved. Another baker with similar symptoms and reacting to cinnamon powder had positive patch tests to the same fragrance materials and to methoxycinnamal 4% pet.

A third baker, who later became cook, had recurrent dermatitis of the hands, arms and face. He was known to react to his wife's perfumes and used fragranced cosmetic products himself. He had no reactions to any spice that he brought in himself, but when tested with a battery of fragrances, there were positive reactions to cinnamyl benzoate 10%, eugenol 8%, dihydrocoumarin 5%, phenylacetaldehyde 2%, and methyl 2-octynoate 0.5%, all in petrolatum. The author was 'inclined' to say that these reactions may have been relevant (1).

Cross-reactions, pseudo-cross-reactions and co-reactions

For general information on cross-/pseudo-cross-/co-reactivity of fragrance chemicals with other fragrances, fragrance markers (fragrance mix I, fragrance mix II, colophonium, Myroxylon pereirae resin [balsam of Peru]) and essential oils see Chapter 1.2 General information on cross-reactions, pseudo-cross-reactions and co-reactions.

Co-reactions have been observed with other cinnamon-derivatives: cinnamyl alcohol, cinnamal, cinnamyl cinnamate, methoxycinnamal, amyl cinnamate (1).

LITERATURE

1   Malten KE. Four bakers showing positive patch tests to a number of fragrance materials, which can also be used as flavors. Acta Derm Venereol 1979;59(suppl.85):117-121

2   De Groot AC. Patch Testing, 4th Edition. Wapserveen, The Netherlands: acdegroot publishing, 2018 (ISBN 978-90-813233-4-5)

3   De Groot AC, Popova MP, Bankova VS. An update on the constituents of poplar-type propolis. Wapserveen, The Netherlands: acdegroot publishing, 2014, 11 pages. ISBN/EAN: 978-90-813233-0-7. Available at: https://www.researchgate.net/publication/262851225_AN_UPDATE_ON_THE_CONSTITUENTS_OF_POPLAR-TYPE_PROPOLIS

4   De Groot AC, Schmidt E. Essential oils: contact allergy and chemical composition. Boca Raton, Fl., USA: CRC Press, Taylor and Francis Group, 2016 (ISBN 9781482246407)

5   Opinion of the Scientific Committee on Cosmetic Products and Non-Food Products Intended for Consumers concerning 'The 1st update of the inventory of ingredients employed in cosmetic products. Section II: Perfume and aromatic raw materials', 24 October 2000, SCCNFP/0389/00, final. Available at: http://ec.europa.eu/health/ph_risk/committees/sccp/documents/out131_en.pdf

Chapter 3.38　CINNAMYL CINNAMATE

IDENTIFICATION

Description/definition : Cinnamyl cinnamate is the aromatic ester that conforms to the structural formula shown below
Chemical class(es) : Aromatic compounds; esters
INCI name USA : Not in the Personal Care Products Council Ingredient Database
Chemical/IUPAC name : 3-Phenylprop-2-enyl 3-phenylprop-2-enoate
Other names : Styracin
CAS registry number(s) : 122-69-0
EC number(s) : 204-566-1
RIFM monograph(s) : Food Chem Toxicol 2007;45(suppl.1):S66-S69; Food Chem Toxicol 2007;45(suppl.1):S1-S23; Food Cosmet Toxicol 1975;13:753 (special issue II)
Merck Index monograph : 3575
Function(s) in cosmetics : EU: perfuming
Patch testing : 5% pet. (1,3)
Molecular formula : $C_{18}H_{16}O_2$

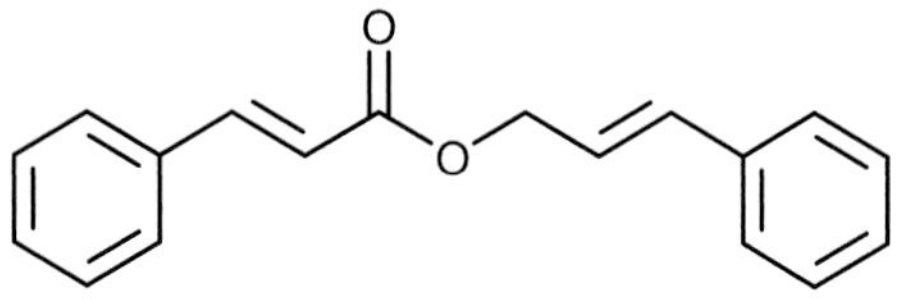

GENERAL

Cinnamyl cinnamate has the appearance of white to pale yellow crystals; its odor type is balsamic and its odor at 100% is described as 'sweet balsam floral cassia cinnamyl' (www.thegoodscentscompany.com).

Presence in essential oils, Myroxylon pereirae resin (balsam of Peru) and propolis

Cinnamyl cinnamate has been identified by chemical analysis in two of 91 essential oils, which have caused contact allergy / allergic contact dermatitis: cinnamon bark oil, Sri Lanka and ginger oil (5). Cinnamyl cinnamate may also be present in Myroxylon pereirae resin (balsam of Peru) (0.5%) (1) and in propolis (4).

CONTACT ALLERGY

Patch testing in groups of patients

Patch testing in consecutive patients suspected of contact dermatitis: routine testing

Studies in which cinnamyl cinnamate was patch tested in consecutive patients suspected of contact dermatitis (routine testing) with positive results have not been found.

Patch testing in groups of selected patients

In 2 studies, patients allergic to Myroxylon pereirae resin (balsam of Peru) have been tested with a battery of its ingredients (1,3); the 12 patients in one of these studies were also allergic to propolis (3).

In Germany, in the period 1995-1998, 102 patients allergic to balsam of Peru were tested with cinnamyl cinnamate 5% and 20 (20%) had a positive reaction (1). In Poland, before 1982, 12 patients allergic to balsam of Peru and propolis were tested with cinnamyl cinnamate 5% pet. and 3 (25%) reacted positively (3). This indicates that cinnamyl cinnamate may be the allergen or an allergen in about one in every five patients allergic to balsam of Peru.

Case reports and case series

Convincing case reports of allergic contact dermatitis from cinnamyl cinnamate have not been found.

A baker had recurrent dyshidrotic eczema of the hands. Routine patch testing was negative, but he reacted to the cinnamon powder he had brought from his work. When tested subsequently with a series of fragrances/flavors, he reacted to cinnamyl cinnamate 8%, cinnamyl alcohol 5%, cinnamal 0.5%, cinnamyl benzoate 10% and benzylidene acetone 0.5%, all in petrolatum. After avoiding skin and mucous membrane contact with cinnamon-containing products and not eating or drinking them, the dermatitis much improved (2).

Another baker with similar symptoms and reacting to cinnamon powder had positive patch tests to the same fragrance materials and to o-methoxycinnamal 4% petrolatum (2). A third baker was patch tested for hand dermatitis and showed positive reactions to cocoao-powder and 'speculaaskruiden', a mixture of unknown composition, which he used at work. When subsequently tested with a series of fragrances and flavors, he had positive reactions to cinnamyl cinnamate 8%, hexyl salicylate 12%, citral 0.5%, cinnamal 0.5%, and amyl cinnamate 32%, all in petrolatum (2). The author was 'inclined' to say that these reactions may have been relevant (2).

Cross-reactions, pseudo-cross-reactions and co-reactions
For general information on cross-/pseudo-cross-/co-reactivity of fragrance chemicals with other fragrances, fragrance markers (fragrance mix I, fragrance mix II, colophonium, Myroxylon pereirae resin [balsam of Peru]) and essential oils see Chapter 1.2 General information on cross-reactions, pseudo-cross-reactions and co-reactions. Co-reactivity with Myroxylon pereirae resin (MP) may be explained by the presence of cinnamyl cinnamate (0.5%) in MP (pseudo-cross-reactions).

Co-reactions have been observed to other cinnamon-derivatives: cinnamyl alcohol, cinnamal, cinnamyl benzoate, methoxycinnamal, and amyl cinnamate (2).

LITERATURE

1   Hausen BM. Contact allergy to Balsam of Peru. II. Patch test results in 102 patients with selected Balsam of Peru constituents. Am J Contact Derm 2001;12:93-102
2   Malten KE. Four bakers showing positive patch tests to a number of fragrance materials, which can also be used as flavors. Acta Derm Venereol 1979;59(suppl.85):117-121
3   Rudzki E, Grzywa Z. Dermatitis from propolis. Contact Dermatitis 1983;9:40-45
4   De Groot AC, Popova MP, Bankova VS. An update on the constituents of poplar-type propolis. Wapserveen, The Netherlands: acdegroot publishing, 2014, 11 pages. ISBN/EAN: 978-90-813233-0-7. Available at: https://www.researchgate.net/publication/262851225_AN_UPDATE_ON_THE_CONSTITUENTS_OF_POPLAR-TYPE_PROPOLIS
5   De Groot AC, Schmidt E. Essential oils: contact allergy and chemical composition. Boca Raton, Fl., USA: CRC Press, Taylor and Francis Group, 2016 (ISBN 9781482246407)

Chapter 3.39 CITRAL

IDENTIFICATION

Description/definition	: Citral is the aldehyde that conforms to the structural formula shown below
Chemical class(es)	: Aldehydes
Chemical/IUPAC name	: 3,7-Dimethyl-2,6-octadienal
Other names	: *trans*-Citral (citral A, α-citral) = geranial; *cis*-citral (citral B; β-citral) = neral; citral is a 2:1 mixture of geranial and neral (1)
CAS registry number(s)	: 5392-40-5
EC number(s)	: 226-394-6
SCCS opinion(s)	: SCCP/1153/08 (9)
RIFM monograph(s)	: Food Cosm Toxicol 1979;17:259
IFRA standard	: Restricted (www.ifraorg.org/en-us/standards-library) (table 3.39.1)
SCCS opinion(s)	: Various (9); SCCS/1459/11 (10); SCCNFP/0389/00, final (69)
Merck Index monograph	: 3591
Function(s) in cosmetics	: EU: flavouring; perfuming. USA: flavoring agents; fragrance ingredients
EU cosmetic restrictions	: Regulated in Annex III/70 of the Regulation (EC) No. 1223/2009, regulated by 2003/15/EC; Must be labeled on cosmetics and detergent products, if present at > 10 ppm (0.001%) in leave-on products and > 100 ppm (0.01%) in rinse-off products
Patch testing	: 2% pet. (SmartPracticeEurope, Chemotechnique, SmartPracticeCanada); 2% pet. has caused irritant reactions (56), although citral 3.5% pet. did not (58); it may be preferable to test the separate ingredients geranial and neral (58); present in the fragrance mix II
Molecular formula	: $C_{10}H_{16}O$

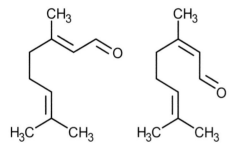

Citral A   Citral B

Table 3.39.1 IFRA restrictions for citral

Category [a]	Limits [b]	Category [a]	Limits [b]	Category [a]	Limits [b]
1	0.04%	5	0.30%	9	5.00%
2	0.05%	6	1.00%	10	2.50%
3	0.20%	7	0.10%	11	not restricted
4	0.60%	8	1.40%		

[a] For explanation of categories see pages 6-8
[b] Limits in the finished products

GENERAL

Citral is a colorless to pale yellow clear liquid; its odor type is citrus and its odor is described as 'fresh, juicy, lemon peel, with a sweet tangy green nuance' (www.thegoodscentscompany.com). Citral is used primarily as a starting material for the manufacturing of other fragrance ingredients (e.g. ionone and methylionone), but is also used *per se* as a fragrance ingredient. As a flavor it has applications in alcoholic and nonalcoholic beverages, baked goods, cheese, chewing gum, condiment (relish), frozen dairy, gelatin (pudding), gravies, hard and soft candy, and meat products for its citrus effect. In addition, it may play a role in the synthesis of vitamin A (U.S. National Library of Medicine).

Citral is the 2:1 combination of the geometric isomers geranial (*trans*-citral) and neral (*cis*-citral). See also Chapter 3.72 Geranial and Chapter 3.128 Neral. It is a constituent of the Fragrance mix II (see Chapter 3.71 Fragrance mix II).

Presence in essential oils

Citral has been identified by chemical analysis in 15 of 91 essential oils, which have caused contact allergy / allergic contact dermatitis. In none of these oils, it belonged to the 'Top-10' of ingredients with the highest concentrations (53). Its 2 components geranial and neral, however, are major ingredients in various essential oils, including lemongrass oil (both the East Indian and West Indian variety), litsea cubeba oil and melissa (lemon balm) oil (see Chapter 3.72 Geranial, Chapter 3.128 Neral and the essential oils chapters).

CONTACT ALLERGY

General

The SCCS (Scientific Committee on Consumer Safety), in a 2012 Opinion on Fragrance allergens in cosmetic products, has marked citral as 'established contact allergen in humans' (10,38). The sensitizing potency of citral was classified as 'moderate' based on an EC3 value of 1.2% in the LLNA (local lymph node assay) in animal experiments (10,38), but also as a strong sensitizer (33). Its component geranial forms oxidation products with increased sensitizing capacity both via spontaneous autoxidization at air exposure and via metabolic oxidation, notably 5,6-epoxygeranial (51). Geranial and neral have been identified as secondary oxidation products when geraniol autoxidizes (49,58) and also as metabolites of geraniol (50,58).

Citral is a constituent of the fragrance mix II. In groups of patients reacting to the mix and tested with its 6 ingredients, citral scored 11.2-19.0% positive patch test reactions (see Chapter 3.71 Fragrance mix II).

Geranial is the main sensitizer in citral (58). It may be preferable to test citral's components separately, as in one study, of 13 patients reacting to geranial 3.5% pet., only 3 (23%) co-reacted to citral 3.5% pet. and of 6 patients reacting to neral 3.5% pet, only 2 (33%) also had positive patch tests to citral 3.5% pet. (58).

General population

In the period 2008-2011, in 5 European countries (Sweden, Germany, Netherlands, Portugal, Italy), a random sample of the general population of 3119 individuals aged 18-74 years were patch tested with the FM I, its 8 ingredients, the FM II, its 6 ingredients and Myroxylon pereirae resin. There were 6 reactions (0.2%) to citral, tested 2% in pet. About half of all positive reactions to fragrances were considered to be relevant based on standardized criteria. Women were affected twice as often as men (46).

Patch testing in groups of patients

Results of studies testing citral in consecutive patients suspected of contact dermatitis (routine testing) are shown in table 3.39.2. Results of testing in groups of *selected* patients (e.g. patients with known or suspected fragrance or cosmetic dermatitis, individuals with eyelid dermatitis) are shown in table 3.39.3.

Patch testing in consecutive patients suspected of contact dermatitis: routine testing

In thirteen studies in which routine testing with citral was performed, frequencies of sensitization have ranged from 0.3% to 3.2% (table 3.39.2). With two exceptions, all rates were 1.2% or lower. In 10/13 investigations, no (specific) data on relevance were provided, but in all 3 addressing the issue, >50% of the reactions were scored as relevant.

Causative products were scented products and essential oils (1) and in one study, of the relevant reactions to any of 26 fragrances tested, 96% were caused by cosmetic products (2).

Table 3.39.2 Patch testing in groups of patients: Routine testing

Years and Country	Test conc. & vehicle	Number of patients tested	positive (%)	Selection of patients (S); Relevance (R); Comments (C)	Ref.
2015-7 Netherlands		821	13 (1.6%)	R: not stated	73
2015-2016 UK	2% pet.	2084	22 (1.1%)	R: not specified for individual fragrances; 25% of patients who reacted to any fragrance or fragrance marker had a positive fragrance history	70
2010-2015 Denmark	2% pet.	6004	(0.39%)	R: present relevance 61%, past relevance 35%	32
2009-2015 Sweden	2% pet.	4430	56 (1.2%)	R: not stated	39
2013-2014 Thailand		312	10 (3.2%)	R: 70%	35
2011-2012 UK	2% pet.	1951	20 (1.0%)	R: not stated	37
2010-2011 Sweden	3.5% pet.	655	6 (0.9%)	R: not specified for individual fragrances; C: this concentration did not cause irritant reactions	58
2008-2010 Denmark	2% pet.	1502	5 (0.3%)	S: mostly routine testing; R:50%; C: 100% co-reactivity of both FM I and FM II; of the relevant reactions to any of the 26 fragrances tested, 96% were caused by cosmetic products	2
2006-2010 Sweden	1.5% pet.	1055	7 (0.7%)	R: high relevance scores; contact with scented products and	1

Table 3.39.2 Patch testing in groups of patients: Routine testing (continued)

Years and Country	Test conc. & vehicle	Number of patients tested | positive (%)		Selection of patients (S); Relevance (R); Comments (C)	Ref.
				essential oils	
2003-2004 IVDK	2% pet.	2021	13 (0.6%)	R: not stated; C: 77% co-reactivity to FM I	4
2002-2003 six Euro-pean countries	1% pet.	1701	6 (0.4%)	R: not specified	7
	2% pet.	1701	12 (0.7%)	R: not specified	
1998-9 Netherlands	2% pet.	1825	19 (1.0%)	R: not stated	12
1997-1998 six Euro-pean countries	2% pet.	1855	21 (1.1%)	R: not stated / specified	22

FM: Fragrance mix; IVDK: Informationsverbund Dermatologischer Kliniken (Germany, Switzerland, Austria)

Patch testing in groups of selected patients

Results of studies patch testing citral in groups of selected patients (e.g. patients with known or suspected fragrance or cosmetic dermatitis, individuals with eyelid dermatitis) are shown in table 3.39.3. In 14 investigations, frequencies of sensitization to citral have ranged from 0.4% to 25%. The highest rates were observed in patients reacting to an experimental fragrance mix containing citral (25% [29]), in patients with allergic reactions to perfumes (10% [68]), in individuals previously reacting to fragrance markers (10.0% [74]) and in physical therapists (9.7% [72]). In most studies, no (specific) relevance data were provided. Some authors considered relevance for all reactions 'possible' (6), others 'assumed' that nearly all positive reactions were of present or past relevance (5). Causative products were not mentioned.

Results of testing in groups of patients reacting to the fragrance mix II are shown in Chapter 3.71 Fragrance mix II.

Table 3.39.3 Patch testing in groups of patients: Selected patient groups

Years and Country	Test conc. & vehicle	Number of patients tested | positive (%)		Selection of patients (S); Relevance (R); Comments (C)	Ref.
2011-2015 Spain	2% pet.	1013	101 (10.0%)	S: patients previously reacting to FM I, FM II, Myroxylon pereirae resin or hydroxyisohexyl 3-cyclohexene carboxaldehyde in the baseline series; R: not stated	74
2007-2011 IVDK	2% pet.	31	3 (9.7%)	S: physical therapists; R: not stated	72
2009-2010 Hungary	2% pet.	565	19 (3.4%)	S: patients with former skin symptoms provoked by scented products in the case history; R: in all cases 'possible'	6
2006-2010 USA	1% pet.	100	5 (5%)	S: patients with eyelid dermatitis; R: not stated	8
2005-10 Netherlands		100	9 (9%)	S: patients with known fragrance sensitivity based on a positive patch test to the FM I and/or the FM II; R: not stated	40
2004-2008 Spain	2% pet.	86	2 (2%)	S: patients previously reacting to the fragrance mix I or Myroxylon pereirae (n=54) or suspected of fragrance contact allergy (n=32); R: not stated	23
2005-7 Netherlands	2% pet.	320	2 (0.6%)	S: patients suspected of fragrance or cosmetic allergy; R: 61% relevance for all positive tested fragrances together	3
2002-2003 Korea	2% pet.	422	5 (1.2%)	S: patients with suspected cosmetic dermatitis; R: not stated	21
2001-2002 Denmark, Sweden	2% pet.	658	28 (4.3%)	S: consecutive patients with hand eczema; R: it was assumed that nearly all positive reactions were of present or past relevance; C: frequency of sensitization to 1% citral: 0.8%; to 0.5% citral: 0.3%; 2% pet. undoubtedly causes irritant reactions (56)	5
<1989 EECDRG	2% pet.	53	13 (25%)	S: patients reacting to an experimental fragrance mix with citral (n=41) or to the FM I but not the experimental mix (n=12)	29
<1986 France	2% pet.	21	2 (10%)	S: patients with dermatitis caused by perfumes; R: not stated	68
1978-1986 Japan	5%	310	8 (2.6%)	S: patients with cosmetic dermatitis; R: unknown (3 articles not read)	61-63
	2%	240	1 (0.4%)		
1983 The Netherlands	2% pet.	182	5 (2.6%)	S: patients suspected of cosmetic allergy; R: not stated	11
<1981 Japan	5% pet.	155	4 (2.6%)	S: patients with cosmetic dermatitis; R: unknown (article not read)	64

Testing in groups of patients reacting to the fragrance mix II

Results of testing citral in groups of patients reacting to the fragrance mix II are shown in Chapter 3.71 Fragrance mix II

EECDRG: European Environmental Contact Dermatitis Research group; FM: Fragrance Mix

Case reports and case series

Case series

Over a period of 2 years, nine beauticians working in the same high-end luxury health spa in the United Kingdom were referred with recent onset of bilateral hand dermatitis. The dermatitis was localized mainly to the dorsum of the hands and fingers; in some patients, there was spread to the wrists and forearms. The dermatitis was reported to improve with work avoidance. All were applying a wide variety of beauty treatments, including massages with essential oils, which were applied to clients' skin by direct, ungloved, hand contact. All had worked at the spa for a minimum of 4 months prior to the onset of their hand dermatitis. Six of the 9 patients had positive patch test reactions, five of who reacted to fragrance mix II 14% pet. All had positive reactions to citral 2.0% pet. (the ingredients of fragrance mix II include citral 1.0% pet.). The predominant brand of product used, termed 'natural and organic', consisted of a large range of essential oils and spa products that all contained citral. Appropriate advice was given, after which no further cases have been referred to the investigators of this study (59).

Citral was stated to be the (or an) allergen in 9 patients in a group of 603 individuals suffering from cosmetic dermatitis, seen in the period 2010-2015 in Leuven, Belgium (30). In the period 1996-2013, in a tertiary referral center in Valencia, Spain, 5419 patients were patch tested. Of these, 628 individuals had allergic contact dermatitis to cosmetics. In this group, citral was the responsible allergen in one case (20).

In the period 2000-2009, in Leuven, Belgium, an unspecified number of patients had positive patch tests or use tests to a total of 344 cosmetic products *and* positive patch tests to FM I, FM II, and/or to one or more of 28 selected specific fragrance ingredients. In 5 of 8 patients reacting to citral, the presence of this fragrance in the cosmetic product(s) was confirmed by reading the product label(s) (41).

Case reports

A young man with dermatitis of the axillae and around the mouth had positive patch test reactions to geraniol, oxidized geraniol, citral, geranial, neral, and the FM I. He used a deodorant which contained both citral and geraniol. The patient also reacted positively to his aftershave, but the incriminated fragrances were not declared on that cosmetic product (1).

A baker was patch tested for hand dermatitis and showed positive reactions to cocoa-powder and 'speculaaskruiden', a mixture of unknown composition, which he used at work. When subsequently tested with a series of fragrances and flavors, he had positive reactions to citral 0.5%, hexyl salicylate 12%, cinnamal 0.5%, amyl cinnamate 32% and cinnamyl cinnamate 8%, all in petrolatum. The author was 'inclined' to say that these reactions may have been relevant (31).

A man had pustular patch test reactions to FM II, citral (which is present in the FM II), oakmoss and an aftershave, which had caused a pustular eruption on the face. It was unknown whether the aftershave contained oakmoss and/or citral (36). A woman had allergic contact dermatitis from several fragrances in an eau de parfum, including citral (42). Another female patient had recurrent allergic contact cheilitis from citral in a lip balm; she also reacted to lemongrass oil, in which citral is the main ingredient (54).

A female bartender with dermatitis of the hands had positive patch tests to the peels of lemon, orange and lime, but not to their constituent limonene. The patient did react, however, to geraniol 5% pet. and to citral 2% and 5% in mineral oil and the hand dermatitis was – albeit not explicitly - ascribed to these chemicals (55). Commercial lemon oils have been found to contain up to 2.1% geranial (*trans*-citral) and up to 1.4% neral (*cis*-citral), but commercial orange oils only contain very low amounts of these chemicals (53).

A patient had contact allergy to bergamot oil from the use of cosmetic products. The individual also reacted to citral and the authors suggested this to be the allergen (43). However, bergamot oil does not contain appreciable amounts of citral or its constituents geranial and neral (53).

Cross-reactions, pseudo-cross-reactions and co-reactions

For general information on cross-/pseudo-cross-/co-reactivity of fragrance chemicals with other fragrances, fragrance markers (fragrance mix I, fragrance mix II, colophonium, Myroxylon pereirae resin [balsam of Peru]) and essential oils see Chapter 1.2 General information on cross-reactions, pseudo-cross-reactions and co-reactions.

Co-reactivity with the fragrance mix II can be expected, as the mix contains citral (pseudo-cross-reactions). Co-reactivity may be expected to geranial and citral (the two constituents of citral), and to the fragrance mix II, which contains 1% citral (59). Simultaneous reactions to citral and (oxidized) geraniol (1,4,58) can be explained by the fact that geranial and neral are secondary oxidation products from geraniol autoxidation (49); they have also been identified as metabolites of geraniol (50). Indeed, in a large study performed by the IVDK in the period 2005-2013, of 111 patients reacting to citral, 50 (45%) co-reacted to geraniol; conversely, of 61 individuals allergic to geraniol, 50 (82%) co-reacted to citral (71).

In a large study performed by the IVDK in the period 2005-2013, eighteen out of 32 patients (56%) reacting to citronellol also reacted to citral; conversely, of 171 citral-positive patients, 18 (11%) co-reacted to citronellol (71). In the same study, of 111 patients reacting to citral, 44 (40%) co-reacted to hydroxycitronellal; conversely, of 112 individuals allergic to hydroxycitronellal, 44 (39%) co-reacted to citral (71).

About 50% of patients reacting to lemongrass oils co-react to citral (52). Neral and geranial, the 2 components of citral, are the major ingredients of these essential oils (53).

Patch test sensitization
One patient patch tested with 8% citral in petrolatum had a positive reaction at day 10 and therefore may have been sensitized by the test, but the patient was not retested for confirmation (31).

Presence in products and chemical analyses
In various studies, the presence of citral in cosmetic and sometimes other products has been investigated. Before 2006, most investigators used chemical analysis, usually GC-MS, for qualitative and quantitative determination. Since then, the presence of the target fragrances was usually investigated by screening the product labels for the 26 fragrances that must be labeled since 2005 on cosmetics and detergent products in the EU, if present at > 10 ppm (0.001%) in leave-on products and > 100 ppm (0.01%) in rinse-off products. This method, obviously, is less accurate and may result in underestimation of the frequency of the fragrances being present in the product. When they are in fact present, but the concentration is lower than mentioned above, labeling is not required and the fragrances' presence will be missed.

The results of the relevant studies for citral are summarized in table 3.39.4. More detailed information can be found in the corresponding text before and following the table. The percentage of products in which citral was found to be present shows wide variations, which can among other be explained by the selection procedure of the products, the method of investigation (false-negatives with information obtained from labels only) and changes in the use of individual fragrance materials over time (fashion).

In 2016, in Sweden, 66 commercially available toothpastes obtained from local pharmacies and supermarkets in Malmö, Sweden were investigated for the presence of flavors by studying the packages and product labels. Citral was found to be present in 1 (2%) of the products (47).

In Denmark, in 2015-2016, 5588 fragranced cosmetic products were examined with a smartphone application for the 26 fragrances that need to be labeled in the EU. Citral was present in 15% of the products (rank number 10) (18).

In Germany, in 2015, fragrance allergens were evaluated based on lists of ingredients in 817 (unique) detergents (all-purpose cleaners, cleaning preparations for special purposes [e.g. bathroom, kitchen, dish-washing] and laundry detergents) present in 131 households. Citral was found to be present in 36 (4%) of the products (70).

Of 179 emollients available in online drugstores in 2014 in Poland, one (0.6%) contained citral, according to information available online (34).

In 2008, 2010 and 2011, 374 deodorants available in German retail shops were randomly selected and their labels checked for the presence of the 26 fragrances that need to be labeled. Citral was found to be present in 69 (17.9%) of the products (48).

In Germany, in the period 2006-2009, 4991 cosmetic products were randomly sampled for an official investigation of conformity of cosmetic products with legal provisions. The labels were inspected for the presence of the 26 fragrances that need to be labeled in the EU. Citral was present in 11% of the products (rank number 9) (17).

Citral was present (as indicated by labeling) in 2% of 204 cosmetic products (92 shampoos, 61 hair conditioners, 34 liquid soaps, 17 wet tissues) and in 5% of 97 detergents in Sweden, 2008 (13).

In 2007, in The Netherlands, twenty-three cosmetic products for children were analyzed for the presence of fragrances that need to be labeled. Citral was identified in 2 of the products (9%) in a concentration range of 109-168 ppm (25). In 2006, of 88 popular perfume containing deodorants purchased in Denmark, 23 (26%) were labeled to contain citral. Analysis of 24 regulated fragrance substances in 23 selected deodorants (19 spray products, 2 deostick and 2 roll-on) was performed by GC-MS. Citral was identified in 10 of the products (44%) with a concentration range of 39–554 ppm (19).

In 2006, in The Netherlands, 52 laundry detergents were investigated for the presence of allergenic fragrances by checking their labels and chemical analyses. Citral was found to be present in one of the products (2%) in a concentration 8 ppm. Citral had rank number 14 in the frequency list (27).

In January 2006, a study of perfumed cosmetic and household products available on the shelves of U.K. retailers was carried out. Products were included if 'parfum' or 'aroma' was listed among the ingredients. Three hundred products were surveyed and any of 26 mandatory labeling fragrances named on the label were recorded. Citral was present in 74 (25%) of the products (rank number 12) (16).

In 2006, the labels of 208 cosmetics for children (especially shampoos, body shampoos and soaps) available in Denmark were checked for the presence of the 26 fragrances that need to be labeled in the EU. Citral was present in 17 products (8.2%), and ranked number 10 in the frequency list (24).

Table 3.39.4 Presence of citral in products [a]

Year	Country	Product type	Nr. investigated	Nr. of products positive [b]	(%)	Method [c]	Ref.
2016	Sweden	Toothpastes	66	1	(2%)	Labeling	47
2015-6	Denmark	Fragranced cosmetic products	5588		(15%)	Labeling	18
2015	Germany	Household detergents	817	36	(4%)	Labeling	44
2014	Poland	Emollients	179	1	(0.6%)	Online info	34
2006-9	Germany	Cosmetic products	4991		(11%)	Labeling	17
2008-11	Germany	Deodorants	374	69	(18%)	Labeling	48
2008	Sweden	Cosmetic products	204		(2%)	Labeling	13
		Detergents	97		(5%)	Labeling	
2007	Netherlands	Cosmetic products for children	23	2	(9%)	Analysis	25
2006	UK	Perfumed cosmetic and house-hold products	300	74	(25%)	Labeling	16
2006	Denmark	Popular perfumed deodorants	88	23	(26%)	Labeling	19
			23	10	(44%)	Analysis	
2006	Netherlands	Laundry detergents	52	1	(2%)	Labeling + analysis	27
2006	Denmark	Rinse-off cosmetics for children	208	17	(8.2%)	Labeling + analysis	24
2004	Denmark, UK, Belgium, Germany	Fragranced products that have caused allergic contact derma-titis used by patients	24	12	(50%)	Labeling	7
2002	Denmark	Home and car air fresheners	19	7	(37%)	Analysis	28
2001	Denmark	Non-cosmetic consumer products	43	7	(16%)	Analysis	26
2000	Denmark, UK, Germany, Italy	Domestic and occupational products	59	15	(25%)	Analysis	14
1997	Denmark, UK, France, Germany, Sweden	Deodorants	71	26	(37%)	Analysis	15
1994	Denmark	Cosmetics that had given a positive patch or use test in FM I allergic patients	23	1	(4%)	Analysis	45

[a] See the corresponding text below for more details
[b] positive = containing the target fragrance
[c] Labeling: information from the ingredient labels on the product / packaging; Analysis: chemical analysis, most often GC-MS

In 2004, in 4 European countries (Denmark, Germany, Belgium, U.K.), of 12 patients allergic to the FM II and one or more of its constituents (hexyl cinnamal 1, citral 3, hydroxyisohexyl 3-cyclohexene carboxaldehyde 11), 24 of the products used by them (deodorant 4, eau de toilette 9, lotion/cream 4, fine perfume 7) that had caused adverse reactions compatible with allergic contact dermatitis, were analyzed for the presence of the six constituents of the fragrance mix II (citral, citronellol, coumarin, farnesol, hexyl cinnamal, hydroxyisohexyl 3-cyclohexene carboxaldehyde). Citral was found in 12/24 (50%), in concentrations of 0.011-0.142% (7).

In 2002, in Denmark, 19 air fresheners (6 for cars, 13 for homes) were analyzed for the presence of fragrances that need to be labeled on cosmetics. Citral was found to be present in 7 products (37%) in a concentration range of 200-26,000 ppm and ranked 14 in the frequency list (28).

In 2001, in Denmark, 43 non-cosmetic consumer products (mainly dish-washing products, laundry detergents, and hard and soft surface cleaners) were analyzed for the 26 fragrances that are regulated for labeling in the EU. Citral was present in 7 products (16%) in a concentration range of 0.00001-0.0501% (m/m) and had rank number 13 in the frequency list (26).

In 2000, fifty-nine domestic and occupational products, purchased in retail outlets in Denmark, England, Germany and Italy were analyzed by GC-MS for the presence of fragrances. The product categories were liquid soap and soap bars (n=13), soft/hard surface cleaners (n=23), fabric conditioners/laundry detergents for hand wash (n=8), dish wash (n=10), furniture polish, car shampoo, stain remover (each n=1) and 2 products used in occupational environments. Citral was present in 15 products (25%) with a mean concentration of 218 ppm and a range of 48-1088 ppm (14).

In 1997, 71 deodorants (22 vapo-spray, 22 aerosol spray and 27 roll-on products) were collected in Denmark, England, France, Germany and Sweden and analyzed by gas chromatography – mass spectrometry (GC-MS) for the presence of fragrances and other materials. Citral was present in 26 (37%) of the products (15).

In Denmark, in 1994, 23 cosmetic products, which had either given a positive patch and/or use test in a total of 11 fragrance-mix-positive patients, and which products completely or partly explained present or past episodes of dermatitis, were analyzed for the presence of the constituents of the FM I (with the exception of oakmoss absolute) and a few other fragrances. Citral was found to be present in one of the 23 products (4) in a concentration of 0.09% v/v (45).

Other information: Quenching

The term 'quenching' was framed to describe the complete abrogation of the sensitizing potential of 3 fragrance chemicals (cinnamal, citral and phenylacetaldehyde) by the presence of certain other fragrance chemicals (notably eugenol and limonene) (66). The conclusions were supported by a summary of human predictive test data. Unfortunately, the absence of any details (numbers tested, reproducibility, etc.) have tended to compromise the credibility of the report (65). Whilst there is some evidence in man for the occurrence of quenching during the induction of skin sensitization, a much more substantial body of work has failed to find supportive evidence in various animals models, at a chemical level or at elicitation in human subjects with existing allergy (65,67). In a thorough review of the subject in 2000, it was therefore concluded that the existence of quenching of these fragrance allergens by other specific fragrance components should be regarded as a hypothesis still lacking substantive proof (65).

OTHER SIDE EFFECTS

Irritant contact dermatitis

In 1976, shortly after the introduction of a new lemon-scented detergent, a cluster of hand eczemas occurred amongst the cleaning personnel of 2 hospitals in the Copenhagen area, Denmark. The patients complained of a burning and stinging sensation when their hands were submerged in hot detergent solutions. Patch testing with the standard series and perfume components were negative and an irritant mechanism was suspected. In identifying the responsible agent, selected perfume components were tested at higher temperatures. Identical tests were placed on both forearms for 20 minutes, one arm being exposed to 43°C, the other to 23-25°C. Little or no reaction was seen on the arm exposed the lower temperature, but the lemon perfume component citral proved to be a strong irritant at higher temperatures. Histological examination of the test sites showed the reaction to be of a toxic (irritant) nature (57).

LITERATURE

1	Hagvall L, Karlberg A-T, Christensson JB. Contact allergy to air-exposed geraniol: clinical observations and report of 14 cases. Contact Dermatitis 2012;67:20-27

2	Heisterberg MV, Menné T, Johansen JD. Contact allergy to the 26 specific fragrance ingredients to be declared on cosmetic products in accordance with the EU cosmetic directive. Contact Dermatitis 2011;65:266-275

3	Oosten EJ van, Schuttelaar ML, Coenraads PJ. Clinical relevance of positive patch test reactions to the 26 EU-labelled fragrances. Contact Dermatitis 2009;61:217-223

4	Schnuch A, Uter W, Geier J, Lessmann H, Frosch PJ. Sensitization to 26 fragrances to be labelled according to current European regulation: Results of the IVDK and review of the literature. Contact Dermatitis 2007;57:1-10

5	Heydorn S, Johansen JD, Andersen KE, Bruze M, Svedman C, White IR, et al. Fragrance allergy in patients with hand eczema – a clinical study. Contact Dermatitis 2003;48:317-323

6	Pónyai G, Németh I, Altmeyer A, Nagy G, Irinyi B, Battya Z, et al. Patch tests with fragrance mix II and its components. Dermatitis 2012;23:71-74

7	Frosch PJ, Rastogi SC, Pirker C, Brinkmeier T, Andersen KE, Bruze M, et al. Patch testing with a new fragrance mix - reactivity to the individual constituents and chemical detection in relevant cosmetic products. Contact Dermatitis 2005;52:216-225

8	Wenk KS, Ehrlich AE. Fragrance series testing in eyelid dermatitis. Dermatitis 2012;23:22-26

9	SCCP (Scientific Committee on Consumer Products). Opinion on Dermal sensitisation quantitative risk assessment (Citral, Farnesol and Phenylacetaldehyde), 24 June 2008, SCCP/1153/08. Available at: http://ec.europa.eu/health/archive/ph_risk/committees/04_sccp/docs/sccp_o_135.pdf

10	SCCS (Scientific Committee on Consumer Safety). Opinion on Fragrance allergens in cosmetic products, 26-27 June 2012, SCCS/1459/11. Available at: https://ec.europa.eu/health/sites/health/files/scientific_committees/consumer_safety/docs/sccs_o_102.pdf

11	Malten KE, van Ketel WG, Nater JP, Liem DH. Reactions in selected patients to 22 fragrance materials. Contact Dermatitis 1984;11:1-10

12 De Groot AC, Coenraads PJ, Bruynzeel DP, Jagtman BA, Van Ginkel CJW, Noz K, et al. Routine patch testing with fragrance chemicals in The Netherlands. Contact Dermatitis 2000;42:184-185

13 Yazar K, Johnsson S, Lind M-L, Boman A, Lidén C. Preservatives and fragrances in selected consumer-available cosmetics and detergents. Contact Dermatitis 2011;64:265-272

14 Rastogi SC, Heydorn S, Johansen JD, Basketter DA. Fragrance chemicals in domestic and occupational products. Contact Dermatitis 2001;45:221-225

15 Rastogi SC, Lepoittevin J-P, Johansen JD, Frosch PJ, Menné T, Bruze M, et al. Fragrances and other materials in deodorants: search for potentially sensitizing molecules using combined GC-MS and structure activity relationship (SAR) analysis. Contact Dermatitis 1998;39:293-303

16 Buckley DA. Fragrance ingredient labelling in products on sale in the UK. Br J Dermatol 2007;157:295-300

17 Uter W, Yazar K, Kratz E-M, Mildau G, Lidén C. Coupled exposure to ingredients of cosmetic products: I. Fragrances. Contact Dermatitis 2013;69:335-341

18 Bennike NH, Oturai NB, Müller S, Kirkeby CS, Jørgensen C, Christensen AB, et al. Fragrance contact allergens in 5588 cosmetic products identified through a novel smartphone application. J Eur Acad Dermatol Venereol 2018;32:79-85

19 Rastogi SC, Hellerup Jensen G, Johansen JD. Survey and risk assessment of chemical substances in deodorants. Survey of Chemical Substances in Consumer Products, No. 86 2007. Danish Ministry of the Environment, Environmental Protection Agency. Available at: https://www2.mst.dk/Udgiv/publications/2007/978-87-7052-625-8/pdf/978-87-7052-626-5.pdf

20 Zaragoza-Ninet V, Blasco Encinas R, Vilata-Corell JJ, Pérez-Ferriols A, Sierra-Talamantes C, Esteve-Martínez A, de la Cuadra-Oyanguren J. Allergic contact dermatitis due to cosmetics: A clinical and epidemiological study in a tertiary hospital. Actas Dermosifiliogr 2016;107:329-336

21 An S, Lee AY, Lee CH, Kim DW, Hahm JH, Kim KJ, et al. Fragrance contact dermatitis in Korea: a joint study. Contact Dermatitis 2005;53:320-323

22 Frosch PJ, Johansen JD, Menné T, Pirker C, Rastogi SC, Andersen KE, et al. Further important sensitizers in patients sensitive to fragrances. I. Reactivity to 14 frequently used chemicals. Contact Dermatitis 2002;47:78-85

23 Cuesta L, Silvestre JF, Toledo F, Lucas A, Perez-Crespo M, Ballester I. Fragrance contact allergy: a 4-year retrospective study. Contact Dermatitis 2010;63:77-84

24 Poulsen PB, Schmidt A. A survey and health assessment of cosmetic products for children. Survey of chemical substances in consumer products, No. 88. Copenhagen: Danish Environmental Protection Agency, 2007. Available at: https://www2.mst.dk/udgiv/publications/2007/978-87-7052-638-8/pdf/978-87-7052-639-5.pdf

25 VWA. Dutch Food and Consumer Product Safety Authority. Cosmetische producten voor kinderen: Inventarisatie van de markt en de veiligheidsborging door producenten en importeurs. Report ND04o065/ND05o170, 2007 (Report in Dutch), 2007. Available at: www.nvwa.nl/documenten/communicatie/inspectieresultaten/ consument/ 2016m/cosmetische- producten-voor-kinderen

26 Rastogi SC. Survey of chemical compounds in consumer products. Contents of selected fragrance materials in cleaning products and other consumer products. Survey no. 8-2002. Copenhagen, Denmark, Danish Environmental Protection Agency. Available at: http://eng.mst.dk/media/mst/69131/8.pdf

27 Bouma K, Van Peursem AJJ. Marktonderzoek naleving detergenten verordening voor textielwasmiddelen. Dutch Food and Consumer Products Safety Authority (VWA) Report ND06K173, 2006 [in Dutch]. Available at: http://docplayer.nl/41524125-Marktonderzoek-naleving-detergenten-verordening-voor-textielwasmiddelen.html

28 Pors J, Fuhlendorff R. Mapping of chemical substances in air fresheners and other fragrance liberating products. Report Danish Ministry of the Environment, Environmental Protection Agency (EPA). Survey of Chemicals in Consumer Products, No 30, 2003. Available at: http://eng.mst.dk/media/mst/69113/30.pdf

29 Wilkinson JD, Andersen K, Camarasa J, Ducombs G, Frosch P, Lahti A, et al. Preliminary results of the effectiveness of two forms of fragrance mix as screening agents for fragrance sensitivity. In: Frosch PJ et al, Eds. Current topics in contact dermatitis. Berlin Heidelberg New York: Springer-Verlag, 1989:127-131

30 Goossens A. Cosmetic contact allergens. Cosmetics 2016, 3, 5; doi:10.3390/cosmetics3010005

31 Malten KE. Four bakers showing positive patch tests to a number of fragrance materials, which can also be used as flavors. Acta Derm Venereol 1979;59(suppl.85):117-121

32 Bennike NH, Zachariae C, Johansen JD. Non-mix fragrances are top sensitizers in consecutive dermatitis patients – a cross-sectional study of the 26 EU-labelled fragrance allergens. Contact Dermatitis 2017;77:270-279

33 Lidén C, Yazar K, Johansen JD, Karlberg A-T, Uter W, White IR. Comparative sensitizing potencies of fragrances, preservatives, and hair dyes. Contact Dermatitis 2016;75:265-275

34 Osinka K, Karczmarz A, Krauze K, Feleszko W. Contact allergens in cosmetics used in atopic dermatitis: analysis of product composition. Contact Dermatitis 2016;75:241-243

35 Vejanurug P, Tresukosol P, Sajjachareonpong P, Puangpet P. Fragrance allergy could be missed without patch testing with 26 individual fragrance allergens. Contact Dermatitis 2016;74:230-235

36 Verma A, Tancharoen C, Tam MM, Nixon R. Pustular allergic contact dermatitis caused by fragrances. Contact Dermatitis 2015;72:245-248

37 Mann J, McFadden JP, White JML, White IR, Banerjee P. Baseline series fragrance markers fail to predict contact allergy. Contact Dermatitis 2014;70:276-281

38 Uter W, Johansen JD, Börje A, Karlberg A-T, Lidén C, Rastogi S, Roberts D, White IR. Categorization of fragrance contact allergens for prioritization of preventive measures: clinical and experimental data and consideration of structure–activity relationships. Contact Dermatitis 2013;69:196-230

39 Mowitz M, Svedman C, Zimerson E, Isaksson M, Pontén A, Bruze M. Simultaneous patch testing with fragrance mix I, fragrance mix II and their ingredients in southern Sweden between 2009 and 2015. Contact Dermatitis 2017;77:280-287

40 Nagtegaal MJC, Pentinga SE, Kuik J, Kezic S, Rustemeyer T. The role of the skin irritation response in polysensitization to fragrances. Contact Dermatitis 2012;67:28-35

41 Nardelli A, Drieghe J, Claes L, Boey L, Goossens A. Fragrance allergens in 'specific' cosmetic products. Contact Dermatitis 2011;64:212-219

42 Nardelli A, Thijs L, Janssen K, Goossens A. *Rosa centifolia* in a 'non-scented' moisturizing body lotion as a cause of allergic contact dermatitis. Contact Dermatitis 2009;61:306-309

43 Zacher KD, Ippen H. Contact dermatitis caused by bergamot oil. Derm Beruf Umwelt 1984;32:95-97 (in German)

44 Wieck S, Olsson O, Kümmerer K, Klaschka U. Fragrance allergens in household detergents. Regul Toxicol Pharmacol 2018;97:163-169

45 Johansen JD, Rastogi SC, Menné T. Exposure to selected fragrance materials: A case study of fragrance-mix-positive eczema patients. Contact Dermatitis 1996;34:106-110

46 Diepgen TL, Ofenloch R, Bruze M, Cazzaniga S, Coenraads PJ, Elsner P, et al. Prevalence of fragrance contact allergy in the general population of five European countries: a cross-sectional study. Br J Dermatol 2015;173:1411-1419

47 Kroona L, Warfvinge G, Isaksson M, Ahlgren C, Dahlin J, Sörensen Ö, Bruze M. Quantification of L-carvone in toothpastes available on the Swedish market. Contact Dermatitis 2017;77:224-230

48 Klaschka U. Contact allergens for armpits - allergenic fragrances specified on deodorants. Int J Hyg Environ Health 2012;215:584-591

49 Hagvall L, Backtorp C, Svensson S, Nyman G, Börje A, Karlberg A-T. Fragrance compound geraniol forms contact allergens on air exposure. Identification and quantification of oxidation products and effect on skin sensitization. Chem Res Toxicol 2007;20:807-814

50 Hagvall L, Baron JM, Börje A, Weidolf L, Merk H, Karlberg A-T. Cytochrome P450-mediated activation of the fragrance compound geraniol forms potent contact allergens. Toxicol Appl Pharmacol 2008;233:308-313

51 Hagvall L. Formation of skin sensitizers from fragrance terpenes via oxidative activation routes. Chemical analysis, structure elucidation and experimental sensitization studies. Thesis, University of Gothenburg, Sweden, 2009. Available at: http://hdl.handle.net/2077/18951).

52 Uter W, Schmidt E, Geier J, Lessmann H, Schnuch A, Frosch P. Contact allergy to essential oils: current patch test results (2000–2008) from the Information Network of Departments of Dermatology (IVDK). Contact Dermatitis 2010;63:277-283

53 De Groot AC, Schmidt E. Essential oils: contact allergy and chemical composition. Boca Raton, Fl., USA: CRC Press, Taylor and Francis Group, 2016 (ISBN 9781482246407)

54 Hindle E, Ashworth J, Beck MH. Chelitis from contact allergy to citral in lip salve. Contact Dermatitis 2007;57:125-126

55 Cardullo AC, Ruszkowski AM, DeLeo VA. Allergic contact dermatitis resulting from sensitivity to citrus peel, geraniol, and citral. J Am Acad Dermatol 1989;21:395-397

56 Heydorn S, Menné T, Andersen KE, Bruze M, Svedman C, White IR, Basketter DA. Citral a fragrance allergen and irritant. Contact Dermatitis 2003;49:32-36

57 Rothenborg HW, Menné T, Sjolin KE. Temperature dependent primary irritant dermatitis from lemon perfume. Contact Dermatitis 1977;3:37-48

58 Hagvall L, Bråred Christensson J. Cross-reactivity between citral and geraniol – can it be attributed to oxidized geraniol? Contact Dermatitis 2014;71:280-288

59 De Mozzi P, Johnston GA. An outbreak of allergic contact dermatitis caused by citral in beauticians working in a health spa. Contact Dermatitis 2014;70:377-379

60 Lalko J, Api AM. Citral: identifying a threshold for induction of dermal sensitization. Regul Toxicol Pharmacol 2008;52:62-73

61 Itoh M, Ishihara M, Hosono K, Kantoh H, Kinoshita M, Yamada K, Nishimura M. Results of patch tests conducted between 1978 and 1985 using cosmetic ingredients. Skin Res 1986;28(suppl.2):110-119 (article in Japanese). Data cited in ref. 60

62 Itoh M, Hosono K, Kantoh H, Kinoshita M, Yamada K, Kurosaka R, Nishimura M. Patch test results with cosmetic ingredients conducted between 1978 and 1986. J Soc Cosmet Sci 1988;12:27-41 (article in Japanese). Data cited in ref. 60

63 Nishimura M, Ishihara M, Itoh M, Hosono K, Kantoh H. Results of patch tests on cosmetic ingredients conducted between 1979 and 1982. Skin Res 1984;26:945-954 (article in Japanese). Data cited in ref. 60

64 Ishihara M, Itoh M, Hosono K, Nishimura M. Some problems with patch tests using fragrance materials. Skin Res 1981;23:808-817 (article in Japanese). Data cited in ref. 60

65 Basketter D. Quenching: fact or fiction? Contact Dermatitis 2000;43:253-258

66 Opdyke DLJ. Inhibition of sensitization reactions induced by certain aldehydes. Fd Cosmet Toxicol 1976;14:197-198

67 Basketter D A, Allenby C F. Studies of the quenching phenomenon in delayed contact hypersensitivity reactions. Contact Dermatitis 1991;25:166-171

68 Meynadier JM, Meynadier J, Peyron JL, Peyron L. Formes cliniques des manifestations cutanées d'allergie aux parfums. Ann Dermatol Venereol 1986;113:31-39

69 Opinion of the Scientific Committee on Cosmetic Products and Non-Food Products Intended for Consumers concerning 'The 1st update of the inventory of ingredients employed in cosmetic products. Section II: Perfume and aromatic raw materials', 24 October 2000, SCCNFP/0389/00, final. Available at: http://ec.europa.eu/health/ph_risk/committees/sccp/documents/out131_en.pdf

70 Ung CY, White JML, White IR, Banerjee P, McFadden JP. Patch testing with the European baseline series fragrance markers: a 2016 update. Br J Dermatol 2018;178:776-780

71 Geier J, Uter W, Lessmann H, Schnuch A. Fragrance mix I and II: results of breakdown tests. Flavour Fragr J 2015;30:264-274

72 Girbig M, Hegewald J, Seidler A, Bauer A, Uter W, Schmitt J. Type IV sensitizations in physical therapists: patch test results of the Information Network of Departments of Dermatology (IVDK) 2007-2011. J Dtsch Dermatol Ges 2013;11:1185-1192

73 Dittmar D, Schuttelaar MLA. Contact sensitization to hydroperoxides of limonene and linalool: Results of consecutive patch testing and clinical relevance. Contact Dermatitis 2018 Oct 31. doi: 10.1111/cod.13137. [Epub ahead of print]

74 Silvestre JF, Mercader P, González-Pérez R, Hervella-Garcés M, Sanz-Sánchez T, Córdoba S, et al. Sensitization to fragrances in Spain: A 5-year multicentre study (2011-2015). Contact Dermatitis. 2018 Nov 14. doi: 10.1111/cod.13152. [Epub ahead of print]

Chapter 3.40   CITRAL DIETHYL ACETAL

IDENTIFICATION

Description/definition	: Citral diethyl acetal is the organic compound that conforms to the structural formula shown below
Chemical class(es)	: Unsaturated organic compounds; acetals
INCI name USA	: Not in the Personal Care Products Council Ingredient Database
Chemical/IUPAC name	: 1,1-Diethoxy-3,7-dimethylocta-2,6-diene
Other names	: 3,7-Dimethyl-2,6-octadienal diethyl acetal; geranial diethyl acetal
CAS registry number(s)	: 7492-66-2
EC number(s)	: 231-323-7
RIFM monograph(s)	: Food Chem Toxicol 1983;21:667
Function(s) in cosmetics	: EU: perfuming
Patch testing	: No data available; based on RIFM data, 4% pet. is probably not irritant (2)
Molecular formula	: $C_{14}H_{26}O_2$

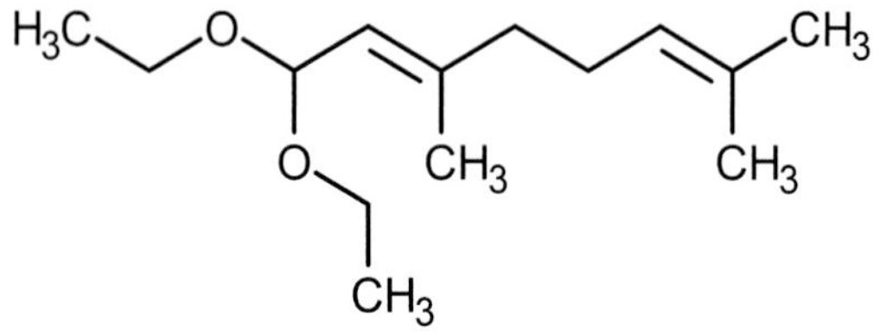

GENERAL

Citral diethyl acetal is a colorless clear liquid; its odor type is citrus and its odor is described as 'sweet citrus, green, floral, waxy, lemon peel' (www.thegoodscentscompany.com).

Presence in essential oils

Citral diethyl acetal is a synthetic fragrance which has not been found in nature thus far (and consequently, not in essential oils) (3).

CONTACT ALLERGY

Patch testing in groups of patients

Pigmented cosmetic dermatitis

While searching for causative ingredients of pigmented cosmetic dermatitis in Japan in the 1970s, both patients with ordinary (nonpigmented) cosmetic dermatitis and women with pigmented cosmetic dermatitis were tested with a large number of fragrance materials. In 1980 the accumulated data enabled the classification of fragrance materials into 4 groups: common sensitizers, rare sensitizers, virtually non-sensitizing fragrances and fragrances considered as non-sensitizers. Citral diethyl acetal was classified in the group of rare sensitizers, indicating that one or more cases of contact allergy / allergic contact dermatitis to it have been observed (1). More specific data are lacking, the results have largely or solely been published in Japanese journals only.

Case reports and case series

Case reports of allergic contact dermatitis from citral diethyl acetal have not been found.

LITERATURE

1   Nakayama H. Fragrance hypersensitivity and its control. In: Frosch PJ, Johansen JD, White IR, Eds. Fragrances - beneficial and adverse effects. Berlin Heidelberg New York: Springer-Verlag, 1998:83-91
2   Research Institute for Fragrance Materials (RIFM). Citral diethyl acetal. Food Chem Toxicol 1983;21:667
3   De Groot AC, Schmidt E. Essential oils: contact allergy and chemical composition. Boca Raton, Fl., USA: CRC Press, Taylor and Francis Group, 2016 (ISBN 9781482246407)

Chapter 3.41   CITRONELLAL

IDENTIFICATION

Description/definition   : Citronellal is the organic compound that conforms to the structural formula shown below
Chemical class(es)   : Aldehydes
Chemical/IUPAC name   : 3,7-Dimethyloct-6-enal
Other names   : 2,3-Dihydrocitral
CAS registry number(s)   : 106-23-0
EC number(s)   : 203-376-6
RIFM monograph(s)   : Food Cosm Toxicol 1975;13:755 (special issue II) (binder, page 233)
Merck Index monograph : 3598
Function(s) in cosmetics : EU: masking. USA: fragrance ingredients
Patch testing   : 2% pet. (SmartPracticeEurope, SmartPracticeCanada)
Molecular formula   : $C_{10}H_{18}O$

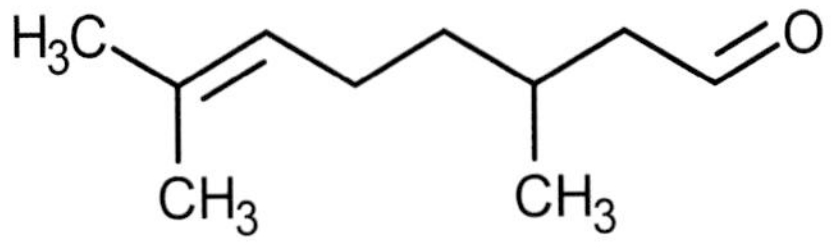

GENERAL

Citronellal is a colorless to pale yellow clear liquid; its odor type is floral and its odor is described as 'sweet, floral rosy waxy and citrus green' (www.thegoodscentscompany.com). Citronellal is used in small amounts for scenting soaps and detergents, is also used as flavor in foods and beverages and is applied as insect repellent. Its principal application, however, is in the preparation of isopulegol, citronellol, and hydroxycitronellol (U.S. National Library of Medicine).

Presence in essential oils

Citronellal has been identified by chemical analysis in 43 of 91 essential oils, which have caused contact allergy / allergic contact dermatitis. In 6 oils, citronellal belonged to the 'Top-10' of ingredients with the highest concentrations which may be expected in commercial essential oils of this type: Eucalyptus citriodora oil (68.6-84.4%), citronella oil Java (31.5-49.6%), melissa oil (0.5-29.2%), citronella oil Sri Lanka (1.0-12%), litsea cubeba oil (0.4-3.8%), and lemongrass oil West Indian (0.2-1.9%) (3).

CONTACT ALLERGY

Patch testing in groups of patients

Studies in which citronellal been patch tested in either consecutive patients suspected of contact dermatitis (routine testing) or in groups of selected patients with positive results have not been found.

Case reports and case series

In the period 1996-2013, in a tertiary referral center in Valencia, Spain, 5419 patients were patch tested. Of these, 628 individuals had allergic contact dermatitis to cosmetics. In this group, citronellal was the responsible allergen in one case (1).

    A woman changed the urinary bag from her child daily and thereby used an ostomy deodorant. She developed dermatitis on the hands and the face. On patch testing she reacted to the deodorant and subsequently to one ingredient, which consisted mainly of citronella oil and citronellal (but according to the manufacturer also pine oil derivatives) (2). Citronellal is the main ingredient of citronella oil present in concentrations of 30-50% (3). The causative role of citronellal in this case, although likely, was not proven.

    Two patients had used oil of citronella for protection against mosquitos and developed dermatitis. They reacted to oil of citronella (pure and 50% in mineral oil, concentrations which are slightly irritant), citronellal, citronellol, hydroxycitronellal, citral and geranyl acetate (4). Citronellal and citronellol are both important components of citronella oils and geranyl acetate may be present in concentrations up to 11% in commercial citronella oil Sri Lanka (3).

Cross-reactions, pseudo-cross-reactions and co-reactions

For general information on cross-/pseudo-cross-/co-reactivity of fragrance chemicals with other fragrances, fragrance markers (fragrance mix I, fragrance mix II, colophonium, Myroxylon pereirae resin [balsam of Peru]) and essential oils see Chapter 1.2 General information on cross-reactions, pseudo-cross-reactions and co-reactions.

Two patients sensitized to oil of citronella reacted to citronellol and citronellal (4); both fragrance chemicals may be present in this essential oil (3). In commercial citronella oils, citronellal has been found in concentrations of 1-49.6% and citronellol in concentrations ranging from 1.7-13.5%, depending on the nature of the citronella oil (Java or Sri Lanka) (see Chapter 6.18 Citronella oil).

When citronellol autoxidizes, low amounts (up to 1%) of citronellal may be formed (5).

LITERATURE

1   Zaragoza-Ninet V, Blasco Encinas R, Vilata-Corell JJ, Pérez-Ferriols A, Sierra-Talamantes C, Esteve-Martínez A, de la Cuadra-Oyanguren J. Allergic contact dermatitis due to cosmetics: A clinical and epidemiological study in a tertiary hospital. Actas Dermosifiliogr 2016;107:329-336

2   Davies MG, Hodgson GA, Evans E. Contact dermatitis from an ostomy deodorant. Contact Dermatitis 1978;4:11-13

3   De Groot AC, Schmidt E. Essential oils: contact allergy and chemical composition. Boca Raton, Fl., USA: CRC Press, Taylor and Francis Group, 2016 (ISBN 9781482246407)

4   Keil H. Contact dermatitis due to oil of citronellal. J Invest Dermatol 1947;8:327-334

5   Rudbäck J, Hagvall L, Börje A, Nilsson U, Karlberg A-T. Characterization of skin sensitizers from autoxidized citronellol – impact of the terpene structure on the autoxidation process. Contact Dermatitis 2014;70:329-339

Chapter 3.42   CITRONELLOL

There are two forms of citronellol: α- and β-citronellol. The terminology and assignment of CAS numbers, EC numbers and synonyms in various chemical databases is very confusing and inconsistent.

α-CITRONELLOL

α-Citronellol is discussed in Chapter 3.144 Rhodinol.

β-CITRONELLOL

IDENTIFICATION

Description/definition	: β-Citronellol is the organic compound that conforms to the structural formula shown below
Chemical class(es)	: Alcohols
INCI name EU and USA	: Citronellol
Chemical/IUPAC name	: 3,7-Dimethyloct-6-en-1-ol
Other names	: Rhodinol; *DL*-citronellol; elenol; cephrol
CAS registry number(s)	: 106-22-9; 68916-43-8; 26489-01-0
EINECS number(s)	: 203-375-0; 247-737-6
RIFM monograph(s)	: Food Chem Toxicol 2008;46(suppl.):S1-S71; Food Chem Toxicol 2008;46(suppl.):S103-S109, S110-S113 (*l*-citronellol, CAS 7540-51-4), and S114-116; Food Cosmet Toxicol 1975;13:757 (special issue II)
IFRA standard	: Restricted (www.ifraorg.org/en-us/standards-library) (table 3.42.1)
SCCS opinion(s)	: Various (9); SCCS/1459/11 (10)
Merck Index monograph	: 9579
Function(s) in cosmetics	: EU: perfuming; USA: fragrance ingredients
EU cosmetic restrictions	: Regulated in Annex III/86 of the Regulation (EC) No. 1223/2009, regulated by 2003/15/EC; Must be labeled on cosmetics and detergent products, if present at > 10 ppm (0.001%) in leave-on products and > 100 ppm (0.01%) in rinse-off products
Patch testing	: 'Citronellol' 1% pet. (SmartPracticeEurope, Chemotechnique, SmartPracticeCanada); also present in the fragrance mix II; some positive reactions to citronellol may be missed when the reactions are not read at D7 (44); it may be preferable to test with oxidized citronellol (51)
Molecular formula	: $C_{10}H_{20}O$

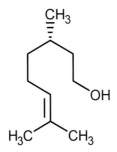

Table 3.42.1 IFRA restrictions for citronellol

Category [a]	Limits [b]	Category [a]	Limits [b]	Category [a]	Limits [b]
1	0.80%	5	7.00%	9	5.00%
2	1.10%	6	21.40%	10	2.50%
3	4.40%	7	2.20%	11	not restricted
4	13.30%	8	2.00%		

[a] For explanation of categories see pages 6-8
[b] Limits in the finished products

GENERAL

Citronellol is a colorless to pale yellow clear liquid; its odor type is floral and its odor is described as 'floral, rosy, sweet, citrus with green fatty terpene nuances' (www.thegoodscentscompany.com). Citronellol occurs naturally in many plant oils and certain fruits. The chemical is a component of citronella oil and is a main component responsible for the insect repellent properties of this essential oil. It is one of the most widely used fragrance materials, particularly for rose notes and for floral compositions in general. Its stability makes it particularly useful in fragrances for soaps, detergents, and other household products. Citronellol, in addition, is important as an intermediate in the synthesis of a number of other fragrance chemicals, including rose oxide, numerous citronellyl esters and hydroxydi-hydrocitronellol. The chemical is also used as a food flavoring and it is an important pesticide on food crops and ornamental plants (U.S. National Library of Medicine).

Presence in essential oils

Citronellol has been identified by chemical analysis in 51 of 91 essential oils, which have caused contact allergy / allergic contact dermatitis. In 6 oils, citronellol belonged to the 'Top-10' of ingredients with the highest concentrations which may be expected in commercial essential oils of this type: geranium oil (20.1-49.4%), rose oil (0.5-44.8%), citronella oil Java (8.7-13.5%), melissa oil (0.05-13.1%), citronella oil Sri Lanka (1.7-9.6%), and Eucalyptus citriodora oil (3.9-8.0%) (49).

CONTACT ALLERGY

General

The SCCS (Scientific Committee on Consumer Safety), in a 2012 Opinion on Fragrance allergens in cosmetic products, has marked citronellol as 'established contact allergen in humans' (10,42). The sensitizing potency of citronellol was classified as 'weak' based on an EC3 value of 43.5% in the LLNA (local lymph node assay) in animal experiments (10, 42). Citronellol is a constituent of the fragrance mix II. In groups of patients reacting to the mix and tested with its 6 ingredients, citronellol scored 0-8.1% positive patch test reactions (see Chapter 3.71 Fragrance mix II).

Pure citronellol is low- or non-sensitizing (51). Indeed, in routine testing of dermatitis patients, reactions to citronellol are very infrequent (Table 3.42.2). However, when exposed to air, citronellol autoxidizes, whereby the content of citronellol decreases over time to 33% after 26 weeks of exposure (51). Several oxidation products have been detected in the oxidation mixture of citronellol: citronellol hydroperoxides (6-hydroperoxy-3,7-dimethyloct-7-ene-1-ol and (E)-7-hydroperoxy-3,7-dimethyloct-5-ene-1-ol), citronellal, citronellyl formate, epoxycitronellal, epoxycitro-nellol, and citronellol diols. Oxidation increased the sensitizing potency of citronellol according to predictive testing with the murine local lymph node assay (LLNA), which is mainly attributable to the hydroperoxides formed (51).

Therefore, is has been suggested that patch testing should be performed with oxidized citronellol (analogous to testing with oxidized limonene, oxidized linalool and oxidized tea tree oil). Indeed, in clinical studies, a high (but unspecified) percentage of consecutive dermatitis patients tested had positive patch test reactions to oxidized citronellol, indicating that more cases will be detected when patch testing is performed with air-exposed citronellol than when it is performed with FM II only (51).

The literature on contact allergy to citronellol up to 2004 has been reviewed (15).

General population

In the period 2008-2011, in 5 European countries (Sweden, Germany, Netherlands, Portugal, Italy), a random sample of the general population of 3119 individuals aged 18-74 years were patch tested with the FM I, its 8 ingredients, the FM II, its 6 ingredients and Myroxylon pereirae resin. There were 3 reactions (0.1%) to citronellol, tested 1% in petrolatum. About half of all positive reactions to fragrances were considered to be relevant based on standardized criteria. Women were affected twice as often as men (47).

Patch testing in groups of patients

Results of studies testing citronellol in consecutive patients suspected of contact dermatitis (routine testing) are shown in table 3.42.2. Results of testing in groups of *selected* patients (e.g. patients with known or suspected fragrance or cosmetic dermatitis, individuals with eyelid dermatitis, patients with hand eczema) are shown in table 3.42.3.

Patch testing in consecutive patients suspected of contact dermatitis: routine testing

In eleven studies in which routine testing with citronellol was performed, frequencies of sensitization were invariably (very) low, ranging from 0.07% to 1% (table 3.42.2). In 7/11 investigations, no (specific) data on relevance were provided; in the other 4 addressing the issue, 0-100% of the positive reactions were scored as relevant, but the numbers of allergic patients were very small. Causative products were usually not mentioned or specified, but in one study, of the relevant reactions to any of 26 fragrances tested, 96% were caused by cosmetic products (1).

Table 3.42.2 Patch testing in groups of patients: Routine testing

Years and Country	Test conc. & vehicle	Number of patients tested	positive (%)		Selection of patients (S); Relevance (R); Comments (C)	Ref.
2015-7 Netherlands		821	7	(0.9%)	R: not stated	55
2015-2016 UK	1% pet.	2084	2	(0.1%)	R: not specified for individual fragrances; 25% of patients who reacted to any fragrance or fragrance marker had a positive fragrance history	57
2010-2015 Denmark	1% pet.	6004	4	(0.07%)	R: present relevance 75%, past relevance 50%	37
2009-2015 Sweden	1% pet.	4175	14	(0.3%)	R: not stated	43
2013-2014 Thailand		312	3	(1.0%)	R: 100%	40
2011-2012 UK	1% pet.	1951	6	(0.3%)	R: not stated	41
2008-2010 Denmark	1% pet.	1503	1	(0.1%)	S: mostly routine testing; R: 100%; C: 100% co-reactivity of both FM I and FM II; C: of the relevant reactions to any of the 26 fragrances tested, 96% were caused by cosmetic products	1
2003-2004 IVDK	1% pet.	2003	9	(0.4%)	R: not stated	3
2002-2003 six European countries	0.5% pet.	1701	2	(0.1%)	R: not specified	6
	1% pet.	1701	4	(0.2%)	R: not specified	
1997-8 six European countries	5% pet.	1855	7	(0.4%)	R: not stated / specified	30
< 1995 Sweden	1% pet.	100	1	(1%)	R: not relevant; C: unknown whether the reactions were in the same patient; a ROAT was negative	29
	5% pet.	100	1	(1%)		

FM: Fragrance mix; IVDK: Informationsverbund Dermatologischer Kliniken (Germany, Switzerland, Austria)

Patch testing in groups of selected patients

Results of studies patch testing citronellol in groups of selected patients (e.g. patients with known or suspected fragrance or cosmetic dermatitis, individuals with eyelid dermatitis, patients with hand eczema) are shown in table 3.42.3.

In 9 investigations, frequencies of sensitization to citronellol have ranged from 0.3% to 35%. The highest rates were observed in patients known to be allergic to fragrances: 35% (13), 8.7% (11) and 5.6% (12).

In 7/9 studies, no (specific) relevance data were provided. Some authors considered relevance for all reactions 'possible' (5), others assumed that nearly all positive reactions were of present or past relevance (4). Causative products were not mentioned.

Results of testing citronellol in groups of patients reacting to the fragrance mix II are shown in Chapter 3.71 Fragrance mix II.

Case reports and case series

Citronellol was stated to be the (or an) allergen in 5 patients in a group of 603 individuals suffering from cosmetic dermatitis, seen in the period 2010-2015 in Leuven, Belgium (36). In the period 2000-2009, also in Leuven, Belgium, an unspecified number of patients had positive patch tests or use tests to a total of 344 cosmetic products *and* positive patch tests to FM I, FM II, and/or to one or more of 28 selected specific fragrance ingredients. In 10 of 17 patients reacting to citronellol, the presence of this fragrance in the cosmetic product(s) was confirmed by reading the product label(s) (45).

In a group of 119 patients with allergic contact dermatitis from cosmetics, investigated in The Netherlands in 1986-1987, 2 cases were caused by citronellol in a skin care product and facial makeup (26,27). In a perfume factory, two bottle fillers developed occupational allergic contact dermatitis from citronellol. Of twenty people working in the same factory who did *not* have dermatitis, one had a positive reaction to this fragrance (8).

Two patients had used oil of citronella for protection against mosquitos and developed dermatitis. They reacted to oil of citronella (pure and 50% in mineral oil, concentrations which are slightly irritant), citronellol, citronellal, hydroxycitronellal, citral and geranyl acetate. Citronellol (8.5-15%) and citronellal (30-50%) are both important components of citronella oils and geranyl acetate may be present in concentrations up to 11% in commercial citronella oil Sri Lanka (49).

One individual had allergic contact dermatitis from citronellol in a skin care product (19). A metal worker suffered from occupational allergic dermatitis of the hands from citronellol in a skin protection cream (53).

Table 3.42.3 Patch testing in groups of patients: Selected patient groups

Years and Country	Test conc. & vehicle	Number of patients tested | positive (%)		Selection of patients (S); Relevance (R); Comments (C)	Ref.
2011-2015 Spain	1% pet.	1013	39 (3.8%)	S: patients previously reacting to FM I, FM II, Myroxylon pereirae resin or hydroxyisohexyl 3-cyclohexene carboxaldehyde in the baseline series; R: not stated	56
2009-2010 Hungary	1% pet.	565	7 (1.2%)	S: patients with former skin symptoms provoked by scented products in the case history; R: in all cases 'possible'	5
2006-2010 USA	0.5% pet.	100	1 (1%)	S: patients with eyelid dermatitis; R: not stated	7
2005-10 Netherlands		100	3 (3%)	S: patients with known fragrance sensitivity based on a positive patch test to the FM I and/or the FM II; R: not stated	44
2005-7 Netherlands	2% pet.	320	1 (0.3%)	S: patients suspected of fragrance or cosmetic allergy; R: 61% relevance for all positive tested fragrances together	2
<2002 Japan, Europe, USA	5% pet.	218	19 (8.7%)	S: patients with known fragrance sensitivity; R: not stated	11
2001-2002 Denmark, Sweden	5% pet.	658	2 (0.3%)	S: consecutive patients with hand eczema; R: it was assumed that nearly all positive reactions were of present or past relevance	4
2000 Japan, Europe, USA	5% pet.	178	10 (5.6%)	S: patients with known fragrance sensitivity; R: not stated; C: the test material was l-citronellol (CAS 7540-51-4)	12
1975 USA	5% pet.	20	7 (35%)	S: fragrance-allergic patients; R: not stated	13

Testing in groups of patients reacting to the fragrance mix II
Results of testing citronellol in groups of patients reacting to the fragrance mix II are shown in Chapter 3.71 Fragrance mix II

FM: Fragrance Mix

Cross-reactions, pseudo-cross-reactions and co-reactions

For general information on cross-/pseudo-cross-/co-reactivity of fragrance chemicals with other fragrances, fragrance markers (fragrance mix I, fragrance mix II, colophonium, Myroxylon pereirae resin [balsam of Peru]) and essential oils see Chapter 1.2 General information on cross-reactions, pseudo-cross-reactions and co-reactions. Co-reactivity with the fragrance mix II can be expected, as the mix contains citronellol (pseudo-cross-reactions).

Two patients sensitized to oil of citronella reacted to citronellol and citronellal (50); these chemicals are both important constituents of this essential oil (49). When citronellol autoxidizes, low amounts (up to 1%) of citronellal may be formed (51).

In a large study performed by the IVDK in the period 2005-2013, eighteen out of 32 patients (56%) reacting to citronellol also reacted to citral; conversely, of 171 citral-positive patients, 18 (11%) co-reacted to citronellol (54).

Presence in products and chemical analyses

In various studies, the presence of citronellol in cosmetic and sometimes other products has been investigated. Before 2006, most investigators used chemical analysis, usually GC-MS, for qualitative and quantitative determination. Since then, the presence of the target fragrances was usually investigated by screening the product labels for the 26 fragrances that must be labeled since 2005 on cosmetics and detergent products in the EU, if present at > 10 ppm (0.001%) in leave-on products and > 100 ppm (0.01%) in rinse-off products. This method, obviously, is less accurate and may result in underestimation of the frequency of the fragrances being present in the product. When they are in fact present, but the concentration is lower than mentioned above, labeling is not required and the fragrances' presence will be missed.

The results of the relevant studies for citronellol are summarized in table 3.42.4. More detailed information can be found in the corresponding text before and following the table. The percentage of products in which citronellol was found to be present shows wide variations, which can among other be explained by the selection procedure of the products, the method of investigation (false-negatives with information obtained from labels only) and changes in the use of individual fragrance materials over time (fashion). Generally speaking, citronellol is one of the more frequently used fragrances.

In 2017, in the USA, the ingredient labels 159 hair-dye kits containing 539 cosmetic products (e.g. colorants, conditioners, shampoos, toners) were screened for the most common sensitizers they contain. Citronellol was found to be present in 54 (10%) of the products (46).

In Denmark, in 2015-2016, 5588 fragranced cosmetic products were examined with a smartphone application for the 26 fragrances that need to be labeled in the EU. Citronellol was present in 29% of the products (rank number 3) (24).

In Germany, in 2015, fragrance allergens were evaluated based on lists of ingredients in 817 (unique) detergents (all-purpose cleaners, cleaning preparations for special purposes [e.g. bathroom, kitchen, dish-washing] and laundry detergents) present in 131 households. Citronellol was found to be present in 93 (11%) of the products (52).

In Sweden, in 2015, contact allergens were identified on the ingredient labels of 26 oxidative hair dye products (from 4 different product series) and on the labels of 35 non-oxidative hair dye products (from 5 different product series, including so-called herbal hair colors). These products were selected on the basis of being advertised as 'organic', 'natural', or similar, or used in hairdressing salons branded with such attributes. Citronellol was present in six (23%) of the 26 oxidative hair dyes and in zero of the 35 non-oxidative hair dye products (39).

Of 179 emollients available in online drugstores in 2014 in Poland, six (3.3%) contained citronellol, according to information available online (38).

Table 3.42.4 Presence of citronellol in products [a]

Year	Country	Product type	Nr. investigated	Nr. of products positive [b]	(%)	Method [c]	Ref.
2017	USA	Cosmetic products in hair-dye kits	539 products in 159 hair-dye kits	54	(10%)	Labeling	46
2015-6	Denmark	Fragranced cosmetic products	5588		(29%)	Labeling	24
2015	Germany	Household detergents	817	93	(11%)	Labeling	52
2015	Sweden	Oxidative hair dye products	26	6	(23%)	Labeling	39
		Non-oxidative	35	0	(0%)	Labeling	
2014	Poland	Emollients	179	6	(3%)	Online info	38
2013	USA	Pediatric cosmetics	187	2	(1%)	Labeling	28
2008-11	Germany	Deodorants	374	153	(41%)	Labeling	48
2006-9	Germany	Cosmetic products	4991		(20%)	Labeling	23
2008	Sweden	Cosmetic products	204		(20%)	Labeling	14
		Detergents	97		(9%)	Labeling	
2007	Netherlands	Cosmetic products for children	23	5	(22%)	Analysis	32
2006	UK	Perfumed cosmetic and household products	300	145	(48%)	Labeling	21
2006	Denmark	Popular perfumed deodorants	88	58	(66%)	Labeling	25
			23	21	(91%)	Analysis	
2006	Netherlands	Laundry detergents	52	11	(21%)	Labeling + analysis	34
2006	Denmark	Rinse-off cosmetics for children	208	22	(11%)	Labeling + analysis	31
2004	Denmark, UK, Belgium, Germany	Fragranced products that had caused allergic contact dermatitis, used by patients	24	21	(88%)	Labeling	6
2002	Denmark	Home and car air fresheners	19	10	(53%)	Analysis	35
2001	Denmark	Non-cosmetic consumer products	43	11	(26%)	Analysis	33
2000	Denmark, UK, Germany, Italy	Domestic and occupational products	59	28	(47%)	Analysis	17
1997-8	Denmark, UK Germany, Sweden	Cosmetics and cosmetic toys for children	25	18	(72%)	Analysis	18
1996	Five European countries	Fragranced deodorants	70	57	(81%)	Analysis	16
1992	Netherlands	Cosmetic products	300		(71%)	Analysis	22
1988	USA	Perfumes used in fine fragrances, household products and soap	400	38-60% (See text)		Analysis	20

[a] See the corresponding text below for more details
[b] positive = containing the target fragrance
[c] Labeling: information from the ingredient labels on the product / packaging; Analysis: chemical analysis, most often GC-MS

In 2013, in the USA, the allergen content of 187 unique pediatric cosmetics from 6 different retailers marketed in the United States as hypoallergenic was evaluated on the basis of labeling. Inclusion criteria were products marketed as pediatric and 'hypoallergenic', 'dermatologist recommended/tested', 'fragrance free', or 'paraben free'. Citronellol was found to be present in 2 (1.1%) of the products (28).

In 2008, 2010 and 2011, 374 deodorants available in German retail shops were randomly selected and their labels checked for the presence of the 26 fragrances that need to be labeled. Citronellol was found to be present in 153 (40.9%) of the products (48).

In Germany, in the period 2006-2009, 4991 cosmetic products were randomly sampled for an official investigation of conformity of cosmetic products with legal provisions. The labels were inspected for the presence of the 26 fragrances that need to be labeled in the EU. Citronellol was present in 20% of the products (rank number 3) (23).

Citronellol was present (as indicated by labeling) in 20% of 204 cosmetic products (92 shampoos, 61 hair conditioners, 34 liquid soaps, 17 wet tissues) and in 9% of 97 detergents in Sweden, 2008 (14).

In 2007, in The Netherlands, twenty-three cosmetic products for children were analyzed for the presence of fragrances that need to be labeled. Citronellol was identified in 5 of the products (22%) in a concentration range of 59-1158 ppm (32).

In 2006, in The Netherlands, 52 laundry detergents were investigated for the presence of allergenic fragrances by checking their labels and chemical analyses. Citronellol was found to be present in 11 of the products (21%) in a concentration range of 13- 516 ppm. Citronellol had rank number 10 in the frequency list (34).

In 2006, of 88 popular perfume containing deodorants purchased in Denmark, 58 (66%) were labeled to contain citronellol. Analysis of 24 regulated fragrance substances in 23 selected deodorants (19 spray products, 2 deostick and 2 roll-on) was performed by GC-MS. Citronellol was identified in 21 of the products (91%) with a concentration range of 1–5848 ppm (25).

In 2006, the labels of 208 cosmetics for children (especially shampoos, body shampoos and soaps) available in Denmark were checked for the presence of the 26 fragrances that need to be labeled in the EU. Citronellol was present in 22 products (10.5%), and ranked number 5 in the frequency list. Seventeen products were analyzed quantitatively for the fragrances. The maximum concentration found for citronellol was 300 mg/kg (31).

In January 2006, a study of perfumed cosmetic and household products available on the shelves of U.K. retailers was carried out. Products were included if 'parfum' or 'aroma' was listed among the ingredients. Three hundred products were surveyed and any of 26 mandatory labeling fragrances named on the label were recorded. Citronellol was present in 145 (48%) of the products (rank number 3) (21).

In 2004, in 4 European countries (Denmark, Germany, Belgium, U.K.), of 12 patients allergic to the FM II and one or more of its constituents (hexyl cinnamal 1, citral 3, hydroxyisohexyl 3-cyclohexene carboxaldehyde 11), 24 of the products used by them (deodorant 4, eau de toilette 9, lotion/cream 4, fine perfume 7) that had caused adverse reactions compatible with allergic contact dermatitis, were analyzed for the presence of the six constituents of the fragrance mix II (citral, citronellol, coumarin, farnesol, hexyl cinnamal, hydroxyisohexyl 3-cyclohexene carboxaldehyde). Citronellol was found in 21/24 (88%) products, in concentrations of 0.031-1.022% (6).

In 2002, in Denmark, 19 air fresheners (6 for cars, 13 for homes) were analyzed for the presence of fragrances that need to be labeled on cosmetics. Citronellol was found to be present in 10 products (53%) in a concentration range of 190-18,000 ppm and ranked 9 in the frequency list (35).

In 2001, in Denmark, 43 non-cosmetic consumer products (mainly dish-washing products, laundry detergents, and hard and soft surface cleaners) were analyzed for the 26 fragrances that are regulated for labeling in the EU. Citronellol was present in 11 products (26%) in a concentration range of 0.00001-0.0763% (m/m) and had rank number 9 in the frequency list (33).

In 2000, fifty-nine domestic and occupational products, purchased in retail outlets in Denmark, England, Germany and Italy were analyzed by GC-MS for the presence of fragrances. The product categories were liquid soap and soap bars (n=13), soft/hard surface cleaners (n=23), fabric conditioners/laundry detergents for hand wash (n=8), dish- wash (n=10), furniture polish, car shampoo, stain remover (each n=1) and 2 products used in occupational environments. Citronellol was present in 28 products (47%) with a mean concentration of 275 ppm and a range of 18-1579 ppm (17).

Twenty-five cosmetics and cosmetic toys for children (5 shampoos and shower gels, 6 perfumes, 1 deodorant (roll-on), 4 baby lotions/creams, 1 baby wipes product, 1 baby oil, 2 lipcare products and 5 toy-cosmetic products: a cosmetic-toy set for blending perfumes and a makeup set) purchased in 1997-1998 in retail outlets in Denmark, Germany, England and Sweden were analyzed in 1998 for the presence of fragrances by GC-MS. Citronellol was found in 18 products (72%) in a concentration range of ≤0.001-0.759% (w/w). For the analytical data in each product category, the original publication should be consulted (18).

Seventy fragranced deodorants, purchased at retail outlets in 5 European countries in 1996, were analyzed by gas chromatography - mass spectrometry (GC-MS) for the determination of the contents of 21 commonly used fragrance materials. Citronellol was identified in 57 products (81%) in a concentration range of 1–5585 ppm (16).

In 1992, in The Netherlands, the presence of fragrances was analyzed in 300 cosmetic products. Citronellol was identified in 71% of the products (rank order 5) (22).

In 1988, in the USA, 400 perfumes used in fine fragrances, household products and soaps (number of products per category not mentioned) were analyzed for the presence of fragrance chemicals in a concentration of at least 1% and a list of the Top-25 (present in the highest number of products) presented. Citronellol was found to be present in 38% of the fine fragrances (rank number 19), 40% of the household product fragrances (rank number 12) and 60% of the fragrances used in soaps (rank number 10) (20).

LITERATURE

1   Heisterberg MV, Menné T, Johansen JD. Contact allergy to the 26 specific fragrance ingredients to be declared on cosmetic products in accordance with the EU cosmetic directive. Contact Dermatitis 2011;65:266-275

2   Oosten EJ van, Schuttelaar ML, Coenraads PJ. Clinical relevance of positive patch test reactions to the 26 EU-labelled fragrances. Contact Dermatitis 2009;61:217-223

3   Schnuch A, Uter W, Geier J, Lessmann H, Frosch PJ. Sensitization to 26 fragrances to be labelled according to current European regulation: Results of the IVDK and review of the literature. Contact Dermatitis 2007;57:1-10

4   Heydorn S, Johansen JD, Andersen KE, Bruze M, Svedman C, White IR, et al. Fragrance allergy in patients with hand eczema – a clinical study. Contact Dermatitis 2003;48:317-323

5   Pónyai G, Németh I, Altmeyer A, Nagy G, Irinyi B, Battya Z, et al. Patch tests with fragrance mix II and its components. Dermatitis 2012;23:71-74

6   Frosch PJ, Rastogi SC, Pirker C, Brinkmeier T, Andersen KE, Bruze M, et al. Patch testing with a new fragrance mix - reactivity to the individual constituents and chemical detection in relevant cosmetic products. Contact Dermatitis 2005;52:216-225

7   Wenk KS, Ehrlich AE. Fragrance series testing in eyelid dermatitis. Dermatitis 2012;23:22-26

8   Schubert HJ. Skin diseases in workers at a perfume factory. Contact Dermatitis 2006;55:81-83

9   Various SCCS opinions on citronellol have been published and are available at: http://ec.europa.eu/growth/tools-databases/cosing/index.cfm?fuseaction=search.details_v2&id=27935&back=1

10 SCCS (Scientific Committee on Consumer Safety). Opinion on Fragrance allergens in cosmetic products, 26-27 June 2012, SCCS/1459/11. Available at: https://ec.europa.eu/health/sites/health/files/scientific_committees/consumer_safety/docs/sccs_o_102.pdf

11 Larsen W, Nakayama H, Fischer T, Elsner P, Frosch P, Burrows D, et al. Fragrance contact dermatitis - a worldwide multicenter investigation (Part III). Contact Dermatitis 2002;46:141-144

12 Larsen W, Nakayama H, Fischer T, Elsner P, Frosch P, Burrows D, et al. Fragrance contact dermatitis: A worldwide multicenter investigation (Part II). Contact Dermatitis 2001;44:344-346

13 Larsen WG. Perfume dermatitis. A study of 20 patients. Arch Dermatol 1977;113:623-626

14 Yazar K, Johnsson S, Lind M-L, Boman A, Lidén C. Preservatives and fragrances in selected consumer-available cosmetics and detergents. Contact Dermatitis 2011;64:265-272

15 Hostýnek JJ, Maibach HI. Sensitization potential of citronellol. Exog Dermatol 2004;3:307-312

16 Rastogi SC, Johansen JD, Frosch P, Menné T, Bruze M, Lepoittevin JP, et al. Deodorants on the European market: quantitative chemical analysis of 21 fragrances. Contact Dermatitis 1998;38:29-35

17 Rastogi SC, Heydorn S, Johansen JD, Basketter DA. Fragrance chemicals in domestic and occupational products. Contact Dermatitis 2001;45:221-225

18 Rastogi SC, Johansen JD, Menné T, Frosch P, Bruze M, Andersen KE, et al. Content of fragrance allergens in children's cosmetics and cosmetic toys. Contact Dermatitis 1999;41:84-88

19 De Groot AC. Contact allergy to cosmetics: causative ingredients. Contact Dermatitis 1987;17:26-34

20 Fenn RS. Aroma chemical usage trends in modern perfumery. Perfumer and Flavorist 1989;14:3-10

21 Buckley DA. Fragrance ingredient labelling in products on sale in the UK. Br J Dermatol 2007;157:295-300

22 Weyland JW. Personal Communication, 1992. Cited in: De Groot AC, Weyland JW, Nater JP. Unwanted effects of cosmetics and drugs used in dermatology, 3rd Ed. Amsterdam: Elsevier, 1994: 579

23 Uter W, Yazar K, Kratz E-M, Mildau G, Lidén C. Coupled exposure to ingredients of cosmetic products: I. Fragrances. Contact Dermatitis 2013;69:335-341

24 Bennike NH, Oturai NB, Müller S, Kirkeby CS, Jørgensen C, Christensen AB, et al. Fragrance contact allergens in 5588 cosmetic products identified through a novel smartphone application. J Eur Acad Dermatol Venereol 2018;32:79-85

25 Rastogi SC, Hellerup Jensen G, Johansen JD. Survey and risk assessment of chemical substances in deodorants. Survey of Chemical Substances in Consumer Products, No. 86 2007. Danish Ministry of the Environment, Environmental Protection Agency. Available at: https://www2.mst.dk/Udgiv/publications/2007/978-87-7052-625-8/pdf/978-87-7052-626-5.pdf

26 De Groot AC, Bruynzeel DP, Bos JD, van der Meeren HL, van Joost T, Jagtman BA, Weyland JW. The allergens in cosmetics. Arch Dermatol 1988;124:1525-1529

27 De Groot AC. Adverse reactions to cosmetics. PhD Thesis, University of Groningen, The Netherlands: 1988, chapter 3.4, pp.105-113

28 Hamann CR, Bernard S, Hamann D, Hansen R, Thyssen JP. Is there a risk using hypoallergenic cosmetic pediatric products in the United States? J Allergy Clin Immunol 2015;135:1070-1071

29 Frosch PJ, Pilz B, Andersen KE, Burrows D, Camarasa JG, Dooms-Goossens A, et al. Patch testing with fragrances: results of a multicenter study of the European Environmental and Contact Dermatitis Research Group with 48 frequently used constituents of perfumes. Contact Dermatitis 1995;33:333-342

30 Frosch PJ, Johansen JD, Menné T, Pirker C, Rastogi SC, Andersen KE, et al. Further important sensitizers in patients sensitive to fragrances. I. Reactivity to 14 frequently used chemicals. Contact Dermatitis 2002;47:78-85

31 Poulsen PB, Schmidt A. A survey and health assessment of cosmetic products for children. Survey of chemical substances in consumer products, No. 88. Copenhagen: Danish Environmental Protection Agency, 2007. Available at: https://www2.mst.dk/udgiv/publications/2007/978-87-7052-638-8/pdf/978-87-7052-639-5.pdf

32 VWA. Dutch Food and Consumer Product Safety Authority. Cosmetische producten voor kinderen: Inventarisatie van de markt en de veiligheidsborging door producenten en importeurs. Report ND04o065/ND05o170, 2007 (Report in Dutch), 2007. Available at: www.nvwa.nl/documenten/communicatie/inspectieresultaten/ consument/2016m/cosmetische- producten-voor-kinderen

33 Rastogi SC. Survey of chemical compounds in consumer products. Contents of selected fragrance materials in cleaning products and other consumer products. Survey no. 8-2002. Copenhagen, Denmark, Danish Environmental Protection Agency. Available at: http://eng.mst.dk/media/mst/69131/8.pdf

34 Bouma K, Van Peursem AJJ. Marktonderzoek naleving detergenten verordening voor textielwasmiddelen. Dutch Food and Consumer Products Safety Authority (VWA) Report ND06K173, 2006 [in Dutch]. Available at: http://docplayer.nl/41524125-Marktonderzoek-naleving-detergenten-verordening-voor- textielwasmiddelen.html

35 Pors J, Fuhlendorff R. Mapping of chemical substances in air fresheners and other fragrance liberating products. Report Danish Ministry of the Environment, Environmental Protection Agency (EPA). Survey of Chemicals in Consumer Products, No 30, 2003. Available at: http://eng.mst.dk/media/mst/69113/30.pdf

36 Goossens A. Cosmetic contact allergens. Cosmetics 2016, 3, 5; doi:10.3390/cosmetics3010005

37 Bennike NH, Zachariae C, Johansen JD. Non-mix fragrances are top sensitizers in consecutive dermatitis patients – a cross-sectional study of the 26 EU-labelled fragrance allergens. Contact Dermatitis 2017;77:270-279

38 Osinka K, Karczmarz A, Krauze K, Feleszko W. Contact allergens in cosmetics used in atopic dermatitis: analysis of product composition. Contact Dermatitis 2016;75:241-243

39 Thorén S, Yazar K. Contact allergens in 'natural' hair dyes. Contact Dermatitis 2016;74:302-304

40 Vejanurug P, Tresukosol P, Sajjachareonpong P, Puangpet P. Fragrance allergy could be missed without patch testing with 26 individual fragrance allergens. Contact Dermatitis 2016;74:230-235

41 Mann J, McFadden JP, White JML, White IR, Banerjee P. Baseline series fragrance markers fail to predict contact allergy. Contact Dermatitis 2014;70:276-281

42 Uter W, Johansen JD, Börje A, Karlberg A-T, Lidén C, Rastogi S, Roberts D, White IR. Categorization of fragrance contact allergens for prioritization of preventive measures: clinical and experimental data and consideration of structure–activity relationships. Contact Dermatitis 2013;69:196-230

43 Mowitz M, Svedman C, Zimerson E, Isaksson M, Pontén A, Bruze M. Simultaneous patch testing with fragrance mix I, fragrance mix II and their ingredients in southern Sweden between 2009 and 2015. Contact Dermatitis 2017;77:280-287

44 Nagtegaal MJC, Pentinga SE, Kuik J, Kezic S, Rustemeyer T. The role of the skin irritation response in polysensitization to fragrances. Contact Dermatitis 2012;67:28-35

45 Nardelli A, Drieghe J, Claes L, Boey L, Goossens A. Fragrance allergens in 'specific' cosmetic products. Contact Dermatitis 2011;64:212-219

46 Hamann D, Kishi P, Hamann CR. Consumer hair dye kits frequently contain isothiazolinones, other common preservatives and fragrance allergens. Dermatitis 2018;29:48-49

47 Diepgen TL, Ofenloch R, Bruze M, Cazzaniga S, Coenraads PJ, Elsner P, et al. Prevalence of fragrance contact allergy in the general population of five European countries: a cross-sectional study. Br J Dermatol 2015;173:1411-1419

48 Klaschka U. Contact allergens for armpits - allergenic fragrances specified on deodorants. Int J Hyg Environ Health 2012;215:584-591

49 De Groot AC, Schmidt E. Essential oils: contact allergy and chemical composition. Boca Raton, Fl., USA: CRC Press, Taylor and Francis Group, 2016 (ISBN 9781482246407)

50 Keil H. Contact dermatitis due to oil of citronellal. J Invest Dermatol 1947;8:327-334

51 Rudbäck J, Hagvall L, Börje A, Nilsson U, Karlberg A-T. Characterization of skin sensitizers from autoxidized citronellol – impact of the terpene structure on the autoxidation process. Contact Dermatitis 2014;70:329-339

52 Wieck S, Olsson O, Kümmerer K, Klaschka U. Fragrance allergens in household detergents. Regul Toxicol Pharmacol 2018;97:163-169

53 Tanko Z, Shab A, Diepgen TL, Weisshaar E. Polyvalent type IV sensitizations to multiple fragrances and a skin protection cream in a metal worker. J Dtsch Dermatol Ges 2009;7:541-543

54 Geier J, Uter W, Lessmann H, Schnuch A. Fragrance mix I and II: results of breakdown tests. Flavour Fragr J 2015;30:264-274

55 Dittmar D, Schuttelaar MLA. Contact sensitization to hydroperoxides of limonene and linalool: Results of consecutive patch testing and clinical relevance. Contact Dermatitis 2018 Oct 31. doi: 10.1111/cod.13137. [Epub ahead of print]

56 Silvestre JF, Mercader P, González-Pérez R, Hervella-Garcés M, Sanz-Sánchez T, Córdoba S, et al. Sensitization to fragrances in Spain: A 5-year multicentre study (2011-2015). Contact Dermatitis. 2018 Nov 14. doi: 10.1111/cod.13152. [Epub ahead of print]

57 Ung CY, White JML, White IR, Banerjee P, McFadden JP. Patch testing with the European baseline series fragrance markers: a 2016 update. Br J Dermatol 2018;178:776-780

Chapter 3.43　COUMARIN

IDENTIFICATION

Description/definition	: Coumarin is the aromatic lactone that conforms to the structural formula shown below
Chemical class(es)	: Heterocyclic compounds
Chemical/IUPAC name	: Chromen-2-one
Other names	: 2H-1-Benzopyran-2-one
CAS registry number(s)	: 91-64-5
EC number(s)	: 202-086-7
RIFM monograph(s)	: Food Cosmet Toxicol 1974;12:385
IFRA standard	: Restricted (www.ifraorg.org/en-us/standards-library) (table 3.43.1)
SCCS opinion(s)	: SCCP/0935/05 (9); SCCS/1459/11 (10)
Merck Index monograph	: 3820
Function(s) in cosmetics	: EU: perfuming. USA: fragrance ingredients
EU cosmetic restrictions	: Regulated in Annex III/77 of the Regulation (EC) No. 1223/2009, regulated by 2003/15/EC; Must be labeled on cosmetics and detergent products, if present at > 10 ppm (0.001%) in leave-on products and > 100 ppm (0.01%) in rinse-off products
Patch testing	: 5% pet. (SmartPracticeEurope, Chemotechnique, SmartPracticeCanada); also present in the fragrance mix II
Molecular formula	: $C_9H_6O_2$

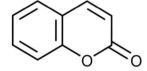

Table 3.43.1 IFRA restrictions for coumarin

Category [a]	Limits [b]	Category [a]	Limits [b]	Category [a]	Limits [b]
1	0.10%	5	0.80%	9	5.00%
2	0.13%	6	2.50%	10	2.50%
3	0.50%	7	0.30%	11	not restricted
4	1.60%	8	2.00%		

[a] For explanation of categories see pages 6-8
[b] Limits in the finished products

GENERAL

Coumarin appears as white crystals; its odor type is tonka and its odor at 10% in dipropylene glycol is described as 'sweet hay tonka new mown hay' (www.thegoodscentscompany.com). Coumarin occurs naturally in fruits, roots, bark, stalks, leaves and branches of a wide variety of plants including Tonka bean, cassie, lavender, lovage, yellow sweet clover, deertongue and woodruff. It is used as a flavoring agent in food, as a fixative and enhancer for the odor of essential oils in perfumes, as a fragrance in toilet soaps, toothpastes and in hair preparations, in tobacco products to enhance and fix the natural taste, flavor and aroma, and in industrial products to mask disagreeable odors (U.S. National Library of Medicine).

Presence in essential oils

Coumarin has been identified by chemical analysis in 14 of 91 essential oils, which have caused contact allergy / allergic contact dermatitis. In one oil, coumarin belonged to the 'Top-10' of ingredients with the highest concentrations which may be expected in commercial essential oils of this type: cassia oil (0.6-2.6%) (34).

CONTACT ALLERGY

General

The SCCS (Scientific Committee on Consumer Safety), in a 2012 Opinion on Fragrance allergens in cosmetic products, has marked coumarin as 'established contact allergen in humans' (10,46). The sensitizing potency of coumarin could not be classified, because no EC3 value was established in the LLNA (local lymph node assay) in animal experiments; higher concentrations should also have been tested (10,46). In other experiments, coumarin was shown to have very weak sensitizing potency, if at all (59,60,61). It has been suggested that positive reactions to coumarin may be due to sensitizing contaminants in commercial (non-pure) coumarin samples, notably dihydrocoumarin, 6-chlorocoumarin and dibenzodioxocin, which were all found to be sensitizers in the murine local lymph node assay (LLNA) (59). However, as the concentration of these impurities are very low, the authors suggested that other coumarin-derivatives may exert synergistic effects with these contaminants to induce sensitization (59).

Coumarin is a constituent of the fragrance mix II. In groups of patients reacting to the mix and tested with its 6 ingredients, coumarin scored 0-8.1% positive patch test reactions (see Chapter 3.71 Fragrance mix II).

General population

In the period 2008-2011, in 5 European countries (Sweden, Germany, Netherlands, Portugal, Italy), a random sample of the general population of 3119 individuals aged 18-74 years were patch tested with the FM I, its 8 ingredients, the FM II, its 6 ingredients and Myroxylon pereirae resin. There were 3 reactions (0.1%) to coumarin, tested 5% in petrolatum. About half of all positive reactions to fragrances were considered to be relevant based on standardized criteria. Women were affected twice as often as men (54).

Patch testing in groups of patients

Results of studies testing coumarin in consecutive patients suspected of contact dermatitis (routine testing) are shown in table 3.43.2. Results of testing in groups of *selected* patients (e.g. patients with known or suspected fragrance or cosmetic dermatitis, individuals with hand eczema) are shown in table 3.43.3.

Patch testing in consecutive patients suspected of contact dermatitis: routine testing

In eleven studies in which routine testing with coumarin was performed, frequencies of sensitization were invariably very low, ranging from 0.05% to 0.7% (table 3.43.2). In 8/11 investigations, no (specific) data on relevance were provided; in the 3 addressing the issue, 67-100% of the positive reactions were scored as relevant, but the numbers of allergic patients were (very) low. Causative products were usually not mentioned or specified, but in one study, of the relevant reactions to any of 26 fragrances tested, 96% were caused by cosmetic products (1).

Table 3.43.2 Patch testing in groups of patients: Routine testing

Years and Country	Test conc. & vehicle	Number of patients tested	positive (%)	Selection of patients (S); Relevance (R); Comments (C)	Ref.
2015-7 Netherlands		821	4 (0.5%)	R: not stated	63
2015-2016 UK	5% pet.	2084	1 (0.05%)	R: not specified for individual fragrances; 25% of patients who reacted to any fragrance or fragrance marker had a positive fragrance history	62
2010-2015 Denmark	5% pet.	6004	8 (0.14%)	R: present relevance 75%, past relevance 63%; C: 192 of the 6004 patients were not tested, of who 2 because of known sensitivity to coumarin	42
2009-2015 Sweden	5% pet.	4175	6 (0.14%)	R: not stated	47
2013-2014 Thailand		312	1 (0.3%)	R: 100%	44
2011-2012 UK	5% pet.	1951	8 (0.4%)	R: not stated	45
2008-2010 Denmark	5% pet.	1503	3 (0.2%)	S: mostly routine testing; R: 67%; no co-reactions to either FM I or FM II; C: of the relevant reactions to any of the 26 fragrances tested, 96% were caused by cosmetic products	1
2003-2004 IVDK	5% pet.	2020	8 (0.4%)	R: not stated	3
1998-9 Netherlands	5% pet.	1825	13 (0.7%)	R: not stated	12
1997-8 six European countries	5% pet.	1855	5 (0.3%)	R: not stated / specified	28
1978-97 Netherlands	5% pet.	14,000	58 (0.4%)	R: not specified, but coumarin was considered to be an indicator of fragrance sensitivity	57

FM: Fragrance mix; IVDK: Informationsverbund Dermatologischer Kliniken (Germany, Switzerland, Austria)

Patch testing in groups of selected patients

Results of studies patch testing coumarin in groups of selected patients (e.g. patients with known or suspected fragrance or cosmetic dermatitis, individuals with hand eczema) are shown in table 3.43.3. In eleven investigations, frequencies of sensitization to coumarin have ranged from 0.5% to 10%. Rates of >5% positive reactions were observed in three studies, two in patients with known fragrance allergy (7,13) and the third in patients suspected to be allergic to cosmetics (11). In most studies, no (specific) relevance data were provided. Some authors considered relevance for all reactions 'possible' (7), others assumed that nearly all positive reactions were of present or past relevance (5). Causative products were not mentioned.

Results of testing coumarin in groups of patients reacting to the fragrance mix II are shown in Chapter 3.71 Fragrance mix II.

Table 3.43.3 Patch testing in groups of patients: Selected patient groups

Years and Country	Test conc. & vehicle	Number of patients tested | positive (%)		Selection of patients (S); Relevance (R); Comments (C)	Ref.
2011-2015 Spain	5% pet.	1013	23 (2.3%)	S: patients previously reacting to FM I, FM II, Myroxylon pereirae resin or hydroxyisohexyl 3-cyclohexene carboxaldehyde in the baseline series; R: not stated	64
2009-2010 Hungary	5% pet.	565	29 (5.1%)	S: patients with former skin symptoms provoked by scented products in the case history; R: in all cases 'possible'	7
2005-10 Netherlands		100	2 (2%)	S: patients with known fragrance sensitivity based on a positive patch test to the FM I and/or the FM II; R: not stated	48
2004-2008 Spain	5% pet.	86	1 (1.2%)	S: patients previously reacting to the fragrance mix I or Myroxylon pereirae (n=54) or suspected of fragrance contact allergy (n=32); R: not stated	29
2005-7 Netherlands	5% pet.	320	2 (0.6%)	S: patients suspected of fragrance or cosmetic allergy; R: 61% relevance for all positive tested fragrances together	2
2005 France	2% pet.	510	1 (0.5%)	S: 379 consecutive dermatitis patients, 101 patients with allergic contact dermatitis and a positive reaction to the FM I and 30 patients with positive reactions to their own perfumes; R: possibly relevant for axillary deodorant contact dermatitis; C: 100 patients were also tested with 10% pet. without irritant reactions; the test concentration may be too low to detect (all) cases of sensitization	59
2001-2 Denmark, Sweden	5% pet.	658	3 (0.5%)	S: consecutive patients with hand eczema; R: it was assumed that nearly all positive reactions were of present or past relevance	5
<1996 Japan, Europe, USA	5% pet.	167	2 (1.2%)	S: patients known or suspected to be allergic to fragrances; R: not stated	6
<1985 Netherlands		242	9 (3.7%)	S: randomly selected patients with proven contact allergy of different origins; R: not stated	52
1983 The Netherlands	6% pet.	182	12 (6.8%)	S: patients suspected of cosmetic allergy; R: not stated	11
1975 USA	5% pet.	20	2 (10%)	S: fragrance-allergic patients; R: not stated	13

Testing in groups of patients reacting to the fragrance mix II
Results of testing coumarin in groups of patients reacting to the fragrance mix II are shown in Chapter 3.71 Fragrance mix II

FM: Fragrance mix

Case reports and case series
Coumarin was stated to be the (or an) allergen in 3 patients in a group of 603 individuals suffering from cosmetic dermatitis, seen in the period 2010-2015 in Leuven, Belgium (41). In the period 2000-2009, in Leuven, Belgium, an unspecified number of patients had positive patch tests or use tests to a total of 344 cosmetic products *and* positive patch tests to FM I, FM II, and/or to one or more of 28 selected specific fragrance ingredients. In 2 patients reacting to coumarin, the presence of this fragrance in the cosmetic product(s) was confirmed by reading the product label(s) (49).

Coumarin was responsible for 4 out of 399 cases of cosmetic allergy where the causal allergen was identified in a study of the NACDG, USA, 1977-1983 (4). In a group of 119 patients with allergic contact dermatitis from cosmetics, investigated in The Netherlands in 1986-1987, one case was caused by coumarin in a perfume (25,26).

A woman developed an axillary rash using a perfumed deodorant. At the same time, she started to use an eau de toilette of the same brand and developed a rash on the neck and the trunk. She was patch tested with the European standard series, including the fragrance mix I 8%, and series of cosmetic allergens, but showed negative results. The patient was then further patch tested with the deodorant, the eau de toilette, and the individual ingredients of both. She reacted only to the products and the perfume concentrate. A repeated open application test (ROAT), done in the antecubital fossa, was positive for both fragranced products. By chemical fractionation of the perfume concentrates with flash column chromatography, ROATs and patch tests, the culprit ingredient was found to be coumarin. This fragrance was present in both products, in the deodorant at a concentration of 0.23% (37).

A man had allergic contact dermatitis from coumarin and vanillin in a topical pharmaceutical preparation used on a traumatic leg ulcer. The patient also reacted to a number of coumarin-derived anticoagulant tablets (powdered and moistened), but there were no reactions to these drugs when tested 10% in petrolatum (55). Another patient had allergic contact dermatitis around leg ulcers. She reacted to Myroxylon pereirae resin (balsam of Peru), cod liver oil (both of which had been used for treatment of leg ulcers) and coumarin, which is present in cod liver oil (35).

Cross-reactions, pseudo-cross-reactions and co-reactions

For general information on cross-/pseudo-cross-/co-reactivity of fragrance chemicals with other fragrances, fragrance markers (fragrance mix I, fragrance mix II, colophonium, Myroxylon pereirae resin [balsam of Peru]) and essential oils see Chapter 1.2 General information on cross-reactions, pseudo-cross-reactions and co-reactions. Co-reactivity with the fragrance mix II can be expected, as the mix contains coumarin (pseudo-cross-reactions).

No cross-sensitivity between coumarin and dihydrocoumarin (60). Possible but unlikely cross-sensitivity to coumarin-derived anticoagulant tablets (55).

Presence in products and chemical analyses

In various studies, the presence of coumarin in cosmetic and sometimes other products has been investigated. Before 2006, most investigators used chemical analysis, usually GC-MS, for qualitative and quantitative determination. Since then, the presence of the target fragrances was usually investigated by screening the product labels for the 26 fragrances that must be labeled since 2005 on cosmetics and detergent products in the EU, if present at > 10 ppm (0.001%) in leave-on products and > 100 ppm (0.01%) in rinse-off products. This method, obviously, is less accurate and may result in underestimation of the frequency of the fragrances being present in the product. When they are in fact present, but the concentration is lower than mentioned above, labeling is not required and the fragrances' presence will be missed.

The results of the relevant studies for coumarin are summarized in table 3.43.4. More detailed information can be found in the corresponding text before and following the table. The percentage of products in which coumarin was found to be present shows wide variations, which can among other be explained by the selection procedure of the products, the method of investigation (false-negatives with information obtained from labels only) and changes in the use of individual fragrance materials over time (fashion).

In 2017, in the USA, the ingredient labels 159 hair-dye kits containing 539 cosmetic products (e.g. colorants, conditioners, shampoos, toners) were screened for the most common sensitizers they contain. Coumarin was found to be present in 20 (2%) of the products (53).

In Denmark, in 2015-2016, 5588 fragranced cosmetic products were examined with a smartphone application for the 26 fragrances that need to be labeled in the EU. Coumarin was present in 13% of the products (rank number 11) (23).

In Germany, in 2015, fragrance allergens were evaluated based on lists of ingredients in 817 (unique) detergents (all-purpose cleaners, cleaning preparations for special purposes [e.g. bathroom, kitchen, dish-washing] and laundry detergents) present in 131 households. Coumarin was found to be present in 25 (3%) of the products (33).

Of 179 emollients available in online drugstores in 2014 in Poland, three (1.6%) contained coumarin, according to information available online (43).

In 2013, in the USA, the allergen content of 187 unique pediatric cosmetics from 6 different retailers marketed in the United States as hypoallergenic was evaluated on the basis of labeling. Inclusion criteria were products marketed as pediatric and 'hypoallergenic', 'dermatologist recommended/tested', 'fragrance free', or 'paraben free'. Coumarin was found to be present in 3 (1.6%) of the products (27).

In 2008, 2010 and 2011, 374 deodorants available in German retail shops were randomly selected and their labels checked for the presence of the 26 fragrances that need to be labeled. Coumarin was found to be present in 106 (28.5%) of the products (56).

In Germany, in the period 2006-2009, 4991 cosmetic products were randomly sampled for an official investigation of conformity of cosmetic products with legal provisions. The labels were inspected for the presence of the 26 fragrances that need to be labeled in the EU. Coumarin was present in 10% of the products (rank number 10) (22).

Coumarin was present (as indicated by labeling) in 6% of 204 cosmetic products (92 shampoos, 61 hair conditioners, 34 liquid soaps, 17 wet tissues) and in 1% of 97 detergents in Sweden, 2008 (14).

In 2007, in The Netherlands, twenty-three cosmetic products for children were analyzed for the presence of fragrances that need to be labeled. Coumarin was identified in 6 of the products (26%) in a concentration range of 77-384 ppm (31).

In 2006, of 88 popular perfume containing deodorants purchased in Denmark, 29 (33%) were labeled to contain coumarin. Analysis of 24 regulated fragrance substances in 23 selected deodorants (19 spray products, 2 deostick and 2 roll-on) was performed by GC-MS. Coumarin was identified in 12 of the products (52%) with a concentration range of 4–1255 ppm (24).

In January 2006, a study of perfumed cosmetic and household products available on the shelves of U.K. retailers was carried out. Products were included if 'parfum' or 'aroma' was listed among the ingredients. Three hundred products were surveyed and any of 26 mandatory labeling fragrances named on the label were recorded. Coumarin was present in 90 (30%) of the products (rank number 9) (20).

Table 3.43.4 Presence of coumarin in products [a]

Year	Country	Product type	Nr. investigated	Nr. of products positive [b]	(%)	Method [c]	Ref.
2017	USA	Cosmetic products in hair-dye kits	539 products in 159 hair-dye kits	20	(2%)	Labeling	53
2015-6	Denmark	Fragranced cosmetic products	5588		(13%)	Labeling	23
2015	Germany	Household detergents	817	25	(31%)	Labeling	33
2014	Poland	Emollients	179	3	(2%)	Online info	43
2013	USA	Pediatric cosmetics	187	3	(2%)	Labeling	27
2008-11	Germany	Deodorants	374	106	(28%)	Labeling	56
2006-9	Germany	Cosmetic products	4991		(10%)	Labeling	22
2008	Sweden	Cosmetic products	204	12	(6%)	Labeling	14
		Detergents	97	1	(1%)	Labeling	
2007	Netherlands	Cosmetic products for children	23	6	(26%)	Analysis	31
2006	UK	Perfumed cosmetic and house-hold products	300	90	(30%)	Labeling	20
2006	Denmark	Popular perfumed deodorants	88	29	(33%)	Labeling	24
			23	12	(52%)	Analysis	
2006	Netherlands	Laundry detergents	52	14	(27%)	Labeling + analysis	38
2006	Denmark	Rinse-off cosmetics for children	208	10	(5%)	Labeling + analysis	30
2004	Denmark, UK, Belgium, Germany	Fragranced products that had caused allergic contact dermatitis, used by patients	24	12	(50%)	Labeling	8
2002	Denmark	Home and car air fresheners	19	9	(47%)	Analysis	39
2001	Denmark	Non-cosmetic consumer products	43	13	(30%)	Analysis	32
2000	Denmark, UK, Germany, Italy	Domestic and occupational products	59	15	(25%)	Analysis	16
1997-8	Denmark, UK Germany, Sweden	Cosmetics and cosmetic toys for children	25	11	(44%)	Analysis	18
1996	Five European countries	Fragranced deodorants	70	40	(57%)	Analysis	15
1995	Denmark	Cosmetic products based on natural ingredients	42	13	(31%)	Analysis	17
1995	Netherlands	Cosmetic products	112		(80%)	Analysis	58
1994	Denmark	Cosmetics that had given a positive patch or use test in FM I allergic patients	23	15	(65%)	Analysis	50
1992	Netherlands	Cosmetic products	300		(44%)	Analysis	21
1988	USA	Perfumes used in fine fragrances, household products and soap	400	?-68% (See text)		Analysis	19

[a] See the corresponding text below for more details
[b] positive = containing the target fragrance
[c] Labeling: information from the ingredient labels on the product / packaging; Analysis: chemical analysis, most often GC-MS

In 2006, the labels of 208 cosmetics for children (especially shampoos, body shampoos and soaps) available in Denmark were checked for the presence of the 26 fragrances that need to be labeled in the EU. Coumarin was present in 10 products (4.8%), and ranked number 17 in the frequency list (30).

In 2006, in The Netherlands, 52 laundry detergents were investigated for the presence of allergenic fragrances by checking their labels and chemical analyses. Coumarin was found to be present in 14 of the products (27%) in a concentration range of 9-90 ppm. Coumarin had rank number 8 in the frequency list (38).

In 2004, in 4 European countries (Denmark, Germany, Belgium, U.K.), of 12 patients allergic to the FM II and one or more of its constituents (hexyl cinnamal 1, citral 3, hydroxyisohexyl 3-cyclohexene carboxaldehyde 11), 24 of the products used by them (deodorant 4, eau de toilette 9, lotion/cream 4, fine perfume 7) that had caused adverse reactions compatible with allergic contact dermatitis, were analyzed for the presence of the six constituents of the fragrance mix II (citral, citronellol, coumarin, farnesol, hexyl cinnamal, hydroxyisohexyl 3-cyclohexene carboxaldehyde). Coumarin was found in 12/24 (50%) products, in concentrations of 0.002-0.140% (8).

In 2002, in Denmark, 19 air fresheners (6 for cars, 13 for homes) were analyzed for the presence of fragrances that need to be labeled on cosmetics. Coumarin was found to be present in 9 products (47%) in a concentration range of 15-13,000 ppm and ranked 11 in the frequency list (39).

In 2001, in Denmark, 43 non-cosmetic consumer products (mainly dish-washing products, laundry detergents, and hard and soft surface cleaners) were analyzed for the 26 fragrances that are regulated for labeling in the EU. Coumarin was present in 13 products (30%) in a concentration range of 0.0027-0.0270% (m/m) and had rank number 7 in the frequency list (32).

In 2000, fifty-nine domestic and occupational products, purchased in retail outlets in Denmark, England, Germany and Italy were analyzed by GC-MS for the presence of fragrances. The product categories were liquid soap and soap bars (n=13), soft/hard surface cleaners (n=23), fabric conditioners/laundry detergents for hand wash (n=8), dish- wash (n=10), furniture polish, car shampoo, stain remover (each n=1) and 2 products used in occupational environments. Coumarin was present in 15 products (25%) with a mean concentration of 149 ppm and a range of 45-309 ppm (16).

Twenty-five cosmetics and cosmetic toys for children (5 shampoos and shower gels, 6 perfumes, 1 deodorant (roll-on), 4 baby lotions/creams, 1 baby wipes product, 1 baby oil, 2 lipcare products and 5 toy-cosmetic products: a cosmetic-toy set for blending perfumes and a makeup set) purchased in 1997-1998 in retail outlets in Denmark, Germany, England and Sweden were analyzed in 1998 for the presence of fragrances by GC-MS. Coumarin was found in 11 products (44%) in a concentration range of ≤0.001-0.018% (w/w). For the analytical data in each product category, the original publication should be consulted (18).

Seventy fragranced deodorants, purchased at retail outlets in 5 European countries in 1996, were analyzed by gas chromatography - mass spectrometry (GC-MS) for the determination of the contents of 21 commonly used fragrance materials. Coumarin was identified in 40 products (57%) in a concentration range of 1–1411 ppm (15).

In 1995, in Denmark, 42 cosmetic products based on natural ingredients from 12 European and US companies (of which 22 were perfumes and 20 various other cosmetics) were investigated by high-resolution gas chromatography-mass spectrometry (GC-MS) for the presence of 11 fragrances. Coumarin was present in 11 (50%) of the 22 perfumes in a concentration range of 0.046-6.043 w/w% ; it was also identified in 2 of the other cosmetics in concentrations of 0.013% (lotion) and 0.0003% (roll-on deo) (17).

In 1995, in a study in The Netherlands, coumarin was found in 80% of the 112 cosmetic products examined, with levels varying from 6-9500 mg/kg; the highest levels were identified in perfumes and aftershaves (58).

In Denmark, in 1994, 23 cosmetic products, which had either given a positive patch and/or use test in a total of 11 fragrance-mix-positive patients, and which products completely or partly explained present or past episodes of dermatitis, were analyzed for the presence of the constituents of the FM I (with the exception of oakmoss absolute) and a few other fragrances. Coumarin was found to be present in 15 of the 23 products (65%) in a concentration range of <0.001-0.2% v/v with a mean concentration of 0.083% v/v. It was also present in one other product, but could not be quantified due to interference (50).

In 1992, in The Netherlands, the presence of fragrances was analyzed in 300 cosmetic products. Coumarin was identified in 44% of the products (rank order 15) (21).

In 1988, in the USA, 400 perfumes used in fine fragrances, household products and soaps (number of products per category not mentioned) were analyzed for the presence of fragrance chemicals in a concentration of at least 1% and a list of the Top-25 (present in the highest number of products) presented. Coumarin was found to be present in 68% of the fine fragrances (rank number 6), an unknown percentage of the household product fragrances and 66% of the fragrances used in soaps (rank number 7) (19).

OTHER SIDE EFFECTS

Photosensitivity

In a group of 50 patients suffering from photosensitivity dermatitis with actinic reticuloid syndrome (PD/AR) patch tested with a battery of fragrances, there were 3 reactions (6%) to coumarin versus 0.2% positive patch tests in a group of 457 routinely tested dermatitis patients (40).

Of four subjects photosensitized to 6-methylcoumarin, two photocross-reacted to coumarin (36).

Immediate-type reactions

Of 565 patients with a history of former skin symptoms provoked by scented products and patch tested with coumarin 5% pet., 8 (1.4%) had a contact urticarial reaction (7). Of 50 individuals who had open tests with coumarin 5% pet. on the forearm, 24 (48%) showed local macular erythema after 45 minutes, termed 'contact urticaria' by the authors (51).

LITERATURE

1   Heisterberg MV, Menné T, Johansen JD. Contact allergy to the 26 specific fragrance ingredients to be declared on cosmetic products in accordance with the EU cosmetic directive. Contact Dermatitis 2011;65:266-275

2   Oosten EJ van, Schuttelaar ML, Coenraads PJ. Clinical relevance of positive patch test reactions to the 26 EU-labelled fragrances. Contact Dermatitis 2009;61:217-223

3   Schnuch A, Uter W, Geier J, Lessmann H, Frosch PJ. Sensitization to 26 fragrances to be labelled according to current European regulation: Results of the IVDK and review of the literature. Contact Dermatitis 2007;57:1-10

4   Adams RM, Maibach HI, for the North American Contact Dermatitis Group. A five-year study of cosmetic reactions. J Am Acad Dermatol 1985;13:1062-1069

5   Heydorn S, Johansen JD, Andersen KE, Bruze M, Svedman C, White IR, et al. Fragrance allergy in patients with hand eczema – a clinical study. Contact Dermatitis 2003;48:317-323

6   Larsen W, Nakayama H, Fischer T, Elsner P, Burrows D, Jordan W, et al. Fragrance contact dermatitis: A worldwide multicenter investigation (Part I). Am J Cont Dermat 1996;7:77-83

7   Pónyai G, Németh I, Altmeyer A, Nagy G, Irinyi B, Battya Z, et al. Patch tests with fragrance mix II and its components. Dermatitis 2012;23:71-74

8   Frosch PJ, Rastogi SC, Pirker C, Brinkmeier T, Andersen KE, Bruze M, et al. Patch testing with a new fragrance mix - reactivity to the individual constituents and chemical detection in relevant cosmetic products. Contact Dermatitis 2005;52:216-225

9   SCCP (Scientific Committee on Consumer Products). Opinion on Coumarin (sensitisation only), 20 June 2006, SCCP/0935/05. Available at:
    http://ec.europa.eu/health/archive/ph_risk/committees/04_sccp/docs/sccp_o_061.pdf

10 SCCS (Scientific Committee on Consumer Safety). Opinion on Fragrance allergens in cosmetic products, 26-27 June 2012, SCCS/1459/11. Available at:
    https://ec.europa.eu/health/sites/health/files/scientific_committees/consumer_safety/docs/sccs_o_102.pdf

11 Malten KE, van Ketel WG, Nater JP, Liem DH. Reactions in selected patients to 22 fragrance materials. Contact Dermatitis 1984;11:1-10

12 De Groot AC, Coenraads PJ, Bruynzeel DP, Jagtman BA, Van Ginkel CJW, Noz K, et al. Routine patch testing with fragrance chemicals in The Netherlands. Contact Dermatitis 2000;42:184-185

13 Larsen WG. Perfume dermatitis. A study of 20 patients. Arch Dermatol 1977;113:623-626

14 Yazar K, Johnsson S, Lind M-L, Boman A, Lidén C. Preservatives and fragrances in selected consumer-available cosmetics and detergents. Contact Dermatitis 2011;64:265-272

15 Rastogi SC, Johansen JD, Frosch P, Menné T, Bruze M, Lepoittevin JP, et al. Deodorants on the European market: quantitative chemical analysis of 21 fragrances. Contact Dermatitis 1998;38:29-35

16 Rastogi SC, Heydorn S, Johansen JD, Basketter DA. Fragrance chemicals in domestic and occupational products. Contact Dermatitis 2001;45:221-225

17 Rastogi SC, Johansen JD, Menné T. Natural ingredients based cosmetics. Content of selected fragrance sensitizers. Contact Dermatitis 1996;34:423-426

18 Rastogi SC, Johansen JD, Menné T, Frosch P, Bruze M, Andersen KE, et al. Content of fragrance allergens in children's cosmetics and cosmetic toys. Contact Dermatitis 1999;41:84-88

19 Fenn RS. Aroma chemical usage trends in modern perfumery. Perfumer and Flavorist 1989;14:3-10

20 Buckley DA. Fragrance ingredient labelling in products on sale in the UK. Br J Dermatol 2007;157:295-300

21 Weyland JW. Personal Communication, 1992. Cited in: De Groot AC, Weyland JW, Nater JP. Unwanted effects of cosmetics and drugs used in dermatology, 3rd Ed. Amsterdam: Elsevier, 1994: 579

22 Uter W, Yazar K, Kratz E-M, Mildau G, Lidén C. Coupled exposure to ingredients of cosmetic products: I. Fragrances. Contact Dermatitis 2013;69:335-341

23 Bennike NH, Oturai NB, Müller S, Kirkeby CS, Jørgensen C, Christensen AB, et al. Fragrance contact allergens in 5588 cosmetic products identified through a novel smartphone application. J Eur Acad Dermatol Venereol 2018;32:79-85

24 Rastogi SC, Hellerup Jensen G, Johansen JD. Survey and risk assessment of chemical substances in deodorants. Survey of Chemical Substances in Consumer Products, No. 86 2007. Danish Ministry of the Environment, Environmental Protection Agency. Available at: https://www2.mst.dk/Udgiv/publications/2007/978-87-7052-625-8/pdf/978-87-7052-626-5.pdf

25   De Groot AC, Bruynzeel DP, Bos JD, van der Meeren HL, van Joost T, Jagtman BA, Weyland JW. The allergens in cosmetics. Arch Dermatol 1988;124:1525-1529

26   De Groot AC. Adverse reactions to cosmetics. PhD Thesis, University of Groningen, The Netherlands: 1988, chapter 3.4, pp.105-113

27   Hamann CR, Bernard S, Hamann D, Hansen R, Thyssen JP. Is there a risk using hypoallergenic cosmetic pediatric products in the United States? J Allergy Clin Immunol 2015;135:1070-1071

28   Frosch PJ, Johansen JD, Menné T, Pirker C, Rastogi SC, Andersen KE, et al. Further important sensitizers in patients sensitive to fragrances. I. Reactivity to 14 frequently used chemicals. Contact Dermatitis 2002;47:78-85

29   Cuesta L, Silvestre JF, Toledo F, Lucas A, Perez-Crespo M, Ballester I. Fragrance contact allergy: a 4-year retrospective study. Contact Dermatitis 2010;63:77-84

30   Poulsen PB, Schmidt A. A survey and health assessment of cosmetic products for children. Survey of chemical substances in consumer products, No. 88. Copenhagen: Danish Environmental Protection Agency, 2007. Available at: https://www2.mst.dk/udgiv/publications/2007/978-87-7052-638-8/pdf/978-87-7052-639-5.pdf

31   VWA. Dutch Food and Consumer Product Safety Authority. Cosmetische producten voor kinderen: Inventarisatie van de markt en de veiligheidsborging door producenten en importeurs. Report ND04o065/ND05o170, 2007 (Report in Dutch), 2007. Available at: www.nvwa.nl/documenten/communicatie/inspectieresultaten/ consument/ 2016m/cosmetische- producten-voor-kinderen

32   Rastogi SC. Survey of chemical compounds in consumer products. Contents of selected fragrance materials in cleaning products and other consumer products. Survey no. 8-2002. Copenhagen, Denmark, Danish Environmental Protection Agency. Available at: http://eng.mst.dk/media/mst/69131/8.pdf

33   Wieck S, Olsson O, Kümmerer K, Klaschka U. Fragrance allergens in household detergents. Regul Toxicol Pharmacol 2018;97:163-169

34   De Groot AC, Schmidt E. Essential oils: contact allergy and chemical composition. Boca Raton, Fl., USA: CRC Press, Taylor and Francis Group, 2016 (ISBN 9781482246407)

35   Hjorth N. Eczematous allergy to balsams. Acta Derm Venereol 1961;41(suppl.46):1-216

36   Kaidbey KH, Kligman AM. Photosensitization by coumarin derivatives. Arch Dermatol 1981;117:258-263

37   Mutterer V, Giménez Arnau E, Lepoittevin J-P, Johansen JD, Frosch PJ, Menné T, et al. Identification of coumarin as the sensitizer in a patient sensitive to her own perfume but negative to the fragrance mix. Contact Dermatitis 1999;40:196-199

38   Bouma K, Van Peursem AJJ. Marktonderzoek naleving detergenten verordening voor textielwasmiddelen. Dutch Food and Consumer Products Safety Authority (VWA) Report ND06K173, 2006 [in Dutch]. Available at: http://docplayer.nl/41524125-Marktonderzoek-naleving-detergenten-verordening-voor-textielwasmiddelen.html

39   Pors J, Fuhlendorff R. Mapping of chemical substances in air fresheners and other fragrance liberating products. Report Danish Ministry of the Environment, Environmental Protection Agency (EPA). Survey of Chemicals in Consumer Products, No 30, 2003. Available at: http://eng.mst.dk/media/mst/69113/30.pdf

40   Addo HA, Ferguson J, Johnson BF, Frain-Bell W. The relationship between exposure to fragrance materials and persistent light reaction in photosensitivity dermatitis with actinic reticuloid syndrome. Br J Dermatol 1982;107:261-274

41   Goossens A. Cosmetic contact allergens. Cosmetics 2016, 3, 5; doi:10.3390/cosmetics3010005

42   Bennike NH, Zachariae C, Johansen JD. Non-mix fragrances are top sensitizers in consecutive dermatitis patients – a cross-sectional study of the 26 EU-labelled fragrance allergens. Contact Dermatitis 2017;77:270-279

43   Osinka K, Karczmarz A, Krauze K, Feleszko W. Contact allergens in cosmetics used in atopic dermatitis: analysis of product composition. Contact Dermatitis 2016;75:241-243

44   Vejanurug P, Tresukosol P, Sajjachareonpong P, Puangpet P. Fragrance allergy could be missed without patch testing with 26 individual fragrance allergens. Contact Dermatitis 2016;74:230-235

45   Mann J, McFadden JP, White JML, White IR, Banerjee P. Baseline series fragrance markers fail to predict contact allergy. Contact Dermatitis 2014;70:276-281

46   Uter W, Johansen JD, Börje A, Karlberg A-T, Lidén C, Rastogi S, Roberts D, White IR. Categorization of fragrance contact allergens for prioritization of preventive measures: clinical and experimental data and consideration of structure–activity relationships. Contact Dermatitis 2013;69:196-230

47   Mowitz M, Svedman C, Zimerson E, Isaksson M, Pontén A, Bruze M. Simultaneous patch testing with fragrance mix I, fragrance mix II and their ingredients in southern Sweden between 2009 and 2015. Contact Dermatitis 2017;77:280-287

48   Nagtegaal MJC, Pentinga SE, Kuik J, Kezic S, Rustemeyer T. The role of the skin irritation response in polysensitization to fragrances. Contact Dermatitis 2012;67:28-35

49   Nardelli A, Drieghe J, Claes L, Boey L, Goossens A. Fragrance allergens in 'specific' cosmetic products. Contact Dermatitis 2011;64:212-219

50 Johansen JD, Rastogi SC, Menné T. Exposure to selected fragrance materials: A case study of fragrance-mix-positive eczema patients. Contact Dermatitis 1996;34:106-110

51 Emmons WW, Marks JG Jr. Immediate and delayed reactions to cosmetic ingredients. Contact Dermatitis 1985;13:258-265

52 Van Joost Th, Stolz E, Van Der Hoek JCS. Simultaneous allergy to perfume ingredients. Contact Dermatitis 1985;12:115-116

53 Hamann D, Kishi P, Hamann CR. Consumer hair dye kits frequently contain isothiazolinones, other common preservatives and fragrance allergens. Dermatitis 2018;29:48-49

54 Diepgen TL, Ofenloch R, Bruze M, Cazzaniga S, Coenraads PJ, Elsner P, et al. Prevalence of fragrance contact allergy in the general population of five European countries: a cross-sectional study. Br J Dermatol 2015;173:1411-1419

55 Van Ketel WG. Allergy to cumarin and cumarin-derivatives. Contact Dermatitis Newsletter 1973;13:355

56 Klaschka U. Contact allergens for armpits - allergenic fragrances specified on deodorants. Int J Hyg Environ Health 2012;215:584-591

57 Kunkeler ACM, Weijland JW, Bruynzeel DP. The rôle of coumarin in patch testing. Contact Dermatitis 1998;39:327-328

58 Rooselaar J, Weijland JW. Coumarine en dihydrocoumarine in kosmetische producten - bepaling en markt survey. Cosmeticarapport 62. Enschede, The Netherlands: Inspectie Gezondheidsbescherming, Keuringsdienst van Waren, 1996

59 Vocanson M, Goujon C, Chabeau G, Castelain M, Valeyrie M, Floch F, et al. The skin allergenic properties of chemicals may depend on contaminants. Evidence from studies on coumarin. Int Arch Allergy Immunol 2006;140:231-238

60 Vocanson M, Valeyrie M, Rozières A, Hennino A, Floch F, Gard A, Nicolas J-F. Lack of evidence for allergenic properties of coumarin in a fragrance allergy mouse model. Contact Dermatitis 2007;57:361-364

61 Hausen BM, Schmieder M. The sensitizing capacity of coumarins (I). Contact Dermatitis 1986;15:157-163

62 Ung CY, White JML, White IR, Banerjee P, McFadden JP. Patch testing with the European baseline series fragrance markers: a 2016 update. Br J Dermatol 2018;178:776-780

63 Dittmar D, Schuttelaar MLA. Contact sensitization to hydroperoxides of limonene and linalool: Results of consecutive patch testing and clinical relevance. Contact Dermatitis 2018 Oct 31. doi: 10.1111/cod.13137. [Epub ahead of print]

64 Silvestre JF, Mercader P, González-Pérez R, Hervella-Garcés M, Sanz-Sánchez T, Córdoba S, et al. Sensitization to fragrances in Spain: A 5-year multicentre study (2011-2015). Contact Dermatitis. 2018 Nov 14. doi: 10.1111/cod.13152. [Epub ahead of print]

Chapter 3.44   CUMINALDEHYDE

IDENTIFICATION

Description/definition   : Cuminaldehyde is the aldehyde that conforms to the structural formula shown below
Chemical class(es)   : Aromatic compounds; aldehydes
INCI name USA   : Not in the Personal Care Products Council Ingredient Database
Chemical/IUPAC name   : 4-Propan-2-ylbenzaldehyde
Other names   : 4-Isopropylbenzaldehyde
CAS registry number(s)   : 122-03-2
EC number(s)   : 204-516-9
RIFM monograph(s)   : Food Cosmet Toxicol 1974;12:395
IFRA standard   : Restricted (www.ifraorg.org/en-us/standards-library) (table 3.44.1)
SCCS opinion(s)   : SCCS/1459/11 (1)
Merck Index monograph   : 3881
Function(s) in cosmetics : EU: perfuming
Patch testing   : 5-15% pet. (5); based on RIFM data, 4% is probably not irritant (5)
Molecular formula   : $C_{10}H_{12}O$

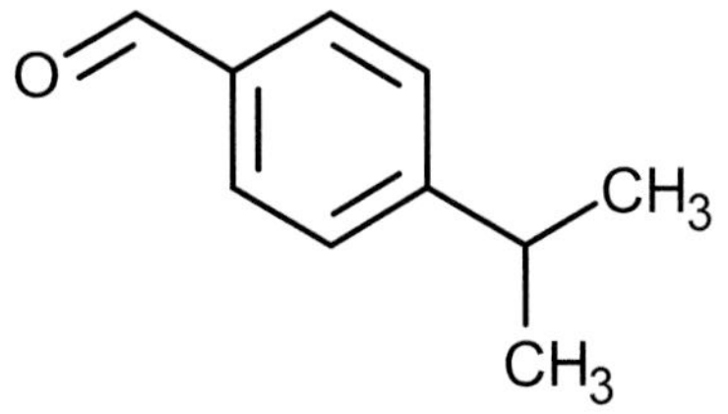

Table 3.44.1 IFRA restrictions for cuminaldehyde

Category [a]	Limits [b]	Category [a]	Limits [b]	Category [a]	Limits [b]
1	0.03%	5	0.26%	9	5.00%
2	0.04%	6	0.80%	10	2.50%
3	0.17%	7	0.08%	11	not restricted
4	0.50%	8	1.11%		

[a] For explanation of categories see pages 6-8
[b] Limits in the finished products

GENERAL

Cuminaldehyde is a colorless to pale yellow clear liquid; its odor type is spicy and its odor is described as 'spicy, green, cumin-like with green herbal spice nuances' (www.thegoodscentscompany.com).

Presence in essential oils

Cuminaldehyde has been identified by chemical analysis in 39 of 91 essential oils, which have caused contact allergy / allergic contact dermatitis. In none of these oils, it belonged to the 'Top-10' of ingredients with the highest concentrations (4).

CONTACT ALLERGY

The SCCS (Scientific Committee on Consumer Safety), in a 2012 Opinion on Fragrance allergens in cosmetic products, has categorized cuminaldehyde as 'likely fragrance contact allergen by combination of evidence' (1,3).

Patch testing in groups of patients

Patch testing in consecutive patients suspected of contact dermatitis: routine testing

Studies in which cuminaldehyde was patch tested in consecutive patients suspected of contact dermatitis (routine testing) with positive results have not been found.

Patch testing in groups of selected patients

In 1984, in The Netherlands, 179 patients suspected of cosmetic allergy were patch tested with a battery of preservatives and fragrances including cuminaldehyde 15% pet. and there were three (1.7%) positive reactions; their relevance was not mentioned (2).

Case reports and case series

Case reports of allergic contact dermatitis from cuminaldehyde have not been found.

LITERATURE

1   SCCS (Scientific Committee on Consumer Safety). Opinion on Fragrance allergens in cosmetic products, 26-27 June 2012, SCCS/1459/11. Available at: https://ec.europa.eu/health/sites/health/files/scientific_committees/consumer_safety/docs/sccs_o_102.pdf

2   De Groot AC, Liem DH, Nater JP, van Ketel WG. Patch tests with fragrance materials and preservatives. Contact Dermatitis 1985;12:87-92

3   Uter W, Johansen JD, Börje A, Karlberg A-T, Lidén C, Rastogi S, Roberts D, White IR. Categorization of fragrance contact allergens for prioritization of preventive measures: clinical and experimental data and consideration of structure–activity relationships. Contact Dermatitis 2013;69:196-230

4   De Groot AC, Schmidt E. Essential oils: contact allergy and chemical composition. Boca Raton, Fl., USA: CRC Press, Taylor and Francis Group, 2016 (ISBN 9781482246407)

5   De Groot AC. Patch Testing, 4th Edition. Wapserveen, The Netherlands: acdegroot publishing, 2018 (ISBN 978-90-813233-4-5)

Chapter 3.45   5-CYCLOHEXADECENONE

IDENTIFICATION

Description/definition   : 5-Cyclohexadecenone is the cyclic ketone that conforms to the structural formula shown
                               below
Chemical class(es)   : Cyclic organic compounds; unsaturated compounds; ketones
INCI name USA   : Not in the Personal Care Products Council Ingredient Database
Chemical/IUPAC name   : Cyclohexadec-5-en-1-one
Other names   : Musk amberol; Ambretone ®
CAS registry number(s)   : 37609-25-9
EC number(s)   : 253-568-9
RIFM monograph(s)   : Food Chem Toxicol 2011;49(suppl.2):S98-S103
Function(s) in cosmetics   : EU: perfuming
Patch testing   : 6% alc. (2)
Molecular formula   : $C_{16}H_{28}O$

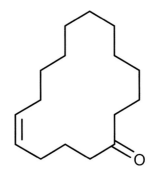

GENERAL

5-Cyclohexadecenone is a colorless to yellow clear viscous liquid; its odor type is musk and its odor at 10% in
dipropylene glycol is described as 'dry powdery musk amber civet' (www.thegoodscentscompany.com).

Presence in essential oils

5-Cyclohexadecenone is a synthetic chemical, not found in nature (and consequently not in essential oils (3)).

CONTACT ALLERGY

Patch testing in groups of patients

Pigmented cosmetic dermatitis

While searching for causative ingredients of pigmented cosmetic dermatitis in Japan in the 1970s, both patients with
ordinary (nonpigmented) cosmetic dermatitis and women with pigmented cosmetic dermatitis were tested with a
large number of fragrance materials. In 1980 the accumulated data enabled the classification of fragrant materials
into 4 groups: common sensitizers, rare sensitizers, virtually non-sensitizing fragrances and fragrances considered as
non-sensitizers. 5-Cyclohexadecenone was classified in the group of rare sensitizers, indicating that one or more
cases of contact allergy / allergic contact dermatitis to it have been observed (1). More specific data are lacking, the
results have largely or solely been published in Japanese journals only.

LITERATURE

1   Nakayama H. Fragrance hypersensitivity and its control. In: Frosch PJ, Johansen JD, White IR, Eds. Fragrances -
    beneficial and adverse effects. Berlin Heidelberg New York: Springer-Verlag, 1998:83-91
2   De Groot AC. Patch Testing, 4th Edition. Wapserveen, The Netherlands: acdegroot publishing, 2018 (ISBN 978-90-
    813233-4-5)
3   De Groot AC, Schmidt E. Essential oils: contact allergy and chemical composition. Boca Raton, Fl., USA: CRC Press,
    Taylor and Francis Group, 2016 (ISBN 9781482246407)

Chapter 3.46   CYCLOHEXYL ACETATE

IDENTIFICATION

Description/definition	: Cyclohexyl acetate is the ester that conforms to the structural formula shown below
Chemical class(es)	: Cyclic organic compounds; esters
INCI name USA	: Not in the Personal Care Products Council Ingredient Database
Chemical/IUPAC name	: Cyclohexyl acetate
CAS registry number(s)	: 622-45-7
EC number(s)	: 210-736-6
RIFM monograph(s)	: Food Chem Toxicol 2008;46(12)(suppl.):S52-S55; Food Cosmet Toxicol 1979;17:751 (special issue V)
SCCS opinion(s)	: SCCS/1459/11 (1)
Function(s) in cosmetics	: EU: perfuming
Patch testing	: 5% pet. (2)
Molecular formula	: $C_8H_{14}O_2$

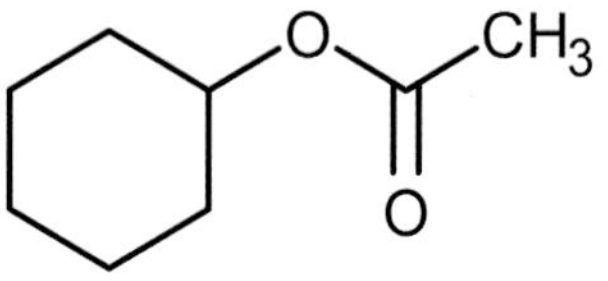

GENERAL

Cyclohexyl acetate is a colorless to pale yellow clear liquid; its odor type is fruity and its odor is described as 'solvent-like and fruity sweet with banana and apple nuances' (www.thegoodscentscompany.com). Cyclohexyl acetate is a synthetic chemical used as a fragrance and flavor. It is also a good solvent for cellulose ethers and nitrocellulose and has powerful solvency for basic dyes, blown oils, raw rubber, metallic soaps, driers, shellac, bitumen, and a wide range of natural and synthetic resins and gums. The chemical is used in spraying and brushing lacquers imparting blush resistance and good flow (U.S. National Library of Medicine).

Presence in essential oils

Cyclohexyl acetate has been identified by chemical analysis in none of 91 essential oils, which have caused contact allergy / allergic contact dermatitis (4).

CONTACT ALLERGY

The SCCS (Scientific Committee on Consumer Safety), in a 2012 Opinion on Fragrance allergens in cosmetic products, has categorized cyclohexyl acetate as 'possible fragrance contact allergen' (1,3).

Patch testing in groups of patients

Studies in which cyclohexyl acetate was patch tested in consecutive patients suspected of contact dermatitis (routine testing) with positive results have not been found. Before 2002, in Japan, European countries and the USA, 218 patients with known fragrance sensitivity were patch tested with cyclohexyl acetate 5% in petrolatum and one positive reaction (0.5%) was observed; its relevancy was not mentioned (2).

Case reports and case series

Case reports of allergic contact dermatitis from cyclohexyl acetate have not been found.

LITERATURE

1   SCCS (Scientific Committee on Consumer Safety). Opinion on Fragrance allergens in cosmetic products, 26-27 June 2012, SCCS/1459/11. Available at:
    https://ec.europa.eu/health/sites/health/files/scientific_committees/consumer_safety/docs/sccs_o_102.pdf
2   Larsen W, Nakayama H, Fischer T, Elsner P, Frosch P, Burrows D, et al. Fragrance contact dermatitis - a worldwide multicenter investigation (Part III). Contact Dermatitis 2002;46:141-144
3   Uter W, Johansen JD, Börje A, Karlberg A-T, Lidén C, Rastogi S, Roberts D, White IR. Categorization of fragrance contact allergens for prioritization of preventive measures: clinical and experimental data and consideration of structure–activity relationships. Contact Dermatitis 2013;69:196-230
4   De Groot AC, Schmidt E. Essential oils: contact allergy and chemical composition. Boca Raton, Fl., USA: CRC Press, Taylor and Francis Group, 2016 (ISBN 9781482246407)

Chapter 3.47   CYCLOPENTADECANONE

IDENTIFICATION

Description/definition   : Cyclopentadecanone is the organic compound that conforms to the structural formula
                                shown below
Chemical class(es)   : Ketones
Chemical/IUPAC name   : Cyclopentadecanone
Other names   : Normuscone
CAS registry number(s)   : 502-72-7
EC number(s)   : 207-951-2
RIFM monograph(s)   : Food Chem Toxicol 2011;49(suppl.2):S142-S148; Food Cosmet Toxicol 1976;14:735
                                (special issue III)
SCCS opinion(s)   : SCCS/1459/11 (1)
Function(s) in cosmetics   : EU: deodorant; masking. USA: deodorant agents; fragrance ingredients
Patch testing   : 5% pet. (2); based on RIFM data, 10% pet. is probably not irritant (4)
Molecular formula   : $C_{15}H_{28}O$

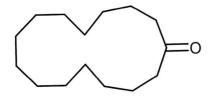

GENERAL

Cyclopentadecanone appears as colorless crystals; its odor type is musk and its odor at 10% in dipropylene glycol is
described as 'powdery musk animal natural greasy' (www.thegoodscentscompany.com).

Presence in essential oils

Cyclopentadecanone has been identified by chemical analysis in none of 91 essential oils, which have caused contact
allergy / allergic contact dermatitis (5). It appears not to be present in plants (www.thegoodscentscompany.com).

CONTACT ALLERGY

The SCCS (Scientific Committee on Consumer Safety), in a 2012 Opinion on Fragrance allergens in cosmetic products,
has categorized cyclopentadecanone as 'likely fragrance contact allergen by combination of evidence' (1,3).

Testing in groups of patients

Studies in which cyclopentadecanone was patch tested in consecutive patients suspected of contact dermatitis
(routine testing) with positive results have not been found. In 2000, in Japan, USA and several European countries,
178 patients with known fragrance sensitivity were tested with a series of fragrances and there were 3 (1.7%)
positive patch test reactions to cyclopentadecanone 5% pet. The relevance of these reactions was not mentioned (2).

Case reports and case series

Case reports of allergic contact dermatitis to cyclopentadecanone have not been found.

LITERATURE

1   SCCS (Scientific Committee on Consumer Safety). Opinion on Fragrance allergens in cosmetic products, 26-27
     June 2012, SCCS/1459/11. Available at:
     https://ec.europa.eu/health/sites/health/files/scientific_committees/consumer_safety/docs/sccs_o_102.pdf
2   Larsen W, Nakayama H, Fischer T, Elsner P, Frosch P, Burrows D, et al. Fragrance contact dermatitis: A worldwide
     multicenter investigation (Part II). Contact Dermatitis 2001;44:344-346
3   Uter W, Johansen JD, Börje A, Karlberg A-T, Lidén C, Rastogi S, Roberts D, White IR. Categorization of fragrance
     contact allergens for prioritization of preventive measures: clinical and experimental data and consideration of
     structure–activity relationships. Contact Dermatitis 2013;69:196-230
4   De Groot AC. Patch Testing, 4th Edition. Wapserveen, The Netherlands: acdegroot publishing, 2018 (ISBN 978-90-
     813233-4-5)
5   De Groot AC, Schmidt E. Essential oils: contact allergy and chemical composition. Boca Raton, Fl., USA: CRC Press,
     Taylor and Francis Group, 2016 (ISBN 9781482246407)

Chapter 3.48   p-CYMENE

IDENTIFICATION

Description/definition   : *p*-Cymene is the aromatic hydrocarbon that conforms to the structural formula shown
                              below
Chemical/IUPAC name   : 1-Methyl-4-propan-2-ylbenzene
Other names   : 4-Isopropyltoluene; *p*-cymol; camphogen; 1-methyl-4-(1-methylethyl)benzene
CAS registry number(s)   : 99-87-6
EC number(s)   : 202-796-7
RIFM monograph(s)   : Food Cosmet Toxicol 1974;12:401
Merck Index monograph   : 4030 (Cymene)
Function(s) in cosmetics   : EU: masking. USA: fragrance ingredients
Patch testing   : 1% alc. (1); based on RIFM data, 4% pet. is probably not irritant (3)
Molecular formula   : $C_{10}H_{14}$

GENERAL

p-Cymene is a colorless to pale yellow clear liquid; its odor type is terpenic and its odor at 1% in dipropylene glycol is described as 'fresh citrus terpene woody spice' (www.thegoodscentscompany.com). *p*-Cymene is used to improve the odor of soaps, detergents and sanitation goods and as a masking odor for industrial products. It also acts as the starting material for the production of *p*-cresol, carvacrol and acetyl hexamethyl tetralin. Other uses include or have included as a solvent for dyes, varnishes and lacquers, as heat-transfer fluid, in metal polishes and in the manufacture of synthetic resins (U.S. National Library of Medicine).

Presence in essential oils, Myroxylon pereirae resin (balsam of Peru) and propolis

p-Cymene has been identified by chemical analysis in 83 of 91 essential oils, which have caused contact allergy / allergic contact dermatitis. In 19 oils, *p*-cymene belonged to the 'Top-10' of ingredients with the highest concentrations. These are shown in table 3.48.1 with the concentration range which may be expected in commercial essential oils of this type (6). *p*-Cymene may also be present in Myroxylon pereirae resin (balsam of Peru) (4) and in propolis (5).

Table 3.48.1 Essential oils containing *p*-cymene in the 'Top-10' and concentration range in commercial oils

Essential oil	Concentration range (min.-max.)	Essential oil	Concentration range (min.-max.)
Angelica root oil	1.3 - 8.4%	Laurel leaf oil	0.04 - 2.7%
Black cumin oil	19.9 - 57.5%	Lemon oil	0.1 - 2.2%
Black pepper oil	0.2 - 6.0%	Mandarin oil	0.3 - 1.2%
Cajeput oil	0.1 - 9.5%	Olibanum oil	2.7 - 4.9%
Carrot seed oil	0.4 - 6.0%	Tangerine oil	0.4 - 1.1%
Cinnamon bark oil Sri Lanka	2.2 - 2.8%	Tea tree oil	0.3 - 19.4%
Coriander fruit oil	0.2 - 7.8%	Thyme oil	0.5 - 25.7%
Dwarf pine oil	0.2 - 4.3%	Thyme oil Spanish	12.8 - 25.4%
Elemi oil	0.9 - 7.1%	Turpentine oil	traces - 2.5%
Eucalyptus globulus oil	1.1 - 3.1%		

CONTACT ALLERGY

GENERAL

p-Cymene is a minor allergen in tea tree oil. Of 64 patients allergic to tea tree oil and tested with a number of its ingredients in various studies, one (1.6%) reacted to *p*-cymene (2).

Patch testing in groups of patients

Patch testing in consecutive patients suspected of contact dermatitis: routine testing
Studies in which *p*-cymene was patch tested in consecutive patients suspected of contact dermatitis (routine testing) with positive results have not been found.

Patch testing in groups of selected patients
In Germany, in the period 1990-1992, 7 patients who had shown a positive patch test reaction to tea tree oil 1% alcohol were tested with a battery of its ingredients and there was one (14%) positive reaction to *p*-cymene 1% in alcohol (1). In several other similar studies, another 57 tea tree oil-allergic individuals were also tested with *p*-cymene, but no positive patch test reactions to it were observed (7,8,9,10,11).

LITERATURE
1   Knight TE, Hausen BM. Melaleuca oil (tea tree oil) dermatitis. J Am Acad Dermatol 1994;30:423-427
2   De Groot AC, Schmidt E. Tea tree oil: contact allergy and chemical composition. Contact Dermatitis 2016;75:129-143
3   De Groot AC. Patch Testing, 4th Edition. Wapserveen, The Netherlands: acdegroot publishing, 2018 (ISBN 978-90-813233-4-5)
4   Mammerler V. Contribution to the analysis and quality control of Peru Balsam. PhD Thesis, University of Vienna, Austria, 2007. Available at: http://othes.univie.ac.at/4056/1/2009-03-23_0201578.pdf
5   De Groot AC, Popova MP, Bankova VS. An update on the constituents of poplar-type propolis. Wapserveen, The Netherlands: acdegroot publishing, 2014, 11 pages. ISBN/EAN: 978-90-813233-0-7. Available at: https://www.researchgate.net/publication/262851225_AN_UPDATE_ON_THE_CONSTITUENTS_OF_POPLAR-TYPE_PROPOLIS
6   De Groot AC, Schmidt E. Essential oils: contact allergy and chemical composition. Boca Raton, Fl., USA: CRC Press, Taylor and Francis Group, 2016 (ISBN 9781482246407)
7   Hausen BM. Evaluation of the main contact allergens in oxidized tea tree oil. Dermatitis 2004;15:213-214
8   Hausen BM, Reichling J, Harkenthal M. Degradation products of monoterpenes are the sensitizing agents in tea tree oil. Am J Cont Derm 1999;10:68-77
9   Pirker C, Hausen BM, Uter W, Hillen U, Brasch J, Bayerl C, et al. Sensitization to tea tree oil in Germany and Austria. A multicenter study of the German Contact Dermatitis group. J Dtsch Dermatol Ges 2003;1:629-634
10   Rubel DM, Freeman S, Southwell I. Tea tree oil allergy: what is the offending agent? Report of three cases of tea tree oil allergy and review of the literature. Australas J Dermatol 1998;39:244-247
11   Lippert U, Walter A, Hausen BM, Fuchs T. Increasing incidence of contact dermatitis to tea tree oil. J Allergy Clin Immunol 2000;105:S43 (abstract 127)

Chapter 3.49   ALPHA-DAMASCONE

IDENTIFICATION

Description/definition   : alpha-Damascone is the organic compound that conforms to the structural formula
                                  shown below
Chemical class(es)   : Ketones
Chemical/IUPAC name   : 1-(2,6,6-Trimethyl-2-cyclohexen-1-yl)-2-buten-1-one
Other names   : Damascone, alpha
CAS registry number(s)   : 23726-94-5; 43052-87-5
EC number(s)   : 245-845-8
RIFM monograph(s)   : Food Chem Toxicol 2007;45(suppl.1):S179-S187 and 188-191 (cis-alpha); Food Chem
                                  Toxicol 2000;38(suppl.3):S199-204
IFRA standard   : Restricted (www.ifraorg.org/en-us/standards-library) (table 3.49.1)
SCCS opinion(s)   : SCCNFP/0392/00 (1); SCCS/1459/11 (2); SCCNFP/0389/00, final (rose ketone-1) (12)
Function(s) in cosmetics   : EU: masking; perfuming. USA: fragrance ingredients
EU cosmetic restrictions   : Regulated in Annex III/157 of the Regulation (EC) No. 344/2013
Patch testing   : 0.2% pet. (3)
Molecular formula   : $C_{13}H_{20}O$

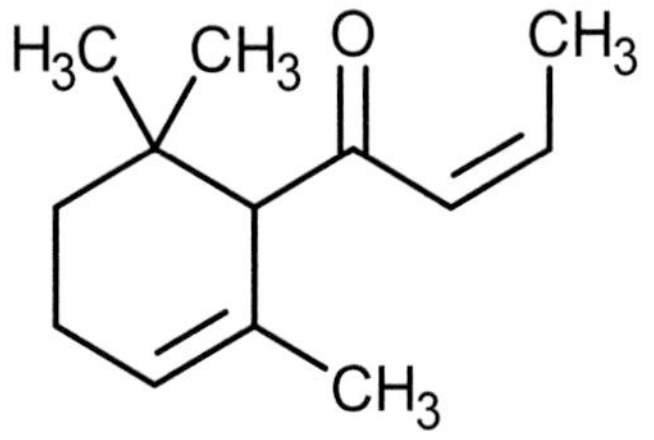

Table 3.49.1 IFRA restrictions for alpha-damascone

Category [a]	Limits [b]	Category [a]	Limits [b]	Category [a]	Limits [b]
1	0.00%	5	0.02%	9	0.02%
2	0.00%	6	0.07%	10	0.02%
3	0.02%	7	0.01%	11	not restricted
4	0.02%	8	0.02%		

[a] For explanation of categories see pages 6-8
[b] Limits in the finished products

GENERAL

alpha-Damascone is a pale yellow clear liquid; its odor type is floral and its odor is described as 'sweet, fruity, floral woody with a green berry nuance' (www.thegoodscentscompany.com).

Presence in essential oils

alpha-Damascone has been identified by chemical analysis in none of 91 essential oils, which have caused contact allergy / allergic contact dermatitis (11).

CONTACT ALLERGY

General

The SCCS (Scientific Committee on Consumer Safety), in a 2012 Opinion on Fragrance allergens in cosmetic products, has marked alpha-damascone as 'established contact allergen in humans' (2,5).

At higher concentrations, alpha-damascone is a potent sensitizer. In thirty patients with malignant tumors (and probably lowered immunity), 30% alpha-damascone in purified lanolin with sodium dodecyl benzene sulphonate as the adjuvant was applied in a patch test unit to the surface of the inner upper arm for 2 days. Two weeks later, alpha-damascone 3% in petrolatum was applied to the other arm and 8/30 (27%) were found to be sensitized. Of 3 healthy volunteers tested in the same manner, all became allergic to alpha-damascone (7). One of these authors ten years later reported that 'Damascone' was found to sensitize volunteers by patch testing; data on the number of volunteers, percentage sensitized, test concentration and vehicle were not provided (4).

Patch testing in groups of patients

In the period 1998-2000, in six European countries, 1606 consecutive patients suspected of contact dermatitis (routine testing) were patch tested with alpha-damascone 0.2% pet. and there were eight (0.5%) positive reactions. The relevance of these reactions was not mentioned. The test material consisted of a mixture of 0.1% alpha- and 0.1% beta-damascone (3).

Case reports and case series

A woman had allergic contact dermatitis from alpha-damascone (tested 2% pet.), hydroxyisohexyl 3-cyclohexene-carboxaldehyde (HICC), hexyl cinnamal and benzophenone-2 in an eau de parfum (6).

Cross-reactions, pseudo-cross-reactions and co-reactions

For general information on cross-/pseudo-cross-/co-reactivity of fragrance chemicals with other fragrances, fragrance markers (fragrance mix I, fragrance mix II, colophonium, Myroxylon pereirae resin [balsam of Peru]) and essential oils see Chapter 1.2 General information on cross-reactions, pseudo-cross-reactions and co-reactions.

Patients sensitized by provocative tests to delta-damascone (8,10) and beta-damascone (10) may cross-react to alpha-damascone.

Patch test sensitization

Patch test sensitization by alpha-damascone is described in the section 'Contact allergy / general' above.

LITERATURE

1   SCCNFP (Scientific Committee on Cosmetic Products and Non-Food Products Intended for Consumers). Opinion of the Scientific Committee on Cosmetic Products and Non-Food Products Intended for Consumers concerning 'An initial list of perfumery materials which must not form part of cosmetic products except subject to the Restrictions and Conditions laid down, 25 September 2001, SCCNFP/0392/00, final. Available at: http://ec.europa.eu/health/archive/ph_risk/committees/sccp/documents/out150_en.pdf

2   SCCS (Scientific Committee on Consumer Safety). Opinion on Fragrance allergens in cosmetic products, 26-27 June 2012, SCCS/1459/11. Available at: https://ec.europa.eu/health/sites/health/files/scientific_committees/consumer_safety/docs/sccs_o_102.pdf

3   Frosch PJ, Johansen JD, Menné T, Pirker C, Rastogi SC, Andersen KE, et al. Further important sensitizers in patients sensitive to fragrances. II. Reactivity to essential oils. Contact Dermatitis 2002;47:279-287

4   Nakayama H. Fragrance hypersensitivity and its control. In: Frosch PJ, Johansen JD, White IR, Eds. Fragrances - beneficial and adverse effects. Berlin Heidelberg New York: Springer-Verlag, 1998:83-91

5   Uter W, Johansen JD, Börje A, Karlberg A-T, Lidén C, Rastogi S, Roberts D, White IR. Categorization of fragrance contact allergens for prioritization of preventive measures: clinical and experimental data and consideration of structure–activity relationships. Contact Dermatitis 2013;69:196-230

6   Gimenez-Arnau A, Gimenez-Arnau E, Serra-Baldrich E, Lepoittevin J-P, Camarasa JG. Principles and methodology for identification of fragrance allergens in consumer products. Contact Dermatitis 2002;47:345-352

7   Takanami I, Nakayama H. TMCHB: A possible alternative to DNCB in skin testing for immune competence. Contact Dermatitis 1988;19:81-83

8   RIFM (Research Institute for Fragrance Materials, Inc.). Evaluation of potential irritation and sensitization hazards of delta-1-(2,6,6-Trimethyl-3-cyclohexen-1-yl)-2-buten-1-one by dermal contact in humans. Unpublished report from IFF Incorporated, 17 November 1982. Report number 15399 (RIFM, Woodcliff Lake, NJ, USA). Data cited in ref. 9

9   Lalko J, Lapczynski A, McGinty D, Bhatia S, Letizia SC, Api AM. Fragrance material review on delta-damascone. Food and Chemical Toxicology 2007;45(suppl.):S205-S210

10 Lapczynski A, Lalko J, McGinty D, Bhatia S, Letizia CS, Api AM. Fragrance material review on α-damascone. Food Chem Toxicol 2007;45(suppl.1):S179-S187

11 De Groot AC, Schmidt E. Essential oils: contact allergy and chemical composition. Boca Raton, Fl., USA: CRC Press, Taylor and Francis Group, 2016 (ISBN 9781482246407)

12 Opinion of the Scientific Committee on Cosmetic Products and Non-Food Products Intended for Consumers concerning 'The 1st update of the inventory of ingredients employed in cosmetic products. Section II: Perfume and aromatic raw materials', 24 October 2000, SCCNFP/0389/00, final. Available at: http://ec.europa.eu/health/ph_risk/committees/sccp/documents/out131_en.pdf

Chapter 3.50   BETA-DAMASCONE *

Not an INCI name

IDENTIFICATION

Description/definition	: beta-Damascone is the cyclic organic compound that conforms to the structural formula shown below
Chemical class(es)	: Ketones; cyclic organic compounds
INCI name USA	: Not in the Personal Care Products Council Ingredient Database
Chemical/IUPAC name	: 1-(2,6,6-Trimethylcyclohexen-1-yl)but-2-en-1-one (*E-* or *Z-*)
Other names	: Rose dihydroketone; rose ketone-2 (*cis-* and *trans-*)
CAS registry number(s)	: 23726-92-3 (*Z-, cis-*); 23726-91-2 (*E-, trans-*)
EC number(s)	: 245-843-7 (*Z-, cis-*); 245-842-1 (*E-, trans-*)
RIFM monograph(s)	: Food Chem Toxicol 2007;45(suppl.1):S192-S198 (*Z-, cis-*); Food Chem Toxicol 2007;45(suppl.1):S199-S204 (*E-, trans-*); Food Chem Toxicol 2000;38(suppl.3):S205-S210 (beta-1-(2,6,6-trimethyl-1-cyclohexen-1-yl)-2-buten-1-one)
IFRA standard	: Restricted (www.ifraorg.org/en-us/standards-library) (table 3.50.1)
SCCS opinion(s)	: SCCNFP/0392/00, final (2); SCCS/1459/11 (3); SCCNFP/0389/00, final (8)
Function(s) in cosmetics	: EU: perfuming
EU cosmetic restrictions	: Regulated in Annex III/162 (*cis-*) and 158 (*trans-*) of the Regulation (EC) No. 344/2013
Patch testing	: 0.1% pet. (1)
Molecular formula	: $C_{13}H_{20}O$

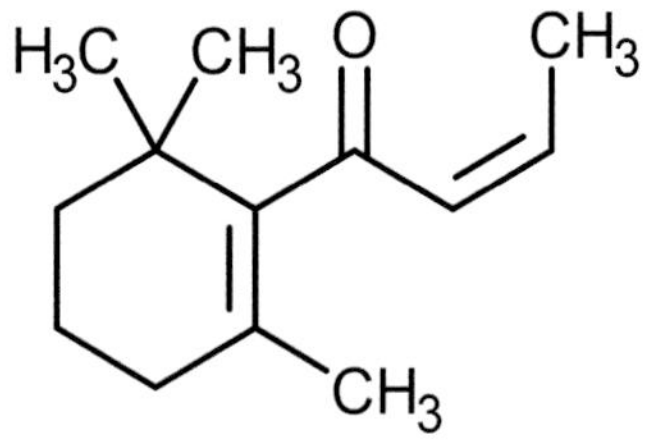

(*Z*)-beta-Damascone 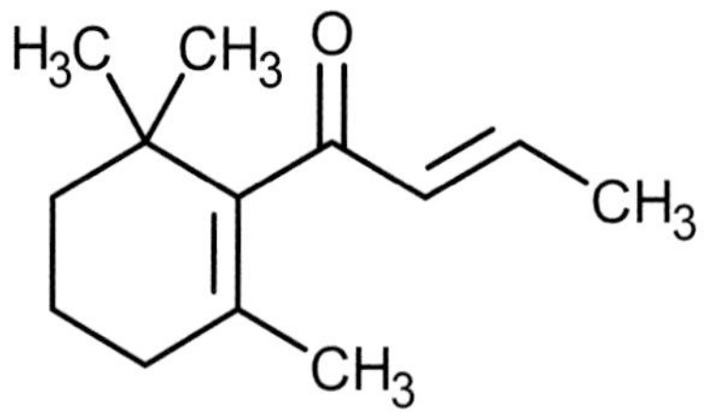   (*E*)-beta-Damascone

Table 3.50.1 IFRA restrictions for beta-damascone

Category [a]	Limits [b]	Category [a]	Limits [b]	Category [a]	Limits [b]
1	0.00%	5	0.02%	9	0.02%
2	0.00%	6	0.07%	10	0.02%
3	0.02%	7	0.01%	11	not restricted
4	0.02%	8	0.02%		

[a] For explanation of categories see pages 6-8
[b] Limits in the finished products

GENERAL

beta-Damascone is a clear yellow liquid; its odor type is fruity and its odor at 1% in dipropylene glycol is described as 'fruity floral black currant plum rose honey tobacco' (www.thegoodscentscompany.com).

Presence in essential oils

beta-Damascone has been identified by chemical analysis in 12 of 91 essential oils, which have caused contact allergy / allergic contact dermatitis. In none of these oils, beta-damascone belonged to the 'Top-10' of ingredients with the highest concentrations which may be expected in commercial essential oils of this type (7).

CONTACT ALLERGY

General

The SCCS (Scientific Committee on Consumer Safety), in a 2012 Opinion on Fragrance allergens in cosmetic products, has marked *cis*-beta-damascone as 'established contact allergen in humans' (3,5).

Patch testing in groups of patients

Patch testing in consecutive patients suspected of contact dermatitis: routine testing
In the period 1998-2000, in six European countries, 1606 consecutive patients were patch tested with damascone 0.2% in petrolatum (a mixture of 0.1% alpha- and 0.1% beta-damascone) and there were 8 (0.5%) positive reactions. The relevance of these reactions was not mentioned (1).

Patch testing in groups of selected patients
Studies in which beta-damascone was patch tested in groups of selected patients with positive results have not been found.

Case reports and case series
Case reports of allergic contact dermatitis from beta-damascone have not been found.

Cross-reactions, pseudo-cross-reactions and co-reactions
For general information on cross-/pseudo-cross-/co-reactivity of fragrance chemicals with other fragrances, fragrance markers (fragrance mix I, fragrance mix II, colophonium, Myroxylon pereirae resin [balsam of Peru]) and essential oils see Chapter 1.2 General information on cross-reactions, pseudo-cross-reactions and co-reactions.

Three patients sensitized to delta-damascone from human repeat insult patch tests (HRIPT) cross-reacted to *Z*-beta-damascone (6).

Patch test sensitization
'Damascone' was found to sensitize volunteers by patch testing (test concentration and vehicle unknown) (4).

LITERATURE

1   Frosch PJ, Johansen JD, Menné T, Pirker C, Rastogi SC, Andersen KE, et al. Further important sensitizers in patients sensitive to fragrances. II. Reactivity to essential oils. Contact Dermatitis 2002;47:279-287

2   SCCNFP (Scientific Committee on Cosmetic Products and Non-Food Products Intended for Consumers). Opinion of the Scientific Committee on Cosmetic Products and Non-Food Products Intended for Consumers concerning 'An initial list of perfumery materials which must not form part of cosmetic products except subject to the Restrictions and Conditions laid down, 25 September 2001, SCCNFP/0392/00, final. Available at: http://ec.europa.eu/health/archive/ph_risk/committees/sccp/documents/out150_en.pdf

3   SCCS (Scientific Committee on Consumer Safety). Opinion on Fragrance allergens in cosmetic products, 26-27 June 2012, SCCS/1459/11. Available at: https://ec.europa.eu/health/sites/health/files/scientific_committees/consumer_safety/docs/sccs_o_102.pdf

4   Nakayama H. Fragrance hypersensitivity and its control. In: Frosch PJ, Johansen JD, White IR, Eds. Fragrances - beneficial and adverse effects. Berlin Heidelberg New York: Springer-Verlag, 1998:83-91

5   Uter W, Johansen JD, Börje A, Karlberg A-T, Lidén C, Rastogi S, Roberts D, White IR. Categorization of fragrance contact allergens for prioritization of preventive measures: clinical and experimental data and consideration of structure–activity relationships. Contact Dermatitis 2013;69:196-230

6   Lalko J, Lapczynski A, Letizia CS, Api AM. Fragrance material review on *cis*-β-damascone. Food Chem Toxicol 2007;45(suppl.1):S192-S198

7   De Groot AC, Schmidt E. Essential oils: contact allergy and chemical composition. Boca Raton, Fl., USA: CRC Press, Taylor and Francis Group, 2016 (ISBN 9781482246407)

8   Opinion of the Scientific Committee on Cosmetic Products and Non-Food Products Intended for Consumers concerning 'The 1st update of the inventory of ingredients employed in cosmetic products. Section II: Perfume and aromatic raw materials', 24 October 2000, SCCNFP/0389/00, final. Available at: http://ec.europa.eu/health/ph_risk/committees/sccp/documents/out131_en.pdf

Chapter 3.51 DEHYDRODIISOEUGENOL

IDENTIFICATION

Description/definition : Dehydrodiisoeugenol is the tricyclic aromatic compound that conforms to the structural formula shown below

Chemical class(es) : Heterocyclic aromatic compounds; ethers; alcohols

INCI name USA : Neither in CosIng nor in the Personal Care Products Council Ingredient Database

Chemical/IUPAC name : 2-Methoxy-4-[7-methoxy-3-methyl-5-[(E)-prop-1-enyl]-2,3-dihydro-1-benzofuran-2-yl]phenol

Other names : Diisoeugenol, dehydro-; isoeugenol, dehydrodi-

CAS registry number (s) : 2680-81-1

EC number(s) : Not available

Patch testing : No data available

Molecular formula : $C_{20}H_{22}O_4$

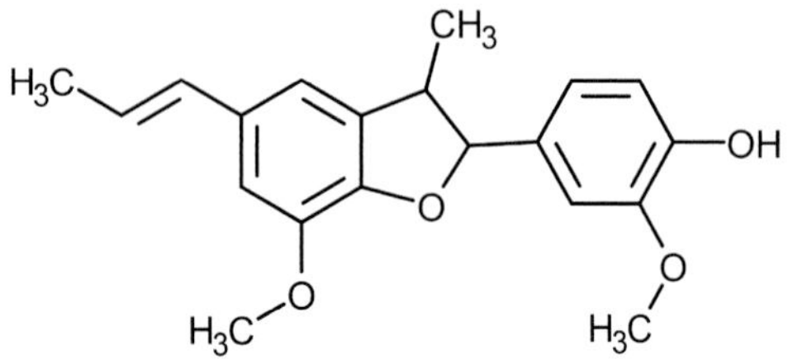

GENERAL

Dehydrodiisoeugenol is not used as fragrance or flavor material and is used for experimental and research use only. Nevertheless, it is discussed here, as it has been termed a main sensitizer in ylang-ylang oil, an essential oil used in perfumery (1). Dehydrodiisoeugenol has a 'characteristic odor' (www.thegoodscentscompany.com). It has been found in several plants, e.g. *Aristolochia taliscana* Hook. & Arn. (4), the seeds of *Myristica fragrans* (nutmeg) (5) and *Nectandra rigida* Nees (6).

Presence in essential oils

Dehydrodiisoeugenol has been identified by chemical analysis in none of 91 essential oils, which have caused contact allergy / allergic contact dermatitis (3).

CONTACT ALLERGY

General

It has been reported that dehydrodiisoeugenol, which is a moderate sensitizer in the murine local lymph node assay (LLNA) and guinea pig maximization test (2), is one of the main sensitizers in ylang-ylang oil (1). However, in a recent in-depth review of the chemical composition of ylang-ylang oil, dehydrodiisoeugenol was not found in these essential oils in any investigation (3).

LITERATURE

1 Sugawara M, et al. Dehydrodiisoeugenol (DDI), one of the main contact sensitizers in ylang-ylang oil. 8th International Symposium on Contact Dermatitis, Cambridge, 1986. Data cited in: Mitchell DM, Beck MH. Contact allergy to benzyl alcohol in a cutting oil reodorant. Contact Dermatitis 1988;18:301-302

2 Takeyoshi M, Iida K, Suzuki K, Yamazaki S. Skin sensitization potency of isoeugenol and its dimers evaluated by a non-radioisotopic modification of the local lymph node assay and guinea pig maximization test. J Appl Toxicol 2008;28:530-504

3 De Groot AC, Schmidt E. Essential oils: contact allergy and chemical composition. Boca Raton, Fl., USA: CRC Press, Taylor and Francis Group, 2016 (ISBN 9781482246407)

4 Ionescu F, Jolad SD, Cole JR. Dehydrodiisoeugenol: a naturally occurring lignan from *Aristolochia taliscana* (Aristolochiaceae). J Pharm Sci 1977;66:1489-1490

5 Cao GY, Yang XW, Xu W, Li F. New inhibitors of nitric oxide production from the seeds of *Myristica fragrans*. Food Chem Toxicol 2013;62:167-171

6 Le Quesne PW, Larrahondo JE, Raffauf RF. Antitumor plants. X. Constituents of *Nectandra rigida*. J Nat Prod 1980;43:353-359

Chapter 3.52   DIETHYL MALEATE

IDENTIFICATION

Description/definition	: Diethyl maleate is the maleic acid ester that conforms to the structural formula shown below
Chemical class(es)	: Unsaturated dicarboxylic acid esters
INCI name USA	: Not in the Personal Care Products Council Ingredient Database
Chemical/IUPAC name	: Diethyl (Z)-but-2-enedioate
Other names	: Ethyl maleate
CAS registry number(s)	: 141-05-9
EC number(s)	: 205-451-9
RIFM monograph(s)	: Food Cosmet Toxicol 1976;14:443
IFRA standard	: Prohibited (www.ifraorg.org/en-us/standards-library)
SCCS Opinion(s)	: SCCNFP/0320/00, final (1)
Merck Index monograph	: 3123
EU cosmetic restrictions	: Regulated in Annex II/426 of the Regulation (EC) No. 1223/2009, regulated by 2002/34/EC; Prohibited
Patch testing	: 0.12% pet. (3)
Molecular formula	: $C_8H_{12}O_4$

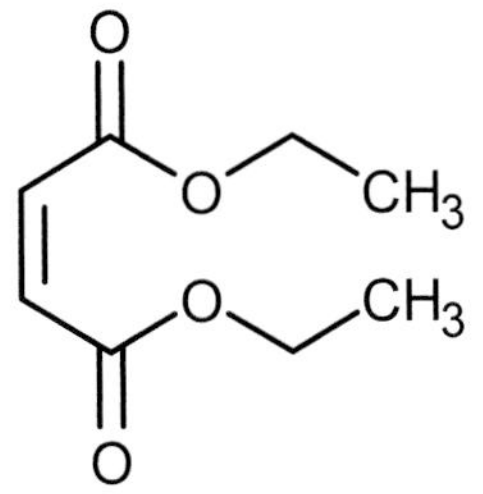

GENERAL

Diethyl maleate is a colorless clear liquid; its odor type is fruity and its odor at 100% is described as 'fruity banana citrus' (www.thegoodscentscompany.com). It is prohibited by IFRA and the EU because of sensitization (8) and is not used anymore as fragrance.

Presence in essential oils

Diethyl maleate has been identified by chemical analysis in none of 91 essential oils, which have caused contact allergy / allergic contact dermatitis (7).

CONTACT ALLERGY

General

The sensitizing potency of diethyl maleate was classified as 'moderate' based on an EC3 value of 5.8% in the LLNA (local lymph node assay) in animal experiments (5,6).

Patch testing in groups of patients

Patch testing in consecutive patients suspected of contact dermatitis: routine testing

Studies in which diethyl maleate was patch tested in consecutive patients suspected of contact dermatitis (routine testing) with positive results have not been found.

Patch testing in groups of selected patients

In 1983, in The Netherlands, 182 patients suspected of cosmetic allergy were patch tested with diethyl maleate 0.1% pet. and there were 6 (3.3%) positive reactions; their relevance was not mentioned (4).

Case reports and case series

Case reports of allergic contact dermatitis from diethyl maleate have not been found.

Cross-reactions, pseudo-cross-reactions and co-reactions
For general information on cross-/pseudo-cross-/co-reactivity of fragrance chemicals with other fragrances, fragrance markers (fragrance mix I, fragrance mix II, colophonium, Myroxylon pereirae resin [balsam of Peru]) and essential oils see Chapter 1.2 General information on cross-reactions, pseudo-cross-reactions and co-reactions.
Diethyl maleate may show cross-reactivity to primary dimethyl fumarate sensitization (3).

Patch test sensitization
Possible patch test sensitization at 5% has been cited in ref. 2.

LITERATURE

1   SCCFNP (Scientific Committee on Cosmetic Products and Non-Food Products Intended for Consumers). Opinion of the Scientific Committee on Cosmetic Products and Non-Food Products Intended for Consumers concerning 'An initial list of perfumery materials which must not form part of fragrances compounds used in cosmetic products', 3 May 2000, SCCNFP/0320/00, final. Available at:
    http://ec.europa.eu/health/archive/ph_risk/committees/sccp/documents/out116_en.pdf
2   De Groot AC. Patch Testing, 4th Edition. Wapserveen, The Netherlands: acdegroot publishing, 2018 (ISBN 978-90-813233-4-5)
3   Lammintausta K, Zimerson E, Winhoven S, Susitaival P, Hasan T, Gruvberger B, Williams J, Beck M, Bruze M. Sensitization to dimethyl fumarate with multiple concurrent patch test reactions. Contact Dermatitis 2010;62:88-96
4   Malten KE, van Ketel WG, Nater JP, Liem DH. Reactions in selected patients to 22 fragrance materials. Contact Dermatitis 1984;11:1-10
5   SCCS (Scientific Committee on Consumer Safety). Opinion on Fragrance allergens in cosmetic products, 26-27 June 2012, SCCS/1459/11. Available at:
    https://ec.europa.eu/health/sites/health/files/scientific_committees/consumer_safety/docs/sccs_o_102.pdf
6   Uter W, Johansen JD, Börje A, Karlberg A-T, Lidén C, Rastogi S, Roberts D, White IR. Categorization of fragrance contact allergens for prioritization of preventive measures: clinical and experimental data and consideration of structure–activity relationships. Contact Dermatitis 2013;69:196-230
7   De Groot AC, Schmidt E. Essential oils: contact allergy and chemical composition. Boca Raton, Fl., USA: CRC Press, Taylor and Francis Group, 2016 (ISBN 9781482246407)
8   Marzulli FN, Maibach HI. Further studies of effects of vehicles and elicitation concentration in experimental contact sensitization testing in humans. Contact Dermatitis 1980;6:131-133

Chapter 3.53   DIHYDROCARVEOL

IDENTIFICATION

Description/definition   : Dihydrocarveol is the cyclohexane derivative that conforms to the structural formula
                                  shown below
Chemical class(es)   : Cyclic organic compounds; unsaturated compounds; alcohols
INCI name USA   : Not in the Personal Care Products Council Ingredient Database
Chemical/IUPAC name   : 2-Methyl-5-prop-1-en-2-ylcyclohexan-1-ol
Other names   : *p*-Menth-8-en-2-ol; 2-methyl-5-(1-methylvinyl)cyclohexanol
CAS registry number(s)   : 619-01-2
EC number(s)   : 210-575-1
RIFM monograph(s)   : Food Chem Toxicol 2008;46(11)(suppl.)S123-S125 and 121-122 (*R,R,R*-); Food Cosmet
                                  Toxicol 1979;17:771 (special issue V)
Function(s) in cosmetics   : EU: perfuming
Patch testing   : No patch test data available; based on RIFM data, 4% pet. is probably not irritant (2)
Molecular formula   : $C_{10}H_{18}O$

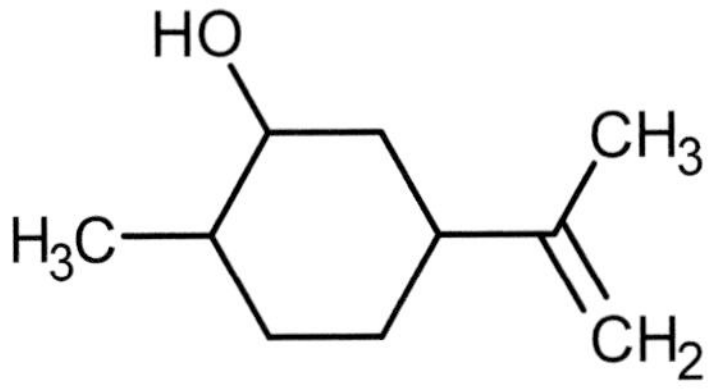

GENERAL

Dihydrocarveol is a pale yellow clear liquid; its odor type is minty and its odor is described as 'minty cooling sweet camphoreous, with fresh terpy nuances' (www.thegoodscentscompany.com).

Presence in essential oils

Dihydrocarveol has been identified by chemical analysis in 15 of 91 essential oils, which have caused contact allergy / allergic contact dermatitis. In one oil, dihydrocarveol belonged to the 'Top-10' of ingredients with the highest concentrations which may be expected in commercial essential oils of this type: spearmint oil (0.05-5.1%) (3).

CONTACT ALLERGY

Patch testing in groups of patients

Patch testing in consecutive patients suspected of contact dermatitis: routine testing

Studies in which dihydrocarveol was patch tested in consecutive patients suspected of contact dermatitis (routine testing) with positive results have not been found.

Patch testing in groups of selected patients

Ten patients allergic to peppermint oil (of who 4 co-reacted to spearmint oil) were patch tested with 24 ingredients. There was one positive reaction to dihydrocarveol, 4 to menthol, 4 to piperitone, 3 to pulegone, 2 to tetrahydro-dimethylbenzofuran (menthofuran), and one to menthyl acetate (1). Further details are lacking (article in Japanese).

Case reports and case series

Case reports of allergic contact dermatitis from dihydrocarveol have not been found.

LITERATURE

1   Saito F, Miyazaki T, Matsuoka Y. Peppermint oil (title incomplete, partly in Japanese). Skin Research 1984;26:636-643 (article in Japanese)

2   De Groot AC. Patch Testing, 4th Edition. Wapserveen, The Netherlands: acdegroot publishing, 2018 (ISBN 978-90-813233-4-5)

3   De Groot AC, Schmidt E. Essential oils: contact allergy and chemical composition. Boca Raton, Fl., USA: CRC Press, Taylor and Francis Group, 2016 (ISBN 9781482246407)

Chapter 3.54   DIHYDROCITRONELLOL

IDENTIFICATION

Description/definition : Dihydrocitronellol is the organic compound that conforms to the formula shown below
Chemical class(es)   : Alcohols
Chemical/IUPAC name   : 3,7-Dimethyl-1-octanol
Other names   : Pelargol; tetrahydrogeraniol; dimethyl octanol
CAS registry number(s) : 106-21-8
EC number(s)   : 203-374-5
RIFM monograph(s)   : Food Chem Toxicol 2017;110 (suppl.1):S412-S420; Food Chem Toxicol 2008;46(11)
                          (suppl.):S139-S141; Food Cosmet Toxicol 1974;12:535 (binder, page 330)
Function(s) in cosmetics : EU: masking; perfuming. USA: fragrance ingredients
Patch testing   : 5% pet. (1); according to RIFM data, 8% pet. is probably not irritant (3)
Molecular formula   : $C_{10}H_{22}O$

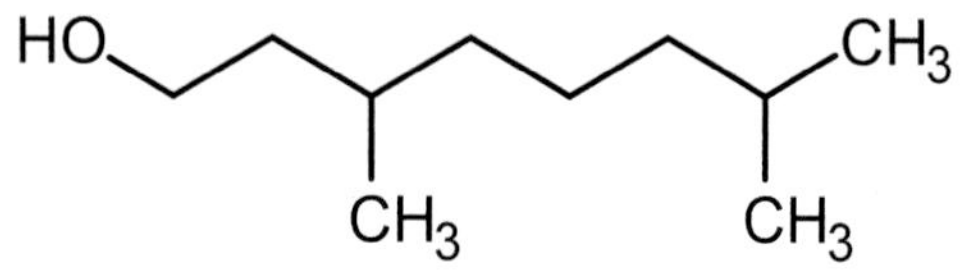

GENERAL

Dihydrocitronellol is a colorless liquid; its odor type is floral and its odor at 100% is described as 'waxy soapy aldehydic leathery musty citrus green' (www.thegoodscentscompany.com).

Presence in essential oils

Dihydrocitronellol has been identified by chemical analysis in 3 of 91 essential oils, which have caused contact allergy / allergic contact dermatitis: bergamot oil, Eucalyptus citriodora oil and geranium oil. In none of these oils, dihydrocitronellol belonged to the 'Top-10' of ingredients with the highest concentrations which may be expected in commercial essential oils of this type (4).

CONTACT ALLERGY

Patch testing in groups of patients

Studies in which dihydrocitronellol has been patch tested in either consecutive patients suspected of contact dermatitis (routine testing) or in groups of selected patients with positive results have not been found.

Case reports and case series

In a group of 119 patients with allergic contact dermatitis from cosmetics, investigated in The Netherlands in 1986-1987, one case was caused by dihydrocitronellol (pelargol) in a skin care product (1,2).

LITERATURE

1   De Groot AC, Bruynzeel DP, Bos JD, van der Meeren HL, van Joost T, Jagtman BA, Weyland JW. The allergens in cosmetics. Arch Dermatol 1988;124:1525-1529
2   De Groot AC. Adverse reactions to cosmetics. PhD Thesis, University of Groningen, The Netherlands: 1988, chapter 3.4, pp.105-113
3   De Groot AC. Patch Testing, 4th Edition. Wapserveen, The Netherlands: acdegroot publishing, 2018 (ISBN 978-90-813233-4-5)
4   De Groot AC, Schmidt E. Essential oils: contact allergy and chemical composition. Boca Raton, Fl., USA: CRC Press, Taylor and Francis Group, 2016 (ISBN 9781482246407)

Chapter 3.55   DIHYDROCOUMARIN

IDENTIFICATION

Description/definition   : Dihydrocoumarin is the heterocyclic compound that conforms to the structural formula
                             shown below
Chemical class(es)   : Ketones
Chemical/IUPAC name   : 3,4-Dihydrochromen-2-one
Other names   : Melilotin; 3,4-dihydro-2*H*-1-benzopyran-2-one
CAS registry number(s)   : 119-84-6
EC number(s)   : 204-354-9
RIFM monograph(s)   : Food Cosmet Toxicol 1974;12:521
IFRA standard   : Restricted (www.ifraorg.org/en-us/standards-library) (table 3.55.1)
SCCS Opinion(s)   : SCCNFP/0320/00, final (1)
Function(s) in cosmetics   : EU: formerly used for masking and perfuming. USA: fragrance ingredients
EU cosmetic restrictions   : Regulated in Annex II/427 of the Regulation (EC) No. 1223/2009, regulated by
                             2002/34/EC (prohibited, delisted in 2004)
Patch testing   : 5% pet.(2,4)
Molecular formula   : $C_9H_8O_2$

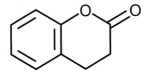

Table 3.55.1 IFRA restrictions for dihydrocoumarin

Category [a]	Limits [b]	Category [a]	Limits [b]	Category [a]	Limits [b]
1	0.03%	5	0.24%	9	5.00%
2	0.04%	6	0.72%	10	2.50%
3	0.15%	7	0.08%	11	not restricted
4	0.45%	8	1.01%		

[a] For explanation of categories see pages 6-8
[b] Limits in the finished products

GENERAL

Dihydrocoumarin is a colorless to pale yellow clear liquid to solid; its odor type is tonka and its odor is described as 'sweet, creamy, coconut, coumarin, vanilla with a slight spice nuance' (www.thegoodscentscompany.com).

Presence in essential oils

Dihydrocoumarin has been identified by chemical analysis in three of 91 essential oils, which have caused contact allergy / allergic contact dermatitis: lavender oil, pine needle oil (Scots pine oil) and spike lavender oil (11).

CONTACT ALLERGY

General

The sensitizing potency of dihydrocoumarin was classified as 'moderate' based on an EC3 value of 5.6% in the LLNA (local lymph node assay) in animal experiments (9,10). In other experiments, it was shown to have moderate to strong sensitizing potency (6,7,12). It has been suggested that dihydrocoumarin is a sensitizing contaminant in commercial coumarin (6).

Patch testing in groups of patients

Studies in which dihydrocoumarin was patch tested in consecutive patients suspected of contact dermatitis (routine testing) with positive results have not been found.

The fragrance has been tested in 2 studies in groups of selected patients (2,4). Before 1989, the members of the European Environmental Contact Dermatitis Research Group (EECDRG) tested 53 patients reacting to an experimental fragrance mix containing dihydrocoumarin (n=41) or to the FM I but not the experimental mix (n=12) with dihydrocoumarin 5% pet. and there were 11 (21%) reactions (4). In 1983, in The Netherlands, 182 patients suspected of cosmetic allergy were tested with dihydrocoumarin 5% pet. and there were 7 (3.7%) positive patch test reactions (2). In neither study was the relevance of these positive reactions mentioned.

Case reports and case series
A baker who later became cook had recurrent dermatitis of the hands, arms and face. He was known to react to his wife's perfumes and used fragranced cosmetic products himself. He had no reactions to any spice that he brought in himself, but when tested with a battery of fragrances, there were positive reactions to dihydrocoumarin 5%, eugenol 8%, phenylacetaldehyde 2%, methyl 2-octynoate 0.5% and cinnamyl benzoate 10%, all in petrolatum. The author was 'inclined' to say that these reactions may have been relevant (5).

Cross-reactions, pseudo-cross-reactions and co-reactions
For general information on cross-/pseudo-cross-/co-reactivity of fragrance chemicals with other fragrances, fragrance markers (fragrance mix I, fragrance mix II, colophonium, Myroxylon pereirae resin [balsam of Peru]) and essential oils see Chapter 1.2 General information on cross-reactions, pseudo-cross-reactions and co-reactions.
    No cross-reactivity to or from coumarin was observed (6).

Patch test sensitization
One patient patch tested with 10% dihydrocoumarin in petrolatum had a positive reaction at D17 and therefore may have been sensitized by the test; he was, however, not retested for confirmation (5).

Presence in products and chemical analyses
In 2008, 66 different fragrance components (including 39 essential oils) were identified in 370 (10% of the total) topical pharmaceutical products marketed in Belgium; 5 of these (1.4%) contained dihydrocoumarin (3). In 1993, in Denmark, dihydrocoumarin was detected in 10 out of 31 cosmetic products (8).

LITERATURE
1   SCCFNP (Scientific Committee on Cosmetic Products and Non-Food Products Intended for Consumers). Opinion of the Scientific Committee on Cosmetic Products and Non-Food Products Intended for Consumers concerning 'An initial list of perfumery materials which must not form part of fragrances compounds used in cosmetic products', 3 May 2000, SCCNFP/0320/00, final. Available at:
    http://ec.europa.eu/health/archive/ph_risk/committees/sccp/documents/out116_en.pdf
2   Malten KE, van Ketel WG, Nater JP, Liem DH. Reactions in selected patients to 22 fragrance materials. Contact Dermatitis 1984;11:1-10
3   Nardelli A, D'Hooge E, Drieghe J, Dooms M, Goossens A. Allergic contact dermatitis from fragrance components in specific topical pharmaceutical products in Belgium. Contact Dermatitis 2009;60:303-313
4   Wilkinson JD, Andersen K, Camarasa J, Ducombs G, Frosch P, Lahti A, et al. Preliminary results of the effectiveness of two forms of fragrance mix as screening agents for fragrance sensitivity. In: Frosch PJ et al, Eds. Current topics in contact dermatitis. Berlin Heidelberg New York: Springer-Verlag, 1989:127-131
5   Malten KE. Four bakers showing positive patch tests to a number of fragrance materials, which can also be used as flavors. Acta Derm Venereol 1979;59(suppl.85):117-121
6   Vocanson M, Valeyrie M, Rozières A, Hennino A, Floch F, Gard A, Nicolas J-F. Lack of evidence for allergenic properties of coumarin in a fragrance allergy mouse model. Contact Dermatitis 2007;57:361-364
7   Hausen BM, Kallweit M. The sensitizing capacity of coumarins (II). Contact Dermatitis 1986;15:289-294
8   Rastogi SC. Analysis of fragrances in cosmetics by gas chromatography-mass spectrometry. In: Sandra P, Devos G, Eds. Proceedings of the 6th International Symposium Capillary Chromatography, Riva del Garda, 27-30 September 1994. Heidelberg: Hüthig, 1994:955-967. Data cited in: Johansen JD, Rastogi SC, Menné T. Exposure to selected fragrance materials: A case study of fragrance-mix-positive eczema patients. Contact Dermatitis 1996;34:106-110
9   SCCS (Scientific Committee on Consumer Safety). Opinion on Fragrance allergens in cosmetic products, 26-27 June 2012, SCCS/1459/11. Available at:
    https://ec.europa.eu/health/sites/health/files/scientific_committees/consumer_safety/docs/sccs_o_102.pdf
10 Uter W, Johansen JD, Börje A, Karlberg A-T, Lidén C, Rastogi S, Roberts D, White IR. Categorization of fragrance contact allergens for prioritization of preventive measures: clinical and experimental data and consideration of structure–activity relationships. Contact Dermatitis 2013;69:196-230
11 De Groot AC, Schmidt E. Essential oils: contact allergy and chemical composition. Boca Raton, Fl., USA: CRC Press, Taylor and Francis Group, 2016 (ISBN 9781482246407)
12 Marzulli FN, Maibach HI. Further studies of effects of vehicles and elicitation concentration in experimental contact sensitization testing in humans. Contact Dermatitis 1980;6:131-133

Chapter 3.56   DIHYDRO PENTAMETHYLINDANONE

IDENTIFICATION

Description/definition   : Dihydro pentamethylindanone is the organic compound that conforms to the structural
                            formula shown below
Chemical class(es)   : Ketones
Chemical/IUPAC name   : 1,1,2,3,3-Pentamethyl-2,5,6,7-tetrahydroinden-4-one
Other names   : 6,7-Dihydro-1,1,2,3,3-pentamethyl-4(5H)-indanone; musk indanone; Cashmeran ®
CAS registry number(s)   : 33704-61-9
EC number(s)   : 251-649-3
IFRA standard   : Restricted (www.ifraorg.org/en-us/standards-library) (table 3.56.1)
Function(s) in cosmetics : EU: masking; perfuming. USA: fragrance ingredients
Patch testing   : 5% pet. (1)
Molecular formula   : $C_{14}H_{22}O$

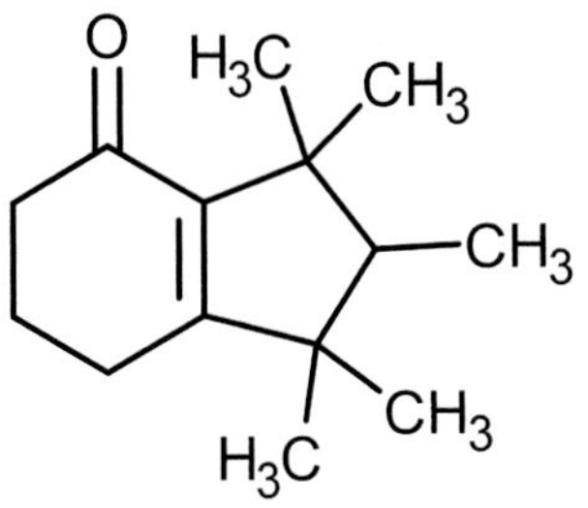

Table 3.56.1 IFRA restrictions for dihydro pentamethylindanone

Category [a]	Limits [b]	Category [a]	Limits [b]	Category [a]	Limits [b]
1	0.34%	5	2.86%	9	5.00%
2	0.44%	6	8.70%	10	2.50%
3	1.81%	7	0.91%	11	not restricted
4	5.43%	8	2.00%		

[a] For explanation of categories see pages 6-8
[b] Limits in the finished products

GENERAL

Dihydro pentamethylindanone is a colorless to pale yellow semi-solid to solid; its odor type is musk and its odor at 10% in dipropylene glycol is described as 'rich spicy musk woody clean' (www.thegoodscentscompany.com). It is a synthetic chemical, not found in nature (and consequently not in essential oils) (2).

CONTACT ALLERGY

Patch testing in consecutive patients suspected of contact dermatitis: routine testing
Studies in which dihydro pentamethylindanone was patch tested in consecutive patients suspected of contact dermatitis (routine testing) with positive results have not been found.

Patch testing in groups of selected patients
Before 1996, in Japan, some European countries and the USA, 167 patients known or suspected to be allergic to fragrances were patch tested with dihydro pentamethylindanone 5% pet. and there was one (0.6%) positive reaction; its relevance was not mentioned (1).

Case reports and case series
Case reports of allergic contact dermatitis from dihydro pentamethylindanone have not been found.

LITERATURE

1   Larsen W, Nakayama H, Fischer T, Elsner P, Burrows D, Jordan W, et al. Fragrance contact dermatitis: A worldwide multicenter investigation (Part I). Am J Cont Dermat 1996;7:77-83
2   De Groot AC, Schmidt E. Essential oils: contact allergy and chemical composition. Boca Raton, Fl., USA: CRC Press, Taylor and Francis Group, 2016 (ISBN 9781482246407)

Chapter 3.57   DIMETHYLBENZYL CARBINYL ACETATE

IDENTIFICATION

Description/definition   : Dimethylbenzyl carbinyl acetate is the aromatic ester that conforms to the structural
                              formula shown below
Chemical class(es)   : Aromatic compounds; esters
INCI name USA   : Not in the Personal Care Products Council Ingredient Database
Chemical/IUPAC name   : (2-Methyl-1-phenylpropan-2-yl) acetate
Other names   : α,α-Dimethylphenethyl acetate; 1,1-dimethyl-2-phenylethyl acetate; benzeneethanol,
                            α,α-dimethyl-, acetate
CAS registry number(s)   : 151-05-3
EC number(s)   : 205-781-3
RIFM monograph(s)   : Food Chem Toxicol 2012;50(suppl.2):S344-349; Food Cosmet Toxicol 1974;12:533
SCCS opinion(s)   : SCCS/1459/11 (1)
Function(s) in cosmetics   : EU: perfuming
Patch testing   : 5% pet. (3,4)
Molecular formula   : $C_{12}H_{16}O_2$

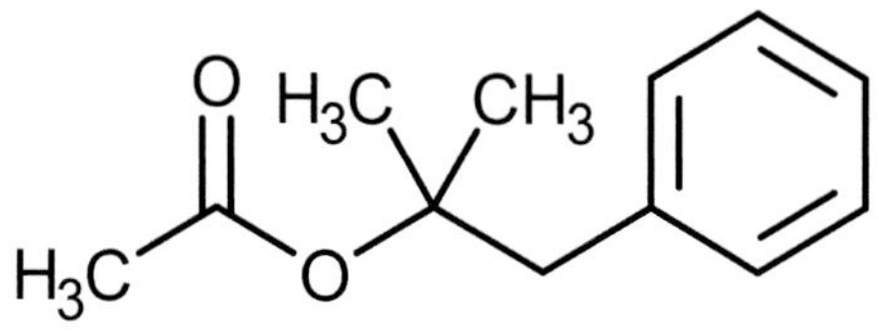

GENERAL

Dimethylbenzyl carbinyl acetate is a white to pale yellow crystalline solid; its odor type is floral and its odor at 100% is described as 'sweet floral fruity rose green pear berry jasmin powdery' (www.thegoodscentscompany.com).

Dimethylbenzyl carbinyl acetate is a synthetic chemical, not found in nature (and consequently not in essential oils (6)).

CONTACT ALLERGY

General

The SCCS (Scientific Committee on Consumer Safety), in a 2012 Opinion on Fragrance allergens in cosmetic products, has marked dimethylbenzyl carbinyl acetate as 'established contact allergen in humans' (1,5).

Patch testing in groups of patients

Patch testing in consecutive patients suspected of contact dermatitis: routine testing

Dimethylbenzyl carbinyl acetate has been patch tested in two studies in consecutive patients suspected of contact dermatitis (routine testing) (3,4). In the period 1997-1998, in six European countries, the fragrance 5% in petrolatum was tested in 1855 patients and there were 3 (0.2%) positive reactions; their relevance was not specified (4).

Before 1995, in the United Kingdom and France, 313 consecutive patients were tested with dimethylbenzyl carbinyl acetate 5% pet. and one individual (0.3%) had a positive patch test reaction; the reaction was not relevant (3).

Patch testing in groups of selected patients

Studies in which groups of selected patients were patch tested with dimethylbenzyl carbinyl acetate have not been found.

Case reports and case series

Case reports of allergic contact dermatitis from dimethylbenzyl carbinyl acetate have not been found.

Presence in products and chemical analyses

In 1988, in the USA, 400 perfumes used in fine fragrances, household products and soaps (number of products per category not mentioned) were analyzed for the presence of fragrance chemicals in a concentration of at least 1% and a list of the Top-25 (present in the highest number of products) presented. Dimethylbenzyl carbinyl acetate was found to be present in an unknown percentage of the fine fragrances, 24% of the household product fragrances (rank number 20) and 40% of the fragrances used in soaps (rank number 18) (2).

LITERATURE

1 SCCS (Scientific Committee on Consumer Safety). Opinion on Fragrance allergens in cosmetic products, 26-27 June 2012, SCCS/1459/11. Available at: https://ec.europa.eu/health/sites/health/files/scientific_committees/consumer_safety/docs/sccs_o_102.pdf

2 Fenn RS. Aroma chemical usage trends in modern perfumery. Perfumer and Flavorist 1989;14:3-10

3 Frosch PJ, Pilz B, Andersen KE, Burrows D, Camarasa JG, Dooms-Goossens A, et al. Patch testing with fragrances: results of a multicenter study of the European Environmental and Contact Dermatitis Research Group with 48 frequently used constituents of perfumes. Contact Dermatitis 1995;33:333-342

4 Frosch PJ, Johansen JD, Menné T, Pirker C, Rastogi SC, Andersen KE, et al. Further important sensitizers in patients sensitive to fragrances. I. Reactivity to 14 frequently used chemicals. Contact Dermatitis 2002;47:78-85

5 Uter W, Johansen JD, Börje A, Karlberg A-T, Lidén C, Rastogi S, Roberts D, White IR. Categorization of fragrance contact allergens for prioritization of preventive measures: clinical and experimental data and consideration of structure–activity relationships. Contact Dermatitis 2013;69:196-230

6 De Groot AC, Schmidt E. Essential oils: contact allergy and chemical composition. Boca Raton, Fl., USA: CRC Press, Taylor and Francis Group, 2016 (ISBN 9781482246407)

Chapter 3.58   DIMETHYL CITRACONATE *

Not an INCI name

IDENTIFICATION

Description/definition   : Dimethyl citraconate is the reaction product of methanol and citraconic anhydride,
                            that conforms to the structural formula shown below
Chemical class(es)   : Unsaturated organic compounds; esters
INCI name USA   : Not in the Personal Care Products Council Ingredient Database
Chemical/IUPAC name   : Dimethyl-2-methylbut-2-enedioate
Other names   : Dimethyl methyl maleate
CAS registry number(s)   : 617-54-9
EC number(s)   : Not available
RIFM monograph(s)   : Food Cosmet Toxicol 1976;14:749 (special issue III)
IFRA standard   : Prohibited (www.ifraorg.org/en-us/standards-library)
SCCS opinion(s)   : SCCNFP/0320/00, final (1)
Function(s) in cosmetics : EU: formerly used for perfuming
EU cosmetic restrictions : Regulated in Annex II/431 of the Regulation (EC) No. 1223/2009, regulated by
                            2002/34/EC; Prohibited since 2002
Patch testing   : 10% pet. (2)
Molecular formula   : $C_7H_{10}O_4$

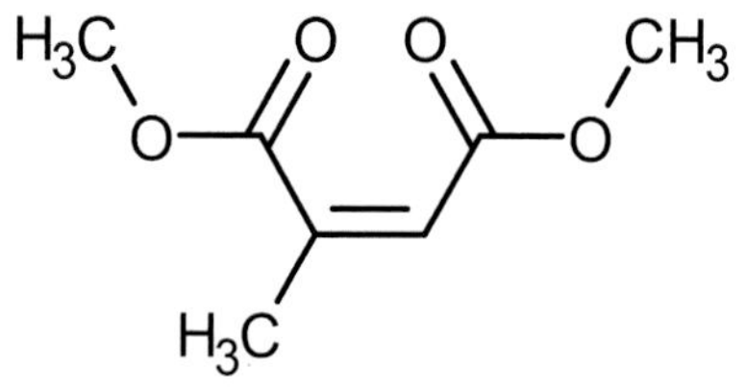

GENERAL

Dimethyl citraconate is a colorless clear liquid. It is a synthetic chemical, not found in nature (and consequently not in essential oils [4]). Dimethyl citraconate is prohibited by IFRA because of sensitization (www.ifraorg.org) and is not used anymore.

CONTACT ALLERGY

Patch testing in groups of patients

Studies in which dimethyl citraconate was patch tested in consecutive patients suspected of contact dermatitis (routine testing) with positive results have not been found. In one investigation, the chemical was tested in a group of selected patients (3). In 1983, in The Netherlands, 182 patients suspected of cosmetic allergy were patch tested with dimethyl citraconate 12% pet. and there were 7 (3.8%) positive reactions. Their relevance was not mentioned and it is likely that some of these reactions have been false-positive, irritant (3).

Case reports and case series

Case reports of allergic contact dermatitis from dimethyl citraconate have not been found.

LITERATURE

1 Opinion of the Scientific Committee on Cosmetic Products and Non-Food Products Intended for Consumers concerning 'An initial list of perfumery materials which must not form part of fragrances compounds used in cosmetic products', 3 May 2000, SCCNFP/0320/00, final. Available at: http://ec.europa.eu/health/archive/ph_risk/committees/sccp/documents/out116_en.pdf
2 De Groot AC. Patch Testing, 4th Edition. Wapserveen, The Netherlands: acdegroot publishing, 2018 (ISBN 978-90-813233-4-5)
3 Malten KE, van Ketel WG, Nater JP, Liem DH. Reactions in selected patients to 22 fragrance materials. Contact Dermatitis 1984;11:1-10
4 De Groot AC, Schmidt E. Essential oils: contact allergy and chemical composition. Boca Raton, Fl., USA: CRC Press, Taylor and Francis Group, 2016 (ISBN 9781482246407)

Chapter 3.59   2,4-DIMETHYL-3-CYCLOHEXENE CARBOXALDEHYDE

IDENTIFICATION

Description/definition : 2,4-Dimethyl-3-cyclohexene carboxaldehyde is the organic compound that conforms to the structural formula shown below

Chemical class(es) : Cyclic organic compounds; aldehydes

Chemical/IUPAC name : 2,4-Dimethylcyclohex-3-ene-1-carbaldehyde

Other names : 4-Formyl-1,3-dimethylcyclohex-1-ene; 2,4-ivy carbaldehyde; Ligustral ®; Triplal ®

CAS registry number(s) : 68039-49-6

EC number(s) : 268-264-1

Function(s) in cosmetics : EU: masking; perfuming; tonic. USA: fragrance ingredients

Patch testing : 5% Schiff's base (1); 5% pet. (3)

Molecular formula : $C_9H_{14}O$

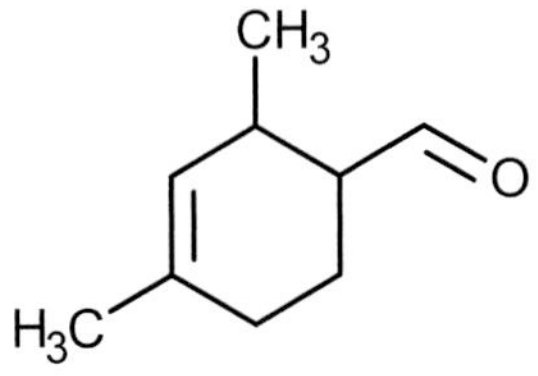

GENERAL

2,4-Dimethyl-3-cyclohexene carboxaldehyde is very similar to dimethyltetrahydro benzaldehyde (Chapter 3.60). Data in various chemical databases such as ChemSpider, ChemIDPlus, PubChem en ECHA are not unambiguous and rather confusing.

2,4-Dimethyl-3-cyclohexene carboxaldehyde is a colorless to pale yellow clear liquid; its odor type is green and its odor at 10% in dipropylene glycol is described as 'green aldehydic leafy cortex tart floral peely' (www.thegood scentscompany.com). It is a synthetic chemical, not found in nature (and consequently not in essential oils (4)).

CONTACT ALLERGY

Patch testing in groups of patients

Before 1996, in Japan, some European countries and the USA, 167 patients known or suspected to be allergic to fragrances were patch tested with 2,4-dimethyl-3-cyclohexene carboxaldehyde and there was one (0.6%) positive reaction; its relevance was not mentioned (1).

Case reports and case series

Case reports of allergic contact dermatitis from 2,4-dimethyl-3-cyclohexene carboxaldehyde have not been found.

Presence in products and chemical analyses

In 2000, fifty-nine domestic and occupational products, purchased in retail outlets in Denmark, England, Germany and Italy were analyzed by GC-MS for the presence of fragrances. The product categories were liquid soap and soap bars (n=13), soft/hard surface cleaners (n=23), fabric conditioners/laundry detergents for hand wash (n=8), dish wash (n=10), furniture polish, car shampoo, stain remover (each n=1) and 2 products used in occupational environments. 2,4-Dimethyl-3-cyclohexene carboxaldehyde (Triplal ®) was present in 5 products; quantification was not performed (2).

LITERATURE

1   Larsen W, Nakayama H, Fischer T, Elsner P, Burrows D, Jordan W, et al. Fragrance contact dermatitis: A worldwide multicenter investigation (Part I). Am J Cont Dermat 1996;7:77-83

2   Rastogi SC, Heydorn S, Johansen JD, Basketter DA. Fragrance chemicals in domestic and occupational products. Contact Dermatitis 2001;45:221-225

3   An S, Lee AY, Lee CH, Kim DW, Hahm JH, Kim KJ, et al. Fragrance contact dermatitis in Korea: a joint study. Contact Dermatitis 2005;53:320-323

4   De Groot AC, Schmidt E. Essential oils: contact allergy and chemical composition. Boca Raton, Fl., USA: CRC Press, Taylor and Francis Group, 2016 (ISBN 9781482246407)

Chapter 3.60   DIMETHYLTETRAHYDRO BENZALDEHYDE

IDENTIFICATION

Description/definition   : Dimethyltetrahydro benzaldehyde is the unsaturated cyclic aldehyde that conforms to the structural formula shown below
Chemical class(es)   : Cyclic organic compounds; aldehydes
INCI name USA   : Not in the Personal Care Products Council Ingredient Database
Chemical/IUPAC name   : 2,4(or 3,5)-Dimethyl-3-cyclohexene-1-carboxaldehyde; Hivertal ®
CAS registry number(s)   : 68737-61-1
EC number(s)   : 272-113-5
RIFM monograph(s)   : Food Chem Toxicol 1992;30(suppl.1):S29 (4)
SCCS opinion(s)   : SCCS/1459/11 (1)
Function(s) in cosmetics : EU: perfuming
Patch testing   : 5% pet. (2)
Molecular formula   : $C_9H_{14}O$

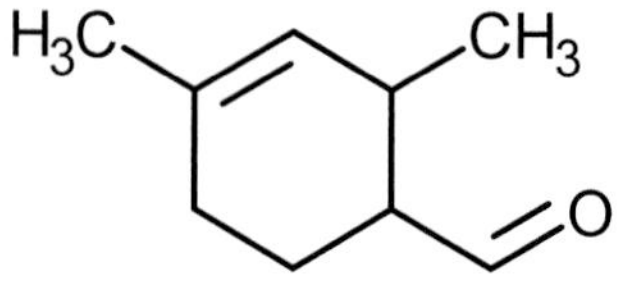

GENERAL

Dimethyltetrahydro benzaldehyde is very similar to 2,4-dimethyl-3-cyclohexene carboxaldehyde (Chapter 3.59). Data in various chemical databases such as ChemSpider, ChemIDPlus, PubChem en ECHA are not unambiguous and rather confusing.

There is no information on the physical properties and odor description of dimethyltetrahydro benzaldehyde on www.thegoodscentscompany.com. It is a synthetic chemical, not found in nature (and consequently not in essential oils). According to RIFM, it is a mixture of isomers, a colorless liquid with a sweet-green, leafy odor (4).

CONTACT ALLERGY

The SCCS (Scientific Committee on Consumer Safety), in a 2012 Opinion on Fragrance allergens in cosmetic products, has categorized dimethyltetrahydro benzaldehyde as 'likely fragrance contact allergen by combination of evidence' (1,3).

Patch testing in consecutive patients suspected of contact dermatitis: routine testing

Studies in which dimethyltetrahydro benzaldehyde was patch tested in consecutive patients suspected of contact dermatitis (routine testing) with positive results have not been found.

Patch testing in groups of selected patients

In 2000, in Japan, USA and several European countries, 178 patients with known fragrance sensitivity were tested with a series of fragrances and there were 4 (2.3%) positive patch test reactions to dimethyltetrahydro benzaldehyde 5% pet. The relevance of these reactions was not mentioned. The test substance was an isomer mixture (2).

Case reports and case series

Case reports of allergic contact dermatitis from dimethyltetrahydro benzaldehyde have not been found.

LITERATURE

1   SCCS (Scientific Committee on Consumer Safety). Opinion on Fragrance allergens in cosmetic products, 26-27 June 2012, SCCS/1459/11. Available at: https://ec.europa.eu/health/sites/health/files/scientific_committees/consumer_safety/docs/sccs_o_102.pdf
2   Larsen W, Nakayama H, Fischer T, Elsner P, Frosch P, Burrows D, et al. Fragrance contact dermatitis: A worldwide multicenter investigation (Part II). Contact Dermatitis 2001;44:344-346
3   Uter W, Johansen JD, Börje A, Karlberg A-T, Lidén C, Rastogi S, Roberts D, White IR. Categorization of fragrance contact allergens for prioritization of preventive measures: clinical and experimental data and consideration of structure–activity relationships. Contact Dermatitis 2013;69:196-230
4   Research Institute for Fragrance Materials (RIFM). Dimethyltetrahydrobenzaldehyde. Food Chem Toxicol 1992;30(suppl.1):S29

Chapter 3.61   ETHYL ANISATE

IDENTIFICATION

Description/definition	: Ethyl anisate is the aromatic compound that conforms to the structural formula shown below
Chemical class(es)	: Aromatic compounds; esters
INCI name USA	: Not in the Personal Care Products Council Ingredient Database
Chemical/IUPAC name	: Ethyl 4-methoxybenzoate
Other names	: Ethyl *p*-methoxybenzoate; ethyl *p*-anisate
CAS registry number(s)	: 94-30-4
EC number(s)	: 202-320-8
RIFM monograph(s)	: Food Cosmet Toxicol 1976;14(suppl.):757
Function(s) in cosmetics	: EU: perfuming
Patch testing	: 4% pet. (2); based on RIFM data, 4% pet. is probably not irritant (1)
Molecular formula	: $C_{10}H_{12}O_3$

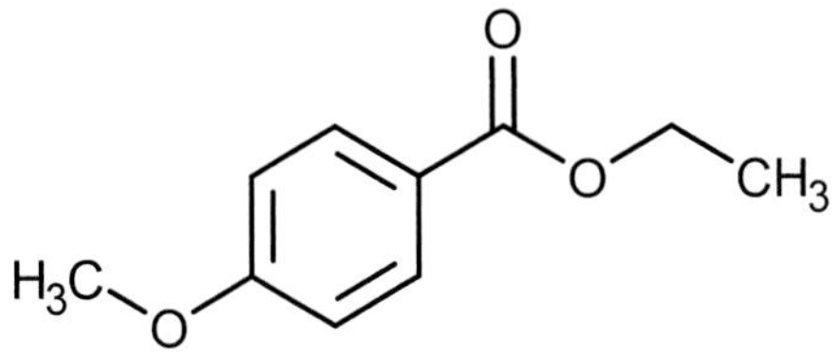

GENERAL

Ethyl anisate is a colorless to pale yellow clear oily liquid; its odor type is anisic and its odor is described as 'sweet anisic, licorice, fruity, spice, cherry, floral and powdery' (www.thegoodscentscompany.com).

Presence in essential oils

Ethyl anisate has been identified by chemical analysis in none of 91 essential oils, which have caused contact allergy / allergic contact dermatitis (3).

CONTACT ALLERGY

Patch testing in groups of patients

Studies in which ethyl anisate was patch tested in either consecutive patients suspected of contact dermatitis (routine testing) or in groups of selected patients with positive results have not been found.

Case reports and case series

A metal grinder who previously suffered from posttraumatic thrombosis developed lower leg ulcers and later a weeping stasis dermatitis. When patch tested, the patient reacted to several allergens, including the paraben-mix, 3 topical pharmaceutical preparations containing parabens, and to methyl and ethyl anisate. The patient denied using perfumes, although – according to the author – perfumes may have been present in some cosmetics or therapeutics used by him. The author further suggested that the reaction to the perfume ingredients should be regarded as group specific reactions (cross-reactions) in a patient contact sensitized to parabens present in topically applied medicaments, because of the chemical similarities between the parabens and the anisates (2).

Cross-reactions, pseudo-cross-reactions and co-reactions

For general information on cross-/pseudo-cross-/co-reactivity of fragrance chemicals with other fragrances, fragrance markers (fragrance mix I, fragrance mix II, colophonium, Myroxylon pereirae resin [balsam of Peru]) and essential oils see Chapter 1.2 General information on cross-reactions, pseudo-cross-reactions and co-reactions.

Possibly to or from methyl *p*-anisate (2); possibly to or more likely from parabens (2).

LITERATURE

1   De Groot AC. Patch Testing, 4th Edition. Wapserveen, The Netherlands: acdegroot publishing, 2018 (ISBN 978-90-813233-4-5)
2   Malten KE. Sensitization to solcoseryl and methylanisate (fragrance ingredient). Contact Dermatitis 1977;3:219
3   De Groot AC, Schmidt E. Essential oils: contact allergy and chemical composition. Boca Raton, Fl., USA: CRC Press, Taylor and Francis Group, 2016 (ISBN 9781482246407)

Chapter 3.62   ETHYLENE DODECANEDIOATE

IDENTIFICATION

Description/definition   : Ethylene dodecanedioate is the organic compound that conforms to the structural
                             formula shown below
Chemical class(es)   : Esters; heterocyclic compounds
Chemical/IUPAC name   : 1,4-Dioxacyclohexadecane-5,16-dione
Other names   : Muskonate
CAS registry number(s)   : 54982-83-1
EC number(s)   : 259-423-6
RIFM monograph(s)   : Food Chem Toxicol 2017;110(suppl.1):S670-S678; Food Chem Toxicol 2011;49(suppl.2):
                             S212-S218; Food Chem Toxicol 1992;30:S31 (special issue VIII)
SCCS opinion(s)   : SCCS/1459/11 (1)
Function(s) in cosmetics   : EU: masking; perfuming. USA: fragrance ingredients
Patch testing   : 5% pet. (2)
Molecular formula   : $C_{14}H_{24}O_4$

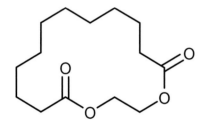

GENERAL

Ethylene dodecanedioate is a pale yellow clear oily liquid; its odor type is musk and its odor at 100% is described as
'sweet clean waxy musk animal' (www.thegoodscentscompany.com). Ethylene dodecanedioate is a synthetic
chemical, not found in nature (and consequently not in essential oils (4)).

CONTACT ALLERGY

The SCCS (Scientific Committee on Consumer Safety), in a 2012 Opinion on Fragrance allergens in cosmetic products,
has categorized ethylene dodecanedioate as 'possible fragrance contact allergen' (1,3).

Patch testing in consecutive patients suspected of contact dermatitis: routine testing

Studies in which ethylene dodecanedioate was patch tested in consecutive patients suspected of contact dermatitis
(routine testing) with positive results have not been found.

Testing in groups of selected patients

Before 2002, in Japan, European countries and the USA, 218 patients with known fragrance sensitivity were patch
tested with ethylene dodecanedioate 5% in petrolatum and two positive reactions (0.9%) were observed; their
relevance was not mentioned (2).

Case reports and case series

Case reports of allergic contact dermatitis from ethylene dodecanedioate have not been found.

LITERATURE

1   SCCS (Scientific Committee on Consumer Safety). Opinion on Fragrance allergens in cosmetic products, 26-27
    June 2012, SCCS/1459/11. Available at:
    https://ec.europa.eu/health/sites/health/files/scientific_committees/consumer_safety/docs/sccs_o_102.pdf
2   Larsen W, Nakayama H, Fischer T, Elsner P, Frosch P, Burrows D, et al. Fragrance contact dermatitis - a
    worldwide multicenter investigation (Part III). Contact Dermatitis 2002;46:141-144
3   Uter W, Johansen JD, Börje A, Karlberg A-T, Lidén C, Rastogi S, Roberts D, White IR. Categorization of fragrance
    contact allergens for prioritization of preventive measures: clinical and experimental data and consideration of
    structure–activity relationships. Contact Dermatitis 2013;69:196-230
4   De Groot AC, Schmidt E. Essential oils: contact allergy and chemical composition. Boca Raton, Fl., USA: CRC Press,
    Taylor and Francis Group, 2016 (ISBN 9781482246407)

Chapter 3.63 ETHYL VANILLIN

IDENTIFICATION

Description/definition	: Ethyl vanillin is the substituted phenolic compound that conforms to the structural formula shown below
Chemical class(es)	: Phenols
Chemical/IUPAC name	: 3-Ethoxy-4-hydroxybenzaldehyde
CAS registry number(s)	: 121-32-4
EC number(s)	: 204-464-7
RIFM monograph(s)	: Food Cosmet Toxicol 1975;13:103 (binder, page 370)
SCCS opinion(s)	: SCCS/1459/11 (1)
Merck Index monograph	: 5178
Function(s) in cosmetics	: EU: masking; soothing. USA: antioxidants; flavoring agents; fragrance Ingredients
Patch testing	: 10% pet. (5, also cited in ref. 4); however, based on RIFM data, 2% pet. may cause irritant reactions (4)
Molecular formula	: $C_9H_{10}O_3$

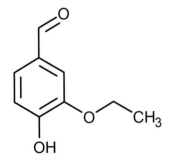

GENERAL

Ethyl vanillin is a white to off-white powder; its odor type is vanilla and its odor is described as 'sweet, creamy, vanilla, with a root berry salicylate-like nuance' (www.thegoodscentscompany.com). It has the odor and taste of vanillin but is much stronger. Ethyl vanillin is an important commercial chemical used in food flavoring, notably in the chocolate industry. In perfumery, it gives a sweet, balsamic note to flowery and fruity fragrance compositions. In addition, it is used as an intermediate to make other chemicals (in U.S. National Library of Medicine). Ethyl vanillin is a synthetic chemical, not found in nature (and consequently not in essential oils (6)).

CONTACT ALLERGY

General
The SCCS (Scientific Committee on Consumer Safety), in a 2012 Opinion on Fragrance allergens in cosmetic products, has categorized ethyl vanillin as 'likely fragrance contact allergen by combination of evidence' (1,2).

Patch testing in groups of patients

Patch testing in consecutive patients suspected of contact dermatitis: routine testing
Studies in which ethyl vanillin was patch tested in consecutive patients suspected of contact dermatitis (routine testing) with positive results have not been found.

Patch testing in groups of selected patients
In a group of 65 patients allergic to Myroxylon pereirae resin (balsam of Peru, MP) and tested with ethyl vanillin 10% pet., there were 9 (14%) positive reactions to ethyl vanillin 10% pet. (which is not present in MP); all also reacted to vanillin (which is present in MP) (5).

Case reports and case series
Case reports of allergic contact dermatitis from ethyl vanillin have not been found.

Cross-reactions, pseudo-cross-reactions and co-reactions

For general information on cross-/pseudo-cross-/co-reactivity of fragrance chemicals with other fragrances, fragrance markers (fragrance mix I, fragrance mix II, colophonium, Myroxylon pereirae resin [balsam of Peru]) and essential oils see Chapter 1.2 General information on cross-reactions, pseudo-cross-reactions and co-reactions.

Vanillin, vanillyl alcohol, coniferyl benzoate (5). Reactions to ethyl vanillin in patients allergic to Myroxylon pereirae resin (balsam of Peru) in one study only occurred in those also reacting to natural vanilla. Conversely, however, patients allergic to vanilla do not necessarily react to ethyl vanillin (5).

OTHER SIDE EFFECTS

Immediate-type reactions

A woman had immediate positive reactions to patch tests with 1% and 2% ethyl vanillin (probably in petrolatum); a similar reaction was seen with Myroxylon pereirae resin (3). She had contact with ethyl vanillin at work and had dermatitis of the flexor aspects of both forearms, but the role of ethyl vanillin in the development of this dermatitis was uncertain (3).

LITERATURE

1   SCCS (Scientific Committee on Consumer Safety). Opinion on Fragrance allergens in cosmetic products, 26-27 June 2012, SCCS/1459/11. Available at:
     https://ec.europa.eu/health/sites/health/files/scientific_committees/consumer_safety/docs/sccs_o_102.pdf
2   Uter W, Johansen JD, Börje A, Karlberg A-T, Lidén C, Rastogi S, Roberts D, White IR. Categorization of fragrance contact allergens for prioritization of preventive measures: clinical and experimental data and consideration of structure–activity relationships. Contact Dermatitis 2013;69:196-230
3   Rudzki E, Grzywa Z. Immediate reactions to balsam of Peru, cassia oil and ethyl vanillin. Contact Dermatitis 1976;2:360-361
4   De Groot AC. Patch Testing, 4th Edition. Wapserveen, The Netherlands: acdegroot publishing, 2018 (ISBN 978-90-813233-4-5)
5   Hjorth N. Eczematous allergy to balsams. Acta Derm Venereol 1961;41(suppl.46):1-216
6   De Groot AC, Schmidt E. Essential oils: contact allergy and chemical composition. Boca Raton, Fl., USA: CRC Press, Taylor and Francis Group, 2016 (ISBN 9781482246407)

Chapter 3.64   EUCALYPTOL

IDENTIFICATION

Description/definition : Eucalyptol is the organic compound that conforms to the structural formula shown below
Chemical class(es)   : Ethers
Chemical/IUPAC name   : 2,2,4-Trimethyl-3-oxabicyclo[2.2.2]octane
Other names   : 1,8-Cineole; cajeputol
CAS registry number(s) : 470-82-6
EC number(s)   : 207-431-5
RIFM monograph(s)   : Food Cosmet Toxicol 1975;13:105
Merck Index monograph   : 5208
Function(s) in cosmetics : EU: denaturant; perfuming; tonic. USA: denaturants; fragrance ingredients; oral
                          health care drugs
Patch testing   : 2% pet. (SmartPracticeEurope)
Molecular formula   : $C_{10}H_{18}O$

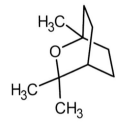

GENERAL

Eucalyptol is a colorless clear liquid; its odor type is herbal and its odor at 10% in dipropylene glycol is described as 'eucalyptus herbal camphor medicinal' (www.thegoodscentscompany.com). Eucalyptol is used as a fragrance and flavoring agent in foods, candies, cough drops, personal care products and medications. It has also been used as a flavor in tobacco. It is present in many consumer products such as mouthwash, waxes for leather, flooring, air fresheners and pine oil-based cleaners (U.S. National Library of Medicine).

Presence in essential oils, Myroxylon pereirae resin (balsam of Peru) and propolis

Eucalyptol has been identified by chemical analysis in 78 of 91 essential oils, which have caused contact allergy / allergic contact dermatitis. In 19 oils, eucalyptol belonged to the 'Top-10' of ingredients with the highest concentrations. These are shown in table 3.64.1 with the concentration range which may be expected in commercial essential oils of this type (7). Eucalyptol may also be present in Myroxylon pereirae resin (balsam of Peru) (9) and in propolis (10).

Table 3.64.1 Essential oils containing eucalyptol in the 'Top-10' and concentration range in commercial oils (7)

Essential oil	Concentration range (min. - max.)	Essential oil	Concentration range (min. - max.)
Basil oil	0.03 - 13.7%	Peppermint oil	0.3 - 9.9%
Cajeput oil	46.0 - 70.2%	Ravensara oil	0.1 - 68.0%
Cardamom oil	23.0 - 35.0%	Rosemary oil	7.6 - 59.8%
Eucalyptus citriodora oil	0.1 - 2.0%	Sage oil Dalmatian	2.1 - 12.1%
Eucalyptus globulus oil	61.6 - 88.7%	Sage oil Spanish	10.0 - 30.0%
Ginger oil	0.4 - 8.9%	Spearmint oil	0.01 - 4.4%
Laurel leaf oil	38.4 - 52.0%	Spike lavender oil	3.2 - 31.2%
Lavandin oil	3.0 - 9.9%	Tea tree oil	0.5 - 18.3%
Lavender oil	0.01 - 2.4%	Thyme oil	0.2 - 36.5%
Niaouli oil	45.3 - 61.2%		

CONTACT ALLERGY

Eucalyptol is a minor allergen in tea tree oil. Of 54 patients allergic to tea tree oil and tested with a number of its ingredients in various studies, 1 (2%) reacted to eucalyptol (5).

Patch testing in groups of patients

Studies in which eucalyptol was patch tested in either consecutive patients suspected of contact dermatitis (routine testing) or in groups of selected patients with positive results have not been found.

Case reports and case series

A man with long-standing atopic dermatitis had been treated by a doctor from a 'Clinical Ecologic Allergy Centre' with tea tree oil applied undiluted to the skin. After initial improvement, the patient suspected that the dermatitis was becoming worse from the medicament. He was then advised to ingest the oil mixed with honey; this resulted in obvious exacerbation of the dermatitis. Patch tests with the European standard series, additional series and the patient's own products gave positive reactions to undiluted tea tree oil only. Later, he was patch tested with its main ingredients, determined by gas chromatography – mass spectrometry: alpha- and beta-pinene, p-cymene, eucalyptol, linalool, terpineol, and beta-caryophyllene. The oil was again positive, as was eucalyptol 5% pet. Twenty controls were negative to both materials (although undiluted tea tree oil may certainly induce irritant reactions) (6). Commercial tea tree oils have been shown to contain up to 18.3% eucalyptol (7).

An athlete developed allergic contact dermatitis from an analgesic and anti-inflammatory cream. When patch tested with its ingredients, he reacted to eucalyptus oil 1% pet. Commercial eucalyptus globulus oils (ex *Eucalyptus globulus* Labill.) may contain up to 88% eucalyptol (7). Although the title of this case reports suggest that eucalyptol was the culprit allergen, its causal role was not proven, as eucalyptol was not tested separately (8).

One case of contact allergy to eucalyptol present in a topical pharmaceutical preparation has been reported from Belgium (2).

Presence in products and chemical analyses

In 2008, 66 different fragrance components (including 39 essential oils) were identified in 370 (10% of the total) topical pharmaceutical products marketed in Belgium; 47 of these 370 products (13%) contained eucalyptol (2).

In 2000, fifty-nine domestic and occupational products, purchased in retail outlets in Denmark, England, Germany and Italy were analyzed by GC-MS for the presence of fragrances. The product categories were liquid soap and soap bars (n=13), soft/hard surface cleaners (n=23), fabric conditioners/laundry detergents for hand wash (n=8), dish wash (n=10), furniture polish, car shampoo, stain remover (each n=1) and 2 products used in occupational environments. Eucalyptol was present in 24 products (41%) with a mean concentration of 76 ppm and a range of 15-446 ppm (3).

In 1997, 71 deodorants (22 vapo-sprays, 22 aerosol sprays and 27 roll-on products) were collected in Denmark, England, France, Germany and Sweden and analyzed by gas chromatography – mass spectrometry (GC-MS) for the presence of fragrances and other materials. Eucalyptol was present in 12 (17%) of the products (4).

OTHER SIDE EFFECTS

Irritant contact dermatitis

In Belgium, nine children of 1 months – 3 years old accidentally received eucalyptol drops in the nose. Immediately thereafter, the parents were alarmed by the child's forceful crying. All children smelled of eucalyptol. Four had irritated nasal mucous membranes and one had tachycardia. In Belgium, eucalyptol and menthol at that time were often sold in the same little bottle as NaCl 0.9%, which led to accidental instillation of the wrong drops (1).

Systemic side effects

In France, two children aged 2 years and 3 months who received a cosmetic baby balm on the skin of their thorax containing eucalyptus, rosemary and lavender essential oils, developed convulsions. As there was no other explanation for this and the 'neurologic toxicity of terpene derivatives is well known' (referring to studies on camphor toxicity), the cosmetic was suspected to be the culprit product. Although no specific terpene ingredient was blamed, the authors discussed the possible role of camphor, menthol and eucalyptol (1,8-cineole). On the basis of these 2 hardly convincing cases, the product was withdrawn from the market (11).

LITERATURE

1   Melis K, Bochner A, Janssens G. Accidental nasal eucalyptol and menthol instillation. Eur J Pediatr 1989;148:786-787

2   Nardelli A, D'Hooge E, Drieghe J, Dooms M, Goossens A. Allergic contact dermatitis from fragrance components in specific topical pharmaceutical products in Belgium. Contact Dermatitis 2009;60:303-313

3   Rastogi SC, Heydorn S, Johansen JD, Basketter DA. Fragrance chemicals in domestic and occupational products. Contact Dermatitis 2001;45:221-225

4   Rastogi SC, Lepoittevin J-P, Johansen JD, Frosch PJ, Menné T, Bruze M, et al. Fragrances and other materials in deodorants: search for potentially sensitizing molecules using combined GC-MS and structure activity relationship (SAR) analysis. Contact Dermatitis 1998;39:293-303

5   De Groot AC, Schmidt E. Tea tree oil: contact allergy and chemical composition. Contact Dermatitis 2016;75:129-143

6   De Groot AC, Weijland JW. Systemic contact dermatitis from tea tree oil. Contact Dermatitis 1992;27:279-280

7   De Groot AC, Schmidt E. Essential oils: contact allergy and chemical composition. Boca Raton, Fl., USA: CRC Press, Taylor and Francis Group, 2016 (ISBN 9781482246407)

8   Vilaplana J, Romaguera C. Allergic contact dermatitis due to eucalyptol in an anti-inflammatory cream. Contact Dermatitis 2000;43:118

9   Mammerler V. Contribution to the analysis and quality control of Peru Balsam. PhD Thesis, University of Vienna, Austria, 2007. Available at: http://othes.univie.ac.at/4056/1/2009-03-23_0201578.pdf

10 De Groot AC, Popova MP, Bankova VS. An update on the constituents of poplar-type propolis. Wapserveen, The Netherlands: acdegroot publishing, 2014, 11 pages. ISBN/EAN: 978-90-813233-0-7. Available at: https://www.researchgate.net/publication/262851225_AN_UPDATE_ON_THE_CONSTITUENTS_OF_POPLAR-TYPE_PROPOLIS

11 Laribière A, Miremont-Salamé G, Bertrand S, François C, Haramburu F. Terpènes dans les cosmétiques: 2 cas d'épilepsie. Thérapie 2005;60: 607-609

Chapter 3.65   EUGENOL

IDENTIFICATION

Description/definition	: Eugenol is the substituted phenol that conforms to the structural formula shown below
Chemical class(es)	: Ethers; phenols
Chemical/IUPAC name	: 2-Methoxy-4-prop-2-enylphenol
CAS registry number(s)	: 97-53-0
EC number(s)	: 202-589-1
RIFM monograph(s)	: Food Chem Toxicol 2016;97(suppl.):S25-S37; Food Cosmet Toxicol 1975;13:545
IFRA standard	: Restricted (www.ifraorg.org/en-us/standards-library) (table 3.65.1)
SCCS opinion(s)	: Various (12); SCCS/1459/11 (13)
Merck Index monograph	: 5210
Function(s) in cosmetics	: EU: denaturant; perfuming; tonic. USA: denaturants; fragrance ingredients
EU cosmetic restrictions	: Regulated in Annex III/71 of the Regulation (EC) No. 1223/2009, regulated by 2003/15/EC; Must be labeled on cosmetics and detergent products, if present at > 10 ppm (0.001%) in leave-on products and > 100 ppm (0.01%) in rinse-off products
Patch testing	: 1% pet. (SmartPracticeEurope, SmartPracticeCanada); 2% pet. (Chemotechnique); also present in the fragrance mix I; TEST ADVICE: 2% pet.
Molecular formula	: $C_{10}H_{12}O_2$

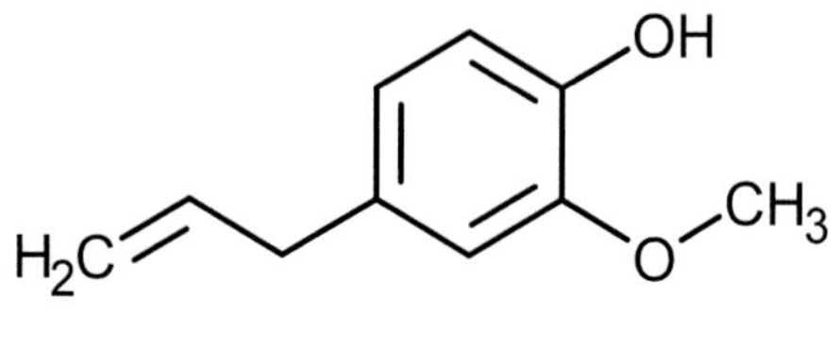

Table 3.65.1 IFRA restrictions for eugenol

Category [a]	Limits [b]	Category [a]	Limits [b]	Category [a]	Limits [b]
1	0.20%	5	0.50%	9	0.50%
2	0.20%	6	4.30%	10	0.50%
3	0.50%	7	0.40%	11	not restricted
4	0.50%	8	0.50%		

[a] For explanation of categories see pages 6-8
[b] Limits in the finished products

GENERAL

Eugenol is a pale yellow to dark yellow clear liquid; its odor type is spicy and its odor at 10% in dipropylene glycol is described as 'sweet spicy clove woody' (www.thegoodscentscompany.com). Eugenol is used in perfumery in clove and carnation compositions as well as for oriental and spicy notes. It is a common component of clove and other aroma compositions. Eugenol from clove leaf oil sources is used as a chemical raw material for conversion to several derivatives, the most important of which is isoeugenol, which in turn is used to produce vanillin. Zinc oxide-eugenol cements have many uses in dentistry; the admixture of powdered zinc oxide and liquid eugenol forms a bland, easily mixed paste having excellent working time but slow-setting antiseptic characteristics that is used in temporary luting and filling material, pulp capping and periodontal packs. Indeed, eugenol is found as a major ingredient in a variety of dental materials such as impression materials, filling materials, dental cements, endodontic sealers, periodontal dressing materials and dry socket dressings (94). In combination with geraniol, eugenol is applied as a kairomone insect attractant which is used widely for monitoring new infestations of the Japanese beetle *Popillia japonica* and for removal trapping in orchards. Eugenol may also be used as a denaturant for alcohol (U.S. National Library of Medicine).

Eugenol is one of the 8 ingredients of the Fragrance mix I (Chapter 3.70 Fragrance mix I).

Presence in essential oils and Myroxylon pereirae resin (balsam of Peru)

Eugenol has been identified by chemical analysis in 54 of 91 essential oils, which have caused contact allergy / allergic contact dermatitis. In 5 oils, eugenol belonged to the 'Top-10' of ingredients with the highest concentrations which may be expected in commercial essential oils of this type: clove bud/leaf/stem oil (75.7-90.4%), cinnamon leaf oil Sri Lanka (72.2-81.6%), bay oil (41.4-54.0%), cinnamon bark oil Sri Lanka (0.2-16.4%), and basil oil (0.03-15.3%) (105). Eugenol may also be present in Myroxylon pereirae resin (balsam of Peru) (0.2% in fraction BP3) (6).

CONTACT ALLERGY

General

The SCCS (Scientific Committee on Consumer Safety), in a 2012 Opinion on Fragrance allergens in cosmetic products, has marked eugenol as 'established contact allergen in humans' (13,60). The sensitizing potency of eugenol was classified as 'moderate' based on an EC3 value of 5.3% in the LLNA (local lymph node assay) in animal experiments (13,60). Eugenol acts as a prohapten, which is a chemical that is itself non-sensitizing or low-sensitizing, but that is transformed into a hapten in the skin (bioactivation), usually via enzymatic catalysis (114).

Eugenol is a constituent of the fragrance mix I. In groups of patients reacting to the mix and tested with its 8 ingredients, eugenol scored 5.0-59.5% positive patch test reactions, median 12.2% and average 16.1%. It has rank number 4/5/6 (with hydroxycitronellal and cinnamyl alcohol) in the list of most frequent reactors in the mix (see Chapter 3.70 Fragrance mix I).

General population

In the period 2008-2011, in 5 European countries (Sweden, Germany, Netherlands, Portugal, Italy), a random sample of the general population of 3119 individuals aged 18-74 years were patch tested with the FM I, its 8 ingredients, the FM II, its 6 ingredients and Myroxylon pereirae resin. There were 6 reactions (0.2%) to eugenol, tested 2% in petrolatum. About half of all positive reactions to fragrances were considered to be relevant based on standardized criteria. Women were affected twice as often as men (85).

Patch testing in groups of patients

Results of studies testing in consecutive patients suspected of contact dermatitis (routine testing) are shown in table 3.65.2. Results of testing in groups of *selected* patients (e.g. patients with known or suspected fragrance or cosmetic dermatitis, individuals with eyelid dermatitis, patients with hand eczema, dentists) are shown in table 3.65.3.

Patch testing in consecutive patients suspected of contact dermatitis: routine testing

In 14 studies in which routine testing with eugenol was performed, frequencies of sensitization have ranged from 0.3% to 3.4%, but were 1.2% or lower in 12 of the 14 investigations. In 10/14 studies, no (specific) relevance data were provided. In the 4 investigations addressing the issue, 38% (54), 67% (57), 75% (2) and 50% (112) of the reactions were scored as relevant. Causative eugenol-containing products were not mentioned in any study, but in one, 96% of the relevant reactions to any of 26 fragrances tested were caused by cosmetic products (2).

Table 3.65.2 Patch testing in groups of patients: Routine testing

Years and Country	Test conc. & vehicle	Number of patients tested	positive (%)	Selection of patients (S); Relevance (R); Comments (C)	Ref.
2015-7 Netherlands		821	8 (1.0%)	R: not stated	126
2015-2016 UK	2% pet.	2084	11 (0.5%)	R: not specified for individual fragrances; 25% of patients who reacted to any fragrance or fragrance marker had a positive fragrance history	117
2010-2015 Denmark	1% pet.	6004	(0.4%)	R: present relevance 38%, past relevance 33%	54
2009-2015 Sweden	2% pet.	4483	26 (0.6%)	R: not stated	61
2013-2014 Thailand		312	3 (1.0%)	R: 67%	57
2011-2012 UK	2% pet.	1951	12 (0.6%)	R: not stated	59
2010-2011 China	2% pet.	296	(3.4%)	R: 67% for all fragrances tested together (excluding FM I)	58
2008-2010 Denmark	1% pet.	1502	4 (0.3%)	S: mostly routine testing; R: 75%; 75% co-reactivity of FM I, 50% of FM II; C: of the relevant reactions to any of the 26 fragrances tested, 96% were caused by cosmetic products	2
2005-2008 IVDK	1% pet.	1214	(0.4%)	R: not stated	64
2003-2004 IVDK	1% pet.	2065	11 (0.5%)	R: not stated; C: 80% co-reactivity of FM I	4
1998-2000 Italy	1% pet.	1754	21 (1.2%)	R: in 12 patients who reacted both the eugenol and FM I, 6 (50%) were considered to have relevant reactions	112
<1995 9 European countries + USA	1% pet.	1072	13 (1.2%)	R: not stated	36
1993 EECDRG	1% pet.	709	6 (0.9%)	R: not stated	72
1991 The Netherlands	5% pet.	677	12 (1.8%)	R: not stated	74

EECDRG: European Environmental and Contact Dermatitis Research Group; FM: Fragrance mix; IVDK: Informationsverbund Dermatologischer Kliniken (Germany, Switzerland, Austria)

Patch testing in groups of selected patients

Results of studies patch testing eugenol in groups of selected patients (e.g. patients with known or suspected fragrance or cosmetic dermatitis, individuals with eyelid dermatitis, patients with hand eczema, dentists) are shown in table 3.65.3. In 15 investigations, frequencies of sensitization to eugenol have ranged from 1.3% to 56%. The highest rates were observed – as expected - in patients previously reacting to fragrances, sometimes to the fragrance mix I, which contains eugenol: 7% (62), 7.9% (127), 14% (38), 20% (15), and 56% (119). The two latter studies were performed in the 1970s and 1980s, in which time periods high concentrations of individual fragrance materials were used. In 12/13 studies no (specific) relevance data were provided; in one, it was assumed that nearly all positive reactions were of present or past relevance (8). Causative products were not mentioned.

In three investigations, patients known to be allergic to Myroxylon pereirae resin (balsam of Peru) were tested with eugenol, an ingredient of the resin. There were 14.1% (118), 19% (6) and 62% (116) positive patch tests to eugenol. The very high 62% frequency was seen in an early Danish study, in which 5% was used for testing eugenol (116). Whether this caused false-positive irritant reactions or that the lower concentrations in the other investigations led to false-negative reactions is unknown. Possibly, the balsam of Peru samples used in the various studies contained different concentrations of eugenol.

Results of testing eugenol in groups of patients reacting to the fragrance mix I (it is one of the 8 ingredients in the mix) are shown in Chapter 3.70 Fragrance mix I.

Table 3.65.3 Patch testing in groups of patients: Selected patient groups

Years and Country	Test conc. & vehicle	Number of patients tested | positive (%)		Selection of patients (S); Relevance (R); Comments (C)	Ref.
2011-2015 Spain	1% or 2% pet.	1013	80 (7.9%)	S: patients previously reacting to FM I, FM II, Myroxylon pereirae resin or hydroxyisohexyl 3-cyclohexene carboxaldehyde in the baseline series; R: not stated; C: the 2% test substances showed a higher rate of positive reactions than the 1% material	127
2007-2011 IVDK	1% pet.	67	3 (4.5%)	S: physical therapists; R: not stated	125
2006-2010 USA	2% pet.	100	2 (2%)	S: patients with eyelid dermatitis; R: not stated	10
2005-10 Netherlands		100	7 (7%)	S: patients with known fragrance sensitivity based on a positive patch test to the FM I and/or the FM II; R: not stated	62
2004-2008 Spain	2% pet.	86	12 (14%)	S: patients previously reacting to the fragrance mix I or Myroxylon pereirae (n=54) or suspected of fragrance contact allergy (n=32); R: not stated	38
2005-7 Netherlands	2% pet.	320	4 (1.3%)	S: patients suspected of fragrance or cosmetic allergy; R: 61% relevance for all positive tested fragrances together	3
<2003 Israel		91	4 (4%)	S: patients with a positive or doubtful reaction to the fragrance mix and/or Myroxylon pereirae resin and/or to one or two commercial fine fragrances; R: not stated	37
2002-2003 Korea	2% pet.	422	8 (1.9%)	S: patients with suspected cosmetic dermatitis; R: not stated	35
2001-2 Denmark, Sweden	5% pet.	658	13 (2.0%)	S: consecutive patients with hand eczema; R: it was assumed that nearly all positive reactions were of present or past relevance	8
1997-2000 Austria	1% pet.	747	19 (2.5%)	S: patients suspected of fragrance allergy: R: not stated	7
<1996 Japan, Europe, USA	5% pet.	167	13 (7.8%)	S: patients known or suspected to be allergic to fragrances; R: not stated	9
1968-1987 Poland	2% pet.	92	5 (5%)	S: dentists; R: not stated	101
1986 France		9	5 (56%)	S: patients with dermatitis caused by perfumes; R: not stated	119
<1985 Netherlands		242	13 (5.4%)	S: randomly selected patients with proven contact allergy of different origins; R: not stated	77
1975 USA	2% pet.	20	4 (20%)	S: fragrance-allergic patients; R: not stated	15

Testing in patients allergic to Myroxylon pereirae resin (balsam of Peru)

1995-1998 Germany	2% pet.	102	19 (19%)	R: ingredient of Balsam of Peru	6
<1976 USA, Canada, Europe		142	20 (14.1%)	R: ingredient of Balsam of Peru	118
1955-1960 Denmark	5% pet.	127	79 (62%)	R: ingredient of balsam of Peru	116

Testing in groups of patients reacting to the fragrance mix I

Results of testing eugenol in groups of patients reacting to the fragrance mix I are shown in Chapter 3.70 Fragrance mix I

FM: Fragrance mix

Case reports and case series

Case series

Eugenol was stated to be the (or an) allergen in 12 patients in a group of 603 individuals suffering from cosmetic dermatitis, seen in the period 2010-2015 in Leuven, Belgium (53).

In the period 1996-2013, in a tertiary referral center in Valencia, Spain, 5419 patients were patch tested. Of these, 628 individuals had allergic contact dermatitis to cosmetics. In this group, eugenol was the responsible allergen in 12 cases (31, overlap with ref. 32).

In the period 2000-2009, in Leuven, Belgium, an unspecified number of patients had positive patch tests or use tests to a total of 344 cosmetic products *and* positive patch tests to FM I, FM II, and/or to one or more of 28 selected specific fragrance ingredients. In 5 of 15 patients reacting to eugenol, the presence of this fragrance in the cosmetic product(s) was confirmed by reading the product labels (63).

In the period 2000-2007, 202 patients with allergic contact dermatitis caused by cosmetics were seen in Valencia, Spain. In this group, eugenol was the allergen in 2 individuals from its presence in cologne (n=1) and in deodorant (n=1) (32, overlap with ref. 31).

In one center in Belgium, between 1985 and 1990, 3970 patients with dermatitis were patch tested. 462 of these reacted positively to patch tests with cosmetic allergens. The reactions were considered to be relevant in 68%, probably relevant in 25% and doubtfully relevant in 7% of the patients. In the list of 'most common allergens' eugenol had rank number 12 with 21 reactions. It should be appreciated that not all patients were patch tested with individual fragrances and that the presence of the allergen in cosmetic products causing dermatitis could not always be verified (at that time, ingredient labeling in the EU was not yet mandatory) (115).

In a group of 119 patients with allergic contact dermatitis from cosmetics, investigated in The Netherlands in 1986-1987, 4 cases were caused by in eugenol in aftershave, perfumes (n=2) and hair cream (29,30).

In Belgium, in the years before 1986, of 5202 consecutive patients with dermatitis patch tested, 156 were diagnosed with pure cosmetic allergy. Eugenol was the 'dermatitic ingredient' in 16 (10.3%) patients (frequency in the entire group: 0.8%). It should be realized, however, that only a very limited number of patients was tested with a fragrance series (75).

Eugenol was responsible for 4 out of 399 cases of cosmetic allergy where the causal allergen was identified in a study of the NACDG, USA, 1977-1983 (5).

Case reports

In a group of 23 patients with (photo)allergic reactions to sunscreens, one had a positive patch test to eugenol, which was an ingredient of a sunscreen product (33). One patient from Japan had allergic contact dermatitis of the covered skin areas from eugenol added to washing detergents (39). Eugenol in chewing gum caused allergic contact dermatitis around the mouth with post-inflammatory hyperpigmentation in a young girl (68).

A man presented with a 12-week history of nonhealing peri-anal erosions. The patient experienced a blistering reaction 10 days after daily self-treatment of his chronic perianal pruritus with an analgesic cream that contained menthol, eugenol and methyl salicylate. He had used the cream intermittently in the past. Sores developed in the area. His primary care provider prescribed a healing spray containing trypsin, Myroxylon pereirae resin (MP) and castor oil and the sores progressed to ulcerations. The spray was discontinued, and the patient was patch tested, which revealed positive reactions to MP (which contains eugenol), eugenol, and the spray. During the patch test, the perianal area became indurated. The authors suggest that this patient became sensitized to the eugenol in the initial analgesic cream and then propagated the reaction with the MP-containing spray aimed at healing the area. The presentation of a nonhealing wound as contact dermatitis may suggest, according to the authors, an aberrant T-cell response in the chronic wound (79).

One or more cases of contact allergy to eugenol in toothpaste(s) (84) were cited in refs. 81 and 82. However, In Fishers' Contact Dermatitis, it is stated that eugenol in *impression paste* and not toothpaste caused allergic cheilitis and stomatitis (83).

A physiotherapist developed occupational allergic contact dermatitis from a massage cream and its ingredients cinnamon oil and clove oil; the patient was also allergic to eugenol (106). Eugenol may well have been the causative allergen, as it is the major ingredient of clove oil and can be present in commercial cinnamon bark oils in a concentration of up to 16% (105).

A man with longstanding oral lichen planus developed painful ulcerations. When treatment with an ointment containing lidocaine, Solcoseryl ® and eugenol was stopped, the pain disappeared and the ulcers healed. Patch testing showed a positive reaction to the ointment and its ingredient eugenol (111).

A woman complained of burning mouth syndrome for 2 years. When patch tested, she reacted to eugenol and a mouthwash containing eugenol. She also consumed large amounts of cinnamon and cloves, which both contain eugenol. After avoiding these products, the burning of the mouth was significantly reduced after 8 weeks (128).

Reactions to eugenol in dentistry

In dentistry, eugenol may be present in a variety of dental materials such as impression materials, filling materials, dental cements, endodontic sealers, periodontal dressing materials and dry socket dressings (94). Oral soft tissue reactions have been classified as follows (94):

1. Eugenol is generally cytotoxic at high concentrations and has an adverse effect on fibroblasts and osteoblast-like cells. Thus, at high concentrations it produces necrosis and reduced healing. This effect is dose-related and will potentially affect all patients.

2. In lower concentrations, eugenol can act as a contact allergen evoking a delayed hypersensitivity reaction (94,95, 96,97,99,100,110).

3. Rarely, eugenol when placed in the mouth, can cause a more significant generalised response including urticaria and anaphylactic shock (92,103).

Adverse effects of eugenol in the oral cavity have been reported in association with its use in surgical and periodontal packs (87,95,96), root canal sealers (97), mouth rinses (99), impression pastes (96,100) and restorative material (110,123). Contact allergy / allergic contact dermatitis to eugenol amongst dental personnel is also well documented (101,102,104,113) .

Case reports and case series

In the 1960s eugenol was a common constituent of dressings used after periodontal surgery (periodontal packs). It was found that 16 of 18 (89%) patients who experienced stomatitis following the placement of a surgical dressing containing 42% colophonium and 7% eugenol, were sensitized to eugenol and/or colophony on patch testing (87,95). When the risk of inducing sensitization to eugenol from the placement of surgical dressings containing eugenol was investigated, a sensitization rate of almost 10% was found and the use of eugenol-free periodontal dressings became favored (96). However, in another publication probably presenting the same data, is was stated that all sensitizations had already been present at the first patch test session (87).

In one individual, contact allergy to eugenol in resin-reinforced zinc oxide-eugenol temporary dressing for root canal treatment caused a painful ulcer with surrounding erythema on the adjacent mucosa (94). In another patient, eugenol in zinc oxide-eugenol cement caused acute pain in the gums, marked erythema and destruction of the interdental papillae (94). In these 2 cases, both allergic and irritant factors of eugenol may have contributed to the clinical picture (94).

A female patient became sensitized to eugenol in a mouthwash and developed inflammation of the oral mucosa with a burning sensation (99). One or more patient had a contact allergic reaction to eugenol in impression paste (100). One or more patients had a contact allergic reaction to eugenol in root canal sealers (97). A dental nurse had vesicular hand dermatitis from contact allergy to eugenol in an intermediate restorative material (104). Another dental assistant developed occupational allergic contact dermatitis from a liquid used in the dental practice containing eugenol (113). A woman had allergic contact gingivitis from eugenol in a restorative dental material (110). Another individual had developed oral lichen planus from contact allergy to eugenol present in cement used for a dental bridge (123).

A dental patient developed an 'allergic reaction' to a zinc oxide-eugenol temporary restoration dental cavity, characterized by irritation and redness of the oral mucosa, complete sloughing of the oral mucosa, bilateral loss of papillae on the tongue, and ulceration at the vermilion border. In addition, mild facial swelling was present. Later, one week following endodontic treatment with a temporary filling containing a lower concentration of eugenol, the patient reported a 'similar allergic reaction with redness of the oral mucosa and altered taste sensation'. It was 'found that the patient had an allergic reaction to the slight amount of eugenol contained in the temporary filling'. However, patch tests were not performed (98).

Pigmented cosmetic dermatitis

In Japan, in the 1960s and 1970s, many female patients developed pigmentation of the face after having facial dermatitis (48). The skin manifestations of this so-called pigmented cosmetic dermatitis consisted of diffuse or patchy brown hyperpigmentation on the cheeks and/or forehead, sometimes the entire face was involved. In severe cases, the pigmentation was black, purple, or blue-black, and in mild cases, it was pale brown. Occasionally, erythematous macules or papules, suggesting a mild contact dermatitis, were observed and itching was also noted at varying times. Pigmented cosmetic dermatitis was shown to be caused by contact allergy to components of cosmetic products, notably essential oils, other fragrance materials, antimicrobials, preservatives and coloring materials (47,48,49). In a group of 620 Japanese patients with this condition investigated between 1970 and 1980, 4-6% had positive patch test reactions to eugenol 5% in petrolatum in various time periods versus 2 to 3% in a control group of patients not suffering from pigmented cosmetic dermatitis (47). The number of patients with pigmented cosmetic dermatitis decreased strongly after 1978, when major cosmetic companies began to eliminate strong contact sensitizers from their products (47). Since 1980, pigmented cosmetic dermatitis became a rare disease in Japan (50).

Cross-reactions, pseudo-cross-reactions and co-reactions

For general information on cross-/pseudo-cross-/co-reactivity of fragrance chemicals with other fragrances, fragrance markers (fragrance mix I, fragrance mix II, colophonium, Myroxylon pereirae resin [balsam of Peru]) and essential oils see Chapter 1.2 General information on cross-reactions, pseudo-cross-reactions and co-reactions. Co-reactivity of eugenol with the fragrance mix I and Myroxylon pereirae resin can be expected, as both contain eugenol (pseudo-cross-reactions) (108).

There is, according to some authors, limited cross-reactivity between isoeugenol and eugenol (34). Of 166 patients with positive reactions to eugenol, 41 (25%) were also allergic to isoeugenol. Conversely, of 219 patients with positive reactions to isoeugenol, 41 (19%) also reacted to eugenol, confirming 'limited' cross-reactivity (51); test concentrations were probably 1% or 2% pet. Previously, however, in an early study from Denmark, a high degree of cross-reactivity between eugenol and isoeugenol, both tested at 5% pet., was found (116). It is conceivable that the differences can be explained by the different concentrations used. Also, in a large study performed by the IVDK in the period 2005-2013, of 203 eugenol-positive patients, 137 (67%) also reacted to isoeugenol; conversely, of 523 individuals allergic to isoeugenol, 137 (26%) co-reacted to eugenol (124).

Pseudo-cross reactions to essential oils containing high concentrations of eugenol, especially clove oil (in which eugenol is the major component) (107,108) and to a lesser degree cinnamon oil (106) can be anticipated.

Of 15 patients reacting to p-allylphenol 2% pet, 14 (93%) co-reacted to eugenol 2% in petrolatum (116).

Patch test sensitization

In 7 patients out of 230 with contact allergy to Myroxylon pereirae resin (balsam of Peru), there was a positive patch test to eugenol 5% pet. that developed 6 days or later after application. Whether these were simply 'delayed' reactions or indicative of patch test sensitization was not well investigated, but one most likely was active sensitization (116).

Serial dilution testing and Repeated Open Application Tests

In 6 patients allergic to eugenol, ROATs with a maximum application time of 3 weeks with eugenol 0.5%, 0.05% and 0.005% wt./vol. in 2:98 diethyl phthalate/alcohol were negative (11). In serial dilution patch testing with concentrations ranging from 0.00006% to 2% vol./vol. in 2:98 diethyl phthalate/alcohol, minimum elicitation concentrations were 0.063% (n=2), 0.5% (n=1), 1% (n=1), 1.32% (n=1) and 2% (n=1) (11).

In a subsequent study by the same authors, five volunteers who had previously tested positive to fragrance mix I and to eugenol 2.0% pet. were studied (1). They were patch tested twice with a serial dilution test of eugenol ranging from 2.0% down to 0.00006% in a vehicle consisting of 2.0% diethyl phthalate and 98.0% ethanol. In addition, ROATs were performed for 4 weeks with four different solutions: three contained eugenol diluted in the same vehicle as used for patch testing at concentrations of 2.7%, 1.0%, and 0.5%, and one solution contained only the vehicle. The ROATs were performed on four sites, two on each arm (3×3 cm each) on the lower volar aspect. Four of the 5 participants who were previously patch test-positive to 2.0% eugenol were positive to concentrations down to 1.32%. This reactivity did not change in the second patch test dilution series. Regarding the ROAT, 4 of 5 became positive to at least the highest concentration of 2.7%, one of them also reacted to the 1% solution after 3 weeks and showed a dubious positive reaction to eugenol 0.5% after 4 weeks (1).

Presence in products and chemical analyses

In various studies, the presence of eugenol in cosmetic and sometimes other products has been investigated. Before 2006, most investigators used chemical analysis, usually GC-MS, for qualitative and quantitative determination. Since then, the presence of the target fragrances was usually investigated by screening the product labels for the 26 fragrances that must be labeled since 2005 on cosmetics and detergent products in the EU, if present at > 10 ppm (0.001%) in leave-on products and > 100 ppm (0.01%) in rinse-off products. This method, obviously, is less accurate and may result in underestimation of the frequency of the fragrances being present in the product. When they are in fact present, but the concentration is lower than mentioned above, labeling is not required and the fragrances' presence will be missed.

The results of the relevant studies for eugenol are summarized in table 3.65.4. More detailed information can be found in the corresponding text following the table. The percentage of products in which eugenol was found to be present shows wide variations, which can among other be explained by the selection procedure of the products, the method of investigation (false-negatives with information obtained from labels only) and changes in the use of individual fragrance materials over time (fashion). Up to 2002, eugenol was frequently found in the products analyzed. Since 2006, however, the use of eugenol appears to have declined considerably, at least in concentrations high enough to require labeling of eugenol.

Table 3.65.4 Presence of eugenol in products [a]

Year	Country	Product type	Nr. investigated	Nr. of products positive [b]	(%)	Method [c]	Ref.
2017	USA	Cosmetic products in hair-dye kits	539 products in 159 hair-dye kits	20	(4%)	Labeling	78
2016	Sweden	Toothpastes	66	5	(8%)	Labeling	88
2015-6	Denmark	Fragranced cosmetic products	5588		(8%)	Labeling	26
2015	Germany	Household detergents	817	20	(2%)	Labeling	120
2015	Sweden	Oxidative hair dye products	26	0	(0%)	Labeling	56
		Non-oxidative	35	5	(14%)	Labeling	
2014	Poland	Emollients	179	5	(3%)	Online info	55
2008-11	Germany	Deodorants	374	45	(12%)	Labeling	109
2006-9	Germany	Cosmetic products	4991		(7%)	Labeling	25
2008	Belgium	Fragranced topical pharmaceutical products	370	15	(4%)	Labeling	14
2008	Sweden	Cosmetic products	204		(2%)	Labeling	16
		Detergents	97		(0%)	Labeling	
2007	Netherlands	Cosmetic products for children	23	1	(4%)	Analysis	43
2006	UK	Perfumed cosmetic and household products	300	80	(27%)	Labeling	23
2006	Denmark	Popular perfumed deodorants	88	24	(27%)	Labeling	28
			23	7	(30%)	Analysis	
2006	Netherlands	Laundry detergents	52	9	(18%)	Labeling + analysis	45
2006	Denmark	Rinse-off cosmetics for children	208	15	(7.2%)	Labeling + analysis	42
2002	Denmark	Home and car air fresheners	19	12	(63%)	Analysis	46
2001	Denmark	Women's fine fragrances	10	7	(70%)	Analysis	27
2001	Denmark	Non-cosmetic consumer products	43	8	(19%)	Analysis	44
2000	Denmark, UK, Germany, Italy	Domestic and occupational products	59	16	(27%)	Analysis	18
<2000	Sweden	Swedish cosmetic products	42	15	(36%)	Analysis	80
1997-8	Denmark, UK Germany, Sweden	Cosmetics and cosmetic toys for children	25	6	(24%)	Analysis	21
1996-7	Denmark	Deodorants that had caused allergic contact dermatitis	19	15	(79%)	Analysis	69
1996	Five European countries	Fragranced deodorants	70	40	(57%)	Analysis	17
1995-6	Denmark	Perfumes from lower-price range cosmetic products	17	8	(47%)	Analysis	70
1995	Denmark	Cosmetic products based on natural ingredients	42	9	(21%)	Analysis	19
1995	Denmark	The 10 most popular women's perfumes	10	9	(90%)	Analysis	20
1994	Denmark	Cosmetics that had given a positive patch or use test in FM I allergic patients	23	17	(74%)	Analysis	71
1992	Netherlands	Cosmetic products	300		(36%)	Analysis	24
1988	USA	Perfumes used in fine fragrances, household products and soap	400	?-40% (See text)		Analysis	22

[a] See the corresponding text below for more details
[b] positive = containing the target fragrance
[c] Labeling: information from the ingredient labels on the product / packaging; Analysis: chemical analysis, most often GC-MS

In 2017, in the USA, the ingredient labels 159 hair-dye kits containing 539 cosmetic products (e.g. colorants, conditioners, shampoos, toners) were screened for the most common sensitizers they contain. Eugenol was found to be present in 20 (4%) of the products (78).

In 2016, in Sweden, 66 commercially available toothpastes obtained from local pharmacies and supermarkets in Malmö, Sweden were investigated for the presence of flavors by studying the packages and product labels. Eugenol was found to be present in 5 (8%) of the products (88).

In Denmark, in 2015-2016, 5588 fragranced cosmetic products were examined with a smartphone application for the 26 fragrances that need to be labeled in the EU. Eugenol was present in 8% of the products (rank number 13) (26).

In Germany, in 2015, fragrance allergens were evaluated based on lists of ingredients in 817 (unique) detergents (all-purpose cleaners, cleaning preparations for special purposes [e.g. bathroom, kitchen, dish-washing] and laundry detergents) present in 131 households. Eugenol was found to be present in 20 (2%) of the products (120).

In Sweden, in 2015, contact allergens were identified on the ingredient labels of 26 oxidative hair dye products (from 4 different product series) and on the labels of 35 non-oxidative hair dye products (from 5 different product series, including so-called herbal hair colors). These products were selected on the basis of being advertised as 'organic', 'natural', or similar, or used in hairdressing salons branded with such attributes. Eugenol was present in zero of the 26 oxidative hair dyes and in five (14%) of the 35 non-oxidative hair dye products (56).

Of 179 emollients available in online drugstores in 2014 in Poland, five (2.8%) contained eugenol, according to information available online (55).

In 2008, 2010 and 2011, 374 deodorants available in German retail shops were randomly selected and their labels checked for the presence of the 26 fragrances that need to be labeled. Eugenol was found to be present in 45 (12.0%) of the products (109).

In Germany, in the period 2006-2009, 4991 cosmetic products were randomly sampled for an official investigation of conformity of cosmetic products with legal provisions. The labels were inspected for the presence of the 26 fragrances that need to be labeled in the EU. Eugenol was present in 7% of the products (rank number 14) (25).

In 2008, 66 different fragrance components (including 39 essential oils) were identified in 370 (10% of the total) topical pharmaceutical products marketed in Belgium; 15 of these (4%) contained eugenol (14).

Eugenol was present (as indicated by labeling) in 2% of 204 cosmetic products (92 shampoos, 61 hair conditioners, 34 liquid soaps, 17 wet tissues) and in none of 97 detergents in Sweden, 2008 (16).

In 2007, in The Netherlands, twenty-three cosmetic products for children were analyzed for the presence of fragrances that need to be labeled. Eugenol was identified in one of the products (4%) in a concentration of 23 ppm (43).

In 2006, in The Netherlands, 52 laundry detergents were investigated for the presence of allergenic fragrances by checking their labels and chemical analyses. Eugenol was found to be present in 9 of the products (18%) in a concentration range of 12-83 ppm. Eugenol had rank number 11 in the frequency list (45).

In 2006, of 88 popular perfume containing deodorants purchased in Denmark, 24 (27%) were labeled to contain eugenol. Analysis of 24 regulated fragrance substances in 23 selected deodorants (19 spray products, 2 deostick and 2 roll-on) was performed by GC-MS. Eugenol was identified in 7 of the products (30%) with a concentration range of 1–514 ppm (28).

In January 2006, a study of perfumed cosmetic and household products available on the shelves of U.K. retailers was carried out. Products were included if 'parfum' or 'aroma' was listed among the ingredients. Three hundred products were surveyed and any of 26 mandatory labeling fragrances named on the label were recorded. Eugenol was present in 80 (27%) of the products (rank number 11) (23).

In 2006, the labels of 208 cosmetics for children (especially shampoos, body shampoos and soaps) available in Denmark were checked for the presence of the 26 fragrances that need to be labeled in the EU. Eugenol was present in 15 products (7.2%), and ranked number 12 in the frequency list (42).

In 2002, in Denmark, 19 air fresheners (6 for cars, 13 for homes) were analyzed for the presence of fragrances that need to be labeled on cosmetics. Eugenol was found to be present in 12 products (63%) in a concentration range of 11-9,000 ppm and ranked 5 in the frequency list (46).

In January 2001, in Denmark, ten women's fine fragrances were purchased; 5 of these had been launched years ago (1921–1990) and 5 were the latest launches by the same companies, introduced 2 months to 4 years before purchase. They were analyzed for the presence and quantity of the 7 well-identified fragrances present in the FM I (see Chapter 3.70 Fragrance mix I). The analysis revealed that the 5 old perfumes contained a mean of 5 of the 7 target allergens of the FM, while the new perfumes contained a mean of 2.8 of the allergens. The mean concentrations of the target allergens were 2.6 times higher in the old perfumes than in the new perfumes, range 2.2-337 ppm. Eugenol was present in all 5 old perfumes, in a concentration range of 0.032-0.738 % (m/m), mean 0.337%; in the new perfumes, it was identified in 2 of the 5 in a concentration of 0.001% (27).

In 2001, in Denmark, 43 non-cosmetic consumer products (mainly dish-washing products, laundry detergents, and hard and soft surface cleaners) were analyzed for the 26 fragrances that are regulated for labeling in the EU. Eugenol was present in 8 products (19%) in a concentration range of 0.00001-0.0119% (m/m) and had rank number 12 in the frequency list (44).

In 2000, fifty-nine domestic and occupational products, purchased in retail outlets in Denmark, England, Germany and Italy were analyzed by GC-MS for the presence of fragrances. The product categories were liquid soap and soap bars (n=13), soft/hard surface cleaners (n=23), fabric conditioners/laundry detergents for hand wash (n=8), dish- wash (n=10), furniture polish, car shampoo, stain remover (each n=1) and 2 products used in occupational environments. Eugenol was present in 16 products (27%) with a mean concentration of 122 ppm and a range of 32-349 ppm (18).

In Sweden, before 2000, 42 cosmetic products of a Swedish manufacturer were investigated for the presence of the ingredients of the FM I by chemical analysis. Eugenol was found to be present in 15 of the products (36%) in a concentration range of 1-107 ppm with a mean of 26 ppm. Data provided by the manufacturer on the qualitative and quantitative presence of the chemicals was quite different from chemical analyses for some of the fragrances (80).

Twenty-five cosmetics and cosmetic toys for children (5 shampoos and shower gels, 6 perfumes, 1 deodorant (roll-on), 4 baby lotions/creams, 1 baby wipes product, 1 baby oil, 2 lipcare products and 5 toy-cosmetic products: a cosmetic-toy set for blending perfumes and a makeup set) purchased in 1997-1998 in retail outlets in Denmark, Germany, England and Sweden were analyzed in 1998 for the presence of fragrances by GC-MS. Eugenol was found in 6 products (24%) in a concentration range of ≤0.001-0.163% (w/w). For the analytical data in each product category, the original publication should be consulted (21).

In Denmark, in 1996-1997, nineteen deodorants that had caused axillary allergic contact dermatitis in 14 patients were analyzed for the presence of the 8 constituents of the FM I and eugenol was found to be present in 15 (79%) of the products in a concentration range of 0.0029-0.1831% (69).

Seventy fragranced deodorants, purchased at retail outlets in 5 European countries in 1996, were analyzed by gas chromatography - mass spectrometry (GC-MS) for the determination of the contents of 21 commonly used fragrance materials. Eugenol was identified in 40 products (57%) in a concentration range of 1–2355 ppm (17).

In Denmark, in 1995-1996, nine perfumes from lower-price cosmetic wash-off products and 8 from stay-on products were analyzed for the presence of the ingredients of the FM I except oakmoss absolute. Eugenol was present in 5 of the 9 (56%) wash-off product perfumes in a concentration range of 0.1028-0.2740% w/v and in 3 of the 8 (38%) stay-on product perfumes in a concentration range of 0.563-0.1090% w/v. In one product, eugenol was detected, but could not be quantified because of interference (70).

In 1995, in Denmark, 42 cosmetic products based on natural ingredients from 12 European and US companies (of which 22 were perfumes and 20 various other cosmetics) were investigated by high-resolution gas chromato-graphy-mass spectrometry (GC-MS) for the presence of 11 fragrances. Eugenol was present in 8 (36%) of the 22 perfumes in a concentration range of 0.035-2.289 w/w%; it was also identified in one of the other cosmetics (an anti-stress gel) in a concentration of 0.0186% (19).

In Denmark, in 1995, the 10 most popular women's perfumes were analyzed with gas chromatography-mass spectrometry for the presence of 7 ingredients of the Fragrance mix I (all except Evernia prunastri extract). Eugenol was identified in 9 of the perfumes (90%) with a mean concentration of 0.31% and in a concentration range of 0.04-0.89% (20).

In Denmark, in 1994, 23 cosmetic products, which had either given a positive patch and/or use test in a total of 11 fragrance-mix-positive patients, and which products completely or partly explained present or past episodes of dermatitis, were analyzed for the presence of the constituents of the FM I (with the exception of oakmoss absolute) and a few other fragrances. Eugenol was found to be present in 17 of the 23 products (74%) in a concentration range of <0.001-0.22% v/v with a mean concentration of 0.066% v/v (71).

In 1992, in The Netherlands, the presence of fragrances was analyzed in 300 cosmetic products. Eugenol was identified in 36% of the products (rank order 18) (24).

In 1988, in the USA, 400 perfumes used in fine fragrances, household products and soaps (number of products per category not mentioned) were analyzed for the presence of fragrance chemicals in a concentration of at least 1% and a list of the Top-25 (present in the highest number of products) presented. Eugenol was found to be present in 26% of the fine fragrances (rank number 21), an unknown percentage of the household product fragrances and 40% of the fragrances used in soaps (rank number 19) (22).

Other information

The term 'quenching' was employed to describe the complete abrogation of the sensitizing potential of 3 fragrance chemicals (cinnamal, citral and phenylacetaldehyde) by the presence of certain other fragrance chemicals, notably eugenol and limonene (90). The conclusions were supported by a summary of human predictive test data. Unfortunately, the absence of any details (numbers tested, reproducibility, etc.) have tended to compromise the credibility of the report (89). Whilst there is some evidence in man for the occurrence of quenching during the induction of skin sensitization, a much more substantial body of work has failed to find supportive evidence in various animals models, at a chemical level or at elicitation in human subjects with existing allergy (89,91). In a thorough review of the subject in 2000, it was therefore concluded that the existence of quenching of these fragrance allergens by other specific fragrance components should be regarded as a hypothesis still lacking substantive proof (89).

OTHER SIDE EFFECTS

Irritant contact dermatitis

Eugenol is generally cytotoxic at high concentrations and has an adverse effect on fibroblasts and osteoblast-like cells. Thus, at high concentrations it produces necrosis and reduced healing. This effect is dose-related and will potentially affect all individuals in contact with such materials on the oral mucosa.

Eugenol and isoeugenol in carnation and spice-type perfumes in the past have apparently caused irritant cosmetic dermatitis which was enhanced by sunburn (photo-irritation) (41).

Photosensitivity

In a group of 50 patients suffering from photosensitivity dermatitis with actinic reticuloid syndrome (PD/AR) patch tested with a battery of fragrances, there were 3 reactions (6%) to eugenol versus 1.5% positive patch tests in a group of 457 routinely tested dermatitis patients. The frequency of reactions to various other fragrances was also elevated in the PD/AR group. In a subgroup of 35 patients (11 with PD/AR, 13 with chronic polymorphic light eruption, 11 with contact dermatitis) who were photopatch tested, there were three reactions to eugenol, some of who also had an immediate-type reaction. These positive photopatch tests were tentatively interpreted as indicating a phototoxic reaction, although the possibility that this phototoxic response may merge subsequently with a delayed allergic type reaction could not be excluded. The authors concluded that in some subjects with PD/AR and persistent light reaction, a significant factor in the latter is likely to be exposure to substances such as fragrance materials which have the ability to produce dermatitis, not only from contact allergic sensitivity but also through photocontact reactions (notably oakmoss, 6-methylcoumarin and musk ambrette) involving either phototoxic or photoallergic mechanisms (52).

Immediate-type reactions

One patient had an immediate contact reaction to eugenol; specific data were not given (65). In Hungary, before 1994, in a group of 50 patients reacting to the FM I and tested with its ingredients (test concentrations unknown), there was one immediate contact reaction to eugenol (73). Of 50 individuals who had open tests with eugenol 4% pet. on the forearm, 18 (36%) showed local macular erythema after 45 minutes, termed 'contact urticaria' by the authors (76).

A woman developed an urticarial rash some 10-12 hours after she had been fitted with a temporary dental bridge, which only subsided after the dental bridge and sealer were removed. There was temporary exacerbation of urticaria at the time of removal. The dental intervention included fixing a polymethyl methacrylate bridge with zinc oxide–eugenol. A skin prick test done 2 weeks later was positive for eugenol (10%) and negative for zinc oxide (10%) and polymethyl methacrylate (10%). No relapse or recurrence was observed during 3 months of follow-up (92).

One eugenol-sensitive patient was reported to have developed anaphylactic-like shock subsequent to a pulpotomy in which zinc-oxide and eugenol cement was used (103).

An 8-year-old boy underwent an extirpation because of chronic irreversible pulpitis; the root canal was medicated with sodium hypochlorite and sealed with zinc oxide eugenol dressing. About 1 minute later, the patient was anxious and excited, with evident erythema on the face, neck, torso, upper limbs, lower limbs and itchiness and redness extending behind the ear. Cutaneous examination revealed extensive weals of various sizes. There was no angioedema or mucosal involvement. Later, he underwent skin prick test for various chemicals which were found to be contained in the root canal disinfectants and zinc oxide eugenol. He showed a positive response to eugenol (10%) and negative responses to zinc oxide (10%), formaldehyde (1% water) and sodium hypochlorite (121).

Other non-eczematous contact reactions

A male hairdresser had developed eczema on his hands and he had suffered from nasal stuffiness and rhinorrhea. Over the last 6 months at work he had also developed episodes of chest tightness, dry cough and shortness of breath upon exposure to perfumes and lacquer. His asthma symptoms worsened progressively but showed a marked improvement away from work. Patch testing with European standard series showed positive results to fragrance mix and isoeugenol. Skin prick testing was performed with common aeroallergens, latex and eugenol 2% w/v and all yielded negative results (one may wonder why eugenol was chosen for further testing). Specific inhalation challenge

(SIC) with eugenol 1/1000 elicited rhinitis symptoms and an isolated late asthmatic response. An increase in sputum eosinophils and lymphocytes was observed 24 hours after the challenge and a methacholine inhalation test became positive. Proliferation tests of peripheral blood showed a 15 times higher (eugenol-induced) proliferation in the patient than in a control at 1/1000 eugenol dilution, whereas no significant difference was observed at 1/100 (why negative?) and 1/10 000 dilutions. According to the authors, these findings supported 'the specificity of the airway reaction (asthma and rhinitis) to eugenol'. How eugenol was chosen for further investigation was not mentioned nor whether the patient was actually exposed to eugenol at work (67).

Miscellaneous side effects

Chronic urticaria in one patient was suspected to be caused by a root canal cement. A causal relationship with eugenol, a cement constituent, could only be established through provocative oral ingestion (93). One of the authors published a similar case of urticaria associated with eugenol in root canal cement some years later. Epicutaneous and intradermal tests were negative and the diagnosis could only be made by oral provocation with eugenol (122, article not read, possibly the same patient as in ref. 93).

OTHER INFORMATION

When eugenol 2% in petrolatum is stored in Finn chambers at room temperature, the concentration of the fragrance decreases by 20% or more within 8 hours, probably from evaporation. This decrease is lower when the test material is stored in a refrigerator. Therefore, application to the test chamber should be performed as close in time to the patch testing as possible and storage in a refrigerator is recommended (86).

LITERATURE

1   Svedman C, Engfeldt M, Api AM, Politano VT, Belsito DV, Isaksson M, Bruze M. A pilot study aimed at finding a suitable eugenol concentration for a leave-on product for use in a repeated open application test. Contact Dermatitis 2012;66:137-139

2   Heisterberg MV, Menné T, Johansen JD. Contact allergy to the 26 specific fragrance ingredients to be declared on cosmetic products in accordance with the EU cosmetic directive. Contact Dermatitis 2011;65:266-275

3   Oosten EJ van, Schuttelaar ML, Coenraads PJ. Clinical relevance of positive patch test reactions to the 26 EU-labelled fragrances. Contact Dermatitis 2009;61:217-223

4   Schnuch A, Uter W, Geier J, Lessmann H, Frosch PJ. Sensitization to 26 fragrances to be labelled according to current European regulation: Results of the IVDK and review of the literature. Contact Dermatitis 2007;57:1-10

5   Adams RM, Maibach HI, for the North American Contact Dermatitis Group. A five-year study of cosmetic reactions. J Am Acad Dermatol 1985;13:1062-1069

6   Hausen BM. Contact allergy to Balsam of Peru. II. Patch test results in 102 patients with selected Balsam of Peru constituents. Am J Contact Derm 2001;12:93-102

7   Wöhrl S, Hemmer W, Focke M, Götz M, Jarisch R. The significance of fragrance mix, balsam of Peru, colophony and propolis as screening tools in the detection of fragrance allergy. Br J Dermatol 2001;145:268-273

8   Heydorn S, Johansen JD, Andersen KE, Bruze M, Svedman C, White IR, et al. Fragrance allergy in patients with hand eczema – a clinical study. Contact Dermatitis 2003;48:317-323

9   Larsen W, Nakayama H, Lindberg M et al. Fragrance contact dermatitis: A worldwide multicenter investigation (Part 1). Am J Cont Derm 1996;7:77–83

10   Wenk KS, Ehrlich AE. Fragrance series testing in eyelid dermatitis. Dermatitis 2012;23:22-26

11   Svedman C, Engfeldt M, Api AM, Politano VT, Belsito DV, Gruvberger B, Bruze M. Does the new standard for eugenol designed to protect against contact sensitization protect those sensitized from elicitation of the reaction? Dermatitis 2012;23:32-38

12   Various SCCS opinions on eugenol have been published and are available at: http://ec.europa.eu/growth/tools-databases/cosing/index.cfm?fuseaction=search.details_v2&id=28322&back=1

13   SCCS (Scientific Committee on Consumer Safety). Opinion on Fragrance allergens in cosmetic products, 26-27 June 2012, SCCS/1459/11. Available at: https://ec.europa.eu/health/sites/health/files/scientific_committees/consumer_safety/docs/sccs_o_102.pdf

14   Nardelli A, D'Hooge E, Drieghe J, Dooms M, Goossens A. Allergic contact dermatitis from fragrance components in specific topical pharmaceutical products in Belgium. Contact Dermatitis 2009;60:303-313

15   Larsen WG. Perfume dermatitis. A study of 20 patients. Arch Dermatol 1977;113:623-626

16   Yazar K, Johnsson S, Lind M-L, Boman A, Lidén C. Preservatives and fragrances in selected consumer-available cosmetics and detergents. Contact Dermatitis 2011;64:265-272

17   Rastogi SC, Johansen JD, Frosch P, Menné T, Bruze M, Lepoittevin JP, et al. Deodorants on the European market: quantitative chemical analysis of 21 fragrances. Contact Dermatitis 1998;38:29-35

18 Rastogi SC, Heydorn S, Johansen JD, Basketter DA. Fragrance chemicals in domestic and occupational products. Contact Dermatitis 2001;45:221-225

19 Rastogi SC, Johansen JD, Menné T. Natural ingredients based cosmetics. Content of selected fragrance sensitizers. Contact Dermatitis 1996;34:423-426

20 Johansen JD, Rastogi SC, Menné T. Contact allergy to popular perfumes: assessed by patch test, use test and chemical analyses. Br J Dermatol 1996;135:419-422

21 Rastogi SC, Johansen JD, Menné T, Frosch P, Bruze M, Andersen KE, et al. Content of fragrance allergens in children's cosmetics and cosmetic toys. Contact Dermatitis 1999;41:84-88

22 Fenn RS. Aroma chemical usage trends in modern perfumery. Perfumer and Flavorist 1989;14:3-10

23 Buckley DA. Fragrance ingredient labelling in products on sale in the UK. Br J Dermatol 2007;157:295-300

24 Weyland JW. Personal Communication, 1992. Cited in: De Groot AC, Weyland JW, Nater JP. Unwanted effects of cosmetics and drugs used in dermatology, 3rd Ed. Amsterdam: Elsevier, 1994: 579

25 Uter W, Yazar K, Kratz E-M, Mildau G, Lidén C. Coupled exposure to ingredients of cosmetic products: I. Fragrances. Contact Dermatitis 2013;69:335-341

26 Bennike NH, Oturai NB, Müller S, Kirkeby CS, Jørgensen C, Christensen AB, et al. Fragrance contact allergens in 5588 cosmetic products identified through a novel smartphone application. J Eur Acad Dermatol Venereol 2018;32:79-85

27 Rastogi SC, Menné T, Johansen JD. The composition of fine fragrances is changing. Contact Dermatitis 2003;48:130-132

28 Rastogi SC, Hellerup Jensen G, Johansen JD. Survey and risk assessment of chemical substances in deodorants. Survey of Chemical Substances in Consumer Products, No. 86 2007. Danish Ministry of the Environment, Environmental Protection Agency. Available at: https://www2.mst.dk/Udgiv/publications/2007/978-87-7052-625-8/pdf/978-87-7052-626-5.pdf

29 De Groot AC, Bruynzeel DP, Bos JD, van der Meeren HL, van Joost T, Jagtman BA, Weyland JW. The allergens in cosmetics. Arch Dermatol 1988;124:1525-1529

30 De Groot AC. Adverse reactions to cosmetics. PhD Thesis, University of Groningen, The Netherlands: 1988, chapter 3.4, pp.105-113

31 Zaragoza-Ninet V, Blasco Encinas R, Vilata-Corell JJ, Pérez-Ferriols A, Sierra-Talamantes C, Esteve-Martínez A, de la Cuadra-Oyanguren J. Allergic contact dermatitis due to cosmetics: A clinical and epidemiological study in a tertiary hospital. Actas Dermosifiliogr 2016;107:329-336

32 Laguna C, de la Cuadra J, Martín-González B, Zaragoza V, Martínez-Casimiro L, Alegre V. Allergic contact dermatitis to cosmetics. Actas Dermosifiliogr 2009;100:53-60

33 Thune P. Contact and photocontact allergy to sunscreens. Photodermatol 1984;1:5-9

34 Buckley DA, Basketter DA, Smith Pease CK, Rycroft RJG, White IR, McFadden JP. Simultaneous sensitivity to fragrances. Br J Dermatol 2006;154:885-888

35 An S, Lee AY, Lee CH, Kim DW, Hahm JH, Kim KJ, et al. Fragrance contact dermatitis in Korea: a joint study. Contact Dermatitis 2005;53:320-323

36 Frosch PJ, Pilz B, Andersen KE, Burrows D, Camarasa JG, Dooms-Goossens A, et al. Patch testing with fragrances: results of a multicenter study of the European Environmental and Contact Dermatitis Research Group with 48 frequently used constituents of perfumes. Contact Dermatitis 1995;33:333-342

37 Trattner A, David M. Patch testing with fine fragrances: comparison with fragrance mix, balsam of Peru and a fragrance series. Contact Dermatitis 2003;49:287-289

38 Cuesta L, Silvestre JF, Toledo F, Lucas A, Perez-Crespo M, Ballester I. Fragrance contact allergy: a 4-year retrospective study. Contact Dermatitis 2010;63:77-84

39 Nakayama H, Hanaoka H, Ohshiro A. Allergen controlled system (ACS). Tokyo: Kanehara Shuppan, 1974:42; data cited in ref. 40

40 Mitchell JC. Contact hypersensitivity to some perfume materials. Contact Dermatitis 1975;1:196-199

41 Klarmann EG. Perfume dermatitis. Annals of Allergy 1958;16:425-434; data cited in ref. 40

42 Poulsen PB, Schmidt A. A survey and health assessment of cosmetic products for children. Survey of chemical substances in consumer products, No. 88. Copenhagen: Danish Environmental Protection Agency, 2007. Available at: https://www2.mst.dk/udgiv/publications/2007/978-87-7052-638-8/pdf/978-87-7052-639-5.pdf

43 VWA. Dutch Food and Consumer Product Safety Authority. Cosmetische producten voor kinderen: Inventarisatie van de markt en de veiligheidsborging door producenten en importeurs. Report ND04o065/ND05o170, 2007 (Report in Dutch), 2007. Available at: www.nvwa.nl/documenten/communicatie/inspectieresultaten/consument/ 2016m/cosmetische- producten-voor-kinderen

44 Rastogi SC. Survey of chemical compounds in consumer products. Contents of selected fragrance materials in cleaning products and other consumer products. Survey no. 8-2002. Copenhagen, Denmark, Danish Environmental Protection Agency. Available at: http://eng.mst.dk/media/mst/69131/8.pdf

45   Bouma K, Van Peursem AJJ. Marktonderzoek naleving detergenten verordening voor textielwasmiddelen. Dutch Food and Consumer Products Safety Authority (VWA) Report ND06K173, 2006 [in Dutch]. Available at: http://docplayer.nl/41524125-Marktonderzoek-naleving-detergenten-verordening-voor-textielwasmiddelen.html

46   Pors J, Fuhlendorff R. Mapping of chemical substances in air fresheners and other fragrance liberating products. Report Danish Ministry of the Environment, Environmental Protection Agency (EPA). Survey of Chemicals in Consumer Products, No 30, 2003. Available at: http://eng.mst.dk/media/mst/69113/30.pdf

47   Nakayama H, Matsuo S, Hayakawa K, Takhashi K, Shigematsu T, Ota S. Pigmented cosmetic dermatitis. Int J Dermatol 1984;23:299-305

48   Nakayama H, Harada R, Toda M. Pigmented cosmetic dermatitis. Int J Dermatol 1976;15:673-675

49   Nakayama H, Hanaoka H, Ohshiro A. Allergen Controlled System. Tokyo: Kanehara Shuppan, 1974

50   Ebihara T, Nakayama H. Pigmented contact dermatitis. Clin Dermatol 1997;15:593-599

51   Buckley DA, Wakelin SH, Seed PT, Holloway D, Rycroft RJ, White IR, et al. The frequency of fragrance allergy in a patch-test population over a 17-year period. Br J Dermatol 2000;142:279-283

52   Addo HA, Ferguson J, Johnson BF, Frain-Bell W. The relationship between exposure to fragrance materials and persistent light reaction in photosensitivity dermatitis with actinic reticuloid syndrome. Br J Dermatol 1982;107:261-274

53   Goossens A. Cosmetic contact allergens. Cosmetics 2016, 3, 5; doi:10.3390/cosmetics3010005

54   Bennike NH, Zachariae C, Johansen JD. Non-mix fragrances are top sensitizers in consecutive dermatitis patients – a cross-sectional study of the 26 EU-labelled fragrance allergens. Contact Dermatitis 2017;77:270-279

55   Osinka K, Karczmarz A, Krauze K, Feleszko W. Contact allergens in cosmetics used in atopic dermatitis: analysis of product composition. Contact Dermatitis 2016;75:241-243

56   Thorén S, Yazar K. Contact allergens in 'natural' hair dyes. Contact Dermatitis 2016;74:302-304

57   Vejanurug P, Tresukosol P, Sajjachareonpong P, Puangpet P. Fragrance allergy could be missed without patch testing with 26 individual fragrance allergens. Contact Dermatitis 2016;74:230-235

58   Liu J, Li L-F. Contact sensitization to fragrances other than fragrance mix I in China. Contact Dermatitis 2015;73:252-253

59   Mann J, McFadden JP, White JML, White IR, Banerjee P. Baseline series fragrance markers fail to predict contact allergy. Contact Dermatitis 2014;70:276-281

60   Uter W, Johansen JD, Börje A, Karlberg A-T, Lidén C, Rastogi S, Roberts D, White IR. Categorization of fragrance contact allergens for prioritization of preventive measures: clinical and experimental data and consideration of structure–activity relationships. Contact Dermatitis 2013;69:196-230

61   Mowitz M, Svedman C, Zimerson E, Isaksson M, Pontén A, Bruze M. Simultaneous patch testing with fragrance mix I, fragrance mix II and their ingredients in southern Sweden between 2009 and 2015. Contact Dermatitis 2017;77:280-287

62   Nagtegaal MJC, Pentinga SE, Kuik J, Kezic S, Rustemeyer T. The role of the skin irritation response in polysensitization to fragrances. Contact Dermatitis 2012;67:28-35

63   Nardelli A, Drieghe J, Claes L, Boey L, Goossens A. Fragrance allergens in 'specific' cosmetic products. Contact Dermatitis 2011;64:212-219

64   Uter W, Geier J, Frosch P, Schnuch A. Contact allergy to fragrances: current patch test results (2005–2008) from the Information Network of Departments of Dermatology. Contact Dermatitis 2010;63:254-261

65   Temesvári E, Németh I, Baló-Banga MJ, Husz S, Kohánka V, Somos Z, et al. Multicentre study of fragrance allergy in Hungary: Immediate and late type reactions. Contact Dermatitis 2002;46:325-330

66   Opdyke DLJ. Inhibition of sensitization reactions induced by certain aldehydes. Fd Cosmet Toxicol 1976;14:197-198

67   Quirce S, Fernandez-Nieto M, del Pozo V, Sastre B, Sastre J. Occupational asthma and rhinitis caused by eugenol in a hairdresser. Allergy 2008;63:137-138

68   Beswick SJ, Ramsay HM, Tan BB. Contact dermatitis from flavourings in chewing gum. Contact Dermatitis 1999;40:49-50

69   Johansen JD, Rastogi SC, Bruze M, Andersen KE, Frosch P, Dreier B, et al. Deodorants: a clinical provocation study in fragrance-sensitive individuals. Contact Dermatitis 1998;39:161-165

70   Johansen JD, Rastogi SC, Andersen KE, Menné T. Content and reactivity to product perfumes in fragrance mix positive and negative eczema patients: A study of perfumes used in toiletries and skin-care products. Contact Dermatitis 1997;36:291-296

71   Johansen JD, Rastogi SC, Menné T. Exposure to selected fragrance materials: A case study of fragrance-mix-positive eczema patients. Contact Dermatitis 1996;34:106-110

72   Frosch PJ, Pilz B, Burrows D, Camarasa JG, Lachapelle J-M, Lahti A, et al. Testing with fragrance mix: Is the addition of sorbitan sesquioleate to the constituents useful? Contact Dermatitis 1995;32:266-272

73 Becker K, Temesvari E, Nemeth I. Patch testing with fragrance mix and its constituents in a Hungarian population. Contact Dermatitis 1994;30:185-186

74 De Groot AC, Van der Kley AMJ, Bruynzeel DP, Meinardi MMHM, Smeenk G, van Joost Th, Pavel S. Frequency of false-negative reactions to the fragrance mix. Contact Dermatitis 1993;28:139-140

75 Broeckx W, Blondeel A, Dooms-Goossens A, Achten G. Cosmetic intolerance. Contact Dermatitis 1987;16:189-194

76 Emmons WW, Marks JG Jr. Immediate and delayed reactions to cosmetic ingredients. Contact Dermatitis 1985;13:258-265

77 Van Joost Th, Stolz E, Van Der Hoek JCS. Simultaneous allergy to perfume ingredients. Contact Dermatitis 1985;12:115-116

78 Hamann D, Kishi P, Hamann CR. Consumer hair dye kits frequently contain isothiazolinones, other common preservatives and fragrance allergens. Dermatitis 2018;29:48-49

79 Hill H, Jacob SE. Peri-anal ulcerations in a patient with essential pruritus. Dermatitis 2015;26:292-293

80 Bárány E, Lodén M. Content of fragrance mix ingredients and customer complaints of cosmetic products. Dermatitis 2000;11:74-79

81 Sainio E-L, Kanerva L. Contact allergens in toothpastes and a review of their hypersensitivity. Contact Dermatitis 1995;33:100-105

82 Millard L. Acute contact sensitivity to a new toothpaste. J Dent 1973;1:168-170

83 Rietschel RL, Fowler JF Jr, Eds. Fisher's Contact Dermatitis. 6th edition. Hamilton: BC Decker Inc; 2008: 418,702,703

84 Göransson K, Karltorp N, Ask H, et al. Nagra fall av eugenoloverkiinslighet (Some cases of eugenol hypersensitivity). Svensk Tandläkaretidskrift 1967;60:545-550 (article in Swedish).

85 Diepgen TL, Ofenloch R, Bruze M, Cazzaniga S, Coenraads PJ, Elsner P, et al. Prevalence of fragrance contact allergy in the general population of five European countries: a cross-sectional study. Br J Dermatol 2015;173:1411-1419

86 Mowitz M, Zimerson E, Svedman C, Bruze M. Stability of fragrance patch test preparations applied in test chambers. Br J Dermatol 2012;167:822-827

87 Magnusson B. The sensitizing effects of eugenol/colophony in surgical dressings. Contact Dermatitis Newsletter 1974;15:454-455

88 Kroona L, Warfvinge G, Isaksson M, Ahlgren C, Dahlin J, Sörensen Ö, Bruze M. Quantification of L-carvone in toothpastes available on the Swedish market. Contact Dermatitis 2017;77:224-230

89 Basketter D. Quenching: fact or fiction? Contact Dermatitis 2000;43:253-258

90 Opdyke DLJ. Inhibition of sensitization reactions induced by certain aldehydes. Fd Cosmet Toxicol 1976;14:197-198

91 Basketter D A, Allenby C F. Studies of the quenching phenomenon in delayed contact hypersensitivity reactions. Contact Dermatitis 1991;25:166-171

92 Bhalla M, Thami GP. Acute urticaria due to dental eugenol. Allergy 2003;58:158

93 Grade AC, Martens BPM. Chronic urticaria due to dental eugenol. Dermatologica 1989;178:217-220

94 Sarrami N, Pemberton MN, Thornhill MH, Theaker ED. Adverse reactions associated with the use of eugenol in dentistry. Br Dent J 2002;193:257-259

95 Koch G, Magnusson B, Nyquist G. Contact allergy to medicaments and materials used in dentistry. II. Sensitivity to eugenol and colophony. Odontol Revy 1971;22:275-289

96 Koch G, Magnusson B, Nobreus N, Nyquist G, Soderholm G. Contact allergy to medicaments and materials used in dentistry. (IV). Sensitizing effect of eugenol-colophony in surgical dressing. Odontol Revy 1973;24:109-114

97 Hensten-Pettersen A, Orstavik D, Wennberg A. Allergenic potential of root canal sealers. Endo Dent Traumatol 1985;1:61-65

98 Barkin ME, Boyd JP, Cohen S. Acute allergic reaction to eugenol. Oral Surg Oral Med Oral Pathol 1984;57:441-442

99 Vilaplana J, Grimalt F, Romaguera C, Conellana F. Contact dermatitis from eugenol in mouthwash. Contact Dermatitis 1991;24:223-224

100 Göransson K, Karltorp N, Ask H, Smedberg O. Nagra fall av eugenoloverkanslighet (some cases of eugenol hypersensitivity). Svensk Tandlakaretidskrift 1967;60:545-549 (article in Swedish). Data cited in ref. 94

101 Rudzki E, Rebandel P, Grzywa Z. Patch tests with occupational contactants in nurses, doctors and dentists. Contact Dermatitis 1989;20:247-250

102 Rudzki E. Occupational dermatitis among health service workers. Derm Beruf Umwelt 1979;27:112-115

103 McCarter RF. An unusual allergy. Midwest Dent 1966;42:20. Data cited in ref. 94

104 Kanerva L, Estlander T, Jolanki R. Dental nurse's occupational allergic contact dermatitis from eugenol used as a restorative dental material with polymethylmethacrylate. Contact Dermatitis 1998;38:339-340

105 De Groot AC, Schmidt E. Essential oils: contact allergy and chemical composition. Boca Raton, Fl., USA: CRC Press, Taylor and Francis Group, 2016 (ISBN 9781482246407

106 Sánchez-Pérez J, García-Díez A. Occupational allergic contact dermatitis from eugenol, oil of cinnamon and oil of cloves in a physiotherapist. Contact Dermatitis 1999;41:346-347

107 Uter W, Schmidt E, Geier J, Lessmann H, Schnuch A, Frosch P. Contact allergy to essential oils: current patch test results (2000–2008) from the Information Network of Departments of Dermatology (IVDK). Contact Dermatitis 2010;63:277-283

108 Steele JC, Bruce AJ, Davis MDP, Torgerson RR, Drage LA, Rogers RS III. Clinically relevant patch test results in patients with burning mouth syndrome. Dermatitis 2012;23:61-70

109 Klaschka U. Contact allergens for armpits - allergenic fragrances specified on deodorants. Int J Hyg Environ Health 2012;215:584-591

110 Silvestre JF, Albares MP, Blanes M, Pascual JC, Pastor N. Allergic contact gingivitis due to eugenol present in a restorative dental material. Contact Dermatitis 2005;52:341

111 Fujita Y, Shimizu T, Nishie W, Shimizu H. Contact dermatitis due to eugenol used to treat oral lichen planus. Contact Dermatitis 2003;48:285

112 Giusti F, Porcaro V, Seidenari S. Evaluation of eugenol allergy in a patch-test population. Contact Dermatitis 2001;44:37-38

113 Ortiz de Frutos FJ, Vergara A, Isarria MJ, del Prado-Sánchez M, Vanaclocha F. Occupational allergic contact eczema in a dental assistant. Actas Dermosifiliogr 2005;96:56-58 (article in Spanish)

114 Karlberg A-T, Börje A, Johansen JD, Lidén C, Rastogi S, Roberts D, et al. Activation of non-sensitizing or low-sensitizing fragrance substances into potent sensitizers – prehaptens and prohaptens. Contact Dermatitis 2013;69:323-334

115 Dooms-Goossens, A, Kerre S, Drieghe J, Bossuyt L, DeGreef H. Cosmetic products and their allergens. Eur J Dermatol 1992;2:465-468

116 Hjorth N. Eczematous allergy to balsams. Acta Derm Venereol 1961;41(suppl.46):1-216

117 Ung CY, White JML, White IR, Banerjee P, McFadden JP. Patch testing with the European baseline series fragrance markers: a 2016 update. Br J Dermatol 2018;178:776-780

118 Mitchell JC, Calnan CD, Clendenning WE, Cronin E, Hjorth N, Magnusson B, et al. Patch testing with some components of balsam of Peru. Contact Dermatitis 1976;2:57-58

119 Meynadier JM, Meynadier J, Peyron JL, Peyron L. Formes cliniques des manifestations cutanées d'allergie aux parfums. Ann Dermatol Venereol 1986;113:31-39

120 Wieck S, Olsson O, Kümmerer K, Klaschka U. Fragrance allergens in household detergents. Regul Toxicol Pharmacol 2018;97:163-169

121 Tammannavar P, Pushpalatha C, Shrenik J, Sowmya SV. An unexpected positive hypersensitive reaction to eugenol. BMJ Case Rep 2013:2013:bcr2013009464

122 Grade AC. Eugenol in wortelkanaalcement. Mogelijke oorzaak voor urticariële reacties. Ned Tijdschr Tandheelkd 1995;102:9-11 (article in Dutch)

123 Behzad M, Michl C, Arweiler N, Pfützner W. Lichenoid contact reaction to eugenol presenting as oral lichen planus. Allergo J Int 2014;23:242-245

124 Geier J, Uter W, Lessmann H, Schnuch A. Fragrance mix I and II: results of breakdown tests. Flavour Fragr J 2015;30:264-274

125 Girbig M, Hegewald J, Seidler A, Bauer A, Uter W, Schmitt J. Type IV sensitizations in physical therapists: patch test results of the Information Network of Departments of Dermatology (IVDK) 2007-2011. J Dtsch Dermatol Ges 2013;11:1185-1192

126 Dittmar D, Schuttelaar MLA. Contact sensitization to hydroperoxides of limonene and linalool: Results of consecutive patch testing and clinical relevance. Contact Dermatitis 2018 Oct 31. doi: 10.1111/cod.13137. [Epub ahead of print]

127 Silvestre JF, Mercader P, González-Pérez R, Hervella-Garcés M, Sanz-Sánchez T, Córdoba S, et al. Sensitization to fragrances in Spain: A 5-year multicentre study (2011-2015). Contact Dermatitis. 2018 Nov 14. doi: 10.1111/cod.13152. [Epub ahead of print]

128 Bui TNPT, Mose KF, Andersen F. Eugenol allergy mimicking burning mouth syndrome. Contact Dermatitis. 2018 Sep 20. doi: 10.1111/cod.13103. [Epub ahead of print]

Chapter 3.66   EVERNIA FURFURACEA (TREEMOSS) EXTRACT

IDENTIFICATION

Description/definition : Evernia furfuracea extract is an extract of the treemoss, *Evernia furfuracea* (L.), Usneaceae (the correct names are *Pseudoevernia furfuracea* and Parmeliaceae)

Chemical class(es) : Botanical products and botanical derivatives

INCI name USA : Evernia furfuracea (tree moss) extract

Other names : Treemoss extract; treemoss absolute

CAS registry number(s) : 90028-67-4; 94944-93-1

EC number(s) : 289-860-8

RIFM monograph(s) : Food Cosmet Toxicol 1975;13:915 (special issue II) (binder, page 711) (Treemoss concrete)

IFRA standard : Restricted (www.ifraorg.org/en-us/standards-library) (table 3.66.1)

SCCS opinion(s) : Various (1); SCCNFP/0389/00, final (29); SCCNFP/0392/00, final (30)

Function(s) in cosmetics : EU: perfuming. USA: fragrance ingredients

EU cosmetic restrictions : Regulated in Annex III/92 of the Regulation (EC) No. 1223/2009, regulated by 2003/15/EC; Must be labeled on cosmetics and detergent products, if present at > 10 ppm (0.001%) in leave-on products and > 100 ppm (0.01%) in rinse-off products; atranol and chloro-atranol are banned from cosmetics in the EU in 2019 (33)

Patch testing : 1% Pet. (SmartPracticeEurope, Chemotechnique, SmartPracticeCanada); recommended test concentration: 1.0% wt./wt. pet. (3)

Table 3.66.1 IFRA restrictions for treemoss extracts

Category [a]	Limits [b]	Category [a]	Limits [b]	Category [a]	Limits [b]
1	0.02%	5	0.10%	9	0.10%
2	0.03%	6	0.50%	10	0.10%
3	0.10%	7	0.10%	11	not restricted
4	0.10%	8	0.10%		

In the presence of oakmoss extracts, the level of treemoss extracts in the respective category has to be reduced accordingly such that the total amount of both extracts does not exceed the maximum permitted level in each category as listed in this table

[a] For explanation of categories see pages 6-8

[b] Limits in the finished products

GENERAL

Treemoss extracts are mostly manufactured from *Pseudevernia furfuracea* (L.) Zopf., a lichen which is particularly common on coniferous trees, mainly pine and cedar trees (20). Treemoss absolute (*Pseudevernia furfuraceae* spp. absolute; CAS numbers 68648-41-9 and 68650-45-3) is a dark brown semi-solid; its odor type is mossy and its odor at 100% is described as 'woody dry forest seaweed herbal green' (www.thegoodscentscompany.com).

Treemoss absolute has both been found 'unlikely' to be a skin sensitizer '(25) and to be a 'moderate skin sensitizer' (26) with the local lymph node assay (LLNA), under the conditions of the tests. In an SCCS opinion, the sensitizing potency of treemoss extract could not be classified, because no EC3 value was established in the LLNA in animal experiments; higher concentrations should also have been tested (27,28).   I

The main sensitizers in treemoss extracts are most likely atranol and chloroatranol. The presence of these chemicals in cosmetic products in the EU will be prohibited from August 2021 on; starting August 2019, cosmetic products containing atranol are not allowed to be placed on the Union market (33). This will probably result in treemoss extract (and oakmoss extract) not being used at all anymore in fragrances.

In most literature on Evernia furfuracea extract (the INCI name), the names treemoss absolute or treemoss extract are used. For convenience sake, in this chapter mostly the term 'treemoss extract' is used. See also the chapters on atranorin, atranol, chloroatranol, physodic acid, physodalic acid and fumarprotocetraric acid, potential allergens found in treemoss extract.

Chemical composition

The chemical composition of treemoss extract is strongly dependent on the geographic origin of the lichen, the source tree, the chemical race (chemotype) of *P. furfuracea*, adulteration with lichens other than *P. furfuracea* and the mode of production. Selected chemicals identified in treemoss extracts of various origins are shown in table 3.66.2 (adapted from ref. 20). Apart from atranorin and chloroatranorin, which represent up to 80% of the depside fraction, olivetonide, physodone and isophysodic acid are considered to be characteristic elements of industrial extracts of *P. furfuracea* (20). In lichen collected on conifers (mainly *P. sylvestris*), tediously separated from any component derived from the host tree, some 40 sterols and triterpenes have been identified by various analytical methods. It is highly probable that these compounds are metabolites from the host tree (*Pinus* spp.), involving a migration from the host to the parasitic lichen (20).

Determining the *quantitative* composition of industrial treemoss and other lichen extracts, either resinoids (first solvent extract from treemoss) or absolutes, is very difficult because of the intense chemical variability of the extracts and, more importantly, the lack of analytical reference compounds that are necessary to perform quantitative measurements by standardization (20). Indeed, the content of defined lichen compounds in *P. furfuracea* has only rarely been measured and quantitative data on the composition of industrial resinoids and other extracts of *P. furfuracea* are even more scarce.

Of chemicals relevant for sensitization, a typical industrial treemoss absolute *oil* (which is also an extract) may contain approximately 0.36% atranol, 0.22% chloroatranol and 5-6% dehydroabietic acid and other resin acids (including the allergenic 7-oxodehydroabietic acid), but undetectable levels of atranorin and chloroatranorin, as these are easily degraded into atranol and chloroatranol (20). The resin acids are not only present in the wood debris from the host pine tree, but they also migrate into the lichen. These are selectively removed from treemoss extracts to lower their concentrations. The IFRA standard specifies that 'treemoss extracts shall not contain more than 0.8% of dehydroabietic acid (DHA) as a marker of 2% of total resin acids. The concentration of DHA (about 40% of the total resin acids) in treemoss can be measured with an HPLC reverse phase-spectrofluorimetry method. Furthermore, levels of atranol and chloroatranol should each be below 100 ppm in treemoss extracts' (www.ifraorg.org/en-us/standards-library).

Table 3.66.2 Selected chemicals identified in treemoss extracts from various origins (adapted from ref. 20)

Monoaryl compounds	Olivetonide [c]	Imbricaric acid
Atranol	Orcinol	Isophysodic acid [c]
Chloroatranol	β-Orcinol	Lecanoric acid
2-Chloro-3,5-dimethoxytoluene	β-Orcinolcarboxylic acid	2'-*O*-Methylphysodic acid
Chlorohaematommic acid	Orcinol monomethylether	2'-*O*-Methylphysodone
Divarinol	5-Pentylresorcinol (= olivetol)	Microphyllinic acid
Ethyl chlorohaematommate	Rhizonic acid	Olivetoric acid
Ethyl haematommate		Perlatolic acid
Haematommic acid	**Depsides and depsidones**	Physodalic acid
Hydroxy-olivetonide	Alectoronic acid	Physodic acid
Isopropyl haematommate [a]	Atranorin [b,c]	Physodone [c]
Methyl haematommate	Chloroatranorin [b,c]	Virensic acid
Methyl β-orcinolcarboxylate	Fumarprotocetraric acid	Vulpinic acid
Methyl orsellinate	Furfuric acid	
Olivetolcarboxylic acid	3-Hydroxyphysodic acid	

[a] artifact formed from atranorin during the extraction with isopropanol (20)

[b] atranorin and chloroatranorin represent up to 80% of the depside fraction (20)

[c] atranorin, chloroatranorin, olivetonide, physodone and isophysodic acid are considered to be characteristic elements of industrial extracts of *P. furfuracea* (20)

CONTACT ALLERGY

General

Treemoss absolute consistently causes >2% positive patch test reactions in routine testing (table 3.66.3). Therefore, it has been suggested to add it to the European baseline series as single fragrance allergen. Up to now, the European Society of Contact Dermatitis (ESCD) nor the EECDRG (European Environmental and Contact Dermatitis Research Group) have reacted to this proposition, probably because 47-80% of the reactions to treemoss absolute are 'picked up' by a positive patch test to the fragrance mix I (2,4,14,16), nearly 60% co-reacts to oakmoss absolute (22) and treemoss is used very infrequently in cosmetic products (see the section 'Presence in products and chemical analyses' below).

There appear to be two subgroups of patients allergic to treemoss extract. The largest group very frequently co-reacts to oakmoss extract, but does not react to colophonium. In this group, the sensitizers are chemicals common to oakmoss and treemoss extract, presumably chloroatranol and atranol. The second subgroup co-reacts infrequently to oakmoss extract but is allergic to colophonium. In these patients, the allergens are oxidized resin acids from pine trees (which are present in treemoss extract), the same as in colophonium. Oakmoss does infrequently co-react in these patients, as the amounts of resin acids in oakmoss are (or at least should be) very low (22).

The presence of atranol and chloroatranol in cosmetic products in the EU will be prohibited from August 2021 on; from August 2019 cosmetic products containing chloroatranol are not allowed to be placed on the Union market (33). This will probably result in a ban of the use of oakmoss extract and tree moss extract (33).

Patch testing in groups of patients
Results of studies testing treemoss extract / absolute in consecutive patients suspected of contact dermatitis (routine testing) and those of testing in groups of *selected* patients (e.g. patients with known or suspected fragrance or cosmetic dermatitis, nurses with occupational contact dermatitis) are shown in table 3.66.3.

Patch testing in consecutive patients suspected of contact dermatitis: routine testing
In seven studies in which routine testing with treemoss extract / absolute was performed, frequencies of sensitization have ranged from 1.5% to 3.3%. In 4/7 investigations, no (specific) data on relevance were provided; in the three other studies addressing the issue, 45-74% of the positive reactions were scored as relevant (2,14,15). Causative products were usually not mentioned or specified, but in one study, of the relevant reactions to any of 26 fragrances tested, 96% were caused by cosmetic products (2).

Patch testing in groups of selected patients
Results of studies patch testing treemoss extract / absolute in groups of selected patients (e.g. patients with known or suspected fragrance or cosmetic dermatitis, nurses with occupational contact dermatitis) are shown in table 3.66.3. In 8 investigations, frequencies of sensitization have ranged from 2.5% to 30%. The highest rates were observed in patients known to be allergic to fragrances (6,17). The frequency of 30% positive reactions was found in a small early study from the USA in a group of 20 fragrance-allergic individuals (6), when presumably high concentrations of fragrances were still used. In none of the 6 studies were (specific) relevance data provided.

Table 3.66.3 Patch testing in groups of patients

Years and Country	Test conc. & vehicle	Number of patients tested | positive (%)		Selection of patients (S); Relevance (R); Comments (C)	Ref.
Routine testing					
2015-7 Netherlands		821	12 (1.5%)	R: not stated	34
2015-2016 UK	1% pet.	2084	44 (2.1%)	R: not specified for individual fragrances; 25% of patients who reacted to any fragrance or fragrance marker had a positive fragrance history	32
2010-2015 Denmark	1% pet.	6004	(3.0%)	R: present relevance 45%, past relevance 29%; C: 47% co-reactivity to FM I	14
2013-2014 Thailand		312	8 (2.6%)	R: 63%	15
2011-2012 UK	1% pet.	1951	44 (2.3%)	R: not stated; 55% co-reactivity to FM I	16
2008-2010 Denmark	1% pet.	1503	50 (3.3%)	S: mostly routine testing; R: 74%; 62% co-reactivity of FM I, 25% of FM II; C: of the relevant reactions to any of the 26 fragrances tested, 96% were caused by cosmetic products	2
2003-2004 IVDK	1% pet.	1658	45 (2.7%)	R: not stated; C: 80% co-reactivity of FM I	4
Testing in groups of selected patients					
2011-2015 Spain	1% pet.	607	27 (4.4%)	S: patients previously reacting to FM I, FM II, Myroxylon pereirae resin or hydroxyisohexyl 3-cyclohexene carboxaldehyde in the baseline series and subsequently tested with a fragrance series; R: not stated	35
2003-2012 IVDK		319	23 (7.2%)	S: nurses with occupational contact dermatitis; R: not stated	12
2006-2011 IVDK	1% pet.	708	46 (6.5%)	S: patients with suspected cosmetic intolerance; R: not stated	13
2003-2010 IVDK	1% pet.	3030	193 (6.4%)	S: unspecified; this was a subgroup that was tested with treemoss, oakmoss and colophonium; R: not stated; C: 58% co-reactivity to oakmoss absolute	22
2005-10 Netherlands		100	19 (19%)	S: patients with known fragrance sensitivity based on a positive patch test to the FM I and/or the FM II; R: not stated	17
2005-2008 IVDK	1% pet.	1947	(6.0%)	S: not specified; R: not stated	18
2005-7 Netherlands	2% pet.	320	8 (2.5%)	S: patients suspected of fragrance or cosmetic allergy; R: 61% relevance for all positive tested fragrances together	5
1975 USA	?% pet.	20	6 (30%)	S: fragrance-allergic patients; R: not stated	6

FM: Fragrance mix; IVDK: Informationsverbund Dermatologischer Kliniken (Germany, Switzerland, Austria)

Case reports and case series
Treemoss absolute was stated to be the (or an) allergen in one patient in a group of 603 individuals suffering from cosmetic dermatitis, seen in the period 2010-2015 in Leuven, Belgium (11).

Cross-reactions, pseudo-cross-reactions and co-reactions
For general information on cross-/pseudo-cross-/co-reactivity of fragrance chemicals with other fragrances, fragrance markers (fragrance mix I, fragrance mix II, colophonium, Myroxylon pereirae resin [balsam of Peru]) and essential oils see Chapter 1.2 General information on cross-reactions, pseudo-cross-reactions and co-reactions.

Treemoss absolutes often contain a considerable amount of resin acids and their oxidation products and therefore may co-react to colophonium, in which the same materials are the sensitizers (22,24).

Of 193 patients allergic to treemoss extract, 112 (58%) co-reacted to oakmoss extract (22). In a subgroup of patients who were negative to colophonium, co-reactivity was 77%, whereas in colophonium-positive patients, co-reactivity to oakmoss extract was only 18%. Moreover, E. furfuracea-sensitized patients showed (strong or extreme) concomitant reactions to colophonium significantly more often if *not* co-sensitized to E. prunastri. It was concluded that two subgroups of E. furfuracea-sensitized patients exist: (i) those with sensitization to (oxidized) resin acids [which are present in treemoss extract but not in oakmoss extract), as indicated by positive patch test reactions also to colophonium, and (ii) those non-sensitized to resin acids, but sensitized to common constituents of E. prunastri and E. furfuracea, presumably chloroatranol and atranol (22).

Of 5 patients reacting to an acetone extract of oakmoss 7% in petrolatum, all co-reacted to treemoss extract, which also contains the oakmoss sensitizers atranorin and chloroatranorin (23).

Presence in products and chemical analyses
As can be seen from the studies below, the use of treemoss extract (in concentrations that require labeling) in fragrances is very limited.

In Denmark, in 2015-2016, 5588 fragranced cosmetic products were examined with a smartphone application for the 26 fragrances that need to be labeled in the EU. Evernia furfuracea extract was present in 0.3% of the products (rank number 22) (9).

In Germany, in 2015, fragrance allergens were evaluated based on lists of ingredients in 817 (unique) detergents (all-purpose cleaners, cleaning preparations for special purposes [e.g. bathroom, kitchen, dish-washing] and laundry detergents) present in 131 households. Evernia furfuracea extract was found to be present in 2 (0.2%) of the products (31).

In 2008, 2010 and 2011, 374 deodorants available in German retail shops were randomly selected and their labels checked for the presence of the 26 fragrances that need to be labeled. Treemoss extract was found to be present in one (0.3%) of the products (19).

In Germany, in the period 2006-2009, 4991 cosmetic products were randomly sampled for an official investigation of conformity of cosmetic products with legal provisions. The labels were inspected for the presence of the 26 fragrances that need to be labeled in the EU. Treemoss extract was present in 0.7% of the products (rank number 21) (8).

In 2006, of 88 popular perfume containing deodorants purchased in Denmark, 2 (2%) were labeled to contain treemoss extract (10).

In January 2006, a study of perfumed cosmetic and household products available on the shelves of U.K. retailers was carried out. Products were included if 'parfum' or 'aroma' was listed among the ingredients. Three hundred products were surveyed and any of 26 mandatory labeling fragrances named on the label were recorded. Treemoss extract was present in 9 (3%) of the products (rank number 23) (7).

Other information
In two commercial treemoss absolutes, the presence of a mixture of resin acids accounting for 11.4% (wt./wt.) and 8.1% (wt./wt.) of the material, respectively, was identified. The major compound was dehydroabietic acid, together with abietic acid and its isomers. Also, the samples proved to contain 1.6% resp. 1.1% of 7-oxo-dehydroabietic acid, an important sensitizer in colophonium (24). To investigate whether patients allergic to colophonium would also react to treemoss, these 2 samples (1% and 2% pet.) were patch tested in 17 patients known to be allergic to colophonium. Twelve patients (71%) reacted to the treemoss samples. It was concluded that treemoss absolute contains enough resin acids and oxidation products to elicit a positive reaction in the great majority of colophonium-allergic patients (24).

LITERATURE

1   Various SCCS opinions on Evernia furfuracea extract have been published and are available at: http://ec.europa.eu/growth/tools-databases/cosing/index.cfm?fuseaction=search.details_v2&id=27941&back=1

2   Heisterberg MV, Menné T, Johansen JD. Contact allergy to the 26 specific fragrance ingredients to be declared on cosmetic products in accordance with the EU cosmetic directive. Contact Dermatitis 2011;65:266-275

3   Bruze M, Svedman C, Andersen KE, Bruynzeel D, Goossens A, Johansen JD, et al. Patch test concentrations (doses in mg/cm2) for the 12 non-mix fragrance substances regulated by European legislation. Contact Dermatitis 2012;66:131-136

4   Schnuch A, Uter W, Geier J, Lessmann H, Frosch PJ. Sensitization to 26 fragrances to be labelled according to current European regulation: Results of the IVDK and review of the literature. Contact Dermatitis 2007;57:1-10

5   Oosten EJ van, Schuttelaar ML, Coenraads PJ. Clinical relevance of positive patch test reactions to the 26 EU-labelled fragrances. Contact Dermatitis 2009;61:217-223

6   Larsen WG. Perfume dermatitis. A study of 20 patients. Arch Dermatol 1977;113:623-626

7   Buckley DA. Fragrance ingredient labelling in products on sale in the UK. Br J Dermatol 2007;157:295-300

8   Uter W, Yazar K, Kratz E-M, Mildau G, Lidén C. Coupled exposure to ingredients of cosmetic products: I. Fragrances. Contact Dermatitis 2013;69:335-341

9   Bennike NH, Oturai NB, Müller S, Kirkeby CS, Jørgensen C, Christensen AB, et al. Fragrance contact allergens in 5588 cosmetic products identified through a novel smartphone application. J Eur Acad Dermatol Venereol 2018;32:79-85

10 Rastogi SC, Hellerup Jensen G, Johansen JD. Survey and risk assessment of chemical substances in deodorants. Survey of Chemical Substances in Consumer Products, No. 86 2007. Danish Ministry of the Environment, Environmental Protection Agency. Available at: https://www2.mst.dk/Udgiv/publications/2007/978-87-7052-625-8/pdf/978-87-7052-626-5.pdf

11 Goossens A. Cosmetic contact allergens. Cosmetics 2016, 3, 5; doi:10.3390/cosmetics3010005

12 Molin S, Bauer A, Schnuch A, Geier J. Occupational contact allergy in nurses: results from the Information Network of Departments of Dermatology 2003–2012. Contact Dermatitis 2015;72:164-171

13 Dinkloh A, Worm M, Geier J, Schnuch A, Wollenberg A. Contact sensitization in patients with suspected cosmetic intolerance: results of the IVDK 2006-2011. J Eur Acad Dermatol Venereol 2015;29:1071-1081

14 Bennike NH, Zachariae C, Johansen JD. Non-mix fragrances are top sensitizers in consecutive dermatitis patients – a cross-sectional study of the 26 EU-labelled fragrance allergens. Contact Dermatitis 2017;77:270-279

15 Vejanurug P, Tresukosol P, Sajjachareonpong P, Puangpet P. Fragrance allergy could be missed without patch testing with 26 individual fragrance allergens. Contact Dermatitis 2016;74:230-235

16 Mann J, McFadden JP, White JML, White IR, Banerjee P. Baseline series fragrance markers fail to predict contact allergy. Contact Dermatitis 2014;70:276-281

17 Nagtegaal MJC, Pentinga SE, Kuik J, Kezic S, Rustemeyer T. The role of the skin irritation response in polysensitization to fragrances. Contact Dermatitis 2012;67:28-35

18 Uter W, Geier J, Frosch P, Schnuch A. Contact allergy to fragrances: current patch test results (2005–2008) from the Information Network of Departments of Dermatology. Contact Dermatitis 2010;63:254-261

19 Klaschka U. Contact allergens for armpits - allergenic fragrances specified on deodorants. Int J Hyg Environ Health 2012;215:584-591

20 Joulain D, Tabacchi R. Lichen extracts as raw materials in perfumery. Part 2: treemoss. Flavour Fragr J 2009;24:105-116

21 Pongpairoj K, Puangpet P, Thaiwat P, McFadden JP. Should Evernia furfuracea be included in a baseline screening series of contact allergens? Contact Dermatitis 2016;74:257-258

22 Uter W, Schmidt E, Lessmann H, Schnuch A. Contact sensitization to tree moss (Evernia furfuracea extract, INCI) is heterogeneous. Contact Dermatitis 2012;67:36-41

23 Fregert S, Dahlquist I. Patch testing with oak moss extract. Contact Dermatitis 1983;9:227

24 Lepoittevin JP, Meschkat E, Huygens S, Goossens A. Presence of resin acids in "Oakmoss" patch test material: a source of misdiagnosis? J Invest Dermatol 2000;115:129-130

25 SCCP (Scientific Committee on Consumer Products). Opinion on Atranol and Chloroatranol present in natural extracts (e.g. oak moss and tree moss extract), 7 December 2004, SCCP/00847/04. Available at: http://ec.europa.eu/health/ph_risk/committees/04_sccp/docs/sccp_o_006.pdf

26 SCCP (Scientific Committee on Consumer Products). Opinion on Oak moss / Tree moss (sensitisation only), 15 April 2008, SCCP/1131/07. Available at: ec.europa.eu/health/ph_risk/committees/04_sccp/docs/sccp_o_131.pdf

27 SCCS (Scientific Committee on Consumer Safety). Opinion on Fragrance allergens in cosmetic products, 26-27 June 2012, SCCS/1459/11. Available at: https://ec.europa.eu/health/sites/health/files/scientific_committees/consumer_safety/docs/sccs_o_102.pdf

28 Uter W, Johansen JD, Börje A, Karlberg A-T, Lidén C, Rastogi S, Roberts D, White IR. Categorization of fragrance contact allergens for prioritization of preventive measures: clinical and experimental data and consideration of structure–activity relationships. Contact Dermatitis 2013;69:196-230

29 Opinion of the Scientific Committee on Cosmetic Products and Non-Food Products Intended for Consumers concerning 'The 1st update of the inventory of ingredients employed in cosmetic products. Section II: Perfume and aromatic raw materials', 24 October 2000, SCCNFP/0389/00, final. Available at: http://ec.europa.eu/health/ph_risk/committees/sccp/documents/out131_en.pdf

30 Opinion of the Scientific Committee on Cosmetic Products and Non-Food Products Intended for Consumers concerning ' An initial list of perfumery materials which must not form part of cosmetic products except subject to the Restrictions and Conditions laid down, 25 September 2001, SCCNFP/0392/00, final. Available at: http://ec.europa.eu/health/archive/ph_risk/committees/sccp/documents/out150_en.pdf

31 Wieck S, Olsson O, Kümmerer K, Klaschka U. Fragrance allergens in household detergents. Regul Toxicol Pharmacol 2018;97:163-169

32 Ung CY, White JML, White IR, Banerjee P, McFadden JP. Patch testing with the European baseline series fragrance markers: a 2016 update. Br J Dermatol 2018;178:776-780

33 Directorate-General for Internal Market, Industry, Entrepreneurship and SMEs (European Commission). Commission Regulation (EU) 2017/1410 of 2 August 2017 amending Annexes II and III to Regulation (EC) No 1223/2009 of the European Parliament and of the Council on cosmetic products. Official J European Union 2017;L202:1-3

34 Dittmar D, Schuttelaar MLA. Contact sensitization to hydroperoxides of limonene and linalool: Results of consecutive patch testing and clinical relevance. Contact Dermatitis 2018 Oct 31. doi: 10.1111/cod.13137. [Epub ahead of print]

35 Silvestre JF, Mercader P, González-Pérez R, Hervella-Garcés M, Sanz-Sánchez T, Córdoba S, et al. Sensitization to fragrances in Spain: A 5-year multicentre study (2011-2015). Contact Dermatitis. 2018 Nov 14. doi: 10.1111/cod.13152. [Epub ahead of print]

Chapter 3.67 EVERNIA PRUNASTRI (OAKMOSS) EXTRACT

IDENTIFICATION

Description/definition : Evernia prunastri extract is an extract of the oakmoss, *Evernia prunastri*, Parmeliaceae

Chemical class(es) : Botanical products and botanical derivatives

INCI name USA : Evernia prunastri (oakmoss) extract

Other names : Oakmoss extract; oakmoss absolute

CAS registry number(s) : 90028-68-5; 68917-10-2; 9000-50-4

EC number(s) : 289-861-3

RIFM monograph(s) : Food Cosmet Toxicol 1975;13:891 (special issue II) (binder, page 599) (oakmoss resinoid)

IFRA standard : Restricted (www.ifraorg.org/en-us/standards-library) (table 3.67.1)

SCCS opinion(s) : Various (1); SCCNFP/0389/00, final (89); SCCNFP/0392/00, final (90)

Function(s) in cosmetics : EU: perfuming. USA: fragrance ingredients

EU cosmetic restrictions : Regulated in Annex III/91 of the Regulation (EC) No. 1223/2009, regulated by 2003/15/EC; Must be labeled on cosmetics and detergent products, if present at > 10 ppm (0.001%) in leave-on products and > 100 ppm (0.01%) in rinse-off products; atranol and chloro-atranol are banned from cosmetics in the EU in 2019 (92)

Patch testing : 1% Pet. (SmartPracticeEurope, SmartPracticeCanada); 2% pet. (Chemotechnique); also present in the fragrance mix I; TEST ADVICE: 2% pet.

Table 3.67.1 IFRA restrictions for oakmoss extracts

Category [a]	Limits [b]	Category [a]	Limits [b]	Category [a]	Limits [b]
1	0.02%	5	0.10%	9	0.10%
2	0.03%	6	0.50%	10	0.10%
3	0.10%	7	0.10%	11	not restricted
4	0.10%	8	0.10%		

Oakmoss extracts used in fragrance compounds must not contain added treemoss, which is a source of resin acids. Traces of resin acids may be carried over to commercial qualities of oakmoss in the manufacturing process. These traces must not exceed 0.1% (1000 ppm) dehydroabietic acid (DHA) in the extract. Further, levels of atranol and chloroatranol should each be below 100 ppm in oakmoss extracts.

[a] For explanation of categories see pages 6-8
[b] Limits in the finished products

GENERAL

Evernia prunastri extract (oakmoss extract) is the extract of the lichen *Evernia prunastri* var. *prunastri* (L.) Ach. (Parmeliaceae), commonly called 'oakmoss'. Oakmoss grows primarily on oak trees all over central and southern Europe, as well as in Morocco and Algeria (70). After being harvested, the lichen is desiccated and then humidified with water prior to the extraction procedure with organic solvents. The solvents used are either hexane or mixtures of hexane and more polar solvents, mainly acetates. The crude solvent extracts, called resinoids, are further treated with alcohol in order to obtain the absolutes (also called soluble resinoids), which are then used in fragrance compositions. The absolutes may also be subjected to physical treatments such as discoloration with charcoal or high-vacuum distillation (50,70,82). Because of its woody aroma and fixative properties, oakmoss absolute is used extensively in perfumery as a natural fragrance, particularly for masculine products such as aftershave lotions, cosmetics and fine perfumes (70).

Freshly harvested oakmoss has substantially no scent. The moss contains various types of depsides, which are non-volatile, odorless, polyfunctional diaryl derivatives, including lecanoric acid, evernic acid, divaricatic acid, barbatic acid, atranorin, chloroatranorin and thamnolic acid (see the section 'Chemical composition' below). The characteristic oakmoss fragrance is only developed after cleavage of the depsides during treatment of the oakmoss resinoid with alcohols to give volatile, scented, monoaryl derivatives (73). Resorcinol derivatives such as methyl-β-orcinol carboxylate and orcinol monomethyl ether are mainly responsible for the characteristic earthy-moss-like odor of the oakmoss products (74).

For oakmoss absolute (Evernia prunastri lichen absolute) (FDA internal no.: 977059-15-6) the following data are provided by www.thegoodscentscompany.com: Oakmoss absolute (Evernia prunastri lichen absolute) is a dark green brown semi-solid; its odor type is mossy and its odor at 100% is described as 'green woody earthy musty mossy oily woody'. In a 2008 SCCS Opinion, it is stated that oakmoss absolute is a dark green, semi-solid to solid mass or a dark brownish-green liquid and oakmoss resinoid is an almost black-green or brownish-green waxy mass (78).

The sensitizing potency of oakmoss extract has been classified as 'moderate' based on an EC3 value of 3.9% in the LLNA (local lymph node assay) in animal experiments (85,86). Most reactions to oakmoss extract are the result of allergy to fragrances, especially aftershave preparations; sensitization from contact with oakmoss lichens themselves are less frequent (43,55,58).

Oakmoss absolute is a constituent of the fragrance mix I. In groups of patients reacting to the mix and tested with its 8 ingredients, oakmoss absolute scored 8.6-44% positive patch test reactions, median 29.3% and average 26.6%. It has rank number 1 in the list of most frequent reactors in the mix (see Chapter 3.70 Fragrance mix I).

In most literature on Evernia prunastri extract (the INCI name), the names oakmoss absolute or oakmoss extract are used. For convenience sake, in this chapter mostly the term 'oakmoss extract' is used, unless the extract discussed was an absolute (for example in the case of patch test results, for which oakmoss absolutes are used).

The presence of atranol and chloroatranol in cosmetic products in the EU will be prohibited from August 2021 on; starting August 2019, cosmetic products containing chloroatranol are not allowed to be placed on the Union market (92). This will probably result in oakmoss extract and treemoss extract not being used at all anymore in fragrances.

See also the chapters on Fragrance mix I, atranol, atranorin, chloroatranol, evernic acid, and usnic acid, potential allergens found in oakmoss extracts.

Chemical composition

The chemical composition of commercial oakmoss extracts is strongly dependent on the mode of production (type of solvent, temperature, duration and number of contacts) and possible intentional or unintentional adulteration with lichens other than Evernia prunastri or biomass (50). In oakmoss of various origins, some 175 constituents have been identified, including 15 depsides, 19 mono-aromatic compounds, 9 chlorinated mono-aromatic compounds, 5 divarinol-derivatives, 26 triterpenes and steroids, 51 terpenoids and 48 other compounds (50). Selected chemicals (the depsides and the terpenoids which are known to have caused contact allergy [from any source]) identified in oakmoss extracts of various origin are shown in table 3.67.2 (adapted from refs. 50,51). The (chlorinated) mono-aromatic compounds and divarinol-derivatives are degradation products of the depsides through hydrolysis or decarboxyla-tion. These include the main sensitizers atranol and chloroatranol, which are derived from the depsides atranorin and chloroatranorin (50).

Determining the *quantitative* composition of industrial oakmoss and other lichen extracts, either resinoids, absolutes or other extracts, is very difficult because of the intense chemical variability of the extracts and, more importantly, the lack of analytical reference compounds that are necessary to perform quantitative measurements by standardization (50). Usnic acid is one of the most common lichen substances. Whereas oakmoss resinoid may contain >15% usnic acid, the absolutes are practically free of it (50). The contents of atranol and chloroatranol in untreated oakmoss absolutes (atranol and chloroatranol not removed) have been reported to be in the ranges of 2.1-2.9% and 0.9-1.4%, respectively (50,70,80).

Table 3.67.2 Selected chemicals identified in oakmoss extracts from various origins (adapted from refs. 50,51)

Depsides	Methyl 3'-methyllecanorate	Geraniol
Atranorin	Prunastric acid	α-Ionone
Barbatic acid	Prunastrin	β-Ionone
Chloroatranorin	Thamnolic acid	Limonene
Divaricatic acid	(+)-Usnic acid [a]	Linalool
Evernic acid		5-Methyl-alpha-ionone
Evernin	**Terpenoids**	Myrcene
Lecanoric acid	Camphor	α-Pinene
Lecanorin	Carvone	β-Pinene
3'-Methylevernic acid	β-Caryophyllene	Terpinen-4-ol
2'-O-Methylevernic acid	Citronellol	Terpinolene
2,2'-di-O-Methylgyrophoric acid	p-Cymene	Thymol
2'',4-di-O-Methylgyrophoric acid	Eucalyptol (1,8-cineole)	

[a] not a depside but a dibenzofuran

Formerly, industrial oakmoss extracts were often mixed with treemoss extracts, both to enhance the characteristic scent and to reduce cost, as treemoss is far cheaper than oakmoss. Currently, the International Fragrance Association's (IFRA) recommendation ('standard') on oakmoss states: 'Oakmoss extracts used in perfume compounds must not contain added treemoss, which is a source of resin acids. Traces of resin acids may be carried over to commercial qualities of oakmoss in the manufacturing process. These traces must not exceed 0.1% (1000 ppm) dehydroabietic acid (DHA) in the extract. Further, levels of atranol and chloroatranol should each be below 100 ppm in oakmoss extracts' (http://www.ifraorg.org/en-us/standards-library).

The allergens in oakmoss extracts

Although oakmoss extract is one of the most frequent causes of fragrance contact allergy, is was found to be only a 'moderate' (79) and 'weak to moderate' (78) sensitizer when analyzed with the local lymph node assay (LLNA), under the conditions of the tests. Experiments in mice, sensitized and challenged with various concentrations of atranol, chloroatranol and oakmoss absolute, in which the immune responses were analyzed as B cell infiltration, T cell proliferation in the draining lymph nodes, and expression of interleukin (IL)-18, IL-1β and tumor necrosis factor-α in skin, have shown that oakmoss induces sensitization when applied in high concentrations. Atranol and chloroatranol, considered to be the most important allergens in oakmoss absolute (see below in this section), elicited challenge reactions following sensitization with oakmoss. It was shown that atranol and chloroatranol can induce both sensitization and challenge reactions, but that the mixture of allergens in oakmoss absolute is more potent than atranol and chloroatranol alone (77). It has been found in animal and human experiments that lowering the concentrations of potential sensitizers in oakmoss absolute (atranol, chloroatranol, ethyl haematommate, ethylchlorohaematommate, see below in this section) decreases the sensitizing potential of oakmoss absolute (50,80).

For many years, when benzene extracts were used, sensitivity to oakmoss was mainly correlated with a sensitivity to atranorin, evernic acid, and usnic acid (43,53,54,55,58,71). Later, compounds formed by trans-esterification of atranorin and chloroatranorin during oakmoss processing, such as ethyl chlorohaematommate, were shown to be allergenic (50,72). Benzene is no longer used for extraction; currently most often pure hexane or mixtures of hexane with more polar solvents (in general acetates) are used to extract the lichen and produce the resinoid. As a consequence, the chemical composition of oakmoss resinoids and their derived absolutes has changed (70).

In 2003, a combination of bioassay-guided chemical fractionation, (repeat) patch testing and analytical and SAR (structure-activity relationship) methods allowed the identification of chloroatranol and atranol, formed by transesterification and decarboxylation of atranorin and chloroatranorin during the oakmoss absolute derivatization, as main sensitizers and to a lesser degree methyl-β-orcinol carboxylate and β-orcinol (70). Pure synthetic chloroatranol and atranol confirmed their strong eliciting potential with some patients reacting strongly at 90 and 210 ppm, respectively (70).

Another indication that chloroatranol and atranol are probably the main sensitizers in oakmoss extract is that patch test reactivity is lower in samples with a reduced content of atranol and chloroatranol than in conventional high content samples (34,82,83,84) (see the section 'Serial dilution testing and ROATS' below). However, it is certain that there are several other sensitizers in the material, as shown by positive patch tests with thin-layer chromatography strips at sites other than the atranol / chloroatranol spots (82).

CONTACT ALLERGY

General population

In the period 2008-2011, in 5 European countries (Sweden, Germany, Netherlands, Portugal, Italy), a random sample of the general population of 3119 individuals aged 18-74 years were patch tested with the FM I, its 8 ingredients, the FM II, its 6 ingredients and Myroxylon pereirae resin. There were 16 reactions (0.5%) to oakmoss absolute and 32 (1.0%) to oakmoss absolute with high chloroatranol and atranol content, both tested 2% in petrolatum. About half of all positive reactions to fragrances were considered to be relevant based on standardized criteria. Women were affected twice as often as men (46).

Patch testing in groups of patients

Results of studies testing oakmoss absolute in consecutive patients suspected of contact dermatitis (routine testing) are shown in table 3.67.3. Results of testing in groups of *selected* patients (e.g. patients with known or suspected fragrance or cosmetic dermatitis, individuals with periorbital dermatitis) are shown in table 3.67.4.

Patch testing in consecutive patients suspected of contact dermatitis: routine testing

In fourteen studies in which routine testing with oakmoss absolute was performed, frequencies of sensitization have ranged from 0.7% to 3.1% (table 3.67.3). In the study with the highest rate, 5% pet. was used for patch testing (40).

In 11/14 investigations, no (specific) data on relevance were provided; in the three studies addressing the issue, 33-67% of the positive reactions were scored as relevant (2,27,28). Causative products were usually not mentioned or specified, but in one study, of the relevant reactions to any of 26 fragrances tested, 96% were caused by cosmetic products (2).

Table 3.67.3 Patch testing in groups of patients: Routine testing

Years and Country	Test conc. & vehicle	Number of patients tested	positive (%)	Selection of patients (S); Relevance (R); Comments (C)	Ref.
2015-7 Netherlands		821	17 (1.2%)	R: not stated	95
2015-2016 UK	2% pet.	2084	36 (1.7%)	R: not specified for individual fragrances; 25% of patients who reacted to any fragrance or fragrance marker had a positive fragrance history	93
2010-2015 Denmark	1% pet.	6004	78 (1.3%)	R: present relevance 59%, past relevance 30%	27
2009-2015 Sweden	2% pet.	4430	79 (1.8%)	R: not stated	32
2013-2014 Thailand		312	3 (1.0%)	R: 67%	28
2011-2012 UK	2% pet.	1951	34 (1.7%)	R: not stated	31
2010-2011 China	2% pet.	296	(0.7%)	R: 67% for all fragrances tested together (excluding FM I)	29
2008-2010 Denmark	1% pet.	1503	31 (2.1%)	S: mostly routine testing; R: 33%; 94% co-reactivity of FM I; C: of the relevant reactions to any of the 26 fragrances tested, 96% were caused by cosmetic products	2
2005-2008 IVDK	1% pet.	1213	(1.8%)	R: not stated	35
2003-2004 IVDK	1% pet.	2063	46 (2.2%)	R: not stated; C: 57% co-reactivity of FM I	3
2000-2001 Denmark	1% pet.	885	28 (3.2%)	R: not stated; C: 100% co-reactivity to FM I, 29% co-reactivity to colophonium; follicular reactions were counted as positive	68
<1995 9 European countries + USA	1% pet.	1072	24 (2.2%)	R: not stated	18
1993 EECDRG	1% pet.	709	18 (2.6%)	R: not stated	39
1991 The Netherlands	5% pet.	677	21 (3.1%)	R: not stated	40

EECDRG: European Environmental and Contact Dermatitis Research Group; FM: Fragrance mix; IVDK: Informationsverbund Dermatologischer Kliniken (Germany, Switzerland, Austria)

Patch testing in groups of selected patients

Results of studies patch testing oakmoss absolute in groups of selected patients (e.g. patients with known or suspected fragrance or cosmetic dermatitis, individuals with periorbital dermatitis) are shown in table 3.67.4.

In 15 investigations, frequencies of sensitization to oakmoss absolute have ranged from 1.9% to 64%. The highest rate (64%) was observed in Norway, in a group of patients with sensitivity to different brands of perfumes, deodorants and aftershave lotions (88). Presumably, in those days (over 30 years ago), the sensitizing capacity of oakmoss extracts were not yet well known and high concentrations of this fragrance material were used.

High percentages of positive reactions to oakmoss absolute were also seen in another group of individuals who had a positive reaction to their own perfume, eau de toilette or shaving product (29% [21]), and – not surprisingly – in groups who had (partly) been selected on the basis of a previous positive patch test reaction to the fragrance mix I (which contains oakmoss absolute) (25% [33], 12.4% [96], 11% [19]). In an early study from the UK, a surprisingly high rate of 44% positive reactions to oakmoss was found in 50 patients with photosensitivity dermatitis with actinic reticuloid syndrome. It was concluded that allergy to oakmoss and other fragrances may be a significant factor in the development of photosensitivity dermatitis with actinic reticuloid syndrome and persistent light reactions (22). In not a single study were (specific) relevance data provided.

Results of testing oakmoss absolute in groups of patients reacting to the fragrance mix I are shown in Chapter 3.70 Fragrance mix I.

Case reports and case series

Case series

Oakmoss absolute was stated to be the (or an) allergen in 48 patients in a group of 603 individuals suffering from cosmetic dermatitis, seen in the period 2010-2015 in Leuven, Belgium (23). In the period 1996-2013, in a tertiary referral center in Valencia, Spain, 5419 patients were patch tested. Of these, 628 individuals had allergic contact dermatitis to cosmetics. In this group, oakmoss absolute was the responsible allergen in 20 cases (14, overlap with ref. 15).

In the period 2000-2009, in Leuven, Belgium, an unspecified number of patients had positive patch tests or use tests to a total of 344 cosmetic products *and* positive patch tests to FM I, FM II, and/or to one or more of 28 selected specific fragrance ingredients. In 2 of 37 patients reacting to oakmoss absolute, the presence of this fragrance in the cosmetic product(s) was confirmed by reading the product label(s) (34).

In the period 2000-2007, 202 patients with allergic contact dermatitis caused by cosmetics were seen in Valencia, Spain. In this group, oakmoss absolute was the allergen in 2 individuals from its presence in gel/soap (n=1) and in cologne (n=1) (15, overlap with ref. 14).

Table 3.67.4 Patch testing in groups of patients: Selected patient groups

Years and Country	Test conc. & vehicle	Number of patients tested	positive (%)	Selection of patients (S); Relevance (R); Comments (C)	Ref.
2011-2015 Spain	1% or 2% pet.	1013	126 (12.4%)	S: patients previously reacting to FM I, FM II, Myroxylon pereirae resin or hydroxyisohexyl 3-cyclohexene carboxaldehyde in the baseline series; R: not stated; C: the 2% test substances showed a higher rate of positive reactions than the 1% material	96
2003-2012 IVDK		607	32 (5.3%)	S: nurses with occupational contact dermatitis; R: not stated	25
2007-2011 IVDK	1% pet.	68	6 (8.8%)	S: physical therapists; R: not stated	94
2005-10 Netherlands		100	25 (25%)	S: patients with known fragrance sensitivity based on a positive patch test to the FM I and/or the FM II; R: not stated	33
2003-2010 IVDK	1% pet.	3030	173 (3.7%)	S: unspecified; this was a subgroup that was tested with treemoss, oakmoss and colophonium; R: not stated; C: co-reaction to treemoss: 65%	56
2000-2010 IVDK		1300	57 (4.5%)	S: patients with periorbital dermatitis; R: not stated; C: the frequency was equal to a control group of routine testing	26
2004-2008 Spain	2% pet.	86	2 (2.3%)	S: patients previously reacting to the fragrance mix I or Myroxylon pereirae (n=54) or suspected of fragrance contact allergy (n=32); R: not stated	20
2005-7 Netherlands	2% pet.	320	6 (1.9%)	S: patients suspected of fragrance or cosmetic allergy; R: 61% relevance for all positive tested fragrances together	4
<2003 Israel		91	10 (11%)	S: patients with a positive or doubtful reaction to the fragrance mix and/or Myroxylon pereirae resin and/or to one or two commercial fine fragrances; R: not stated	19
2002-2003 Korea	2% pet.	422	6 (1.4%)	S: patients with suspected cosmetic dermatitis; R: not stated	17
1998-2002 IVDK	1% pet.	28	8 (29%)	S: patients who had a positive reaction to their own perfume, eau de toilette or shaving product; R: not stated; C: there was a significant difference in percentage positive reactions compared with a control group of dermatitis patients who had *not* reacted to their own cosmetic products of this type	21
1997-2000 Austria	1% pet.	747	37 (5.0%)	S: patients suspected of fragrance allergy; R: not stated	5
1990-1994 IVDK		163	16 (9.8%)	S: patients with periorbital eczema; R: not stated	24
<1987 Norway	2% pet.	55	35 (64%)	S: patients with sensitivity to different brands of perfumes, deodorants, aftershave lotions etc. verified by repeated questioning, and/or testing; R: not stated; C: the authors concluded that 'the present study has shown that plant extract particularly from lichens are important allergenic constituents in cosmetics'	88
<1982 UK	2% pet.	50	22 (44%)	S: patients with photosensitivity dermatitis with actinic reticuloid syndrome; R: it was concluded that allergy to oakmoss and other fragrances may be a significant factor in the development of photosensitivity dermatitis with actinic reticuloid syndrome and persistent light reactions; C: there were no positive reactions to oakmoss absolute in 32 patients with polymorphic light eruption and 2.4% reactions in 457 routinely tested patients with dermatitis	22

Testing in groups of patients reacting to the fragrance mix I
Results of testing oakmoss absolute in groups of patients reacting to the fragrance mix I are shown in Chapter 3.70 Fragrance mix I

FM: Fragrance mix; IVDK: Informationsverbund Dermatologischer Kliniken (Germany, Switzerland, Austria)

In Bologna, Italy, 12 cases of contact dermatitis to lichens were observed in the period 1990-1996. Five individuals reacted to oakmoss absolute. All co-reacted to the FM I (which contains oakmoss absolute) and to atranorin (a constituent of oakmoss absolute). In 3 patients, the reactions were caused by aftershave preparations, in the other 2, the source of sensitization remained unknown, but was probably also related to cosmetics (38).

In one center in Belgium, between 1985 and 1990, 3970 patients with dermatitis were patch tested. 462 of these reacted positively to patch tests with cosmetic allergens. The reactions were considered to be relevant in 68%, probably relevant in 25% and doubtfully relevant in 7% of the patients. In the list of 'most common allergens', 'oak moss' had rank number 5 with 44 reactions. It should be appreciated that not all patients were patch tested with individual fragrances and that the presence of the allergen in cosmetic products causing dermatitis could not always be verified (at that time, ingredient labeling in the EU was not yet mandatory) (87).

In Belgium, in the years before 1986, of 5202 consecutive patients with dermatitis patch tested, 156 were diagnosed with pure cosmetic allergy. Oakmoss absolute was the 'dermatitic ingredient' in 7 (4.5%) patients (frequency in the entire group: 0.3%). It should be realized, however, that only a very limited number of patients was tested with a fragrance series (41).

In Portugal, in the period 1960-1986, 69 patients reacting to the FM I (test concentration not mentioned) were tested with its ingredients and there were 31 (45%) reactions to oakmoss extract. In 20, the origin of sensitization were perfumes, in 7 lichens themselves and in 4 patients the sensitization source was unknown (58).

In the period 1980-1982, in a clinic in Norway, 7 of 2000 routinely tested patients revealed contact allergy to oakmoss absolute in perfumes. In three, the reactions to the perfumes were positive, in the others, they were not tested. The authors suggested that cosmetics containing lichen extracts are a much more important source of contact allergy than lichens encountered in nature (43).

Case reports and case series

In a male patient, an aftershave caused a pustular eruption on the face. When patch tested, there were positive reactions to the aftershave, oakmoss absolute, citral and the fragrance mix II (which contains citral); the reactions were all pustular. Whether the aftershave contained oakmoss absolute remained unknown (30). A man had acute dermatitis from his aftershave lotion. The individual fragrances, obtained from the manufacturer were tested and he reacted to 'Mousse de Chênes', which is oakmoss (48). A female patient developed allergic contact dermatitis of the face from oakmoss absolute and hydroxycitronellal in a foundation lotion (49).

A man had suffered from a mild itchy, erythematous eruption above the sternum for the last 18 months. His dermatitis increased and spread over the sides of the neck during the summer months. The patient had a long beard and had been using an eau de cologne every day for the past 18 months. The day before his consultation, he developed a spread with a drop-like configuration to the xiphoid area suggesting that the lotion applied was the cause. Patch testing and photopatch testing showed photocontact allergy to the eau de cologne and evernic acid and photoaggravated contact allergy to oakmoss absolute and atranorin (52). This patient was later retested, he now had plain contact allergy to oakmoss extract, oakmoss (lichen, pure), treemoss (lichen, pure) and atranorin, but photocontact allergy to evernic acid. Whether the eau de cologne contained oakmoss extract was not mentioned (57).

An unconvincing case of possible pigmented cosmetic dermatitis from moisturizing cream was reported from Spain. There were positive patch tests to oakmoss extract and atranorin, but not to any cosmetic product. Use tests or ROATs were apparently not performed and it was unknown whether the cream actually contained oakmoss extract (59).

A woman presented with acute facial eczema within a few weeks of using a new moisturizer. Patch testing gave positive reactions to musk ambrette in the face series, oakmoss absolute in the fragrance series, the facial moisturizer as is, and the perfume in the moisturizer tested 5% and 10% pet. Further patch testing to the individual ingredients of the perfume revealed positive reactions to oakmoss absolute 2% pet. and musk moskene 5% pet. Photopatch tests were not performed (61).

A male patient had a 3-year history of dermatitis of his hands, forearms and face. He had worked as an engineer grinding components for printing presses for 24 years. During an enforced absence from work, he noticed that his rash resolved, but relapsed within 2 days. When the coolant used during the grinding process was withdrawn, the patient's rash subsequently resolved and he has remained symptom-free ever since. Patch testing gave positive reactions to the coolant at 10% aq., fragrance mix, Myroxylon pereirae resin, diethanolamine, oakmoss absolute and his own soluble oil. Further patch tests were then carried out with the constituents of the coolant plus the individual components of the fragrance used within it, which yielded positive reactions to oakmoss resin and monoethanol-amine (63).

A hairdresser developed occupational contact dermatitis of the hands from contact allergy to oakmoss absolute in a permanent waving solution. Using the solution on her own hair resulted in scalp dermatitis (62). A female patient had allergic contact dermatitis from oakmoss absolute in her husband's aftershave lotion (which is termed connubial or consort contact dermatitis) (64).

A male patient, who had allergic contact dermatitis from oakmoss absolute in aftershave lotions, experienced exacerbations of his hand dermatitis when handling firewood or trees in the forest (presumably containing lichens), and he had allergic reactions to atranorin and evernic acid on patch testing (65). A woman was patch tested for pruritus vulvae. She strongly reacted to the FM I, oakmoss absolute, a cream and its perfume 1% pet., but the presence of oakmoss absolute in the perfume of the cream could not be ascertained (81).

A male patient, who had an ileostomy secondary to underlying Crohn's disease, developed allergic contact dermatitis inferior to the stoma bag from oakmoss extract and limonene in a deodorizer sprayed into the bag (91). It has been shown that limonene and other fragrance components can permeate polythene and citrus aroma can be detected by smell a few minutes after some deodorizer drops have been placed in the stoma bag. It was postulated that exposure occurred via fragrance penetrating the stoma bag to affect the skin (91).

In a group of 23 patients with (photo)allergic reactions to sunscreens, 2 had positive patch tests to the ingredient oakmoss absolute (16).

Cross-reactions, pseudo-cross-reactions and co-reactions

For general information on cross-/pseudo-cross-/co-reactivity of fragrance chemicals with other fragrances, fragrance markers (fragrance mix I, fragrance mix II, colophonium, Myroxylon pereirae resin [balsam of Peru]) and essential oils see Chapter 1.2 General information on cross-reactions, pseudo-cross-reactions and co-reactions. Co-reactivity with the fragrance mix I can be expected, as the mix contains oakmoss extract (pseudo-cross-reactions).

Treemoss extract

All 5 patients tested in Sweden, before 1983, and reacting to an oakmoss acetone extract 7% in petrolatum, co-reacted to treemoss (55). Of 173 patients reacting to oakmoss extract, 65% co-reacted to treemoss extract (56).

Atranorin

Of 5 patients reacting to oakmoss absolute, all co-reacted to atranorin (38). In 7 other patients allergic to oakmoss, there were 4 reactions to atranorin (43). In Sweden, before 1983, of 10 patients reacting to an acetone extract of oakmoss, 7% in petrolatum, all co-reacted to atranorin (55). Of 20 patients allergic to oakmoss extract (identified by ingredient testing of the fragrance mix I), 10 co-reacted to atranorin (58). Of 15 patients allergic to oakmoss absolute, 4 also reacted to atranorin (82).

Of 10 patients reacting to atranorin 0.1% pet. seen in Sweden before 1981, all co-reacted to oakmoss perfume and 9/10 to acetone oakmoss extract 7% pet. (54). Of 7 patients reacting to atranorin 1% pet., all co-reacted to Evernia prunastri (oakmoss) extract and an oakmoss perfume 1% (53).

Colophonium

Co-reactivity between oakmoss absolute and colophonium is discussed in the section 'Other information: resin acids in commercial oakmoss absolute' below.

Other co-reactions

In 7 patients allergic to oakmoss extract, patch tests were also performed with lichen acids and there were 5 reactions to usnic acid, 4 to evernic acid, and 3 to physodic/physodalic acid (not present in oakmoss but in treemoss) (43). In Sweden, before 1983, in patients reacting to an acetone extract of oakmoss, 7% in petrolatum, the following co-reactions were observed: fumarprotocetraric acid 7/7 (not present in oakmoss but in treemoss), evernic acid 4/7, d-usnic acid 2/10, and reindeer lichen (Cladonia alpestris, contains atranorin) 5/5 (55).

Of 20 patients allergic to oakmoss extract (identified by ingredient testing of the fragrance mix I), 8 co-reacted to usnic acid, 6 to evernic acid, and 3 to fumarprotocetraric acid (not present in oakmoss but in treemoss); of 25 such patients, 20 co-reacted to a lichen-mix and 16 to Frullania (58).

Of 15 patients allergic to oakmoss absolute, 2 co-reacted to evernic acid and one to usnic acid (82). Of 27 patients allergic to Frullania, 10 (37%) reacted to the fragrance mix, in 8 of these cases from allergy to Evernia prunastri (oakmoss) extract (42). These were considered not to be cross-reactions but multiple specific allergies (42).

Presence in products and chemical analyses

In various studies, the presence oakmoss absolute in cosmetic and sometimes other products has been investigated. Before 2006, most investigators used chemical analysis, usually GC-MS, for qualitative and quantitative determination. Since then, the presence of the target fragrances was usually investigated by screening the product labels for the 26 fragrances that must be labeled since 2005 on cosmetics and detergent products in the EU, if present at > 10 ppm (0.001%) in leave-on products and > 100 ppm (0.01%) in rinse-off products. This method, obviously, is less accurate and may result in underestimation of the frequency of the fragrances being present in the product. When they are in fact present, but the concentration is lower than mentioned above, labeling is not required and the fragrances' presence will be missed.

The results of the relevant studies for oakmoss absolute are summarized in table 3.67.5. More detailed information can be found in the corresponding text before and following the table. Generally speaking it can be stated that Evernia prunastri extract is (currently) a very little used fragrance material.

In Denmark, in 2015-2016, 5588 fragranced cosmetic products were examined with a smartphone application for the 26 fragrances that need to be labeled in the EU. Oakmoss extract was present in 0.1% of the products (rank number 24) (12).

In Germany, in 2015, fragrance allergens were evaluated based on lists of ingredients in 817 (unique) detergents (all-purpose cleaners, cleaning preparations for special purposes [e.g. bathroom, kitchen, dish-washing] and laundry detergents) present in 131 households. Evernia prunastri extract was found to be present in one (0.1%) of the products (7).

Table 3.67.5 Presence of Evernia prunastri extract in products [a]

Year	Country	Product type	Nr. investigated	Nr. of products positive [b]	(%)	Method [c]	Ref.
2015-6	Denmark	Fragranced cosmetic products	5588		(0.1%)	Labeling	12
2015	Germany	Household detergents	817	1	(0.1%)	Labeling	7
2008-11	Germany	Deodorants	374	2	(0.5%)	Labeling	47
2006-9	Germany	Cosmetic products	4991		(0.7%)	Labeling	11
2008	Sweden	Cosmetic products	204	1	(0.5%)	Labeling	6
		Detergents	97	0	(0%)	Labeling	
2006	UK	Perfumed cosmetic and house-hold products	300	13	(4%)	Labeling	10
2006	Denmark	Popular perfumed deodorants	88	4	(5%)	Labeling	13
2000	Denmark, UK, Germany, Italy	Domestic and occupational products	59	1	(3%)	Analysis	8
<2000	Sweden	Swedish cosmetic products	42	13	(31%)	Analysis	45
1997	Denmark, UK, France, Germa-ny, Sweden	Deodorants	71	10	(14%)	Analysis	9
1996-7	Denmark	Deodorants that had caused allergic contact dermatitis	19	2	(11%)	Analysis	37

[a] See the corresponding text below for more details
[b] positive = containing the target fragrance
[c] Labeling: information from the ingredient labels on the product / packaging; Analysis: chemical analysis, most often GC-MS

In 2008, 2010 and 2011, 374 deodorants available in German retail shops were randomly selected and their labels checked for the presence of the 26 fragrances that need to be labeled. Oakmoss extract was found to be present in 2 (0.5%) of the products (47).

In Germany, in the period 2006-2009, 4991 cosmetic products were randomly sampled for an official investigation of conformity of cosmetic products with legal provisions. The labels were inspected for the presence of the 26 fragrances that need to be labeled in the EU. Evernia prunastri extract was present in 0.7% of the products (rank number 21) (11).

Oakmoss extract was present (as indicated by labeling) in 0.5% of 204 cosmetic products (92 shampoos, 61 hair conditioners, 34 liquid soaps, 17 wet tissues) and in none of 97 detergents in Sweden, 2008 (6).

In 2006, of 88 popular perfume containing deodorants purchased in Denmark, 4 (4.6%) were labeled to contain Evernia prunastri extract (13).

In January 2006, a study of perfumed cosmetic and household products available on the shelves of U.K. retailers was carried out. Products were included if 'parfum' or 'aroma' was listed among the ingredients. Three hundred products were surveyed and any of 26 mandatory labeling fragrances named on the label were recorded. Evernia prunastri extract was present in 13 (4%) of the products (rank number 21) (10).

In 2000, fifty-nine domestic and occupational products, purchased in retail outlets in Denmark, England, Germany and Italy were analyzed by GC-MS for the presence of fragrances. The product categories were liquid soap and soap bars (n=13), soft/hard surface cleaners (n=23), fabric conditioners/laundry detergents for hand wash (n=8), dish- wash (n=10), furniture polish, car shampoo, stain remover (each n=1) and 2 products used in occupational environments. Evernia prunastri extract (as indicated by the presence of evernic acid methyl ester) was present in one product; quantification was not performed (8).

In Sweden, before 2000, 42 cosmetic products of a Swedish manufacturer were investigated for the presence of the ingredients of the FM I by chemical analysis. Oakmoss absolute was found to be present in 13 of the products (31%) in a concentration range of 2.6-39 ppm with a mean of 13 ppm. Data provided by the manufacturer on the qualitative and quantitative presence of the chemicals was quite different from chemical analyses for some of the fragrances (45).

In 1997, 71 deodorants (22 vapo-spray, 22 aerosol spray and 27 roll-on products) were collected in Denmark, England, France, Germany and Sweden and analyzed by gas chromatography – mass spectrometry (GC-MS) for the presence of fragrances and other materials. Evernic acid methyl ester (marker for oakmoss absolute) was present in 10 (14%) of the products (9).

In Denmark, in 1996-1997, nineteen deodorants that had caused axillary allergic contact dermatitis in 14 patients were analyzed for the presence of the 8 constituents of the FM I and oakmoss absolute was found to be present in 2 (11%) of the products. The absolute was only detected qualitatively, but had a high detection limit of 0.2% (37).

Serial dilution patch testing and Repeated Open Application Tests

From the experiments described below using serial dilution patch tests and repeated open application tests (ROATs) with samples of oakmoss extracts containing either high or low concentrations of atranol and chloroatranol it can be concluded that:

1 reducing the concentration of atranol and chloroatranol results in a significantly lowered patch test reactivity to oakmoss extracts

2 this does not apply to reactivity to ROATs, though the time required to elicit a positive reaction is significantly lower with reduced content of atranol and chloroatranol

3 concentrations of atranol and chloroatranol less than 10 ppm, may elicit allergic reactions in individuals previously sensitized to oakmoss extract and are therefore unsafe for the consumer

4 there are several other sensitizers in oak moss besides atranol and chloroatranol

Study 1 Serial dilution patch testing In the period 2004-2006, in Belgium, a study investigated whether chemically modified extracts of oakmoss with low concentrations of chloroatranol and atranol would produce positive patch test reactions in previously sensitized subjects. A sample of oakmoss extract was treated by a polymer-based method to reduce the content of atranol and chloroatranol from 3.4% to less than 75 ppm and from 1.8% to less than 25 ppm, respectively. Fourteen subjects with positive reactions to oakmoss absolute were patch tested to this sample, diluted 1% in petrolatum. The chemically modified sample reacted negatively in six but gave still positive reactions in eight subjects, with the same intensity as the commercially available oakmoss patch test materials. It was concluded that concentrations of atranol and chloroatranol less than 75 ppm and 25 ppm, respectively, may elicit allergic reactions in individuals previously sensitized to oakmoss extract and are therefore unsafe for the consumer (75).

These positive reactions may have 2 explanations: 1. The reactions are caused by chloroatranol and/or atranol. Indeed, with regard to elicitation, chloroatranol has been shown to cause reactions at the ppm level (0.0005%, i.e. 5 ppm) by repeated open exposure and at the ppb (parts per billion) level on patch testing, 50% reacting to an extreme low concentration of 0.000015%, i.e. 150 ppb, 0.15 ppm) (76). Judged from this elicitation profile, chloroatranol is considered to be the most potent allergen present in consumer products today. The second explanation is that the reactions are caused by methyl-β-orcinol carboxylate, which was previously shown to be a sensitizer in oakmoss absolute (70), and which was not removed by the method used to decrease the content of chloroatranol and atranol (75), or by other allergens.

Study 2 Serial dilution patch testing In a patch test study in Sweden, performed between 2006 and 2008, 15 patients allergic to oakmoss absolute were patch tested with serial dilution tests of 2 samples of oakmoss absolute (82). Sample A (high content) contained approximately 2.5% (25,000 ppm) of atranol and 0.93% (9300 ppm) of chloroatranol; sample B (low content, current commercial quality) contained 90 ppm of atranol and 20 ppm of chloroatranol. Concentrations ranged from 2.0% (wt./vol.) in acetone down 0.000063% (wt./vol.). Atranol and chloroatranol were each dissolved and diluted in acetone to a concentration of 0.010% (wt./vol.).

Subjects reacting positively to the 0.010% preparations of atranol and/or chloroatranol on D3 or D4 were additionally tested with dilutions of atranol and/or chloroatranol at 0.0032%, 0.0010%, 0.00032%, and 0.00010% (wt./vol.). Subjects who were negative to the 0.010% preparations of atranol and/or chloroatranol on D3 or D4 were tested with 0.050% (wt./vol.) preparations of atranol and/or chloroatranol. Furthermore, all subjects were patch tested with 0.1% (wt./vol.) petrolatum preparations of the lichen allergens atranorin (plus dilution series if positive), usnic acid, and evernic acid. The patients were also patch tested with TLC strips (Thin-Layer Chromatography) of oakmoss absolute.

Results Sample A (high content atranol/chloroatranol): All 15 individuals reacted to 2.0%, 12 to 0.63%, 13 to 0.20%, 8 to 0.063%, 5 to 0.020%, 1 to 0.0063%, 1 to 0.0020% and none to 0.00063% oakmoss absolute in alcohol. Results Sample B (low content atranol/chloroatranol): Only 2 reacted to 2%, none to lower concentrations. Eleven patients not reacting to 2% were tested with 6.3% oakmoss absolute in acetone and 4 now had a positive reaction. Results atranol: There were 4 positive reactions to 0.050% (negative to 0.010%), 2 to 0.01% and one of these reacted down to 0.00032% atranol in acetone.

Results chloroatranol: There were 4 positive reactions to 0.050% (negative to 0.010%), 3 to 0.010%, 2 to 0.0032% and one to 0.0010% chloroatranol in acetone.

Results other lichen allergens: Two subjects reacted to evernic acid, one to usnic acid, and 4 to atranorin 0.1% pet. Of 2 who reacted to atranorin and were tested with a dilution series, one reacted to 0.032% in acetone as lower threshold and the other down to 0.0032% atranorin in acetone.

Results TLC strips: Positive reactions to the TLC strips of sample A were observed in 13 of 15 subjects. Only 1 of 11 subjects tested with TLC strips of sample B showed a positive reaction. The reactions to the TLC strips of sample A were distributed all over the area where the components of the oakmoss absolute had migrated. Eleven subjects reacted to spots within this region, and, in total, 11 subjects showed positive reactions to other areas of the chromatograms.

This study showed a statistically significant lowering of the patch test reactivity to the oakmoss absolute with a reduced content of atranol and chloroatranol as compared with a conventional high content sample. In addition, the TLC patch tests indicate the presence of several other sensitizers in oakmoss absolute (82).

Study 3 Serial dilution patch testing and ROATs Fifteen subjects with contact allergy to oakmoss absolute underwent a repeated open application test (ROAT) using solutions of an untreated oakmoss absolute (sample A) and an oakmoss absolute with reduced content of atranol and chloroatranol, <100 ppm each (sample B). ROAT solutions of samples A and B were each prepared in a concentration of 0.10% (w/v). Furthermore a sample of a 0.00020% (w/v) dilution of sample A with atranol and chloroatranol concentrations in the same order of magnitude as in the 0.10% preparation of sample B were used in the ROAT. All subjects were in addition patch-tested with serial dilutions of samples A and B, concentrations ranging from 2.0% w/v down to 0.000061% w/v. The vehicle used was 2.0% (v/v) diethyl phthalate (DEP) and 98.0% (v/v) ethanol.

In patch testing, 14/15 subjects had positive reactions to sample A and 8/15 to sample B. Thirteen subjects were found to be more reactive towards sample A, and 2 were equally reactive to samples A and B. The MEC (minimum eliciting concentration, lowest concentration to give a positive reaction) of sample A ranged between 0.00049% and 2.0% and the MEC of sample B ranged between 0.13% and 2.0% (83).

In the ROATs, 11/15 were positive to sample A and 8/15 to sample B. This difference is not statistically significant. Eight had a positive ROAT to sample A 0.00020%, the exact same number as positive to sample B, in which the concentration of atranol and chloroatranol are about the same. The average time required for the ROAT to become positive was 6.5 days for sample A (high content) and 16.5 days for sample B (commercial sample, low content of atranol and chloroatranol) (83).

It was concluded that statistically significantly more subjects react to oakmoss absolute with higher content than to the sample with the lower content. No corresponding difference was observed in the ROAT, though there was a significant difference in the time required to elicit a positive reaction. The ROAT indicates that the use of a cosmetic product containing oakmoss absolute with reduced levels of atranol and chloroatranol is capable of eliciting an allergic reaction in previously sensitized individuals (83).

Study 4 Serial dilution patch testing and ROATs In a similar, larger study, serial patch testing and ROATs were performed in 30 oakmoss-allergic patients and 30 controls. ROATS were performed with 0.1% classic oakmoss (COM) containing 27,000 ppm atranol and 15,000 ppm chloroatranol in the neat extract and 0.1% new oakmoss (NOM) containing 48 ppm atranol and 37 ppm chloro-atranol each in the neat extract (84). For the serial dilution patch tests, concentrations of both COM and NOM were prepared in the range of 2.0% down to 0.00003% (wt./vol.). The vehicle used was 2% diethyl phthalate and 98% ethanol. In the ROAT, twenty-two of 30 oakmoss-sensitive subjects had a positive reaction to COM; of these, only 6 reacted to NOM. No subjects reacted to NOM only. COM caused significantly more reactions than NOM. Among the subjects who had a positive ROAT result, the mean numbers of applications needed to elicit a positive reaction were 15 for COM and 26 for NOM. In patch testing, COM caused significantly more reactions than NOM and to a significantly lower concentration of COM than of NOM. It was concluded that reactivity to NOM is significantly lower than reactivity to COM, and that NOM is less likely to induce sensitivity than COM (84).

Other information: resin acids in commercial oakmoss absolute

Formerly, oakmoss absolute from commercial suppliers for patch testing contained varying amounts of resin acids and their oxidation products. These chemicals, which are sensitizers in colophonium (i.e. the oxidation products), are not present in pure oakmoss absolute, but were the result of contamination with treemoss. In a number of patients allergic to colophonium, especially when highly reactive, the amount of resin acids and oxidation products was high enough to induce a positive patch test reaction to oakmoss absolute, also in patients *not* allergic to oakmoss itself. This also explains the significant association between positive patch test reactions to colophonium and oakmoss absolute found in several studies. These are conclusions drawn from the studies described below.

Seventeen patients allergic to colophonium were tested with commercial patch test materials containing 1% (sample T from company T) resp. 2% (sample C from company C) oakmoss absolute. Nine (53%) co-reacted to the oakmoss from company T and 2 (12%) to that from company C. This was unexpected, as pure oakmoss absolute does not contain resin acids and their oxidation products, which are the sensitizers in colophonium. Samples of oakmoss absolute used to prepare the commercial patch test materials were analyzed and it was found that sample T (9 positive reactions) contained 5.6% (wt./wt.) resin acids and 0.7% (wt./wt.) of 7-dehydroabietic acid, whereas sample C (2 positive reactions) contained only 0.4% resin acids. Moreover, the chemical distribution of resin acids present in sample T was very similar to the one found in treemoss, suggesting contamination of oakmoss absolute by treemoss absolute. Thus, the authors suggested that the presence of resin acids in oakmoss patch test materials could be responsible for a positive reaction in patients allergic to colophonium and a misdiagnosis in some patients (i.e., the patient is allergic to colophonium but not to oakmoss) (66).

In a large IVDK study of 12,614 patients tested with both colophonium and oakmoss absolute 1% from company T, 27.0% of all persons allergic to colophonium reacted positively to oakmoss, whereas only 5.5% positive reactions to oakmoss were found in the rest, pointing at a substantial degree of association between the two patch tests (relative risk: 4.89). The proportion of oakmoss positive patients increased from 5.4% in patients not reacting to colophonium, to 14.7% in those reacting with erythema only (?+), to 19.4% in those with a + reaction, to 30.0% in those with a ++ reaction, and to 53.3% in those with very strong (+++) reactions to colophonium. This strongly suggests that small amounts of resin acids oxidation products (the sensitizers in colophonium) present in the oakmoss absolute 1% are indeed able to elicit positive patch test reactions to 'oakmoss', and more so in patients with stronger allergy to colophonium (67). Therefore, these data corroborate the findings of the authors of ref. 66, although the conclusion of the IVDK study was different, based on a low Cohen's kappa value (67).

In Denmark, two more studies were performed to clarify this issue. In the first one, of 885 consecutive patients tested, 42 (4.7%) reacted to colophonium and 28 (3.2%) to oakmoss absolute 1% from company T, containing resin acids. Co-reactivity to colophonium was found in 8/28 (29%) of the patients reacting to oakmoss absolute, while a co-reaction to oakmoss was seen in 19% of the patients reacting to colophonium. The relationship between reactions to oakmoss absolute and colophonium was statistically significant (68). In the second study there were no differences between oakmoss absolute from company T and an oakmoss preparation without abietic acid in their ability to give positive, doubtful or irritant reactions, but this was performed in 119 patients only and therefore has limited value (68).

Finally, In London, in the period 1984-2000, 1203 patients were tested to the constituents of the fragrance mix. 342 of these were allergic to oakmoss absolute. There was a highly statistically significant association between allergy to oakmoss absolute and allergy to colophonium, 73 (21.3%) of 342 oakmoss-positive patients being allergic to colophonium versus 115 (13.4%) of 861 oakmoss-negative patients. The authors confirmed the association between allergy to oakmoss absolute and colophonium, which was ascribed to the presence of contaminating resin acids (abietic, dehydroabietic and 7-oxo-dehydroabietic acids) in the oakmoss absolute patch test material from company T (69).

The manufacturer of sample T oakmoss confirmed (cited in ref. 69) that they had found contaminating resin acids in their oakmoss absolute patch test material subsequent to the results of the first study of this issue (66) and that they had changed their supplier to one who guarantees pure oakmoss and whose samples consistently test negative for abietic acid at a detection limit of 0.1%.

Currently, the International Fragrance Association's (IFRA) recommendation ('standard') on oakmoss extracts states: 'Oakmoss extracts used in perfume compounds must not contain added treemoss, which is a source of resin acids. Traces of resin acids may be carried over to commercial qualities of oakmoss in the manufacturing process. These traces must not exceed 0.1% (1000 ppm) dehydroabietic acid (DHA) in the extract'.

OTHER SIDE EFFECTS

Photosensitivity

Photopatch testing in groups of patients
In a group of 35 patients (11 with photosensitivity dermatitis with actinic reticuloid syndrome[PD/AR], 13 with chronic polymorphic light eruption, 11 with contact dermatitis) who were photopatch tested, there were 6 patients with positive reactions to oakmoss absolute, 3 of who also had an immediate-type reaction. These positive photopatch tests were tentatively interpreted as indicating a phototoxic reaction, although the possibility that this phototoxic response may merge subsequently with a delayed allergic type reaction could not be excluded. On the basis of these results and of 'plain' patch tests with oakmoss absolute and other fragrances in patients with PD/AR, polymorphic light eruption and consecutive patients suspected of contact dermatitis (see table 3.67.4), the authors concluded that in some subjects with PD/AR and persistent light reaction, a significant factor in the latter is likely to be exposure to substances such as fragrance materials which have the ability to produce dermatitis, not only from contact allergic sensitivity but also through photocontact reactions (notably oakmoss absolute, 6-methylcoumarin and musk ambrette) involving either phototoxic or photoallergic mechanisms (22).

Case reports and case series
A man had suffered from a mild itchy, erythematous eruption above the sternum for the last 18 months. His dermatitis increased and spread over the sides of the neck during the summer months. The patient had a long beard and had been using an eau de cologne every day for the past 18 months. Patch testing and photopatch testing showed photocontact allergy to the eau de cologne and evernic acid and photoaggravated contact allergy to oakmoss absolute and atranorin (52). However, the patient was later retested, he now had plain contact allergy to oakmoss extract, oakmoss, treemoss and atranorin, but photocontact allergy only to evernic acid (57).

Immediate-type reactions

In a group of 160 patients with a positive patch test to fragrance mix I, two (1.2%) had an immediate contact reaction to oakmoss absolute (36). In a group of 35 patients, mostly with photosensitive disorders, who were photopatch tested, there were 6 patients with positive reactions to oakmoss absolute, 3 of who also had an immediate-type reaction (22).

LITERATURE

1   Various SCCS opinions on Evernia prunastri extract have been published and are available at: http://ec.europa.eu/growth/tools-databases/cosing/index.cfm?fuseaction=search.details_v2&id=27940&back=1

2   Heisterberg MV, Menné T, Johansen JD. Contact allergy to the 26 specific fragrance ingredients to be declared on cosmetic products in accordance with the EU cosmetic directive. Contact Dermatitis 2011;65:266-275

3   Schnuch A, Uter W, Geier J, Lessmann H, Frosch PJ. Sensitization to 26 fragrances to be labelled according to current European regulation: Results of the IVDK and review of the literature. Contact Dermatitis 2007;57:1-10

4   Oosten EJ van, Schuttelaar ML, Coenraads PJ. Clinical relevance of positive patch test reactions to the 26 EU-labelled fragrances. Contact Dermatitis 2009;61:217-223

5   Wöhrl S, Hemmer W, Focke M, Götz M, Jarisch R. The significance of fragrance mix, balsam of Peru, colophony and propolis as screening tools in the detection of fragrance allergy. Br J Dermatol 2001;145:268-273

6   Yazar K, Johnsson S, Lind M-L, Boman A, Lidén C. Preservatives and fragrances in selected consumer-available cosmetics and detergents. Contact Dermatitis 2011;64:265-272

7   Wieck S, Olsson O, Kümmerer K, Klaschka U. Fragrance allergens in household detergents. Regul Toxicol Pharmacol 2018;97:163-169

8   Rastogi SC, Heydorn S, Johansen JD, Basketter DA. Fragrance chemicals in domestic and occupational products. Contact Dermatitis 2001;45:221-225

9   Rastogi SC, Lepoittevin J-P, Johansen JD, Frosch PJ, Menné T, Bruze M, et al. Fragrances and other materials in deodorants: search for potentially sensitizing molecules using combined GC-MS and structure activity relationship (SAR) analysis. Contact Dermatitis 1998;39:293-303

10 Buckley DA. Fragrance ingredient labelling in products on sale in the UK. Br J Dermatol 2007;157:295-300

11 Uter W, Yazar K, Kratz E-M, Mildau G, Lidén C. Coupled exposure to ingredients of cosmetic products: I. Fragrances. Contact Dermatitis 2013;69:335-341

12 Bennike NH, Oturai NB, Müller S, Kirkeby CS, Jørgensen C, Christensen AB, et al. Fragrance contact allergens in 5588 cosmetic products identified through a novel smartphone application. J Eur Acad Dermatol Venereol 2018;32:79-85

13 Rastogi SC, Hellerup Jensen G, Johansen JD. Survey and risk assessment of chemical substances in deodorants. Survey of Chemical Substances in Consumer Products, No. 86 2007. Danish Ministry of the Environment, Environmental Protection Agency. Available at: https://www2.mst.dk/Udgiv/publications/2007/978-87-7052-625-8/pdf/978-87-7052-626-5.pdf

14 Zaragoza-Ninet V, Blasco Encinas R, Vilata-Corell JJ, Pérez-Ferriols A, Sierra-Talamantes C, Esteve-Martínez A, de la Cuadra-Oyanguren J. Allergic contact dermatitis due to cosmetics: A clinical and epidemiological study in a tertiary hospital. Actas Dermosifiliogr 2016;107:329-336

15 Laguna C, de la Cuadra J, Martín-González B, Zaragoza V, Martínez-Casimiro L, Alegre V. Allergic contact dermatitis to cosmetics. Actas Dermosifiliogr 2009;100:53-60

16 Thune P. Contact and photocontact allergy to sunscreens. Photodermatol 1984;1:5-9

17 An S, Lee AY, Lee CH, Kim DW, Hahm JH, Kim KJ, et al. Fragrance contact dermatitis in Korea: a joint study. Contact Dermatitis 2005;53:320-323

18 Frosch PJ, Pilz B, Andersen KE, Burrows D, Camarasa JG, Dooms-Goossens A, et al. Patch testing with fragrances: results of a multicenter study of the European Environmental and Contact Dermatitis Research Group with 48 frequently used constituents of perfumes. Contact Dermatitis 1995;33:333-342

19 Trattner A, David M. Patch testing with fine fragrances: comparison with fragrance mix, balsam of Peru and a fragrance series. Contact Dermatitis 2003;49:287-289

20 Cuesta L, Silvestre JF, Toledo F, Lucas A, Perez-Crespo M, Ballester I. Fragrance contact allergy: a 4-year retrospective study. Contact Dermatitis 2010;63:77-84

21 Uter W, Geier J, Schnuch A, Frosch PJ. Patch test results with patients' own perfumes, deodorants and shaving lotions: results of the IVDK 1998-2002. J Eur Acad Dermatol Venereol 2007;21:374-379

22 Addo HA, Ferguson J, Johnson BF, Frain-Bell W. The relationship between exposure to fragrance materials and persistent light reaction in photosensitivity dermatitis with actinic reticuloid syndrome. Br J Dermatol 1982;107:261-274

23 Goossens A. Cosmetic contact allergens. Cosmetics 2016, 3, 5; doi:10.3390/cosmetics3010005

24 Ockenfels H, Seemann U, Goos M. Contact allergy in patients with periorbital eczema: an analysis of allergens. Dermatology 1997;195:119-124

25 Molin S, Bauer A, Schnuch A, Geier J. Occupational contact allergy in nurses: results from the Information
    Network of Departments of Dermatology 2003–2012. Contact Dermatitis 2015;72:164-171
26 Landeck L, John SM, Geier J. Periorbital dermatitis in 4779 patients – patch test results during a 10-year period.
    Contact Dermatitis 2014;70:205-212
27 Bennike NH, Zachariae C, Johansen JD. Non-mix fragrances are top sensitizers in consecutive dermatitis
    patients – a cross-sectional study of the 26 EU-labelled fragrance allergens. Contact Dermatitis 2017;77:270-279
28 Vejanurug P, Tresukosol P, Sajjachareonpong P, Puangpet P. Fragrance allergy could be missed without patch
    testing with 26 individual fragrance allergens. Contact Dermatitis 2016;74:230-235
29 Liu J, Li L-F. Contact sensitization to fragrances other than fragrance mix I in China. Contact Dermatitis
    2015;73:252-253
30 Verma A, Tancharoen C, Tam MM, Nixon R. Pustular allergic contact dermatitis caused by fragrances. Contact
    Dermatitis 2015;72:245-248
31 Mann J, McFadden JP, White JML, White IR, Banerjee P. Baseline series fragrance markers fail to predict contact
    allergy. Contact Dermatitis 2014;70:276-281
32 Mowitz M, Svedman C, Zimerson E, Isaksson M, Pontén A, Bruze M. Simultaneous patch testing with fragrance
    mix I, fragrance mix II and their ingredients in southern Sweden between 2009 and 2015. Contact Dermatitis
    2017;77:280-287
33 Nagtegaal MJC, Pentinga SE, Kuik J, Kezic S, Rustemeyer T. The role of the skin irritation response in
    polysensitization to fragrances. Contact Dermatitis 2012;67:28-35
34 Nardelli A, Drieghe J, Claes L, Boey L, Goossens A. Fragrance allergens in 'specific' cosmetic products. Contact
    Dermatitis 2011;64:212-219
35 Uter W, Geier J, Frosch P, Schnuch A. Contact allergy to fragrances: current patch test results (2005–2008) from
    the Information Network of Departments of Dermatology. Contact Dermatitis 2010;63:254-261
36 Temesvári E, Németh I, Baló-Banga MJ, Husz S, Kohánka V, Somos Z, et al. Multicentre study of fragrance allergy
    in Hungary: Immediate and late type reactions. Contact Dermatitis 2002;46:325-330
37 Johansen JD, Rastogi SC, Bruze M, Andersen KE, Frosch P, Dreier B, et al. Deodorants: a clinical provocation study
    in fragrance-sensitive individuals. Contact Dermatitis 1998;39:161-165
38 Stinchi C, Gulrrini V, Guetti E, Tosti A. Contact dermatitis from lichens. Contact Dermatitis 1997;36:309-310
39 Frosch PJ, Pilz B, Burrows D, Camarasa JG, Lachapelle J-M, Lahti A, et al. Testing with fragrance mix: Is the
    addition of sorbitan sesquioleate to the constituents useful? Contact Dermatitis 1995;32:266-272
40 De Groot AC, Van der Kley AMJ, Bruynzeel DP, Meinardi MMHM, Smeenk G, van Joost Th, Pavel S. Frequency of
    false-negative reactions to the fragrance mix. Contact Dermatitis 1993;28:139-140
41 Broeckx W, Blondeel A, Dooms-Goossens A, Achten G. Cosmetic intolerance. Contact Dermatitis 1987;16:189-
    194
42 Gonçalo S. Contact sensitivity to lichens and Compositae in Frullania dermatitis. Contact Dermatitis 1987;16: 84-
    86
43 Thune P, Solberg Y, McFadden N, Stærfeet F, Sandberg M. Perfume allergy due to oak moss and other lichens.
    Contact Dermatitis 1982;8:396-400
44 Strauss RM, Orton DI. Allergic contact cheilitis in the United Kingdom: a retrospective study. Dermatitis
    2003;14:75-77
45 Bárány E, Lodén M. Content of fragrance mix ingredients and customer complaints of cosmetic products.
    Dermatitis 2000;11:74-79
46 Diepgen TL, Ofenloch R, Bruze M, Cazzaniga S, Coenraads PJ, Elsner P, et al. Prevalence of fragrance contact
    allergy in the general population of five European countries: a cross-sectional study. Br J Dermatol
    2015;173:1411-1419
47 Klaschka U. Contact allergens for armpits - allergenic fragrances specified on deodorants. Int J Hyg Environ
    Health 2012;215:584-591
48 Hannuksela M, Kousa M, Pirilä V. Allergy to ingredients of vehicles. Contact Dermatitis 1976;2:105-110
49 Calnan CD. Perfume dermatitis from the cosmetic ingredients oakmoss and hydroxycitronellal. Contact
    Dermatitis 1979;5:194
50 Joulain D, Tabacchi R. Lichen extracts as raw materials in perfumery. Part 1: oakmoss. Flavour Fragr J 2009;24:49-
    61
51 Joulain D, Tabacchi R. Lichen extracts as raw materials in perfumery. Part 2: treemoss. Flavour Fragr J
    2009;24:105-116
52 Fernández de Corres L, Muñoz D, Leaniz-Barrutia I, Corrales JL. Photocontact dermatitis from oak moss. Contact
    Dermatitis 1983;9:528-529
53 Dahlquist I, Fregert S. Contact allergy to atranorin in lichens and perfumes. Contact Dermatitis 1980;6:111-119
54 Dahlquist I, Fregert S. Atranorin and oak moss contact allergy. Contact Dermatitis 1981;7:168-169
55 Fregert S, Dahlquist I. Patch testing with oak moss extract. Contact Dermatitis 1983;9:227

56 Uter W, Schmidt E, Lessmann H, Schnuch A. Contact sensitization to tree moss (Evernia furfuracea extract, INCI) is heterogeneous. Contact Dermatitis 2012;67:36-41

57 Fernández de Corres L. Photosensitivity to oak moss. Contact Dermatitis 1986;15:118

58 Gonçalo S, Cabral F, Gonçalo M. Contact sensitivity to oak moss. Contact Dermatitis 1988;19:355-357

59 Romaguera C, Vilaplana J, Grimalt F. Contact dermatitis from oak moss. Contact Dermatitis 1991;24:224-225

60 Ford RA, Api AM. An investigation of the potential for allergic contact sensitization of several oakmoss preparations. Contact Dermatitis 1990;23:249

61 Parry EJ, Beck MH. Contact allergy to musk moskene in a perfumed moisturizing cream. Contact Dermatitis 1997;37:236

62 Kanerva L, Jolanki R, Estlander T. Hairdresser's dermatitis caused by oak moss in permanent waving solution. Contact Dermatitis 1999;41:55-56

63 Owen CM, August PJ, Beck MH. Contact allergy to oak moss resin in a soluble oil. Contact Dermatitis 2000;43:112

64 Held JL. Ruszkowski AM, DeLeo VA. Consort contact dermatitis due to oak moss. Arch Dermatol 1988;124:261-262

65 Aalto-Korte K, Lauerma A, Alanko K. Occupational allergic contact dermatitis from lichens in present-day Finland. Contact Dermatitis 2005;52:36-38

66 Lepoittevin JP, Meschkat E, Huygens S, Goossens A. Presence of resin acids in "Oakmoss" patch test material: a source of misdiagnosis? J Invest Dermatol 2000;115:129-130

67 Uter W, Gefeller O, Geier J, Schnuch A. Limited concordance between 'oakmoss' and colophony in clinical patch testing. J Invest Dermatol 2001;116:478-480

68 Johansen JD, Heydorn S, Menné T. Oak moss extracts in the diagnosis of fragrance contact allergy. Contact Dermatitis 2002;46:157-161

69 Buckley DA, Rycroft RJ, White IR, McFadden JP. Contaminating resin acids have not caused the high rate of sensitivity to oak moss. Contact Dermatitis 2002;47:19-20

70 Bernard G, Giménez-Arnau E, Rastogi SC, Heydorn S, Johansen JD, Menné T, et al. Contact allergy to oak moss: search for sensitizing molecules using combined bioassay-guided chemical fractionation, GC-MS, and structure-activity relationship analysis. Arch Dermatol Res 2003;295:229-235

71 Sandberg M, Thune P. The sensitizing capacity of atranorin. Contact Dermatitis 1984;11:168-173

72 Terajima Y, Ichikawa H, Tokuda K, Nakamura S, Quantitative analysis of oak moss oil. In: Lawrence BM, Mookerjee BD, Willis BJ, Eds. Flavors and fragrances: a world perspective. Amsterdam: Elsevier Science, 1988:685-695

73 Boelens MH. Formation of volatile compounds from oakmoss. Perfumer Flavorist 1993;18:27-30

74 Bauer K, Garbe D, Surburg H. Common fragrance and flavor materials: preparation, properties and uses, 3rd Ed. Weinheim, Germany: Wiley-VCH Verlag, 1997

75 Nardelli A, Giménez-Arnau E, Bernard G, Lepoittevin J-P, Goossens A. Is a low content in atranol/chloroatranol safe in oak moss-sensitized individuals? Contact Dermatitis 2009;60:91-95

76 Johansen JD, Andersen KE, Svedman C, Bruze M, Bernard G, Giménez-Arnau E, Rastogi SC, Lepoittevin JP, Menné T. Chloroatranol, an extremely potent allergen hidden in perfumes: a dose–response elicitation study. Contact Dermatitis 2003;49:180-184

77 Menné Bonefeld C, Nielsen MM, Gimenéz-Arnau E, Lang M, Vennegaard T, et al. An immune response study of oakmoss absolute and its constituents atranol and chloroatranol. Contact Dermatitis 2014;70:282-290

78 SCCP (Scientific Committee on Consumer Products). Opinion on Oak moss / Tree moss (sensitisation only), 15 April 2008, SCCP/1131/07. Available at: http://ec.europa.eu/health/ph_risk/committees/04_sccp/docs/sccp_o_131.pdf

79 SCCP (Scientific Committee on Consumer Products). Opinion on Atrranol and Chloroatranol present in natural extracts (e.g. oak moss and tree moss extract), 7 December 2004, SCCP/00847/04. Available at: http://ec.europa.eu/health/ph_risk/committees/04_sccp/docs/sccp_o_006.pdf

80 Ehret C, Maupetit P, Petrzilka M, Klecak G. Preparation of oak moss absolute with reduced allergenic potential. Int J Cosmetic Sci 1992;14:121-130

81 Garioch JJ, Forsyth A, Chapman RS. Allergic contact dermatitis from perfume in Locan® cream. Contact Dermatitis 1989;20:61-62

82 Mowitz M, Zimerson E, Svedman C, Bruze M. Patch testing with serial dilutions and thin-layer chromatograms of oak moss absolutes containing high and low levels of atranol and chloroatranol. Contact Dermatitis 2013;69:342-349

83 Mowitz M, Svedman C, Zimerson E, Bruze M. Usage tests of oak moss absolutes containing high and low levels of atranol and chloroatranol. Acta Derm Venereol 2014;94:398-402

84 Andersen F, Andersen KH, Bernois A, Brault C, Bruze M, Eudes H, et al. Reduced content of chloroatranol and atranol in oak moss absolute significantly reduces the elicitation potential of this fragrance material. Contact Dermatitis 2015;72:75-83

85 Uter W, Johansen JD, Börje A, Karlberg A-T, Lidén C, Rastogi S, Roberts D, White IR. Categorization of fragrance contact allergens for prioritization of preventive measures: clinical and experimental data and consideration of structure–activity relationships. Contact Dermatitis 2013;69:196-230

86 SCCS (Scientific Committee on Consumer Safety). Opinion on Fragrance allergens in cosmetic products, 26-27 June 2012, SCCS/1459/11. Available at:
https://ec.europa.eu/health/sites/health/files/scientific_committees/consumer_safety/docs/sccs_o_102.pdf

87 Dooms-Goossens, A, Kerre S, Drieghe J, Bossuyt L, DeGreef H. Cosmetic products and their allergens. Eur J Dermatol 1992;2:465-468

88 Thune P, Sandberg M. Allergy to lichen and compositae compounds in perfumes. Investigations on the sensitizing, toxic and mutagenic potential. Acta Derm Venereol 1987;134(suppl.):87-89

89 Opinion of the Scientific Committee on Cosmetic Products and Non-Food Products Intended for Consumers concerning 'The 1st update of the inventory of ingredients employed in cosmetic products. Section II: Perfume and aromatic raw materials', 24 October 2000, SCCNFP/0389/00, final. Available at:

90 http://ec.europa.eu/health/ph_risk/committees/sccp/documents/out131_en.pdf
Opinion of the Scientific Committee on Cosmetic Products and Non-Food Products Intended for Consumers concerning 'An initial list of perfumery materials which must not form part of cosmetic products except subject to the Restrictions and Conditions laid down, 25 September 2001, SCCNFP/0392/00, final. Available at:
http://ec.europa.eu/health/archive/ph_risk/committees/sccp/documents/out150_en.pdf

91 Elshimy N, Sheraz F, Lyon C. The secret sensitizer gets out of the bag. Contact Dermatitis 2018;79:54-55

92 Directorate-General for Internal Market, Industry, Entrepreneurship and SMEs (European Commission). Commission Regulation (EU) 2017/1410 of 2 August 2017 amending Annexes II and III to Regulation (EC) No 1223/2009 of the European Parliament and of the Council on cosmetic products. Official J European Union 2017;L202:1-3

93 Ung CY, White JML, White IR, Banerjee P, McFadden JP. Patch testing with the European baseline series fragrance markers: a 2016 update. Br J Dermatol 2018;178:776-780

94 Girbig M, Hegewald J, Seidler A, Bauer A, Uter W, Schmitt J. Type IV sensitizations in physical therapists: patch test results of the Information Network of Departments of Dermatology (IVDK) 2007-2011. J Dtsch Dermatol Ges 2013;11:1185-1192

95 Dittmar D, Schuttelaar MLA. Contact sensitization to hydroperoxides of limonene and linalool: Results of consecutive patch testing and clinical relevance. Contact Dermatitis 2018 Oct 31. doi: 10.1111/cod.13137. [Epub ahead of print]

96 Silvestre JF, Mercader P, González-Pérez R, Hervella-Garcés M, Sanz-Sánchez T, Córdoba S, et al. Sensitization to fragrances in Spain: A 5-year multicentre study (2011-2015). Contact Dermatitis. 2018 Nov 14. doi: 10.1111/cod.13152. [Epub ahead of print]

Chapter 3.68   FARNESOL

IDENTIFICATION

Description/definition	: Farnesol is the organic compound that conforms to the structural formula shown below
Chemical class(es)	: Alcohols
Chemical/IUPAC name	: 3,7,11-Trimethyldodeca-2,6,10-trien-1-ol
Other names	: Farnesyl alcohol
CAS registry number(s)	: 4602-84-0
EC number(s)	: 225-004-1
RIFM monograph(s)	: Food Chem Toxicol 2008;46(11)(suppl.):S1-S71; Food Chem Toxicol 2008;46(11)(suppl.): S149-S156
IFRA standard	: Restricted (www.ifraorg.org/en-us/standards-library) (table 3.68.1)
SCCS opinion(s)	: SCCP/1153/08 (10); SCCS/1459/11 (11); SCCNFP/0389/00, final (49)
Merck Index monograph	: 5245
Function(s) in cosmetics	: EU: deodorant; perfuming; solvent; soothing. USA: fragrance ingredients
EU cosmetic restrictions	: Regulated in Annex III/82 of the Regulation (EC) No. 1223/2009, regulated by 2003/15/EC; Must be labeled on cosmetics and detergent products, if present at > 10 ppm (0.001%) in leave-on products and > 100 ppm (0.01%) in rinse-off products
Patch testing	: 5% Pet. (SmartPracticeEurope, Chemotechnique, SmartPracticeCanada); also present in the fragrance mix II; some positive reactions to farnesol may be missed when the reactions are not read at D7 (30)
Molecular formula	: $C_{15}H_{26}O$

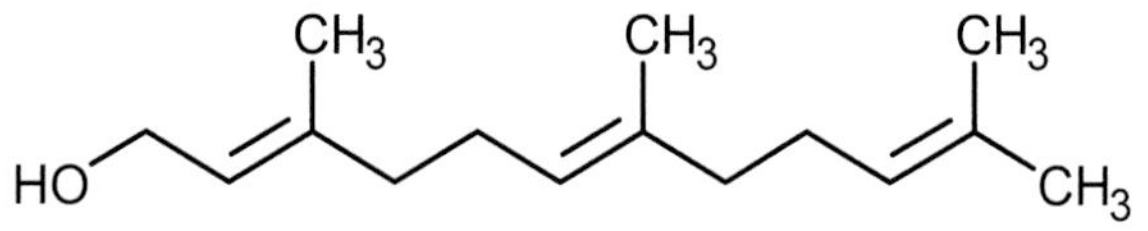

Table 3.68.1 IFRA restrictions for farnesol

Category [a]	Limits [b]	Category [a]	Limits [b]	Category [a]	Limits [b]
1	0.08%	5	0.60%	9	5.00%
2	0.11%	6	2.00%	10	2.50%
3	0.40%	7	0.20%	11	not restricted
4	1.20%	8	2.00%		

[a] For explanation of categories see pages 6-8
[b] Limits in the finished products

GENERAL

Farnesol is a colorless to pale yellow clear oily liquid; its odor type is floral and its odor at 100% is described as 'mild fresh sweet linden floral angelica' (www.thegoodscentscompany.com). In perfumery it is used to emphasize odor of sweet floral perfumes, such as lilac and cyclamen. It is present in many deodorants and antiperspirants, not only as a fragrance, but also as a natural microbiocide (38). Other uses are as flavoring agent in foods and beverages and as insect attractant (U.S. National Library of Medicine, 36).

Presence in essential oils and Myroxylon pereirae resin (balsam of Peru)

Farnesol (any isomer) has been identified by chemical analysis in 39 of 91 essential oils, which have caused contact allergy / allergic contact dermatitis. In 4 oils, farnesol belonged to the 'Top-10' of ingredients with the highest concentrations which may be expected in commercial essential oils of this type: sandalwood oil ((E,E)-, 1.4-18.4%), ylang-ylang oil ((E,E)-, 0.1-4.0%), neroli oil ((E,E)-, 0.3-3.5%), and palmarosa oil ((Z,E)-, 0.5-1.5%) (44). Farnesol may also be present in traces in Myroxylon pereirae resin (balsam of Peru) (5).

CONTACT ALLERGY

General

The SCCS (Scientific Committee on Consumer Safety), in a 2012 Opinion on Fragrance allergens in cosmetic products, has marked farnesol as 'established contact allergen in humans' (11,28). The sensitizing potency of farnesol was classified as 'moderate' based on an EC3 value of 4.1% in the LLNA (local lymph node assay) in animal experiments (11,28).

Farnesol is a constituent of the fragrance mix II. In groups of patients reacting to the mix and tested with its 6 ingredients, farnesol scored 2.7-13.9% positive patch test reactions (see Chapter 3.71 Fragrance mix II).

The literature up to 2010, including published and unpublished studies on the sensitization potential of farnesol, has been reviewed (46).

General population

In the period 2008-2011, in 5 European countries (Sweden, Germany, Netherlands, Portugal, Italy), a random sample of the general population of 3119 individuals aged 18-74 years were patch tested with the FM I, its 8 ingredients, the FM II, its 6 ingredients and Myroxylon pereirae resin. There were 14 reactions (0.4%) to farnesol, tested 5% in petrolatum. About half of all positive reactions to fragrances were considered to be relevant based on standardized criteria. Women were affected twice as often as men (33).

Patch testing in groups of patients

Results of studies testing farnesol in consecutive patients suspected of contact dermatitis (routine testing) are shown in table 3.68.2. Results of testing in groups of *selected* patients (e.g. patients with known or suspected fragrance or cosmetic dermatitis, individuals with eyelid dermatitis or dermatitis of the face, patients allergic to balsam of Peru) are shown in table 3.68.3.

Patch testing in consecutive patients suspected of contact dermatitis: routine testing

In twelve studies in which routine testing with farnesol was performed, frequencies of sensitization have ranged from 0.2% to 2.5% (table 3.68.2). With two exceptions, all rates were 1.1% or lower. In the (early) study with 2.5% positive patch tests (50), the test material contained 50% farnesol, which may have resulted in some irritant reactions. In 9/12 investigations, no (specific) data on relevance were provided; in the three studies addressing the issue, 54-80% of the positive reactions were scored as relevant (1,24,26). Causative products were usually not mentioned or specified, but in one study, of the relevant reactions to any of 26 fragrances tested, 96% were caused by cosmetic products (1).

Table 3.68.2 Patch testing in groups of patients: Routine testing

Years and Country	Test conc. & vehicle	Number of patients tested	positive (%)	Selection of patients (S); Relevance (R); Comments (C)	Ref.
2015-7 Netherlands		821	5 (0.6%)	R: not stated	53
2015-2016 UK	5% pet.	2084	5 (0.2%)	R: not specified for individual fragrances; 25% of patients who reacted to any fragrance or fragrance marker had a positive fragrance history	52
2010-2015 Denmark	5% pet.	6004	49 (0.82%)	R: present relevance 54%, past relevance 29%	24
2009-2015 Sweden	5% pet.	4430	27 (0.6%)	R: not stated	29
2013-2014 Thailand		312	5 (1.6%)	R: 80%	26
2011-2012 UK	5% pet.	1951	8 (0.4%)	R: not stated	27
2008-2010 Denmark	5% pet.	1502	6 (0.4%)	S: mostly routine testing; R: 60%; C: 60% co-reactivity of FM I, 80% of FM II; C: of the relevant reactions to any of the 26 fragrances tested, 96% were caused by cosmetic products	1
2003-2004 IVDK	5% pet.	4238	38 (0.9%)	R: not stated; C: co-reactivity of FM I: 25%	3
2003 IVDK	5% pet.	2021	22 (1.1%)	R: not stated; C: co-reactivity to FM I: 23%; 2 co-reactions to propolis (odds ratio: 6.2)	41
2002-2003 six Euro-pean countries	2.5% pet.	1701	4 (0.2%)	R: not specified	7
	5% pet.	1701	6 (0.4%)	R: not specified	
1997-1998 six Euro-pean countries	5% pet.	1855	10 (0.5%)	R: not stated / specified	19
<1973 Poland	50% pet.	200	5 (2.5%)	R: not stated; C: probably some irritant reactions	50

FM: Fragrance mix; IVDK: Informationsverbund Dermatologischer Kliniken (Germany, Switzerland, Austria)

Patch testing in groups of selected patients

Results of studies patch testing farnesol in groups of selected patients (e.g. patients with known or suspected fragrance or cosmetic dermatitis, individuals with eyelid dermatitis or dermatitis of the face, patients allergic to balsam of Peru) are shown in table 3.68.3. In 13 investigations, frequencies of sensitization to farnesol have ranged from 0.9% to 10%, but most were low. The highest rate (10%) was observed in a group of 100 patients with known fragrance sensitivity based on a positive reaction to the fragrance mix I and/or the fragrances mix II, the latter of which containing farnesol (30). In most studies, no (specific) relevance data were provided, were not applicable (in the case of testing patients allergic to balsam of Peru, which may contain traces of farnesol) or data were lacking (in the case of early Japanese studies published in Japanese journals only). The authors of one study considered relevance for all reactions 'possible' (6). Causative products were not mentioned.

Results of testing farnesol in groups of patients reacting to the fragrance mix II are shown in Chapter 3.71 Fragrance mix II.

Table 3.68.3 Patch testing in groups of patients: Selected patient groups

Years and Country	Test conc. & vehicle	Number of patients tested | positive (%)		Selection of patients (S); Relevance (R); Comments (C)	Ref.
2011-2015 Spain	5% pet.	1013	28 (2.8%)	S: patients previously reacting to FM I, FM II, Myroxylon pereirae resin or hydroxyisohexyl 3-cyclohexene carboxaldehyde in the baseline series; R: not stated	54
2009-2010 Hungary	5% pet.	565	14 (2.5%)	S: patients with former skin symptoms provoked by scented products in the case history; R: in all cases 'possible'	6
2006-2010 USA	2.5% pet.	100	3 (3%)	S: patients with eyelid dermatitis; R: not stated	8
2005-10 Netherlands		100	10 (10%)	S: patients with known fragrance sensitivity based on a positive patch test to the FM I and/or the FM II; R: not stated	30
2004-2008 Spain	5% pet.	86	1 (1.2%)	S: patients previously reacting to the fragrance mix I or Myroxylon pereirae (n=54) or suspected of fragrance contact allergy (n=32); R: not stated	20
2005-7 Netherlands	5% pet.	320	3 (0.9%)	S: patients suspected of fragrance or cosmetic allergy; R: 61% relevance for all positive tested fragrances together	2
1995-1998 Germany	5% pet.	102	4 (3.9%)	S: patients allergic to Myroxylon pereirae resin	5
1990-1998 Japan	5% pet.	1483	16 (1.1%)	S: patients suspected of cosmetic contact dermatitis, virtually all were women; range of annual frequency of sensitization: 0-2.3%; R: not stated	9
1984-1987 Japan	20% pet.	573	7 (1.2%)	S: patients with 'cosmetic dermatitis or eczema'; R: unknown	40
1977-1985 Japan	5% pet.	456	(1.5%)	S: patients suspected of fragrance sensitivity; R: unknown	35
1984 Japan	2%, 5% and 10% pet.	1367	? (?)	S: patients with dermatitis of the face; R: unknown; C: sensitization reactions were observed at all concentrations	46
1983 The Netherlands	4% pet.	182	2 (1.1%)	S: patients suspected of cosmetic allergy; R: not stated	37
1955-1960 Denmark	50% o.o.	53	1 (2%)	S: patients allergic to balsam of Peru	47

Testing in groups of patients reacting to the fragrance mix II
Results of testing farnesol in groups of patients reacting to the fragrance mix II are shown in Chapter 3.71 Fragrance mix II

FM: Fragrance mix; IVDK: Informationsverbund Dermatologischer Kliniken (Germany, Switzerland, Austria); o.o.: Olive oil

Case reports and case series
Farnesol was stated to be the (or an) allergen in 11 patients in a group of 603 individuals suffering from cosmetic dermatitis, seen in the period 2010-2015 in Leuven, Belgium (23). In the period 1996-2013, in a tertiary referral center in Valencia, Spain, 5419 patients were patch tested. Of these, 628 individuals had allergic contact dermatitis to cosmetics. In this group, farnesol was the responsible allergen in two cases (17).

Farnesol was responsible for 6 out of 959 cases of cosmetic allergy where the causal allergen was identified, Belgium, 2000-2010 (used as an antimicrobial) (4). In the period 2000-2009, in Leuven, Belgium, an unspecified number of patients had positive patch tests or use tests to a total of 344 cosmetic products *and* positive patch tests to FM I, FM II, and/or to one or more of 28 selected specific fragrance ingredients. In 7 of 14 patients reacting to farnesol, the presence of this fragrance in the cosmetic product(s) was confirmed by reading the product label(s) (31).

A woman with axillary dermatitis had positive patch tests to a deodorant. When tested with its ingredients, she reacted to farnesol (1% pet.) and the perfume (38). Another female patient had allergic contact dermatitis from several fragrances in an eau de parfum, including farnesol (32).

Cross-reactions, pseudo-cross-reactions and co-reactions
For general information on cross-/pseudo-cross-/co-reactivity of fragrance chemicals with other fragrances, fragrance markers (fragrance mix I, fragrance mix II, colophonium, Myroxylon pereirae resin [balsam of Peru]) and essential oils see Chapter 1.2 General information on cross-reactions, pseudo-cross-reactions and co-reactions. Co-reactivity with the fragrance mix II can be expected, as the mix contains farnesol (pseudo-cross-reactions).

Of 7 patients with contact allergy to farnesol, 5 (71%) co-reacted to Myroxylon pereirae resin (MP) (39), in which it may be present, albeit in very low concentrations (5,42). In some samples of MP, farnesol could not be detected at all (43). According to the manufacturer of patch test materials, the concentration of farnesol, if present in the patch-test preparation of M. pereirae resin, would have been too low to elicit a positive reaction. Indeed, in another study, only 2 out of 22 farnesol-allergic patients reacted to MP (43). Cases of concurrent reactions to farnesol and MP, therefore, should be regarded as independent sensitizations (43). Conversely, of 102 patients sensitized to MP, 4 (4%) co-reacted to farnesol (5).

In 22 patients reacting to farnesol, there were 2 co-reactions to propolis (odds ratio: 6.2) (43). Farnesol has not been demonstrated in propolis (42,45), but has been found in poplar buds, the source material for propolis (42).

Presence in products and chemical analyses

In various studies, the presence of farnesol in cosmetic and sometimes other products has been investigated. Before 2006, most investigators used chemical analysis, usually GC-MS, for qualitative and quantitative determination of various fragrances. Since then, the presence of the target fragrances was usually investigated by screening the product labels for the 26 fragrances that must be labeled since 2005 on cosmetics and detergent products in the EU, if present at > 10 ppm (0.001%) in leave-on products and > 100 ppm (0.01%) in rinse-off products. This method, obviously, is less accurate and may result in underestimation of the frequency of the fragrances being present in the product. When they are in fact present, but the concentration is lower than mentioned above, labeling is not required and the fragrances' presence will be missed.

The results of the relevant studies for farnesol are summarized in table 3.68.4. More detailed information can be found in the corresponding text following the table. The percentage of products in which farnesol was found to be present shows wide variations, which can among other be explained by the selection procedure of the products, the method of investigation (false-negatives with information obtained from labels only) and changes in the use of individual fragrance materials over time (fashion). However, most percentages are low and farnesol appears to be one of the lesser used fragrances (in concentrations which need labeling).

Table 3.68.4 Presence of farnesol in products [a]

Year	Country	Product type	Nr. investigated	Nr. of products positive [b]	(%)	Method [c]	Ref.
2015-6	Denmark	Fragranced cosmetic products	5588		(3%)	Labeling	15
2015	Germany	Household detergents	817	2	(0.2%)	Labeling	51
2014	Poland	Emollients	179	1	(0.6%)	Online info	25
2013	USA	Pediatric cosmetics	187	1	(0.5%)	Labeling	18
2008-11	Germany	Deodorants	374	12	(3%)	Labeling	34
2006-9	Germany	Cosmetic products	4991		(3%)	Labeling	14
2008	Sweden	Cosmetic products	204		(0.5%)	Labeling	12
		Detergents	97		(0%)	Labeling	
2007	Netherlands	Cosmetic products for children	23	1	(4%)	Analysis	22
2006	UK	Perfumed cosmetic and house-hold products	300	23	(8%)	Labeling	13
2006	Denmark	Popular perfumed deodorants	88	13	(15%)	Labeling	16
			23	9	(39%)	Analysis	
2006	Denmark	Rinse-off cosmetics for children	208	6	(3%)	Labeling + analysis	21
2004	Denmark, UK, Belgium, Germany	Fragranced products that had caused allergic contact derma-titis, used by patients	24	0	(0%)	Labeling	7

[a] See the corresponding text below for more details
[b] positive = containing the target fragrance
[c] Labeling: information from the ingredient labels on the product / packaging; Analysis: chemical analysis, most often GC-MS

In Denmark, in 2015-2016, 5588 fragranced cosmetic products were examined with a smartphone application for the 26 fragrances that need to be labeled in the EU. Farnesol was present in 3% of the products (rank number 17) (15).

In Germany, in 2015, fragrance allergens were evaluated based on lists of ingredients in 817 (unique) detergents (all-purpose cleaners, cleaning preparations for special purposes [e.g. bathroom, kitchen, dish-washing] and laundry detergents) present in 131 households. Farnesol was found to be present in two (0.2%) of the products (51).

Of 179 emollients available in online drugstores in 2014 in Poland, one (0.6%) contained farnesol, according to information available online (25).

In 2013, in the USA, the allergen content of 187 unique pediatric cosmetics from 6 different retailers marketed in the United States as hypoallergenic was evaluated on the basis of labeling. Inclusion criteria were products marketed as pediatric and 'hypoallergenic', 'dermatologist recommended/tested', 'fragrance free', or 'paraben free'. Farnesol was found to be present in one (0.5%) of the products (18).

In 2008, 2010 and 2011, 374 deodorants available in German retail shops were randomly selected and their labels checked for the presence of the 26 fragrances that need to be labeled. Farnesol was found to be present in 12 (3.2%) of the products (34).

In Germany, in the period 2006-2009, 4991 cosmetic products were sampled for an official investigation of conformity of cosmetic products with legal provisions. The labels were inspected for the presence of the 26 fragrances that need to be labeled in the EU. Farnesol was present in 3% of the products (rank number 16) (14).

Farnesol was present in 0.5% of 204 cosmetic products (92 shampoos, 61 hair conditioners, 34 liquid soaps, 17 wet tissues) and in none of 97 detergents in Sweden, 2008 (12).

In 2007, in The Netherlands, twenty-three cosmetic products for children were analyzed for the presence of fragrances that need to be labeled. Farnesol was identified in one of the products (4%) in a concentration of 524 ppm (22).

In 2006, the labels of 208 cosmetics for children (especially shampoos, body shampoos and soaps) available in Denmark were checked for the presence of the 26 fragrances that need to be labeled in the EU. Farnesol was present in 6 products (2.9%), and ranked number 20 in the frequency list (21).

In 2006, of 88 popular perfume containing deodorants purchased in Denmark, 13 (15%) were labeled to contain farnesol. Analysis of 24 regulated fragrance substances in 23 selected deodorants (19 spray products, 2 deostick and 2 roll-on) was performed by GC-MS. Farnesol was identified in 9 of the products (39%) with a concentration range of 9–1791 ppm (16).

In January 2006, a study of perfumed cosmetic and household products available on the shelves of U.K. retailers was carried out. Products were included if 'parfum' or 'aroma' was listed among the ingredients. Three hundred products were surveyed and any of 26 mandatory labeling fragrances named on the label were recorded. Farnesol was present in 23 (8%) of the products (rank number 18) (13).

In 2004, in 4 European countries (Denmark, Germany, Belgium, U.K.), of 12 patients allergic to the FM II and one or more of its constituents (hexyl cinnamal 1, citral 3, hydroxyisohexyl 3-cyclohexene carboxaldehyde 11), 24 of the products used by them (deodorant 4, eau de toilette 9, lotion/cream 4, fine perfume 7) that had caused adverse reactions compatible with allergic contact dermatitis, were analyzed for the presence of the six constituents of the fragrance mix II (citral, citronellol, coumarin, farnesol, hexyl cinnamal, hydroxyisohexyl 3-cyclohexene carboxaldehyde). Farnesol was not detected in any product (7).

LITERATURE

1   Heisterberg MV, Menné T, Johansen JD. Contact allergy to the 26 specificc fragrance ingredients to be declared on cosmetic products in accordance with the EU cosmetic directive. Contact Dermatitis 2011;65:266-275
2   Oosten EJ van, Schuttelaar ML, Coenraads PJ. Clinical relevance of positive patch test reactions to the 26 EU-labelled fragrances. Contact Dermatitis 2009;61:217-223
3   Schnuch A, Uter W, Geier J, Lessmann H, Frosch PJ. Sensitization to 26 fragrances to be labelled according to current European regulation: Results of the IVDK and review of the literature. Contact Dermatitis 2007;57:1-10
4   Travassos AR, Claes L, Boey L, Drieghe J, Goossens A. Non-fragrance allergens in specific cosmetic products. Contact Dermatitis 2011;65:276-285
5   Hausen BM. Contact allergy to Balsam of Peru. II. Patch test results in 102 patients with selected Balsam of Peru constituents. Am J Contact Derm 2001;12:93-102
6   Pónyai G, Németh I, Altmeyer A, Nagy G, Irinyi B, Battya Z, et al. Patch tests with fragrance mix II and its components. Dermatitis 2012;23:71-74
7   Frosch PJ, Rastogi SC, Pirker C, Brinkmeier T, Andersen KE, Bruze M, et al. Patch testing with a new fragrance mix - reactivity to the individual constituents and chemical detection in relevant cosmetic products. Contact Dermatitis 2005;52:216-225
8   Wenk KS, Ehrlich AE. Fragrance series testing in eyelid dermatitis. Dermatitis 2012;23:22-26
9   Sugiura M, Hayakawa R, Kato Y, Sugiura K, Hashimoto R. Results of patch testing with lavender oil in Japan. Contact Dermatitis 2000;43:157-160
10 SCCP (Scientific Committee on Consumer Products). Opinion on Dermal sensitisation quantitative risk assessment (Citral, Farnesol and Phenylacetaldehyde), 24 June 2008, SCCP/1153/08. Available at: http://ec.europa.eu/health/archive/ph_risk/committees/04_sccp/docs/sccp_o_135.pdf
11 SCCS (Scientific Committee on Consumer Safety). Opinion on Fragrance allergens in cosmetic products, 26-27 June 2012, SCCS/1459/11. Available at: https://ec.europa.eu/health/sites/health/files/scientific_committees/consumer_safety/docs/sccs_o_102.pdf
12 Yazar K, Johnsson S, Lind M-L, Boman A, Lidén C. Preservatives and fragrances in selected consumer-available cosmetics and detergents. Contact Dermatitis 2011;64:265-272
13 Buckley DA. Fragrance ingredient labelling in products on sale in the UK. Br J Dermatol 2007;157:295-300
14 Uter W, Yazar K, Kratz E-M, Mildau G, Lidén C. Coupled exposure to ingredients of cosmetic products: I. Fragrances. Contact Dermatitis 2013;69:335-341

15 Bennike NH, Oturai NB, Müller S, Kirkeby CS, Jørgensen C, Christensen AB, et al. Fragrance contact allergens in 5588 cosmetic products identified through a novel smartphone application. J Eur Acad Dermatol Venereol 2018;32:79-85

16 Rastogi SC, Hellerup Jensen G, Johansen JD. Survey and risk assessment of chemical substances in deodorants. Survey of Chemical Substances in Consumer Products, No. 86 2007. Danish Ministry of the Environment, Environmental Protection Agency. Available at: https://www2.mst.dk/Udgiv/publications/2007/978-87-7052-625-8/pdf/978-87-7052-626-5.pdf

17 Zaragoza-Ninet V, Blasco Encinas R, Vilata-Corell JJ, Pérez-Ferriols A, Sierra-Talamantes C, Esteve-Martínez A, de la Cuadra-Oyanguren J. Allergic contact dermatitis due to cosmetics: A clinical and epidemiological study in a tertiary hospital. Actas Dermosifiliogr 2016;107:329-336

18 Hamann CR, Bernard S, Hamann D, Hansen R, Thyssen JP. Is there a risk using hypoallergenic cosmetic pediatric products in the United States? J Allergy Clin Immunol 2015;135:1070-1071

19 Frosch PJ, Johansen JD, Menné T, Pirker C, Rastogi SC, Andersen KE, et al. Further important sensitizers in patients sensitive to fragrances. I. Reactivity to 14 frequently used chemicals. Contact Dermatitis 2002;47:78-85

20 Cuesta L, Silvestre JF, Toledo F, Lucas A, Perez-Crespo M, Ballester I. Fragrance contact allergy: a 4-year retrospective study. Contact Dermatitis 2010;63:77-84

21 Poulsen PB, Schmidt A. A survey and health assessment of cosmetic products for children. Survey of chemical substances in consumer products, No. 88. Copenhagen: Danish Environmental Protection Agency, 2007. Available at: https://www2.mst.dk/udgiv/publications/2007/978-87-7052-638-8/pdf/978-87-7052-639-5.pdf

22 VWA. Dutch Food and Consumer Product Safety Authority. Cosmetische producten voor kinderen: Inventarisatie van de markt en de veiligheidsborging door producenten en importeurs. Report ND04o065/ND05o170, 2007 (Report in Dutch), 2007. Available at: www.nvwa.nl/documenten/communicatie/inspectieresultaten/ consument/ 2016m/cosmetische- producten-voor-kinderen

23 Goossens A. Cosmetic contact allergens. Cosmetics 2016, 3, 5; doi:10.3390/cosmetics3010005

24 Bennike NH, Zachariae C, Johansen JD. Non-mix fragrances are top sensitizers in consecutive dermatitis patients – a cross-sectional study of the 26 EU-labelled fragrance allergens. Contact Dermatitis 2017;77:270-279

25 Osinka K, Karczmarz A, Krauze K, Feleszko W. Contact allergens in cosmetics used in atopic dermatitis: analysis of product composition. Contact Dermatitis 2016;75:241-243

26 Vejanurug P, Tresukosol P, Sajjachareonpong P, Puangpet P. Fragrance allergy could be missed without patch testing with 26 individual fragrance allergens. Contact Dermatitis 2016;74:230-235

27 Mann J, McFadden JP, White JML, White IR, Banerjee P. Baseline series fragrance markers fail to predict contact allergy. Contact Dermatitis 2014;70:276-281

28 Uter W, Johansen JD, Börje A, Karlberg A-T, Lidén C, Rastogi S, Roberts D, White IR. Categorization of fragrance contact allergens for prioritization of preventive measures: clinical and experimental data and consideration of structure–activity relationships. Contact Dermatitis 2013;69:196-230

29 Mowitz M, Svedman C, Zimerson E, Isaksson M, Pontén A, Bruze M. Simultaneous patch testing with fragrance mix I, fragrance mix II and their ingredients in southern Sweden between 2009 and 2015. Contact Dermatitis 2017;77:280-287

30 Nagtegaal MJC, Pentinga SE, Kuik J, Kezic S, Rustemeyer T. The role of the skin irritation response in polysensitization to fragrances. Contact Dermatitis 2012;67:28-35

31 Nardelli A, Drieghe J, Claes L, Boey L, Goossens A. Fragrance allergens in 'specific' cosmetic products. Contact Dermatitis 2011;64:212-219

32 Nardelli A, Thijs L, Janssen K, Goossens A. *Rosa centifolia* in a 'non-scented' moisturizing body lotion as a cause of allergic contact dermatitis. Contact Dermatitis 2009;61:306-309

33 Diepgen TL, Ofenloch R, Bruze M, Cazzaniga S, Coenraads PJ, Elsner P, et al. Prevalence of fragrance contact allergy in the general population of five European countries: a cross-sectional study. Br J Dermatol 2015;173:1411-1419

34 Klaschka U. Contact allergens for armpits - allergenic fragrances specified on deodorants. Int J Hyg Environ Health 2012;215:584-591

35 Sugai T. Group Study IV - farnesol and lily aldehyde. Environ Dermatol 1994;1:213-214 (article in Japanese)

36 Gilpin S, Maibach H. Allergic contact dermatitis caused by farnesol: clinical relevance. Cutan Ocul Toxicol 2010;29:278-287

37 Malten KE, van Ketel WG, Nater JP, Liem DH. Reactions in selected patients to 22 fragrance materials. Contact Dermatitis 1984;11:1-10

38 Hemmer W, Focke M, Leitner B, Götz M, Jarisch R. Axillary dermatitis from farnesol in a deodorant. Contact Dermatitis 2000;42:168-169

39 Goossens A, Merckx L. Allergic contact dermatitis from farnesol in a deodorant. Contact Dermatitis 1997;37:179-180

40 Hirose O, Arima Y, Hosokawa K, Suzuki M, Matsunaga K, Hayakawa R. Patch test results of cosmetic allergens during recent 30 months. Skin Research 1987;29: 95-100 (article in Japanese). Data cited in ref. 48

41 Schnuch A, Uter W, Geier J, Lessmann H, Frosch PJ. Contact allergy to farnesol in 2021 consecutively patch tested patients. Results of the IVDK. Contact Dermatitis 2004;50:117-121

42 Hausen BM, Evers P, Stüwe HT, König WA, Wollenweber E. Propolis allergy (IV). Studies with further sensitizers from propolis and constituents common to propolis, poplar buds and balsam of Peru. Contact Dermatitis 1992;26:34-44

43 Hausen BM, Simatupang T, Bruhn G, Evers P, Koenig WA. Identification of new allergenic constituents and proof of evidence for coniferyl benzoate in balsam of Peru. Am J Contact Dermat 1995;6:199-208

44 De Groot AC, Schmidt E. Essential oils: contact allergy and chemical composition. Boca Raton, Fl., USA: CRC Press, Taylor and Francis Group, 2016 (ISBN 9781482246407)).

45 De Groot AC, Popova MP, Bankova VS. An update on the constituents of poplar-type propolis. Wapserveen, The Netherlands: acdegroot publishing, 2014, 11 pages (ISBN/EAN: 978-90-813233-0-7)

46 Yamamoto, S. Japan Patch Test Research Group, 1985. An approach to determine the optimal concentration of farnesol in patch-testing and the incidence of positive reactions of benzyl salicylate in new patients with facial melanosis in 1984. Skin Research 1985;28(suppl.2):135-141 (article in Japanese). Data cited in ref. 48

47 Hjorth N. Eczematous allergy to balsams. Acta Derm Venereol 1961;41(suppl.46):1-216

48 Lapczynski A, Bhatia SP, Letizia CS, Api AM. Fragrance material review on farnesol. Food Chem Toxicol 2008;46(11)(suppl.):S149-S156

49 Opinion of the Scientific Committee on Cosmetic Products and Non-Food Products Intended for Consumers concerning 'The 1st update of the inventory of ingredients employed in cosmetic products. Section II: Perfume and aromatic raw materials', 24 October 2000, SCCNFP/0389/00, final. Available at: http://ec.europa.eu/health/ph_risk/committees/sccp/documents/out131_en.pdf

50 Rudzki E, Kielak D. Sensitivity to some compounds related to Balsam of Peru. Contact Dermatitis Newsletter 1972;nr.13:335-336

51 Wieck S, Olsson O, Kümmerer K, Klaschka U. Fragrance allergens in household detergents. Regul Toxicol Pharmacol 2018;97:163-169

52 Ung CY, White JML, White IR, Banerjee P, McFadden JP. Patch testing with the European baseline series fragrance markers: a 2016 update. Br J Dermatol 2018;178:776-780

53 Dittmar D, Schuttelaar MLA. Contact sensitization to hydroperoxides of limonene and linalool: Results of consecutive patch testing and clinical relevance. Contact Dermatitis 2018 Oct 31. doi: 10.1111/cod.13137. [Epub ahead of print]

54 Silvestre JF, Mercader P, González-Pérez R, Hervella-Garcés M, Sanz-Sánchez T, Córdoba S, et al. Sensitization to fragrances in Spain: A 5-year multicentre study (2011-2015). Contact Dermatitis. 2018 Nov 14. doi: 10.1111/cod.13152. [Epub ahead of print]

Chapter 3.69   FERULA GALBANIFLUA GUM

IDENTIFICATION

Description/definition   : Ferula galbaniflua gum is a gum obtained from the galbanum, *Ferula galbaniflua*,
                            Apiaceae
Chemical class(es)   : Botanical products and botanical derivatives
INCI name USA   : Not in the Personal Care Products Council Ingredient Database
Other names   : Galbanum resin; galbanum gum
CAS registry number(s)   : 93165-40-3
EC number(s)   : 296-925-4
RIFM monograph(s)   : Food Chem Toxicol 1992;30(suppl.1):S39
Function(s) in cosmetics : EU: perfuming
Patch testing   : 2% pet. (1)

GENERAL

Galbanum is an aromatic gum resin and a product of certain umbelliferous Persian plant species in the genus Ferula, chiefly *Ferula galbaniflua* (synonym *F. gummosa*) and *Ferula rubricaulis*. Galbanum-yielding plants grow plentifully on the slopes of the mountain ranges of northern Iran. The gum occurs at the roots usually in hard or soft, irregular, more or less translucent and shining lumps, or occasionally in separate tears. These have a light-brown, yellowish or greenish-yellow color, and a disagreeable, bitter taste, a peculiar, somewhat musky odor, and an intense green scent (Wikipedia).

CONTACT ALLERGY

Patch testing in groups of patients

Patch testing in consecutive patients suspected of contact dermatitis: routine testing
Studies in which Ferula galbaniflua gum was patch tested in consecutive patients suspected of contact dermatitis (routine testing) with positive results have not been found.

Patch testing in groups of selected patients
Before 1996, in Japan, some European countries and the USA, 167 patients known or suspected to be allergic to fragrances were patch tested with 'galbanum resin' 2% pet. and there were eight (4.8%) positive reactions; their relevance was not mentioned (1).

Case reports and case series
Case reports of allergic contact dermatitis from Ferula galbaniflua gum have not been found.

Cross-reactions, pseudo-cross-reactions and co-reactions
For general information on cross-/pseudo-cross-/co-reactivity of fragrance chemicals with other fragrances, fragrance markers (fragrance mix I, fragrance mix II, colophonium, Myroxylon pereirae resin [balsam of Peru]) and essential oils see Chapter 1.2 General information on cross-reactions, pseudo-cross-reactions and co-reactions.

A man developed acute eczematous contact dermatitis in response to the application of tincture of benzoin to the skin under a cast. This was followed within 48 hours by the appearance of generalized non-eczematous exanthem, which was ascribed to absorption of benzoin through the skin. Patch tests were performed with tincture of benzoin, benzoin gum and 16 other gums (test concentrations and vehicles not mentioned). The patient reacted not only to benzoin but also to 4 other gums including galbanum gum, which were considered to be a cross-reactions (2).

A series of resins and balsams was tested 10% in alcohol in 11 patients allergic to Myroxylon pereirae resin (balsam of Peru) and 3 reacted to galbanum (Ferula galbaniflua gum) (3).

LITERATURE

1   Larsen W, Nakayama H, Fischer T, Elsner P, Burrows D, Jordan W, et al. Fragrance contact dermatitis: A
     worldwide multicenter investigation (Part I). Am J Cont Dermat 1996;7:77-83
2   Spott DA, Shelley WB. Exanthem due to contact allergen (benzoin) absorbed through skin. JAMA 1970;214:1881
3   Hjorth N. Eczematous allergy to balsams. Acta Derm Venereol 1961;41(suppl.46):1-216

Chapter 3.70 FRAGRANCE MIX I

IDENTIFICATION

Description/definition : The fragrance mix I (FM I) is a mixture of fragrance materials for patch testing; it contains 8 chemicals in petrolatum, each in a concentration of 1%: amyl cinnamal, cinnamal, cinnamyl alcohol, eugenol, Evernia prunastri (oakmoss) extract, geraniol, isoeugenol and hydroxycitronellal; see the individual chapters of these chemicals for their specific data

Patch testing : 8% Pet. (SmartPracticeEurope, Chemotechnique, SmartPracticeCanada); the use of preparations from different suppliers affects the patch test results (122); it is well known that the sensitivity of the TRUE test in detecting fragrance allergy is lower than FM I in petrolatum (105,115,167,170,188,209,212); the FM I TRUE test has apparently been reformulated to overcome this problem (203); when patch tests are performed with the 8 ingredients of the mix in FM 1-positive patients ('breakdown testing'), the emulsifier sorbitan sesquioleate must also be tested, as some reactions to the mix (and its ingredients) are not caused by fragrance allergy but by contact allergy to sorbitan sesquioleate present in the test substances (101); in fact, sorbitan sesquioleate should preferably always be tested in the baseline series in order to interpret a positive reaction to the FM I correctly

GENERAL

The fragrance mix I (FM I) was developed in the late 1970s, based on the important work of Larsen (32). It consists of amyl cinnamal, cinnamal, cinnamyl alcohol, eugenol, geraniol, hydroxycitronellal, isoeugenol, and Evernia prunastri extract (oakmoss absolute) in petrolatum. At first, these 8 ingredients each had a concentration of 2% (8x2%, total 16%). This mix was used routinely in the late 1970s and early 1980s to screen for contact sensitization to fragrances and, in particular, to its eight ingredients. At that time, it had an estimated sensitivity of 70-80%, but it also caused many false-positive, irritant, reactions (200). In 1984, the concentration of its ingredients, therefore, was reduced to 8% (8x1%) (149).

During the 1990s, 5% sorbitan sesquioleate (SSO) was added as an emulsifier in order to ensure a stable, homogenous distribution of the fragrance compounds in the petrolatum vehicle. This resulted in more cases of sensitivity being detected (133,140), but also increased the irritancy of the test preparation (133). SSO can also cause sensitization and may be the cause of a positive patch test to the FM I in up to 5-10% of the reactions (101,133,150). Therefore, in order to prevent that such patients are unduly advised to avoid all fragrances, the members of the European Environmental and Contact Dermatitis Research Group (EECDRG) already in 1995 advised to add SSO to the European standard series (133), which has, however, not been implemented, possibly because it was thought that contact allergy to SSO is infrequent. In 2015, however, the IVDK convincingly showed that reactivity to SSO markedly affects the outcome of patch testing with FM I and its single constituents. The authors advised that SSO must be an obligatory part of the full FM I breakdown test, and should ideally be included in the baseline series (101).

Even now, 40 years after its introduction, the qualitative composition of the FM I has remained virtually unchanged (see below in this section) and it is included in almost all patch test baseline series throughout the world as a marker (indicator) of fragrance sensitivity. It still is very useful, although we now know that the mix may fail to detect from 40 up to 65% of all cases of fragrance sensitization (1,2).

The FM I 8% pet. with 5% SSO causes many (up to 25% [170]) dubious (?+) reactions, some of which may be 'non-specific' (170) and are likely to be rated as irritant by many investigators. In addition, also a large portion of weak-positive (+) reactions to FM I are considered to be false-positive (i.e., irritant) by some authors (60,185). Others, however, have shown that nearly 60% of patients with a ?+ reaction to FM I have a positive retest and many are considered to be relevant (150). Other problems with the FM I are discussed below in the section 'Testing with the constituents of fragrance mix I in patients reacting to mix'.

It has convincingly been shown that the fragrance mix in the TRUE Test is (considerably) less sensitive in detecting fragrance contact allergy than patch testing with petrolatum-based test material in Finn Chambers or Van der Bend chambers (105,115,167,170,188). However, the TRUE test does identify a number of fragrance-allergic individuals that are not identified by the 8x1% petrolatum-based materials (170) and patch testing with FM I TRUE Test has a slightly higher specificity and a higher positive predictive value (188).

As a historical note, in the early years, the FM I contained amylcinnamyl alcohol (149,68). It was replaced with amyl cinnamal, but no one seems to know why and when and there is no article that describes the creation of the fragrance mix I (149).

CONTACT ALLERGY

Contact allergy in the general population
There have been several investigations, especially in Europe, in which random samples of the population of certain age groups have been patch tested with the fragrance mix I. In a 2018 meta-analysis of 19 studies covering 19,440 patch tested individuals from the general population, the pooled prevalence for sensitization to the fragrance mix I was 3.5% (women 3.4%, men 2.9%) (27). Ten years earlier, based on data from a systematic literature review up to 2008, the median prevalence of FM I sensitization among adults was found to be 2.3% (women, 1.7%; men, 1.3%). The weighted average prevalence of FM I sensitization among adults was 3.7% (184).

Estimates of the 10-year prevalence (1997-2006) of contact allergy to FM I in the general population of Denmark based on the CE-DUR method ranged from 1.25 to 1.69% (59). In a similar study from Germany, the estimated prevalence in the general population in the period 1992-2000 ranged from 1.8 to 4.2% (60,73).

Patch testing in groups of patients
Results of patch testing FM I in consecutive patients suspected of contact dermatitis (routine testing) back to 2000 are shown in table 3.70.1. Results of testing in groups of *selected* patients (e.g. nurses with occupational contact dermatitis, individuals with eyelid dermatitis, patients with allergic contact cheilitis, individuals with stasis dermatitis / leg ulcers, patients suspected of cosmetic intolerance or fragrance allergy, patients with hand dermatitis) are shown in table 3.70.2. Women are more frequently allergic to (ingredients of) the FM I than men (generally women: men = 1.3 - 1.6) and fragrance sensitization is more prevalent in older age groups (122,173,184,189,216).

Patch testing in consecutive patients suspected of contact dermatitis: routine testing
As the FM I is present in most, if not all, baseline / routine / screening / standard series tested worldwide, data on testing FM I in consecutive patients (routine testing) is abundant. The results of nearly 60 such published investigations back to 2000 are shown in table 3.70.1.

USA
In fourteen studies from the USA, 10 of which were performed by the North American Contact Dermatitis Group (NACDG), frequencies of sensitization have ranged from 5.9% to 12.1% (9,10,11,12,40,41,46,49,54,57,64,151,217, 218). The average of all studies excepted the one with the low 5.9% rate was 10.3%. The study scoring only 5.9% was performed in 2003 in 5 centers participating in the NACDG (151). The results of the *entire* NACDG in 2003-2004 was a frequency of sensitization of 9.1% (12). From European multinational and multicenter studies it is well known that there can be great variability between countries and centers. Generally speaking, in the USA, between 9 and 12% of patients routinely tested react to the fragrance mix I. In various NACDG studies, 'definite' + 'probable' relevance was usually 30-35%. In two non-NACDG centers, relevance was scored in 60% (54) and 71% (10) of the positive patch test reactions.

Europe, multicenter studies
In nine multinational multicenter studies performed in Europe (European Surveillance System on Contact Allergy network, European Environmental and Contact Dermatitis Research Group, other parties) frequencies of sensitization have ranged from 6.6 to 11.4% (3,14,23,39,45,52,55,58,105). Rates were generally lower than in the USA. In some, there was a significant variability in the results per center or country: 0-16% (58), 4.8-14.7% (105), 3.7-10.4% (14), 4.8-7.7% (55), 1.9-17.5% (39), 3.7-10.4% (45) and 5.0-12.8% (52). The rates of sensitizations are the highest in central Europe and appear to be lower in the south. Relevance data were not provided in any of the 9 investigations.

IVDK (Informationsverbund Dermatologischer Kliniken: Germany, Switzerland, Austria)
The results of testing large groups of patients with FM I by the IVDK have been reported in 5 publications (13,34, 43,64,111) with overlapping study periods and populations. Rates of sensitization have ranged from 6.6 to 9.5%. Since 2007 there is a clear increase in their frequencies (34,64). Relevance data were not provided.

Denmark
The results of testing patients in Denmark have been reported in 8 publications with overlapping study periods and populations. Rates of sensitization in seven have ranged from 6.0 to 9.3% (1,44,117,169,170,174,189). In a review of nearly 25,000 patients tested between 1986 and 2015 (overall frequency of sensitization: 7.8%), rates per year ranged from 4.7 to 10.6%. The was an increase in prevalence of FM sensitization in men in the years 2006-2015 and in women throughout the period of investigation, indicating, according to the authors, continued exposure to well-established fragrance allergens causing sensitization to FM I (189). Relevance rates, where provided, were usually high with 65-80% (1,169,170,174,189). Culprit products were not mentioned.

In one investigation (115), the TRUE test was used for patch testing and 4.6% positive reactions were observed. It is well known that the sensitivity of the TRUE test in detecting fragrance allergy is lower than FM I in petrolatum (105, 115,167,170,188,209,212)

Table 3.70.1 Patch testing in groups of patients: Routine testing

Years and Country	Test conc. & vehicle	Number of patients tested	positive (%)	Selection of patients (S); Relevance (R); Comments (C)	Ref.
2015-2017 NACDG	8% pet.	5595	632 (11.3%)	R: definite + probable relevance: 24%	217
2015-2016 UK	8% pet.	2084	107 (5.1%)	R: not specified for individual fragrances; 25% of patients who reacted to any fragrance or fragrance marker had a positive fragrance history	62
2011-2015 Spain	8% pet.	19,588	924 (4.7%)	R: not stated; C: 71% of the patients were tested with the TRUE test, which has a low sensitivity in detecting fragrance allergy	216
2011-2015 USA	8% pet.	2575	173 (6.7%)	R: not stated	218
2010-2015 Denmark	8% pet.	6004	(9.3%)	R: present relevance 66%, past relevance 34%; current and/or past relevance: 80%; C: 15.4% doubtful positive reactions	174
2009-2015 Sweden	8% pet.	4430	288 (6.5%)	R: not stated; C: the use of preparations from different suppliers affected the patch test results	122
1986-2015 Denmark	8% pet.	24,168	(7.8%)	R: 78% in the period 2006-2015; C: range per year: 4.7-10.6%; increase in prevalence of FM sensitization in men in the last 10 years and in women throughout the period of investigation	189
2013-2014 NACDG	8% pet.	4858	576 (11.9%)	R: definite + probable relevance: 34%	57
2013-2014 Twelve European countries, 46 departments [a]	8% pet.	18,145	(7.8%)	R: not stated; C: results of 6 occupational dermatology clinics and one pediatric clinic not included in these figures; range of positive reactions: 0%-16%	58
2013-2014 Thailand		312	57 (18.3%)	R: 83%	102
2010-2014 IVDK	8% pet.	48,956	4652 (9.5%)	R: not stated	64
2009-2014 NACDG	8% pet.	13,398	1453 (10.8%)	R: not stated	64
2008-2014 UK	8% pet.	3541	195 (5.5%)	R: not stated; C: there were 2.2% ?+ and 2.3% irritant reactions	100
2009-2013 Singapore	8% pet.	2598	(6.7%)	R: present + past relevance: 37%; C: range of positive reactions per year 5.0-8.0%	96
2011-2012 UK	8% pet.	1951	124 (6.4%)	R: not stated	106
2011-2012 NACDG	8% pet.	4232	511 (12.1%)	R: definite + probable relevance: 32%	40
2009-2012 Twelve European countries [a]	8% pet.	56,813	(7.4%)	R: not stated; C: range per country: 4.8-14.7%; C: the TRUE ® test system is less sensitive for detecting sensitivity to FM I than the pet.-based chamber systems	105
1999-2012 IVDK	8% pet.	130,325	(8.7%)	R: not stated ; C: significant decrease from 1999-2005/2006 followed by a significant increase	34
2010-2011 China	8% pet.	296	(9.1%)	R: 89%	104
1990-2011 Belgium	8% pet.	13,332	1259 (9.4%)	R: not stated	185
2009-2010 NACDG	8% pet.	4303	(8.5%)	R: definite + probable relevance: 33%	41
2008-2010 Denmark	8% pet.	1503	110 (7.3%)	R: 76%; C: *mostly* routine testing	1
2006-2010 USA	8% pet.	3092	(10.4%)	R: 60%	54
2001-2010 Australia	8% pet.	5228	605 (11.6%)	R: 38%	56
2009 Sweden	8% pet.	3112	(5.2%)	R: not stated	53
2007-2009 Sweden	8% pet.	1187	81 (6.8%)	R: not stated	171
2004-2009 China	8% pet.	2758	(6.9%)	R: 41% relevance for all positive patch test reactions together	109
1998-2009 Denmark	8% pet.	5006	464 (9.3%)	R: 64%; C: patients were also tested with the FM I TRUE test, which showed 4.4% positive reactions; of patients with a stronger reaction to FM I TRUE Test almost all reacted to FM I in petrolatum, whereas the reverse situation showed a lower association	170
2007-2008 NACDG	8% pet.	5079	(9.4%)	R: definite + probable relevance: 35%	9
2007-2008 Eleven European countries [a]	8% pet.	25,181	(6.6%)	R: not stated; C: prevalences ranged from 3.7% (Lithuania) to 10.4% (Austria)	14
2005-2008 Denmark	8% pet.	12,302	737 (6.0%)	R: 71%	169
2005-2008 IVDK	8% pet.	36,961	(6.6%)	R: not stated	111
2004-2008 Spain	8% pet.	1253	56 (4.5%)	R: 93%	26
2004-2008 Iran	8% pet.	1105	41 (3.7%)	R: 82% of all reactions to FM I, FM II, Myroxylon pereirae resin, hydroxyisohexyl 3-cyclohexene carboxaldehyde and/or turpentine were clinically relevant	5
1995-2007 Denmark	TRUE test	6115	(4.6%)	R: not stated; C: testing with the TRUE test usually yields fewer positive reactions than the FM pet. test material	115
1985-2007 Denmark	8% pet.	16,173	(7.2%)	R: not stated; C: significant decline of positive reactions to	117

Table 3.70.1 Patch testing in groups of patients: Routine testing (continued)

Years and Country	Test conc. & vehicle	tested	positive (%)	Selection of patients (S); Relevance (R); Comments (C)	Ref.
2005-2006 Ten European countries [a]	8% pet.	18,542	1300 (7.0%)	FM I from 1997 to 2007 in women but not in men R: not stated; C: prevalences were 7.7% in Central Europe, 6.8% in West, 5.7% in Northeast and 4.8% in South Europe	55
2005-2006 NACDG	8% pet.	4439	(11.5%)	R: definite + probable relevance: 31%	11
2001-2006 China	8% pet.	1354	(22.2%)	R: not stated; C: all other tested haptens also had very high prevalence scores, suggesting that the patients were highly selected for (routine) patch testing	108
2001-2005 USA	8% pet.	3844	(11.3%)	R: 71%	10
1990-2005 Belgium	8% pet.	10,128	924 (9.1%)	R: not stated	82
1985-2005 Denmark	8% pet.	14,971	(7.7%)	R: not stated	44
2004, Eleven European countries [a]	8% pet.	9941	758 (7.6%)	R: not stated; C: range positives per center: 1.9-17.5%	39
2003-2004 NACDG	8% pet.	5140	468 (9.1%)	R: not stated	12
2001-2004 IVDK	8% pet.	30,933	(8.8%)	R: not stated	43
2000-4 Switzerland	8% pet.	4094	427 (10.4%)	R: not stated	112
1998-2004 Israel	8% pet.	2156	154 (7.1%)	R: not stated	42
1992-2004 Turkey	8% pet.	1038	22 (2.1%)	R: not stated	50
2003 NACDG	8% pet.	1603	94 (5.9%)	R: definite + probable relevance: 34%	151
<2003 Israel	8% pet.	641	60 (9.4%)	R: not stated	25
2002-2003, Six European countries	8% pet.	1701	111 (6.5%)	R: not stated	3
2002-2003 Europe [a]	8% pet.	9663	(7.1%)	R: not stated; C: 17 centers in 9 European countries; range per center: 3.7-10.4%	45
2001-2002 UK	8% pet.	766	91 (11.8%)	R: not stated	15
2001-2002 NACDG	8% pet.	4896	(10.4%)	R: definite + probable relevance: 19%	46
2000-2002 Finland	8% pet.	11,708	(6.9%)	R: not stated	47
1996-2002 IVDK	8% pet.	59,298		R: not stated; C: range per year: 8.9-13.5%; significant increase in the frequency between 1996 and 1998, and a significant decline from 1999 to 2002	13
1999-2001 Sweden	8% pet.	3790	(6.9%)	R: not stated	48
1997-2001 Czech Rep.	8% pet.	12,058	697 (5.8%)	R: not stated	51
2000 Sweden	8% pet.	3825	(6.9%)	R: not stated	53
1998-2000 Six European countries	8% pet.	1606	184 (11.4%)	R: not stated	23
1998-2000 USA	8% pet.	1323	(10.4%)	R: not stated	49
1996-2000 Europe	8% pet.	26,210	(9.7%)	R: not stated; C: ten centers, seven countries, EECDRG study; range per center 5.0-12.8%	52

[a] Study of the ESSCA (European Surveillance System on Contact Allergy network)
IVDK: Informationsverbund Dermatologischer Kliniken (Germany, Switzerland, Austria)
NACDG: North American Contact Dermatitis Group (USA, Canada)

Other European countries
Prevalence rates of sensitization in various European countries published after 2000 are shown in table 3.70.2. High rates (>9%) have been observed in Belgium and Switzerland. The other countries generally had scores ranging from 5.1 to 6.9%. The only country where the frequency of sensitization was lower than 5% is Spain (4.5%, [26]). Relevance data were hardly ever provided. In the Spanish study, 93% of 56 positive patch tests to the FM I were considered to be relevant. Culprit products were not mentioned.

Non-European countries
Prevalence rates of sensitization in various non-European countries published after 2000 are shown in table 3.70.2. High rates have been observed in Australia (11.6% [56]) and extremely high ones in China (22.2% [108]) and Thailand (18.3% [102]). In the two latter investigations, other haptens also scored very high frequencies, so possibly only patients strongly suspected of allergic contact dermatitis were selected for routine testing. Low scores were observed in Iran (3.7% [5]) and Turkey (2.1% [50]). In a few studies addressing relevance, 38 to 89% of the positive patch test reactions to FM I were considered to be relevant (56,102,104). Culprit products were not mentioned.

The relevance of reactions to FM I increases significantly with the strength of the reactions. In one study, the percentages of relevant ?+, +, ++, and +++ reactions were 25%, 41%, 71%, and 75%, respectively (150).

Table 3.70.2 Frequencies of sensitization in other European and in non-European countries

Country	Years of investigation, frequencies of sensitization and (references)
European countries	
Belgium	1990-2011: 9.4% (185); 1990-2005: 9.1% (82)
Czech Republic	1997-2001: 5.8% (51)
Finland	2000-2002: 6.9% (47)
Spain	2004-2008: 4.5% (26); 2011-2015: 4.7% (216) [a]
Sweden	2009-2015: 6.5% (122); 2009: 5.2% (53); 2007-2009: 6.8% (171); 1999-2001: 6.9% (48); 2000: 6.9% (53)
Switzerland	2000-2004: 10.4% (117)
United Kingdom	2015-2016: 5.1% (62); 2008-2014: 5.5% (100); 2011-2012: 6.4% (106); 2001-2002: 11.8% (15)
Non-European countries	
Australia	2001-2010: 11.6% (56)
China	2010-2011: 9.1% (104); 2004-2009: 6.9% (109); 2001-2006: 22.2% (108)
Iran	2004-2008: 3.7% (5)
Israel	1998-2004: 7.1% (42); before 2003: 9.4% (25)
Singapore	2009-2013: 6.7% (96)
Thailand	2013-2014: 18.3% (102) (in this study, most individual fragrances also had high scores)
Turkey	1992-2004: 2.1% (50)

[a] 71% of the patients were tested with the TRUE test, which has a low sensitivity in detecting fragrance allergy

Patch testing in groups of selected patients

Results of testing in groups of selected patients (e.g. nurses with occupational contact dermatitis, individuals with eyelid dermatitis, patients with allergic contact cheilitis, individuals with stasis dermatitis / leg ulcers, patients suspected of cosmetic intolerance or fragrance allergy, patients with hand dermatitis) are shown in table 3.70.3. The studies shown are selected, and the table does not provide a full literature review. Studies in groups of hairdressers are not included, as the prevalence of fragrance sensitization in most investigations is not or only slightly elevated (87,88,89,90,95); however, adequate control groups are largely lacking.

Patients with eyelid dermatitis / periorbital dermatitis

In 9 studies, in which patients with eyelid dermatitis / periorbital dermatitis were patch tested with the FM I, frequencies of sensitization have ranged from 6.2 to 19% (4,38,66,76,78,82,93,136,205). In a tenth investigation, the frequency was 28%, but this included 'other fragrances' (not specified [77]). In 4 investigations where relevance was addressed, rates of relevant reactions ranged from 19% to 100%; in only one study were culprit products mentioned: 'most frequently cosmetics' (93). In 4 of the 5 studies with a control group, the frequency of sensitization to FM I was significantly *lower* than in routine testing (76,78,82,205).

Patients with stasis dermatitis / leg ulcers

In 4 studies performed after 2004 testing patients with stasis dermatitis / leg ulcers, frequencies of sensitization ranged from 11.4% to 26.5% (85,113,118,210). Relevance was mentioned in one study only: 'definite' zero per cent, 'probable' 18% (210). In the study with the highest rate (26.5% [113]) from France it was mentioned that, at the time of the study, wound dressings with Myroxylon pereirae resin (balsam of Peru, MP) were still used there, so a large number of reactions to FM I may in fact have been (pseudo)-cross reactions to MP (113).

Previously, in a meta-analysis, 26 studies investigating sensitization in leg ulcer / stasis dermatitis patients published between 1975 and 2003 had been analyzed. In the period 1975-1990, the average percentage of positive reactions (unadjusted for sample size) in 15 studies to FM I was 10.7% (range 5.6-14.0%) and in the period 1991-2003 in 11 investigations was 18.8% (range 2.9-28.0%), indicating a strong increase in sensitization in time. It should be realized, however, that the percentage of positive reactions was in some studies not significantly higher than in control groups of routinely tested patients. In addition, the high percentages found in three French studies may partly have been the result of primary sensitization to Myroxylon pereirae resin (154).

Patients suspected of fragrance or cosmetic allergy

In 8 studies in groups of patients suspected of cosmetic or fragrance allergy (2,6,8,21,30,86,123,131) frequencies of sensitization have ranged from 5.8% to 18%. Relevance was mentioned in one study only (97%), but this investigation had certain weaknesses (8). There was a control group in only one study; the frequency of sensitization in the group suspected of cosmetic / fragrance allergy (9%) was significantly higher than in a control group of routine testing (86).

Patients with cosmetic allergy including allergic contact cheilitis

In 7 studies in groups of patients with cosmetic allergy (allergic contact cheilitis, patients known to be allergic to cosmetics, patients with previous positive patch tests to deodorant, perfume, eau de toilette, aftershave, bath or shower products, skin creams or 'cosmetics') frequencies of sensitization to FM I ranged from 20 to 57% (28,74,79, 119,132,152,204). These high frequencies are hardly surprizing considering the selection criteria. Relevance in four studies addressing this issue were 90-100% (79,132,152,204), but causative products were not mentioned.

Miscellaneous indications for patch testing

No obviously elevated rates of sensitization to FM I have been found in patients with difficult-to-treat atopic dermatitis (9% [202]), with psoriasis (4.5%, lower than in routine testing [201]), with burning mouth syndrome (9.8% [37]), with pure allergic contact dermatitis of the hands (11.3% [207]), with possible scalp dermatitis (9.5%, lower than in routine testing [92]), and individuals with hand dermatitis (9.5%, lower than in routine testing [211]).

In an IVDK study, geriatric nurses with occupational contact dermatitis had a higher rate of sensitization to FM I than geriatric nurses without occupational dermatitis (but the diagnosis of occupational contact dermatitis may have been *on the basis* of a positive FM I reaction) (61), but generally speaking, nurses and other health care workers do not have a significantly elevated rate of sensitization to the fragrance mix (75,97,98).

(Possibly) elevated sensitization rates have been observed in patients suspected of airborne contact dermatitis (12.2%, significantly higher than in a control group [103]), individuals with poikiloderma of Civatte (12.5%, but this was to all fragrances tested together [155]), patients with allergic contact dermatitis of the face (18%, reactions to FM I were probably a diagnostic criterium [80]), women with vulval problems (13.2% [83], 18% [135], no control groups), patients suspected of facial allergic contact dermatitis (15% [91]), coal miners with eczematous dermatitis, most of who used a highly perfumed body lotion provided at the pit-head baths (26% [141]) and physical therapists (12.2%, significantly higher than in routine testing [215]).

Table 3.70.3 Patch testing in groups of patients: Selected patient groups

Years and Country	Test conc. & vehicle	Number of patients		Selection of patients (S); Relevance (R); Comments (C)	Ref.
		tested	positive (%)		
2014-2016 France		264	20 (7.6%)	S: patients suspected of eyelid allergic contact dermatitis; R: 8/20 (40%)	66
2012-5 Netherlands	8%pet.	44	4 (9%)	S: patients with difficult-to-treat atopic dermatitis; R: 100%	202
1996-2015 IVDK	8% pet.	2230	96 (4.5%)	S: patients with psoriasis; R: not stated; C: the percentage of positive reactions was significantly lower than in the control group of consecutive dermatitis patients (8.4%)	201
2005-2014 IVDK	8% pet.	644	80 (11.6%)	S: geriatric nurses with occupational contact dermatitis; R: not stated; C: the frequency was significantly higher than in a control group of geriatric nurses without occupational contact dermatitis (5.9%)	61
2003-2014 IVDK	8% pet.	5202	(11.4%)	S: patients with stasis dermatitis / chronic leg ulcers; R: not stated; C: percentage of reactions significantly higher than in a control group of routine testing	85
1996-2013 Netherlands	8% pet.	1008	100 (9.9%)	S: children aged 0-17 years; R: not stated; significantly more reactions in children with atopic dermatitis (12.1%) than in those without atopic dermatitis (8.1%)	84
1994-2013 IVDK	8% pet.	1203	(12.2%)	S: patients suspected of airborne contact dermatitis; R: not specified, but the reactions were ascribed to perfumes and spray deodorants; C: the frequency in a control group was 9.7%; the difference was statistically significant	103
2008-2012 Canada	8% pet.	132	13 (9.8%)	S: patients with burning mouth syndrome; R: 74% relevance for all allergens together	37
2007-2011 IVDK	8% pet.	115	14 (12.2%)	S: physical therapists; R: not stated; C: the frequency of sensitization was 'distinctly' higher than in routine testing (5.0%)	215
2006-2011 IVDK	8% pet.	10,124	859 (9.0%)	S: patients with suspected cosmetic intolerance; R: not stated; C: the prevalence was significantly higher than in a control group matched for sex and age	86
2001-2011 USA	8% pet.	41	11 (27%)	S: patients with allergic contact cheilitis; R: 100%	204
2006-2010 USA	8% pet.	100	17 (17%)	S: patients with eyelid dermatitis; R: not stated	4
2000-2010 IVDK		4394	306 (6.2%)	S: patients with periorbital dermatitis; R: not stated; C: the frequency was lower than in a control group of routine testing	76
2005-2008 France	8% pet.	423	112 (26.5%)	S: patients with leg ulcers; R: not stated, but is was mentioned that, at that time, wound dressings with Myroxylon pereirae resin were still used in France for leg ulcers; hence, the high frequency of sensitization to the FM I may be the result of	113

Table 3.70.3 Patch testing in groups of patients: Selected patient groups (continued)

Years and Country	Test conc. & vehicle	Number of patients tested	positive (%)	Selection of patients (S); Relevance (R); Comments (C)	Ref.
2005-7 Netherlands	8% pet.	227	17 (5.8%)	(pseudo)cross-reactivity to balsam of Peru S: patients suspected of fragrance or cosmetic allergy; R: 61% relevance for all positive tested fragrances together	2
2000-2007 USA	8% pet.	940	106 (11.3%)	S: patients who were tested with a supplemental cosmetic screening series; R: 97%; C: weak study: a. high rate of macular erythema and weak reactions; b. relevance figures included 'questionable' and 'past' relevance	8
1990-2006 USA	8% pet.	266	35 (13.2%)	S: patients with periorbital dermatitis; R: 19/35 (54%); C: the frequency was lower than in controls (16.3%)	205
<2005 India	8% pet.	50	9 (18%)	S: patients suspected of cosmetic dermatitis; R: not stated	30
<2005 Poland	8% pet.	50	10 (20%)	S: patients with chronic venous leg ulcers; R: not stated	118
<2004 USA, Canada	8% pet.	54	11 (20%)	S: patients with past or present leg ulcers with or without dermatitis; R: definite zero, probable 18%	210
2001-2004 NACDG	8% pet.	60	18 (30%)	S: patients with allergic contact cheilitis and relevant contact allergies to allergens in the NACDG series; R: these reactions were probably all relevant, but the causative products were not mentioned	79
1999-2004 Germany	8% pet.	88	10 (11.4%)	S: patients with periorbital eczema; R: in 48 patients with allergic contact dermatitis, 9 reactions to FM I (19%) were considered to be relevant; cosmetics were the most frequent causative products	93
1994-2004 USA	8% pet.	46	13 (28%)	S: patients with allergic contact dermatitis of the eyelids; R: these were relevant reactions, but the causative products were not mentioned; C: this number included 'other fragrances'	77
1994-2004 NACDG	8% pet.	959	(11.3%)	S: patients with pure allergic contact dermatitis of the hands; R: the patients were selected on the basis of relevant reactions	207
2002-2003 Korea	8% pet.	422	41 (9.7%)	S: patients with suspected cosmetic dermatitis; R: not stated	21
1993-2003 IVDK	8% pet.	1234	117 (9.5%)	S: patients patch tested to confirm of rule out (secondary) allergic contact dermatitis of the scalp; R: not stated; C: the frequency was lower than in the total IVDK test population	92
2001-2002 NACDG	8% pet.	2193	440 (20.1%)	S: patients with (presumed) cosmetic allergy; R: not stated	74
1998-2002 IVDK	8% pet.	61	25 (38%)	S: patients who had a positive reaction to their own deodorant; R: not stated; C: there was a significant difference in percentage positive reactions compared with a control group of dermatitis patients who had *not* reacted to their own deodorant	28
		56	32 (57%)	S: patients who had a positive reaction to their own perfume, eau de toilette or shaving product; R: not stated; C: there was a significant difference in percentage positive reactions compared with a control group of dermatitis patients who had *not* reacted to their own cosmetic products of this type	
1998-2002 IVDK	8% pet.	70	21 (30%)	S: patients with a positive patch test to one or more bath and shower products; R: not stated; C: the frequency was signify-cantly higher than in a control group of patients not reacting to bath and shower products (13%)	119
1998-2002 IVDK	8% pet.	304	101 (31.4%)	S: patients with a positive patch test to one or more skin care cream products; R: not stated; C: the frequency was signifi-cantly higher than in a control group of patients not reacting to skin care cream products (11.9%)	119
1999-2001 China	8% pet.	105	10 (9.5%)	S: patients with hand dermatitis; R: not stated; C: the frequency was lower than in a control group of routinely tested patients (12.7%)	211
1982-2001 UK	8% pet.	22	9 (41%)	S: patients with allergic contact cheilitis; R: all reactions were considered to be relevant	152
1997-2000 Austria	8% pet.	747	126 (16.9%)	S: patients suspected of fragrance allergy; R: not stated	6
1997-2000 Israel	8% pet.	244	30 (12.3%)	S: patients suspected of cosmetic allergic contact dermatitis; R: 64% for all allergens together	123
1995-1999 IVDK	8% pet.	972	(9.4%)	S: patients with allergic periorbital contact dermatitis; R: not stated; C: the rate was significantly lower than in a control group of routine testing	82
1995-1998 Greece	8% pet.	32	4 (12.5%)	S: patients with Poikiloderma of Civatte; R: it was suggested that fragrances play an etiological role; C: the frequency of	155

Table 3.70.3 Patch testing in groups of patients: Selected patient groups (continued)

Years and Country	Test conc. & vehicle	Number of patients tested | positive (%)		Selection of patients (S); Relevance (R); Comments (C)	Ref.
1994-1998 UK	8% pet.	232	14 (6.0%)	sensitization to *all* fragrances was significantly higher than in a control group of patients suspected of contact dermatitis. S: patients with eyelid dermatitis; R: all were currently relevant, but causative products were not mentioned; C: the frequency was lower than in a controls group of routine testing	78
1994-8 Netherlands	8% pet.	757	112 (14.8%)	S: patients suspected of cosmetic allergy; R: not stated	131
1995-1997 USA	8% pet.	57	10 (18%)	S: patients with facial allergic contact dermatitis; R: only relevant reactions were mentioned, causative products were not mentioned	80
1994-1996 Denmark	8% pet.	40	11 (28%)	S: patients with a positive reaction to one or more of their personal cosmetics; R: 8 relevant, 2 partly relevant, one not relevant; C: the frequency was significantly higher than in a control group of individuals with ?+ reactions to their cosmetics (8.5%) and a control group of dermatitis patients (6.7%)	132
1991-1995 UK		121	16 (13.2%)	S: women with pruritus vulvae and primary vulval dermatoses suspected of secondary allergic contact dermatitis; R: 49% for all positive reactions together	83
1992-1994 UK		69	12 (18%)	S: women with 'vulval problems'; R: 58% for all allergens together	135
1990-1994 IVDK		588	84 (14.1%)	S: patients with periorbital eczema; R: not stated	38
<1991 China	8% pet.	107	16 (15%)	S: patients suspected of facial contact dermatitis; R: an unspecified number were caused by fragrances in cosmetic creams, mainly cinnamyl alcohol and hydroxycitronellal	91
1990-1991 Italy	8% pet.	150	12 (8.0%)	S: patients with eyelid dermatitis; R: not stated; C: the rate of positive reactions in a control dermatitis group without eyelid involvement was 4.6%	136
1986-1987 UK	8% pet.	35	9 (26%)	S: coal miners with eczematous skin problems; R: not specified; however, there was a relationship with the use of a highly perfumed body lotion provided at the pit-head baths; only 7 miners admitted to using it, but of these, 5 were fragrance sensitive; C: the rate of sensitization was significantly (almost two times) higher than in control groups of non-miner consecutive patients with dermatitis	141

IVDK: Informationsverbund Dermatologischer Kliniken (Germany, Switzerland, Austria)
NACDG: North American Contact Dermatitis Group (USA, Canada)

Testing with the constituents of fragrance mix I in patients reacting to the mix

Fragrance mix I positive, testing with ingredients ('breakdown') negative

In many studies, the 8 ingredients of the FM I have been patch tested separately in patients showing a positive reaction to the fragrance mix, either at the same time or later. The results of these investigations are shown in table 3.70.4. The second column from the right shows the percentages of FM I-positive individuals who displayed positive patch tests to one or more of the 8 ingredients. These data clearly show that a large portion of FM I-positive individuals have a 'negative breakdown', i.e. that they do *not* react to any ingredient. The range of negative breakdowns is 10% to 57%, median 40%, and average (unadjusted for sample size) 34% (table 3.70.4). Thus, about 1/3 of patients with a positive patch test to FM I have a negative breakdown.

Possible explanations for this apparent discrepancy include:

1   false-positive (irritant) reactions to the mix

2   false-negative reactions to the individual constituents. In most studies, these have been tested at 1% in petrolatum, which is the same as in the mix. That the FM *does* react despite having the same concentration as the constituents that are negative separately may be related to:

a.   enhancement of elicitation of contact allergic reactions by allergen mixtures (22,157,158,172) or irritants

b.   increased skin penetration caused by the (combined) irritancy of other constituents of the mix including sorbitan sesquioleate, or

c.   the formation of new allergens in the mix (compound allergy); no evidence for this latter scenario is as yet available.

The extreme variability of the percentages of FM I-allergic individuals with a negative breakdown (7% (140) to 67% (174)) (table 3.70.4) is not easy to explain completely, but several parameters may influence the results:

1. test concentrations. Most investigators have used 8x1%, three studies tested at 2% and two others used higher concentrations for the ingredients ranging from 3 to 5%. This item is discussed below in the section 'Influence of test concentrations on the results'.

2. the presence or absence of sorbitan sesquioleate (SSO) as emulsifier in the ingredients. In older studies (SSO was introduced in the mid-1990s), testing with constituents without the addition of SSO yielded less positive reactions (133,140).

Table 3.70.4 Results of testing with the 8 ingredients of the fragrance mix I in patients reacting to the mix [n]

Years and Country	Nr. pat. pos. to FM I	Percentage of positive reactions to ingredients								Pos.%	Ref.
		Oakmos	Isoeug	Hydrox	CinAld	CinAlc	Eugen	Geran	AmylCin		
Patch test data of all patients reacting to FM I and tested with its ingredients											
1998-2013 IVDK [a, g]	2952	29.3	20.4	12.6	12.2	10.0	9.0	7.0	3.3	58%	101
1998-2013 IVDK [a]	2798	27.2	18.7	10.9	10.6	8.4	7.3	5.5	1.5	57%	35
2006-2011 IVDK [a]	405	31.9	19.3	14.6	12.6	11.1	9.6	7.4	4.4	ns	86
1990-2011 Belgium	940	24.6	17.0	2.6	7.0	13.7	12.6	5.5	3.2	ns	185
2005-2009 Croatia	157	24.2	?	?	?	34.4	55.4	?	?	?	63
1998-2009 Denmark	348	23.6	14.9	16.1	16.4	12.6	8.3	4.9	2.9	54%	170
2005-2008 IVDK [a]	655	29.8	18.0	12.8	11.6	9.6	6.7	4.7	2.8	61%	111
2006-2007 Belgium, The Netherlands [c, g]	121	9.9	15.7	11.8	17.4	1.7	12.4	16.5	6.6	90%	150
1996-2002 IVDK [a]	1549-1701	29.9	18.9	13.0	10.4	7.9	8.3	5.9	3.2	ns	13
1998-1999 Hungary [f]	160	13.1	14.8	2.5	8.1	20.6	8.8	7.5	5.0	71%	124
1989-1999 Portugal	226	22.1	19.9	6.6	13.3	7.9	14.6	8.4	4.4	59%	127
1984-1998 UK	1112	34.0	20.8	8.0	14.8	12.5	14.3	6.0	2.8	84%	126
1985-1996 Greece	38	36.8	23.7	18.4	31.6	42.1	18.4	13.2	7.9	84%	156
1994-1995 UK [f]	40	30	20	2.5	12.5	10	5	0	0	ns	130
1994-8 Netherlands [d]	50	44	32	20	20	16	12	6	0	45%	131
1991 The Netherlands	61	34.4	24.6	19.7	34.4	31.1	19.7	13.1	4.9	ns	193
1987 Germany [e]	162	8.6	16.7	6.2	21.0	5.6	6.8	2.5	1.2	43%	139
<1986 Poland [f]	42	16.7	45.2	14.3	38.1	23.8	59.5	23.8	14.3	ns	145
1984-1985 Italy [b]	54	35.2	22.2	16.7	5.6	9.3	16.7	7.4	1.9	83%	144
Range		8.6-44	14.8-45.2	2.5-20	7.0-38.1	1.7-42.1	5-59.5	0-23.8	0-14.3	43-90	
Median		29.3	19.6	12.9	12.9	11.1	12.2	6.8	3.2	60	
Average (unadjusted for sample size)		26.6	21.2	11.6	16.5	15.2	16.1	8.0	3.7	66	
Different data presented											
2010-2015 Denmark [i]	529	40.4	31.7	25.4	42.7	19.7	9.8	7.5	4.6	33%	174
2009-2015 Sweden [j]	288									55%	122
2008-2011 five European countries [j]	82									63%	167
2005-10 Netherlands [f]	75									65%	180
<1995 EECDRG	53									42-55% [k]	133
1979-1992 Denmark [h, i]	367	38.4	30.4	12.1	27.7	17.9	13.4	6.7	4.5	61%	134
<1991 Germany	39-53									51-93% [m]	140

AmylCin: Amyl cinnamal; CinAlc: Cinnamyl alcohol; CinAld: Cinnamal (cinnamaldehyde); Eugen: Eugenol; Geran: Geraniol; Hydrox: Hydroxycitronellal; Isoeug: Isoeugenol; Oakmos: Oakmoss absolute (Evernia prunastri extract)

EECDRG: European Environmental and Contact Dermatitis Research Group

IVDK: Informationsverbund Dermatologischer Kliniken (Germany, Switzerland, Austria)

ns: not stated

Pos.%: percentage of patients reacting to the FM I who have a positive patch test to one or more of its ingredients

[a] there is an important overlap in the various IVDK studies, i.e. that partly data from the same patient groups are reported; [b] oakmoss absolute, cinnamyl alcohol, geraniol and amyl cinnamal 3%, eugenol, isoeugenol and hydroxycitronellal 5%, cinnamal 2%; [c] 2% pet. for cinnamal, 5% pet. for all other ingredients; [d] all constituents tested at 2% pet.; [e] for (some) constituents, the low rate of positive reactions may be explained by the fact that they did not contain sorbitan sesquioleate (139); [f] test concentrations unknown; [g] there were many positive reactions to sorbitan sesquioleate; [h] in the period 1979-1983, the constituents were tested at 2% pet., thereafter at 1% pet; from that moment on, the frequency of cinnamal-positives dropped; [i] percentages of ingredients do not relate to the number of FM I-allergic patients tested with the ingredients, but of patients who reacted to at least one ingredient; [j] all constituents 2% pet. except for cinnamal (1% pet.); [k] 42% positive reactions to the 8 constituents without sorbitan sesquioleate (SSO), 55% to constituents containing 1% SSO; [m] 51% positive to ingredients without sorbitan sesquioleate (SSO), 93% to ingredients with 1% SSO; [n] 1% pet. for each ingredient unless indicated otherwise

3. varying frequencies of allergic reactions to SSO (101). In some studies, a low frequency of SSO sensitization (around 1%) was found, but others have documented 5-10% positive patch tests to SSO in patients reacting to FM I (101,133,150), which is both present in the mix (at 5%) and in the individual constituents test materials (1% each). In a number of studies, SSO has not been tested separately. Allergy to SSO, if undetected, results in higher frequencies of positive reactions to the ingredients and also to a larger number of positive reactions per individual. If these are not excluded, incorrect data are presented. Indeed, in 2015, the IVDK convincingly showed that reactivity to SSO markedly affects the outcome of patch testing with FM I and its single constituents. Therefore, SSO must be an obligatory part of the full FM I breakdown test, and should ideally be included in the baseline series, in order to prevent that patients reacting to FM I, who are allergic to SSO (but not to fragrances) are advised to avoid all fragrances and fragranced products (101). In fact, the members of the European Environmental and Contact Dermatitis Research Group (EECDRG) already in 1995 advised to add SSO to the European standard series (133), which has, however, thus far not been implemented.

4. study period. Some studies were performed >25 years earlier than recent ones, in which time period the relative use of fragrances may have changed by fashion or as a result of increased knowledge, e.g. the lowering of the concentration of the allergens (chloro)atranol in Evernia prunastri (oakmoss) extract.

5. there probably is a large variability between clinics and individual investigators in the interpretation of patch test reactions to the mix. The FM I induces quite a few dubious (?+) and many weak-positive (+) reactions. Many reactions may be in between the ?+ (which should formally be counted as negative) and + reactions (which are usually considered to be allergic), e.g. faint erythema with minimal infiltration. Some authors even consider a large portion of weak-positive (+) reactions to FM I to be false-positive (i.e., irritant) (60,185). If these weak reactions are interpreted as 'FM-positive', the subsequent testing with the ingredients should result in far lower frequencies of positive reactions, as it has been well documented that strong reactions (++ or +++) are far more often followed by positive ingredient patch tests that the weaker (?+ or +) ones. This is discussed in more detail in the section 'Relationship between strength of the reaction to FM I and the percentage of individuals reacting to ingredients' below.

Influence of test concentrations on the results

The studies in table 3.70.4 can be used to determine the effects of the concentration of the individual ingredients on the percentage of positive reactions to at least one ingredient. Investigations in which the concentrations used were unknown are excluded as are the studies not mentioning the percentages of negative breakdowns.

In 12 studies, in which 1% was used for all 8 constituents (35,101,111,126,127,133,134,139,140,156,170,174), the percentages of individuals with at least one positive reaction ranged from 33 to 93%, average 62% and median 58.5%. In three studies in which 2% concentrations were used (1% for cinnamal) for ingredient patch testing, scores of positive reactions were 45% (131), 55% (122) and 63% (167) of the FM I-positive individuals, which is not higher than in the studies where 1% pet. was used for testing. However, most recent data from Spain (ref. 216, November 2018) have shed new light on this issue. In a multicenter study, some clinics did a breakdown with each ingredient at 1% and others with each ingredient at 2% except cinnamal, which was tested at 1% (216). Of 258 patients reacting to FM I and tested with its ingredients at 2% (except cinnamal), only 67 (26%) had a negative breakdown. Of 178 FM I-allergic patients tested with its ingredients 1% each, on the other hand, 117 (66%) had a negative breakdown. This provides clear evidence that testing with the higher concentrations is preferable. One may argue that the fact that the materials came from two different commercial suppliers may have influenced the results independent of concentration. However, in the case of the fragrance mix II, where both providers used the same concentrations for its 6 ingredients, the percentages negative breakdowns were virtually identical (216).

There are two investigations in which the ingredients of the mix were tested at still higher concentrations (144,150). In an older Italian study, in which oakmoss absolute, cinnamyl alcohol, geraniol and amyl cinnamal were tested at 3%, eugenol, isoeugenol and hydroxycitronellal at 5% and cinnamal at 2%, the breakdown tests were positive in 83% of 54 FM-positive individuals (144). In the other investigation, performed in 2006-2007 in Belgium and The Netherlands, and in which 2% pet. was used for cinnamal and 5% pet. for all other ingredients, there was at least one positive reaction to an ingredient in 90% of 121 FM I-positive individuals (150). Possibly, though, some reactions to cinnamal 2% pet. may have been false-positive.

On the basis of theoretical considerations and these data, it can be concluded that it is preferable to test the individual ingredients, cinnamal excepted, with a concentration of 2% (216), and possibly even higher concentrations. Previously, 5% has been suggested (72,186) and some investigators have used 5% concentrations (or higher) for the ingredients without reporting obvious irritancy or patch test sensitization (191-198) and sometimes having performed 60-100 controls (193,197). Geraniol should additionally be tested as oxidized material, for which 11% in petrolatum has been suggested (190, Chapter 3.73 Geraniol).

Relationship between strength of the reaction to FM I and the percentage of individuals reacting to ingredients
There is a strong relationship between the strength of the reaction to FM I and the percentage of patients reacting to at least one of its single constituents, and vice versa (167). Individuals with stronger FM reactions also more often have positive reactions to 2 or more ingredients (101,111). The results of relevant studies are shown in table 3.70.5. In 7 investigations, the percentages of patients with a positive breakdown increase for +, ++ and +++ FM I-reactivity as follows. Patients with + reactions to FM I: range 15-76%, median 46%, average 46%; patients with ++ reactions to FM I: range 46-100%, median 74%, average 73%; and patients with +++ reactions to FM I: range 83-100%, median 90%, average 87%. It should be realized that the three IVDK studies have major overlaps and therefore provide virtually identical data, which unduly influence the overall results.

Table 3.70.5 Relationship between strength of the reaction to FM I and percentage of patients reacting to at least one ingredient

Years and Country	Nr. pat.	Percentage of patients reacting with different strengths of FM I reactions (?+, +, ++, +++)					Ref.
		All reactions	?+	+	++	+++	
2010-2015 Denmark	529	33%		15%	46%	83%	174
2009-2015 Sweden	288	55%		42%	67% [d]	67% [d]	122
1998-2013 IVDK [a]	2952	58%		46%	74%	91%	101
1998-2013 IVDK [a]	2798	57%		44%	74%	91%	35
2005-2008 IVDK [c]	655	61%		48%	78%	90%	111
2006-2007 Belgium, NL	121	90%	28%	76%	100%	100%	150
??	82	63%		53%	72%	88%	[b]
Range				**15-76%**	**46-100%**	**83-100%**	
Median				**46%**	**74%**	**90%**	
Average (unadjusted for sample size)				**46%**	**73%**	**87%**	

[a] virtually the same population and results; [b] reference lost during writing; [c] subgroup of the other IVDK populations; [d] ++ and +++ combined; IVDK: Informationsverbund Dermatologischer Kliniken (Germany, Switzerland, Austria); NL: The Netherlands
Nr. pat.: number of patients positive to FM I and tested with its ingredients

Negative reactions to the fragrance mix I in patients reacting to one or more of its ingredients
It has been shown that a portion of fragrance-allergic patients react positively to the individual ingredients of the fragrance mix I but not to the mix itself, suggesting a false-negative reaction to the mix (assuming that the reactions

Table 3.70.6 Negative reactions to fragrance mix I in patients reacting to one or more constituents

Years and country	Nr. pat. pos. to ingredients	Nr. pat. pos. to FM I (%)	Test conc. of ingredients	Comments	Ref.
2010-2015 Denmark	188	173 (92.0%)	all 1% pet.	FM was doubtful positive in in 9 (4.8%) and negative in only 6 (3.2%) individuals	174
2009-2015 Sweden	214	157 (73.4%)	seven 2% pet., cinnamal 1%		122
2008-2011 Five European countries	86	52 (60.5%)	seven 2% pet., cinnamal 1%	Study in general population	167
	69	27 (39.1%)	TRUE test	It is well known that the sensitivity of the TRUE test for detecting fragrance allergy is lower than FM I in petrolatum (105,115,167,170,188)	
1984-1998 UK	934	826 (88.4%)	all 1% pet.		187
1991 Netherlands	67	61 (91.0%)	seven 5% pet., cinnamal 2%	the ingredient test materials did not contain SSO, which may have resulted in false-negative reactions to the ingredients despite their high concentrations	193

to the ingredients are not false-positive) (122,167,174,187,193) (table 3.70.6). In some studies, this may be explained by the use of concentrations higher those in the mix (1% for each ingredient) (122,167,193), but in the studies where 1% was used (174,187), negative reactions to the mix are difficult to explain.

In the 4 most recent studies, the percentages of reactions to the mix were far higher (92.0% [174], 88.4% [187]) when 1% was used for the ingredients than when the ingredients were tested at 2% (73.4% [122] and 60.5% [167]). This may indicate that testing with 2% detects more cases of sensitization (weak sensitivities, not reacting to the 1% in the FM I) and to the ingredients than 1% and, therefore, a concentration higher than 1% may be preferable. The Dutch 1991 study would not seem to support this suggestion, as 91% of all ingredient reactions tested at 2% (cinnamal) or 5% (the other 7) were picked up by the FM 8x1%. However, these test materials did not contain SSO, the absence of which may well have resulted in false-negative reactions despite the higher concentrations of the fragrance ingredients (133,140).

Frequency of reactions to the 8 ingredients in patients allergic to the fragrance mix I

The results of studies testing the 8 ingredients of the FM I in patients reacting to the FM I (breakdown testing) are shown in table 3.70.4. In the first part (Patch test data of all patients reacting to FM I and tested with their ingredients), the percentages shown for the 8 ingredients relate to the total number of patients tested, i.e., including those with a negative breakdown. In the second part (Different data presented), the percentages from the two Danish studies relate to the number of patients with at least one positive reaction in the breakdown test and are not comparable therefore with the other investigations.

In the assessment of these data, it should be noted that 5 of the 19 studies were performed by the IVDK, and that these were often overlapping in study period and population investigated. Hence, their results are very similar and strongly influence the overall results. In addition, comparison of the study results is difficult because of the variability in test substances used, concentrations (ranging from 1% to 5%), large time frame (possible shift in use of certain fragrances), absence of sorbitan sesquioleate (SSO) in the test substances in some older studies and great variability in sample sizes, ranging from 38 to 2952 FM I-positive individuals.

A summary of these data, i.e., range of positive reactions, median percentage, average percentage and average of rank numbers is provided in table 3.70.7. below. From these data it is clear that oakmoss absolute is the most frequent sensitizer in the FM I, followed by isoeugenol (rank numbers 1 and 2). The least frequent sensitizers (rank numbers 7 and 8) are clearly geraniol and amyl cinnamal. In between are cinnamal, cinnamyl alcohol, hydroxycitronellal and eugenol with medians in a small range of 11.1% to 12.9% and averages of 11.6% to 16.5%. Cinnamal may be slightly more often positive than the other 3. A serious limitation of course is that the data presented in table 3.70.7 are not adjusted for sample size, test concentrations, overlapping data (IVDK) and presence or absence of sorbitan sesquioleate. In addition, cinnamal was sometimes tested at 2% in petrolatum, which causes irritant reactions and the role of geraniol may be underestimated as testing with oxidized geraniol will detect many more cases of sensitization (Chapter 3.73 Geraniol).

Table 3.70.7 Ranking sensitizers in the fragrance mix I [a]

Ingredient	Range pos. reactions	Median	Average	Average of rank numbers [b]
Oakmoss absolute	8.6 - 44%	29.3%	26.6%	1.8
Isoeugenol	14.8 - 45.2%	19.6%	21.2%	2.4
Cinnamal	7.0 - 38.1%	12.9%	16.5%	3.6
Cinnamyl alcohol	1.7 - 42.1%	11.1%	15.2%	4.6
Hydroxycitronellal	2.5 - 20%	12.9%	11.6%	4.6
Eugenol	5.0 - 59.5%	12.2%	16.1%	4.8
Geraniol	0 - 23.8%	6.8%	8.0%	6.3
Amyl cinnamal	0 - 14.3%	3.2%	3.7%	7.8

[a] Unadjusted for sample size, test concentrations, overlapping data (IVDK) and presence or absence of sorbitan sesquioleate
[b] Highest frequency is rank number 1, lowest is rank number 8, all rank numbers added up and divided by number of publications; the lower the average number, the higher the frequency of positive reactions

Data are insufficient to relate parameters such as test substance, test concentration, presence or absence of SSO, time period of study etc. to the differences in study results. However, it is remarkable that the 2006-2007 study from Belgium and The Netherlands (150) shows atypical results from both the general picture and from other studies from these same countries (131,185,193). This may be related to the concentrations used, which was 2% for cinnamal and 5% for the 7 other constituents. The highest percentage of positive reactions was seen to cinnamal. This may be caused by the use of 2% pet. test material for cinnamal, which is known to cause irritant reactions (and therefore, sometimes incorrectly scored as positive). Oakmoss and cinnamyl alcohol, however, had a very low score relative to others, notably to geraniol and amyl cinnamal, which are usually the least frequent reactors. This may indicate that the extra yield of positive reactions, by increasing the test concentration from 1% to 5%, is high for geraniol and amyl cinnamal, but low for oakmoss absolute and for cinnamyl alcohol, thereby altering the relative frequencies of sensitization.

Case reports and case series

In several reports, fragrance mix I was stated to be the responsible allergen in patients with allergic contact dermatitis, notably from cosmetics (18,19,36,67,142). As the FM I *per se* is not used in cosmetics, this statement is not quite correct. What is probably meant in these studies is that one or more of FM's ingredients were the allergens or were *supposed to be* the allergens, without verification by patch testing and ascertaining their presence in causative products. It is plausible, though, that in a number of these patients, individual ingredients have been patch tested and were positive, but that FM was also counted as allergen.

A small number of case reports, in which the patient reacted to the FM I, and where one or more of its ingredients may have been responsible for allergic contact dermatitis, but not proven by ingredient patch testing and identification of a specific sensitizer in culprit products, are also shown here.

Case series

FM I was stated to be the (or an) allergen in 158 patients in a group of 603 individuals suffering from cosmetic dermatitis, seen in the period 2010-2015 in Leuven, Belgium (36).

In the period 1996-2013, in a tertiary referral center in Valencia, Spain, 5419 patients were patch tested. Of these, 628 individuals had allergic contact dermatitis to cosmetics. In this group, FM I was stated to be the responsible allergen in 122 cases (18, overlap with ref. 19).

In the period 2000-2009, in Leuven, Belgium, an unspecified number of patients had positive patch tests or use tests to a total of 344 cosmetic products *and* positive patch tests to FM I, FM II, and/or to one or more of 28 selected specific fragrance ingredients. In 23 of 140 patients reacting to FM I, the presence of one or more of its components in the cosmetic products was confirmed by reading the product labels (110).

In the period 2000-2007, 202 patients with allergic contact dermatitis caused by cosmetics were seen in Valencia, Spain. In this group, the fragrance mix I was the allergen in 22 individuals from its presence in perfume (n=9), gel/soap (n=5), moisturizing cream (n=5), shampoo (n=2), deodorant (n=1) and hair gel (n=1) (19, overlap with ref. 18).

In one center in Belgium, between 1985 and 1990, 3970 patients with dermatitis were patch tested. 462 of these reacted positively to patch tests with cosmetic allergens. The reactions were considered to be relevant in 68%, probably relevant in 25% and doubtfully relevant in 7% of the patients. In the list of 'most common allergens' FM I had rank number 1 with 141 reactions. It should be appreciated that the presence of the allergen in cosmetic products causing dermatitis could not always be verified (at that time, ingredient labeling in the EU was not yet mandatory) (67).

In Belgium, in the years before 1986, of 5202 consecutive patients with dermatitis patch tested, 156 were diagnosed with pure cosmetic allergy. FM I was the 'dermatitic ingredient' in 49 (31.4%) patients (frequency in the entire group: 4.2%) (142).

Case reports

A man was referred with pruritic impetiginized dermatitis in the beard region of the face. The eruption arose after 3 weeks of using a new electric shaver that released a scented lotion onto the skin during the shaving process. Positive patch test reactions were observed to Myroxylon pereirae resin and fragrance mix I with sorbitan sesquioleate, 'which were found in the product' (the latter statement is of course incorrect). It was concluded that the eruption was caused by fragrances in the scented lotion, but no attempts were made to identify the allergenic culprit (107).

A woman with vulval dermatitis had positive patch test reactions to the FM I, hydroxyisohexyl 3-cyclohexene carboxaldehyde (HICC) and a body milk which she applied to the vulva. It was stated that these sensitizations were clinically relevant for her vulval dermatitis. Avoiding perfumed products including her own perfumed body milk led to a marked improvement of the vulval complaints. However, it was not specifically stated that the milk contained either HICC and/or one or more of the FM I ingredients (116).

Another female patient, known to be allergic to fragrances and therefore avoiding fragranced products, had connubial contact dermatitis from the deodorants of her husband. She reacted to FM I, FM II, Myroxylon pereirae resin and 2 deodorant sprays. After the husband stopped using fragranced products, the dermatitis quickly disappeared. Unfortunately, no attempt was made to identify the sensitizer(s) (148).

A female individual had extensive edema of the labia minora which led to urinary retention. When patch tested later, she reacted to a lubricant, the fragrance mix I and (later) to 6 of its components: cinnamyl alcohol, cinnamal, eugenol, isoeugenol, geraniol and hydroxycitronellal. The lubricant was perfumed, but the manufacturer did not respond to a request for disclosing its ingredients (65).

A woman had a history of episodes of gastrointestinal disorders and sometimes angioedema of the lips which appeared within 2 hours from the ingestion of packed food like biscuits, cereals or fruit juice. A patch test with the

European baseline series and with food preservatives was positive to the fragrances mix I only. The avoidance of packed food labeled as containing flavors among the ingredients led to disappearance of the patient's symptoms; details are lacking (article not read) (183).

Cross-reactions, pseudo-cross-reactions and co-reactions

For general information on cross-/pseudo-cross-/co-reactivity of fragrance chemicals with other fragrances, fragrance markers (fragrance mix I, fragrance mix II, colophonium, Myroxylon pereirae resin [balsam of Peru]) and essential oils see Chapter 1.2 General information on cross-reactions, pseudo-cross-reactions and co-reactions.

In patients reacting to FM I, co-reactions are frequently observed (only a few references provided) to Myroxylon pereirae resin (13,24,82,124,145,146,150,185,206,213), colophonium (24,82,120,145), FM II (111,122,169), essential oils, individual fragrances present in the FM I, other fragrances, sometimes to propolis (99,145), the Compositae-mix (29), the sesquiterpene lactone mix (214) and – when tested – commercial fine fragrances (125).

FM I is reported to be a good indicator for contact allergy to spices (69,70,71).

Other co-reactions

In patients with polysensitization (defined as at least 3 positive patch test reactions), the following allergens were particularly associated with the FM I: Myroxylon pereirae resin (odds ratio [OR] 17.3), FM II (OR 25.4), nickel sulfate (OR 18.1), cobalt chloride (OR 35.8), propolis (OR 38.9), colophonium (OR 36.9), oil of turpentine (OR 44.7), methyldibromo glutaronitrile (OR 44.6) and lanolin alcohols (OR 43.5) (94). It was concluded that (combinations of/with) fragrances are the main driving forces of multiple sensitization, possibly because exposure to fragrances is both ubiquitous and multiple (94).

Positive patch test reactions to FM I and/or FM II have a statistically significant association with positive reactions to MCI/MI and/or MI and with positive reactions to formaldehyde (99,206). Presumably, fragrances and preservatives are often present in the same consumer products (99).

In some studies, a significant association between positive reactions to the FM I and to epoxy resin has been found (114,115). Supplementary testing with fragrance mix ingredients showed that the association was related to positive reactions to amyl cinnamal and isoeugenol (115). The clinical implications are not clarified, and the association, which has not been found in several other studies, may be coincidental.

Of 27 patients allergic to *Frullania*, 10 (37%) reacted to the fragrance mix, in 8 of these cases from allergy to Evernia prunastri (oakmoss) extract; these were considered not to be cross-reactions but multiple specific allergies (143). Of 12 patients with occupational sensitization to *Frullania*, 5 (42%) co-reacted to the FM I (153). Of 21 patients allergic to tincture of benzoin, 14 (67%) co-reacted to the FM I (219).

In various studies a significant association between photocontact allergy to the NSAID ketoprofen and contact sensitization to the fragrance mix I (FM I) and Myroxylon pereirae resin (balsam of Peru) (159,164) has been observed (159-164,166). In the studies in which the ingredients of the FM I were tested, by far most reactions were observed to cinnamyl alcohol (163,164,166). It has been suggested that this may be due to cross-reactivity, as computerized conformational analysis has shown that there is a strong similarity between the standard structure of cinnamyl alcohol and the UV-A–excited ketoprofen structure (166). Indeed, in patients with a reaction to the FM I, who were patch and photopatch tested with ketoprofen and a number of other NSAIDs, there were 23% positive photopatch tests to ketoprofen and 31% to the related NSAID tiaprofenic acid. There was a clear association with contact allergy to cinnamyl alcohol but not with any other ingredient of the FM I. It was concluded that sensitization to cinnamyl alcohol (which is tested as part of the fragrance mix I) may be considered a marker or even a risk factor for photocontact allergy to ketoprofen and tiaprofenic acid (165).

A statistically significant overrepresentation has been found of simultaneous patch test reactions to FM I and phenol-formaldehyde resins (146). Of 72 patients with a positive patch test to FM I, 11 (15%) co-reacted to hydroabietyl alcohol (146). Of 10 patients reacting to atranorin 0.1% pet. seen in Sweden before 1981, all co-reacted to fragrance mix I (containing 2% oakmoss extract, in which atranol is one of the main sensitizers) (168).

Patch test sensitization

In 2 studies, in which groups of patients were tested with FM I twice, a marked increase in net gain of positivity on the second test compared with the first has been observed. One of the possible explanations is active sensitization from the first test in a number of the patients (181,182).

OTHER SIDE EFFECTS

Photosensitivity

Photopatch tests with FM I have been performed in several studies, usually for suspected photoallergic contact dermatitis or other photosensitivity disorders (table 3.70.8). Rates of photocontact sensitization were invariably low, ranging from 0.4% to 3.1%. In five of seven investigations, no (specific) relevance data were provided

(7,16,20,176,208). In the other two studies, one of 8 (13% [177]) and 5/7 (71% [175]) were considered to be relevant, but culprit products were not mentioned. Photoallergic reactions to the fragrance mix have also been reported in refs 178 and 179 (articles not read). Some positive photopatch tests were considered to be phototoxic rather than photoallergic (16,179) and some were photoaggravated contact allergic reactions (177).

Table 3.70.8 Photopatch testing in groups of patients

Years and Country	Test conc. & vehicle	Number of patients		Selection of patients (S); Relevance (R); Comments (C)	Ref.
		tested	positive (%)		
<2007 India	8% pet.	70	1 (1%)	S: patients with dermatitis of photo-exposed areas or dermatitis with photosensitivity; R: not stated	208
2004-2006 Italy		1082	8 (0.7%)	S: patients with histories and clinical features suggestive of photoallergic contact dermatitis; R: one reaction was relevant; C: of the 8 photoallergic reactions, 3 were photoaggravated (photoaugmented) contact allergic reactions	177
2004-2005 Spain	8% pet.	224	7 (3.1%)	S: not stated; R: 5/7 (71%); C: is was not mentioned whether these patients also had positive photopatch tests to ketoprofen (see the section 'Cross-reactions, pseudo-cross-reactions and co-reactions' above)	175
1994-9 Netherlands	8% pet.	55	1 (1.8%)	S: patients suspected of photosensitivity disorders; R: not stated	176
1990-1994 France	8% pet.	<370	7 (>1.9%)	S: patients with suspected photodermatitis; R: not stated; C: the FM was tested in 1993-1994 only, but it was not stated how many of the total of 370 patients were tested in that period; (some of) the reactions were considered to be photo-toxic rather than photoallergic	16
1985-1993 Italy		1050	23 (2.2%)	S: patients suspected of photoallergic contact dermatitis; R: not specified (78% for all photoallergens together)	7
1980-85 Germany, Austria, Switzerland	8% pet.	1129	4 (0.4%)	S: patients suspected of photoallergy, polymorphic light eruption, phototoxicity and skin problems with photo-distribution; R: not stated	20

Immediate-type reactions

Some 10-55% of individuals patch tested with FM I for immediate contact reactions have been found show a positive response (121,126,137,156). This is most likely due to the ingredient cinnamal, which is a well-known inducer of non-immune immediate contact reactions (Chapter 3.34 Cinnamal).

In a study performed in Greece, in the period 1996-1998, 664 consecutive dermatitis patients were patch tested and the reactions were read at 30 minutes to detect immediate contact reactions. The FM mix was positive in 112 individuals (16.9%). Of these, 15 (13%) later also proved to have delayed-type allergy to the FM. The percentage was significantly higher than in patients with negative immediate reactions and also than in the entire group, suggesting, according to the authors, that allergen-specific immune responses may in fact be involved in immediate contact reactions (128,156). However, in a group of 60 patients with a positive patch test reaction to FM I and/or MP, 7 (12%) had immediate contact reactions to FM I 8% pet. In a control group of 50 non-allergic patients, the percentage of immediate reactions was also 12. It was concluded that these results underline the non-immunological nature of the immediate contact reactions (121).

In 18 subjects not allergic to fragrances tested for non-immune immediate contact reactions, the fragrance mix (16% pet.) caused an urticarial reaction in two subjects (11%) (33). Sixteen patients with atopic dermatitis were patch tested with FM I and the reactions were read at 30 minutes; 9 (56%) showed erythema, termed 'immediate positive reactions' by the authors (137).

A female patient had recurrent episodes of widespread urticaria. When patch tested, she showed a local response to the fragrance mix and Myroxylon pereirae resin at both 30 and 60 minutes. Moreover, at 60 minutes, the patient developed widespread urticaria, not associated with respiratory or other systemic symptoms, which lasted for about 6 hours before spontaneously disappearing. When the patient was instructed to strictly avoid further contact with such substances, this resulted in rapid and complete remission of symptoms, which lasted for 6 months of follow-up (129).

Other non-eczematous contact reactions

A consistent and significant association has been found between perfume contact allergy diagnosed by positive patch tests to the fragrance mix I and/or Myroxylon pereirae resin and symptoms elicited by fragrance products from the eyes and airways. The symptoms are mostly reported as occurring within seconds or minutes after airborne exposure to fragrance products. However, contact eczema in sensitized individuals usually develops hours to days after exposure to an allergen and immediate responses are not in agreement with a type IV immunological reaction. As yet, the mechanism remains undetermined (17).

LITERATURE

1   Heisterberg MV, Menné T, Johansen JD. Contact allergy to the 26 specific fragrance ingredients to be declared on cosmetic products in accordance with the EU cosmetic directive. Contact Dermatitis 2011;65:266-275

2   Oosten EJ van, Schuttelaar ML, Coenraads PJ. Clinical relevance of positive patch test reactions to the 26 EU-labelled fragrances. Contact Dermatitis 2009;61:217-223

3   Frosch PJ, Pirker C, Rastogi SC, Andersen KE, Bruze M, Svedman C, et al. Patch testing with a new fragrance mix detects additional patients sensitive to perfumes and missed by the current fragrance mix. Contact Dermatitis 2005;52:207-215

4   Wenk KS, Ehrlich AE. Fragrance series testing in eyelid dermatitis. Dermatitis 2012;23:22-26

5   Firooz A, Nassiri-Kashani M, Khatami A, Gorouhi F, Babakoohi S, Montaser-Kouhsari L, et al. Fragrance contact allergy in Iran. J Eur Acad Dermatol Venereol 2010;24:1437-1441

6   Wöhrl S, Hemmer W, Focke M, Götz M, Jarisch R. The significance of fragrance mix, balsam of Peru, colophony and propolis as screening tools in the detection of fragrance allergy. Br J Dermatol 2001;145:268-273

7   Pigatto PD, Legori A, Bigardi AS,Guarrera M, Tosti A, Santucci B, et al. Gruppo Italiano recerca dermatiti da contatto ed ambientali Italian multicenter study of allergic contact photodermatitis: epidemiological aspects. Am J Contact Dermatitis 1996;7:158-163

8   Wetter DA, Yiannias JA, Prakash AV, Davis MDP, Farmer SA, el-Azhary RA. Results of patch testing to personal care product allergens in a standard series and a supplemental cosmetic series: an analysis of 945 patients from the Mayo Clinic Contact Dermatitis Group, 2000-2007. J Am Acad Dermatol 2010;63:789-798

9   Fransway AF, Zug KA, Belsito DV, Deleo VA, Fowler JF Jr, Maibach HI, et al. North American Contact Dermatitis Group patch test results for 2007-2008. Dermatitis 2013;24:10-21

10 Davis MDP, Scalf LA, Yiannias JA, Cheng JF, El-Azhary RA, Rohlinger AL, et al. Changing trends and allergens in the patch test standard series. Arch Dermatol 2008;144:67-72

11 Zug KA, Warshaw EM, Fowler JF jr, Maibach HI, Belsito DL, Pratt MD, et al. Patch-test results of the North American Contact Dermatitis Group 2005-2006. Dermatitis 2009;20:149-160

12 Warshaw EM, Belsito DV, DeLeo VA, Fowler JF Jr, Maibach HI, Marks JG, et al. North American Contact Dermatitis Group patch-test results, 2003-2004 study period. Dermatitis 2008;19:129-136

13 Schnuch A, Lessmann H, Geier J, Frosch PJ, Uter W. Contact allergy to fragrances: frequencies of sensitization from 1996 to 2002. Results of the IVDK. Contact Dermatitis 2004;50:65-76

14 Uter W, Aberer W, Armario-Hita JC, Fernandez-Vozmediano JM, Ayala F, Balato A, et al. Current patch test results with the European baseline series and extensions to it from the 'European Surveillance System on Contact Allergy' network, 2007-2008. Contact Dermatitis 2012;67:9-19

15 Baxter KF, Wilkinson SM, Kirk SJ. Hydroxymethyl pentylcyclohexene-carboxaldehyde (Lyral) as a fragrance allergen in the UK. Contact Dermatitis 2003;48:117-118

16 Journe F, Marguery M-C, Rakotondrazafy J, El Sayed F, Bazex J. Sunscreen sensitization: a 5-year study. Acta Derm Venereol 1999;79:211-213

17 Elberling J, Linneberg A, Mosbech H, Dirksen A, Frolund L, Madsen F, et al. A link between skin and airways regarding sensitivity to fragrance products? Br J Dermatol 2004;151:1197-1203

18 Zaragoza-Ninet V, Blasco Encinas R, Vilata-Corell JJ, Pérez-Ferriols A, Sierra-Talamantes C, Esteve-Martínez A, de la Cuadra-Oyanguren J. Allergic contact dermatitis due to cosmetics: A clinical and epidemiological study in a tertiary hospital. Actas Dermosifiliogr 2016;107:329-336

19 Laguna C, de la Cuadra J, Martín-González B, Zaragoza V, Martínez-Casimiro L, Alegre V. Allergic contact dermatitis to cosmetics. Actas Dermosifiliogr 2009;100:53-60

20 Hölzle E, Neumann N, Hausen B, Przybilla B, Schauder S, Hönigsmann H, et al. Photopatch testing: the 5-year experience of the German, Austrian and Swiss Photopatch Test Group. J Am Acad Dermatol 1991;25:59-68

21 An S, Lee AY, Lee CH, Kim DW, Hahm JH, Kim KJ, et al. Fragrance contact dermatitis in Korea: a joint study. Contact Dermatitis 2005;53:320-323

22 McLelland J, Shuster S. Contact dermatitis with negative patch tests: the additive effect of allergens in combination. Br J Dermatol 1990;122:623-630

23 Frosch PJ, Johansen JD, Menné T, Pirker C, Rastogi SC, Andersen KE, et al. Further important sensitizers in patients sensitive to fragrances. II. Reactivity to essential oils. Contact Dermatitis 2002;47:279-287

24 Brasch J, Uter W, Geier J, Schnuch A. Associated positive patch test reactions to standard contact allergens. Am J Contact Dermat 2001;12:197-202

25 Trattner A, David M. Patch testing with fine fragrances: comparison with fragrance mix, balsam of Peru and a fragrance series. Contact Dermatitis 2003:49:287-289

26 Cuesta L, Silvestre JF, Toledo F, Lucas A, Perez-Crespo M, Ballester I. Fragrance contact allergy: a 4-year retrospective study. Contact Dermatitis 2010;63:77-84

27 Alinaghi F, Bennike NH, Egeberg A, Thyssen JP, Johansen JD. Prevalence of contact allergy in the general population: A systematic review and meta-analysis. Contact Dermatitis 2018 Oct 29. doi: 10.1111/cod.13119. [Epub ahead of print]

28 Uter W, Geier J, Schnuch A, Frosch PJ. Patch test results with patients' own perfumes, deodorants and shaving lotions: results of the IVDK 1998-2002. J Eur Acad Dermatol Venereol 2007;21:374-379

29 Paulsen E, Andersen KE. Colophonium and Compositae mix as markers of fragrance allergy: cross-reactivity between fragrance terpenes, colophonium and Compositae plant extracts. Contact Dermatitis 2005;53:285-291

30 Tomar J, Jain VK, Aggarwal K, Dayal S, Guptaet S. Contact allergies to cosmetics: testing with 52 cosmetic ingredients and personal products. J Dermatol 2005;32:951-955

31 Buckley DA, Wakelin SH, Seed PT, Holloway D, Rycroft RJ, White IR, et al. The frequency of fragrance allergy in a patch-test population over a 17-year period. Br J Dermatol 2000;142:279-283

32 Larsen WG. Perfume dermatitis. A study of 20 patients. Arch Dermatol 1977;113:623-626

33 Safford RJ, Basketter DA, Allenby CF, Goodwin BF. Immediate contact reactions to chemicals in the fragrance mix and a study of the quenching action of eugenol. Br J Dermatol 1990;123:595-606

34 Uter W, Fießler C, Gefeller O, Geier J, Schnuch A. Contact sensitization to fragrance mix I and II, to *Myroxylon pereirae* resin and oil of tupentine: multifactorial analysis of risk factors based on data of the IVDK network. Flavour Fragr J 2015;30:255-263

35 Geier J, Uter W, Lessmann H, Schnuch A. Fragrance mix I and II: results of breakdown tests. Flavour Fragr J 2015;30:264-274

36 Goossens A. Cosmetic contact allergens. Cosmetics 2016, 3, 5; doi:10.3390/cosmetics3010005

37 Lynde CB, Grushka M, Walsh SR. Burning mouth syndrome: patch test results from a large case series. J Cutan Med Surg 2014;18:174-179

38 Ockenfels H, Seemann U, Goos M. Contact allergy in patients with periorbital eczema: an analysis of allergens. Dermatology 1997;195:119-124

39 ESSCA Writing Group. The European Surveillance System of Contact Allergies (ESSCA): results of patch testing the standard series, 2004. J Eur Acad Dermatol Venereol 2008;22:174-181

40 Warshaw EM, Maibach HI, Taylor JS, Sasseville D, DeKoven JG, Zirwas MJ, et al. North American Contact Dermatitis Group patch test results: 2011-2012. Dermatitis 2015;26:49-59

41 Warshaw EM, Belsito DV, Taylor JS, Sasseville D, DeKoven JG, Zirwas MJ, et al. North American Contact Dermatitis Group patch test results: 2009 to 2010. Dermatitis 2013;24:50-59

42 Lazarov A. European Standard Series patch test results from a contact dermatitis clinic in Israel during the 7-year period from 1998 to 2004. Contact Dermatitis 2006;55:73-76

43 Worm M, Brasch J, Geier J, Uter W, Schnuch A. Epikutantestung mit der DKG-Standardreihe 2001-2004. Hautarzt 2005;56:1114-1124

44 Carlsen BC, Menné T, Johansen JD. 20 Years of standard patch testing in an eczema population with focus on patients with multiple contact allergies. Contact Dermatitis 2007;57:76-83

45 Uter W, Hegewald J, Aberer W, Ayala F, Bircher AJ, Brasch J, et al. The European standard series in 9 European countries, 2002/2003 – First results of the European Surveillance System on Contact Allergies. Contact Dermatitis 2005;53:136-145

46 Pratt MD, Belsito DV, DeLeo VA, Fowler JF Jr, Fransway AF, Maibach HI, et al. North American Contact Dermatitis Group patch-test results, 2001-2002 study period. Dermatitis 2004;15:176-183

47 Hasan T, Rantanen T, Alanko K, Harvima RJ, Jolanki R, Kalimo K, et al. Patch test reactions to cosmetic allergens in 1995-1997 and 2000-2002 in Finland – a multicentre study. Contact Dermatitis 2005;53:40-45

48 Lindberg M, Edman B, Fischer T, Stenberg B. Time trends in Swedish patch test data from 1992 to 2000. A multi-centre study based on age- and sex-adjusted results of the Swedish standard series. Contact Dermatitis 2007;56:205-210

49 Wetter DA, Davis MDP, Yiannias JA, Cheng JF, Connolly SM, el-Azhary RA, et al. Patch test results from the Mayo Contact Dermatitis Group, 1998–2000. J Am Acad Dermatol 2005;53:416-421

50 Akyol A, Boyvat A, Peksari Y, Gurgey E. Contact sensitivity to standard series allergens in 1038 patients with contact dermatitis in Turkey. Contact Dermatitis 2005;52:333-337

51 Machovcova A, Dastychova E, Kostalova D, et al. Common contact sensitizers in the Czech Republic. Patch test results in 12,058 patients with suspected contact dermatitis. Contact Dermatitis 2005;53:162-166

52 Bruynzeel DP, Diepgen TL, Andersen KE, Brandão FM, Bruze M, Frosch PJ, et al (EECDRG). Monitoring the European Standard Series in 10 centres 1996–2000. Contact Dermatitis 2005;53:146-152

53 Fall S, Bruze M, Isaksson M, Lidén C, Matura M, Stenberg B, Lindberg M. Contact allergy trends in Sweden – a retrospective comparison of patch test data from 1992, 2000, and 2009. Contact Dermatitis 2015;72:297-304

54 Wentworth AB, Yiannias JA, Keeling JH, Hall MR, Camilleri MJ, Drage LA, et al. Trends in patch-test results and allergen changes in the standard series: a Mayo Clinic 5-year retrospective review (January 1, 2006, to December 31, 2010). J Am Acad Dermatol 2014;70:269-275

55 Uter W, Rämsch C, Aberer W, Ayala F, Balato A, Beliauskiene A, et al. The European baseline series in 10 European Countries, 2005/2006 – Results of the European Surveillance System on Contact Allergies (ESSCA). Contact Dermatitis 2009;61:31-38

56 Toholka R, Wang Y-S, Tate B, Tam M, Cahill J, Palmer A, Nixon R. The first Australian Baseline Series: Recommendations for patch testing in suspected contact dermatitis. Australas J Dermatol 2015;56:107-115

57 DeKoven JG, Warshaw EM, Belsito DV, Sasseville D, Maibach HI, Taylor JS, et al. North American Contact Dermatitis Group Patch Test Results: 2013-2014. Dermatitis 2017;28:33-46

58 Uter W, Amario-Hita JC, Balato A, Ballmer-Weber B, Bauer A, Belloni Fortina A, et al. European Surveillance System on Contact Allergies (ESSCA): results with the European baseline series, 2013/14. J Eur Acad Dermatol Venereol 2017;31:1516-1525

59 Thyssen JP, Uter W, Schnuch A, Linneberg A, Johansen JD. 10-year prevalence of contact allergy in the general population in Denmark estimated through the CE-DUR method. Contact Dermatitis 2007;57:265-272

60 Schnuch A, Uter W, Geier J, Gefeller O (for the IVDK study group). Epidemiology of contact allergy: an estimation of morbidity employing the clinical epidemiology and drug-utilization research (CE-DUR) approach. Contact Dermatitis 2002;47:32-39

61 Schubert S, Bauer A, Molin S, Skudlik C, Geier J. Occupational contact sensitization in female geriatric nurses: Data of the Information Network of Departments of Dermatology (IVDK) 2005-2014. J Eur Acad Dermatol Venereol 2017;31:469-476

62 Ung CY, White JML, White IR, Banerjee P, McFadden JP. Patch testing with the European baseline series fragrance markers: a 2016 update. Br J Dermatol 2018;178:776-780

63 Turić P, Lipozencić J, Milavec-Puretić V, Kulisić SM. Contact allergy caused by fragrance mix and Myroxylon pereirae (balsam of Peru)--a retrospective study. Coll Antropol 2011;35:83-87

64 Warshaw EM, Zug KA, Belsito DV, Fowler JF Jr, DeKoven JG, Sasseville D, et al. Positive patch-test reactions to essential oils in consecutive patients: Results from North America and Central Europe. Dermatitis 2017;28:246-252

65 Ljubojević Hadžavdić S, Jović A, Hadžavdić A, Ljubojević Grgec D. Vulvar oedema. Contact Dermatitis 2018;78:226-227

66 Assier H, Tetart F, Avenel-Audran M, Barbaud A, Ferrier-le Bouëdec MC, Giordano-Labadie F, et al. Is a specific eyelid patch test series useful? Results of a French prospective study. Contact Dermatitis 2018;79:157-161

67 Dooms-Goossens, A, Kerre S, Drieghe J, Bossuyt L, DeGreef H. Cosmetic products and their allergens. Eur J Dermatol 1992;2:465-468

68 Calnan CD, Cronin E, Rycroft RJ. Allergy to perfume ingredients. Contact Dermatitis 1980;6:500-501

69 Niinimäki A. Double-blind placebo-controlled peroral challenges in patients with delayed-type allergy to balsam of Peru. Contact Dermatitis 1995;33:78-83

70 Bruynzeel DP, Prevoo RLMA. Patch tests with some spices. Dermatol Clin 1990;8:85-87

71 Van den Akker Th , Roesyanto-Mahadi ID, van Toorenenbergen AW, van Joost Th. Contact allergy to spices. Contact Dermatitis 1990;22:267-272

72 Larsen W. Perfume dermatitis. J Am Acad Dermatol 1985;12:1-9

73 Brasch J, Becker D, Aberer W, Bircher A, Kränke B, Denzer-Fürst S, Schnuch A. Contact Dermatitis. J Dtsch Dermatol Ges 2007;5: 943-951

74 Warshaw EM, Buchholz HJ, Belsito DV et al. Allergic patch test reactions associated with cosmetics: Retrospective analysis of cross-sectional data from the North American Contact Dermatitis Group, 2001-2004. J Am Acad Dermatol 2009;60:23-38

75 Molin S, Bauer A, Schnuch A, Geier J. Occupational contact allergy in nurses: results from the Information Network of Departments of Dermatology 2003–2012. Contact Dermatitis 2015;72:164-171

76 Landeck L, John SM, Geier J. Periorbital dermatitis in 4779 patients – patch test results during a 10-year period. Contact Dermatitis 2014;70:205-212

77 Amin KA, Belsito DV. The aetiology of eyelid dermatitis: a 10-year retrospective analysis. Contact Dermatitis 2006;55:280-285

78 Cooper SM, Shaw S. Eyelid dermatitis: an evaluation of 232 patch test patients over 5 years. Contact Dermatitis 2000;42:291-293

79 Zug KA, Kornik R, Belsito DV, DeLeo VA, Fowler JF Jr, Maibach HI, et al. Patch-testing North American lip dermatitis patients: Data from the North American Contact Dermatitis Group, 2001 to 2004. Dermatitis 2008;19:202-208

80 Katz AS, Sherertz EF. Facial dermatitis: Patch test results and final diagnoses. Am J Cont Dermat 1999;10:153-156

81 Herbst RA, Uter W, Pirker C, Geier J, Frosch PJ. Allergic and non-allergic periorbital dermatitis: patch test results of the Information Network of the Departments of Dermatology during a 5-year period. Contact Dermatitis 2004;51:13-19

82 Nardelli A, Carbonez A, Ottoy W, Drieghe J, Goossens A. Frequency of and trends in fragrance allergy over a 15-year period. Contact Dermatitis 2008;58:134-141

83 Lewis FM, Shah M, Gawkrodger DJ. Contact sensitivity in pruritus vulvae: patch test results and clinical outcome. Dermatitis 1997;8:137-140

84 Lubbes S, Rustemeyer T, Sillevis Smitt JH, Schuttelaar ML, Middelkamp-Hup MA. Contact sensitization in Dutch children and adolescents with and without atopic dermatitis - a retrospective analysis. Contact Dermatitis 2017;76:151-159

85 Erfurt-Berge C, Geier J, Mahler V. The current spectrum of contact sensitization in patients with chronic leg ulcers or stasis dermatitis - new data from the Information Network of Departments of Dermatology (IVDK). Contact Dermatitis 2017;77:151-158

86 Dinkloh A, Worm M, Geier J, Schnuch A, Wollenberg A. Contact sensitization in patients with suspected cosmetic intolerance: results of the IVDK 2006-2011. J Eur Acad Dermatol Venereol 2015;29:1071-1081

87 Schwensen JF, Johansen JD, Veien NK, Funding AT, Avnstorp C, Østerballe M, et al. Occupational contact dermatitis in hairdressers: an analysis of patch test data from the Danish Contact Dermatitis Group, 2002–2011. Contact Dermatitis 2014;70:233-237

88 Uter W, Lessmann H, Geier J, Schnuch A. Contact allergy to ingredients of hair cosmetics in female hairdressers and clients: an 8-year analysis of IVDK data. Contact Dermatitis 2003;49:236-240

89 Uter W, Lessmann H, Geier J, Schnuch A. Contact allergy to hairdressing allergens in female hairdressers and clients – current data from the IVDK 2003–2006. J Dtsch Dermatol Ges 2007;5:993-1001

90 Uter W, Gefeller O, John SM, Schnuch A, Geier J. Contact allergy to ingredients of hair cosmetics – a comparison of female hairdressers and clients based on IVDK 2007–2012 data. Contact Dermatitis 2014;71:13-20

91 Zhao B, Fan WX. Facial contact dermatitis. Pathogenetic factors in China. Int J Dermatol 1991;30:485-486

92 Hillen U, Grabbe S, Uter W. Patch test results in patients with scalp dermatitis: analysis of data of the Information Network of Departments of Dermatology. Contact Dermatitis 2007;56:87-93

93 Feser A, Plaza T, Vogelgsang L, Mahler V. Periorbital dermatitis – a recalcitrant disease: causes and differential diagnoses. Brit J Dermatol 2008;159:858-863

94 Adler W, Gefeller O, Uter W. Positive reactions to pairs of allergens associated with polysensitization: analysis of IVDK data with machine-learning techniques. Contact Dermatitis 2017;76:247-251

95 Carøe TK, Ebbehøj NE, Agner T. Occupational dermatitis in hairdressers – influence of individual and environmental factors. Contact Dermatitis 2017;76:146-150

96 Ochi H, Cheng SWN, Leow YH, Goon ATJ. Contact allergy trends in Singapore – a retrospective study of patch test data from 2009 to 2013. Contact Dermatitis 2017;76:49-50

97 Higgins CL, Palmer AM, Cahill JL, Nixon RL. Occupational skin disease among Australian healthcare workers: a retrospective analysis from an occupational dermatology clinic, 1993–2014. Contact Dermatitis 2016;75:213-222

98 Ibler KS, Jemec GBE, Garvey LH, Agner T. Prevalence of delayed-type and immediate-type hypersensitivity in healthcare workers with hand eczema. Contact Dermatitis 2016;75:223-229

99 Pontén A, Bruze M, Engfeldt M, Hauksson I, Isaksson M. Concomitant contact allergies to formaldehyde, methylchloroisothiazolinone/methylisothiazolinone, methylisothiazolinone, and fragrance mixes I and II. Contact Dermatitis 2016;75:285-289

100 Sabroe RA, Holden CR, Gawkrodger DJ. Contact allergy to essential oils cannot always be predicted from allergy to fragrance markers in the baseline series. Contact Dermatitis 2016;74:236-241

101 Geier J, Schnuch A, Lessmann H, Uter W. Reactivity to sorbitan sesquioleate affects reactivity to fragrance mix I. Contact Dermatitis 2015;73:296-304

102 Vejanurug P, Tresukosol P, Sajjachareonpong P, Puangpet P. Fragrance allergy could be missed without patch testing with 26 individual fragrance allergens. Contact Dermatitis 2016;74:230-235

103 Breuer K, Uter W, Geier J. Epidemiological data on airborne contact dermatitis – results of the IVDK. Contact Dermatitis 2015;73:239-247

104 Liu J, Li L-F. Contact sensitization to fragrances other than fragrance mix I in China. Contact Dermatitis 2015;73:252-253

105 Frosch PJ, Johansen JD, Schuttelaar M-LA, Silvestre JF, Sánchez-Pérez J, Weisshaar E, et al. (on behalf of the ESSCA network). Patch test results with fragrance markers of the baseline series – analysis of the European Surveillance System on Contact Allergies (ESSCA) network 2009–2012. Contact Dermatitis 2015;73:163-171

106 Mann J, McFadden JP, White JML, White IR, Banerjee P. Baseline series fragrance markers fail to predict contact allergy. Contact Dermatitis 2014;70:276-281

107 Jensen P, Menné T, Johansen JD, Thyssen JP. Facial allergic contact dermatitis caused by fragrance ingredients released by an electric shaver. Contact Dermatitis 2012;67:380-381

108 Cheng S, Cao M, Zhang Y, Peng S, Dong J, Zhang D, et al. Time trends of contact allergy to a modified European baseline series in Beijing between 2001 and 2006. Contact Dermatitis 2011;65:22-27

109 Yin R, Huang XY, Zhou XF, Hao F. A retrospective study of patch tests in Chongqing, China from 2004 to 2009. Contact Dermatitis 2011;65:28-33

110 Nardelli A, Drieghe J, Claes L, Boey L, Goossens A. Fragrance allergens in 'specific' cosmetic products. Contact Dermatitis 2011;64:212-219

111 Uter W, Geier J, Frosch P, Schnuch A. Contact allergy to fragrances: current patch test results (2005–2008) from the Information Network of Departments of Dermatology. Contact Dermatitis 2010;63:254-261

112 Janach M, Kühne A, Seifert B, French FE, Ballmer-Weber B, Hofbauer GFL. Changing delayed-type sensitizations to the baseline series allergens over a decade at the Zurich University Hospital. Contact Dermatitis 2010;63:42-48

113 Barbaud A, Collet E, Le Coz CJ, Meaume S, Gillois P. Contact allergy in chronic leg ulcers: results of a multicentre study carried out in 423 patients and proposal for an updated series of patch tests. Contact Dermatitis 2009;60:279-287

114 Pontén A, Björk J, Carstensen O, Gruvberger B, Isaksson M, Rasmussen K, Bruze M. Associations between contact allergy to epoxy resin and fragrance mix. Acta Derm Venereol 2004;84:151-152

115 Andersen KE, Porskjær Christensen L, Vølund A, Johansen JD, Paulsen E. Association between positive patch tests to epoxy resin and fragrance mix I ingredients. Contact Dermatitis 2009;60:155-157

116 Vermaat H, Smienk F, Rustemeyer T, Bruynzeel DP, Kirtschig G. Anogenital allergic contact dermatitis, the role of spices and flavour allergy. Contact Dermatitis 2008;59:233-237

117 Thyssen JP, Carlsen BC, Menné T, Johansen JD. Trends of contact allergy to fragrance mix I and Myroxylon pereirae among Danish eczema patients tested between 1985 and 2007. Contact Dermatitis 2008;59:238-244

118 Zmudzinska M, Czarnecka-Operacz M, Silny W, Kramer L. Contact allergy in patients with chronic venous leg ulcers – possible role of chronic venous insufficiency. Contact Dermatitis 2006;54:100-105

119 Uter W, Balzer C, Geier J, Frosch PJ, Schnuch A. Patch testing with patients' own cosmetics and toiletries – results of the IVDK, 1998–2002. Contact Dermatitis 2005;53:226-233

120 Lu X, Li L-F, Wang W, Wang J. A clinical and patch test study of patients with positive patch test reactions to fragrance mix in China. Contact Dermatitis 2005;52:188-191

121 Tanaka S, Matsumoto Y, Dlova N, Ostlere LS, Goldsmith PC, Rycroft RJG, et al. Immediate contact reactions to fragrance mix constituents and Myroxylon pereirae resin. Contact Dermatitis 2004;51:20-21

122 Mowitz M, Svedman C, Zimerson E, Isaksson M, Pontén A, Bruze M. Simultaneous patch testing with fragrance mix I, fragrance mix II and their ingredients in southern Sweden between 2009 and 2015. Contact Dermatitis 2017;77:280-287

123 Trattner A, Farchi Y, David M. Cosmetics patch tests: first report from Israel. Contact Dermatitis 2002;47:180-181

124 Temesvári E, Németh I, Baló-Banga MJ, Husz S, Kohánka V, Somos Z, et al. Multicentre study of fragrance allergy in Hungary: Immediate and late type reactions. Contact Dermatitis 2002;46:325-330

125 Johansen JD, Frosch PJ, Rastogi SC, Menné T. Testing with fine fragrances in eczema patients: Results and test methods. Contact Dermatitis 2001;44:304-307

126 Buckley DA, Rycroft RJG, White IR, McFadden JP. Contact allergy to individual fragrance mix constituents in relation to primary site of dermatitis. Contact Dermatitis 2000;43:304-305

127 Brites MM, Gonçalo M, Figueiredo A. Contact allergy to fragrance mix--a 10-year study. Contact Dermatitis 2000;43:181-182

128 Katsarou A, Armenaka M, Ale I, Koufou V, Kalogeromitros D. Frequency of immediate reactions to the European standard series. Contact Dermatitis 1999;41:276-279

129 Cancian M, Belloni Fortini A, Peserico A. Contact urticaria syndrome from constituents of balsam of Peru and fragrance mix in a patient with chronic urticaria. Contact Dermatitis 1999;41:300

130 Katsarma G, Gawkrodger DJ. Suspected fragrance allergy requires extended patch testing to individual fragrance allergens. Contact Dermatitis 1999;41:193-197

131 Hendriks SA, van Ginkel CJW. Evaluation of the fragrance mix in the European standard series. Contact Dermatitis 1999;41:161-162

132 Held E, Johansen JD, Agner T, Menné T. Contact allergy to cosmetics: testing with patients' own products. Contact Dermatitis 1999;40:310-315

133 Frosch PJ, Pilz B, Burrows D, Camarasa JG, Lachapelle J-M, Lahti A, et al. Testing with fragrance mix: Is the addition of sorbitan sesquioleate to the constituents useful? Contact Dermatitis 1995;32:266-272

134 Johansen JD, Menné T. The fragrance mix and its constituents: a 14-year material. Contact Dermatitis 1995;32:18-23

135 Lewis FM, Harrington CI, Gawkrodger DJ. Contact sensitivity in pruritus vulvae: a common and manageable problem. Contact Dermatitis 1994;31:264-265

136 Valsecchi R, Imberti G, Martino D, Cainelli T. Eyelid dermatitis: an evaluation of 150 patients. Contact Dermatitis 1992;27:143-147

137 Abifadel R, Mortureux P, Perromat M, Ducombs G, Taier A. Contact sensitivity to flavourings and perfumes in atopic dermatitis. Contact Dermatitis 1992;27:43-46

138 van den Akker ThW, Roesyanto-Mahadi D, van Toorenbergen AW, van Joost Th. Contact allergy to spices. Contact Dermatitis 1990;22:267-272

139 Enders F, Przybilla B, Ring J. Patch testing with fragrance mix at 16% and 8%, and its individual constituents. Contact Dermatitis 1989;20:237-238

140 Enders F, Przybilla B, Ring J. Patch testing with fragrance-mix and its constituents: discrepancies are largely due to the presence or absence of sorbitan sesquioleate. Contact Dermatitis 1991;24:238-239

141 Goodfield MJD, Saihan EM. Fragrance sensitivity in coal miners. Contact Dermatitis 1988;18:81-83

142 Broeckx W, Blondeel A, Dooms-Goossens A, Achten G. Cosmetic intolerance. Contact Dermatitis 1987;16:189-194

143 Gonçalo S. Contact sensitivity to lichens and compositae in *Frullania* dermatitis. Contact Dermatitis 1987;16: 84-86

144 Santucci B, Cristaudo A, Cannistraci C, Picardo M. Contact dermatitis to fragrances. Contact Dermatitis 1987;16:93-95

145 Rudzki E, Grzywa Z. Allergy to perfume mixture. Contact Dermatitis 1986;15:115-116

146 Bruze M. Simultaneous reactions to phenol-formaldehyde resins colophony/hydroabietyl alcohol and balsam of Peru/perfume mixture. Contact Dermatitis 1986;14:119-120

147 Shi Y, Nedorost S, Scheman L, Scheman A. Propolis, colophony, and fragrance cross-reactivity and allergic contact dermatitis. Dermatitis 2016;27:123-126

148 Jensen P, Ortiz PG, Hartmann-Petersen S, Sandby-Møller J, Menné T, Thyssen JP. Connubial allergic contact dermatitis caused by fragrance ingredients. Dermatitis 2012;23:e1-e2

149 Storrs FJ. Fragrance. Dermatitis 2007;18:3-7

150 Devos SA, Constandt L, Tupker RA, Noz KC, Lucker GPH, Bruynzeel DP, et al. Relevance of positive patch-test reactions to fragrance mix. Dermatitis 2008;19:43-47

151 Belsito DV, Fowler JF Jr, Sasseville D, Marks JG Jr, De Leo VA, Storrs FJ. Delayed-type hypersensitivity to fragrance materials in a select North American population. Dermatitis 2006;17:23-28

152 Strauss RM, Orton DI. Allergic contact cheilitis in the United Kingdom: a retrospective study. Dermatitis 2003;14:75-77

153 Gonçalo S. Occupational contact dermatitis to *Frullania*. Contact Dermatitis 1984;11:54-55

154 Machet L, Couhe C, Perrinaud A, Hoarau C, Lorette G, Vaillant L. A high prevalence of sensitization still persists in leg ulcer patients: a retrospective series of 106 patients tested between 2001 and 2002 and a meta-analysis of 1975-2003. Br J Dermatol 2004;150:929-935

155 Katoulis AC, Stavrianeas NG, Katsarou A, Antoniou C, Georgala S, Rigopoulos D, et al. Evaluation of the role of contact sensitization and photosensitivity in the pathogenesis of poikiloderma of Civatte. Br J Dermatol 2002;147:493-497

156 Katsarou A, Armenaka M, Kalogeromitros D, Koufou V, Georgala S. Contact reactions to fragrances. Ann Allergy Asthma Immunol 1999;82:449-455

157 Bonefeld CM, Nielsen MM, Rubin IM, Vennegaard MT, Dabelsteen S, Gimenéz-Arnau E, et al. Enhanced sensitization and elicitation responses caused by mixtures of common fragrance allergens. Contact Dermatitis 2011;65:336-342

158 Johansen JD, Skov L, Vølund A, Andersen K, Menné T. Allergens in combination have a synergistic effect on the elicitation response: a study of fragrance-sensitized individuals. Br J Dermatol 1998;139:264-270

159 Matthieu L, Meuleman L, Van Hecke E, Blondeel A, Dezfoulian B, Constandt L, Goossens A. Contact and photocontact allergy to ketoprofen. The Belgian experience. Contact Dermatitis 2004;50:238-241

160 Durieu C, Marguery M-C, Giordano-Labadie F, Journe F, Loche F, Bazex J. Allergies de contact photoaggravées et photoallergies de contact au kétoprofène: 19 Cas. Ann Dermatol Venereol 2001;128:1020-1024

161 Girardin P, Vigan M, Humbert P, Aubin F. Cross-reactions in patch testing with ketoprofen, fragrance mix and cinnamic derivatives. Contact Dermatitis 2006;55:126-128

162 Pigatto P, Bigardi A, Legori A, Valsecchi R, Picardo M. Cross-reactions in patch testing and photopatch testing with ketoprofen, thiaprophenic acid, and cinnamic aldehyde. Am J Contact Dermat 1996;7:220-223

163 Durbize E, Vigan M, Puzenat E, Girardin P, Adessi B, Desprez PH, et al. Spectrum of cross-photosensitization in 18 consecutive patients with contact photoallergy to ketoprofen: associated photoallergies to non-benzophenone-containing molecules. Contact Dermatitis 2003;48:144-149

164 Devleeschouwer V, Roelandts R, Garmyn M, Goossens A. Allergic and photoallergic contact dermatitis from ketoprofen: results of (photo) patch testing and follow-up of 42 patients. Contact Dermatitis 2008;58:159-166

165 Stingeni L, Foti C, Cassano N, Bonamonte D, Vonella M, Vena GA, et al. Photocontact allergy to arylpropionic acid non-steroidal anti-inflammatory drugs in patients sensitized to fragrance mix I. Contact Dermatitis 2010;63:108-110

166 Foti C, Bonamonte D, Conserva A, Stingeni L, Lisi P, Lionetti N, et al. Allergic and photoallergic contact dermatitis from ketoprofen: evaluation of cross-reactivities by a combination of photopatch testing and computerized conformational analysis. Curr Pharm Des 2008;14:2833-2839

167 Diepgen TL, Ofenloch R, Bruze M, Cazzaniga S, Coenraads PJ, Elsner P, et al. Prevalence of fragrance contact allergy in the general population of five European countries: a cross-sectional study. Br J Dermatol 2015;173:1411-1419

168 Dahlquist I, Fregert S. Atranorin and oak moss contact allergy. Contact Dermatitis 1981;7:168-169

169 Heisterberg MV, Andersen KE, Avnstorp C, Kristensen B, Kristensen O, Kaaber K, et al. Fragrance mix II in the baseline series contributes significantly to detection of fragrance allergy. Contact Dermatitis 2010;63:270-276

170 Mortz CG, Andersen KE. Fragrance mix I patch test reactions in 5006 consecutive dermatitis patients tested simultaneously with TRUE Test ® and Trolab ® test material. Contact Dermatitis 2010;63:248-253

171 Bråred Christensson J, Hellsén S, Börje A, Karlberg A-T. Limonene hydroperoxide analogues show specific patch test reactions. Contact Dermatitis 2014;70:291-299

172 Kynemund Pedersen L, Johansen JD, Held E, Agner T. Augmentation of skin response by exposure to a combination of allergens and irritants – a review. Contact Dermatitis 2004;50:265-273

173 Buckley DA, Rycroft RJG, White IR, McFadden JP. The frequency of fragrance allergy in patch-tested patients increases with their age. Br J Dermatol 2003;149:986-989

174 Bennike NH, Zachariae C, Johansen JD. Non-mix fragrances are top sensitizers in consecutive dermatitis patients – a cross-sectional study of the 26 EU-labelled fragrance allergens. Contact Dermatitis 2017;77:270-279

175 De La Cuadra-Oyanguren J, Perez-Ferriols A, Lecha-Carrelero M, Giménez-Arnau AM, Fernández-Redondo V, Ortiz de Frutos FJ, et al. Results and assessment of photopatch testing in Spain: towards a new standard set of photoallergens. Actas Dermosfiliogr 2007;98:96-101

176 Bakkum RS, Heule F. Results of photopatch testing in Rotterdam during a 10-year period. Br J Dermatol 2002;146:275-279

177 Pigatto PD, Guzzi G, Schena D, Guarrera M, Foti C, Francalanci S, et al. Photopatch tests: an Italian multicentre study from 2004 to 2006. Contact Dermatitis 2008;59:103-108

178 Szczurko C, Dompmartin A, Michel M, Moreau A, Leroy D. Photocontact allergy to oxybenzone: ten years of experience. Photodermatol Photoimmunol Photomed 1994;10:144-147

179 Leonard F, Kalis B, Journe F. The standard battery for photopatch tests in France. Prospective study by the French Society for Photodermatology. Nouv Dermatol 1994;13:305-314

180 Nagtegaal MJC, Pentinga SE, Kuik J, Kezic S, Rustemeyer T. The role of the skin irritation response in polysensitization to fragrances. Contact Dermatitis 2012;67:28-35

181 White JML, McFadden JP, White IR. A review of 241 subjects who were patch tested twice: could fragrance mix I cause active sensitization? Br J Dermatol 2008;158:518-521

182 Carlsen BC, Menné T, Johansen JD. 20 years of standard patch testing in an eczema population with focus on patients with multiple contact allergies. Contact Dermatitis 2007;57:76-83

183 Ricciardi L, Saitta S, Isola S, Aglio M, Gangemi S. Fragrances as a cause of food allergy. Allergol Immunopathol (Madr) 2007;35:276-277

184 Thyssen J P, Menné T, Linneberg A, Johansen JD. Contact sensitization to fragrances in the general population: a Koch's approach may reveal the burden of disease. Br J Dermatol 2009;160:729-735

185 Nardelli A, Carbonez A, Drieghe J, Goossens A. Results of patch testing with fragrance mix 1, fragrance mix 2, and their ingredients, and Myroxylon pereirae and colophonium, over a 21-year period. Contact Dermatitis 2013;68:307-313

186 Larsen WG. Fragrance testing in the 21st century. Contact Dermatitis 2002;47:60-61

187 Buckley DA, Basketter DA, Smith Pease CK, Rycroft RJG, White IR, McFadden JP. Simultaneous sensitivity to fragrances. Br J Dermatol 2006;154:885-888

188 Schollhammer L, Andersen KE, Gotthard Mortz C. The diagnostic value of patch tests with two fragrance mix I preparations for detection of clinically relevant perfume allergy. Contact Dermatitis 2012;66:350-352

189 Bennike NH, Zachariae C, Johansen DJ. Trends in contact allergy to fragrance mix I in consecutive Danish eczema patients over three decades; a cross-sectional study from 1986 to 2015. Br J Dermatol 2017;176:1035-1041

190 Hagvall L, Bruze M, Engfeldt M, Isaksson M, Lindberg M, Ryberg K, et al. Contact allergy to oxidized geraniol among Swedish dermatitis patients - A multicentre study by the Swedish Contact Dermatitis Research Group. Contact Dermatitis 2018;79:232-238

191 Larsen W, Nakayama H, Lindberg M, Fischer T, Elsner P, Burrows D, et al. Fragrance contact dermatitis: A worldwide multicenter investigation (Part 1). Am J Cont Derm 1996;7:77-83

192 Larsen W, Nakayama H, Fischer T, Elsner P, Frosch P, Burrows D, et al. Fragrance contact dermatitis: A worldwide multicenter investigation (Part II). Contact Dermatitis 2001;44:344-346

193 De Groot AC, Van der Kley AMJ, Bruynzeel DP, Meinardi MMHM, Smeenk G, van Joost Th, Pavel S. Frequency of false-negative reactions to the fragrance mix. Contact Dermatitis 1993;28:139-140

194 Heydorn S, Johansen JD, Andersen KE, Bruze M, Svedman C, White IR, et al. Fragrance allergy in patients with hand eczema – a clinical study. Contact Dermatitis 2003;48:317-323

195 Sugiura M, Hayakawa R, Kato Y, Sugiura K, Hashimoto R. Results of patch testing with lavender oil in Japan. Contact Dermatitis 2000;43:157-160

196 Cuesta L, Silvestre JF, Toledo F, Lucas A, Perez-Crespo M, Ballester I. Fragrance contact allergy: a 4-year retrospective study. Contact Dermatitis 2010;63:77-84

197 De Groot AC, Liem DH, Nater JP, Van Ketel WG. Patch tests with fragrance materials and preservatives. Contact Dermatitis 1985;12:87-92

198 Malten KE, van Ketel WG, Nater JP, Liem DH. Reactions in selected patients to 22 fragrance materials. Contact Dermatitis 1984;11:1-10

199 De Groot AC. Propolis: a review of properties, applications, chemical composition, contact allergy, and other adverse effects. Dermatitis 2013;24:263-82

200 Lynde CW, Mitchell JC. Patch testing with balsam of Peru and fragrance mix. Contact Dermatitis 1982;8:274-277

201 Claßen A, Buhl T, Schubert S, Worm M, Bauer A, Geier J, Molin S; Information Network of Departments of Dermatology (IVDK) study group. The frequency of specific contact allergies is reduced in patients with psoriasis. Br J Dermatol 2018 Aug 12. doi: 10.1111/bjd.17080. [Epub ahead of print]

202 Boonstra M, Rustemeyer T, Middelkamp-Hup MA. Both children and adult patients with difficult-to-treat atopic dermatitis have high prevalences of concomitant allergic contact dermatitis and are frequently polysensitized. J Eur Acad Dermatol Venereol 2018;32:1554-1561

203 Hamann C. New fragrance mix I formulation in TRUE test. Br J Dermatol 2016;175:824

204 O'Gorman SM, Torgerson RR. Contact allergy in cheilitis. Int J Dermatol 2016;55:e386-e391

205 Landeck L, Schalock PC, Baden LA, Gonzalez E. Periorbital contact sensitization. Am J Ophthalmol 2010;150:366-370

206 Landeck L, González E, Baden L, Neumann K, Schalock P. Positive concomitant test reactions to allergens in the standard patch test series. Int J Dermatol 2010;49:517-519.

207 Warshaw EM, Ahmed RL, Belsito DV, DeLeo VA, Fowler JF Jr, Maibach HI, et al. Contact dermatitis of the hands: cross-sectional analyses of North American Contact Dermatitis Group Data, 1994-2004. J Am Acad Dermatol 2007;57:301-314

208 Sharma VK, Sethuraman G, Bansal A. Evaluation of photopatch test series in India. Contact Dermatitis 2007;56:168-169

209 Lazarov A, David M, Abraham D, Trattner A. Comparison of reactivity to allergens using the TRUE Test and IQ chamber system. Contact Dermatitis 2007;56:140-145

210 Saap L, Fahim S, Arsenault E, Pratt M, Pierscianowski T, Falanga V, Pedvis-Leftick A. Contact sensitivity in patients with leg ulcerations: a North American study. Arch Dermatol 2004;140:1241-1246

211 Li LF, Wang J. Contact hypersensitivity in hand dermatitis. Contact Dermatitis 2002;47:206-209

212 Sherertz EF, Fransway AF, Belsito DV, DeLeo VA, Fowler JF Jr, Maibach HI, et al. Patch testing discordance alert: false-negative findings with rubber additives and fragrances. J Am Acad Dermatol 2001;45:313-314

213 Albert MR, Chang Y, González E. Concomitant positive reactions to allergens in a patch testing standard series from 1988-1997. Am J Contact Dermat 1999;10:219-223

214 Paulsen E, Andersen KE, Brandão FM, Bruynzeel DP, Ducombs G, Frosch PJ, et al. Routine patch testing with the sesquiterpene lactone mix in Europe: a 2-year experience. A multicentre study of the EECDRG. Contact Dermatitis 1999;40:72-76

215 Girbig M, Hegewald J, Seidler A, Bauer A, Uter W, Schmitt J. Type IV sensitizations in physical therapists: patch test results of the Information Network of Departments of Dermatology (IVDK) 2007-2011. J Dtsch Dermatol Ges 2013;11:1185-1192

216 Silvestre JF, Mercader P, González-Pérez R, Hervella-Garcés M, Sanz-Sánchez T, Córdoba S, et al. Sensitization to fragrances in Spain: A 5-year multicentre study (2011-2015). Contact Dermatitis. 2018 Nov 14. doi: 10.1111/cod.13152. [Epub ahead of print]

217 DeKoven JG, Warshaw EM, Zug KA, Maibach HI, Belsito DV, Sasseville D, et al. North American Contact Dermatitis Group patch test results: 2015-2016. Dermatitis 2018;29:297-309

218 Veverka KK, Hall MR, Yiannias JA, Drage LA, El-Azhary RA, Killian JM, et al. Trends in patch testing with the Mayo Clinic standard series, 2011-2015. Dermatitis 2018;29:310-315

219 Gilissen L, Huygens S, Goossens A. Allergic contact dermatitis caused by topical herbal remedies: importance of patch testing with the patients' own products. Contact Dermatitis 2018;78:177-184

Chapter 3.71   FRAGRANCE MIX II

IDENTIFICATION

Description/definition   : The fragrance mix II is a mixture of fragrance materials for patch testing. It contains 6
chemicals in a total concentration of 14% in petrolatum: citral (1%), citronellol (0.5%),
coumarin (2.5%), farnesol (2.5%), hexyl cinnamal (5%) and hydroxyisohexyl 3-cyclohexene
carboxaldehyde (2.5%). See the individual chapters of these chemicals for their specific
data

Patch testing   : 14% Pet. (SmartPracticeEurope, Chemotechnique, SmartPracticeCanada)

GENERAL

At the end of the 20th century it became increasingly clear that a considerable number of clinically relevant cases of
sensitization to fragrances were not 'picked up' by the fragrance indicators (fragrance markers) fragrance mix I and
Myroxylon pereirae resin (balsam of Peru) in the European baseline series. Therefore, a new mixture of fragrances,
the fragrance mix II (FM II), was constituted by the EECDRG (European Environmental and Contact Dermatitis
Research Group) (5). It contained six chemicals that had given most positive reactions in a previously performed
European multicenter trial with 14 frequently used chemicals: hydroxyisohexyl 3-cyclohexene carboxaldehyde (Lyral
®), citral, farnesol, citronellol, hexyl cinnamal and coumarin (65). In a dose-finding study, the results of testing with
FM II with total concentrations of 2.8%, 14% and 28% in petrolatum were compared and it was decided that the 14%
preparation was the most appropriate diagnostic screening tool (4,5). It was found that this mix identified additional
fragrance-sensitive patients who did not react to the fragrance mix I, the FM I being negative in about 1/3 of
individuals reacting to the FM II (5).

In a German study performed in 2005, 535 of 6968 (7.7%) patients reacted to fragrance mix I and 321 of 6968
(4.6%) patients to fragrance mix II. One hundred and fifty of them reacted to both allergens; 171 patients (2.5% of
the test population and 53% of subjects reacting to the FM II) tested negatively to fragrance mix I but positively to
fragrance mix II (66). This study showed that the fragrance mix II at 14.0% in pet. has acceptable diagnostic qualities
and is helpful as an additional marker for fragrance allergy (11).

The 14% fragrance mix II was added to the European baseline series in 2008 as advised by the EECDRG (11). It
was recommended, whenever there is a positive reaction to fragrance mix II, to perform additional patch testing
with the 6 ingredients, or 5 if there are simultaneous positive reactions to hydroxyisohexyl 3-cyclohexene
carboxaldehyde (HICC) and FM II (HICC was also added at the same time to the baseline series as single chemical).
Soon thereafter, in subsequent studies by the ESSCA (European Surveillance System on Contact Allergy network)
(22), the IVDK (Informationsverbund Dermatologischer Kliniken; Germany, Switzerland, Austria) (45) and in a
multicenter Danish study (54) testing the FM II in larger populations of patients with dermatitis, equally high rates of
4.7% (22), 4.6% (45) and 4.5% (54) positive reactions to the mix were observed, many of those in individuals with a
negative reaction to the FM I, thereby confirming the usefulness of the FM II.

CONTACT ALLERGY

General population

In the period 2008-2011, in 5 European countries (Sweden, Germany, Netherlands, Portugal, Italy), a random sample
of the general population of 3119 individuals aged 18-74 years were patch tested with the FM II and its 6 ingredients.
There were 60 reactions (1.9%) to FM II, tested 14% in petrolatum. About half of all positive reactions to fragrances
were considered to be relevant based on standardized criteria. Women were affected twice as often (2.5%) as men
(1.3%) (18,58).

Patch testing in groups of patients

Results of patch testing FM II in consecutive patients suspected of contact dermatitis (routine testing) are shown in
table 3.71.1. Results of testing in groups of *selected* patients (e.g. geriatric nurses with occupational contact
dermatitis, individuals with eyelid dermatitis, patients with stasis dermatitis, female hairdressers and their clients,
patients suspected of fragrance or cosmetic allergy) are shown in table 3.71.2.

Patch testing in consecutive patients suspected of contact dermatitis: routine testing

In 37 studies published since the fragrance mix II was first used for patch testing in 2002-2003 (5), frequencies of
sensitization have ranged from 1.4% to 8.0%. The high rate of 8% was seen in a small study performed in Thailand in
2013-2014, in which most other fragrances also had high scores of positive patch test reactions (39). Most studies
found sensitization rates of 3-5.2%, but a Dutch 2015-2017 study scored 6.8% positive reactions (69). There are no

major differences between Europe, the USA, Australia and Singapore, but Thailand had a higher rate (8% [39]) and Iran a far lower frequency of reactions to the FM II (1.1% [7]).

Table 3.71.1 Patch testing in groups of patients: Routine testing

Years and Country	Test conc. & vehicle	Number of patients tested	positive (%)	Selection of patients (S); Relevance (R); Comments (C)	Ref.
2015-2017 NACDG	14% pet.	5594	299 (5.3%)	R: definite + probable relevance: 37%	71
2015-7 Netherlands		821	56 (6.8%)	R: not stated	69
2015-2016 UK	14% pet.	2084	61 (2.9%)	R: not specified for individual fragrances; 25% of patients who reacted to any fragrance or fragrance marker had a positive fragrance history	14
2011-2015 Spain	14% pet.	19,588	661 (3.3%)	R: not stated	70
2011-2015 USA	14% pet.	2572	67 (2.6%)	R: not stated	72
2010-2015 Denmark	14% pet.	6004	(4.4%)	R: present relevance 68%, past relevance 35%; current and/or past relevance: 82%	60
2009-2015 Sweden	14% pet.	4430	143 (3.2%)	R: not stated; C: the use of preparations from different suppliers affected the patch test results	49
2013-2014 NACDG	14% pet.	4859	277 (5.7%)	R: definite + probable relevance: 39%	24
2013-2014 Twelve European countries, 46 departments [a]	14% pet.	28,145	(4.0%)	R: not stated; C: results of 6 occupational dermatology clinics and one pediatric clinic not included in these figures; range of positive reactions: 0.4%-9.1%	25
2013-2014 Thailand		312	25 (8.0%)	R: 84%	39
2013-2014 Sweden	14% pet.	2118	68 (3.2%)	R: not stated; C: range per center: 0.8-6.4%; a FM II mix containing 5% HICC (instead of the usual 2.5%) did not detect significantly more positive patients, but also did not increase the irritancy of the mix	57
2010-2014 IVDK	14% pet.	48,956	2535 (5.2%)	R: not stated	62
2009-2014 NACDG	14% pet.	13,398	695 (5.2%)	R: not stated	62
2008-2014 UK	14% pet.	3537	51 (1.4%)	R: not stated; C: there were 0.7% ?+ and 0.8% irritant reactions	38
2009-2013 Singapore	14% pet.	2598	(3.9%)	R: present + past relevance 26%; C: range of positive reactions per year 2.5-5.4%	36
2011-2012 NACDG	14% pet.	4237	219 (5.2%)	R: definite + probable relevance: 38%	19
2011-2012 UK	14% pet.	1951	64 (3.3%)	R: not stated	43
2009-2012 Twelve European countries [a]	14% pet.	51,477	(4.0%)	R: not stated; C: range per country: 1.5-7.8%	41
2005-2012 IVDK	14% pet.	81,290	(4.9%)	R: not stated	15
2005-2011 Belgium	14% pet.	3416	205 (6.0%)	R: not stated	59
2008-2010 Denmark	14% pet.	1503	60 (4.0%)	S: mostly routine testing; R: 83%	1
2006-2011 Sweden	14% pet.	10,001	337 (3.4%)	R: not stated; C: range per center: 2.1-6.3%	56
2009-2010 NACDG	14% pet.	4307	(4.7%)	R: definite + probable relevance: 42%	29
2006-2010 USA	14% pet.	2713	(6.1%)	R: 53%	21
2001-2010 Australia	14% pet.	855	37 (4.3%)	R: 43%	23
2007-2009 Sweden	14% pet.	1178	21 (1.8%)	R: not stated	50
2007-2009 Hungary	14% pet.	1555	105 (6.8%)	R: not stated	55
2007-2008 NACDG	14% pet.	5071	(3.6%)	R: definite + probable relevance: 40%	9
2004-2008 Spain	14% pet.	450	7 (1.6%)	R: not stated	13
2007-2008 10 European countries [a]	14% pet.	22,243	866 (3.9%)	R: not stated; prevalences ranged from 1.9% (Spain) to 7.9% (Austria) [a]	10
2005-2008 Denmark	14% pet.	12,302	553 (4.5%)	R: 72%	54
2005-2008 IVDK	14% pet.	35,738	(4.6%)	R: not stated; C: same population as in ref. 53	45
2005-2008 IVDK	14% pet.	35,633	1742 (4.9%)	R: not stated; C: same population as in ref. 45	53
2004-2008 Iran	14% pet.	267	3 (1.1%)	R: 82% of all reactions to FM I, FM II, *Myroxylon pereirae* resin, hydroxyisohexyl 3-cyclohexene carboxaldehyde and/or turpentine were clinically relevant	7
2005-2006 Ten European countries [a]	14% pet.	5402	255 (4.7%)	R: not stated; C: prevalences were 5.5% in Central Europe, 2.5% in West, 4.0% in Northeast and 1.8% in South Europe	22
2005 Germany	14% pet.	7014	329 (4.7%)	R: not stated; C: in a subgroup of 7002 patients tested with both FM II and its ingredient HICC, 85% of HICC-positives co-reacted to FM II and 46% of FM II-positives co-reacted to HICC	66
2002-2003, Six European countries	14% pet.	1701	50 (2.9%)	R: not stated	5

[a] study of the ESSCA (European Surveillance System on Contact Allergy)
FM: Fragrance Mix; IVDK: Informationsverbund Dermatologischer Kliniken (Germany, Switzerland, Austria); NACDG: North American Contact Dermatitis Group (USA, Canada)

However, the differences in rates of sensitization between countries in the studies of the ESSCA (European Surveillance System on Contact Allergy) are striking, ranging from 0.4 to 9.1% (25), 1.5 to 7.8% (41), 1.9 to 7.9% (10) and 1.8 to 5.5% (large geographical areas [22]). The highest prevalences appear to occur in Central Europe (Germany, Austria, Switzerland), the lowest in southern Europe including Spain (10,13,22,70). Large variations are even seen in different clinics in one country, Sweden: 0.8-6.4% (57) and 2.1-6.3% (56).

Table 3.71.2 Patch testing in groups of patients: Selected patient groups

Years and Country	Test conc. & vehicle	Number of patients tested	positive (%)	Selection of patients (S); Relevance (R); Comments (C)	Ref.
2014-2017 USA		502	14 (2.8%)	S: consecutive adult patients with dermatitis; R: not stated; C: the prevalence of sensitization in patients with active atopic dermatitis (5.6%) was significantly higher than in those without (2.0%) which was ascribed to the use of personal care products	63
2014-2016 France		264	5 (1.9%)	S: patients suspected of eyelid allergic contact dermatitis; R: 1/5 (20%)	61
1996-2015 IVDK	14% pet.	1474	26 (1.7%)	S: patients with psoriasis; R: not stated; C: the percentage of positive reactions was significantly lower than in the control group of consecutive dermatitis patients (4.5%)	67
2005-2014 IVDK	14% pet.	650	60 (8.2%)	S: geriatric nurses with occupational contact dermatitis; R: not stated; C: the frequency was significantly higher than in a control group of geriatric nurses without occupational contact dermatitis (4.0%)	64
2003-2014 IVDK	14% pet.	5202	(6.8%)	S: patients with stasis dermatitis / chronic leg ulcers; R: not stated; C: percentage of reactions significantly higher than in a control group of routine testing	30
1996-2013 Nether-Lands	14% pet.	574	28 (4.9%)	S: children aged 0-17 years; R: not stated; *not* significantly more reactions in children with atopic dermatitis (5.3%) than in those without atopic dermatitis (4.3%)	29
1994-2013 IVDK	14% pet.	1203	(6.3%)	S: patients suspected of airborne contact dermatitis; R: not stated; C: the frequency in a control group was 5.1%; the difference was not statistically significant	40
2007-2012 IVDK	14% pet.	698	33 (4.7%)	S: female hairdressers with current or previous occupational contact dermatitis; R: not stated	34
		1895	86 (4.5%)	S: female patients, clients of hairdressers, in who hair cosmetics were regarded as a cause of dermatitis, and who had never worked as hairdressers; R: not stated	
2003-2012 IVDK	14% pet.	1625	121 (7.4%)	S: nurses with occupational contact dermatitis; R: not stated	26
2007-2011 IVDK	14% pet.	115	15 (13.0%)	S: physical therapists; R: not stated; C: the frequency of sensitization was 'distinctly' higher than in routine testing (7.4%)	68
2006-2011 IVDK	14% pet.	10,124	559 (5.9%)	S: patients with suspected cosmetic intolerance; R: not stated; C: the prevalence was significantly higher than in a control group matched for sex and age	33
2009-2010 Hungary	14% pet.	565	97 (17.2%)	S: patients with former skin symptoms provoked by scented products in the case history; R: not specified	3
2006-2010 USA	14% pet.	100	19 (19%)	S: patients with eyelid dermatitis; R: not stated	6
2000-2010 IVDK		3007	148 (4.5%)	S: patients with periorbital dermatitis; R: not stated; C: the frequency was equal to a control group of routine testing	27
1994-2010 NACDG	1% water	432	? (?)	S: hairdressers / cosmetologists; R: in the group of 57 patients who had at least one relevant occupationally related reaction, 2 (3.5%) reacted to FM II	28
2005-7 Netherlands	14% pet.	227	21 (9.3%)	S: patients suspected of fragrance or cosmetic allergy; R: 61% relevance for all positive tested fragrances together	2
2000-2007 USA	14% pet.	192	10 (5.2%)	S: patients who were tested with a supplemental cosmetic screening series; R: 100%; C: weak study: a. high rate of macular erythema and weak reactions; b. relevance figures included 'questionable' and 'past' relevance	8
2005-2006 IVDK	14% pet.	151	(6.3%)	S: female hairdressers with suspected occupational contact dermatitis; R: not stated	32
2003-2006 IVDK	14% pet.	316	(3.8%)	S: women with suspected reactions to hair cosmetics; R: not stated	32

NACDG: North American Contact Dermatitis Group (USA, Canada)

In 24/37 investigations no (specific) relevance data were provided. In the studies performed by the NACDG (North American Contact Dermatitis Group), about 40% of the positive patch tests to FM II were considered to have definite or probable relevance (9,19,24,29,71). In the other studies addressing the issue of relevance, scores ranged from 26% to 84% (1,21,23,36,39,54,60). Culprit products were never mentioned.

Patch testing in groups of selected patients

Results of testing in groups of selected patients (e.g. geriatric nurses with occupational contact dermatitis, individuals with eyelid dermatitis, patients with stasis dermatitis, female hairdressers and their clients, patients suspected of fragrance or cosmetic allergy) are shown in table 3.71.2. Frequencies of sensitization have ranged from 1.7% to 19%. The latter high rate was observed in patients with eyelid dermatitis (6). Other high frequencies of sensitization were observed in patients with former skin symptoms provoked by scented products in the case history (17.2% [3]), physical therapists (13.0% [68]), patients suspected of fragrance or cosmetic allergy (9.3% [2]), geriatric nurses with occupational contact dermatitis (8.2% [64]) and nurses with occupational contact dermatitis (7.4% [26]). Prevalence rates of sensitization to FM II were significantly higher than in control groups in patients with adult atopic dermatitis (63), geriatric nurses (64), patients with stasis dermatitis / chronic leg ulcers (30), and physical therapists (68). Specific causative products were never mentioned.

The relationship between reactivity to the fragrance mix II and its 6 constituents

The fragrance mix II has 6 ingredients. When patients reacting to the mix are patch tested at the same time or later with its composing fragrances, one might expect all patients to react at least to one of the constituents, especially as these are tested separately at twice the concentrations they have in the mix. However, just as with the fragrance mix I, quite a few FM II-allergic individuals (17-52%, table 3.71.3) do not react to any constituent at all. The reverse situation also occurs: in patients with positive patch tests to one or more constituents, there is no allergic reaction to the mix.

Fragrance mix II positive, ingredients negative

Data on a negative 'breakdown' (no reactions to any ingredient) in patients reacting to the fragrance mix II are shown in table 3.71.3. The percentage of negative reactions to any ingredient ranged from 17% to 52% (median 35%). It is clear that the strength of the reaction to the FM II determines the rate of negatives to the ingredients: the stronger the patch test, the lower the percentage of negative reactions to any ingredient (16,49,53,58,60). In patients with a weak positive (+) patch test reaction to the FM II, a negative breakdown was seen in 24-67%, decreasing to <8.5-28% for ++ reactions and 0-7% for extreme positive (+++) reactions (the 26% shown in the table refers to ++ and +++ reactions together, data not specified). Possible explanations for negative reactions to any ingredient include false-positive reactions to the mix, enhancement of elicitation of contact allergic reactions by allergen mixtures (indicating false-negative reactions to single ingredients (51,52)), increased skin penetration caused by the (combined) irritancy of other constituents of the mix, or the formation of new allergens in the mix.

Table 3.71.3 Negative reactions to any constituent in fragrance mix II-allergic individuals

Years	Country	Nr. Pat. FM II +	Nr. Pat. Neg. to ingredients (percentage)	Negative reactions to ingredients and strength of reaction to fragrance mix II			Ref.
				+ reaction	++ reaction	+++ reaction	
2011-2015	Spain	419	164 (39%)				70
2010-2015	Denmark	256	110 (43%)	67%	28%	0%	60
2009-2015	Sweden	143	50 (35%)	44%	26% [a]	26% [a]	49
2005-2013	IVDK	1058	380 (36%)	47%	11%	7%	16
2008-2011	Sweden, Germany, Italy, Netherlands, Portugal	60	10 (17%)	24%	10%	0%	58
2005-2010	The Netherlands	33	12 (36%)				48
2005-2008	IVDK	367	(32%)	59%	8.5% [a]	8.5% [a]	53
2005-2007	Hungary	37	10 (27%)				5
2002-2003	Germany, Belgium, France, UK, Denmark, Sweden	50	26 (52%)				4

[a] ++ and +++ reactions together
IVDK: Informationsverbund Dermatologischer Kliniken (Germany, Switzerland, Austria)

Ingredients positive, fragrance mix II negative

The reverse situation, positive reactions to one or more ingredients of the FM II but a negative reaction to the mix itself also occurs. In a study from Denmark, performed in the period 2010-2015, positive reactions to the constituents in 194 patients were in about 88% accompanied by a positive (75.3%) or doubtful positive (12.4%)

reaction to the mix. The percentage of concomitant positive reactions to the mix (excluding doubtful positive reactions) was the lowest for farnesol (50%) and coumarin (57%) and the highest for hydroxyisohexyl 3-cyclohexene carboxaldehyde (92%) and citronellol (100%) (60). In a Swedish investigation, 36% of the patients who showed positive reactions to one or more of the ingredients of FM II were FM II-negative (49).

The incomplete co-reactivity of individual ingredients and the fragrance mix II may (to some extent) be explained by the fact that the concentrations used for ingredient patch testing are twice those used in the FM II.

Testing with the 6 constituents in fragrance mix II-reactive individuals

The results of studies testing the individual ingredients of the mix in FM II-positive patients (tested either concurrently or later) are show in table 3.71.4. By far most reactions were to hydroxyisohexyl 3-cyclohexene carboxaldehyde with percentages positive reactions ranging from 28.3% to 47.7%. Second comes citral (11.2-19.0%), followed by farnesol (2.7-13.9%). Coumarin and citronellol least frequency give positive reactions. Ranges of positive reactions, medians and average rates (unadjusted for sample sizes) for all 6 components are shown in table 3.71.4.

As concerns hydroxyisohexyl 3-cyclohexene carboxaldehyde, a significant downward trend from 48% positive reactions in 2007-2008 to 28% in 2013 has been noted in a large IVDK study (16). Undoubtedly this indicates a reduction in its use or use concentrations by manufacturers as a result of the vast amount on publications on contact allergy to and allergic contact dermatitis from this fragrance (Chapter 3.84 Hydroxyisohexyl 3-cyclohexene carboxaldehyde). It should be realized that the 4 IVDK studies shown in table 3.71.4 have overlapping populations and test results, thereby unduly influencing the average and median concentrations.

Table 3.71.4 Testing with the 6 ingredients (or only HICC) in patients reacting to the fragrance mix

Years and Country	Nr. pat.	Percentage of positive reactions to ingredients						Ref.
		HICC 5% pet	Citral 2% pet.	Farnesol 5% pet.	Hexyl cin 10% pet.	Coumarin 5% pet.	Citronellol 1% pet.	
2013-2014 Sweden [d]	68	37						57
2005-2013 IVDK [c]	1058	40.2 [a]	16.2	12.4	4.9 [b]	3.4	3.0	16
2006-2011 IVDK [c]	137	46.7	19.0	13.9	7.3	4.4	5.8	31
2006-2011 Sweden [d]	337	44						56
2005-2011 Belgium	205	28.3	11.2	13.2	9.7	4.4	5.4	59
2005-2008 IVDK [c]	367	47.7	16.1	11.4	3.8	2.7	2.5	53
2005-2008 Denmark [d]	553	44						54
2005-2007 Hungary	37	43.2	13.5	2.7	8.1	8.1	8.1	55
2005 IVDK [c]	65	38.5	16.9	10.8	0	4.6	0	66
2005 Six European countries	50	36	12	8	2	0	2	4
2005 Germany [d]	324	46						66
Range		36-47.7	11.2-19.0	2.7-13.9	0-9.7	0-8.1	0-8.1	
Median		40.2	16.1	11.4	4.9	4.4	3.0	
Average (unadjusted for sample size)		43.2	15.0	10.3	5.1	3.9	3.8	

[a] Significant downward trend from 48% positive reactions in 2007-2008 to 28% in 2013
[b] Increase from 3% positive reactions in 2005-2006 to 11% in 2011-2012
[c] Overlap in data with other IVDK studies
[d] Only hydroxyisohexyl 3-cyclohexene carboxaldehyde was tested
Hexyl cin: Hexyl cinnamal; HICC: Hydroxyisohexyl 3-cyclohexene carboxaldehyde
IVDK: Informationsverbund Dermatologischer Kliniken (Germany, Switzerland, Austria)

Most patients with positive reactions to FM II who also react to one or more ingredients showed co-reactivity to one single constituent, most often hydroxyisohexyl 3-cyclohexene carboxaldehyde. Of 1058 patients reacting to the FM II, 543 (51.3%) reacted to a single constituent, 90 (8.5%) to two, 33 (3.1%) to three, 10 (0.9%) to 4 and 2 (0.2%) had positive patch tests to 5 of the 6 ingredients of the mix (16).

Case reports and case series

FM II was stated to be the (or an) allergen in 82 patients in a group of 603 individuals suffering from cosmetic dermatitis, seen in the period 2010-2015 in Leuven, Belgium (17). As the FM II *per se* is not an allergen in cosmetics, this statement is not quite correct. Possibly, one or more of its constituents were considered to be the allergen, for example when found to be present by labeling on products used by the patient and considered to be relevant.

In the period 1996-2013, in a tertiary referral center in Valencia, Spain, 5419 patients were patch tested. Of these, 628 individuals had allergic contact dermatitis to cosmetics. In this group, FM II was considered to be the responsible allergen in 21 cases (12), which is equally incorrect.

In the period 2000-2009, in Leuven, Belgium, an unspecified number of patients had positive patch tests or use tests to a total of 344 cosmetic products *and* positive patch tests to FM I, FM II, and/or to one or more of 28 selected specific fragrance ingredients. In 44 of 73 patients reacting to FM II, the presence of one or more of its components in the cosmetic product(s) was confirmed by reading the product label(s) (44).

A man had pustular patch test reactions to FM II, citral (an ingredient of FM II), oakmoss and an aftershave, which had caused a pustular eruption on the face. It was unknown whether the aftershave contained oakmoss and/or citral (42). A woman, known to be allergic to fragrances and therefore avoiding fragranced products, had connubial contact dermatitis from the deodorants of her husband. She reacted to FM I, FM II, Myroxylon pereirae resin and 2 deodorant sprays. After the husband stopped using fragranced products, the dermatitis quickly disappeared. Unfortunately, no attempt was made to identify the sensitizer(s) (47).

Cross-reactions, pseudo-cross-reactions and co-reactions

General
For general information on cross-/pseudo-cross-/co-reactivity of fragrance chemicals with other fragrances, fragrance markers (fragrance mix I, fragrance mix II, colophonium, Myroxylon pereirae resin [balsam of Peru]) and essential oils see Chapter 1.2 General information on cross-reactions, pseudo-cross-reactions and co-reactions. Co-reactivity of citral, citronellol, coumarin, farnesol, hexyl cinnamal and hydroxyisohexyl 3-cyclohexene carboxaldehyde can be expected, as these are ingredients of the Fragrance mix II (pseudo-cross-reactions).

Fragrance mix I
Co-reactivity to fragrance mix I in FM II-positive patients is frequent, as shown by the following studies. In a large study by the IVDK, concomitant reactions to FM I were observed in 42% of 1742 patients reacting to FM II (53). In a group of 553 patients reacting to FM II, 217 (39%) co-reacted to FM I (54). In a cohort of 105 individuals with positive patch tests to FM II, there were 35 (33%) co-reactions to the FM I (55). In Belgium, 106 of 205 patients (52%) allergic to FM II co-reacted to FM I (59). Fifty-one per cent of the patients who were FM II-positive were also FM I-positive (49). In a group of 59 patients allergic to FM II seen in The Netherlands, 26 (44%) co-reacted to FM I (48).

In patients with polysensitization (defined as at least 3 positive patch test reactions), the following allergens were particularly associated with the FM II: Myroxylon pereirae resin (odds ratio [OR] 34.2) and FM I (OR 25.4) (35).

Other co-reactions
Positive patch test reactions to FM I and/or FM II have a statistically significant association with positive reactions to methylchloroisothiazolinone/methylisothiazolinone (MCI/MI) and/or methylisothiazolinone (MI) and with positive reactions to formaldehyde. Presumably, fragrances and preservatives are often present in the same consumer products. The association between allergies to these two groups of chemicals might be explained either by the use of a range of products containing different combinations of allergens, or different products with different combinations of allergens being used by the same person (37).

OTHER SIDE EFFECTS

Immediate-type reactions
Of 565 patients with a history of former skin symptoms provoked by scented products and patch tested with the fragrance mix II, 12 (2.1%) had a contact urticarial reaction to the mix (3).

LITERATURE

1   Heisterberg MV, Menné T, Johansen JD. Contact allergy to the 26 specific fragrance ingredients to be declared on cosmetic products in accordance with the EU cosmetic directive. Contact Dermatitis 2011;65:266-275
2   Oosten EJ van, Schuttelaar ML, Coenraads PJ. Clinical relevance of positive patch test reactions to the 26 EU-labelled fragrances. Contact Dermatitis 2009;61:217-223
3   Pónyai G, Németh I, Altmeyer A, Nagy G, Irinyi B, Battya Z, et al. Patch tests with fragrance mix II and its components. Dermatitis 2012;23:71-74
4   Frosch PJ, Rastogi SC, Pirker C, Brinkmeier T, Andersen KE, Bruze M, et al. Patch testing with a new fragrance mix - reactivity to the individual constituents and chemical detection in relevant cosmetic products. Contact Dermatitis 2005;52:216-225

5   Frosch PJ, Pirker C, Rastogi SC, Andersen KE, Bruze M, Svedman C, et al. Patch testing with a new fragrance mix detects additional patients sensitive to perfumes and missed by the current fragrance mix. Contact Dermatitis 2005;52:207-215

6   Wenk KS, Ehrlich AE. Fragrance series testing in eyelid dermatitis. Dermatitis 2012;23:22-26

7   Firooz A, Nassiri-Kashani M, Khatami A, Gorouhi F, Babakoohi S, Montaser-Kouhsari L, et al. Fragrance contact allergy in Iran. J Eur Acad Dermatol Venereol 2010;24:1437-1441

8   Wetter DA, Yiannias JA, Prakash AV, Davis MDP, Farmer SA, el-Azhary RA. Results of patch testing to personal care product allergens in a standard series and a supplemental cosmetic series: an analysis of 945 patients from the Mayo Clinic Contact Dermatitis Group, 2000-2007. J Am Acad Dermatol 2010;63:789-798

9   Fransway AF, Zug KA, Belsito DV, Deleo VA, Fowler JF Jr, Maibach HI, et al. North American Contact Dermatitis Group patch test results for 2007-2008. Dermatitis 2013;24:10-21

10   Uter W, Aberer W, Armario-Hita JC, Fernandez-Vozmediano JM, Ayala F, Balato A, et al. Current patch test results with the European baseline series and extensions to it from the 'European Surveillance System on Contact Allergy' network, 2007-2008. Contact Dermatitis 2012;67:9-19

11   Bruze M, Andersen KE, Goossens A. Recommendation to include fragrance mix 2 and hydroxyisohexyl 3-cyclohexene carboxaldehyde (Lyral) in the European baseline patch test series. Contact Dermatitis 2008;58:129-133

12   Zaragoza-Ninet V, Blasco Encinas R, Vilata-Corell JJ, Pérez-Ferriols A, Sierra-Talamantes C, Esteve-Martínez A, de la Cuadra-Oyanguren J. Allergic contact dermatitis due to cosmetics: A clinical and epidemiological study in a tertiary hospital. Actas Dermosifiliogr 2016;107:329-336

13   Cuesta L, Silvestre JF, Toledo F, Lucas A, Perez-Crespo M, Ballester I. Fragrance contact allergy: a 4-year retrospective study. Contact Dermatitis 2010;63:77-84

14   Ung CY, White JML, White IR, Banerjee P, McFadden JP. Patch testing with the European baseline series fragrance markers: a 2016 update. Br J Dermatol 2018;178:776-780

15   Uter W, Fießler C, Gefeller O, Geier J, Schnuch A. Contact sensitization to fragrance mix I and II, to *Myroxylon pereirae* resin and oil of tupentine: multifactorial analysis of risk factors based on data of the IVDK network. Flavour and Fragrance Journal 2015;30:255-263

16   Geier J, Uter W, Lessmann H, Schnuch A. Fragrance mix I and II: results of breakdown tests. Flavour Fragr J 2015;30:264-274

17   Goossens A. Cosmetic contact allergens. Cosmetics 2016, 3, 5; doi:10.3390/cosmetics3010005

18   Diepgen TL, Ofenloch RF, Bruze M, Bertuccio P, Cazzaniga S, Coenraads P-J, et al. Prevalence of contact allergy in the general population in different European regions. Br J Dermatol 2016;174:319-329

19   Warshaw EM, Maibach HI, Taylor JS, Sasseville D, DeKoven JG, Zirwas MJ, et al. North American Contact Dermatitis Group patch test results: 2011-2012. Dermatitis 2015;26:49-59

20   Warshaw EM, Belsito DV, Taylor JS, Sasseville D, DeKoven JG, Zirwas MJ, et al. North American Contact Dermatitis Group patch test results: 2009 to 2010. Dermatitis 2013;24:50-59

21   Wentworth AB, Yiannias JA, Keeling JH, Hall MR, Camilleri MJ, Drage LA, et al. Trends in patch-test results and allergen changes in the standard series: a Mayo Clinic 5-year retrospective review (January 1, 2006, to December 31, 2010). J Am Acad Dermatol 2014;70:269-275

22   Uter W, Rämsch C, Aberer W, Ayala F, Balato A, Beliauskiene A, et al. The European baseline series in 10 European Countries, 2005/2006 – Results of the European Surveillance System on Contact Allergies (ESSCA). Contact Dermatitis 2009;61:31-38

23   Toholka R, Wang Y-S, Tate B, Tam M, Cahill J, Palmer A, Nixon R. The first Australian Baseline Series: Recommendations for patch testing in suspected contact dermatitis. Australas J Dermatol 2015;56:107-115

24   DeKoven JG, Warshaw EM, Belsito DV, Sasseville D, Maibach HI, Taylor JS, et al. North American Contact Dermatitis Group Patch Test Results: 2013-2014. Dermatitis 2017;28:33-46

25   Uter W, Amario-Hita JC, Balato A, Ballmer-Weber B, Bauer A, Belloni Fortina A, et al. European Surveillance System on Contact Allergies (ESSCA): results with the European baseline series, 2013/14. J Eur Acad Dermatol Venereol 2017;31:1516-1525

26   Molin S, Bauer A, Schnuch A, Geier J. Occupational contact allergy in nurses: results from the Information Network of Departments of Dermatology 2003–2012. Contact Dermatitis 2015;72:164-171

27   Landeck L, John SM, Geier J. Periorbital dermatitis in 4779 patients – patch test results during a 10-year period. Contact Dermatitis 2014;70:205-212

28   Warshaw EM, Wang MZ, Mathias CGT, Maibach HI, Belsito DV, Zug KA, et al. Occupational contact dermatitis in hairdressers/cosmetologists; retrospective analysis of North American Contact Dermatitis Group data, 1994 to 2010. Dermatitis 2012;23:258-268

29   Lubbes S, Rustemeyer T, Sillevis Smitt JH, Schuttelaar ML, Middelkamp-Hup MA. Contact sensitization in Dutch children and adolescents with and without atopic dermatitis - a retrospective analysis. Contact Dermatitis 2017;76:151-159

30 Erfurt-Berge C, Geier J, Mahler V. The current spectrum of contact sensitization in patients with chronic leg ulcers or stasis dermatitis - new data from the Information Network of Departments of Dermatology (IVDK). Contact Contact Dermatitis 2017;77:151-158

31 Dinkloh A, Worm M, Geier J, Schnuch A, Wollenberg A. Contact sensitization in patients with suspected cosmetic intolerance: results of the IVDK 2006-2011. J Eur Acad Dermatol Venereol 2015;29:1071-1081

32 Uter W, Lessmann H, Geier J, Schnuch A. Contact allergy to hairdressing allergens in female hairdressers and clients – current data from the IVDK 2003–2006. J Dtsch Dermatol Ges 2007;5:993-1001

33 Dinkloh A, Worm M, Geier J, Schnuch A, Wollenberg A. Contact sensitization in patients with suspected cosmetic intolerance: results of the IVDK 2006-2011. J Eur Acad Dermatol Venereol 2015;29:1071-1081

34 Uter W, Gefeller O, John SM, Schnuch A, Geier J. Contact allergy to ingredients of hair cosmetics – a comparison of female hairdressers and clients based on IVDK 2007–2012 data. Contact Dermatitis 2014;71:13-20

35 Adler W, Gefeller O, Uter W. Positive reactions to pairs of allergens associated with polysensitization: analysis of IVDK data with machine-learning techniques. Contact Dermatitis 2017;76:247-251

36 Ochi H, Cheng SWN, Leow YH, Goon ATJ. Contact allergy trends in Singapore – a retrospective study of patch test data from 2009 to 2013. Contact Dermatitis 2017;76:49-50

37 Pontén A, Bruze M, Engfeldt M, Hauksson I, Isaksson M. Concomitant contact allergies to formaldehyde, methylchloroisothiazolinone/methylisothiazolinone, methylisothiazolinone, and fragrance mixes I and II. Contact Dermatitis 2016;75:285-289

38 Sabroe RA, Holden CR, Gawkrodger DJ. Contact allergy to essential oils cannot always be predicted from allergy to fragrance markers in the baseline series. Contact Dermatitis 2016;74:236-241

39 Vejanurug P, Tresukosol P, Sajjachareonpong P, Puangpet P. Fragrance allergy could be missed without patch testing with 26 individual fragrance allergens. Contact Dermatitis 2016;74:230-235

40 Breuer K, Uter W, Geier J. Epidemiological data on airborne contact dermatitis – results of the IVDK. Contact Dermatitis 2015;73:239-247

41 Frosch PJ, Johansen JD, Schuttelaar M-LA, Silvestre JF, Sánchez-Pérez J, Weisshaar E, et al. (on behalf of the ESSCA network). Patch test results with fragrance markers of the baseline series – analysis of the European Surveillance System on Contact Allergies (ESSCA) network 2009–2012. Contact Dermatitis 2015;73:163-171

42 Verma A, Tancharoen C, Tam MM, Nixon R. Pustular allergic contact dermatitis caused by fragrances. Contact Dermatitis 2015;72:245-248

43 Mann J, McFadden JP, White JML, White IR, Banerjee P. Baseline series fragrance markers fail to predict contact allergy. Contact Dermatitis 2014;70:276-281

44 Nardelli A, Drieghe J, Claes L, Boey L, Goossens A. Fragrance allergens in 'specific' cosmetic products. Contact Dermatitis 2011;64:212-219

45 Uter W, Geier J, Frosch P, Schnuch A. Contact allergy to fragrances: current patch test results (2005–2008) from the Information Network of Departments of Dermatology. Contact Dermatitis 2010;63:254-261

46 Shi Y, Nedorost S, Scheman L, et al. Propolis, colophony, and fragrance cross-reactivity and allergic contact dermatitis. Dermatitis 2016;27:123-126

47 Jensen P, Ortiz PG, Hartmann-Petersen S, et al. Connubial allergic contact dermatitis caused by fragrance ingredients. Dermatitis 2012;23:e1-e2

48 Nagtegaal MJC, Pentinga SE, Kuik J, Kezic S, Rustemeyer T. The role of the skin irritation response in polysensitization to fragrances. Contact Dermatitis 2012;67:28-35

49 Mowitz M, Svedman C, Zimerson E, Isaksson M, Pontén A, Bruze M. Simultaneous patch testing with fragrance mix I, fragrance mix II and their ingredients in southern Sweden between 2009 and 2015. Contact Dermatitis 2017;77:280-287

50 Bråred Christensson J, Hellsén S, Börje A, Karlberg A-T. Limonene hydroperoxide analogues show specific patch test reactions. Contact Dermatitis 2014;70:291-299

51 Bonefeld CM, Nielsen MM, Rubin IM, Vennegaard MT, Dabelsteen S, Gimenéz-Arnau E, et al. Enhanced sensitization and elicitation responses caused by mixtures of common fragrance allergens. Contact Dermatitis 2011;65:336-342

52 Johansen JD, Skov L, Vølund A, Andersen K, Menné T. Allergens in combination have a synergistic effect on the elicitation response: a study of fragrance-sensitized individuals. Br J Dermatol 1998;139:264-270

53 Krautheim A, Uter W, Frosch P, Schnuch A, Geier J. Patch testing with fragrance mix II: results of the IVDK 2005-2008. Contact Dermatitis 2010;63:262-269

54 Heisterberg MV, Andersen KE, Avnstorp C, Kristensen B, Kristensen O, Kaaber K, et al. Fragrance mix II in the baseline series contributes significantly to detection of fragrance allergy. Contact Dermatitis 2010;63:270-276

55 Pónyai G, Németh I, Temesvári E. Patch-testing with fragrance mix II. Dermatitis 2011;22:169-170

56 Isaksson M, Inerot A, Lidén C, Lindberg M, Matura M, Möller H, et al. Multicentre patch testing with fragrance mix II and hydroxyisohexyl 3-cyclohexene carboxaldehyde by the Swedish Contact Dermatitis Research Group. Contact Dermatitis 2014;70:187-189

57 Engfeldt M, Hagvall L, Isaksson M, Matura M, Mowitz M, Ryberg K, et al. Patch testing with hydroxyisohexyl 3-cyclohexene carboxaldehyde (HICC) – a multicentre study of the Swedish Contact Dermatitis Research Group. Contact Dermatitis 2017;76:34-39

58 Diepgen TL, Ofenloch R, Bruze M, Cazzaniga S, Coenraads PJ, Elsner P, et al. Prevalence of fragrance contact allergy in the general population of five European countries: a cross-sectional study. Br J Dermatol 2015;173:1411-1419

59 Nardelli A, Carbonez A, Drieghe J, Goossens A. Results of patch testing with fragrance mix 1, fragrance mix 2, and their ingredients, and Myroxylon pereirae and colophonium, over a 21-year period. Contact Dermatitis 2013;68:307-313

60 Bennike NH, Zachariae C, Johansen JD. Non-mix fragrances are top sensitizers in consecutive dermatitis patients – a cross-sectional study of the 26 EU-labelled fragrance allergens. Contact Dermatitis 2017;77:270-279

61 Assier H, Tetart F, Avenel-Audran M, Barbaud A, Ferrier-le Bouëdec MC, Giordano-Labadie F, et al. Is a specific eyelid patch test series useful? Results of a French prospective study. Contact Dermatitis 2018;79:157-161

62 Warshaw EM, Zug KA, Belsito DV, Fowler JF Jr, DeKoven JG, Sasseville D, et al. Positive patch-test reactions to essential oils in consecutive patients: Results from North America and Central Europe. Dermatitis 2017;28:246-252

63 Rastogi S, Patel KR, Singam V, Silverberg JI. Allergic contact dermatitis to personal care products and topical medications in adults with atopic dermatitis. J Am Acad Dermatol. 2018 Jul 25. pii: S0190-9622(18)32316-8. doi: 10.1016/j.jaad.2018.07.017. [Epub ahead of print]

64 Schubert S, Bauer A, Molin S, Skudlik C, Geier J. Occupational contact sensitization in female geriatric nurses: Data of the Information Network of Departments of Dermatology (IVDK) 2005-2014. J Eur Acad Dermatol Venereol 2017;31:469-476

65 Frosch PJ, Johansen JD, Menné T, Pirker C, Rastogi SC, Andersen KE, et al. Further important sensitizers in patients sensitive to fragrances. I. Reactivity to 14 frequently used chemicals. Contact Dermatitis 2002;47:78-85

66 Geier J, Lessmann H, Uter W, Schnuch A. Experiences with the fragrance mix II – the German perspective. Contact Dermatitis 2006;55(suppl.1):12 (Abstract)

67 Claßen A, Buhl T, Schubert S, Worm M, Bauer A, Geier J, Molin S; Information Network of Departments of Dermatology (IVDK) study group. The frequency of specific contact allergies is reduced in patients with psoriasis. Br J Dermatol. 2018 Aug 12. doi: 10.1111/bjd.17080. [Epub ahead of print]

68 Girbig M, Hegewald J, Seidler A, Bauer A, Uter W, Schmitt J. Type IV sensitizations in physical therapists: patch test results of the Information Network of Departments of Dermatology (IVDK) 2007-2011. J Dtsch Dermatol Ges 2013;11:1185-1192

69 Dittmar D, Schuttelaar MLA. Contact sensitization to hydroperoxides of limonene and linalool: Results of consecutive patch testing and clinical relevance. Contact Dermatitis 2018 Oct 31. doi: 10.1111/cod.13137. [Epub ahead of print]

70 Silvestre JF, Mercader P, González-Pérez R, Hervella-Garcés M, Sanz-Sánchez T, Córdoba S, et al. Sensitization to fragrances in Spain: A 5-year multicentre study (2011-2015). Contact Dermatitis. 2018 Nov 14. doi: 10.1111/cod.13152. [Epub ahead of print]

71 DeKoven JG, Warshaw EM, Zug KA, Maibach HI, Belsito DV, Sasseville D, et al. North American Contact Dermatitis Group patch test results: 2015-2016. Dermatitis 2018;29:297-309

72 Veverka KK, Hall MR, Yiannias JA, Drage LA, El-Azhary RA, Killian JM, et al. Trends in patch testing with the Mayo Clinic standard series, 2011-2015. Dermatitis 2018;29:310-315

Chapter 3.72 GERANIAL

IDENTIFICATION

Description/definition	: Geranial is the aldehyde that conforms to the structural formula shown below; it is the *trans*-isomer of citral
Chemical class(es)	: Aldehydes
INCI name USA	: Not in the Personal Care Products Council Ingredient Database
Chemical/IUPAC name	: (2*E*)-3,7-Dimethyl-2,6-octadienal
Other names	: *trans*-Citral; α-citral; citral A
CAS registry number(s)	: 141-27-5
EC number(s)	: 205-476-5
RIFM monograph(s)	: Food Cosmet Toxicol 1979;17:259 (citral)
SCCS opinion(s)	: SCCNFP/0389/00, final (9)
Merck Index monograph	: 3591 (Citral)
Function(s) in cosmetics	: EU: perfuming
Patch testing	: 3.5% pet. (5)
Molecular formula	: $C_{10}H_{16}O$

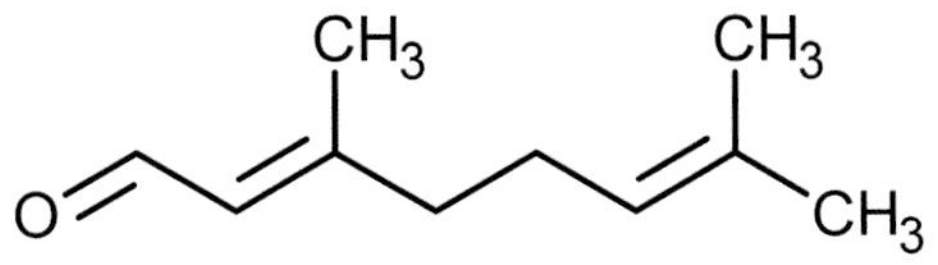

GENERAL

Geranial is a colorless to yellow clear liquid; its odor type is citrus and its odor at 100% is described as 'citrus lemon' (www.thegoodscentscompany.com).

Geranial is itself a hapten with moderate sensitizing potency, but can be activated to more potent sensitizers. Indeed, geranial acting as prehapten is transformed into a hapten outside the skin by chemical transformation (autoxidation) from air exposure (7). The most important oxidation products thus formed are 5,6-epoxygeranial and a dioxolan hydroperoxide (4,6). Both chemicals are strong sensitizers and are considered to be the compounds mainly responsible for the skin sensitization potency of air-exposed geranial (6).

Geranial (*trans*-citral) in a 2:1 isomeric mixture with neral (*cis*-citral) forms citral (1). See also Chapter 3.39 Citral, where much information on geranial (as part of citral) can be found. Geranial has (just as neral) also been identified as a secondary oxidation product when geraniol autoxidizes (2,5) and as metabolite of geraniol (3,5).

Presence in essential oils

Geranial has been identified by chemical analysis in 47 of 91 essential oils, which have caused contact allergy / allergic contact dermatitis. In 9 oils, geranial belonged to the 'Top-10' of ingredients with the highest concentrations which may be expected in commercial essential oils of this type: lemongrass oil West Indian (41.8-46.3%), lemongrass oil East Indian (35.8-46.3%), litsea cubeba oil (35.0-42.3%), melissa oil (0.2-41.7%), ginger oil (0.06-12.6%), citronella oil Sri Lanka (0.5-11.3%), geranium oil (0.1-10.3%), lemon oil (0.6-2.1%), and palmarosa oil (0.2-0.7%) (8).

CONTACT ALLERGY

Patch testing in groups of patients

Patch testing in consecutive patients suspected of contact dermatitis: routine testing

Results of two studies, both from Sweden, testing geranial in consecutive patients suspected of contact dermatitis (routine testing) are shown in table 3.72.1 (1,5). Depending on the concentration, the frequencies of sensitization ranged from 0.4% to 0.6% when the test material contained 1-1.5% geranial (1) to 2.0% in a group of 655 patients tested with geranial 3.5% pet. (5). There were high relevance scores from contact with scented products and essential oils for all tested fragrances together, but data were not specified for individual fragrances (1,5).

Patch testing in groups of selected patients

Studies in which geranial was patch tested in groups of selected patients have not been found.

Table 3.72.1 Patch testing in groups of patients: Routine testing

Years and Country	Test conc. & vehicle	Number of patients tested	positive (%)		Selection of patients (S); Relevance (R); Comments (C)	Ref.
2010-2011 Sweden	3.5% pet.	655	13	(2.0%)	R: not specified for individual fragrances	5
2008-2010 Sweden	1% pet.	948	6	(0.6%)	R: high relevance scores from contact with scented products	1
2006-2007	1.5% pet.	1204	5	(0.4%)	and essential oils for all fragrances together	

Case reports and case series

A male patient had eczema of the axillae and the perioral region following the use of fragranced hygiene products. There were positive patch tests to an aftershave, a deodorant stick, oxidized geraniol, geranial, neral, and citral. The deodorant stick contained citral and geraniol. As citral is composed of geranial and neral, both these positive patch tests were relevant (1).

A female patient working as a masseuse presented with a 5-year history of hand eczema. Upon patch testing, she reacted to a massage oil, geranial, oxidized geraniol and the fragrance mix II. According to the manufacturer, the massage oil contained a high concentration of citral. As citral is composed of neral and geranial, the positive test to geranial was relevant (1).

Cross-reactions, pseudo-cross-reactions and co-reactions

For general information on cross-/pseudo-cross-/co-reactivity of fragrance chemicals with other fragrances, fragrance markers (fragrance mix I, fragrance mix II, colophonium, Myroxylon pereirae resin [balsam of Peru]) and essential oils see Chapter 1.2 General information on cross-reactions, pseudo-cross-reactions and co-reactions.

Co-reactivity to (oxidized) geraniol, neral and citral (which contains geranial) has been observed (1,5). Most patients who react to geranial, however, do not react to neral, indicating that there is no general cross-reactivity between geranial and neral. Although the only difference between the two molecules is the *cis/trans*-conformation of the α,β-double bond, this is most likely enough to induce separate immunological responses (5).

LITERATURE

1   Hagvall L, Karlberg A-T, Christensson JB. Contact allergy to air-exposed geraniol: clinical observations and report of 14 cases. Contact Dermatitis 2012;67:20-27
2   Hagvall L, Backtorp C, Svensson S, Nyman G, Börje A, Karlberg A-T. Fragrance compound geraniol forms contact allergens on air exposure. Identification and quantification of oxidation products and effect on skin sensitization. Chem Res Toxicol 2007;20:807-814
3   Hagvall L, Baron JM, Börje A, Weidolf L, Merk H, Karlberg A-T. Cytochrome P450-mediated activation of the fragrance compound geraniol forms potent contact allergens. Toxicol Appl Pharmacol 2008;233:308-313
4   Hagvall L. Formation of skin sensitizers from fragrance terpenes via oxidative activation routes. Chemical analysis, structure elucidation and experimental sensitization studies. Thesis, University of Gothenburg, Sweden, 2009. Available at: http://hdl.handle.net/2077/18951).
5   Hagvall L, Bråred Christensson J. Cross-reactivity between citral and geraniol – can it be attributed to oxidized geraniol? Contact Dermatitis 2014;71:280-288
6   Hagvall L, Backtorp C, Norrby PO, Karlberg AT, Börje A. Experimental and theoretical investigations of the autoxidation of geranial: a dioxolane hydroperoxide identified as a skin sensitizer. Chem Res Toxicol 2011;24:1507-1515
7   Karlberg A-T, Börje A, Johansen JD, Lidén C, Rastogi S, Roberts D, et al. Activation of non-sensitizing or low-sensitizing fragrance substances into potent sensitizers – prehaptens and prohaptens. Contact Dermatitis 2013;69:323-334
8   De Groot AC, Schmidt E. Essential oils: contact allergy and chemical composition. Boca Raton, Fl., USA: CRC Press, Taylor and Francis Group, 2016 (ISBN 9781482246407)
9   Opinion of the Scientific Committee on Cosmetic Products and Non-Food Products Intended for Consumers concerning 'The 1st update of the inventory of ingredients employed in cosmetic products. Section II: Perfume and aromatic raw materials', 24 October 2000, SCCNFP/0389/00, final. Available at: http://ec.europa.eu/health/ph_risk/committees/sccp/documents/out131_en.pdf

Chapter 3.73   GERANIOL

IDENTIFICATION

Description/definition : Geraniol is the terpene alcohol that conforms to the structural formula shown below
Chemical class(es) : Alcohols
Chemical/IUPAC name : (2*E*)-3,7-Dimethylocta-2,6-dien-1-ol
Other names : Geranyl alcohol; *trans*-3,7-dimethyl-2,6-octadien-1-ol
CAS registry number(s) : 106-24-1
EC number(s) : 203-377-1
RIFM monograph(s) : Food Chem Toxicol 2008:46(11)(suppl.):S1-S71; Food Chem Toxicol 2008;46(11)(suppl.): S160-S170; Food Cosmet Toxicol 1974;12:881
IFRA standard : Restricted (www.ifraorg.org/en-us/standards-library) (table 3.73.1)
SCCS opinion(s) : Various (16); SCCS/1459/11 (17)
Merck Index monograph : 5707
Function(s) in cosmetics : EU: perfuming; tonic. USA: fragrance ingredients
EU cosmetic restrictions : Regulated in Annex III/78 of the Regulation (EC) No. 1223/2009, regulated by 2003/15/EC; Must be labeled on cosmetics and detergent products, if present at > 10 ppm (0.001%) in leave-on products and > 100 ppm (0.01%) in rinse-off products
Patch testing : 1% Pet. (SmartPracticeEurope, SmartPracticeCanada); 2% pet. (Chemotechnique); also present in the fragrance mix I; oxidized geraniol is more sensitizing than pure geraniol and is more suitable for patch testing (1,95,103); oxidized geraniol 11% has been recommended for patch testing (103); there can be little doubt that the currently used test concentrations of 1% and 2% in commercially available test materials are (far) too low
Molecular formula : $C_{10}H_{18}O$

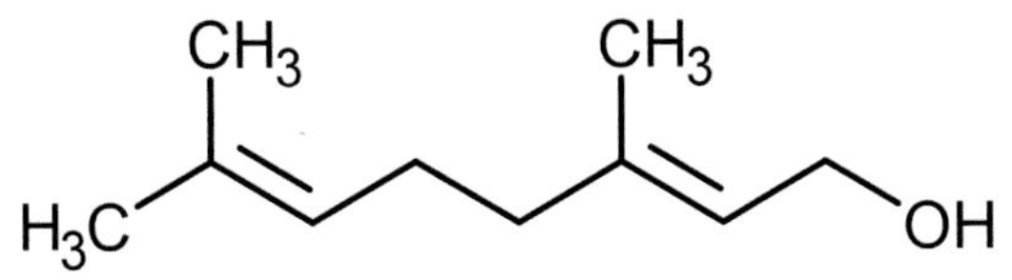

Table 3.73.1 IFRA restrictions for geraniol

Category [a]	Limits [b]	Category [a]	Limits [b]	Category [a]	Limits [b]
1	0.30%	5	2.80%	9	5.00%
2	0.40%	6	8.60%	10	2.50%
3	1.80%	7	0.90%	11	not restricted
4	5.30%	8	2.00%		

[a] For explanation of categories see pages 6-8
[b] Limits in the finished products

GENERAL

Geraniol is a colorless clear liquid; its odor type is floral and its odor at 100% is described as 'sweet floral fruity rose waxy citrus' (www.thegoodscentscompany.com). Geraniol occurs naturally in over 200 plants, including tea, grapes, apricots and plums. It is an important commercial chemical used in perfumery and food flavoring. Geraniol is also used in insect attractant formulations that are applied on fruits, vegetables, ornamentals, homes and garbage dumps. It is an ingredient in some natural tick repellents, pesticides, and animal repellents (U.S. National Library of Medicine).

Geraniol is one of the eight ingredients of the Fragrance mix I (Chapter 3.70 Fragrance mix I)

Presence in essential oils

Geraniol has been identified by chemical analysis in 71 of 91 essential oils, which have caused contact allergy / allergic contact dermatitis. In 15 oils, geraniol belonged to the 'Top-10' of ingredients with the highest concentrations. These are shown in table 3.73.2 with the concentration range which may be expected in commercial essential oils of this type (21).

CONTACT ALLERGY

General

The SCCS (Scientific Committee on Consumer Safety), in a 2012 Opinion on Fragrance allergens in cosmetic products, has marked geraniol as 'established contact allergen in humans' (17,68). The sensitizing potency of geraniol (in one test with low levels of oxidation, in the other pure) was classified as 'moderate' based on an EC3 value of 5.6% and as weak based on an EC3 value of 22.4% in the LLNA (local lymph node assay) in animal experiments; however, geraniol oxidized for 10 weeks and geraniol oxidized for 45 weeks were moderate sensitizers based on EC3 values of 4.4% and 5.8%, respectively (17,68).

Table 3.73.2 Essential oils containing geraniol in the 'Top-10' and concentration range in commercial oils (21)

Essential oil	Concentration range (min.-max.)	Essential oil	Concentration range (min.-max.)
Palmarosa oil	74.2 - 86.9%	Coriander fruit oil	0.2 - 7.0%
Citronella oil Sri Lanka	18.0 - 48.7%	Lemongrass oil East Indian	1.5 - 6.6%
Geranium oil	5.6 - 31.8%	Petitgrain bigarade oil	0.9 - 4.4%
Thyme oil	0 - 26.0%	Neroli oil	2.0 - 3.6%
Citronella oil Java	17.3 - 25.2%	Clary sage oil	0.2 - 3.6%
Rose oil	4.9 - 23.8%	Ylang-ylang oil	trace - 3.0%
Melissa oil	0.2 - 22.2%	Rosewood oil	0.7 - 2.3%
Lemongrass oil West Indian	3.0 - 7.9%		

Geraniol acts both as a prehapten (a chemical that is itself non-sensitizing or low-sensitizing, but that is transformed into a hapten outside the skin by chemical transformation (air oxidation; photoactivation) and without the requirement for specific enzymatic systems) and as a prohapten (a chemical that is itself non-sensitizing or low-sensitizing, but that is transformed into a hapten in the skin (bioactivation), usually via enzymatic catalysis (91).

The sensitizing potency of geraniol increases considerably by air exposure. The autoxidation of geraniol follows two paths, originating from allylic hydrogen abstraction near the two double bonds (2). From geraniol, hydrogen peroxide is primarily formed together with the aldehydes geranial and neral. In addition, small amounts of a hydroperoxide are formed, as are geranyl formate, epoxygeraniol and 3,7-dimethylocta-2,5-diene-1,7-diol (2). The autoxidation of geraniol greatly influences its sensitizing effect. The oxidized samples had moderate sensitizing capacity in the local lymph node assay (LLNA) whereas pure geraniol had weak sensitizing capacity. Geraniol hydroperoxide (7-hydroperoxy-3,7-dimethylocta-2,5-dien-1-ol) is believed to be the major contributor to allergenic activity, together with the aldehydes geranial and neral; the hydrogen peroxide was found to be non-sensitizing (2). The two isomeric aldehydes (geranial [*trans*-citral] and neral [*cis*-citral] = citral), are stable secondary oxidation products from a very unstable hydroxyhydroperoxide.

In the skin, geraniol may be metabolized into geranial, neral, 2,3-epoxygeraniol, 6,7-epoxygeraniol and 6,7-epoxygeranial (3). Geranial is the main metabolite formed followed by 6,7-epoxygeraniol. In the murine local lymph node assay (LLNA), geranial, neral and 6,7-epoxygeraniol were shown to be moderate sensitizers, and 6,7-epoxygeranial a strong sensitizer (3).

Geraniol is a constituent of the fragrance mix I. In groups of patients reacting to the mix and tested with its 8 ingredients, geraniol scored 0-23.8% positive patch test reactions, median 6.8% and average 8.0%. It has rank number 7 in the list of most frequent reactors in the mix (see Chapter 3.70 Fragrance mix I).

The literature on contact allergy to geraniol up to 2003 has been reviewed (29). The literature on patch testing with geraniol in selected and unselected groups of patients published between 1979 and 2003 has been reviewed in ref. 97, including a number of Japanese studies which have been published in Japanese journals only (97).

General population

In the period 2008-2011, in five European countries (Sweden, Germany, Netherlands, Portugal, Italy), a random sample of the general population of 3119 individuals aged 18-74 years were patch tested with the FM I, its 8 ingredients, the FM II, its 6 ingredients and Myroxylon pereirae resin. There were 13 reactions (0.4%) to geraniol, tested 2% in petrolatum. About half of all positive reactions to fragrances were considered to be relevant based on standardized criteria. Women were affected twice as often as men (84).

Patch testing in groups of patients

Results of studies testing geraniol in consecutive patients suspected of contact dermatitis (routine testing) are shown in table 3.73.3. Results of testing geraniol in groups of *selected* patients (e.g. patients with known or suspected fragrance or cosmetic dermatitis, individuals with eyelid dermatitis, patients with hand eczema) are shown in table 3.73.4.

Patch testing in consecutive patients suspected of contact dermatitis: routine testing

In fourteen studies in which routine testing with geraniol was performed, frequencies of sensitization were generally low, ranging from 0.2% to 2.6% (table 3.73.3). In 12/14 investigations, rates were 1% or lower. The high percentage of 2.6 was seen in a study from Thailand, where also other fragrances had high prevalence scores (66). Test concentrations used were 1%, 2%, 4%, 5%, 6% pet. and 11% pet., but mostly, the concentration had no apparent influence on the sensitization scores. In one study, however, in which patients were tested with geraniol 4%, 6% and 11% pet., the percentage positive reactions rose from 0.2% with the lowest concentration to 1.1% with the highest (95).

In three studies from Sweden, *oxidized* geraniol was used for patch testing in concentrations of 2%, 4% , 6% and 11% in petrolatum (1,95,103). With the higher concentrations of these test substances, far more cases of sensitization were detected, with rates of 2.3% and 2.8% with 6% oxidized geraniol and 4.6% and 8.2% with the 11% test material (95,103). In the most recent study, oxidized geraniol 11% was suggested as test concentration for routine patch testing (103).

Relevance data were provided in 2 studies only: 75% (66) and 53% (present relevance) resp. 40% (past relevance (64). Culprit products were hardly ever mentioned. In one study, a high relevance score was suggested for all positively tested fragrances together, from contact with fragranced products and essential oils (1).

Table 3.73.3 Patch testing in groups of patients: Routine testing

Years and Country	Test conc. & vehicle	Number of patients tested | positive (%)		Selection of patients (S); Relevance (R); Comments (C)	Ref.
2015-7 Netherlands		821	8 (1.0%)	R: not stated	106
2015-2016 UK	2% pet.	2084	10 (0.5%)	R: not specified for individual fragrances; 25% of patients who reacted to any fragrance or fragrance marker had a positive fragrance history	6
2010-2015 Denmark	1% pet.	6004	(0.26%)	R: present relevance 53%, past relevance 40%	64
2009-2015 Sweden	2% pet.	4483	22 (0.5%)	R: not stated	69
2013-2014 Thailand		312	8 (2.6%)	R: 75%	66
2012 Sweden	6% pet.	1476	15 (1.0%)	R: not stated; C: the oxidation mixture of geraniol contained geraniol 59%, geranial 4.6%, neral 1.2%, and geraniol-7-hydroperoxide 3.7%; 3.5% of the patients showed doubtful reactions to oxidized geraniol 6.0% pet., and 4.9% to oxidized geraniol 11% pet.; 52 patients had doubtful test reactions to oxidized geraniol 6.0% pet.; of these, 27 had positive patch test reactions to oxidized geraniol 11.0% pet.	103
	6% ox.	1476	42 (2.8%)		
	11% ox.	1476	122 (8.2%)		
2011-2012 UK	2% pet.	1951	9 (0.5%)	R: not stated	67
2010-2011 Sweden	4% pet.	655	1 (0.2%)	R: not stated for any concentration, oxidized or non-oxidized ('pure'); a test concentration of geraniol 6% oxidized was re-commended; as some patients react to pure geraniol but not to oxidized material, testing with a 'high concentration', together with 6% oxidized, was recommended	95
	6% pet.	649	3 (0.5%)		
	11% pet.	655	7 (1.1%)		
	4% pet. ox.	655	6 (0.9%)		
	6% pet. ox.	655	15 (2.3%)		
	11% pet. ox.	655	30 (4.6%)		
2006-2010 Sweden	2% pet. air oxidized	2227	3 (0.1%)	R: high relevance scores; contact with scented products and essential oils	1
	2% pet.	2179	12 (0.6%)		
2005-2008 IVDK	1% pet.	1214	(0.4%)	R: not stated	72
2003-2004 IVDK	1% pet.	2063	10 (0.5%)	R: not stated; C: 67% co-reactivity to FM I	5
<1995 Nine European countries + USA	1% pet.	1072	8 (0.8%)	R: not stated	48
1993 EECDRG	1% pet.	709	5 (0.7%)	R: not stated	77
1991 The Netherlands	5% pet.	677	8 (1.2%)	R: not stated	79

EECDRG: European Environmental and Contact Dermatitis Research Group; FM: Fragrance mix; IVDK: Informationsverbund; Dermatologischer Kliniken (Germany, Switzerland, Austria); ox: air oxidized

Patch testing in groups of selected patients

Results of testing in groups of selected patients (e.g. patients with known or suspected fragrance or cosmetic dermatitis, individuals with eyelid dermatitis, patients with hand eczema) are shown in table 3.73.4. In 13 investigations, frequencies of sensitization to geraniol ranged from 0.6% to 30%. The higher rates of positive reactions of 9% (70), 10% (99), 15% (107), 20% (50) and 30% (18) were – not unexpectedly – observed in groups of patients with proven fragrance allergy, sometimes by a positive patch test to the fragrance mix I, of which geraniol is one of the eight constituents.

In nearly all studies, relevance data were not provided; in one, the authors assumed that nearly all reactions to fragrances were of present or past relevance. Causative products were not mentioned in any investigation.

Results of testing geraniol in groups of patients reacting to the fragrance mix I are shown in Chapter 3.70 Fragrance mix I.

Table 3.73.4 Patch testing in groups of patients: Selected patient groups

Years and Country	Test conc. & vehicle	Number of patients tested | positive (%)		Selection of patients (S); Relevance (R); Comments (C)	Ref.
2011-2015 Spain	1% or 2% pet.	1013	152 (15.0%)	S: patients previously reacting to FM I, FM II, Myroxylon pereirae resin or hydroxyisohexyl 3-cyclohexene carboxaldehyde in the baseline series; R: not stated; C: the 2% test substance showed a higher rate of positive reactions than the 1% material	107
2006-2010 USA	2% pet.	100	5 (5%)	S: patients with eyelid dermatitis; R: not stated	14
2005-10 Netherlands		100	9 (9%)	S: patients with known fragrance sensitivity based on a positive patch test to the FM I and/or the FM II; R: not stated	70
2004-2008 Spain	2% pet.	86	17 (20%)	S: patients previously reacting to the fragrance mix I or Myroxylon pereirae resin (n=54) or suspected of fragrance contact allergy (n=32); R: not stated	50
2005-7 Netherlands	2% pet.	320	2 (0.6%)	S: patients suspected of fragrance or cosmetic allergy; R: 61% relevance for all positive tested fragrances together	4
<2003 Israel		91	4 (4%)	S: patients with a positive or doubtful reaction to the fragrance mix and/or Myroxylon pereirae resin and/or to one or two commercial fine fragrances; R: not specified	49
2001-2 Denmark, Sweden	3% pet.	658	6 (0.9%)	S: consecutive patients with hand eczema; R: it was assumed that nearly all positive reactions were of present or past relevance	12
1998-2002 IVDK	1% pet.	29	2 (7%)	S: patients who had a positive reaction to their own deodorant; R: not stated; C: there was no significant difference in percentage positive reactions compared with a control group of dermatitis patients who had *not* reacted to their own deodorant	51
1997-2000 Austria	1% pet.	747	7 (0.9%)	S: patients suspected of fragrance allergy; R: not stated	11
1990-1998 Japan	5% pet.	1483	5 (0.3%)	S: patients suspected of cosmetic contact dermatitis, virtually all were women; R: not stated; C: range of annual frequency of sensitization: 0-1.5%	20
<1996 Japan, Europe, USA	5% pet.	167	5 (3.0%)	S: patients known or suspected to be allergic to fragrances; R: not stated	13
<1986 France	3% pet.	21	2 (10%)	S: patients with dermatitis caused by perfumes; R: not stated	99
<1982 UK		50	4 (8%)	S: patients with photosensitivity dermatitis with actinic reticuloid syndrome (PD/AR); R: not specified for individual fragrances, but the authors concluded that in some subjects with PD/AR and persistent light reaction, a significant factor in the latter is likely to be exposure to substances such as fragrance materials; C: in a control group of 457 dermatitis patients, only 0.7% reacted positively to geraniol	62
1975 USA	5% pet.	20	6 (30%)	S: fragrance-allergic patients; R: not stated	18

Testing in groups of patients reacting to the fragrance mix I
Results of testing geraniol in groups of patients reacting to the fragrance mix I are shown in Chapter 3.70 Fragrance mix I

FM: Fragrance mix; IVDK: Informationsverbund Dermatologischer Kliniken (Germany, Switzerland, Austria)

Case reports and case series

Case series
Geraniol was stated to be the (or an) allergen in 10 patients in a group of 603 individuals suffering from cosmetic dermatitis, seen in the period 2010-2015 in Leuven, Belgium (63).

In the period 1996-2013, in a tertiary referral center in Valencia, Spain, 5419 patients were patch tested. Of these, 628 individuals had allergic contact dermatitis to cosmetics. In this group, geraniol was the responsible allergen in 18 cases (43, overlap with ref. 44).

In the period 2000-2009, in Leuven, Belgium, an unspecified number of patients had positive patch tests or use tests to a total of 344 cosmetic products *and* positive patch tests to FM I, FM II, and/or to one or more of 28 selected specific fragrance ingredients. In 18 of 34 patients reacting to geraniol, the presence of this fragrance in the cosmetic product(s) was confirmed by reading the product label(s) (71).

In the period 2000-2007, 202 patients with allergic contact dermatitis caused by cosmetics were seen in Valencia, Spain. In this group, geraniol was the allergen in 7 individuals from its presence in cologne (n=3), gel/soap (n=2), shampoo (n=2) and moisturizing cream (n=1) (44, overlap with ref. 43).

In one center in Belgium, between 1985 and 1990, 3970 patients with dermatitis were patch tested. 462 of these reacted positively to patch tests with cosmetic allergens. The reactions were considered to be relevant in 68%, probably relevant in 25% and doubtfully relevant in 7% of the patients. In the list of 'most common allergens' geraniol had rank number 17 with 11 reactions. It should be appreciated that not all patients were patch tested with individual fragrances and that the presence of the allergen in cosmetic products causing dermatitis could not always be verified (at that time, ingredient labeling in the EU was not yet mandatory) (98).

In a group of 119 patients with allergic contact dermatitis from cosmetics, investigated in The Netherlands in 1986-1987, two cases were caused by geraniol in shaving foam and facial makeup (41,42).

In Belgium, in the years before 1986, of 5202 consecutive patients with dermatitis patch tested, 156 were diagnosed with pure cosmetic allergy. Geraniol was the 'dermatitic ingredient' in 2 (1.3%) patients (frequency in the entire group: 0.2%). It should be realized, however, that only a very limited number of patients was tested with a fragrance series (80).

Geraniol was responsible for 8 out of 399 cases of cosmetic allergy where the causal allergen was identified in a study of the NACDG, USA, 1977-1983 (10).

In a perfume factory, six bottle fillers developed occupational allergic contact dermatitis from geraniol. Of twenty people working in the same factory who did *not* have dermatitis, 6 also had positive reactions to geraniol (15).

Case reports

A woman using lipstick, lip balm and toothpaste was patch tested for suspected allergic contact cheilitis. She reacted to geraniol, the FM I (in which geraniol is one of the 8 ingredients) and rose oil (which may contain up to 23.8% geraniol) (21). The lipstick, lip balm, and toothpaste did not contain geraniol, and therefore contact allergy to geraniol present in food was suspected. Subsequent avoidance of ice cream, candy and gum containing geraniol caused a significant improvement of the symptoms within 2 weeks (22).

A woman developed dermatitis from application of an eau de cologne. When patch tested, she reacted to the fragrance mix I, geraniol 2% pet. and Bulgarian rose oil 2% pet. Chromatographic analysis showed the Bulgarian rose oil patch test material to contain approximately 20% geraniol. Quite curiously, it was not attempted to analyse the perfume, which was apparently not patch tested, for the presence of geraniol (23).

Two patients had allergic contact dermatitis from geraniol in topical pharmaceutical preparations (24, probably also presented in ref. 104). One individual had allergic contact dermatitis from geraniol in an ointment used to stimulate new tissue growth in leg ulcers (25). A dentist developed hand dermatitis from contact allergy to geraniol in a washing-up liquid he used at work; apparently, the geraniol had been added for its antimicrobial properties (26).

A female bartender with dermatitis of the hands had positive patch tests to the peels of lemon, orange and lime, but not to their main constituent limonene. The patient did react, however, to geraniol 5% pet. and to citral 2% and 5% in mineral oil and the hand dermatitis seemed to be – albeit not explicitly - ascribed to these chemicals (27). However, commercial lemon oils have been found to contain up to 0.2% geraniol only and orange oil hardly contains any of this chemical (21).

One individual had allergic contact dermatitis from geraniol in a shaving foam (32). Two professional aroma-therapists reacted upon patch testing to multiple essential oils. They were also patch tested with geraniol (2% pet.), which was found to be present in many of the essential oils by GC-MS and both had positive reactions to this fragrance (33). In a group of 23 patients with (photo)allergic reactions to sunscreens, 2 had positive patch tests to the ingredient geraniol (45).

One patient developed disseminated allergic contact dermatitis from geraniol and lavender essence in a pharmaceutical cream applied to the lower leg; the patient also reacted to geranium oil Bourbon and Bulgarian rose oil, both of which contain high concentrations of geraniol (89). A patient with hand dermatitis reacted to rose oil, geraniol and several other fragrances and essential oils; she used a 'fragrance-free' hand soap containing rose oil (92); commercial rose oils may contain up to 23.8% geraniol (21).

A young girl developed a rash on the lips and around the mouth. She reacted to a lip salve and geraniol, which was present in the fragrance of the lip salve in a concentration of 2.5% (93). A woman had cheilitis, which was caused by geranium oil in a sunblock lip balm. The title of the publication indicates geraniol to have been the culprit, but in the text only geranium oil is mentioned, not geraniol (which may be present in high concentrations in geranium oil) (94).

A metal worker suffered from occupational allergic dermatitis of the hands from geraniol in a skin protection cream (101). A female patient working in a company for baking ingredients, who had been handling grated lemon peel and lemon oil for several years, developed allergic contact dermatitis of the fingers of both her hands. By means of thin-layer chromatography geraniol was identified in both lemon peel and lemon oil and this proved it to be the only source of the allergic reaction (102). More specific data are not available (article not read). It should be realized that pure commercial lemon peel oil will contain a maximum of 0.2% geraniol (21).

Pigmented cosmetic dermatitis
In Japan, in the 1960s and 1970s, many female patients developed pigmentation of the face after having facial dermatitis (58). The skin manifestations of this so-called pigmented cosmetic dermatitis consisted of diffuse or patchy brown hyperpigmentation on the cheeks and/or forehead, sometimes the entire face was involved. In severe cases, the pigmentation was black, purple, or blue-black, and in mild cases, it was pale brown. Occasionally, erythematous macules or papules, suggesting a mild contact dermatitis, were observed and itching was also noted at varying times. Pigmented cosmetic dermatitis was shown to be caused by contact allergy to components of cosmetic products, notably essential oils, other fragrance materials, antimicrobials, preservatives and coloring materials (57,58,59). In a group of 620 Japanese patients with this condition investigated between 1970 and 1980, 3-4% had positive patch test reactions to geraniol 20% in petrolatum in various time periods versus 1 to 2% in a control group of patients not suffering from pigmented cosmetic dermatitis (57). The number of patients with pigmented cosmetic dermatitis decreased strongly after 1978, when major cosmetic companies began to eliminate strong contact sensitizers from their products (57). Since 1980, pigmented cosmetic dermatitis became a rare disease in Japan (60).

Cross-reactions, pseudo-cross-reactions and co-reactions
For general information on cross-/pseudo-cross-/co-reactivity of fragrance chemicals with other fragrances, fragrance markers (fragrance mix I, fragrance mix II, colophonium, Myroxylon pereirae resin [balsam of Peru]) and essential oils see Chapter 1.2 General information on cross-reactions, pseudo-cross-reactions and co-reactions. Co-reactivity with the fragrance mix I can be expected, as the mix contains geraniol (pseudo-cross-reactions).

Geraniol is converted into neral and geranial both in the skin by skin metabolism and by autoxidation from air exposure; both are strong allergens (95). This explains the co-reactivity between geraniol and geranial (2,96), neral (2,96) and citral (which is a mixture of geranial and neral [2,5,96]). As to citral, in a large study performed by the IVDK in the period 2005-2013, of 111 patients reacting to citral, 50 (45%) co-reacted to geraniol; conversely, of 61 individuals allergic to geraniol, 50 (82%) co-reacted to citral (105).

Geraniol is an important ingredient of many essential oils and co-reactions with rose oil (21,23,89,92) and geranium oil (89) have been observed and are not unexpected.

Patch test sensitization
A patient tested with geraniol in 2 sessions was negative in the first session, but positive in the second. In the first session, he had been tested with geraniol 5% pet. and the fragrance mix, containing geraniol at 2%. In the second session, the patient reacted to geraniol 1% pet., albeit stronger after 24 hours (++) than after 48 hours (+) (87).

Presence in products and chemical analyses
In various studies, the presence of geraniol in cosmetic and sometimes other products has been investigated. Before 2006, most investigators used chemical analysis, usually GC-MS, for qualitative and quantitative determination. Since then, the presence of the target fragrances was usually investigated by screening the product labels for the 26 fragrances that must be labeled since 2005 on cosmetics and detergent products in the EU, if present at > 10 ppm (0.001%) in leave-on products and > 100 ppm (0.01%) in rinse-off products. This method, obviously, is less accurate and may result in underestimation of the frequency of the fragrances being present in the product. When they are in fact present, but the concentration is lower than mentioned above, labeling is not required and the fragrances' presence will be missed.

The results of the relevant studies for geraniol are summarized in table 3.73.5. More detailed information can be found in the corresponding text before and following the table. The percentage of products in which geraniol was found to be present shows wide variations, which can among other be explained by the selection procedure of the products, the method of investigation (false-negatives with information obtained from labels only) and changes in the use of individual fragrance materials over time (fashion). Geraniol is a frequently used fragrance, especially in fine fragrances, deodorants and fragranced cosmetic products.

In 2017, in the USA, the ingredient labels 159 hair-dye kits containing 539 cosmetic products (e.g. colorants, conditioners, shampoos, toners) were screened for the most common sensitizers they contain. Geraniol was found to be present in 28 (5%) of the products (82).

In Denmark, in 2015-2016, 5588 fragranced cosmetic products were examined with a smartphone application for the 26 fragrances that need to be labeled in the EU. Geraniol was present in 24% of the products (rank number 4) (38).

Table 3.73.5 Presence of geraniol in products [a]

Year	Country	Product type	Nr. investigated	Nr. of products positive [b]	(%)	Method [c]	Ref.
2017	USA	Cosmetic products in hair-dye kits	539 products in 159 hair-dye kits	28	(5%)	Labeling	82
2015-6	Denmark	Fragranced cosmetic products	5588		(24%)	Labeling	38
2015	Germany	Household detergents	817	70	(9%)	Labeling	100
2014	Poland	Emollients	179	4	(2.2%)	Online info	65
2013	USA	Pediatric cosmetics	187	3	(1.6%)	Labeling	46
2008-11	Germany	Deodorants	374	162	(43%)	Labeling	86
2009	Italy	Liquid household washing and cleaning products	291	47	(16%)	Labeling and website info	73
2006-9	Germany	Cosmetic products	4991		(18%)	Labeling	37
2008	Sweden	Cosmetic products	204		(11%)	Labeling	19
		Detergents	97		(3%)	Labeling	
2007	Netherlands	Cosmetic products for children	23	12	(52%)	Analysis	53
2006	UK	Perfumed cosmetic and house-hold products	300	126	(42%)	Labeling	35
2006	Denmark	Popular perfumed deodorants	88	43	(49%)	Labeling	40
			23	20	(87%)	Analysis	
2006	Netherlands	Laundry detergents	52	22	(42%)	Labeling + analysis	55
2006	Denmark	Rinse-off cosmetics for children	208	25	(12%)	Labeling + analysis	52
2002	Denmark	Home and car air fresheners	19	8	(42%)	Analysis	56
2001	Denmark	Women's fine fragrances	10	10	(100%)	Analysis	39
2001	Denmark	Non-cosmetic consumer products	43	9	(21%)	Analysis	54
2000	Denmark, UK, Germany, Italy	Domestic and occupational products	59	24	(41%)	Analysis	8
<2000	Sweden	Swedish cosmetic products	42	33	(79%)	Analysis	83
1997-8	Denmark, UK, Germany, Sweden	Cosmetics and cosmetic toys for children	25	14	(56%)	Analysis	31
1996-7	Denmark	Deodorants that had caused allergic contact dermatitis	19	15	(79%)	Analysis	74
1996	Five European countries	Fragranced deodorants	70	53	(76%)	Analysis	7
1995-6	Denmark	Perfumes from lower-price range cosmetic products	17	12	(71%)	Analysis	75
1995	Denmark	Cosmetic products based on natural ingredients	42	15	(36%)	Analysis	9
1995	Denmark	The 10 most popular women's perfumes	10	9	(90%)	Analysis	30
1994	Denmark	Cosmetics that had given a positive patch or use test in FM I allergic patients	23	12	(52%)	Analysis	76
1992	Netherlands	Cosmetic products	300		(50%)	Analysis	36
1988	USA	Perfumes used in fine fragrances, household products and soap	400	36-43% (see text)		Analysis	34

[a] See the corresponding text below for more details
[b] Positive = containing the target fragrance
[c] Labeling: information from the ingredient labels on the product / packaging; Analysis: chemical analysis, most often GC-MS

In Germany, in 2015, fragrance allergens were evaluated based on lists of ingredients in 817 (unique) detergents (all-purpose cleaners, cleaning preparations for special purposes [e.g. bathroom, kitchen, dish-washing] and laundry detergents) present in 131 households. Geraniol was found to be present in 70 (9%) of the products (100).

Of 179 emollients available in online drugstores in 2014 in Poland, four (2.2%) contained geraniol according to information available online (65).

In 2013, in the USA, the allergen content of 187 unique pediatric cosmetics from 6 different retailers marketed in the United States as hypoallergenic was evaluated on the basis of labeling. Inclusion criteria were products marketed as pediatric and 'hypoallergenic', 'dermatologist recommended/tested', 'fragrance free', or 'paraben free'. Geraniol was found to be present in 3 (1.6%) of the products (46).

In 2008, 2010 and 2011, 374 deodorants available in German retail shops were randomly selected and their labels checked for the presence of the 26 fragrances that need to be labeled. Geraniol was found to be present in 162 (43.4%) of the products (86).

In Italy, in 2009, the labels and website product information of 291 liquid household washing and cleaning products were studied for the presence of potential allergens. Geraniol was found to be present in 47 (16%) of the products (73).

In Germany, in the period 2006-2009, 4991 cosmetic products were randomly sampled for an official investigation of conformity of cosmetic products with legal provisions. The labels were inspected for the presence of the 26 fragrances that need to be labeled in the EU. Geraniol was present in 18% of the products (rank number 4) (37).

Geraniol was present (as indicated by labeling) in 11% of 204 cosmetic products (92 shampoos, 61 hair conditioners, 34 liquid soaps, 17 wet tissues) and in 3% of 97 detergents in Sweden, 2008 (19).

In 2007, in The Netherlands, twenty-three cosmetic products for children were analyzed for the presence of fragrances that need to be labeled. Geraniol was identified in 12 of the products (52%) in a concentration range of 50-492 ppm (53).

In 2006, of 88 popular perfume containing deodorants purchased in Denmark, 43 (49%) were labeled to contain geraniol. Analysis of 24 regulated fragrance substances in 23 selected deodorants (19 spray products, 2 deostick and 2 roll-on) was performed by GC-MS. Geraniol was identified in 20 of the products (87%) with a concentration range of 1–399 ppm (40).

In January 2006, a study of perfumed cosmetic and household products available on the shelves of U.K. retailers was carried out. Products were included if 'parfum' or 'aroma' was listed among the ingredients. Three hundred products were surveyed and any of 26 mandatory labeling fragrances named on the label were recorded. Geraniol was present in 126 (42%) of the products (rank number 4) (35).

In 2006, the labels of 208 cosmetics for children (especially shampoos, body shampoos and soaps) available in Denmark were checked for the presence of the 26 fragrances that need to be labeled in the EU. Geraniol was present in 25 products (12%), and ranked number 3 in the frequency list. Seventeen products were analyzed quantitatively for the fragrances. The maximum concentration found for geraniol was 180 mg/kg (52).

In 2006, in The Netherlands, 52 laundry detergents were investigated for the presence of allergenic fragrances by checking their labels and chemical analyses. Geraniol was found to be present in 22 of the products (42%) in a concentration range of 10-319 ppm. Geraniol had rank number 2 in the frequency list (55).

In 2002, in Denmark, 19 air fresheners (6 for cars, 13 for homes) were analyzed for the presence of fragrances that need to be labeled on cosmetics. Geraniol was found to be present in 8 products (42%) in a concentration range of 390-8900 ppm and ranked 13 in the frequency list (56).

In January 2001, in Denmark, ten women's fine fragrances were purchased; 5 of these had been launched years ago (1921–1990) and 5 were the latest launches by the same companies, introduced 2 months to 4 years before purchase. They were analyzed for the presence and quantity of the 7 well-identified fragrances present in the FM I (see Chapter 3.70 Fragrance mix I). The analysis revealed that the 5 old perfumes contained a mean of 5 of the 7 target allergens of the FM, while the new perfumes contained a mean of 2.8 of the allergens. The mean concentrations of the target allergens were 2.6 times higher in the old perfumes than in the new perfumes, range 2.2-337 ppm.

Geraniol was present in all 5 old perfumes, in a concentration range of 0.072-0.432% (m/m), mean 0.340%; in the new perfumes, it was identified in all 5 in a concentration range of 0.090-0.236% (m/m), mean 0.156% (39).

In 2001, in Denmark, 43 non-cosmetic consumer products (mainly dish-washing products, laundry detergents, and hard and soft surface cleaners) were analyzed for the 26 fragrances that are regulated for labeling in the EU. Geraniol was present in 9 products (21%) in a concentration range of 0.0001-0.1454% (m/m) and had rank number 11 in the frequency list (54).

In 2000, fifty-nine domestic and occupational products, purchased in retail outlets in Denmark, England, Germany and Italy were analyzed by GC-MS for the presence of fragrances. The product categories were liquid soap and soap bars (n=13), soft/hard surface cleaners (n=23), fabric conditioners/laundry detergents for hand wash (n=8), dish- wash (n=10), furniture polish, car shampoo, stain remover (each n=1) and 2 products used in occupational environments. Geraniol was present in 24 products (41%) with a mean concentration of 234 ppm and a range of 53-1758 ppm (8).

In Sweden, before 2000, 42 cosmetic products of a Swedish manufacturer were investigated for the presence of the ingredients of the FM I by chemical analysis. Geraniol was found to be present in 33 of the products (79%) in a concentration range of 1-107 ppm with a mean of 26 ppm. Data provided by the manufacturer on the qualitative and quantitative presence of the chemicals was quite different from chemical analyses for some of the fragrances (83).

Twenty-five cosmetics and cosmetic toys for children (5 shampoos and shower gels, 6 perfumes, 1 deodorant (roll-on), 4 baby lotions/creams, 1 baby wipes product, 1 baby oil, 2 lipcare products and 5 toy-cosmetic products: a cosmetic-toy set for blending perfumes and a makeup set) purchased in 1997-1998 in retail outlets in Denmark, Germany, England and Sweden were analyzed in 1998 for the presence of fragrances by GC-MS. Geraniol was found in 14 products (56%) in a concentration range of ≤0.001-1.764% (w/w). For the analytical data in each product category, the original publication should be consulted (31).

In Denmark, in 1996-1997, nineteen deodorants that had caused axillary allergic contact dermatitis in 14 patients were analyzed for the presence of the 8 constituents of the FM I and geraniol was found to be present in 15 (79%) of the products in a concentration range of 0.0022-0.0703% (74).

Seventy fragranced deodorants, purchased at retail outlets in 5 European countries in 1996, were analyzed by gas chromatography - mass spectrometry (GC-MS) for the determination of the contents of 21 commonly used fragrance materials. Geraniol was identified in 53 products (76%) in a concentration range of 1–1178 ppm (7).

In Denmark, in 1995-1996, nine perfumes from lower-price cosmetic wash-off products and 8 from stay-on products were analyzed for the presence of the ingredients of the FM I except oakmoss absolute. Geraniol was present in 7 of the 9 (78%) wash-off product perfumes in a concentration range of 0.05-0.1187% w/v and in 5 of the 8 (63%) stay-on product perfumes in a concentration in one product of 0.1866% w/v. In 7 products, geraniol was detected, but could not be quantified because of interference (75).

In 1995, in Denmark, 42 cosmetic products based on natural ingredients from 12 European and US companies (of which 22 were perfumes and 20 various other cosmetics) were investigated by high-resolution gas chromatography-mass spectrometry (GC-MS) for the presence of 11 fragrances. Geraniol was present in 14 (64%) of the 22 perfumes in a concentration of 1.191 w/w% in one product (quantification of geraniol in remaining products was not possible due to overlapping by a large GC-peak of linalyl acetate); it was also identified in one of the other cosmetics (a lotion) in a concentration of 0.0163% (geraniol identification in the other products was not possible due to overlapping by a large GC peak of linalyl acetate) (9).

In Denmark, in 1995, the 10 most popular women's perfumes were analyzed with gas chromatography-mass spectrometry for the presence of 7 ingredients of the Fragrance mix I (all except Evernia prunastri extract). Geraniol was identified in 9 of the perfumes (90%) with a mean concentration of 0.22% and in a concentration range of 0.08-0.48% (30).

In Denmark, in 1994, 23 cosmetic products, which had either given a positive patch and/or use test in a total of 11 fragrance-mix-positive patients, and which products completely or partly explained present or past episodes of dermatitis, were analyzed for the presence of the constituents of the FM I (with the exception of oakmoss absolute) and a few other fragrances. Geraniol was found to be present in 12 of the 23 products (52%) in a concentration range of <0.001-0.62% v/v with a mean concentration of 0.105% v/v. It was also present in three other products, but could not be quantified due to interference (76).

In 1992, in The Netherlands, the presence of fragrances was analyzed in 300 cosmetic products. Geraniol was identified in 50% of the products (rank order 10) (36).

In 1988, in the USA, 400 perfumes used in fine fragrances, household products and soaps (number of products per category not mentioned) were analyzed for the presence of fragrance chemicals in a concentration of at least 1% and a list of the Top-25 (present in the highest number of products) presented. Geraniol was found to be present in 43% of the fine fragrances (rank number 14), 36% of the household product fragrances (rank number 13) and 40% of the fragrances used in soaps (rank number 16) (34).

OTHER SIDE EFFECTS

Immediate-type reactions

A woman with a history of atopic dermatitis developed edematous erythema on her lips, cheeks, eyelids and neck. She also had noticed urticaria. With open and closed patch tests read after 20 minutes, 7 cosmetics provoked erythema or erythema plus edema. They all contained 2 perfume mixtures that also reacted positively after 20 minutes. The 48-h closed test with the perfume mixtures revealed a wheal with both substances. One day later, the patient developed generalized urticaria. The ingredients were unknown (uncooperative manufacturer), but the investigators tested some fragrances and obtained positive direct tests with geraniol, the fragrance mix I, Myroxylon pereirae resin and cinnamal. The manufacturer then confirmed the presence of geraniol in both perfumes (28).

In 18 subjects not allergic to fragrances tested for non-immune immediate contact reactions (NIICR), geraniol (2% pet.) caused erythema in one (61). In Hungary, before 1994, in a group of 50 patients reacting to the FM I and tested with its ingredients (test concentrations unknown), there was one immediate contact reaction to geraniol (78).

Of 50 individuals who had open tests with geraniol 5% on the forearm, 35 (70%) showed local macular erythema after 45 minutes, termed 'contact urticaria' by the authors (81).

Other non-eczematous contact reactions

A 27-year-old woman presented with a patchy, dark brown hyperpigmentation on the face. Patch tests were positive to lemon oil, geraniol and hydroxycitronellal, but negative to a cosmetic she used, a compact face powder. A ROAT with this product, however, was positive. The face powder contained lemon oil and geraniol. The hyperpigmentation disappeared within 6 months after the patient avoided contact with cosmetics containing these fragrances. The diagnosis was pigmented cosmetic dermatitis, which the authors called Riehl's melanosis. It was ascribed to geraniol contact allergy, but a phototoxicity reaction to lemon oil was not excluded (47).

OTHER INFORMATION

When geraniol 2% in petrolatum is stored in Finn chambers at room temperature, the concentration of the fragrance decreases by nearly 30% within 8 hours, probably from evaporation. This decrease is lower when the test material is stored in a refrigerator. Therefore, application to the test chamber should be performed as close in time to the patch testing as possible and storage in a refrigerator is recommended (85).

LITERATURE

1   Hagvall L, Karlberg A-T, Christensson JB. Contact allergy to air-exposed geraniol: clinical observations and report of 14 cases. Contact Dermatitis 2012;67:20-27
2   Hagvall L, Backtorp C, Svensson S, Nyman G, Börje A, Karlberg AT. Fragrance compound geraniol forms contact allergens on air exposure. Identification and quantification of oxidation products and effect on skin sensitization. Chem Res Toxicol 2007;20:807-814
3   Hagvall L, Baron JM, Börje A, Weidolf L, Merk H, Karlberg AT. Cytochrome P450-mediated activation of the fragrance compound geraniol forms potent contact allergens. Toxicol Appl Pharmacol 2008;233:308-313
4   Oosten EJ van, Schuttelaar ML, Coenraads PJ. Clinical relevance of positive patch test reactions to the 26 EU-labelled fragrances. Contact Dermatitis 2009;61:217-223
5   Schnuch A, Uter W, Geier J, Lessmann H, Frosch PJ. Sensitization to 26 fragrances to be labelled according to current European regulation: Results of the IVDK and review of the literature. Contact Dermatitis 2007;57:1-10
6   Ung CY, White JML, White IR, Banerjee P, McFadden JP. Patch testing with the European baseline series fragrance markers: a 2016 update. Br J Dermatol 2018;178:776-780
7   Rastogi SC, Johansen JD, Frosch P, Menné T, Bruze M, Lepoittevin JP, et al. Deodorants on the European market: quantitative chemical analysis of 21 fragrances. Contact Dermatitis 1998;38:29-35
8   Rastogi SC, Heydorn S, Johansen JD, Basketter DA. Fragrance chemicals in domestic and occupational products. Contact Dermatitis 2001;45:221-225
9   Rastogi SC, Johansen JD, Menné T. Natural ingredients based cosmetics. Content of selected fragrance sensitizers. Contact Dermatitis 1996;34:423-426
10 Adams RM, Maibach HI, for the North American Contact Dermatitis Group. A five-year study of cosmetic reactions. J Am Acad Dermatol 1985;13:1062-1069
11 Wöhrl S, Hemmer W, Focke M, Götz M, Jarisch R. The significance of fragrance mix, balsam of Peru, colophony and propolis as screening tools in the detection of fragrance allergy. Br J Dermatol 2001;145:268-273
12 Heydorn S, Johansen JD, Andersen KE, Bruze M, Svedman C, White IR, et al. Fragrance allergy in patients with hand eczema – a clinical study. Contact Dermatitis 2003;48:317-323
13 Larsen W, Nakayama H, Fischer T, Elsner P, Burrows D, Jordan W, et al. Fragrance contact dermatitis: A worldwide multicenter investigation (Part I). Am J Cont Dermat 1996;7:77-83
14 Wenk KS, Ehrlich AE. Fragrance series testing in eyelid dermatitis. Dermatitis 2012;23:22-26
15 Schubert HJ. Skin diseases in workers at a perfume factory. Contact Dermatitis 2006;55:81-83
16 Various SCCS opinions on geraniol have been published and are available at: http://ec.europa.eu/growth/tools-databases/cosing/index.cfm?fuseaction=search.details_v2&id=28329&back=1
17 SCCS (Scientific Committee on Consumer Safety). Opinion on Fragrance allergens in cosmetic products, 26-27 June 2012, SCCS/1459/11. Available at: https://ec.europa.eu/health/sites/health/files/scientific_committees/consumer_safety/docs/sccs_o_102.pdf

18 Larsen WG. Perfume dermatitis. A study of 20 patients. Arch Dermatol 1977;113:623-626

19 Yazar K, Johnsson S, Lind M-L, Boman A, Lidén C. Preservatives and fragrances in selected consumer-available cosmetics and detergents. Contact Dermatitis 2011;64:265-272

20 Sugiura M, Hayakawa R, Kato Y, Sugiura K, Hashimoto R. Results of patch testing with lavender oil in Japan. Contact Dermatitis 2000;43:157-160

21 De Groot AC, Schmidt E. Essential oils: contact allergy and chemical composition. Boca Raton, Fl., USA: CRC Press, Taylor and Francis Group, 2016 (ISBN 9781482246407)

22 Tamagawa-Mineoka R, Katoh N, Kishimoto S. Allergic contact cheilitis due to geraniol in food. Contact Dermatitis 2007;56:242-243

23 Vilaplana J, Romaguera C, Grimalt F. Contact dermatitis from geraniol in Bulgarian rose oil. Contact Dermatitis 1991;24:301

24 Romaguera C, Grimalt F, Vilaplana J. Geraniol dermatitis. Contact Dermatitis 1986;14:185-186

25 Guerra P, Aguilar A, Urbina F, Cristobal MC, Garcia-Perez A. Contact dermatitis to geraniol in a leg ulcer. Contact Dermatitis 1987;16:298-299

26 Murphy LA, White IR. Contact dermatitis from geraniol in washing-up liquid. Contact Dermatitis 2003;49:52

27 Cardullo AC, Ruszkowski AM, DeLeo VA. Allergic contact dermatitis resulting from sensitivity to citrus peel, geraniol, and citral. J Am Acad Dermatol 1989;21:395-397

28 Yamamoto A, Morita A, Tsuji T, Suzuki K, Matsunaga K. Contact urticaria from geraniol. Contact Dermatitis 2002;46:52

29 Hostynek JJ, Maibach HI. Is there evidence that geraniol causes allergic contact dermatitis? Exog Dermatol 2004;3:318-331

30 Johansen JD, Rastogi SC, Menné T. Contact allergy to popular perfumes: assessed by patch test, use test and chemical analyses. Br J Dermatol 1996;135:419-422

31 Rastogi SC, Johansen JD, Menné T, Frosch P, Bruze M, Andersen KE, et al. Content of fragrance allergens in children's cosmetics and cosmetic toys. Contact Dermatitis 1999;41:84-88

32 De Groot AC. Contact allergy to cosmetics: causative ingredients. Contact Dermatitis 1987;17:26-34

33 Dharmagunawardena B, Takwale A, Sanders KJ, Cannan S, Rodger A, Ilchyshyn A. Gas chromatography: an investigative tool in multiple allergies to essential oils. Contact Dermatitis 2002;47:288-292

34 Fenn RS. Aroma chemical usage trends in modern perfumery. Perfumer and Flavorist 1989;14:3-10

35 Buckley DA. Fragrance ingredient labelling in products on sale in the UK. Br J Dermatol 2007;157:295-300

36 Weyland JW. Personal Communication, 1992. Cited in: De Groot AC, Weyland JW, Nater JP. Unwanted effects of cosmetics and drugs used in dermatology, 3rd Ed. Amsterdam: Elsevier, 1994: 579

37 Uter W, Yazar K, Kratz E-M, Mildau G, Lidén C. Coupled exposure to ingredients of cosmetic products: I. Fragrances. Contact Dermatitis 2013;69:335-341

38 Bennike NH, Oturai NB, Müller S, Kirkeby CS, Jørgensen C, Christensen AB, et al. Fragrance contact allergens in 5588 cosmetic products identified through a novel smartphone application. J Eur Acad Dermatol Venereol 2018;32:79-85

39 Rastogi SC, Menné T, Johansen JD. The composition of fine fragrances is changing. Contact Dermatitis 2003;48:130-132

40 Rastogi SC, Hellerup Jensen G, Johansen JD. Survey and risk assessment of chemical substances in deodorants. Survey of Chemical Substances in Consumer Products, No. 86 2007. Danish Ministry of the Environment, Environmental Protection Agency. Available at: https://www2.mst.dk/Udgiv/publications/2007/978-87-7052-625-8/pdf/978-87-7052-626-5.pdf

41 De Groot AC, Bruynzeel DP, Bos JD, van der Meeren HL, van Joost T, Jagtman BA, Weyland JW. The allergens in cosmetics. Arch Dermatol 1988;124:1525-1529

42 De Groot AC. Adverse reactions to cosmetics. PhD Thesis, University of Groningen, The Netherlands: 1988, chapter 3.4, pp.105-113

43 Zaragoza-Ninet V, Blasco Encinas R, Vilata-Corell JJ, Pérez-Ferriols A, Sierra-Talamantes C, Esteve-Martínez A, de la Cuadra-Oyanguren J. Allergic contact dermatitis due to cosmetics: A clinical and epidemiological study in a tertiary hospital. Actas Dermosifiliogr 2016;107:329-336

44 Laguna C, de la Cuadra J, Martín-González B, Zaragoza V, Martínez-Casimiro L, Alegre V. Allergic contact dermatitis to cosmetics. Actas Dermosifiliogr 2009;100:53-60

45 Thune P. Contact and photocontact allergy to sunscreens. Photodermatol 1984;1:5-9

46 Hamann CR, Bernard S, Hamann D, Hansen R, Thyssen JP. Is there a risk using hypoallergenic cosmetic pediatric products in the United States? J Allergy Clin Immunol 2015;135:1070-1071

47 Serrano G, Pujol C, Cuadra J, Gallo S, Aliaga A. Riehl's melanosis: pigmented contact dermatitis caused by fragrances. J Am Acad Dermatol 1989;21:1057-1060

48 Frosch PJ, Pilz B, Andersen KE, Burrows D, Camarasa JG, Dooms-Goossens A, et al. Patch testing with fragrances: results of a multicenter study of the European Environmental and Contact Dermatitis Research Group with 48 frequently used constituents of perfumes. Contact Dermatitis 1995;33:333-342

49 Trattner A, David M. Patch testing with fine fragrances: comparison with fragrance mix, balsam of Peru and a fragrance series. Contact Dermatitis 2003:49:287-289

50 Cuesta L, Silvestre JF, Toledo F, Lucas A, Perez-Crespo M, Ballester I. Fragrance contact allergy: a 4-year retrospective study. Contact Dermatitis 2010;63:77-84

51 Uter W, Geier J, Schnuch A, Frosch PJ. Patch test results with patients' own perfumes, deodorants and shaving lotions: results of the IVDK 1998-2002. J Eur Acad Dermatol Venereol 2007;21:374-379

52 Poulsen PB, Schmidt A. A survey and health assessment of cosmetic products for children. Survey of chemical substances in consumer products, No. 88. Copenhagen: Danish Environmental Protection Agency, 2007. Available at: https://www2.mst.dk/udgiv/publications/2007/978-87-7052-638-8/pdf/978-87-7052-639-5.pdf

53 VWA. Dutch Food and Consumer Product Safety Authority. Cosmetische producten voor kinderen: Inventarisatie van de markt en de veiligheidsborging door producenten en importeurs. Report ND04o065/ND05o170, 2007 (Report in Dutch), 2007. Available at: www.nvwa.nl/documenten/communicatie/inspectieresultaten/ consument/2016m/cosmetische- producten-voor-kinderen

54 Rastogi SC. Survey of chemical compounds in consumer products. Contents of selected fragrance materials in cleaning products and other consumer products. Survey no. 8-2002. Copenhagen, Denmark, Danish Environmental Protection Agency. Available at: http://eng.mst.dk/media/mst/69131/8.pdf

55 Bouma K, Van Peursem AJJ. Marktonderzoek naleving detergenten verordening voor textielwasmiddelen. Dutch Food and Consumer Products Safety Authority (VWA) Report ND06K173, 2006 [in Dutch]. Available at: http://docplayer.nl/41524125-Marktonderzoek-naleving-detergenten-verordening-voor-textielwasmiddelen. html

56 Pors J, Fuhlendorff R. Mapping of chemical substances in air fresheners and other fragrance liberating products. Report Danish Ministry of the Environment, Environmental Protection Agency (EPA). Survey of Chemicals in Consumer Products, No 30, 2003. Available at: http://eng.mst.dk/media/mst/69113/30.pdf

57 Nakayama H, Matsuo S, Hayakawa K, Takhashi K, Shigematsu T, Ota S. Pigmented cosmetic dermatitis. Int J Dermatol 1984;23:299-305

58 Nakayama H, Harada R, Toda M. Pigmented cosmetic dermatitis. Int J Dermatol 1976;15:673-675

59 Nakayama H, Hanaoka H, Ohshiro A. Allergen Controlled System. Tokyo: Kanehara Shuppan, 1974

60 Ebihara T, Nakayama H. Pigmented contact dermatitis. Clin Dermatol 1997;15:593-599

61 Safford RJ, Basketter DA, Allenby CF, Goodwin BF. Immediate contact reactions to chemicals in the fragrance mix and a study of the quenching action of eugenol. Br J Dermatol 1990;123:595-606

62 Addo HA, Ferguson J, Johnson BF, Frain-Bell W. The relationship between exposure to fragrance materials and persistent light reaction in photosensitivity dermatitis with actinic reticuloid syndrome. Br J Dermatol 1982;107:261-274

63 Goossens A. Cosmetic contact allergens. Cosmetics 2016, 3, 5; doi:10.3390/cosmetics3010005

64 Bennike NH, Zachariae C, Johansen JD. Non-mix fragrances are top sensitizers in consecutive dermatitis patients – a cross-sectional study of the 26 EU-labelled fragrance allergens. Contact Dermatitis 2017;77:270-279

65 Osinka K, Karczmarz A, Krauze K, Feleszko W. Contact allergens in cosmetics used in atopic dermatitis: analysis of product composition. Contact Dermatitis 2016;75:241-243

66 Vejanurug P, Tresukosol P, Sajjachareonpong P, Puangpet P. Fragrance allergy could be missed without patch testing with 26 individual fragrance allergens. Contact Dermatitis 2016;74:230-235

67 Mann J, McFadden JP, White JML, White IR, Banerjee P. Baseline series fragrance markers fail to predict contact allergy. Contact Dermatitis 2014;70:276-281

68 Uter W, Johansen JD, Börje A, Karlberg A-T, Lidén C, Rastogi S, Roberts D, White IR. Categorization of fragrance contact allergens for prioritization of preventive measures: clinical and experimental data and consideration of structure–activity relationships. Contact Dermatitis 2013;69:196-230

69 Mowitz M, Svedman C, Zimerson E, Isaksson M, Pontén A, Bruze M. Simultaneous patch testing with fragrance mix I, fragrance mix II and their ingredients in southern Sweden between 2009 and 2015. Contact Dermatitis 2017;77:280-287

70 Nagtegaal MJC, Pentinga SE, Kuik J, Kezic S, Rustemeyer T. The role of the skin irritation response in polysensitization to fragrances. Contact Dermatitis 2012;67:28-35

71 Nardelli A, Drieghe J, Claes L, Boey L, Goossens A. Fragrance allergens in 'specific' cosmetic products. Contact Dermatitis 2011;64:212-219

72 Uter W, Geier J, Frosch P, Schnuch A. Contact allergy to fragrances: current patch test results (2005–2008) from the Information Network of Departments of Dermatology. Contact Dermatitis 2010;63:254-261

73 Magnano M, Silvani S, Vincenzi C, Nino M, Tosti A. Contact allergens and irritants in household washing and cleaning products. Contact Dermatitis 2009;61:337-341

74 Johansen JD, Rastogi SC, Bruze M, Andersen KE, Frosch P, Dreier B, et al. Deodorants: a clinical provocation study in fragrance-sensitive individuals. Contact Dermatitis 1998;39:161-165

75 Johansen JD, Rastogi SC, Andersen KE, Menné T. Content and reactivity to product perfumes in fragrance mix positive and negative eczema patients: A study of perfumes used in toiletries and skin-care products. Contact Dermatitis 1997;36:291-296

76 Johansen JD, Rastogi SC, Menné T. Exposure to selected fragrance materials: A case study of fragrance-mix-positive eczema patients. Contact Dermatitis 1996;34:106-110

77 Frosch PJ, Pilz B, Burrows D, Camarasa JG, Lachapelle J-M, Lahti A, et al. Testing with fragrance mix: Is the addition of sorbitan sesquioleate to the constituents useful? Contact Dermatitis 1995;32:266-272

78 Becker K, Temesvari E, Nemeth I. Patch testing with fragrance mix and its constituents in a Hungarian population. Contact Dermatitis 1994;30:185-186

79 De Groot AC, Van der Kley AMJ, Bruynzeel DP, Meinardi MMHM, Smeenk G, van Joost Th, Pavel S. Frequency of false-negative reactions to the fragrance mix. Contact Dermatitis 1993;28:139-140

80 Broeckx W, Blondeel A, Dooms-Goossens A, Achten G. Cosmetic intolerance. Contact Dermatitis 1987;16:189-194

81 Emmons WW, Marks JG Jr. Immediate and delayed reactions to cosmetic ingredients. Contact Dermatitis 1985;13:258-265

82 Hamann D, Kishi P, Hamann CR. Consumer hair dye kits frequently contain isothiazolinones, other common preservatives and fragrance allergens. Dermatitis 2018;29:48-49

83 Bárány E, Lodén M. Content of fragrance mix ingredients and customer complaints of cosmetic products. Dermatitis 2000;11:74-79

84 Diepgen TL, Ofenloch R, Bruze M, Cazzaniga S, Coenraads PJ, Elsner P, et al. Prevalence of fragrance contact allergy in the general population of five European countries: a cross-sectional study. Br J Dermatol 2015;173:1411-1419

85 Mowitz M, Zimerson E, Svedman C, Bruze M. Stability of fragrance patch test preparations applied in test chambers. Br J Dermatol 2012;167:822-827

86 Klaschka U. Contact allergens for armpits - allergenic fragrances specified on deodorants. Int J Hyg Environ Health 2012;215:584-591

87 Larsen WG. Allergic contact dermatitis to the fragrance material lilial. Contact Dermatitis 1983;9:158-159

88 Meynadier JM, Meynadier J, Peyron JL, Peyron L. Formes cliniques des manifestations cutanées d'allergie aux parfums. Ann Dermatol Venereol 1986;113:31-39

89 Juarez A, Goiriz R, Sanchez-Perez J, Garcia-Diez A. Disseminated allergic contact dermatitis after exposure to a topical medication containing geraniol. Dermatitis 2008;19:163

90 Thomson MA, Preston PW, Prais L, Foulds IS. Lime dermatitis from gin and tonic with a twist of lime. Contact Dermatitis 2007;56:114-115

91 Karlberg A-T, Börje A, Johansen JD, Lidén C, Rastogi S, Roberts D, et al. Activation of non-sensitizing or low-sensitizing fragrance substances into potent sensitizers – prehaptens and prohaptens. Contact Dermatitis 2013;69:323-334

92 Scheinman PL. Is it really fragrance free? Am J Cont Derm 1997;8:239-242

93 Calnan CD, Cronin E, Rycroft RJ. Allergy to phenyl salicylate. Contact Dermatitis 1981;7:208-211

94 Chang Y-C, Maibach HI. Pseudo flautist's lip: allergic contact cheilitis from geraniol. Contact Dermatitis 1997;37:39

95 Hagvall L, Karlberg A-T, Christensson JB. Finding the optimal patch test material and test concentration to detect contact allergy to geraniol. Contact Dermatitis 2013;68:224-231

96 Hagvall L, Bråred Christensson J. Cross-reactivity between citral and geraniol – can it be attributed to oxidized geraniol? Contact Dermatitis 2014;71:280-288

97 Lapczynski A, Bhatia SP, Foxenberg RJ, Letizia CS, Api AM. Fragrance material review on geraniol. Food Chem Toxicol 2008;46(11)(suppl.):S160-S170

98 Dooms-Goossens, A, Kerre S, Drieghe J, Bossuyt L, DeGreef H. Cosmetic products and their allergens. Eur J Dermatol 1992;2:465-468

99 Meynadier JM, Meynadier J, Peyron JL, Peyron L. Formes cliniques des manifestations cutanées d'allergie aux parfums. Ann Dermatol Venereol 1986;113:31-39

100 Wieck S, Olsson O, Kümmerer K, Klaschka U. Fragrance allergens in household detergents. Regul Toxicol Pharmacol 2018;97:163-169

101 Tanko Z, Shab A, Diepgen TL, Weisshaar E. Polyvalent type IV sensitizations to multiple fragrances and a skin protection cream in a metal worker. J Dtsch Dermatol Ges 2009;7:541-543

102 Hausen BM, Kulenkamp D. Geraniol contact allergy. Z Hautkr 1990;65:492-494 (Article in German)

103 Hagvall L, Bruze M, Engfeldt M, Isaksson M, Lindberg M, Ryberg K, et al. Contact allergy to oxidized geraniol among Swedish dermatitis patients - A multicentre study by the Swedish Contact Dermatitis Research Group. Contact Dermatitis 2018;79:232-238

104 Romaguera C, Grimalt F, Vilaplana J, Mascaro JM. Contact dermatitis caused by perfumes and essences contained in various preparations for topical use. Med Cutan Ibero Lat Am 1987;15:367-370 (Article in Spanish)

105 Geier J, Uter W, Lessmann H, Schnuch A. Fragrance mix I and II: results of breakdown tests. Flavour Fragr J 2015;30:264-274

106 Dittmar D, Schuttelaar MLA. Contact sensitization to hydroperoxides of limonene and linalool: Results of consecutive patch testing and clinical relevance. Contact Dermatitis 2018 Oct 31. doi: 10.1111/cod.13137. [Epub ahead of print]

107 Silvestre JF, Mercader P, González-Pérez R, Hervella-Garcés M, Sanz-Sánchez T, Córdoba S, et al. Sensitization to fragrances in Spain: A 5-year multicentre study (2011-2015). Contact Dermatitis. 2018 Nov 14. doi: 10.1111/cod.13152. [Epub ahead of print]

Chapter 3.74   GERANYL ACETATE

IDENTIFICATION

Description/definition   : Geranyl acetate is the ester of geraniol and acetic acid
Chemical class(es)   : Esters
Chemical/IUPAC name   : [(2E)-3,7-Dimethylocta-2,6-dienyl] acetate
Other names   : Geraniol acetate
CAS registry number(s)   : 105-87-3
EC number(s)   : 203-341-5
RIFM monograph(s)   : Food Cosmet Toxicol 1974;12:885 (special issue I) (binder, page 399)
Function(s) in cosmetics   : EU: perfuming; tonic. USA: fragrance ingredients
Patch testing   : 1% acetone (1); based on RIFM data, 4% pet. is probably not irritant (3)
Molecular formula   : $C_{12}H_{20}O_2$

GENERAL

Geranyl acetate is a colorless clear liquid; its odor type is floral and its odor at 100% is described as 'floral rose lavender green waxy' (www.thegoodscentscompany.com).

Presence in essential oils

Geranyl acetate has been identified by chemical analysis in 69 of 91 essential oils, which have caused contact allergy / allergic contact dermatitis. In 12 oils, geranyl acetate belonged to the 'Top-10' of ingredients with the highest concentrations which may be expected in commercial essential oils of this type: thyme oil (0-21.8%), ylang-ylang oil (0.4-15.0%), palmarosa oil (3.4-12.5%), citronella oil Java (1.9-8.7%), lemongrass oil, East Indian (1.0-6.0%), coriander fruit oil (1.4-5.0%), petitgrain bigarade oil (2.5-4.8%), lemongrass oil, West Indian (1.0-4.3%), clary sage oil (0.5-4.0%), neroli oil (1.7-3.7%), cananga oil (1.0-3.0%), and lemon oil (0.1-1.3%) (4).

CONTACT ALLERGY

Patch testing in groups of patients

Studies in which geranyl acetate was patch tested in either consecutive patients suspected of contact dermatitis (routine testing) or in groups of selected patients with positive results have not been found.

Case reports

Two patients had used oil of citronella for protection against mosquitos and developed dermatitis. They reacted to oil of citronella (pure and 50% in mineral oil, concentrations are slightly irritant), citronellal, citronellol, hydroxycitronellal, citral and geranyl acetate. Citronellal (30-50%) and citronellol (8.5-15%) are both important components of citronella oils and geranyl acetate may be present in concentrations up to 8.7% in commercial citronella oil Java and up to 5.2% in commercial citronella oil Sri Lanka samples (4).

Presence in products and chemical analyses

In 1992, in The Netherlands, the presence of fragrances was analyzed in 300 cosmetic products. Geranyl acetate was identified in 35% of the products (rank order 20) (2).

LITERATURE

1   Keil H. Contact dermatitis due to oil of citronellal. J Invest Dermatol 1947;8:327-334
2   Weyland JW. Personal Communication, 1992. Cited in: De Groot AC, Weyland JW, Nater JP. Unwanted effects of cosmetics and drugs used in dermatology, 3rd Ed. Amsterdam: Elsevier, 1994: 579
3   De Groot AC. Patch Testing, 4th Edition. Wapserveen, The Netherlands: acdegroot publishing, 2018 (ISBN 978-90-813233-4-5)
4   De Groot AC, Schmidt E. Essential oils: contact allergy and chemical composition. Boca Raton, Fl., USA: CRC Press, Taylor and Francis Group, 2016 (ISBN 9781482246407)

Chapter 3.75   HELIOTROPINE

IDENTIFICATION

Description/definition   : Heliotropine is the organic compound that conforms to the structural formula shown
                             below
Chemical class(es)   : Aldehydes; heterocyclic compounds
Chemical/IUPAC name   : 1,3-Benzodioxole-5-carbaldehyde
Other names   : Piperonal
CAS registry number(s)   : 120-57-0
EC number(s)   : 204-409-7
RIFM monograph(s)   : Food Cosmet Toxicol 1974;12:907 (special issue I)
SCCS opinion(s)   : SCCS/1459/11 (3)
Merck Index monograph   : 8858
Function(s) in cosmetics   : EU: masking; perfuming; skin conditioning. USA: fragrance ingredients
Patch testing   : 5% pet. (8)
Molecular formula   : $C_8H_6O_3$

GENERAL

Heliotropine is a white crystalline powder; its odor type is floral and its odor is described as 'cherry, vanilla, sweet cherry pit notes and creamy with cinnamic nuances' (www.thegoodscentscompany.com).

Presence in essential oils

Heliotropine has been identified by chemical analysis in three of 91 essential oils, which have caused contact allergy / allergic contact dermatitis: black pepper oil, cypress oil and lemongrass oil West Indian (13).

CONTACT ALLERGY

General

The SCCS (Scientific Committee on Consumer Safety), in a 2012 Opinion on Fragrance allergens in cosmetic products, has categorized heliotropine as 'likely fragrance contact allergen by combination of evidence' (3,9).

Patch testing in groups of patients

Results of studies testing heliotropine in consecutive patients suspected of contact dermatitis (routine testing) and those of testing in groups of *selected* patients (patients with known fragrance contact allergy) are shown in table 3.75.1. In routine testing, only 0.4% and 0.1% positive reactions were observed in one study with test concentrations of 5% and 1% in petrolatum, respectively (8). In a small group of 20 fragrance-allergic individuals patch tested with a battery of individual fragrance chemicals, one (5%) reacted to heliotropine (1). Relevance was not mentioned in either study.

Table 3.75.1 Patch testing in groups of patients

Years and Country	Test conc. & vehicle	Number of patients tested	positive (%)		Selection of patients (S); Relevance (R); Comments (C)	Ref.
Routine testing						
1998-2000 six Euro-	5% pet.	1606	6	(0.4%)	R: not stated	8
pean countries	1% pet.	1606	2	(0.1%)	R: not stated	
Testing in groups of selected patients						
1975 USA	5% pet.	20	1	(5%)	S: fragrance-allergic patients; R: not stated	1

Case reports

A woman had allergic contact dermatitis from the perfume in an eye cream. Subsequently, she was tested with 94 individual liquid fragrance materials from this perfume (test concentration not stated). The patient at day 5 had 12 positive patch test reactions, including to heliotropine. Three controls were negative. She was not retested, so false-positive reactions due to the excited skin syndrome (there was an additional strong reaction to allyl cyclohexyl propionate which proved to be irritant) cannot be excluded (1). Indeed, two years later, in a Letter to the Editor, the author mentioned that he had retested the patient with the 12 fragrances to which she had previously shown a positive patch test. Only hydroxycitronellal had again given a positive reaction (11).

One case of contact allergy to heliotropine from its presence in a topical pharmaceutical preparation was reported from Belgium (2).

One patient allergic to Myroxylon pereirae resin (balsam of Peru) and with a history of sensitivity to perfumes had a positive patch test to heliotropine 5% pet. (12).

Presence in products and chemical analyses

In 2008, 66 different fragrance components (including 39 essential oils) were identified in 370 (10% of the total) topical pharmaceutical products marketed in Belgium; one of these (0.3%) contained heliotropine (2).

In 2000, fifty-nine domestic and occupational products, purchased in retail outlets in Denmark, England, Germany and Italy were analyzed by GC-MS for the presence of fragrances. The product categories were liquid soap and soap bars (n=13), soft/hard surface cleaners (n=23), fabric conditioners/laundry detergents for hand wash (n=8), dish wash (n=10), furniture polish, car shampoo, stain remover (each n=1) and 2 products used in occupational environments. Heliotropine was present in 13 products (22%) with a mean concentration of 76 ppm and a range of 18-150 ppm (5).

Twenty-five cosmetics and cosmetic toys for children (5 shampoos and shower gels, 6 perfumes, 1 deodorant (roll-on), 4 baby lotions/creams, 1 baby wipes product, 1 baby oil, 2 lipcare products and 5 toy-cosmetic products: a cosmetic-toy set for blending perfumes and a makeup set) purchased in 1997-1998 in retail outlets in Denmark, Germany, England and Sweden were analyzed in 1998 for the presence of fragrances by GC-MS. Heliotropine (piperonal) was found in 15 products (60%) in a concentration range of ≤0.001-2.482% (w/w). For the analytical data in each product category, the original publication should be consulted (6).

Seventy fragranced deodorants, purchased at retail outlets in 5 European countries in 1996, were analyzed by gas chromatography - mass spectrometry (GC-MS) for the determination of the contents of 21 commonly used fragrance materials. Heliotropine (piperonal) was identified in 28 products (40%) in a concentration range of 1-612 ppm (4).

In 1988, in the USA, 400 perfumes used in fine fragrances, household products and soaps (number of products per category not mentioned) were analyzed for the presence of fragrance chemicals in a concentration of at least 1% and a list of the Top-25 (present in the highest number of products) presented. Heliotropine was found to be present in 43% of the fine fragrances (rank number 15), an unknown percentage of the household product fragrances and 39% of the fragrances used in soaps (rank number 20) (7).

LITERATURE

1   Larsen WG. Perfume dermatitis. A study of 20 patients. Arch Dermatol 1977;113:623-626
2   Nardelli A, D'Hooge E, Drieghe J, Dooms M, Goossens A. Allergic contact dermatitis from fragrance components in specific topical pharmaceutical products in Belgium. Contact Dermatitis 2009;60:303-313
3   SCCS (Scientific Committee on Consumer Safety). Opinion on Fragrance allergens in cosmetic products, 26-27 June 2012, SCCS/1459/11. Available at:
    https://ec.europa.eu/health/sites/health/files/scientific_committees/consumer_safety/docs/sccs_o_102.pdf
4   Rastogi SC, Johansen JD, Frosch P, Menné T, Bruze M, Lepoittevin JP, et al. Deodorants on the European market: quantitative chemical analysis of 21 fragrances. Contact Dermatitis 1998;38:29-35
5   Rastogi SC, Heydorn S, Johansen JD, Basketter DA. Fragrance chemicals in domestic and occupational products. Contact Dermatitis 2001;45:221-225
6   Rastogi SC, Johansen JD, Menné T, Frosch P, Bruze M, Andersen KE, et al. Content of fragrance allergens in children's cosmetics and cosmetic toys. Contact Dermatitis 1999;41:84-88
7   Fenn RS. Aroma chemical usage trends in modern perfumery. Perfumer and Flavorist 1989;14:3-10
8   Frosch PJ, Johansen JD, Menné T, Pirker C, Rastogi SC, Andersen KE, et al. Further important sensitizers in patients sensitive to fragrances. II. Reactivity to essential oils. Contact Dermatitis 2002;47:279-287
9   Uter W, Johansen JD, Börje A, Karlberg A-T, Lidén C, Rastogi S, Roberts D, White IR. Categorization of fragrance contact allergens for prioritization of preventive measures: clinical and experimental data and consideration of structure–activity relationships. Contact Dermatitis 2013;69:196-230
10 Larsen WG. Cosmetic dermatitis due to a perfume. Contact Dermatitis 1975;1:142-145
11 Larsen WG. Perfume dermatitis revisited. Contact Dermatitis 1977;3:98
12 Hjorth N. Eczematous allergy to balsams. Acta Derm Venereol 1961;41(suppl.46):1-216
13 De Groot AC, Schmidt E. Essential oils: contact allergy and chemical composition. Boca Raton, Fl., USA: CRC Press, Taylor and Francis Group, 2016 (ISBN 9781482246407)

Chapter 3.76   HEPTANAL

IDENTIFICATION

Description/definition	: Heptanal is the aliphatic aldehyde that conforms to the structural formula shown below
Chemical class(es)	: Aliphatic organic compounds; aldehydes
INCI name USA	: Not in the Personal Care Products Council Ingredient Database
Chemical/IUPAC name	: Heptanal
Other names	: Aldehyde C-7; heptaldehyde
CAS registry number(s)	: 111-71-7
EC number(s)	: 203-898-4
RIFM monograph(s)	: Food Cosmet Toxicol 1975;13:701 (special issue II) (binder, page 48)
Merck Index monograph	: 5963
Function(s) in cosmetics	: EU: perfuming
Patch testing	: No patch test data available; based on RIFM data, 4% pet. is probably not irritant (3)
Molecular formula	: $C_7H_{14}O$

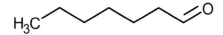

GENERAL

Heptanal is a colorless clear liquid; its odor type is green and its odor at 1% in dipropylene glycol is described as 'fresh aldehydic fatty green herbal wine-lee ozone' (www.thegoodscentscompany.com). The chemical is or has been used in the manufacture of 1-heptanol, organic synthesis, perfumery, pharmaceuticals, and flavoring (U.S. National Library of Medicine).

Presence in essential oils

Heptanal has been identified by chemical analysis in 21 of 91 essential oils, which have caused contact allergy / allergic contact dermatitis. In none of these oils, it belonged to the 'Top-10' of ingredients with the highest concentrations (4).

CONTACT ALLERGY

Patch testing in groups of patients

Studies in which heptanal was patch tested in either consecutive patients suspected of contact dermatitis (routine testing) or in groups of selected patients with positive results have not been found.

Case reports and case series

A woman had allergic contact dermatitis from the perfume in an eye cream. Subsequently, she was tested with 94 individual liquid fragrance materials from this perfume (test concentrations not stated). The patient at day 5 had 12 positive patch test reactions, including to heptanal (aldehyde C-7). Three controls were negative. She was not retested, so false-positive reactions due to the excited skin syndrome (there was an additional strong reaction to allyl cyclohexyl propionate which proved to be irritant) cannot be excluded (1).

Indeed, two years later, in a Letter to the Editor, the author mentioned that he had retested the patient with the 12 fragrances to which she had previously shown a positive patch test. Only hydroxycitronellal had again given a positive reaction (2). This means that, in fact, contact allergy to heptanal has not been demonstrated thus far beyond doubt.

LITERATURE

1   Larsen WG. Cosmetic dermatitis due to a perfume. Contact Dermatitis 1975;1:142-145
2   Larsen WG. Perfume dermatitis revisited. Contact Dermatitis 1977;3:98
3   De Groot AC. Patch Testing, 4th Edition. Wapserveen, The Netherlands: acdegroot publishing, 2018 (ISBN 978-90-813233-4-5)
4   De Groot AC, Schmidt E. Essential oils: contact allergy and chemical composition. Boca Raton, Fl., USA: CRC Press, Taylor and Francis Group, 2016 (ISBN 9781482246407)

Chapter 3.77   HEXADECANOLACTONE

IDENTIFICATION

Description/definition   : Hexadecanolactone is the organic compound that conforms to the structural formula
                              shown below
Chemical class(es)   : Ketones
Chemical/IUPAC name   : Oxacycloheptadecan-2-one
Other names   : Hexadecanolide; dihydroambrettolide; juniperolactone
CAS registry number(s)   : 109-29-5
EC number(s)   : 203-662-0
RIFM monograph(s)   : Food Chem Toxicol 2011;49(suppl.2):S183-S188; Food Cosmet Toxicol 1975;13:452
SCCS opinion(s)   : SCCS/1459/11 (1)
Function(s) in cosmetics   : EU: masking; perfuming. USA: fragrance ingredients
Patch testing   : 5% pet. (2,3)
Molecular formula   : $C_{16}H_{30}O_2$

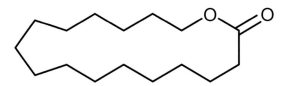

GENERAL

Hexadecanolactone is a colorless solid; its odor type is musk and its odor at 10% in dipropylene glycol is described as
'sweet musk balsam amber animal' (www.thegoodscentscompany.com).

Presence in essential oils

Hexadecanolactone has been identified by chemical analysis in two of 91 essential oils, which have caused contact
allergy / allergic contact dermatitis: angelica root oil and vetiver oil (5). However, the chemical is apparently not
found in plants (www.thegoodscentscompany.com) and therefore, the analytical identification of this chemical may
have been erroneous.

CONTACT ALLERGY

General

The SCCS (Scientific Committee on Consumer Safety), in a 2012 Opinion on fragrance allergens in cosmetic products,
has marked hexadecanolactone as 'established contact allergen in humans' (1,4).

Patch testing in groups of patients

Patch testing in consecutive patients suspected of contact dermatitis: routine testing

Studies in which hexadecanolactone was patch tested in consecutive patients suspected of contact dermatitis
(routine testing) with positive results have not been found.

Patch testing in groups of selected patients

Results of two studies patch testing hexadecanolactone in groups of selected patients are shown in table 3.77.1. In
Korea, in the period 2002-2003, 422 patients with suspected cosmetic dermatitis were patch tested with
hexadecanolacto-ne 5% pet. and there were 6 (1.4%) positive reactions (3). In the year 2000, in Japan, some
European countries and the USA, 178 patients with known fragrance sensitivity were patch tested with this
fragrance, also 5% in petrolatum, and one patient (0.6%) had a positive patch test reaction (2). In neither study were
relevance data provided (2,3).

Table 3.77.1 Patch testing in groups of patients: Selected patient groups

Years and Country	Test conc. & vehicle	Number of patients tested	positive (%)	Selection of patients (S); Relevance (R); Comments (C)	Ref.
2002-2003 Korea	5% pet.	422	6 (1.4%)	S: patients with suspected cosmetic dermatitis; R: not stated	3
2000 Japan, Europe, USA	5% pet.	178	1 (0.6%)	S: patients with known fragrance sensitivity; R: not stated	2

Case reports

Case reports of allergic contact dermatitis from hexadecanolactone have not been found.

LITERATURE

1   SCCS (Scientific Committee on Consumer Safety). Opinion on Fragrance allergens in cosmetic products, 26-27 June 2012, SCCS/1459/11. Available at: https://ec.europa.eu/health/sites/health/files/scientific_committees/consumer_safety/docs/sccs_o_102.pdf

2   Larsen W, Nakayama H, Fischer T, Elsner P, Frosch P, Burrows D, et al. Fragrance contact dermatitis: A worldwide multicenter investigation (Part II). Contact Dermatitis 2001;44:344-346

3   An S, Lee AY, Lee CH, Kim DW, Hahm JH, Kim KJ, et al. Fragrance contact dermatitis in Korea: a joint study. Contact Dermatitis 2005;53:320-323

4   Uter W, Johansen JD, Börje A, Karlberg A-T, Lidén C, Rastogi S, Roberts D, White IR. Categorization of fragrance contact allergens for prioritization of preventive measures: clinical and experimental data and consideration of structure–activity relationships. Contact Dermatitis 2013;69:196-230

5   De Groot AC, Schmidt E. Essential oils: contact allergy and chemical composition. Boca Raton, Fl., USA: CRC Press, Taylor and Francis Group, 2016 (ISBN 9781482246407)

Chapter 3.78 HEXAMETHYLINDANOPYRAN

IDENTIFICATION

Description/definition	: Hexamethylindanopyran is the organic compound that conforms to the structural formula shown below
Chemical class(es)	: Ethers
Chemical/IUPAC name	: 4,6,6,7,8,8-Hexamethyl-1,3,4,7-tetrahydrocyclopenta[g]isochromene
Other names	: 1,3,4,6,7,8-Hexahydro-4,6,6,7,8,8-hexamethylindeno(5,6-c)pyran; Galaxolide ®
CAS registry number(s)	: 1222-05-5
EC number(s)	: 214-946-9
SCCS opinion(s)	: SCCFNP 0403/00 (2); SCCNFP/0610/02, final (3); SCCS/1459/11 (4)
RIFM monograph(s)	: Food Cosmet Toxicol 1976;14:793 (special issue III)
Function(s) in cosmetics	: EU: perfuming. USA: fragrance ingredients
Patch testing	: 10% in isopropyl myristate (1,10); 5% pet. (9); 7% pet. (6); based on RIFM data, 15% pet. is probably not irritant (12)
Molecular formula	: $C_{18}H_{26}O$

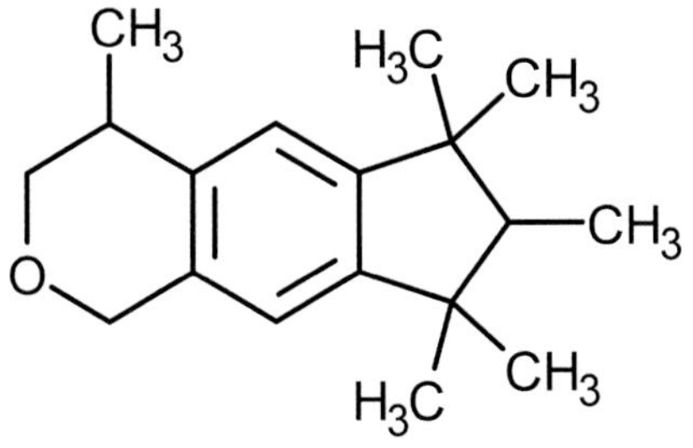

GENERAL

Hexamethylindanopyran is a colorless clear viscous liquid; its odor type is musk and its odor at 100% is described as 'strong diffusive sweet floral musk' (www.thegoodscentscompany.com). It is a synthetic artificial musk fragrance that has not been found in nature (and consequently, not in essential oils (13)). Hexamethylindanopyran is a fragrance ingredient in perfumes, soaps, cosmetics, and detergents. As a laundry detergent fragrance, it is sufficiently substantive to provide residual fragrance on cloth (U.S. National Library of Medicine).

CONTACT ALLERGY

General

The SCCS (Scientific Committee on Consumer Safety), in a 2012 Opinion on Fragrance allergens in cosmetic products, has marked hexamethylindanopyran as 'established contact allergen in humans' (4,11).

Patch testing in groups of patients

Results of studies testing hexamethylindanopyran in consecutive patients suspected of contact dermatitis (routine testing) and those of testing in groups of *selected* patients (patients with known or suspected fragrance or cosmetic dermatitis) are shown in table 3.78.1. In one study in which routine testing with hexamethylindanopyran was performed in six European countries in 1997-1998, a frequency of sensitization of 0.2% was observed; the relevance of positive reactions was not mentioned (10).

Rates of positive reactions in 4 studies testing the fragrance in selected patient groups ranged from 0.3% to 3.4% (1,5,6,9), the latter frequency having been observed in a group of 178 patients with known fragrance sensitivity (6). The relevance of positive reactions was either not mentioned or not specified (1,5,6,9).

Case reports and case series

Case reports of allergic contact dermatitis from hexamethylindanopyran have not been found.

Presence in products and chemical analyses

In 2000, fifty-nine domestic and occupational products, purchased in retail outlets in Denmark, England, Germany and Italy were analyzed by GC-MS for the presence of fragrances. The product categories were liquid soap and soap bars (n=13), soft/hard surface cleaners (n=23), fabric conditioners/laundry detergents for hand wash (n=8), dish wash (n=10), furniture polish, car shampoo, stain remover (each n=1) and 2 products used in occupational environments. Hexamethylindanopyran was present in 21 products (36%) with a mean concentration of 111.8 ppm and a range of 6-346 ppm (7).

In 1988, in the USA, 400 perfumes used in fine fragrances, household products and soaps (number of products per category not mentioned) were analyzed for the presence of fragrance chemicals in a concentration of at least 1% and a list of the Top-25 (present in the highest number of products) presented. Hexamethylindanopyran was found to be present in 41% of the fine fragrances (rank number 16), 31% of the household product fragrances (rank number 16) and 28% of the fragrances used in soaps (rank number 24) (8).

Table 3.78.1 Patch testing in groups of patients

Years and Country	Test conc. & vehicle	Number of patients tested | positive (%)		Selection of patients (S); Relevance (R); Comments (C)	Ref.
Routine testing					
1997-8 Six European countries	10% isopropyl myristate	1855	3 (0.2%)	R: not stated / specified	10
Testing in groups of selected patients					
2002-2003 Korea	5% pet.	422	5 (1.2%)	S: patients with suspected cosmetic dermatitis; R: not stated	9
2001-2002 Denmark, Sweden	10% isopropyl myristate	658	2 (0.3%)	S: consecutive patients with hand eczema; R: it was assumed that nearly all positive reactions in the study were of present or past relevance	1
2000 Japan, Europe, USA	7% pet.	178	6 (3.4%)	S: patients with known fragrance sensitivity; R: not stated	6
1984 The Netherlands	25% pet.	179	3 (1.7%)	S: patients suspected of cosmetic allergy; R: not stated; C: false-positive reactions due to excited skin syndrome could not be excluded in some cases	5

LITERATURE

1   Heydorn S, Johansen JD, Andersen KE, Bruze M, Svedman C, White IR, et al. Fragrance allergy in patients with hand eczema – a clinical study. Contact Dermatitis 2003;48:317-323

2   SCCFNP (Scientific Committee on Cosmetic Products and Non-Food Products Intended for Consumers). Opinion of the Scientific Committee on Cosmetic Products and Non-Food Products Intended for Consumers concerning Hexahydro-hexamethyl-cyclopenta (g)-2-benzopyran (HHCB), 24 October2000, SCCFNP 0403/00. Available at: http://ec.europa.eu/health/scientific_committees/consumer_safety/opinions/ sccnfp_opinions_97_04/ sccp_out125_en.htm

3   SCCFNP (Scientific Committee on Cosmetic Products and Non-Food Products Intended for Consumers). Opinion of the Scientific Committee on Cosmetic Products and Non-Food Products Intended for Consumers concerning Hexahydro-hexamethyl-cyclopenta (γ)-2-benzopyran, (HHCB), 17 September 2002, SCCNFP/0610/02, final. Available at: http://ec.europa.eu/health/ph_risk/committees/sccp/documents/out179_en.pdf

4   SCCS (Scientific Committee on Consumer Safety). Opinion on Fragrance allergens in cosmetic products, 26-27 June 2012, SCCS/1459/11. Available at: https://ec.europa.eu/health/sites/health/files/scientific_committees/consumer_safety/docs/sccs_o_102.pdf

5   De Groot AC, Liem DH, Nater JP, van Ketel WG. Patch tests with fragrance materials and preservatives. Contact Dermatitis 1985;12:87-92

6   Larsen W, Nakayama H, Fischer T, Elsner P, Frosch P, Burrows D, et al. Fragrance contact dermatitis: A worldwide multicenter investigation (Part II). Contact Dermatitis 2001;44:344-346

7   Rastogi SC, Heydorn S, Johansen JD, Basketter DA. Fragrance chemicals in domestic and occupational products. Contact Dermatitis 2001;45:221-225

8   Fenn RS. Aroma chemical usage trends in modern perfumery. Perfumer and Flavorist 1989;14:3-10

9   An S, Lee AY, Lee CH, Kim DW, Hahm JH, Kim KJ, et al. Fragrance contact dermatitis in Korea: a joint study. Contact Dermatitis 2005;53:320-323

10 Frosch PJ, Johansen JD, Menné T, Pirker C, Rastogi SC, Andersen KE, et al. Further important sensitizers in patients sensitive to fragrances. I. Reactivity to 14 frequently used chemicals. Contact Dermatitis 2002;47:78-85

11 Uter W, Johansen JD, Börje A, Karlberg A-T, Lidén C, Rastogi S, Roberts D, White IR. Categorization of fragrance contact allergens for prioritization of preventive measures: clinical and experimental data and consideration of structure–activity relationships. Contact Dermatitis 2013;69:196-230

12 De Groot AC. Patch Testing, 4th Edition. Wapserveen, The Netherlands: acdegroot publishing, 2018 (ISBN 978-90-813233-4-5)

13 De Groot AC, Schmidt E. Essential oils: contact allergy and chemical composition. Boca Raton, Fl., USA: CRC Press, Taylor and Francis Group, 2016 (ISBN 9781482246407)

Chapter 3.79   cis-3-HEXENYL SALICYLATE

IDENTIFICATION

Description/definition	: cis-3-Hexenyl salicylate is the unsaturated salicylic acid ester that conforms to the structural formula shown below
Chemical class(es)	: Aromatic compounds; esters; unsaturated organic compounds
INCI name USA	: Not in the Personal Care Products Council Ingredient Database
Chemical/IUPAC name	: [(Z)-Hex-3-enyl] 2-hydroxybenzoate
CAS registry number(s)	: 65405-77-8
EC number(s)	: 265-745-8
RIFM monograph(s)	: Food Chem Toxicol 2007;45(suppl.1):S402-S405; Food Chem Toxicol 2007;45(suppl.1): S318-S361; Food Cosmet Toxicol 1979;17:373
Function(s) in cosmetics	: EU: perfuming
Patch testing	: 3% pet.
Molecular formula	: $C_{13}H_{16}O_3$

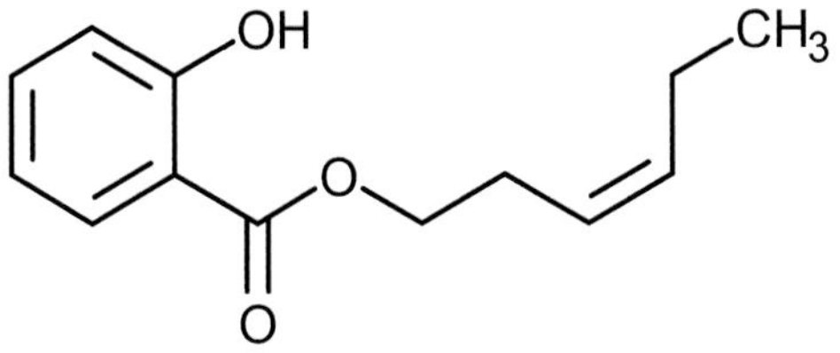

GENERAL

cis-3-Hexenyl salicylate is a colorless clear oily liquid; its odor type is floral and its odor at 100% is described as 'floral green metallic herbal balsam' (www.thegoodscentscompany.com).

Presence in essential oils

cis-3-Hexenyl salicylate has been identified by chemical analysis in none of 91 essential oils, which have caused contact allergy / allergic contact dermatitis (5).

CONTACT ALLERGY

Patch testing in groups of patients

While searching for causative ingredients of pigmented cosmetic dermatitis in Japan in the 1970s, both patients with ordinary (nonpigmented) cosmetic dermatitis and women with pigmented cosmetic dermatitis were tested with a large number of fragrance materials. In 1980 the accumulated data enabled the classification of fragrant materials into 4 groups: common sensitizers, rare sensitizers, virtually non-sensitizing fragrances and fragrances considered as non-sensitizers. cis-3-Hexenyl acetate was classified in the group of rare sensitizers, indicating that one or more cases of contact allergy / allergic contact dermatitis to it have been observed (2). More specific data are lacking, the results have largely or solely been published in Japanese journals only.

Other studies in which cis-3-hexenyl salicylate was patch tested in either consecutive patients suspected of contact dermatitis (routine testing) or in groups of selected patients with positive results have not been found.

Case reports and case series

A woman had experienced recurrent severe dermatitis on sun-exposed skin. She always wore sunscreens before being exposed to sunlight. She also had a history of contact dermatitis from some fragrances, fragranced products, and jewelry. When patch tested, there were positive reactions to nickel sulfate, Myroxylon pereirae resin, a commercial eau de toilette used by the patient, ethylhexyl salicylate (octisalate) 5% pet., and a sunscreen containing this UV-absorber. Photopatch tests gave the same results as those seen in the sunscreens not exposed to UVA. A ROAT with ethylhexyl salicylate was positive after 4 days. The patient declined subsequent patch testing with other salicylates. However, she agreed to a double-blinded right-versus-left antecubital provocative use test with plain petrolatum versus cis-3-hexenyl salicylate 3% pet., which was chosen because it was present in the eau de toilette to which the patient reacted and it was also a salicylate. After 3 days of twice-daily applications, the patient developed contact dermatitis at the cis-3-hexenyl salicylate application site. She had no further dermatitis after 1 year of follow-up while using fragrance-free and ethylhexyl salicylate-free skin care products (4).

A female patient developed an itchy dermatitis on the trunk after applying a perfumed toilet lotion. Patch testing with the ICDRG series revealed a positive reaction to fragrance mix (16% pet.) and to hydroxycitronellal (2% pet.). By infrared spectroscopy and gas chromatography in combination with mass spectrometry, the following ingredients were found (Laboratory of Food Inspection Service, Cosmetics Section, Enschede, The Netherlands): *d*-limonene, benzyl acetate, linalool, linalyl acetate, geranyl acetate, diethyl phthalate, *cis*-3-hexenyl salicylate, celestolide, α-hexylcinnamic aldehyde (hexyl cinnamal), acetyl cedrene, benzyl salicylate, musk ketone and geraniol. All these ingredients were patch tested in concentrations varying from 3 to 35% in petrolatum. The only positive patch test reaction was to *cis*-3-hexenyl salicylate, tested 3% pet. In 10 control persons, the reaction to this compound was negative (3).

Cross-reactions, pseudo-cross-reactions and co-reactions
For general information on cross-/pseudo-cross-/co-reactivity of fragrance chemicals with other fragrances, fragrance markers (fragrance mix I, fragrance mix II, colophonium, Myroxylon pereirae resin [balsam of Peru]) and essential oils see Chapter 1.2 General information on cross-reactions, pseudo-cross-reactions and co-reactions.

No cross-sensitivity to hexyl salicylate, methyl salicylate, phenyl salicylate or benzyl salicylate (3). Possible cross-reaction to ethylhexyl salicylate (4).

Presence in products and chemical analyses
In 2000, fifty-nine domestic and occupational products, purchased in retail outlets in Denmark, England, Germany and Italy were analyzed by GC-MS for the presence of fragrances. The product categories were liquid soap and soap bars (n=13), soft/hard surface cleaners (n=23), fabric conditioners/laundry detergents for hand wash (n=8), dish wash (n=10), furniture polish, car shampoo, stain remover (each n=1) and 2 products used in occupational environments. 3-Hexenyl salicylate was present in one product; quantification was not performed (1).

LITERATURE
1   Rastogi SC, Heydorn S, Johansen JD, Basketter DA. Fragrance chemicals in domestic and occupational products. Contact Dermatitis 2001;45:221-225
2   Nakayama H. Fragrance hypersensitivity and its control. In: Frosch PJ, Johansen JD, White IR, Eds. Fragrances - beneficial and adverse effects. Berlin Heidelberg New York: Springer-Verlag, 1998:83-91
3   Van Ketel WG. Sensitization to *cis*-3-hexenyl salicylate. Contact Dermatitis 1983;9:154
4   Shaw DW. Allergic contact dermatitis from octisalate and *cis*-3-hexenyl salicylate. Dermatitis 2006;17:152-155
5   De Groot AC, Schmidt E. Essential oils: contact allergy and chemical composition. Boca Raton, Fl., USA: CRC Press, Taylor and Francis Group, 2016 (ISBN 9781482246407)

Chapter 3.80   HEXYL CINNAMAL

IDENTIFICATION

Description/definition : Hexyl cinnamal is the organic compound that conforms to the structural formula shown below
Chemical class(es) : Aldehydes
Chemical/IUPAC name : 2-Benzylideneoctanal
Other names : α-Hexylcinnamaldehyde; hexyl cinnamic aldehyde
CAS registry number(s) : 101-86-0
EC number(s) : 202-983-3
RIFM monograph(s) : Food Cosmet Toxicol 1974;12:915 (special issue I)
IFRA standard : Restricted (www.ifraorg.org/en-us/standards-library) (table 3.80.1)
SCCS opinion(s) : Various (7); SCCS/1459/11 (8)
Function(s) in cosmetics : EU: perfuming. USA: fragrance ingredients
EU cosmetic restrictions : Regulated in Annex III/87 of the Regulation (EC) No. 1223/2009, regulated by 2003/15/EC; Must be labeled on cosmetics and detergent products, if present at > 10 ppm (0.001%) in leave-on products and > 100 ppm (0.01%) in rinse-off products
Patch testing : 10% Pet. (SmartPracticeEurope, Chemotechnique, SmartPracticeCanada); also present in the fragrance mix II
Molecular formula : $C_{15}H_{20}O$

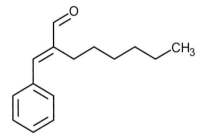

Table 3.80.1 IFRA restrictions for hexyl cinnamal

Category [a]	Limits [b]	Category [a]	Limits [b]	Category [a]	Limits [b]
1	0.70%	5	5.60%	9	5.00%
2	0.90%	6	17.10%	10	2.50%
3	3.60%	7	1.80%	11	not restricted
4	10.70%	8	2.00%		

[a] For explanation of categories see pages 6-8
[b] Limits in the finished products

GENERAL

Hexyl cinnamal is a pale yellow to yellow clear liquid to solid; its odor type is floral and its odor is described as 'sweet, floral, green, citrus and fruity with powdery tropical spicy notes' (www.thegoodscentscompany.com).

Presence in essential oils

Hexyl cinnamal has been identified by chemical analysis in three of 91 essential oils, which have caused contact allergy / allergic contact dermatitis: cinnamon leaf oil, Sri Lanka, neem oil and valerian oil (45).

CONTACT ALLERGY

General

The SCCS (Scientific Committee on Consumer Safety), in a 2012 Opinion on Fragrance allergens in cosmetic products, has marked hexyl cinnamal as 'established contact allergen in humans' (8,35). The sensitizing potency of hexyl cinnamal was classified as 'moderate' based on an EC3 value of 5.3% in the LLNA (local lymph node assay) in animal experiments (8,35). However, using Globally Harmonized Scheme criteria and applying a precautionary approach, hexyl cinnamal would classify as a weaker skin sensitizer than predicted by the local lymph node assay (47).

Hexyl cinnamal is a constituent of the fragrance mix II. In groups of patients reacting to the mix and tested with its 6 ingredients, hexyl cinnamal scored 0-9.7% positive patch test reactions (see Chapter 3.71 Fragrance mix II).

General population
In the period 2008-2011, in 5 European countries (Sweden, Germany, Netherlands, Portugal, Italy), a random sample of the general population of 3119 individuals aged 18-74 years were patch tested with the FM I, its 8 ingredients, the FM II, its 6 ingredients and Myroxylon pereirae resin. There were 8 reactions (0.3%) to hexyl cinnamal, tested 10% in petrolatum. About half of all positive reactions to fragrances were considered to be relevant based on standardized criteria. Women were affected twice as often as men (43).

Patch testing in groups of patients
Results of studies testing hexyl cinnamal in consecutive patients suspected of contact dermatitis (routine testing) and results of testing in groups of *selected* patients (e.g. patients with known or suspected fragrance or cosmetic dermatitis, individuals with hand eczema) are shown in table 3.80.2.

Patch testing in consecutive patients suspected of contact dermatitis: routine testing
In nine studies in which routine testing with hexyl cinnamal was performed, frequencies of sensitization were invariably (very) low, ranging from 0.06% to 0.6% (table 3.80.2). In 7/9 investigations, no (specific) data on relevance were provided; in the two studies addressing the issue, some 2/3 of the positive reactions were scored as relevant (1,31). Causative products were not mentioned.

Table 3.80.2 Patch testing in groups of patients

Years and Country	Test conc. & vehicle	Number of patients tested	positive (%)	Selection of patients (S); Relevance (R); Comments (C)	Ref.
Routine testing					
2015-7 Netherlands		821	3 (0.4%)	R: not stated	50
2015-2016 UK	10% pet.	2084	7 (0.3%)	R: not specified for individual fragrances; 25% of patients who reacted to any fragrance or fragrance marker had a positive fragrance history	48
2010-2015 Denmark	8% pet.	6004	(0.45%)	R: present relevance 62%, past relevance 31%	31
2009-2015 Sweden	10% pet.	4175	9 (0.2%)	R: not stated	36
2011-2012 UK	10% pet.	1951	9 (0.5%)	R: not stated	34
2008-2010 Denmark	10% pet.	1503	9 (0.6%)	S: mostly routine testing; R: 67%; C: 33% co-reactivity of FM I, 78% of FM II; C: of the relevant reactions to any of the 26 fragrances tested, 96% were caused by cosmetic products	1
2003-2004 IVDK	10% pet.	2019	3 (0.1%)	R: not stated	3
2002-2003 six European countries	5% pet.	1701	1 (0.06%)	R: not specified	6
	10% pet.	1701	2 (0.1%)	R: not specified	
1997-1998 six European countries	10% pet.	1855	6 (0.3%)	R: not stated / specified	24
Testing in groups of selected patients					
2011-2015 Spain	10% pet.	1013	21 (2.1%)	S: patients previously reacting to FM I, FM II, Myroxylon pereirae resin or hydroxyisohexyl 3-cyclohexene carboxaldehyde in the baseline series; R: not stated	51
2009-2010 Hungary	10% pet.	565	20 (3.5%)	S: patients with former skin symptoms provoked by scented products in the case history; R: in all cases 'possible'	5
2005-10 Netherlands		100	7 (7%)	S: patients with known fragrance sensitivity based on a positive patch test to the FM I and/or the FM II; R: not stated	37
2005-7 Netherlands	5% pet.	320	2 (0.6%)	S: patients suspected of fragrance or cosmetic allergy; R: 61% relevance for all positive tested fragrances together	2
2001-2002 Denmark, Sweden	10% pet.	658	3 (0.5%)	S: consecutive patients with hand eczema; R: it was assumed that nearly all positive reactions were of present or past relevance	4
1975 USA	5% pet.	20	1 (5%)	S: fragrance-allergic patients; R: not stated	9

Testing in groups of patients reacting to the fragrance mix II
Results of testing hexyl cinnamal in groups of patients reacting to the fragrance mix II are shown in Chapter 3.71 Fragrance mix II

FM: Fragrance mix; IVDK: Informationsverbund Dermatologischer Kliniken (Germany, Switzerland, Austria)

Patch testing in groups of selected patients
Results of studies patch testing hexyl cinnamal in groups of selected patients (e.g. patients with known or suspected fragrance or cosmetic dermatitis, individuals with hand eczema) are shown in table 3.80.2. In eight investigations, frequencies of sensitization to hexyl cinnamal have ranged from 0.5% to 7%. The highest rates (5% and 7%) were

observed in groups of patients known to be allergic to fragrances (9,37). In one of these, with 7% positive reactions, patients were (partly) selected on the basis of a reaction to the fragrance mix II, which contains hexyl cinnamal (37). In most studies, no (specific) relevance data were provided. Some authors considered relevance for all reactions 'possible' (5), others 'assumed' that nearly all positive reactions were of present or past relevance (4). Causative products were usually not mentioned or specified, but in one study, of the relevant reactions to any of 26 fragrances tested, 96% were caused by cosmetic products (1).

Results of testing hexyl cinnamal in groups of patients reacting to the fragrance mix II are shown in Chapter 3.71 Fragrance mix II.

Case reports and case series

Hexyl cinnamal was stated to be the (or an) allergen in 7 patients in a group of 603 individuals suffering from cosmetic dermatitis, seen in the period 2010-2015 in Leuven, Belgium (30).

In the period 2000-2009, in Leuven, Belgium, an unspecified number of patients had positive patch tests or use tests to a total of 344 cosmetic products *and* positive patch tests to FM I, FM II, and/or to one or more of 28 selected specific fragrance ingredients. In 8 of 10 patients reacting to hexyl cinnamal, the presence of this fragrance in the cosmetic product(s) was confirmed by reading the product label(s) (38).

In a group of 119 patients with allergic contact dermatitis from cosmetics, investigated in The Netherlands in 1986-1987, one case was caused by hexyl cinnamal in a skin care product (21,22).

A woman had allergic contact dermatitis from hexyl cinnamal, hydroxyisohexyl 3-cyclohexenecarboxaldehyde, alpha-damascone and benzophenone-2 in an eau de parfum (40). Another patient had axillary dermatitis from contact allergy to hexyl cinnamal in a deodorant (6).

Cross-reactions, pseudo-cross-reactions and co-reactions

For general information on cross-/pseudo-cross-/co-reactivity of fragrance chemicals with other fragrances, fragrance markers (fragrance mix I, fragrance mix II, colophonium, Myroxylon pereirae resin [balsam of Peru]) and essential oils see Chapter 1.2 General information on cross-reactions, pseudo-cross-reactions and co-reactions. Co-reactivity with the fragrance mix II can be expected, as the mix contains hexyl cinnamal (pseudo-cross-reactions).

In a large study performed by the IVDK in the period 2005-2013, of 26 patients reacting to hexyl cinnamal, five (19%) co-reacted to amyl cinnamal. Conversely, of 11 individuals allergic to amyl cinnamal, five (45%) co-reacted to hexyl cinnamal (49). In the same investigation, of 39 patients reacting to cinnamal, 3 (7.7%) had a positive reaction to hexyl cinnamal (49).

Presence in products and chemical analyses

In various studies, the presence of hexyl cinnamal in cosmetic and sometimes other products has been investigated. Before 2006, most investigators used chemical analysis, usually GC-MS, for qualitative and quantitative determination. Since then, the presence of the target fragrances was usually investigated by screening the product labels for the 26 fragrances that must be labeled since 2005 on cosmetics and detergent products in the EU, if present at > 10 ppm (0.001%) in leave-on products and > 100 ppm (0.01%) in rinse-off products. This method, obviously, is less accurate and may result in underestimation of the frequency of the fragrances being present in the product. When they are in fact present, but the concentration is lower than mentioned above, labeling is not required and the fragrances' presence will be missed.

The results of the relevant studies for hexyl cinnamal are summarized in table 3.80.3. More detailed information can be found in the corresponding text before and following the table. The percentage of products in which hexyl cinnamal was found to be present shows wide variations, but generally speaking it can be stated that hexyl cinnamal is a frequently used fragrance.

In 2017, in the USA, the ingredient labels 159 hair-dye kits containing 539 cosmetic products (e.g. colorants, conditioners, shampoos, toners) were screened for the most common sensitizers they contain. Hexyl cinnamal was found to be present in 32 (6%) of the products (42).

In Denmark, in 2015-2016, 5588 fragranced cosmetic products were examined with a smartphone application for the 26 fragrances that need to be labeled in the EU. Hexyl cinnamal was present in 22% of the products (rank number 6) (19).

In Germany, in 2015, fragrance allergens were evaluated based on lists of ingredients in 817 (unique) detergents (all-purpose cleaners, cleaning preparations for special purposes [e.g. bathroom, kitchen, dish-washing] and laundry detergents) present in 131 households. Hexyl cinnamal was found to be present in 117 (14%) of the products (46).

In Sweden, in 2015, contact allergens were identified on the ingredient labels of 26 oxidative hair dye products (from 4 different product series) and on the labels of 35 non-oxidative hair dye products (from 5 different product series, including so-called herbal hair colors). These products were selected on the basis of being advertised as 'organic', 'natural', or similar, or used in hairdressing salons branded with such attributes. Hexyl cinnamal was present in six (23%) of the 26 oxidative hair dyes and in zero of the 35 non-oxidative hair dye products (33).

Table 3.80.3 Presence of hexyl cinnamal in products [a]

Year	Country	Product type	Nr. investigated	Nr. of products positive [b]	(%)	Method [c]	Ref.
2017	USA	Cosmetic products in hair-dye kits	539 products in 159 hair-dye kits	32	(6%)	Labeling	42
2015-6	Denmark	Fragranced cosmetic products	5588		(22%)	Labeling	19
2015	Germany	Household detergents	817	117	(14%)	Labeling	46
2015	Sweden	Oxidative hair dye products	26	6	(23%)	Labeling	33
		Non-oxidative	35	0	(0%)	Labeling	
2014	Poland	Emollients	179	5	(3%)	Online info	32
2013	USA	Pediatric cosmetics	187	1	(0.5%)	Labeling	23
2008-11	Germany	Deodorants	374	103	(28%)	Labeling	44
2009	Italy	Liquid household washing and cleaning products	291	83	(29%)	Labeling & website information	39
2006-9	Germany	Cosmetic products	4991		(13%)	Labeling	18
2008	Sweden	Cosmetic products	204		(32%)	Labeling	10
		Detergents	97		(13%)	Labeling	
2007	Netherlands	Cosmetic products for children	23	13	(43%)	Analysis	26
2006	UK	Perfumed cosmetic and house-hold products	300	125	(42%)	Labeling	16
2006	Denmark	Popular perfumed deodorants	88	29	(33%)	Labeling	20
			23	11	(48%)	Analysis	
2006	Netherlands	Laundry detergents	52	29	(56%)	Labeling + analysis	28
2006	Denmark	Rinse-off cosmetics for children	208	21	(10%)	Labeling + analysis	25
2004	Denmark, UK, Belgium, Germany	Fragranced products that had caused allergic contact derma-titis, used by patients	24	14	(58%)	Labeling	6
2002	Denmark	Home and car air fresheners	19	13	(68%)	Analysis	29
2001	Denmark	Non-cosmetic consumer pro-ducts	43	17	(40%)	Analysis	27
2000	Denmark, UK, Germany, Italy	Domestic and occupational products	59	19	(32%)	Analysis	12
1997-8	Denmark, UK Germany, Sweden	Cosmetics and cosmetic toys for children	25	12	(48%)	Analysis	14
1996	Five European countries	Fragranced deodorants	70	50	(71%)	Analysis	11
1995	Denmark	Cosmetic products based on natural ingredients	42	26	(62%)	Analysis	13
1994	Denmark	Cosmetics that had given a po-sitive patch or use test in FM I allergic patients	23	15	(65%)	Analysis	41
1992	Netherlands	Cosmetic products	300		(48%)	Analysis	17
1988	USA	Perfumes used in fine fragran-ces, household products and soap	400	40-51% (see text)		Analysis	15

[a] See the corresponding text below for more details
[b] Positive = containing the target fragrance
[c] Labeling: information from the ingredient labels on the product / packaging; Analysis: chemical analysis, most often GC-MS

Of 179 emollients available in online drugstores in 2014 in Poland, five (2.8%) contained hexyl cinnamal, according to information available online (32).

In 2013, in the USA, the allergen content of 187 unique pediatric cosmetics from 6 different retailers marketed in the United States as hypoallergenic was evaluated on the basis of labeling. Inclusion criteria were products marketed as pediatric and 'hypoallergenic', 'dermatologist recommended/tested', 'fragrance free', or 'paraben free'. Hexyl cinnamal was found to be present in one (0.5%) of the products (23).

In 2008, 2010 and 2011, 374 deodorants available in German retail shops were randomly selected and their labels checked for the presence of the 26 fragrances that need to be labeled. Hexyl cinnamal was found to be present in 103 (27.5%) of the products (44).

In Italy, in 2009, the labels and website product information of 291 liquid household washing and cleaning products were studied for the presence of potential allergens. Hexyl cinnamal was found to be present in 83 (29%) of the products (39).

In Germany, in the period 2006-2009, 4991 cosmetic products were randomly sampled for an official investigation of conformity of cosmetic products with legal provisions. The labels were inspected for the presence of the 26 fragrances that need to be labeled in the EU. Hexyl cinnamal was present in 13% of the products (rank number 6) (18).

Hexyl cinnamal was present (as indicated by labeling) in 32% of 204 cosmetic products (92 shampoos, 61 hair conditioners, 34 liquid soaps, 17 wet tissues) and in 13% of 97 detergents in Sweden, 2008 (10).

In 2007, in The Netherlands, twenty-three cosmetic products for children were analyzed for the presence of fragrances that need to be labeled. Hexyl cinnamal was identified in 10 of the products (43%) in a concentration range of 29-4124 ppm (26).

In 2006, of 88 popular perfume containing deodorants purchased in Denmark, 29 (33%) were labeled to contain hexyl cinnamal. Analysis of 24 regulated fragrance substances in 23 selected deodorants (19 spray products, 2 deostick and 2 roll-on) was performed by GC-MS. Hexyl cinnamal was identified in 11 of the products (48%) with a concentration range of 1–4434 ppm (20).

In 2006, the labels of 208 cosmetics for children (especially shampoos, body shampoos and soaps) available in Denmark were checked for the presence of the 26 fragrances that need to be labeled in the EU. Hexyl cinnamal was present in 21 products (10.1%), and ranked number 4 in the frequency list. Seventeen products were analyzed quantitatively for the fragrances. Seventeen products were analyzed quantitatively for the fragrances. The maximum concentration found for hexyl cinnamal was 170 mg/kg (25).

In January 2006, a study of perfumed cosmetic and household products available on the shelves of U.K. retailers was carried out. Products were included if 'parfum' or 'aroma' was listed among the ingredients. Three hundred products were surveyed and any of 26 mandatory labeling fragrances named on the label were recorded. Hexyl cinnamal was present in 125 (42%) of the products (rank number 6) (16).

In 2006, in The Netherlands, 52 laundry detergents were investigated for the presence of allergenic fragrances by checking their labels and chemical analyses. Hexyl cinnamal was found to be present in 29 of the products (56%) in a concentration range of 8-744 ppm. Hexyl cinnamal had rank number 1 in the frequency list (28).

In 2004, in 4 European countries (Denmark, Germany, Belgium, U.K.), of 12 patients allergic to the FM II and one or more of its constituents (hexyl cinnamal 1, citral 3, hydroxyisohexyl 3-cyclohexene carboxaldehyde 11), 24 of the products used by them (deodorant 4, eau de toilette 9, lotion/cream 4, fine perfume 7) that had caused adverse reactions compatible with allergic contact dermatitis, were analyzed for the presence of the six constituents (citral, citronellol, coumarin, farnesol, hexyl cinnamal, hydroxyisohexyl 3-cyclohexene carboxaldehyde). Hexyl cinnamal was found in 14/24 products (58%) in concentrations ranging from 0.010–1.087% (6).

In 2002, in Denmark, 19 air fresheners (6 for cars, 13 for homes) were analyzed for the presence of fragrances that need to be labeled on cosmetics. Hexyl cinnamal was found to be present in 13 products (68%) in a concentration range of 39-22,000 ppm and ranked 3 in the frequency list (29).

In 2001, in Denmark, 43 non-cosmetic consumer products (mainly dish-washing products, laundry detergents, and hard and soft surface cleaners) were analyzed for the 26 fragrances that are regulated for labeling in the EU. Hexyl cinnamal was present in 17 products (40%) in a concentration range of 0.0001-0.0492% (m/m) and had rank number 3 in the frequency list (27).

In 2000, fifty-nine domestic and occupational products, purchased in retail outlets in Denmark, England, Germany and Italy were analyzed by GC-MS for the presence of fragrances. The product categories were liquid soap and soap bars (n=13), soft/hard surface cleaners (n=23), fabric conditioners/laundry detergents for hand wash (n=8), dish- wash (n=10), furniture polish, car shampoo, stain remover (each n=1) and 2 products used in occupational environments. Hexyl cinnamal was present in 19 products (32%) with a mean concentration of 328 ppm and a range of 53-674 ppm (12).

Twenty-five cosmetics and cosmetic toys for children (5 shampoos and shower gels, 6 perfumes, 1 deodorant (roll-on), 4 baby lotions/creams, 1 baby wipes product, 1 baby oil, 2 lipcare products and 5 toy-cosmetic products: a cosmetic-toy set for blending perfumes and a makeup set) purchased in 1997-1998 in retail outlets in Denmark, Germany, England and Sweden were analyzed in 1998 for the presence of fragrances by GC-MS. Hexyl cinnamal was found in 12 products (48%) in a concentration range of 0.002-0.333% (w/w). For the analytical data in each product category, the original publication should be consulted (14).

Seventy fragranced deodorants, purchased at retail outlets in 5 European countries in 1996, were analyzed by gas chromatography - mass spectrometry (GC-MS) for the determination of the contents of 21 commonly used fragrance materials. Hexyl cinnamal was identified in 50 products (71%) in a concentration range of 2–1684 ppm (11).

In 1995, in Denmark, 42 cosmetic products based on natural ingredients from 12 European and US companies (of which 22 were perfumes and 20 various other cosmetics) were investigated by high-resolution gas chromatography-mass spectrometry (GC-MS) for the presence of 11 fragrances. Hexyl cinnamal was present in 8 (36%) of the 22 perfumes in a concentration range of 0.105-7.706 w/w%; it was also identified in 4 of the other cosmetics in a concentration range of 0.0007-0.0820 % (13).

In Denmark, in 1994, 23 cosmetic products, which had either given a positive patch and/or use test in a total of 11 fragrance-mix-positive patients, and which products completely or partly explained present or past episodes of dermatitis, were analyzed for the presence of the constituents of the FM I (with the exception of oakmoss absolute) and a few other fragrances. Hexyl cinnamal was found to be present in 15 of the 23 products (65%) in a concentration range of <0.001-0.66% v/v with a mean concentration of 0.127% v/v (41).

In 1992, in The Netherlands, the presence of fragrances was analyzed in 300 cosmetic products. Hexyl cinnamal was identified in 48% of the products (rank order 13) (17).

In 1988, in the USA, 400 perfumes used in fine fragrances, household products and soaps (number of products per category not mentioned) were analyzed for the presence of fragrance chemicals in a concentration of at least 1% and a list of the Top-25 (present in the highest number of products) presented. Hexyl cinnamal was found to be present in 51% of the fine fragrances (rank number 9), 46% of the product fragrances (rank number 10) and 40% of the fragrances used in soaps (rank number 15) (15).

LITERATURE

1   Heisterberg MV, Menné T, Johansen JD. Contact allergy to the 26 specific fragrance ingredients to be declared on cosmetic products in accordance with the EU cosmetic directive. Contact Dermatitis 2011;65:266-275

2   Oosten EJ van, Schuttelaar ML, Coenraads PJ. Clinical relevance of positive patch test reactions to the 26 EU-labelled fragrances. Contact Dermatitis 2009;61:217-223

3   Schnuch A, Uter W, Geier J, Lessmann H, Frosch PJ. Sensitization to 26 fragrances to be labelled according to current European regulation: Results of the IVDK and review of the literature. Contact Dermatitis 2007;57:1-10

4   Heydorn S, Johansen JD, Andersen KE, Bruze M, Svedman C, White IR, et al. Fragrance allergy in patients with hand eczema – a clinical study. Contact Dermatitis 2003;48:317-323

5   Pónyai G, Németh I, Altmeyer A, Nagy G, Irinyi B, Battya Z, et al. Patch tests with fragrance mix II and its components. Dermatitis 2012;23:71-74

6   Frosch PJ, Rastogi SC, Pirker C, Brinkmeier T, Andersen KE, Bruze M, et al. Patch testing with a new fragrance mix - reactivity to the individual constituents and chemical detection in relevant cosmetic products. Contact Dermatitis 2005;52:216-225

7   Various SCCS opinions on hexyl cinnamal have been published and are available at: http://ec.europa.eu/growth/tools-databases/cosing/index.cfm?fuseaction=search.details_v2&id=27936

8   SCCS (Scientific Committee on Consumer Safety). Opinion on Fragrance allergens in cosmetic products, 26-27 June 2012, SCCS/1459/11. Available at: https://ec.europa.eu/health/sites/health/files/scientific_committees/consumer_safety/docs/sccs_o_102.pdf

9   Larsen WG. Perfume dermatitis. A study of 20 patients. Arch Dermatol 1977;113:623-626

10   Yazar K, Johnsson S, Lind M-L, Boman A, Lidén C. Preservatives and fragrances in selected consumer-available cosmetics and detergents. Contact Dermatitis 2011;64:265-272

11   Rastogi SC, Johansen JD, Frosch P, Menné T, Bruze M, Lepoittevin JP, et al. Deodorants on the European market: quantitative chemical analysis of 21 fragrances. Contact Dermatitis 1998;38:29-35

12   Rastogi SC, Heydorn S, Johansen JD, Basketter DA. Fragrance chemicals in domestic and occupational products. Contact Dermatitis 2001;45:221-225

13   Rastogi SC, Johansen JD, Menné T. Natural ingredients based cosmetics. Content of selected fragrance sensitizers. Contact Dermatitis 1996;34:423-426

14   Rastogi SC, Johansen JD, Menné T, Frosch P, Bruze M, Andersen KE, et al. Content of fragrance allergens in children's cosmetics and cosmetic toys. Contact Dermatitis 1999;41:84-88

15   Fenn RS. Aroma chemical usage trends in modern perfumery. Perfumer and Flavorist 1989;14:3-10

16   Buckley DA. Fragrance ingredient labelling in products on sale in the UK. Br J Dermatol 2007;157:295-300

17   Weyland JW. Personal Communication, 1992. Cited in: De Groot AC, Weyland JW, Nater JP. Unwanted effects of cosmetics and drugs used in dermatology, 3rd Ed. Amsterdam: Elsevier, 1994:579

18   Uter W, Yazar K, Kratz E-M, Mildau G, Lidén C. Coupled exposure to ingredients of cosmetic products: I. Fragrances. Contact Dermatitis 2013;69:335-341

19   Bennike NH, Oturai NB, Müller S, Kirkeby CS, Jørgensen C, Christensen AB, et al. Fragrance contact allergens in 5588 cosmetic products identified through a novel smartphone application. J Eur Acad Dermatol Venereol 2018;32:79-85

20 Rastogi SC, Hellerup Jensen G, Johansen JD. Survey and risk assessment of chemical substances in deodorants. Survey of Chemical Substances in Consumer Products, No. 86 2007. Danish Ministry of the Environment, Environmental Protection Agency. Available at: https://www2.mst.dk/Udgiv/publications/2007/978-87-7052-625-8/pdf/978-87-7052-626-5.pdf

21 De Groot AC, Bruynzeel DP, Bos JD, van der Meeren HL, van Joost T, Jagtman BA, Weyland JW. The allergens in cosmetics. Arch Dermatol 1988;124:1525-1529

22 De Groot AC. Adverse reactions to cosmetics. PhD Thesis, University of Groningen, The Netherlands: 1988, chapter 3.4, pp.105-113

23 Hamann CR, Bernard S, Hamann D, Hansen R, Thyssen JP. Is there a risk using hypoallergenic cosmetic pediatric products in the United States? J Allergy Clin Immunol 2015;135:1070-1071

24 Frosch PJ, Johansen JD, Menné T, Pirker C, Rastogi SC, Andersen KE, et al. Further important sensitizers in patients sensitive to fragrances. I. Reactivity to 14 frequently used chemicals. Contact Dermatitis 2002;47:78-85

25 Poulsen PB, Schmidt A. A survey and health assessment of cosmetic products for children. Survey of chemical substances in consumer products, No. 88. Copenhagen: Danish Environmental Protection Agency, 2007. Available at: https://www2.mst.dk/udgiv/publications/2007/978-87-7052-638-8/pdf/978-87-7052-639-5.pdf

26 VWA. Dutch Food and Consumer Product Safety Authority. Cosmetische producten voor kinderen: Inventarisatie van de markt en de veiligheidsborging door producenten en importeurs. Report ND04o065/ND05o170, 2007 (Report in Dutch), 2007. Available at: www.nvwa.nl/documenten/communicatie/inspectieresultaten/ consument/ 2016m/cosmetische- producten-voor-kinderen

27 Rastogi SC. Survey of chemical compounds in consumer products. Contents of selected fragrance materials in cleaning products and other consumer products. Survey no. 8-2002. Copenhagen, Denmark, Danish Environmental Protection Agency. Available at: http://eng.mst.dk/media/mst/69131/8.pdf

28 Bouma K, Van Peursem AJJ. Marktonderzoek naleving detergenten verordening voor textielwasmiddelen. Dutch Food and Consumer Products Safety Authority (VWA) Report ND06K173, 2006 [in Dutch]. Available at: http://docplayer.nl/41524125-Marktonderzoek-naleving-detergenten-verordening-voor-textielwasmiddelen.html

29 Pors J, Fuhlendorff R. Mapping of chemical substances in air fresheners and other fragrance liberating products. Report Danish Ministry of the Environment, Environmental Protection Agency (EPA). Survey of Chemicals in Consumer Products, No 30, 2003. Available at: http://eng.mst.dk/media/mst/69113/30.pdf

30 Goossens A. Cosmetic contact allergens. Cosmetics 2016, 3, 5; doi:10.3390/cosmetics3010005

31 Bennike NH, Zachariae C, Johansen JD. Non-mix fragrances are top sensitizers in consecutive dermatitis patients – a cross-sectional study of the 26 EU-labelled fragrance allergens. Contact Dermatitis 2017;77:270-279

32 Osinka K, Karczmarz A, Krauze K, Feleszko W. Contact allergens in cosmetics used in atopic dermatitis: analysis of product composition. Contact Dermatitis 2016;75:241-243

33 Thorén S, Yazar K. Contact allergens in 'natural' hair dyes. Contact Dermatitis 2016;74:302-304

34 Mann J, McFadden JP, White JML, White IR, Banerjee P. Baseline series fragrance markers fail to predict contact allergy. Contact Dermatitis 2014;70:276-281

35 Uter W, Johansen JD, Börje A, Karlberg A-T, Lidén C, Rastogi S, Roberts D, White IR. Categorization of fragrance contact allergens for prioritization of preventive measures: clinical and experimental data and consideration of structure–activity relationships. Contact Dermatitis 2013;69:196-230

36 Mowitz M, Svedman C, Zimerson E, Isaksson M, Pontén A, Bruze M. Simultaneous patch testing with fragrance mix I, fragrance mix II and their ingredients in southern Sweden between 2009 and 2015. Contact Dermatitis 2017;77:280-287

37 Nagtegaal MJC, Pentinga SE, Kuik J, Kezic S, Rustemeyer T. The role of the skin irritation response in polysensitization to fragrances. Contact Dermatitis 2012;67:28-35

38 Nardelli A, Drieghe J, Claes L, Boey L, Goossens A. Fragrance allergens in 'specific' cosmetic products. Contact Dermatitis 2011;64:212-219

39 Magnano M, Silvani S, Vincenzi C, Nino M, Tosti A. Contact allergens and irritants in household washing and cleaning products. Contact Dermatitis 2009;61:337-341

40 Giménez-Arnau A, Giménez-Arnau E, Serra-Baldrich E, Lepoittevin J-P, Camarasa JG. Principles and methodology for identification of fragrance allergens in consumer products. Contact Dermatitis 2002;47:345-352

41 Johansen JD, Rastogi SC, Menné T. Exposure to selected fragrance materials: A case study of fragrance-mix-positive eczema patients. Contact Dermatitis 1996;34:106-110

42 Hamann D, Kishi P, Hamann CR. Consumer hair dye kits frequently contain isothiazolinones, other common preservatives and fragrance allergens. Dermatitis 2018;29:48-49

43 Diepgen TL, Ofenloch R, Bruze M, Cazzaniga S, Coenraads PJ, Elsner P, et al. Prevalence of fragrance contact allergy in the general population of five European countries: a cross-sectional study. Br J Dermatol 2015;173:1411-1419

44 Klaschka U. Contact allergens for armpits - allergenic fragrances specified on deodorants. Int J Hyg Environ Health 2012;215:584-591

45 De Groot AC, Schmidt E. Essential oils: contact allergy and chemical composition. Boca Raton, Fl., USA: CRC Press, Taylor and Francis Group, 2016 (ISBN 9781482246407)

46 Wieck S, Olsson O, Kümmerer K, Klaschka U. Fragrance allergens in household detergents. Regul Toxicol Pharmacol 2018;97:163-169

47 Basketter D, White IR, McFadden JP, Kimber I. Hexyl cinnamal: consideration of skin-sensitizing properties and suitability as a positive control. Cutan Ocul Toxicol 2015;34:227-231

48 Ung CY, White JML, White IR, Banerjee P, McFadden JP. Patch testing with the European baseline series fragrance markers: a 2016 update. Br J Dermatol 2018;178:776-780

49 Geier J, Uter W, Lessmann H, Schnuch A. Fragrance mix I and II: results of breakdown tests. Flavour Fragr J 2015;30:264-274

50 Dittmar D, Schuttelaar MLA. Contact sensitization to hydroperoxides of limonene and linalool: Results of consecutive patch testing and clinical relevance. Contact Dermatitis 2018 Oct 31. doi: 10.1111/cod.13137. [Epub ahead of print]

51 Silvestre JF, Mercader P, González-Pérez R, Hervella-Garcés M, Sanz-Sánchez T, Córdoba S, et al. Sensitization to fragrances in Spain: A 5-year multicentre study (2011-2015). Contact Dermatitis. 2018 Nov 14. doi: 10.1111/cod.13152. [Epub ahead of print]

Chapter 3.81   HEXYL SALICYLATE

IDENTIFICATION

Description/definition : Hexyl salicylate is the organic compound that conforms to the structural formula shown below

Chemical class(es) : Esters; phenols

Chemical/IUPAC name : Hexyl 2-hydroxybenzoate

Other names : Benzoic acid, 2-hydroxy-, hexyl ester

CAS registry number(s) : 6259-76-3

EC number(s) : 228-408-6

RIFM monograph(s) : Food Chem Toxicol 2007;45(suppl.1):S410-S417; Food Chem Toxicol 2007;45(suppl.1): S318-S361; Food Cosmet Toxicol 1975;13:807 (special issue II)

IFRA standard : Restricted (www.ifraorg.org/en-us/standards-library) (table 3.81.1)

Function(s) in cosmetics : EU: masking; perfuming. USA: fragrance ingredients

Patch testing : 12% pet. (2); based on RIFM data, 3% pet. is probably not irritant (4)

Molecular formula : $C_{13}H_{18}O_3$

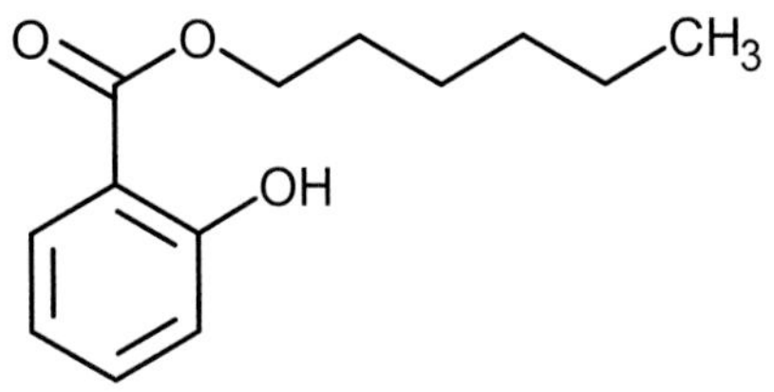

Table 3.81.1 IFRA restrictions for hexyl salicylate

Category [a]	Limits [b]	Category [a]	Limits [b]	Category [a]	Limits [b]
1	1.00%	5	8.40%	9	5.00%
2	1.30%	6	25.70%	10	2.50%
3	5.30%	7	2.70%	11	not restricted
4	16.00%	8	2.00%		

[a] For explanation of categories see pages 6-8
[b] Limits in the finished products

GENERAL

Hexyl salicylate is a colorless clear oily liquid; its odor type is herbal and its odor at 100% is described as 'fresh herbal orchid green' (www.thegoodscentscompany.com).

Presence in essential oils

Hexyl salicylate has been identified by chemical analysis in none of 91 essential oils, which have caused contact allergy / allergic contact dermatitis (6).

CONTACT ALLERGY

General

Hexyl salicylate was found to be an 'extreme' sensitizer in the murine local lymph node assay (LLNA) (3). In another report, the sensitizing potency of hexyl salicylate was classified as 'strong' based on an EC3 value of 0.18% in the LLNA in animal experiments (5).

Patch testing in groups of patients

Patch testing in consecutive patients suspected of contact dermatitis: routine testing

Studies in which hexyl salicylate was patch tested in consecutive patients suspected of contact dermatitis (routine testing) with positive results have not been found.

Patch testing in groups of selected patients

Before 2002, in Japan, European countries and the USA, 218 patients with known fragrance sensitivity were patch tested with hexyl salicylate 5% in petrolatum and there were no positive reactions (7).

Case reports and case series

A baker was patch tested for hand dermatitis and showed positive reactions to cocoa-powder and 'speculaas-kruiden', a mixture of unknown composition, which he used at work. When subsequently tested with a series of fragrances and flavors, he had positive reactions to hexyl salicylate 12%, citral 0.5%, cinnamal 0.5%, amyl cinnamate 32% and cinnamyl cinnamate 8%, all in petrolatum. The author was 'inclined' to say that these reactions may have been relevant (2).

Presence in products and chemical analyses

In 2000, fifty-nine domestic and occupational products, purchased in retail outlets in Denmark, England, Germany and Italy were analyzed by GC-MS for the presence of fragrances. The product categories were liquid soap and soap bars (n=13), soft/hard surface cleaners (n=23), fabric conditioners/laundry detergents for hand wash (n=8), dish wash (n=10), furniture polish, car shampoo, stain remover (each n=1) and 2 products used in occupational environments. Hexyl salicylate was present in 11 products (19%) with a mean concentration of 634 ppm and a range of 61-4060 ppm (1).

LITERATURE

1   Rastogi SC, Heydorn S, Johansen JD, Basketter DA. Fragrance chemicals in domestic and occupational products. Contact Dermatitis 2001;45:221-225

2   Malten KE. Four bakers showing positive patch tests to a number of fragrance materials, which can also be used as flavors. Acta Derm Venereol 1979;59(suppl.85):117-121

3   Lidén C, Yazar K, Johansen JD, Karlberg A-T, Uter W, White IR. Comparative sensitizing potencies of fragrances, preservatives, and hair dyes. Contact Dermatitis 2016;75:265-275

4   De Groot AC. Patch Testing, 4th Edition. Wapserveen, The Netherlands: acdegroot publishing, 2018 (ISBN 978-90-813233-4-5)

5   SCCS (Scientific Committee on Consumer Safety). Opinion on Fragrance allergens in cosmetic products, 26-27 June 2012, SCCS/1459/11. Available at: https://ec.europa.eu/health/sites/health/files/scientific_committees/consumer_safety/docs/sccs_o_102.pdf

6   De Groot AC, Schmidt E. Essential oils: contact allergy and chemical composition. Boca Raton, Fl., USA: CRC Press, Taylor and Francis Group, 2016 (ISBN 9781482246407)

7   Larsen W, Nakayama H, Fischer T, Elsner P, Frosch P, Burrows D, et al. Fragrance contact dermatitis - a worldwide multicenter investigation (Part III). Contact Dermatitis 2002;46:141-144

Chapter 3.82   HYDROXYCITRONELLAL

IDENTIFICATION

Description/definition	: Hydroxycitronellal is the aldehyde that conforms to the structural formula shown below
Chemical class(es)	: Aldehydes
Chemical/IUPAC name	: 7-Hydroxy-3,7-dimethyloctanal
CAS registry number(s)	: 107-75-5
EC number(s)	: 203-518-7
RIFM monograph(s)	: Food Chem Toxicol 1988;26:921-926; Food Cosmet Toxicol 1974;12:921 (special issue 1)
IFRA standard	: Restricted (www.ifraorg.org/en-us/standards-library) (table 3.82.1)
SCCS opinion(s)	: SCCNFP/0392/00 (8); SCCS/1459/11 (9); SCCNFP/0389/00, final (89)
Function(s) in cosmetics	: EU: perfuming. USA: fragrance ingredients
EU cosmetic restrictions	: Regulated in Annex III/72 of the Regulation (EC) No. 1223/2009, regulated by 2003/15/EC; Must be labeled on cosmetics and detergent products, if present at > 10 ppm (0.001%) in leave-on products and > 100 ppm (0.01%) in rinse-off products
Patch testing	: 1% Pet. (SmartPracticeEurope, SmartPracticeCanada); 2% pet. (Chemotechnique); also present in the fragrance mix I; TEST ADVICE: 2% pet.
Molecular formula	: $C_{10}H_{20}O_2$

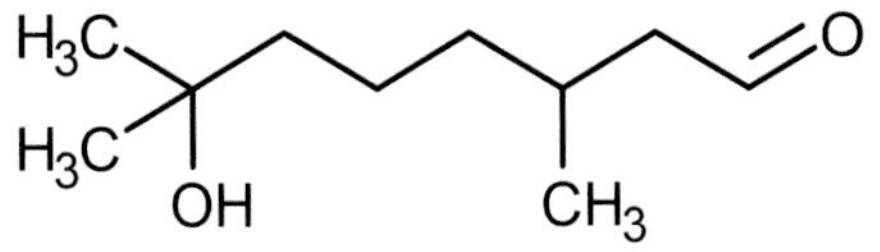

Table 3.82.1 IFRA restrictions for hydroxycitronellal

Category [a]	Limits [b]	Category [a]	Limits [b]	Category [a]	Limits [b]
1	0.10%	5	1.00%	9	1.00%
2	0.20%	6	3.60%	10	1.00%
3	0.80%	7	0.40%	11	not restricted
4	1.00%	8	1.00%		

[a] For explanation of categories see pages 6-8
[b] Limits in the finished products

GENERAL

Hydroxycitronellal is a colorless to pale yellow clear oily liquid; its odor type is floral and its odor is described as 'sweet floral perfume-like notes with green citrus and melon undertones' (www.thegoodscentscompany.com). Hydroxycitronellal is a synthetic fragrance and has not been found in nature (and consequently not in essential oils [87]).

CONTACT ALLERGY

General

The SCCS (Scientific Committee on Consumer Safety), in a 2012 Opinion on Fragrance allergens in cosmetic products, has marked hydroxycitronellal as 'established contact allergen in humans' (9,59). The sensitizing potency of hydroxycitronellal was classified as 'weak' based on an EC3 value of 19.3% in the LLNA (local lymph node assay) in animal experiments (9,59). Nevertheless, concentrations as low as 2.5% hydroxycitronellal have been shown to induce sensitization in the human repeated insult patch test and 5% hydroxycitronellal was found to sensitize 36% of healthy volunteers (77,86).

Hydroxycitronellal is a constituent of the fragrance mix I. In groups of patients reacting to the mix and tested with its 8 ingredients, hydroxycitronellal scored 2.5-20% positive patch test reactions, median 12.9% and average 11.6%. It has rank number 4/5/6 (with cinnamyl alcohol and eugenol) in the list of most frequent reactors in the mix (see Chapter 3.70 Fragrance mix I).

General population

In the period 2008-2011, in 5 European countries (Sweden, Germany, Netherlands, Portugal, Italy), a random sample of the general population of 3119 individuals aged 18-74 years were patch tested with the FM I, its 8 ingredients, the FM II, its 6 ingredients and Myroxylon pereirae resin. There were 15 (0.5%) reactions to hydroxycitronellal, tested 2%

in petrolatum. About half of all positive reactions to fragrances were considered to be relevant based on standardized criteria. Women were affected twice as often as men (74).

Patch testing in groups of patients
Results of studies testing hydroxycitronellal in consecutive patients suspected of contact dermatitis (routine testing) are shown in table 3.82.2. Results of testing in groups of *selected* patients (e.g. patients with known or suspected fragrance or cosmetic dermatitis, individuals with hand eczema, individuals who had previously had positive patch tests to their own perfumes) are shown in table 3.82.3.

Patch testing in consecutive patients suspected of contact dermatitis: routine testing
In thirteen studies in which routine testing with hydroxycitronellal was performed, frequencies of sensitization have ranged from 0.4% to 3.8% (table 3.82.2). The very high rate of 3.8% was observed in a small study from Thailand, in which virtually all fragrances had higher scores than in other investigations (56).

In 10/13 investigations, no (specific) data on relevance were provided; in the three studies addressing the issue, 50-83% of the positive reactions were scored as relevant (1,54,56). Causative products were usually not mentioned or specified, but in one study, of the relevant reactions to any of 26 fragrances tested, 96% were caused by cosmetic products (1).

Table 3.82.2 Patch testing in groups of patients: Routine testing

Years and Country	Test conc. & vehicle	Number of patients tested	positive (%)	Selection of patients (S); Relevance (R); Comments (C)	Ref.
2015-7 Netherlands		821	14 (1.7%)	R: not stated	93
2015-2016 UK	2% pet.	2084	22 (1.1%)	R: not specified for individual fragrances; 25% of patients who reacted to any fragrance or fragrance marker had a positive fragrance history	91
2010-2015 Denmark	1% pet.	6004	55 (0.92%)	R: present relevance 50%, past relevance 41%	54
2009-2015 Sweden	2% pet.	4483	22 (0.5%)	R: not stated	61
2013-2014 Thailand		312	12 (3.8%)	R: 83%	56
2011-2012 UK	2% pet.	1951	20 (1.0%)	R: not stated	58
2010-2011 China	2% pet.	296	(1.4%)	R: 67% for all fragrances tested together (excluding FM I)	57
2008-2010 Denmark	1% pet.	1498	13 (0.9%)	S: mostly routine testing; R: 67%; 100% co-reactivity of FM I, 89% of FM II; C: of the relevant reactions to any of the 26 fragrances tested, 96% were caused by cosmetic products	1
2005-2008 IVDK	1% pet.	1214	(1.2%)	R: not stated	64
2003-2004 IVDK	1% pet.	2063	21 (1.0%)	R: not stated; C: 67% co-reactivity of FM I	3
<1995 9 European countries + USA	1% pet.	1072	8 (0.8%)	R: not stated	33
1993 EECDRG	1% pet.	709	3 (0.4%)	R: not stated	68
1991 The Netherlands	5% pet.	677	12 (1.8%)	R: not stated	69

EECDRG: European Environmental and Contact Dermatitis Research Group; FM: Fragrance Mix; IVDK: Informationsverbund Dermatologischer Kliniken (Germany, Switzerland, Austria)

Patch testing in groups of selected patients
Results of studies patch testing hydroxycitronellal in groups of selected patients (e.g. patients with known or suspected fragrance or cosmetic dermatitis, individuals with hand eczema, individuals who had previously had positive patch tests to their own perfumes) are shown in table 3.82.3.

In 14 investigations, frequencies of sensitization to hydroxycitronellal have ranged from 1.0% to 45%. The latter extremely high rate of 45% was observed in an early small study from the USA among 20 patients with fragrance allergy (12), when very high concentrations of hydroxycitronellal were still used in fragrances. Frequencies of 7-14% positive reactions to hydroxycitronellal were observed in patients known or suspected to be fragrance-allergic. In 13/14 studies, no (specific) relevance data were provided; the authors of the one investigation addressing the issue 'assumed' that nearly all positive reactions were of present or past relevance (6). Causative products were not mentioned.

Results of testing hydroxycitronellal in groups of patients reacting to the fragrance mix I are shown in Chapter 3.70 Fragrance mix I.

Table 3.82.3 Patch testing in groups of patients: Selected patient groups

Years and Country	Test conc. & vehicle	Number of patients tested	positive (%)	Selection of patients (S); Relevance (R); Comments (C)	Ref.
2011-2015 Spain	1% or 2% pet.	1013	71 (7.0%)	S: patients previously reacting to FM I, FM II, Myroxylon pereirae resin or hydroxyisohexyl 3-cyclohexene carboxaldehyde in the baseline series; R: not stated; C: the 2% test substances showed a higher rate of positive reactions than the 1% material	94
2003-2012 IVDK		607	26 (4.3%)	S: nurses with occupational contact dermatitis; R: not stated	53
2005-10 Netherlands		100	8 (8%)	S: patients with known fragrance sensitivity based on a positive patch test to the FM I and/or the FM II; R: not stated	62
2004-2008 Spain	5% pet.	86	6 (7%)	S: patients previously reacting to the fragrance mix I or Myroxylon pereirae (n=54) or suspected of fragrance contact allergy (n=32); R: not stated	35
2005-7 Netherlands	2% pet.	320	7 (2.2%)	S: patients suspected of fragrance or cosmetic allergy; R: 61% relevance for all positive tested fragrances together	2
<2003 Israel		91	3 (3%)	S: patients with a positive or doubtful reaction to the fragrance mix and/or Myroxylon pereirae resin and/or to one or two commercial fine fragrances; R: not stated	34
2001-2002 Denmark, Sweden	5% pet.	658	20 (3.0%)	S: consecutive patients with hand eczema; R: it was assumed that nearly all positive reactions were of present or past relevance	6
1998-2002 IVDK	1% pet.	33	4 (12%)	S: patients who had a positive reaction to their own deodorant; R: not stated	38
		31	4 (13%)	S: patients who had a positive reaction to their own perfume, eau de toilette or shaving product; R: not stated; C: there was a significant difference in percentage positive reactions compared with a control group of dermatitis patients who had *not* reacted to their own cosmetic products of this type	
1997-2000 Austria	1% pet.	747	11 (1.5%)	S: patients suspected of fragrance allergy; R: not stated	5
1990-1998 Japan	5% pet.	1483	15 (1.0%)	S: patients suspected of cosmetic contact dermatitis, virtually all were women; range of annual frequency of sensitization: 0-2.3%; R: not stated	80
<1996 Japan, Europe, USA	4% pet.	167	23 (13.8%)	S: patients known or suspected to be allergic to fragrances; R: not stated; C: also 13.8% reactivity to hydroxycitronellal 7%	7
<1986 France	5% pet.	21	2 (10%)	S: patients with dermatitis caused by perfumes; R: not stated	88
<1985 Netherlands		242	11 (4.5%)	S: randomly selected patients with proven contact allergy of different origins; R: not stated	71
1975 USA	5% pet.	20	9 (45%)	S: fragrance-allergic patients; R: not stated	12

Testing in groups of patients reacting to the fragrance mix I
Results of testing hydroxycitronellal in groups of patients reacting to the fragrance mix I are shown in Chapter 3.70 Fragrance mix I

FM: Fragrance Mix; IVDK: Informationsverbund Dermatologischer Kliniken (Germany, Switzerland, Austria)

Case reports and case series

Case series
Hydroxycitronellal was stated to be the (or an) allergen in 13 patients in a group of 603 individuals suffering from cosmetic dermatitis, seen in the period 2010-2015 in Leuven, Belgium (52). In the period 1996-2013, in a tertiary referral center in Valencia, Spain, 5419 patients were patch tested. Of these, 628 individuals had allergic contact dermatitis to cosmetics. In this group, hydroxycitronellal was the responsible allergen in 8 cases (31, overlap with ref. 32).

In the period 2000-2009, in Leuven, Belgium, an unspecified number of patients had positive patch tests or use tests to a total of 344 cosmetic products *and* positive patch tests to FM I, FM II, and/or to one or more of 28 selected specific fragrance ingredients. In 10 of 43 patients reacting to hydroxycitronellal, the presence of this fragrance in the cosmetic product(s) was confirmed by reading the product label(s) (63).

In the period 2000-2007, 202 patients with allergic contact dermatitis caused by cosmetics were seen in Valencia, Spain. In this group, hydroxycitronellal was the allergen in 4 individuals from its presence in cologne (n=3), shampoo (n=1) and moisturizing cream (n=1) (32, overlap with ref. 31). In a group of 119 patients with allergic contact dermatitis from cosmetics, investigated in The Netherlands in 1986-1987, 4 cases were caused by hydroxycitronellal in skin care products (n=2), deodorant and perfume (29,30).

In Belgium, in the years before 1986, of 5202 consecutive patients with dermatitis patch tested, 156 were diagnosed with pure cosmetic allergy. Hydroxycitronellal was the 'dermatitic ingredient' in 6 (3.8%) patients (frequency in the entire group: 0.5%). It should be realized, however, that only a very limited number of patients was tested with a fragrance series (70). Hydroxycitronellal was responsible for 11 out of 399 cases of cosmetic allergy where the causal allergen was identified in a study of the NACDG, USA, 1977-1983 (4).

Three individuals had allergic contact dermatitis from hydroxycitronellal in skin care products, and 3 others from this fragrance in hair lotion, deodorant cream and aftershave, respectively (20). Three other patients from Japan had allergic contact dermatitis of the covered skin areas from hydroxycitronellal added to washing detergents (36). Eight patients had allergic contact dermatitis from a topical pharmaceutical product and all reacted to its ingredient ethylenediamine (a stabilizer) and to the perfume 5% pet. When tested with the 28 individual fragrances of the perfume, there were 2 reactions to hydroxycitronellal, 5 to amyl cinnamal, 4 to cinnamyl alcohol, 2 to benzyl alcohol, and one to oakmoss synthetic (43).

Case reports

A female patient had allergic contact dermatitis from hydroxycitronellal in an eye cream (60). A man suffering from psoriasis developed allergic contact dermatitis from hydroxycitronellal and linalool in an aftershave, that evolved into facial psoriasis (Köbner-phenomenon) (21). One individual working in a perfume factory developed occupational contact allergy to hydroxycitronellal (44).

A barber had contact dermatitis localized to the dorsa of the fingers. Upon patch testing, he reacted to an aftershave only. Further patch testing with 22 perfume ingredients showed positive reactions to hydroxycitronellal (10% pet.), methyl 2-octynoate (0.5% pet.), and cinnamyl alcohol (5% pet.). By thin layer chromatography, column chromatography and gas chromatography all three fragrances were demonstrated in the aftershave. Whether this was the cause of the dermatitis of his hands was not stated (72).

A man had longstanding partly airborne dermatitis from contact allergy to hydroxycitronellal in a bubble bath and from his wife's spray perfumes and colognes used as air fresheners (45). A female patient had allergic contact dermatitis of the face from hydroxycitronellal in a cream make-up and a foundation lotion (78).

A man presented with follicular pustules and papules and large turgid red plaques in the beard area resembling folliculitis barbae, but mycological and bacterial studies were negative. Patch tests were positive to hydroxycitronellal, cinnamal, cinnamyl alcohol, FM I, Myroxylon pereirae resin, an aftershave and 2 colognes used by his wife. The patient often used a surgeon's mask in his work as dentist and would regularly spray this with perfume (which was patch test-negative). When all perfumes and perfumed products were stopped by him and his wife, the facial eruption subsided completely except for some mild folliculitis barbae. The author stated that 'It is clear that this man had an allergic contact dermatitis of the face due to cinnamyl alcohol, cinnamal and hydroxycitronellal. It was aggravated by his use of a surgeon's mask. The primary source may have been one of his wife's perfumes or one of his own aftershaves'. However, the presence of hydroxycitronellal, cinnamal and cinnamyl alcohol was not verified in any of the products (79).

A young atopic boy developed widespread itching eczematous dermatitis involving his trunk and limbs. The child's mother stated that she had applied insect repellent wipes on the days before the onset of dermatitis. Patch tests were positive to MCI/MI, hydroxycitronellal 5% pet. and the wipe 'as is'. The wipes, as declared on the packaging, contained DEET as the active principle, citriodiol, ethanol, and 'perfume'. They were analysed with liquid chromatography and mass spectroscopy (LCMS). MCI and MI were not identified, but a peak in accordance with DEET was observed and another peak that corresponded to the molecular weights of both hydroxycitronellal and citriodiol (81).

Pigmented cosmetic dermatitis

In Japan, in the 1960s and 1970s, many female patients developed pigmentation of the face after having facial dermatitis (47). The skin manifestations of this so-called pigmented cosmetic dermatitis consisted of diffuse or patchy brown hyperpigmentation on the cheeks and/or forehead, sometimes the entire face was involved. In severe cases, the pigmentation was black, purple, or blue-black, and in mild cases, it was pale brown. Occasionally, erythematous macules or papules, suggesting a mild contact dermatitis, were observed and itching was also noted at varying times. Pigmented cosmetic dermatitis was shown to be caused by contact allergy to components of cosmetic products, notably essential oils, other fragrance materials, antimicrobials, preservatives and coloring materials (46,47,48).

In a group of 575 Japanese patients with this condition investigated between 1970 and 1980, 5-8% had positive patch test reactions to hydroxycitronellal 10% in purified lanolin in various time periods versus 0 to 1% in a control group of patients not suffering from pigmented cosmetic dermatitis. The corresponding figures for patch testing with hydroxycitronellal 10% in hydrophilic ointment (Japanese preparation) were 18-21% and 3-10% (46).

The number of patients with pigmented cosmetic dermatitis decreased strongly after 1978, when major cosmetic companies began to eliminate strong contact sensitizers from their products (46). Since 1980, pigmented cosmetic dermatitis became a rare disease in Japan (49).

A female patient from Spain had developed pigmented contact dermatitis from a face compact powder. She showed positive patch test reactions to lemon oil, geraniol and hydroxycitronellal; two of these were present in the cosmetic, hydroxycitronellal probably not, but the authors did not make a clear statement about it. A ROAT with the face powder was positive and became pigmented (14).

Cross-reactions, pseudo-cross-reactions and co-reactions

For general information on cross-/pseudo-cross-/co-reactivity of fragrance chemicals with other fragrances, fragrance markers (fragrance mix I, fragrance mix II, colophonium, Myroxylon pereirae resin [balsam of Peru]) and essential oils see Chapter 1.2 General information on cross-reactions, pseudo-cross-reactions and co-reactions. Co-reactivity with the fragrance mix I can be expected, as the mix contains hydroxycitronellal (pseudo-cross-reactions).

In a large study performed by the IVDK in the period 2005-2013, of 111 patients reacting to citral, 44 (40%) co-reacted to hydroxycitronellal; conversely, of 112 individuals allergic to hydroxycitronellal, 44 (39%) co-reacted to citral (92).

Possibly there may be cross-reactivity to and from methoxycitronellal (76).

Presence in products and chemical analyses

In various studies, the presence of hydroxycitronellal in cosmetic and sometimes other products has been investigated. Before 2006, most investigators used chemical analysis, usually GC-MS, for qualitative and quantitative determination. Since then, the presence of the target fragrances was usually investigated by screening the product labels for the 26 fragrances that must be labeled since 2005 on cosmetics and detergent products in the EU, if present at > 10 ppm (0.001%) in leave-on products and > 100 ppm (0.01%) in rinse-off products. This method, obviously, is less accurate and may result in underestimation of the frequency of the fragrances being present in the product. When they are in fact present, but the concentration is lower than mentioned above, labeling is not required and the fragrances' presence will be missed.

The results of the relevant studies for hydroxycitronellal are summarized in table 3.82.4. More detailed information can be found in the corresponding text before and following the table. The percentage of products in which hydroxycitronellal was found to be present shows wide variations, which can among other be explained by the selection procedure of the products, the method of investigation (false-negatives with information obtained from labels only) and changes in the use of individual fragrance materials over time (fashion). The use of hydroxycitronellal appears to be decreasing in the last decade; before that, it appears to have been used frequently, especially in perfumes and deodorants.

In Denmark, in 2015-2016, 5588 fragranced cosmetic products were examined with a smartphone application for the 26 fragrances that need to be labeled in the EU. Hydroxycitronellal was present in 7% of the products (rank number 14) (26).

In Germany, in 2015, fragrance allergens were evaluated based on lists of ingredients in 817 (unique) detergents (all-purpose cleaners, cleaning preparations for special purposes [e.g. bathroom, kitchen, dish-washing] and laundry detergents) present in 131 households. Hydroxycitronellal was found to be present in 10 (1%) of the products (90).

Of 179 emollients available in online drugstores in 2014 in Poland, five (2.8%) contained hydroxycitronellal, according to information available online (55).

In 2008, 2010 and 2011, 374 deodorants available in German retail shops were randomly selected and their labels checked for the presence of the 26 fragrances that need to be labeled. Hydroxycitronellal was found to be present in 23 (6.1%) of the products (75).

In Germany, in the period 2006-2009, 4991 cosmetic products were randomly sampled for an official investigation of conformity of cosmetic products with legal provisions. The labels were inspected for the presence of the 26 fragrances that need to be labeled in the EU. Hydroxycitronellal was present in 7% of the products (rank number 14) (25).

In 2008, 66 different fragrance components (including 39 essential oils) were identified in 370 (10% of the total) topical pharmaceutical products marketed in Belgium; 5 of these (1.4%) contained hydroxycitronellal (11).

Hydroxycitronellal was present in 2% of 204 cosmetic products (92 shampoos, 61 hair conditioners, 34 liquid soaps, 17 wet tissues) and in 1% of 97 detergents in Sweden, 2008 (13).

In January 2001, in Denmark, ten women's fine fragrances were purchased; 5 of these had been launched years ago (1921–1990) and 5 were the latest launches by the same companies, introduced 2 months to 4 years before purchase. They were analyzed for the presence and quantity of the 7 well-identified fragrances present in the FM I (see Chapter 3.70 Fragrance mix I). The analysis revealed that the 5 old perfumes contained a mean of 5 of the 7 target allergens of the FM, while the new perfumes contained a mean of 2.8 of the allergens. The mean concentrations of the target allergens were 2.6 times higher in the old perfumes than in the new perfumes, range 2.2-337 ppm.

Table 3.82.4 Presence of hydroxycitronellal in products [a]

Year	Country	Product type	Nr. investigated	Nr. of products positive [b]	(%)	Method [c]	Ref.
2015-6	Denmark	Fragranced cosmetic products	5588		(7%)	Labeling	26
2015	Germany	Household detergents	817	10	(1%)	Labeling	90
2014	Poland	Emollients	179	3	(3%)	Online info	55
2008-11	Germany	Deodorants	374	23	(6%)	Labeling	75
2006-9	Germany	Cosmetic products	4991		(7%)	Labeling	25
2008	Belgium	Fragranced topical pharmaceutical products	370	5	(1%)	Labeling	11
2008	Sweden	Cosmetic products	204		(2%)	Labeling	13
		Detergents	97		(1%)	Labeling	
2007	Netherlands	Cosmetic products for children	23	10	(43%)	Analysis	40
2006	UK	Perfumed cosmetic and household products	300	52	(17%)	Labeling	23
2006	Denmark	Popular perfumed deodorants	88	24	(27%)	Labeling	28
			23	16	(70%)	Analysis	
2006	Denmark	Rinse-off cosmetics for children	208	13	(6%)	Labeling + analysis	39
2002	Denmark	Home and car air fresheners	19	5	(26%)	Analysis	42
2001	Denmark	Women's fine fragrances	10	10	(100%)	Analysis	27
2001	Denmark	Non-cosmetic consumer products	43	3	(7%)	Analysis	41
2000	Denmark, UK, Germany, Italy	Domestic and occupational products	59	7	(12%)	Analysis	16
<2000	Sweden	Swedish cosmetic products	42	20	(48%)	Analysis	73
1997-8	Denmark, UK Germany, Sweden	Cosmetics and cosmetic toys for children	25	10	(40%)	Analysis	19
1996-7	Denmark	Deodorants that had caused allergic contact dermatitis	19	10	(53%)	Analysis	65
1996	Five European countries	Fragranced deodorants	70	35	(50%)	Analysis	15
1995-6	Denmark	Perfumes from lower-price range cosmetic products	17	6	(35%)	Analysis	66
1995	Denmark	Cosmetic products based on natural ingredients	42	5	(12%)	Analysis	17
1995	Denmark	The 10 most popular women's perfumes	10	9	(90%)	Analysis	18
1994	Denmark	Cosmetics that had given a positive patch or use test in FM I allergic patients	23	20	(87%)	Analysis	67
1992	Netherlands	Cosmetic products	300		(49%)	Analysis	24
1988	USA	Perfumes used in fine fragrances, household products and soap	400	?-21% (see text)		Analysis	22

[a] See the corresponding text below for more details
[b] positive = containing the target fragrance
[c] Labeling: information from the ingredient labels on the product / packaging; Analysis: chemical analysis, most often GC-MS

Hydroxycitronellal was present in all 5 old perfumes, in a concentration range of 0.222-0.979 % (m/m), mean 0.615%; in the new perfumes, it was identified in all 5 in a concentration range of 0.015-0.478% (m/m), mean 0.169% (27).

In 2007, in The Netherlands, twenty-three cosmetic products for children were analyzed for the presence of fragrances that need to be labeled. Hydroxycitronellal was identified in 10 of the products (43%) in a concentration range of 21-873 ppm (40).

In 2006, the labels of 208 cosmetics for children (especially shampoos, body shampoos and soaps) available in Denmark were checked for the presence of the 26 fragrances that need to be labeled in the EU. Hydroxycitronellal was present in 13 products (6.3%), and ranked number 14 in the frequency list (39).

In 2006, of 88 popular perfume containing deodorants purchased in Denmark, 24 (27%) were labeled to contain hydroxycitronellal. Analysis of 24 regulated fragrance substances in 23 selected deodorants (19 spray products, 2 deostick and 2 roll-on) was performed by GC-MS. Hydroxycitronellal was identified in 16 of the products (70%) with a concentration range of 1–1747 ppm (28).

In January 2006, a study of perfumed cosmetic and household products available on the shelves of U.K. retailers was carried out. Products were included if 'parfum' or 'aroma' was listed among the ingredients. Three hundred products were surveyed and any of 26 mandatory labeling fragrances named on the label were recorded. Hydroxycitronellal was present in 52 (17%) of the products (rank number 15) (23).

In 2002, in Denmark, 19 air fresheners (6 for cars, 13 for homes) were analyzed for the presence of fragrances that need to be labeled on cosmetics. Hydroxycitronellal was found to be present in 5 products (26%) in a concentration range of 440-2600 ppm and ranked 16 in the frequency list (42).

In 2001, in Denmark, 43 non-cosmetic consumer products (mainly dish-washing products, laundry detergents, and hard and soft surface cleaners) were analyzed for the 26 fragrances that are regulated for labeling in the EU. Hydroxycitronellal was present in 3 products (7%) in a concentration range of 0.0025-0.0078% (m/m) and had rank number 15 in the frequency list (41).

In 2000, fifty-nine domestic and occupational products, purchased in retail outlets in Denmark, England, Germany and Italy were analyzed by GC-MS for the presence of fragrances. The product categories were liquid soap and soap bars (n=13), soft/hard surface cleaners (n=23), fabric conditioners/laundry detergents for hand wash (n=8), dish- wash (n=10), furniture polish, car shampoo, stain remover (each n=1) and 2 products used in occupational environments. Hydroxycitronellal was present in 7 products (12%) with a mean concentration of 69 ppm and a range of 15-140 ppm (16).

In Sweden, before 2000, 42 cosmetic products of a Swedish manufacturer were investigated for the presence of the ingredients of the FM I by chemical analysis. Hydroxycitronellal was found to be present in 20 of the products (48%) in a concentration range of 0.6-770 ppm with a mean of 112 ppm. Data provided by the manufacturer on the qualitative and quantitative presence of the chemicals was quite different from chemical analyses for some of the fragrances (73).

Twenty-five cosmetics and cosmetic toys for children (5 shampoos and shower gels, 6 perfumes, 1 deodorant (roll-on), 4 baby lotions/creams, 1 baby wipes product, 1 baby oil, 2 lipcare products and 5 toy-cosmetic products: a cosmetic-toy set for blending perfumes and a makeup set) purchased in 1997-1998 in retail outlets in Denmark, Germany, England and Sweden were analyzed in 1998 for the presence of fragrances by GC-MS. Hydroxycitronellal was found in 10 products (40%) in a concentration range of ≤0.001-1.180% (w/w). For the analytical data in each product category, the original publication should be consulted (19).

In Denmark, in 1996-1997, nineteen deodorants that had caused axillary allergic contact dermatitis in 14 patients were analyzed for the presence of the 8 constituents of the FM I and hydroxycitronellal was found to be present in 10 (53%) of the products in a concentration range of 0.0001-0.0769% (65).

Seventy fragranced deodorants, purchased at retail outlets in 5 European countries in 1996, were analyzed by gas chromatography - mass spectrometry (GC-MS) for the determination of the contents of 21 commonly used fragrance materials. Hydroxycitronellal was identified in 35 products (50%) in a concentration range of 1–1023 ppm (15).

In Denmark, in 1995-1996, nine perfumes from lower-price cosmetic wash-off products and 8 from stay-on products were analyzed for the presence of the ingredients of the FM I except oakmoss absolute. Hydroxycitronellal was present in 2 of the 9 (22%) wash-off product perfumes in a concentration of 0.0990% w/v and in 4 of the 8 (50%) stay-on product perfumes in a concentration range of 0.007-0.2444% w/v. In one product, hydroxycitronellal was detected, but could not be quantified because of interference (66).

In 1995, in Denmark, 42 cosmetic products based on natural ingredients from 12 European and US companies (of which 22 were perfumes and 20 various other cosmetics) were investigated by high-resolution gas chromatography-mass spectrometry (GC-MS) for the presence of 11 fragrances. Hydroxycitronellal was present in 5 (23%) of the 22 perfumes in a concentration range of 0.135-6.044 w/w% ; it was not identified in any of the other cosmetics (17).

In Denmark, in 1995, the 10 most popular women's perfumes were analyzed with gas chromatography-mass spectrometry for the presence of 7 ingredients of the Fragrance mix I (all except Evernia prunastri extract). Hydroxycitronellal was identified in 9 of the perfumes (90%) with a mean concentration of 0.76% and in a concentration range of 0.25-1.19% (18).

In Denmark, in 1994, 23 cosmetic products, which had either given a positive patch and/or use test in a total of 11 fragrance-mix-positive patients, and which products completely or partly explained present or past episodes of dermatitis, were analyzed for the presence of the constituents of the FM I (with the exception of oakmoss absolute) and a few other fragrances. Hydroxycitronellal was found to be present in 20 of the 23 products (87%) in a concentration range of <0.001-0.54% v/v with a mean concentration of 0.102% v/v. The content of hydroxycitronellal was, on average, 5x higher in cosmetics from hydroxycitronellal-sensitive patients, compared to cosmetics from hydroxycitronellal-negative patients (67).

In 1992, in The Netherlands, the presence of fragrances was analyzed in 300 cosmetic products. Hydroxycitronellal was identified in 49% of the products (rank order 11) (24).

In 1988, in the USA, 400 perfumes used in fine fragrances, household products and soaps (number of products per category not mentioned) were analyzed for the presence of fragrance chemicals in a concentration of at least 1% and a list of the Top-25 (present in the highest number of products) presented. Hydroxycitronellal was found to be present in 21 % of the fine fragrances (rank number 25), an unknown percentage of the household product fragrances and an unknown percentage of the fragrances used in soaps (22).

Serial dilution testing and Repeated Open Application Tests

Seven patients contact allergic to hydroxycitronellal were patch tested with a dilution series of hydroxycitronellal in alcohol, in concentrations ranging from 2% to 0.00006% w/v, with deodorants containing hydroxycitronellal 0.032%, 0.1% and 0.32% w/v in alcohol and with alcohol and unscented deodorants as controls. In addition, they performed ROATS in the axilla with the deodorants for 2 weeks with one or more of the 3 concentrations, beginning with the lowest. Higher concentrations were used after 2 weeks only when the ROAT with lower concentration was negative. Seven non-allergic patients served as controls (82).The lowest concentration of alcoholic hydroxycitronellal to which the patients had a positive patch test was 0.00012% in one individual, 0.125% in one, 0.25% in one, 0.5% in two, 1% in one and 4% in one. Three reacted to the scented deodorants with as lowest concentrations 0.032% (n=1), 0.1% (n=1) and 0.32% (n=1). The ROATs were positive in all 7 patients to the scented deodorants, none to the unscented. Four reacted to the lowest concentration (0.032%), one was negative to the lowest but reacted to the medium concentration (0.1%) and the other 2 were negative to the 2 lower concentrations but had positive ROATS to the deodorant containing 0.32% hydroxycitronellal. There was a correlation between threshold concentrations of hydroxycitronellal ethanol solutions on patch testing and the outcome of ROAT. All tests in individuals not allergic to hydroxycitronellal were negative (82).

Repeated skin exposure to a fragrance allergen in 15 patients previously diagnosed with hand eczema and contact allergy to the fragrance was used to explore whether immersion of fingers in a solution with or without the patch-test-positive fragrance allergen would cause or exacerbate hand eczema on the exposed finger. The study was double blinded and randomized. All participants had a positive patch test to either hydroxycitronellal (n=13) or hydroxyisohexyl 3-cyclohexenecarboxaldehyde (Lyral ®, HICC). Each participant immersed a finger from each hand, once a day for 10 minutes, in a 10% alcoholic solution containing the fragrance allergen or placebo. During the first 2 weeks, the concentration of fragrance allergen in the solution was low (approximately 10 ppm), whilst during the following 2 weeks, the concentration was relatively high (approximately 250 ppm), imitating real-life exposure to a household product like dishwashing liquid diluted in water and the undiluted product, respectively. Evaluation was made using a clinical scale and laser Doppler flow meter. In the 13 patients with allergy to hydroxycitronellal, there were 4 reactions to the placebo solution and 5 clinically visible reactions on a finger immersed in the fragrance solution. Thus, no clear association between immersion of a finger in a solution containing hydroxycitronellal to which the subject was allergic and development of clinically visible eczema was found (84).

A perfume prepared from equal amounts of hydroxycitronellal, geraniol, and hydroxyisohexyl 3-cyclohexenecarboxaldehyde (HICC, Lyral ®) was added at various levels to an unperfumed shampoo and distributed for *ad libitum* use to 12 test subjects with preexisting contact hypersensitivities to either hydroxycitronellal or geraniol. At 2-week intervals shampoo perfume levels were increased threefold if no subjective or visible skin reactions occurred. Five percent of each perfume ingredient (15% total) was the maximum level used. Two of the 12 subjects (both presensitized to hydroxycitronellal) showed evidence of allergic responses upon shampoo use at the 5% level, but not at the 3% level. The 3% level was resp. 30 and 120 times higher than the two subjects' 48-hr closed patch lowest threshold to hydroxycitronellal (85).

Daily use of a soap bar containing a perfume with 0.05% hydroxycitronellal, and later a lotion with 0.03% hydroxycitronellal for several months, gave no clinical symptoms in 41 subjects previously sensitized to hydroxycitronellal by a human repeated insult patch test. When 31 of these subjects proceeded to use a cologne containing 0.05% hydroxycitronellal 3 times daily for a month, one subject reacted. Another 3 sensitized individuals developed dermatitis after having used a cologne containing 1% hydroxycitronellal (50,77).

Other information

Patch testing with hydroxycitronellal in 10% alcohol, to which 0.2% of the irritant sodium lauryl sulfate had been added, gave stronger reactions than patch tests with hydroxycitronellal in alcohol alone (83).

OTHER SIDE EFFECTS

Photosensitivity

In a group of 50 patients suffering from photosensitivity dermatitis with actinic reticuloid syndrome (PD/AR) patch tested with a battery of fragrances, there were 8 reactions (16%) to hydroxycitronellal versus 1.8% positive patch tests in a group of 457 routinely tested dermatitis patients. The frequency of reactions to various other fragrances was also elevated in the PD/AR group. In a subgroup of 35 patients (11 with PD/AR, 13 with chronic polymorphic light eruption, 11 with contact dermatitis) who were photopatch tested, there were positive reactions to hydroxycitronellal in 2 patients, one of who also had an immediate-type reaction. These positive photopatch tests were tentatively interpreted as indicating a phototoxic reaction, although the possibility that this phototoxic response may merge subsequently with a delayed allergic type reaction could not be excluded. The authors concluded that in some subjects with PD/AR and persistent light reaction, a significant factor in the latter is likely to be exposure to substances such as fragrance materials which have the ability to produce dermatitis, not only from contact allergic sensitivity but also through photocontact reactions (notably oakmoss, 6-methylcoumarin and musk ambrette) involving either phototoxic or photoallergic mechanisms (51).

LITERATURE

1   Heisterberg MV, Menné T, Johansen JD. Contact allergy to the 26 specific fragrance ingredients to be declared on cosmetic products in accordance with the EU cosmetic directive. Contact Dermatitis 2011;65:266-275

2   Oosten EJ van, Schuttelaar ML, Coenraads PJ. Clinical relevance of positive patch test reactions to the 26 EU-labelled fragrances. Contact Dermatitis 2009;61:217-223

3   Schnuch A, Uter W, Geier J, Lessmann H, Frosch PJ. Sensitization to 26 fragrances to be labelled according to current European regulation: Results of the IVDK and review of the literature. Contact Dermatitis 2007;57:1-10

4   Adams RM, Maibach HI, for the North American Contact Dermatitis Group. A five-year study of cosmetic reactions. J Am Acad Dermatol 1985;13:1062-1069

5   Wöhrl S, Hemmer W, Focke M, Götz M, Jarisch R. The significance of fragrance mix, balsam of Peru, colophony and propolis as screening tools in the detection of fragrance allergy. Br J Dermatol 2001;145:268-273

6   Heydorn S, Johansen JD, Andersen KE, Bruze M, Svedman C, White IR, et al. Fragrance allergy in patients with hand eczema – a clinical study. Contact Dermatitis 2003;48:317-323

7   Larsen W, Nakayama H, Fischer T, Elsner P, Burrows D, Jordan W, et al. Fragrance contact dermatitis: A worldwide multicenter investigation (Part I). Am J Cont Dermat 1996;7:77-83

8   SCCNFP (Scientific Committee on Cosmetic Products and Non-Food Products Intended for Consumers). Opinion of the Scientific Committee on Cosmetic Products and Non-Food Products Intended for Consumers concerning 'An initial list of perfumery materials which must not form part of cosmetic products except subject to the Restrictions and Conditions laid down, 25 September 2001, SCCNFP/0392/00, final. Available at: http://ec.europa.eu/health/archive/ph_risk/committees/sccp/documents/out150_en.pdf

9   SCCS (Scientific Committee on Consumer Safety). Opinion on Fragrance allergens in cosmetic products, 26-27 June 2012, SCCS/1459/11. Available at: https://ec.europa.eu/health/sites/health/files/scientific_committees/consumer_safety/docs/sccs_o_102.pdf

10 Larsen WG. Cosmetic dermatitis due to a perfume. Contact Dermatitis 1975;1:142-145

11 Nardelli A, D'Hooge E, Drieghe J, Dooms M, Goossens A. Allergic contact dermatitis from fragrance components in specific topical pharmaceutical products in Belgium. Contact Dermatitis 2009;60:303-313

12 Larsen WG. Perfume dermatitis. A study of 20 patients. Arch Dermatol 1977;113:623-626

13 Yazar K, Johnsson S, Lind M-L, Boman A, Lidén C. Preservatives and fragrances in selected consumer-available cosmetics and detergents. Contact Dermatitis 2011;64:265-272

14 Serrano G, Pujol C, Cuadra J, Gallo S, Aliaga A. Riehl's melanosis: Pigmented contact dermatitis caused by fragrances. J Am Acad Dermatol 1989;21:1057-1060

15 Rastogi SC, Johansen JD, Frosch P, Menné T, Bruze M, Lepoittevin JP, et al. Deodorants on the European market: quantitative chemical analysis of 21 fragrances. Contact Dermatitis 1998;38:29-35

16 Rastogi SC, Heydorn S, Johansen JD, Basketter DA. Fragrance chemicals in domestic and occupational products. Contact Dermatitis 2001;45:221-225

17 Rastogi SC, Johansen JD, Menné T. Natural ingredients based cosmetics. Content of selected fragrance sensitizers. Contact Dermatitis 1996;34:423-426

18 Johansen JD, Rastogi SC, Menné T. Contact allergy to popular perfumes: assessed by patch test, use test and chemical analyses. Br J Dermatol 1996;135:419-422

19 Rastogi SC, Johansen JD, Menné T, Frosch P, Bruze M, Andersen KE, et al. Content of fragrance allergens in children's cosmetics and cosmetic toys. Contact Dermatitis 1999;41:84-88

20 De Groot AC. Contact allergy to cosmetics: causative ingredients. Contact Dermatitis 1987;17:26-34

21 De Groot AC, Liem DH. Facial psoriasis caused by contact allergy to linalool and hydroxycitronellal in an aftershave. Contact Dermatitis 1983;9:230-232

22 Fenn RS. Aroma chemical usage trends in modern perfumery. Perfumer and Flavorist 1989;14:3-10

23 Buckley DA. Fragrance ingredient labelling in products on sale in the UK. Br J Dermatol 2007;157:295-300

24 Weyland JW. Personal Communication, 1992. Cited in: De Groot AC, Weyland JW, Nater JP. Unwanted effects of cosmetics and drugs used in dermatology, 3rd Ed. Amsterdam: Elsevier, 1994: 579

25 Uter W, Yazar K, Kratz E-M, Mildau G, Lidén C. Coupled exposure to ingredients of cosmetic products: I. Fragrances. Contact Dermatitis 2013;69:335-341

26 Bennike NH, Oturai NB, Müller S, Kirkeby CS, Jørgensen C, Christensen AB, et al. Fragrance contact allergens in 5588 cosmetic products identified through a novel smartphone application. J Eur Acad Dermatol Venereol 2018;32:79-85

27 Rastogi SC, Menné T, Johansen JD. The composition of fine fragrances is changing. Contact Dermatitis 2003;48:130-132

28 Rastogi SC, Hellerup Jensen G, Johansen JD. Survey and risk assessment of chemical substances in deodorants. Survey of Chemical Substances in Consumer Products, No. 86 2007. Danish Ministry of the Environment, Environmental Protection Agency. Available at: https://www2.mst.dk/Udgiv/publications/2007/978-87-7052-625-8/pdf/978-87-7052-626-5.pdf

29 De Groot AC, Bruynzeel DP, Bos JD, van der Meeren HL, van Joost T, Jagtman BA, Weyland JW. The allergens in cosmetics. Arch Dermatol 1988;124:1525-1529

30 De Groot AC. Adverse reactions to cosmetics. PhD Thesis, University of Groningen, The Netherlands: 1988, chapter 3.4, pp.105-113

31 Zaragoza-Ninet V, Blasco Encinas R, Vilata-Corell JJ, Pérez-Ferriols A, Sierra-Talamantes C, Esteve-Martínez A, de la Cuadra-Oyanguren J. Allergic contact dermatitis due to cosmetics: A clinical and epidemiological study in a tertiary hospital. Actas Dermosifiliogr 2016;107:329-336

32 Laguna C, de la Cuadra J, Martín-González B, Zaragoza V, Martínez-Casimiro L, Alegre V. Allergic contact dermatitis to cosmetics. Actas Dermosifiliogr 2009;100:53-60

33 Frosch PJ, Pilz B, Andersen KE, Burrows D, Camarasa JG, Dooms-Goossens A, et al. Patch testing with fragrances: results of a multicenter study of the European Environmental and Contact Dermatitis Research Group with 48 frequently used constituents of perfumes. Contact Dermatitis 1995;33:333-342

34 Trattner A, David M. Patch testing with fine fragrances: comparison with fragrance mix, balsam of Peru and a fragrance series. Contact Dermatitis 2003;49:287-289

35 Cuesta L, Silvestre JF, Toledo F, Lucas A, Perez-Crespo M, Ballester I. Fragrance contact allergy: a 4-year retrospective study. Contact Dermatitis 2010;63:77-84

36 Nakayama H, Hanaoka H, Ohshiro A. Allergen controlled system (ACS). Tokyo: Kanehara Shuppan, 1974:42; data cited in ref. 37.

37 Mitchell JC. Contact hypersensitivity to some perfume materials. Contact Dermatitis 1975;1:196-199

38 Uter W, Geier J, Schnuch A, Frosch PJ. Patch test results with patients' own perfumes, deodorants and shaving lotions: results of the IVDK 1998-2002. J Eur Acad Dermatol Venereol 2007;21:374-379

39 Poulsen PB, Schmidt A. A survey and health assessment of cosmetic products for children. Survey of chemical substances in consumer products, No. 88. Copenhagen: Danish Environmental Protection Agency, 2007. Available at: https://www2.mst.dk/udgiv/publications/2007/978-87-7052-638-8/pdf/978-87-7052-639-5.pdf

40 VWA. Dutch Food and Consumer Product Safety Authority. Cosmetische producten voor kinderen: Inventarisatie van de markt en de veiligheidsborging door producenten en importeurs. Report ND04o065/ND05o170, 2007 (Report in Dutch), 2007. Available at: www.nvwa.nl/documenten/communicatie/inspectieresultaten/consument/2016m/cosmetische- producten-voor-kinderen

41 Rastogi SC. Survey of chemical compounds in consumer products. Contents of selected fragrance materials in cleaning products and other consumer products. Survey no. 8-2002. Copenhagen, Denmark, Danish Environmental Protection Agency. Available at: http://eng.mst.dk/media/mst/69131/8.pdf

42 Pors J, Fuhlendorff R. Mapping of chemical substances in air fresheners and other fragrance liberating products. Report Danish Ministry of the Environment, Environmental Protection Agency (EPA). Survey of Chemicals in Consumer Products, No 30, 2003. Available at: http://eng.mst.dk/media/mst/69113/30.pdf

43 Larsen WG. Allergic contact dermatitis to the perfume in Mycolog cream. J Am Acad Dermatol 1979;1:131-133

44 Saito F. A case of perfume dermatitis. Hifuka Rinsho 1960;2:930 (article in Japanese). Data cited in ref. 46

45 Mathias VG, Cram D, Ragsdale J, Maibach HI. Contact dermatitis caused by spouse's perfume and cologne. Can Med Assoc J 1978;119:257-258

46 Nakayama H, Matsuo S, Hayakawa K, Takhashi K, Shigematsu T, Ota S. Pigmented cosmetic dermatitis. Int J Dermatol 1984;23:299-305

47 Nakayama H, Harada R, Toda M. Pigmented cosmetic dermatitis. Int J Dermatol 1976;15:673-675

48 Nakayama H, Hanaoka H, Ohshiro A. Allergen Controlled System. Tokyo: Kanehara Shuppan, 1974

49 Ebihara T, Nakayama H. Pigmented contact dermatitis. Clin Dermatol 1997;15:593-599

50 Suskind RR. The Hydroxycitronellal story: What can we learn from it? In: Frosch PJ, Johansen JD, White IR, Eds. Fragrances - beneficial and adverse effects. Berlin Heidelberg New York: Springer-Verlag, 1998:159-165

51 Addo HA, Ferguson J, Johnson BF, Frain-Bell W. The relationship between exposure to fragrance materials and persistent light reaction in photosensitivity dermatitis with actinic reticuloid syndrome. Br J Dermatol 1982;107:261-274

52 Goossens A. Cosmetic contact allergens. Cosmetics 2016, 3, 5; doi:10.3390/cosmetics3010005

53 Molin S, Bauer A, Schnuch A, Geier J. Occupational contact allergy in nurses: results from the Information Network of Departments of Dermatology 2003–2012. Contact Dermatitis 2015;72:164-171

54 Bennike NH, Zachariae C, Johansen JD. Non-mix fragrances are top sensitizers in consecutive dermatitis patients – a cross-sectional study of the 26 EU-labelled fragrance allergens. Contact Dermatitis 2017;77:270-279

55 Osinka K, Karczmarz A, Krauze K, Feleszko W. Contact allergens in cosmetics used in atopic dermatitis: analysis of product composition. Contact Dermatitis 2016;75:241-243

56 Vejanurug P, Tresukosol P, Sajjachareonpong P, Puangpet P. Fragrance allergy could be missed without patch testing with 26 individual fragrance allergens. Contact Dermatitis 2016;74:230-235

57 Liu J, Li L-F. Contact sensitization to fragrances other than fragrance mix I in China. Contact Dermatitis 2015;73:252-253

58 Mann J, McFadden JP, White JML, White IR, Banerjee P. Baseline series fragrance markers fail to predict contact allergy. Contact Dermatitis 2014;70:276-281

59 Uter W, Johansen JD, Börje A, Karlberg A-T, Lidén C, Rastogi S, Roberts D, White IR. Categorization of fragrance contact allergens for prioritization of preventive measures: clinical and experimental data and consideration of structure–activity relationships. Contact Dermatitis 2013;69:196-230

60 Larsen WG. Perfume dermatitis revisited. Contact Dermatitis 1977;3:98

61 Mowitz M, Svedman C, Zimerson E, Isaksson M, Pontén A, Bruze M. Simultaneous patch testing with fragrance mix I, fragrance mix II and their ingredients in southern Sweden between 2009 and 2015. Contact Dermatitis 2017;77:280-287

62 Nagtegaal MJC, Pentinga SE, Kuik J, Kezic S, Rustemeyer T. The role of the skin irritation response in polysensitization to fragrances. Contact Dermatitis 2012;67:28-35

63 Nardelli A, Drieghe J, Claes L, Boey L, Goossens A. Fragrance allergens in 'specific' cosmetic products. Contact Dermatitis 2011;64:212-219

64 Uter W, Geier J, Frosch P, Schnuch A. Contact allergy to fragrances: current patch test results (2005–2008) from the Information Network of Departments of Dermatology. Contact Dermatitis 2010;63:254-261

65 Johansen JD, Rastogi SC, Bruze M, Andersen KE, Frosch P, Dreier B, et al. Deodorants: a clinical provocation study in fragrance-sensitive individuals. Contact Dermatitis 1998;39:161-165

66 Johansen JD, Rastogi SC, Andersen KE, Menné T. Content and reactivity to product perfumes in fragrance mix positive and negative eczema patients: A study of perfumes used in toiletries and skin-care products. Contact Dermatitis 1997;36:291-296

67 Johansen JD, Rastogi SC, Menné T. Exposure to selected fragrance materials: A case study of fragrance-mix-positive eczema patients. Contact Dermatitis 1996;34:106-110

68 Frosch PJ, Pilz B, Burrows D, Camarasa JG, Lachapelle J-M, Lahti A, et al. Testing with fragrance mix: Is the addition of sorbitan sesquioleate to the constituents useful? Contact Dermatitis 1995;32:266-272

69 De Groot AC, Van der Kley AMJ, Bruynzeel DP, Meinardi MMHM, Smeenk G, van Joost Th, Pavel S. Frequency of false-negative reactions to the fragrance mix. Contact Dermatitis 1993;28:139-140

70 Broeckx W, Blondeel A, Dooms-Goossens A, Achten G. Cosmetic intolerance. Contact Dermatitis 1987;16:189-194

71 Van Joost Th, Stolz E, Van Der Hoek JCS. Simultaneous allergy to perfume ingredients. Contact Dermatitis 1985;12:115-116

72 Van Ketel WG. Dermatitis from an aftershave. Contact Dermatitis 1978;4:117

73 Bárány E, Lodén M. Content of fragrance mix ingredients and customer complaints of cosmetic products. Dermatitis 2000;11:74-79

74 Diepgen TL, Ofenloch R, Bruze M, Cazzaniga S, Coenraads PJ, Elsner P, et al. Prevalence of fragrance contact allergy in the general population of five European countries: a cross-sectional study. Br J Dermatol 2015;173:1411-1419

75 Klaschka U. Contact allergens for armpits - allergenic fragrances specified on deodorants. Int J Hyg Environ Health 2012;215:584-591

76 Nakayama H, cited in Nethercott JR, Larsen WG. Contact allergens - what's new? Fragrances. Clin Dermatol 1997;15:499-504

77 Suskind RR. Hydroxycitronellal. "The whole and final story". RIFM proceedings from the 6th International Information Exchange, 1992:75-83. Data cited in refs. 17 and 67

78 Calnan CD. Perfume dermatitis from the cosmetic ingredients oakmoss and hydroxycitronellal. Contact Dermatitis 1979;5:194

79 Calnan CD. Unusual hydroxycitronellal perfume dermatitis. Contact Dermatitis 1979;5:123

80 Sugiura M, Hayakawa R, Kato Y, Sugiura K, Hashimoto R. Results of patch testing with lavender oil in Japan. Contact Dermatitis 2000;43:157-160

81 Corazza M, Virgili A, Bertoldi AM, Benetti S, Borghi A. Allergic contact dermatitis caused by insect repellent wipes. Contact Dermatitis 2016;74:295-296

82 Svedman C, Bruze M, Johansen JD, Andersen KE, Goossens A, Frosch PJ, et al. Deodorants: an experimental provocation study with hydroxycitronellal. Contact Dermatitis 2003;48:217-223

83 Heydorn S, Andersen KE, Johansen JD, Menné T. A stronger patch test elicitation reaction to the allergen hydroxycitronellal plus the irritant sodium lauryl sulfate. Contact Dermatitis 2003;49:133-139

84 Heydorn S, Menné T, Andersen KE, Bruze M, Svedman C, Basketter D, Johansen JD. The fragrance hand immersion study – an experimental model simulating real-life exposure for allergic contact dermatitis on the hands. Contact Dermatitis 2003;48:324-330

85 Benke GM, Larsen WG. Safety evaulation of perfumes shampoos: dose/response relationships for products and testing by presensitized subjects. J Toxicol Cut Ocul Toxicol 1984;3:65-72

86 Ford RA, Api AM, Suskind RR. Allergic contact sensitization potential of hydroxycitronellal in humans. Food Chem Toxicol 1988;26:921-926

87 De Groot AC, Schmidt E. Essential oils: contact allergy and chemical composition. Boca Raton, Fl., USA: CRC Press, Taylor and Francis Group, 2016 (ISBN 9781482246407)

88 Meynadier JM, Meynadier J, Peyron JL, Peyron L. Formes cliniques des manifestations cutanées d'allergie aux parfums. Ann Dermatol Venereol 1986;113:31-39

89 Opinion of the Scientific Committee on Cosmetic Products and Non-Food Products Intended for Consumers concerning 'The 1st update of the inventory of ingredients employed in cosmetic products. Section II: Perfume and aromatic raw materials', 24 October 2000, SCCNFP/0389/00, final. Available at: http://ec.europa.eu/health/ph_risk/committees/sccp/documents/out131_en.pdf

90 Wieck S, Olsson O, Kümmerer K, Klaschka U. Fragrance allergens in household detergents. Regul Toxicol Pharmacol 2018;97:163-169

91 Ung CY, White JML, White IR, Banerjee P, McFadden JP. Patch testing with the European baseline series fragrance markers: a 2016 update. Br J Dermatol 2018;178:776-780

92 Geier J, Uter W, Lessmann H, Schnuch A. Fragrance mix I and II: results of breakdown tests. Flavour Fragr J 2015;30:264-274

93 Dittmar D, Schuttelaar MLA. Contact sensitization to hydroperoxides of limonene and linalool: Results of consecutive patch testing and clinical relevance. Contact Dermatitis 2018 Oct 31. doi: 10.1111/cod.13137. [Epub ahead of print]

94 Silvestre JF, Mercader P, González-Pérez R, Hervella-Garcés M, Sanz-Sánchez T, Córdoba S, et al. Sensitization to fragrances in Spain: A 5-year multicentre study (2011-2015). Contact Dermatitis. 2018 Nov 14. doi: 10.1111/cod.13152. [Epub ahead of print]

Chapter 3.83   HYDROXYCITRONELLOL

IDENTIFICATION

Description/definition   : Hydroxycitronellol is the polyvalent alcohol (diol) that conforms to the structural formula
                              shown below
Chemical class(es)   : Aliphatic organic compounds; alcohols
INCI name USA   : Not in the Personal Care Products Council Ingredient Database
Chemical/IUPAC name   : 3,7-Dimethyloctane-1,7-diol
CAS registry number(s)   : 107-74-4
EC number(s)   : 203-517-1
RIFM monograph(s)   : Food Chem Toxicol 2008;46(11)(suppl.):S1-S71; Food Chem Toxicol 2008;46(11)(suppl.):
                              S179-S181; Food Cosmet Toxicol 1974;12:923 (special issue I) (binder, page 442)
SCCS opinion(s)   : SCCS/1459/11 (1)
Function(s) in cosmetics   : EU: perfuming
Patch testing   : 7% pet. (2); based on RIFM data, 10% pet. is probably not irritant (4)
Molecular formula   : $C_{10}H_{22}O_2$

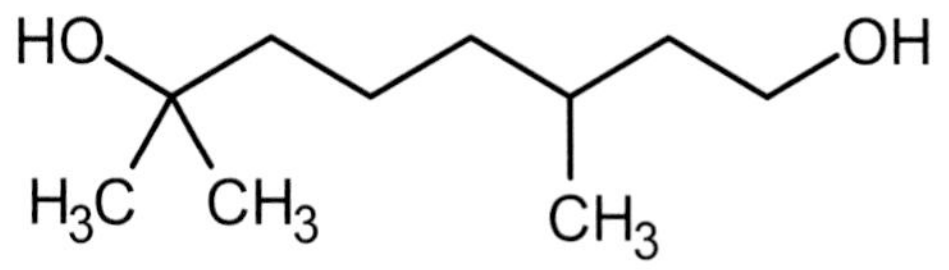

GENERAL

Hydroxycitronellol is a colorless clear viscous liquid; its odor type is floral and its odor at 100% is described as 'mild clean floral lily green peony' (www.thegoodscentscompany.com).

Presence in essential oils

Hydroxycitronellol has been identified by chemical analysis in 1 of 91 essential oils, which have caused contact allergy / allergic contact dermatitis: Eucalyptus citriodora oil (4).

CONTACT ALLERGY

The SCCS (Scientific Committee on Consumer Safety), in a 2012 Opinion on Fragrance allergens in cosmetic products, has categorized hydroxycitronellol as 'possible fragrance contact allergen' (1,3).

Patch testing in consecutive patients suspected of contact dermatitis: routine testing

Studies in which hydroxycitronellol was patch tested in consecutive patients suspected of contact dermatitis (routine testing) with positive results have not been found.

Patch testing in groups of selected patients

Before 2002, in Japan, European countries and the USA, 218 patients with known fragrance sensitivity were patch tested with hydroxycitronellol 7% in petrolatum and thirteen positive reactions (6.0%) were observed; their relevance was not mentioned (2).

Case reports and case series

Case reports of allergic contact dermatitis from hydroxycitronellol have not been found.

LITERATURE

1   SCCS (Scientific Committee on Consumer Safety). Opinion on Fragrance allergens in cosmetic products, 26-27
    June 2012, SCCS/1459/11. Available at:
    https://ec.europa.eu/health/sites/health/files/scientific_committees/consumer_safety/docs/sccs_o_102.pdf
2   Larsen W, Nakayama H, Fischer T, Elsner P, Frosch P, Burrows D, et al. Fragrance contact dermatitis - a
    worldwide multicenter investigation (Part III). Contact Dermatitis 2002;46:141-144
3   Uter W, Johansen JD, Börje A, Karlberg A-T, Lidén C, Rastogi S, Roberts D, White IR. Categorization of fragrance
    contact allergens for prioritization of preventive measures: clinical and experimental data and consideration of
    structure–activity relationships. Contact Dermatitis 2013;69:196-230
4   De Groot AC, Schmidt E. Essential oils: contact allergy and chemical composition. Boca Raton, Fl., USA: CRC Press,
    Taylor and Francis Group, 2016 (ISBN 9781482246407)

Chapter 3.84   HYDROXYISOHEXYL 3-CYCLOHEXENE CARBOXALDEHYDE

IDENTIFICATION

Description/definition	: Hydroxyisohexyl 3-cyclohexene carboxaldehyde (HICC) is the organic compound that conforms to the structural formula shown below
Chemical class(es)	: Alcohols; aldehydes
Chemical/IUPAC name	: 3 and 4-(4-Hydroxy-4-methylpentyl)cyclohex-3-ene-1-carbaldehyde
Other names	: Lyral ®
CAS registry number(s)	: 31906-04-4; 51414-25-6
EC number(s)	: 250-863-4; 257-187-9
RIFM monograph(s)	: Food Chem Toxicol 1992;30(suppl.1):S49-S51
IFRA standard	: Restricted (www.ifraorg.org/en-us/standards-library) (92) (table 3.84.1)
SCCS opinion(s)	: SCCS/1456/11 (25); SCCS/1459/11 (26)
Function(s) in cosmetics	: EU: masking; perfuming. USA: fragrance ingredients
EU cosmetic restrictions	: Must be labeled on cosmetics and detergent products, if present at > 10 ppm (0.001%) in leave-on products and > 100 ppm (0.01%) in rinse-off products; from 23 August 2019 on, cosmetic products containing HICC shall not be placed on the Union market; from 23 August 2021 on, cosmetic products containing HICC shall not be made available on the Union market (Annex II/1380) (99)
Patch testing	: 5% Pet. (SmartPracticeEurope, Chemotechnique, SmartPracticeCanada); some positive reactions to HICC may be missed when the patient is not seen at D7 (101); also present in the fragrance mix II
Molecular formula	: $C_{13}H_{22}O_2$

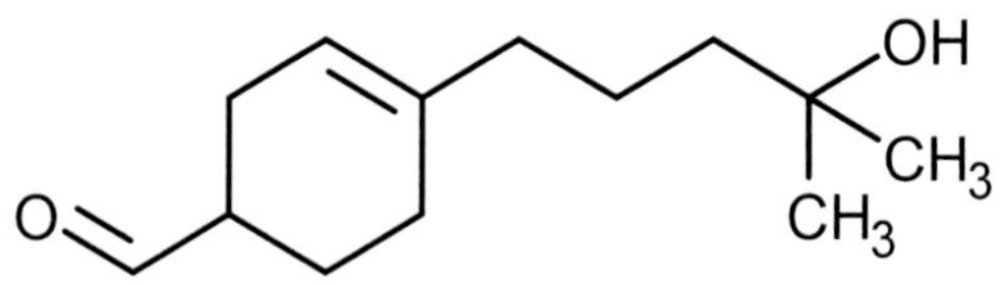

Table 3.84.1 IFRA restrictions for hydroxyisohexyl 3-cyclohexene carboxaldehyde

Category [a]	Limits [b]	Category [a]	Limits [b]	Category [a]	Limits [b]
1	0.02%	5	0.20%	9	0.20%
2	0.02%	6	0.20%	10	0.20%
3	0.20%	7	0.02%	11	not restricted
4	0.20%	8	0.20%		

[a] For explanation of categories see pages 6-8
[b] Limits in the finished products

GENERAL

Hydroxyisohexyl 3-cyclohexene carboxaldehyde (HICC) is a colorless to pale yellow clear viscous liquid; its odor type is floral and its odor at 100% is described as 'floral muguet cyclamen rhubarb woody' (www.thegoodscentscompany. com). It is a synthetic fragrance not found in nature, and consequently not in essential oils (96).

CONTACT ALLERGY

General

Hydroxyisohexyl 3-cyclohexene carboxaldehyde (HICC) was created and introduced in 1960 by the International Flavors and Fragrances Company. This aromatic chemical is formed through the reaction of myrcenol and acrolein (84). HICC is used in consumer products such as deodorants, lotions, perfumes and household products.

The initial testing of the allergenic potential of HICC in animal and human studies by the Research Institute for Fragrance Materials (RIFM) was negative (10) and later, HICC was identified as a weak (11) to moderate (25) sensitizer in the local lymph node assay in animal experiments. The SCCS (Scientific Committee on Consumer Safety) 2012 Opinion on Fragrance allergens in cosmetic products, although marking HICC as 'established contact allergen in humans', classified the sensitizing potency of hydroxyisohexyl 3-cyclohexene carboxaldehyde as 'weak' based on an EC3 value of 17.1% in the LLNA (local lymph node assay) in animal experiments (26,71). That HICC would nevertheless become one of the most important fragrance allergens has been attributed to its widespread use and sometimes high concentration in fragrances and use on occluded skin including axillae promoting sensitization (95).

Case reports of contact allergy to HICC began to appear in the 1980s and 90s (12,13,17,45). Risk factors for HICC sensitization are polysensitization and dermatitis of the axillae (91). From 1998 on, prevalences of sensitization to this fragrance material generally rose to 1.5-2.5% in European countries (Table 3.84.2). In contrast, in North America, the prevalence was found to be only 0.4% in 2003 (32), which was considered to be mainly because of the presence of the ingredient in higher concentrations in deodorants in the EU compared with the USA (20).

Consequently, HICC was included in the German baseline series already in 2002 (9) and was added to the European baseline series in 2008 in a concentration of 5% in petrolatum (16). Hydroxyisohexyl 3-cyclohexene carboxaldehyde is also present in the Fragrance mix II in a concentration of 2.5%, wherein it is the most frequent sensitizer (21) with 36-47.7% positive reactions in groups of patients reacting to the FM II and tested with its ingredients (Chapter 3.71 Fragrance mix II).

In Sweden, in 2014, HICC 5% pet. was removed from the Swedish baseline series, as it was argued that separate testing with HICC does not detect a sufficient proportion of patients who react only to HICC without concomitant reactions to FM II (in the order of 0% to 0.2-0.4% [69,86,87,88,89]), to warrant its inclusion in a baseline series (86,87).

As HICC has caused large numbers of sensitization, from 23 August 2019 on it will be prohibited to place cosmetic products containing HICC on the European Union market and from 23 August 2021 on, such cosmetic products should not be available at all on the Union market (99).

The older literature on contact allergy to HICC was briefly reviewed in 2005 (93).

General population
In the period 2008-2011, in 5 European countries (Sweden, Germany, Netherlands, Portugal, Italy), a random sample of the general population of 3119 individuals aged 18-74 years were patch tested with the FM I, its 8 ingredients, the FM II, its 6 ingredients and Myroxylon pereirae resin. There were 46 reactions (1.5%) to HICC, tested 5% in petrolatum. About half of all positive reactions to fragrances were considered to be relevant based on standardized criteria. Women were affected twice as often as men (55,80).

In Germany, the 10 year prevalence (1998-2007) of sensitization in the general population of Germany to HICC, based on the 'Clinical Epidemiology–Drug Utilization Research' (CE-DUR) method, has been estimated to be 0.82% (95).

Patch testing in groups of patients
Results of patch testing HICC in consecutive patients suspected of contact dermatitis (routine testing) are shown in table 3.84.2. Results of testing in groups of selected patients (e.g. nurses with occupational contact dermatitis, individuals with eyelid dermatitis, female hairdressers and their clients, individuals with known or suspected fragrance or cosmetic dermatitis) are shown in table 3.84.3.

Patch testing in consecutive patients suspected of contact dermatitis: routine testing
In 35 studies performed between 1997 and 2016 in which HICC was tested in consecutive patients, frequencies of sensitization have ranged from 0.4% to 4.8%. The lower concentrations of 0.4% were observed in the UK in 2008-2014 (67) and in 2003 in North America (32); Iran is the only other country where a rate lower than 1% (0.7%) has been observed (23). The highest frequencies of positive patch test reactions to HICC in routine testing of 4.8% and 3.2% were recently observed in The Netherlands (107) resp. in a 2013-2014 study from Thailand (68), where other fragrances also score high prevalence rates. In all other investigations (all but an Australian study (59) performed in (one or more) European countries), the rates were generally between 1% and 2.5% (table 3.84.2).

In 26/35 studies, either no relevance data or no specific data were provided. In the other nine addressing the issue of relevance, generally a high percentage of all positive patch test reactions to HICC were considered to be relevant: 94% (90), 92% (4), 90% (68), 77% (102), 63% (14), 51% (3), 49% (15), 40% (7), and 33% (59). Causative products were hardly ever mentioned, but in one study, of the relevant reactions to any of the 26 fragrances (including HICC) tested, 96% were caused by cosmetic products (4).

Table 3.84.2 Patch testing in groups of patients: Routine testing

Years and Country	Test conc. & vehicle	Number of patients tested | positive (%)		Selection of patients (S); Relevance (R); Comments (C)	Ref.
2015-7 Netherlands		821	39 (4.8%)	R: not stated	107
2015-2016 UK	5% pet.	2084	30 (1.4%)	R: not specified for individual fragrances; 25% of patients who reacted to any fragrance or fragrance marker had a positive fragrance history	100
2011-2015 Spain	5% pet.	19,588	224 (1.1%)	R: not stated	108

Table 3.84.2 Patch testing in groups of patients: Routine testing (continued)

Years and Country	Test conc. & vehicle	Number of patients tested	positive (%)	Selection of patients (S); Relevance (R); Comments (C)	Ref.
2010-2015 Denmark	5% pet.	6004	(2.1%)	R: present relevance 38%, past relevance 83%	66
2009-2015 Sweden	5% pet.	4430	56 (1.2%)	R: not stated	72
2013-2014 Sweden	5% pet.	2118	32 (1.5%)	R: not stated; C: range per center: 0.4-3.0%; by testing HICC in duplicate, the number of allergic patients increased by 29% with the prevalence of positive reactions to HICC rising to 1.9%	86
2013-2014 Twelve European countries, 46 departments [a]	5% pet.	27,225	(1.7%)	R: not stated; C: results of 6 occupational dermatology clinics and one pediatric clinic not included in these figures; C: range of positive reactions: 0.4%-4.7%	60
2013-2014 Thailand		312	10 (3.2%)	R: 90%	68
2008-2014 UK	5% pet.	3517	14 (0.4%)	R: not stated	67
2011-2012 UK	5% pet.	1951	25 (1.3%)	R: not stated	70
2009-2012 Twelve European countries [a]	5% pet.	50,675	(1.8%)	R: not stated; C: range per country: 1.0-3.0%	69
2006-2011 Sweden	5% pet.	10,010	171 (1.7%)	R: not stated; only 0.2% of HICC positive patients did *not* co-react to FM II	87
2003-2011 Denmark	5% pet.	37,860	928 (2.5%)	R: >80% (present relevance 51%); yearly prevalence rate ranged from 2.1% to 2.8%	3
2002-2011 IVDK	5% pet.	95,452	(2.1%)	R: not stated; yearly prevalence rates ranged from 1.75% to 2.46%; slight decrease from 2006 to 2011	2
2002-2011 Belgium	5% pet.	3927	82 (2.1%)	R: not stated	88
2008-2010 Denmark	5% pet.	1502	34 (2.3%)	S: mostly routine testing; R: 92%; C: 54% co-reactivity of FM I, 96% of FM II; C: of the relevant reactions to any of the 26 fragrances tested, 96% were caused by cosmetic products	4
2001-2010 Australia	5% pet.	4804	99 (2.1%)	R: 33%	59
2007-2009 Portugal	5% pet.	629	17 (2.7%)	R: 16/17 (94%); all co-reacted to FM II	90
2007-2008 Ten European countries [a]	5% pet.	21,993	330 (1.5%)	R: not stated; C: prevalences ranged from 0-2.9%; highest rate in Switzerland (2.9%), lowest in Poland (0%) and Italy (0.8%)	1
2005-2008 Denmark	5% pet.	12,302	292 (2.4%)	R: 77%	102
2004-2008 Spain	5% pet.	852	9 (1.1%)	R: not stated	44
2005-2008 IVDK	5% pet.	37,270	(2.4%)	R: not stated	75
2004-2008 Iran		1137	8 (0.7%)	R: 82% of all reactions to FM I, FM II, Myroxylon pereirae resin, hydroxyisohexyl 3-cyclohexene carboxaldehyde and/or turpentine were clinically relevant	23
2003-2007 Denmark	5% pet.	18,789		R: 49% currently relevant; C: the yearly prevalence ranged from 2.1% in 2003 to 2.8% in 2007	15
2005-2006 Ten European countries [a]	5% pet.	11,790	222 (1.9%)	R: not stated; C: prevalences were 2.7% in Central Europe, 1.8% in West, 1.2% in Northeast and 0.5% in South Europe	58
2005 Germany	5% pet.	8046	205 (2.5%)	R: not stated; C: in a subgroup of 7002 patients tested with both HICC and FM II, 46% of patients allergic to FM II co-reacted to HICC and, of patients reacting to HICC, 85% were also allergic to FM II	104
2002-2005 Belgium	5% pet.	2901	62 (2.1%)	R: not stated	77
2003-2004 IVDK	5% pet.	21,325	502 (2.4%)	R: not stated; C: 51% co-reactivity of FM I	6
2001-2004 IVDK	5% pet.	25,676	(2.3%)	R: not stated	56
2003 NACDG	5% pet.	1603	7 (0.4%)	R: definite + probable relevance 0%	32
2002-2003 Europe [a]	5% pet.	3862	(2.2%)	R: not stated; C: range per center: 1.6-4.9%	57
2002-2003 Six European countries	2.5% pet. 5% pet.	1701 1701	20 (1.2%) 28 (1.6%)	R: not specified	22
2001-2002 UK	5% pet.	766	16 (2.1%)	R: 10 of 16 (63%) currently relevant; C: 63% co-reactivity to FM I	14
2000-2001 IVDK	5% pet.	3245	62 (1.9%)	R: 49% had a history of adverse reactions to perfumes, after-shave, or deodorants	9
1998 Six European countries	5% pet.	1855	(2.7%)	R: 40% relevance 'certain', 24% 'probable'; 58% co-reactivity to FM I	7
1997-8 Six European countries	5% pet.	1855	50 (2.7%)	R: not stated / specified	43

[a] study of the ESSCA (European Surveillance System on Contact Allergy Network)
FM: Fragrance mix; IVDK: Informationsverbund Dermatologischer Kliniken (Germany, Switzerland, Austria): NACDG: North American Contact Dermatitis Group (USA, Canada)

Relevance was hardly ever addressed. In one study, one of 4 reactions (25%) was considered to be relevant (97), another investigation from the US considered all 8 reactions to be relevant, but this had certain flaws: high rate of macular erythema (which was counted as positive) and weak reactions, and relevance figures included 'questionable' and 'past' relevance (27). Results of testing HICC in groups of patients reacting to the fragrance mix II are shown in Chapter 3.71 Fragrance mix II.

Patch testing in groups of selected patients

Results of testing HICC in groups of selected patients (e.g. nurses with occupational contact dermatitis, individuals with eyelid dermatitis, female hairdressers and their clients, individuals with known or suspected fragrance or cosmetic dermatitis) are shown in table 3.84.3. In twenty investigations, frequencies of sensitization to HICC ranged from 0.9% to 40%. As expected, the higher and highest rates were found in groups of patients known to be allergic to fragrances: 7.3% (21), 8.1% (44), 14.5% (108), 17% (73) and 27 resp. 40% (46). The high 27% and 40% positive reactions were found in small groups of patients who had a positive reaction to their own deodorant resp. a positive patch test to their own perfume, eau de toilette of shaving product (46).

Contrary to what might be expected, female hairdressers had no elevated frequencies of sensitization (64,82). Patients with stasis dermatitis / chronic leg ulcers had significantly lower percentages than a control group (65), but in an IVDK study, geriatric nurses with occupational dermatitis had significantly more frequently positive reactions (6.2%) than their colleagues without occupational contact dermatitis (2.9%) (103).

Table 3.84.3 Patch testing in groups of patients: Selected patient groups

Years and Country	Test conc. & vehicle	Number of patients tested	positive (%)	Selection of patients (S); Relevance (R); Comments (C)	Ref.
2014-2016 France		264	4 (1.5%)	S: patients suspected of eyelid allergic contact dermatitis; R: 1/4 (25%)	97
2011-2015 Spain	5% pet.	1013	147 (14.5%)	S: patients previously reacting to FM I, FM II, Myroxylon pereirae resin or hydroxyisohexyl 3-cyclohexene carboxaldehyde in the baseline series; R: not stated	108
1996-2015 IVDK	5% pet.	1709	15 (0.9%)	S: patients with psoriasis; R: not stated; C: the percentage of positive reactions was significantly lower than in the control group of consecutive dermatitis patients (1.9%)	105
2005-2014 IVDK	5% pet.	666	46 (6.2%)	S: geriatric nurses with occupational contact dermatitis; R: not stated; C: the frequency was significantly higher than in a control group of geriatric nurses without occupational contact dermatitis (2.9%)	103
2003-2014 IVDK	5% pet.	5202	(0.9%)	S: patients with stasis dermatitis / chronic leg ulcers; R: not stated; C: percentage of reactions far lower than in a control group of routine testing (2.7%)	65
2007-2012 IVDK	5% pet.	704	13 (1.8%)	S: female hairdressers with current or previous occupational contact dermatitis; R: not stated	64
		1905	53 (2.8%)	S: female patients, clients of hairdressers, in who hair cosmetics were regarded as a cause of dermatitis, and who had never worked as hairdressers; R: not stated	
2003-2012 IVDK		2043	93 (4.6%)	S: nurses with occupational contact dermatitis; R: not stated	61
2007-2011 IVDK	5% pet.	116	4 (3.5%)	S: physical therapists; R: not stated	106
2006-2011 IVDK	5% pet.	10,124	242 (2.5%)	S: patients with suspected cosmetic intolerance; R: not stated; C: the prevalence was *not* significantly higher than in a control group matched for sex and age	63
2002-2011 Denmark		399	6 (1.5%)	S: hairdressers with contact dermatitis; R: not stated; C: the frequency of sensitization to HICC, but also that of FM I and Myroxylon pereirae resin was lower than in a control group of consecutive patients routinely tested	82
2009-2010 Hungary	5% pet.	565	41 (7.3%)	S: patients with former skin symptoms provoked by scented products in the case history; R: in all cases 'possible'	21
2006-2010 USA	2.5% pet.	100	4 (4%)	S: patients with eyelid dermatitis; R: not stated	24
2005-10 Netherlands		100	17 (17%)	S: patients with known fragrance sensitivity based on a positive patch test to the FM I and/or the FM II; R: not stated	73
2000-2010 IVDK		4222	97 (2.0%)	S: patients with periorbital dermatitis; R: not stated; C: the frequency was lower than in a control group of routine testing	62
2004-2008 Spain	5% pet.	86	7 (8.1%)	S: patients previously reacting to the fragrance mix I or Myroxylon pereirae (n=54) or suspected of fragrance contact allergy (n=32); R: not stated	44
2005-7 Netherlands	2% pet.	320	10 (3.1%)	S: patients suspected of fragrance or cosmetic allergy; R: 61% relevance for all positive tested fragrances together	5
2000-2007 USA	5% pet.	354	8 (2.3%)	S: patients who were tested with a supplemental cosmetic	27

Table 3.84.3 Patch testing in groups of patients: Selected patient groups (continued)

Years and Country	Test conc. & vehicle	Number of patients tested | positive (%)		Selection of patients (S); Relevance (R); Comments (C)	Ref.
				screening series; R: 100%; C: weak study: a. high rate of macular erythema and weak reactions; b. relevance figures included 'questionable' and 'past' relevance	
2002-2003 Korea	5% pet.	422	7 (1.7%)	S: patients with suspected cosmetic dermatitis; R: not stated	42
2001-2002 Denmark, Sweden	5% pet.	658	14 (2.1%)	S: consecutive patients with hand eczema; R: it was assumed that nearly all positive reactions were of present or past relevance	8
1998-2002 IVDK	5% pet.	26	7 (27%)	S: patients who had a positive reaction to their own deodorant; R: not stated; C: there was a significant difference in percentage positive reactions compared with a control group of dermatitis patients who had *not* reacted to their own deodorant	46
		20	8 (40%)	S: patients who had a positive reaction to their own perfume, eau de toilette or shaving product; R: not stated; C: there was a significant difference in percentage positive reactions compared with a control group of dermatitis patients who had *not* reacted to their own cosmetic products of this type	

Testing in groups of patients reacting to the fragrance mix II
Results of testing HICC in groups of patients reacting to the fragrance mix II are shown in Chapter 3.71 Fragrance mix II

FM: Fragrance mix; IVDK: Informationsverbund Dermatologischer Kliniken (Germany, Switzerland, Austria)

Case reports and case series

Case series
HICC was stated to be the (or an) allergen in 44 patients in a group of 603 individuals suffering from cosmetic dermatitis, seen in the period 2010-2015 in Leuven, Belgium (54).

In the period 1996-2013, in a tertiary referral center in Valencia, Spain, 5419 patients were patch tested. Of these, 628 individuals had allergic contact dermatitis from cosmetics. In this group, HICC was the responsible allergen in 15 cases (40, overlap with ref. 41).

In the period 2000-2009, in Leuven, Belgium, an unspecified number of patients had positive patch tests or use tests to a total of 344 cosmetic products *and* positive patch tests to FM I, FM II, and/or to one or more of 28 selected specific fragrance ingredients. In 48 of 120 patients reacting to HICC, the presence of this fragrance in the cosmetic product(s) was confirmed by reading the product label(s) (74).

In the period 2000-2007, 202 patients with allergic contact dermatitis caused by cosmetics were seen in Valencia, Spain. In this group, HICC was the allergen in 3 individuals from its presence in deodorant (n=2) and in gel/soap (n=1) (41, overlap with ref. 40).

In a group of 119 patients with allergic contact dermatitis from cosmetics, investigated in The Netherlands in 1986-1987, one case was caused by HICC in deodorant (38,39).

Four patients with allergic contact dermatitis from HICC were presented in one study (7). A male student had itching eczematous patches on the neck and cheeks. He had positive reactions to 3 aftershaves and to HICC 5% pet. In all 3 aftershaves, HICC was identified with GC-MS. A female nurse had allergic contact dermatitis from HICC in a perfume. A man developed dermatitis of the face, presumably from an aftershave. He reacted to HICC 5% pet., but the cosmetic product itself was not tested. However, the presence of the fragrance in the aftershave was shown by chemical analysis and the dermatitis resolved when the incriminated product ceased to be used. A woman developed axillary dermatitis from 4 deodorants. She reacted to HICC 5% pet.; the deodorants themselves were not tested, but in all, HICC was identified by GC-MS. The products from these 4 patients contained HICC in concentrations ranging from 0.02% to 2.34% (7).

Case reports
A woman presented with a 5-month history of severe dermatitis in both axillae, related to the use of her underarm deodorant. Both a repeated application test and patch test with this deodorant were positive, whereas the European standard series was negative. Subsequently, patch testing with all the ingredients of the deodorant was positive to HICC and the fragrance of the deodorant, which contained HICC. Switching to a fragrance-free deodorant resolved the axillary dermatitis completely (45).

A man had bilateral contact dermatitis presenting as indurated plaques with satellite peripheral erythematous papules caused by contact allergy to HICC in a deodorant spray (84). One patient had allergic contact dermatitis from HICC in a deodorant cream (12). Another individual had allergic contact dermatitis from HICC in 2 deodorants (13). A woman also developed allergic contact dermatitis of the axillae from HICC in a deodorant (52). Another female patient had allergic contact dermatitis of the face and neck from HICC in her perfume (53).

A woman with vulval dermatitis had positive patch test reactions to the FM I, HICC and a body milk which she applied to the vulva. It was stated that these sensitizations were clinically relevant for her vulval dermatitis. Avoiding perfumed products including her own perfumed body milk led to a marked improvement of the vulval complaints. However, it was not specifically stated that the milk contained either HICC and/or one or more of the FM I ingredients (76).

Another female individual had allergic contact dermatitis from HICC, hexyl cinnamal, alpha-damascone and benzophenone-2 in an eau de parfum (78).

Cross-reactions, pseudo-cross-reactions and co-reactions

For general information on cross-/pseudo-cross-/co-reactivity of fragrance chemicals with other fragrances, fragrance markers (fragrance mix I, fragrance mix II, colophonium, Myroxylon pereirae resin [balsam of Peru]) and essential oils see Chapter 1.2 General information on cross-reactions, pseudo-cross-reactions and co-reactions. Co-reactivity with the fragrance mix II can be expected, as the mix contains hydroxyisohexyl 3-cyclohexene carbox-aldehyde (pseudo-cross-reactions). Indeed, in a group of 175 patients allergic to HICC, seen in Germany in 2005, 149 (85%) co-reacted to the FM II (104).

Presence in products and chemical analyses

In various studies, the presence of HICC in cosmetic and sometimes other products has been investigated. Before 2006, most investigators used chemical analysis, usually GC-MS, for qualitative and quantitative determination. Since then, the presence of the target fragrances was usually investigated by screening the product labels for the 26 fragrances that must be labeled since 2005 on cosmetics and detergent products in the EU, if present at > 10 ppm (0.001%) in leave-on products and > 100 ppm (0.01%) in rinse-off products. This method, obviously, is less accurate and may result in underestimation of the frequency of the fragrances being present in the product. When they are in fact present, but the concentration is lower than mentioned above, labeling is not required and the fragrances' presence will be missed.

The results of the relevant studies for HICC are summarized in table 3.84.4. More detailed information can be found in the corresponding text before and following the table. The percentage of products in which HICC was found to be present shows wide variations, which can among other be explained by the selection procedure of the products, the method of investigation (false-negatives with information obtained from labels only) and changes in the use of individual fragrance materials over time (fashion). Over the last decade, undoubtedly as a result of increasing knowledge on the sensitizing properties of this fragrance, its use appears to have declined strongly.

In 2017, in the USA, the ingredient labels 159 hair-dye kits containing 539 cosmetic products (e.g. colorants, conditioners, shampoos, toners) were screened for the most common sensitizers they contain. HICC was found to be present in 5 (1%) of the products (79).

In Denmark, in 2015-2016, 5588 fragranced cosmetic products were examined with a smartphone application for the 26 fragrances that need to be labeled in the EU. HICC was present in 7% of the products (rank number 14) (36).

In Germany, in 2015, fragrance allergens were evaluated based on lists of ingredients in 817 (unique) detergents (all-purpose cleaners, cleaning preparations for special purposes [e.g. bathroom, kitchen, dish-washing] and laundry detergents) present in 131 households. HICC was found to be present in 12 (1.5%) of the products (98).

In 2008, 2010 and 2011, 374 deodorants available in German retail shops were randomly selected and their labels checked for the presence of the 26 fragrances that need to be labeled. HICC was found to be present in 47 (12.6%) of the products (81).

Hydroxyisohexyl 3-cyclohexene carboxaldehyde was present (as indicated by labeling) in 7% of 204 cosmetic products (92 shampoos, 61 hair conditioners, 34 liquid soaps, 17 wet tissues) and in none of 97 detergents in Sweden, 2008 (28).

In 2007, in The Netherlands, twenty-three cosmetic products for children were analyzed for the presence of fragrances that need to be labeled. HICC was identified in 12 of the products (52%) in a concentration range of 44-2790 ppm (48).

In 2006, of 88 popular perfume containing deodorants purchased in Denmark, 29 (33%) were labeled to contain HICC. Analysis of 24 regulated fragrance substances in 23 selected deodorants (19 spray products, 2 deostick and 2 roll-on) was performed by GC-MS. HICC was identified in 17 of the products (74%) with a concentration range of 1–4431 ppm (37).

In Denmark, in 2006, 25 perfume products (13 eau de parfum, 8 eau de toilette, one parfum spray, one parfum, and 2 after-shave lotions) for both men and women were purchased from Danish retail outlets and investigated for the presence of isoeugenol, hydroxyisohexyl 3-cyclohexenecarboxaldehyde, atranol and chloroatranol. HICC was present in 18 products (72%) in a concentration range of 59-2058 ppm (51).

In January 2006, a study of perfumed cosmetic and household products available on the shelves of U.K. retailers was carried out. Products were included if 'parfum' or 'aroma' was listed among the ingredients. Three hundred products were surveyed and any of 26 mandatory labeling fragrances named on the label were recorded. HICC was present in 88 (29%) of the products (rank number 10) (34).

Table 3.84.4 Presence of hydroxyisohexyl 3-cyclohexene carboxaldehyde in products [a]

Year	Country	Product type	Nr. investigated	Nr. of products positive [b]	(%)	Method [c]	Ref.
2017	USA	Cosmetic products in hair-dye kits	539 products in 159 hair-dye kits	5	(1%)	Labeling	79
2015-6	Denmark	Fragranced cosmetic products	5588		(7%)	Labeling	36
2015	Germany	Household detergents	817	12	(1%)	Labeling	98
2008-11	Germany	Deodorants	374	47	(13%)	Labeling	81
2008	Sweden	Cosmetic products	204		(7%)	Labeling	28
		Detergents	97		(0%)	Labeling	
2007	Netherlands	Cosmetic products for children	23	12	(52%)	Analysis	48
2006	UK	Perfumed cosmetic and house-hold products	300	88	(29%)	Labeling	34
2006	Denmark	Popular perfumed deodorants	88	29	(33%)	Labeling	37
			23	17	(74%)	Analysis	
2006	Denmark	Rinse-off cosmetics for children	208	12	(6%)	Labeling + analysis	47
2006	Denmark	Perfume products	25	18	(72%)	Analysis	51
2004	Denmark, UK, Belgium, Germany	Fragranced products that had caused allergic contact dermatitis, used by patients	24	19	(79%)	Labeling	22
2002	Denmark	Home and car air fresheners	19	9	(47%)	Analysis	50
2001	Denmark	Non-cosmetic consumer products	43	3	(7%)	Analysis	49
2000	Denmark, UK, Germany, Italy	Domestic and occupational products	59	6	(10%)	Analysis	30
1997-8	Denmark, UK Germany, Sweden	Cosmetics and cosmetic toys for children	25	8	(32%)	Analysis	31
1996	Five European countries	Fragranced deodorants	70	37	(53%)	Analysis	29
1992	Netherlands	Cosmetic products	300		(33%)	Analysis	25
1988	USA	Perfumes used in fine fragrances, household products and soap'	400	?-46% (See text)		Analysis	33

[a] See the corresponding text below for more details
[b] positive = containing the target fragrance
[c] Labeling: information from the ingredient labels on the product / packaging; Analysis: chemical analysis, most often GC-MS

In 2006, the labels of 208 cosmetics for children (especially shampoos, body shampoos and soaps) available in Denmark were checked for the presence of the 26 fragrances that need to be labeled in the EU. HICC was present in 12 products (5.8%), and ranked number 16 in the frequency list. Seventeen products were analyzed quantitatively for the fragrances. The maximum concentration found for HICC was 2700 mg/kg (47).

In 2004, in 4 European countries (Denmark, Germany, Belgium, U.K.), of 12 patients allergic to the FM II and one or more of its constituents (hexyl cinnamal 1, citral 3, hydroxyisohexyl 3-cyclohexene carboxaldehyde 11), 24 of the products used by them (deodorant 4, eau de toilette 9, lotion/cream 4, fine perfume 7) that had caused adverse reactions compatible with allergic contact dermatitis, were analyzed for the presence of the six constituents (citral, citronellol, coumarin, farnesol, hexyl cinnamal, hydroxyisohexyl 3-cyclohexene carboxaldehyde). Hydroxyisohexyl 3-cyclohexene carboxaldehyde was found in 19/24 products (79%) in concentrations ranging from 0.017-3.832% (22).

In 2002, in Denmark, 19 air fresheners (6 for cars, 13 for homes) were analyzed for the presence of fragrances that need to be labeled on cosmetics. HICC was found to be present in 9 products (47%) in a concentration range of 310-62,000 ppm and ranked 12 in the frequency list (50).

In 2001, in Denmark, 43 non-cosmetic consumer products (mainly dish-washing products, laundry detergents, and hard and soft surface cleaners) were analyzed for the 26 fragrances that are regulated for labeling in the EU. HICC was present in 3 products (7%) in a concentration range of 0.0053-0.0110% (m/m) and had rank number 16 in the frequency list (49).

In 2000, fifty-nine domestic and occupational products, purchased in retail outlets in Denmark, England, Germany and Italy were analyzed by GC-MS for the presence of fragrances. The product categories were liquid soap and soap bars (n=13), soft/hard surface cleaners (n=23), fabric conditioners/laundry detergents for hand wash (n=8), dish-wash (n=10), furniture polish, car shampoo, stain remover (each n=1) and 2 products used in occupational environments. Hydroxyisohexyl 3-cyclohexene carboxaldehyde (Lyral ®) was present in 6 products (10%) with a mean concentration of 75 ppm and a range of 36-103 ppm (30).

Twenty-five cosmetics and cosmetic toys for children (5 shampoos and shower gels, 6 perfumes, 1 deodorant (roll-on), 4 baby lotions/creams, 1 baby wipes product, 1 baby oil, 2 lipcare products and 5 toy-cosmetic products: a cosmetic-toy set for blending perfumes and a makeup set) purchased in 1997-1998 in retail outlets in Denmark, Germany, England and Sweden were analyzed in 1998 for the presence of fragrances by GC-MS. Hydroxyisohexyl 3-cyclohexene carboxaldehyde (Lyral ®) was found in 8 products (32%) in a concentration range of ≤0.001-0.630% (w/w). For the analytical data in each product category, the original publication should be consulted (31).

Seventy fragranced deodorants, purchased at retail outlets in 5 European countries in 1996, were analyzed by gas chromatography - mass spectrometry (GC-MS) for the determination of the contents of 21 commonly used fragrance materials. Hydroxyisohexyl 3-carboxaldehyde was identified in 37 products (53%) in a concentration range of 1-1874 ppm (29).

In 1992, in The Netherlands, the presence of fragrances was analyzed in 300 cosmetic products. HICC was identified in 33% of the products (rank order 24) (25).

In 1988, in the USA, 400 perfumes used in fine fragrances, household products and soaps (number of products per category not mentioned) were analyzed for the presence of fragrance chemicals in a concentration of at least 1% and a list of the Top-25 (present in the highest number of products) presented. HICC was found to be present in 46% of the fine fragrances (rank number 13), an unknown percentage of the household product fragrances and an unknown percentage of the fragrances used in soaps (33).

Serial dilution testing and Repeated Open Application Tests

Eighteen patients with dermatitis who previously had given a positive patch test to HICC 5% petrolatum and 7 control subjects were tested with a serial dilution of HICC in alcohol from 6% (60,000 ppm) w/v down to 0.0006% (6 ppm). One or more reactions to the dilution patch series were found in all patients but one (17/18). From the dose–response curve is was calculated that the dose of HICC eliciting a reaction in 10% of the group was 29 ppm and 50% elicited to 662 ppm, corresponding to 0.9 mg/cm^2 and 20 mg/cm^2, respectively (19). In addition, the patients performed a 2-week repeated open application test (ROAT) on the volar aspect of the forearm with a 0.5% w/v concentration of HICC in alcohol. In the case of no reaction, this was followed by another 2 weeks of testing with a 3% alcoholic solution of HICC. In 16 of 18 patients (89%), a positive use test developed, 11 reacting to the low and 5 only to the high concentration. None reacted to the vehicle control of ethanol applied to the contralateral arm and all controls were negative to both the test solutions of HICC and the ethanol control (19).

In a study aimed at determining elicitation thresholds for HICC under simulated conditions of deodorant use, 15 patients with previously diagnosed contact allergy to HICC were patch tested with 5 solutions of HICC (0.0006%, 0.006%, 0.06%, 0.6%, and 6% in ethanol), ethanol, unscented deodorant, 3 scented deodorants containing 200, 600, and 1800 ppm HICC, respectively, and standard HICC 5% in petrolatum (20). All fourteen patients who completed the study reacted to HICC 6% in ethanol at patch testing, one though showing only a weak reaction (?+). The lowest observed threshold concentration was 0.0006% (6 ppm) seen in one patient. From the fitted dose–response curves it was estimated that about 10% of sensitized individuals will react to 25 ppm, 50% to 610 ppm and 90% to 15,000 ppm (1.5%). Simultaneous positive patch test reactions to one or more of the scented deodorants were seen in 7 patients, of who 2 had positive patch tests to the deodorant with 200 ppm, further 2 reacted to the deodorant containing 600 ppm and 3 to deodorant with 1800 ppm HICC only. None of the controls had positive patch tests. The 15 patients and 10 healthy controls also performed a use test in the axillae using deodorants scented with HICC in increasing concentrations and unscented deodorants as control. The concentration of HICC was increased every second week (200, 600, and 1800 ppm) until either a reaction developed or for 6 weeks. Fourteen patients completed the study, and all developed unilateral eczema from the HICC-containing deodorant, while controls were all negative. In 9/14 patients, a positive use test developed during the first 2 weeks to the deodorant containing 200 ppm HICC. It was concluded that HICC elicits allergic contact dermatitis in a high proportion of sensitized individuals at common usage concentrations (200 ppm or higher) in deodorants (20).

In another investigation performing serial dilution patch testing in 17 patients allergic to HICC with amounts ranging from 1500 - 0.0022 µg HICC cm^{-2}, the lowest dose to which all 17 patients reacted was 100 µg HICC cm^{-2} (18). The calculated dose with a response frequency of 50% (ED$_{50}$) was 11.1 µg HICC cm^{-2} and the ED$_{10}$ was 0.66 µg HICC cm^{-2} (18). In the same study, ROATS were positive within three weeks in 15/16 patients (94%) with a dose/application of 35.7 µg HICC cm^{-2}, 12/16 (75%) with a dose/application of 3.57 µg HICC cm^{-2} and 3/16 (19%) with a dose/application of 0.357 µg HICC cm^{-2} (18).

Repeated skin exposure to a fragrance allergen in 15 patients previously diagnosed with hand eczema and contact allergy to the fragrance was used to explore whether immersion of fingers in a solution with or without the patch-test-positive fragrance allergen would cause or exacerbate hand eczema on the exposed finger. The study was double-blinded and randomized. All participants had a positive patch test to either hydroxycitronellal (n=13) or hydroxyisohexyl 3-cyclohexene carboxaldehyde (Lyral ®, HICC). Each participant immersed a finger from each hand, once a day for 10 minutes, in a 10% alcoholic solution containing the fragrance allergen or placebo. During the first 2 weeks, the concentration of fragrance allergen in the solution was low (approximately 10 ppm), whilst during the following 2 weeks, the concentration was relatively high (approximately 250 ppm), imitating real-life exposure to a household product like dishwashing liquid diluted in water and the undiluted product, respectively. Evaluation was made using a clinical scale and laser Doppler flow meter. Three of 15 hand eczema patients developed eczema on the finger immersed in the fragrance-containing solution, 3 of 15 on the placebo finger and 3 of 15 on both fingers. Thus, no association between immersion of a finger in a solution containing fragrance to which the subject was allergic and development of clinically visible eczema was found. In the 2 patients with allergy to HICC, there were 2 reactions to the placebo solution and one clinically visible reaction on a finger immersed in the fragrance solution (83).

To investigate whether patients allergic to HICC could develop skin reactions from HICC residues on fabrics deposited by washing powder and fabric softener, 17 HICC-allergic individuals were patch tested with a dilution series of HICC and with pieces of cotton containing HICC (94). For the dose–response patch tests, the concentration of allergens used was between 0.00001 and 0.01% (v/v), equivalent to 0.00045–0.00049 to 0.45–0.49 µg/cm^2 which is for the latter more than 20-fold higher than the likely skin exposure levels associated with a fabric washed with washing powder and a fabric softener. The dose HICC in the fabric for patch testing was 0.1 µg/cm^2 (0.63 µg/ml), which is 6-fold higher than the likely skin exposure levels associated with a washed fabric The vehicle for HICC in the dilution series and in the fabric (ethanol/diethyl phthalate 3:1 v/v) and an untreated piece of cotton served as controls (94). None of the panellists had a positive reaction to the patch tests with HICC solution, indicating that their lower threshold for elicitation is >0.01%, which (0.01%) is 20-fold higher than the likely skin exposure levels associated with a fabric washed with washing powder and a fabric softener. Patch testing with the fabric containing HICC at D4 showed 6 irritant reactions (5 in de control without HICC), 2 ?+ reactions (2 in controls) and one + reaction (2 in controls). In the patient with a + reaction, the vehicle control fabric also showed a + reaction. It was concluded that HICC residues present on fabric do not appear to present a risk of the elicitation of contact allergic skin reactions on individuals already sensitized to HICC (94).

In a study performed by the IVDK between December 2006 and March 2007, 64 patients previously shown to be allergic to HICC performed ROATs on their underarm with two products: an alcoholic solution with five different concentrations of HICC (0.005%, 0.01%, 0.1%, 0.5% and 2.5%) and a cream containing 15% glyceryl stearate in water as vehicle, containing HICC in the same concentrations. The vehicles without HICC (ethanol 96% and 15% glyceryl stearate in water, respectively) served as negative controls. The panelists started with the lowest concentrations and would, if after 2 weeks no reaction was observed, continue with the two products in the next (higher) concentration. In total, 56 patients (88%) reacted to the cream and 53 (83%) to the perfume. With the cream, 3 reacted to 0.005% (50 ppm), 5 to 0.01% (100 ppm), 19 to 0.1%, 15 to 0.5% and 14 to 2.5% as lowest concentrations. With the lotion, one reacted to 0.005%, one to 0.01%, 17 to 0.1%, 18 to 0.5% and 16 to 2.5% as lowest concentrations. Investigating the relationship between the cumulative response and increasing amounts as µg/cm^2 of perfume and cream, it was shown that the 10% thresholds for no response were 1.2 µg/cm^2 for the perfume and 4.9 µg/cm^2 for the cream. The concentrations being tolerated by 90% of those sensitized to HICC were thus estimated as <88.2 ppm for the cream and <270 ppm for the perfume. The panelists, after performing the ROATS, were patch tested with 4 HICC preparations (2.5% pet., Fragrance mix II, and two 5% pet. preparations of different suppliers). Of 52 who reacted to the cream-ROAT, 50 (96%) reacted to at least one of the HICC patch tests; of 49 with a positive perfume ROAT, 48 (98%) also reacted to the patch test(s). There was a substantial inverse correlation between the ROAT concentrations and the reaction strength in patch testing. The lower the ROAT concentrations leading to reactions, i.e. the lower the individual elicitation threshold, the stronger were the reactions in confirmatory patch testing (95).

Other information

Hydroxyisohexyl 3-cyclohexene carboxaldehyde concentrations are stable in petrolatum in IQ Chambers and Finn Chambers with covers at 5, 25 and 35°C for 8 hours; only when exposed to ambient air or heat for prolonged periods, decreasing concentrations are observed. After 9 days, HICC concentrations were found to fall approximately 30% when stored at 35°C, 10% at 25°C, and less than 5% at 5°C (85).

LITERATURE

1   Uter W, Aberer W, Armario-Hita JC, Fernandez-Vozmediano JM, Ayala F, Balato A, et al. Current patch test results with the European baseline series and extensions to it from the 'European Surveillance System on Contact Allergy' network, 2007-2008. Contact Dermatitis 2012;67:9-19

2   Schnuch A, Geier J, Uter W. Is hydroxyisohexyl 3-cyclohexene carboxaldehyde sensitization declining in central Europe? Contact Dermatitis 2012;67:47-49

3   Heisterberg MV, Laurberg G, Veien N, Menné T, Avnstorp C, Kaaber K, et al. Prevalence of allergic contact dermatitis caused by hydroxyisohexyl 3-cyclohexene carboxaldehyde has not changed in Denmark. Contact Dermatitis 2012;67:49-51

4   Heisterberg MV, Menné T, Johansen JD. Contact allergy to the 26 specificc fragrance ingredients to be declared on cosmetic products in accordance with the EU cosmetic directive. Contact Dermatitis 2011;65:266-275

5   Oosten EJ van, Schuttelaar ML, Coenraads PJ. Clinical relevance of positive patch test reactions to the 26 EU-labelled fragrances. Contact Dermatitis 2009;61:217-223

6   Schnuch A, Uter W, Geier J, Lessmann H, Frosch PJ. Sensitization to 26 fragrances to be labelled according to current European regulation: Results of the IVDK and review of the literature. Contact Dermatitis 2007;57:1-10

7   Frosch PJ, Johansen JD, Menné T, Rastogi SC, Bruze M, Andersen KE, et al. Lyral ® is an important sensitizer in patients sensitive to fragrances. Br J Dermatol 1999;141:1076-1083

8   Heydorn S, Johansen JD, Andersen KE, Bruze M, Svedman C, White IR, et al. Fragrance allergy in patients with hand eczema – a clinical study. Contact Dermatitis 2003;48:317-323

9   Geier J, Brasch J, Schnuch A, Lessmann H, Pirker C, Frosch PJ; Information Network of Departments of Dermatology (IVDK) and the German Contact Dermatitis Research Group (DKG). Lyral has been included in the patch test standard series in Germany. Contact Dermatitis 2002;46:295-297

10 Ford RA, Api AM, Letizia CS. Monographs on fragrance raw materials. Food Chem Toxicol 1992;30(suppl.):S49-S51

11 Patlewicz GY, Wright ZM, Basketter DA, Pease CK, Lepoittevin JP, Giménez Arneau E. Structure-activity relationships for selected fragrance allergens. Contact Dermatitis 2002;47:219-226

12 De Groot AC. Contact allergy to cosmetics: causative ingredients. Contact Dermatitis 1987;17:26-34

13 Handley J, Burrows D. Allergic contact dermatitis from the synthetic fragrances Lyral and acetyl cedrene in separate underarm deodorant preparations. Contact Dermatitis 1994;31:288-290

14 Baxter KF, Wilkinson SM, Kirk SJ. Hydroxymethyl pentylcyclohexene-carboxaldehyde (Lyral) as a fragrance allergen in the UK. Contact Dermatitis 2003;48:117-118

15 Braendstrup P, Johansen JD on behalf of the Danish Contact Dermatitis Group. Hydroxyisohexyl 3-cyclohexene carboxaldehyde (Lyral) is still a frequent allergen. Contact Dermatitis 2008;59:187-188

16 Bruze M, Andersen KE, Goossens A. Recommendation to include fragrance mix 2 and hydroxyisohexyl 3-cyclohexene carboxaldehyde (Lyral) in the European baseline patch test series. Contact Dermatitis 2008;58:129-133

17 De Groot AC. Adverse reactions to cosmetics. PhD Thesis, Groningen, State University of Groningen, 1988

18 Fischer LA, Menné T, Avnstorp C Kasting GB, Johansen JD. Hydroxyisohexyl 3-cyclohexene carboxaldehyde allergy: relationship between patch test and repeated open application test thresholds. Br J Dermatol 2009;161:560-567

19 Johansen JD, Frosch PJ, Svedman C, Andersen KE, Bruze M, Pirker C, Menné T. Hydroxyisohexyl 3-cyclohexene carboxaldehyde known as Lyral: quantitative aspects and risk assessment of an important fragrance allergen. Contact Dermatitis 2003;48:310-316

20 Jorgensen PH, Jensen CD, Rastogi S, Andersen KE, Johansen JD. Experimental elicitation with hydroxyisohexyl-3-cyclohexene carboxaldehyde-containing deodorants. Contact Dermatitis 2007;56:146-150

21 Pónyai G, Németh I, Altmeyer A, Nagy G, Irinyi B, Battya Z, et al. Patch tests with fragrance mix II and its components. Dermatitis 2012;23:71-74

22 Frosch PJ, Rastogi SC, Pirker C, Brinkmeier T, Andersen KE, Bruze M, et al. Patch testing with a new fragrance mix - reactivity to the individual constituents and chemical detection in relevant cosmetic products. Contact Dermatitis 2005;52:216-225

23 Firooz A, Nassiri-Kashani M, Khatami A, Gorouhi F, Babakoohi S, Montaser-Kouhsari L, et al. Fragrance contact allergy in Iran. J Eur Acad Dermatol Venereol 2010;24:1437-1441

24 Wenk KS, Ehrlich AE. Fragrance series testing in eyelid dermatitis. Dermatitis 2012;23:22-26

25 SCCP (Scientific Committee on Consumer Products), Opinion on hydroxyisohexyl 3-cyclohexene carboxaldehyde (HICC), 13-14 December 2011, SCCS/1456/11. Available at:
    https://ec.europa.eu/health/sites/health/files/scientific_committees/consumer_safety/docs/sccs_o_074.pdf

26 SCCS (Scientific Committee on Consumer Safety). Opinion on Fragrance allergens in cosmetic products, 26-27 June 2012, SCCS/1459/11. Available at:
    https://ec.europa.eu/health/sites/health/files/scientific_committees/consumer_safety/docs/sccs_o_102.pdf

27 Wetter DA, Yiannias JA, Prakash AV, Davis MDP, Farmer SA, el-Azhary RA. Results of patch testing to personal care product allergens in a standard series and a supplemental cosmetic series: an analysis of 945 patients from the Mayo Clinic Contact Dermatitis Group, 2000-2007. J Am Acad Dermatol 2010;63:789-798

28 Yazar K, Johnsson S, Lind M-L, Boman A, Lidén C. Preservatives and fragrances in selected consumer-available cosmetics and detergents. Contact Dermatitis 2011;64:265-272

29 Rastogi SC, Johansen JD, Frosch P, Menné T, Bruze M, Lepoittevin JP, et al. Deodorants on the European market: quantitative chemical analysis of 21 fragrances. Contact Dermatitis 1998;38:29-35

30 Rastogi SC, Heydorn S, Johansen JD, Basketter DA. Fragrance chemicals in domestic and occupational products. Contact Dermatitis 2001;45:221-225

31 Rastogi SC, Johansen JD, Menné T, Frosch P, Bruze M, Andersen KE, et al. Content of fragrance allergens in children's cosmetics and cosmetic toys. Contact Dermatitis 1999;41:84-88

32 Belsito DV, Fowler JF Jr, Sasseville D, Marks JG Jr, DeLeo VA, Storrs FJ. Delayed-type hypersensitivity to fragrance materials in a select North American population. Dermatitis 2006;17:23-28

33 Fenn RS. Aroma chemical usage trends in modern perfumery. Perfumer and Flavorist 1989;14:3-10

34 Buckley DA. Fragrance ingredient labelling in products on sale in the UK. Br J Dermatol 2007;157:295-300

35 Weyland JW. Personal Communication, 1992. Cited in: De Groot AC, Weyland JW, Nater JP. Unwanted effects of cosmetics and drugs used in dermatology, 3rd Ed. Amsterdam: Elsevier, 1994: 579

36 Bennike NH, Oturai NB, Müller S, Kirkeby CS, Jørgensen C, Christensen AB, et al. Fragrance contact allergens in 5588 cosmetic products identified through a novel smartphone application. J Eur Acad Dermatol Venereol 2018;32:79-85

37 Rastogi SC, Hellerup Jensen G, Johansen JD. Survey and risk assessment of chemical substances in deodorants. Survey of Chemical Substances in Consumer Products, No. 86 2007. Danish Ministry of the Environment, Environmental Protection Agency. Available at: https://www2.mst.dk/Udgiv/publications/2007/978-87-7052-625-8/pdf/978-87-7052-626-5.pdf

38 De Groot AC, Bruynzeel DP, Bos JD, van der Meeren HL, van Joost T, Jagtman BA, Weyland JW. The allergens in cosmetics. Arch Dermatol 1988;124:1525-1529

39 De Groot AC. Adverse reactions to cosmetics. PhD Thesis, University of Groningen, The Netherlands: 1988, chapter 3.4, pp.105-113

40 Zaragoza-Ninet V, Blasco Encinas R, Vilata-Corell JJ, Pérez-Ferriols A, Sierra-Talamantes C, Esteve-Martínez A, de la Cuadra-Oyanguren J. Allergic contact dermatitis due to cosmetics: A clinical and epidemiological study in a tertiary hospital. Actas Dermosifiliogr 2016;107:329-336

41 Laguna C, de la Cuadra J, Martín-González B, Zaragoza V, Martínez-Casimiro L, Alegre V. Allergic contact dermatitis to cosmetics. Actas Dermosifiliogr 2009;100:53-60

42 An S, Lee AY, Lee CH, Kim DW, Hahm JH, Kim KJ, et al. Fragrance contact dermatitis in Korea: a joint study. Contact Dermatitis 2005;53:320-323

43 Frosch PJ, Johansen JD, Menné T, Pirker C, Rastogi SC, Andersen KE, et al. Further important sensitizers in patients sensitive to fragrances. I. Reactivity to 14 frequently used chemicals. Contact Dermatitis 2002;47:78-85

44 Cuesta L, Silvestre JF, Toledo F, Lucas A, Perez-Crespo M, Ballester I. Fragrance contact allergy: a 4-year retrospective study. Contact Dermatitis 2010;63:77-84

45 Hendriks SA, Bousema MT, van Ginkel CJW. Allergic contact dermatitis from the fragrance ingredient Lyral in underarm deodorant. Contact Dermatitis 1999;41:119

46 Uter W, Geier J, Schnuch A, Frosch PJ. Patch test results with patients' own perfumes, deodorants and shaving lotions: results of the IVDK 1998-2002. J Eur Acad Dermatol Venereol 2007;21:374-379

47 Poulsen PB, Schmidt A. A survey and health assessment of cosmetic products for children. Survey of chemical substances in consumer products, No. 88. Copenhagen: Danish Environmental Protection Agency, 2007. Available at: https://www2.mst.dk/udgiv/publications/2007/978-87-7052-638-8/pdf/978-87-7052-639-5.pdf

48 VWA. Dutch Food and Consumer Product Safety Authority. Cosmetische producten voor kinderen: Inventarisatie van de markt en de veiligheidsborging door producenten en importeurs. Report ND04o065/ND05o170, 2007 (Report in Dutch), 2007. Available at: www.nvwa.nl/documenten/communicatie/inspectieresultaten/consument/2016m/cosmetische-producten-voor-kinderen

49 Rastogi SC. Survey of chemical compounds in consumer products. Contents of selected fragrance materials in cleaning products and other consumer products. Survey no. 8-2002. Copenhagen, Denmark, Danish Environmental Protection Agency. Available at: http://eng.mst.dk/media/mst/69131/8.pdf

50 Pors J, Fuhlendorff R. Mapping of chemical substances in air fresheners and other fragrance liberating products. Report Danish Ministry of the Environment, Environmental Protection Agency (EPA). Survey of Chemicals in Consumer Products, No 30, 2003. Available at: http://eng.mst.dk/media/mst/69113/30.pdf

51 Rastogi SC, Johansen JD, Bossi R. Selected important fragrance sensitizers in perfumes: current exposures. Contact Dermatitis 2007;56:201-204

52 Heras F, Díaz-Recuero JL, Cabello MJ, Conde-Salazar L. Sensitization to Lyral. Actas Dermosifiliogr 2006;97:374-378 (article in Spanish)

53 Zirwas MJ, Bechtel M. Allergic contact dermatitis to a perfume containing Lyral. J Am Acad Dermatol 2008;58(5 suppl.1):S97-S98

54 Goossens A. Cosmetic contact allergens. Cosmetics 2016, 3, 5; doi:10.3390/cosmetics3010005

55 Diepgen TL, Ofenloch RF, Bruze M, Bertuccio P, Cazzaniga S, Coenraads P-J, et al. Prevalence of contact allergy in the general population in different European regions. Br J Dermatol 2016;174:319-329

56 Worm M, Brasch J, Geier J, Uter W, Schnuch A. Epikutantestung mit der DKG-Standardreihe 2001-2004. Hautarzt 2005;56:1114-1124

57 Uter W, Hegewald J, Aberer W, Ayala F, Bircher AJ, Brasch J, et al. The European standard series in 9 European countries, 2002/2003 – First results of the European Surveillance System on Contact Allergies. Contact Dermatitis 2005;53:136-145

58 Uter W, Rämsch C, Aberer W, Ayala F, Balato A, Beliauskiene A, et al. The European baseline series in 10 European Countries, 2005/2006 – Results of the European Surveillance System on Contact Allergies (ESSCA). Contact Dermatitis 2009;61:31-38

59 Toholka R, Wang Y-S, Tate B, Tam M, Cahill J, Palmer A, Nixon R. The first Australian Baseline Series: Recommendations for patch testing in suspected contact dermatitis. Australas J Dermatol 2015;56:107-115

60 Uter W, Amario-Hita JC, Balato A, Ballmer-Weber B, Bauer A, Belloni Fortina A, et al. European Surveillance System on Contact Allergies (ESSCA): results with the European baseline series, 2013/14. J Eur Acad Dermatol Venereol 2017;31:1516-1525

61 Molin S, Bauer A, Schnuch A, Geier J. Occupational contact allergy in nurses: results from the Information Network of Departments of Dermatology 2003–2012. Contact Dermatitis 2015;72:164-171

62 Landeck L, John SM, Geier J. Periorbital dermatitis in 4779 patients – patch test results during a 10-year period. Contact Dermatitis 2014;70:205-212

63 Dinkloh A, Worm M, Geier J, Schnuch A, Wollenberg A. Contact sensitization in patients with suspected cosmetic intolerance: results of the IVDK 2006-2011. J Eur Acad Dermatol Venereol 2015;29:1071-1081

64 Uter W, Gefeller O, John SM, Schnuch A, Geier J. Contact allergy to ingredients of hair cosmetics – a comparison of female hairdressers and clients based on IVDK 2007–2012 data. Contact Dermatitis 2014;71:13-20

65 Erfurt-Berge C, Geier J, Mahler V. The current spectrum of contact sensitization in patients with chronic leg ulcers or stasis dermatitis - new data from the Information Network of Departments of Dermatology (IVDK). Contact Dermatitis 2017;77:151-158

66 Bennike NH, Zachariae C, Johansen JD. Non-mix fragrances are top sensitizers in consecutive dermatitis patients –a cross-sectional study of the 26 EU-labelled fragrance allergens. Contact Dermatitis 2017;77:270-279

67 Sabroe RA, Holden CR, Gawkrodger DJ. Contact allergy to essential oils cannot always be predicted from allergy to fragrance markers in the baseline series. Contact Dermatitis 2016;74:236-241

68 Vejanurug P, Tresukosol P, Sajjachareonpong P, Puangpet P. Fragrance allergy could be missed without patch testing with 26 individual fragrance allergens. Contact Dermatitis 2016;74:230-235

69 Frosch PJ, Johansen JD, Schuttelaar M-LA, Silvestre JF, Sánchez-Pérez J, Weisshaar E, et al. (on behalf of the ESSCA network). Patch test results with fragrance markers of the baseline series – analysis of the European Surveillance System on Contact Allergies (ESSCA) network 2009–2012. Contact Dermatitis 2015;73:163-171

70 Mann J, McFadden JP, White JML, White IR, Banerjee P. Baseline series fragrance markers fail to predict contact allergy. Contact Dermatitis 2014;70:276-281

71 Uter W, Johansen JD, Börje A, Karlberg A-T, Lidén C, Rastogi S, Roberts D, White IR. Categorization of fragrance contact allergens for prioritization of preventive measures: clinical and experimental data and consideration of structure–activity relationships. Contact Dermatitis 2013;69:196-230

72 Mowitz M, Svedman C, Zimerson E, Isaksson M, Pontén A, Bruze M. Simultaneous patch testing with fragrance mix I, fragrance mix II and their ingredients in southern Sweden between 2009 and 2015. Contact Dermatitis 2017;77:280-287

73 Nagtegaal MJC, Pentinga SE, Kuik J, Kezic S, Rustemeyer T. The role of the skin irritation response in polysensitization to fragrances. Contact Dermatitis 2012;67:28-35

74 Nardelli A, Drieghe J, Claes L, Boey L, Goossens A. Fragrance allergens in 'specific' cosmetic products. Contact Dermatitis 2011;64:212-219

75 Uter W, Geier J, Frosch P, Schnuch A. Contact allergy to fragrances: current patch test results (2005–2008) from the Information Network of Departments of Dermatology. Contact Dermatitis 2010;63:254-261

76 Vermaat H, Smienk F, Rustemeyer T, Bruynzeel DP, Kirtschig G. Anogenital allergic contact dermatitis, the role of spices and flavour allergy. Contact Dermatitis 2008;59:233-237

77 Nardelli A, Carbonez A, Ottoy W, Drieghe J, Goossens A. Frequency of and trends in fragrance allergy over a 15-year period. Contact Dermatitis 2008;58:134-141

78   Giménez-Arnau A, Giménez-Arnau E, Serra-Baldrich E, Lepoittevin J-P, Camarasa JG. Principles and methodology for identification of fragrance allergens in consumer products. Contact Dermatitis 2002;47:345-352

79   Hamann D, Kishi P, Hamann CR. Consumer hair dye kits frequently contain isothiazolinones, other common preservatives and fragrance allergens. Dermatitis 2018;29:48-49

80   Diepgen TL, Ofenloch R, Bruze M, Cazzaniga S, Coenraads PJ, Elsner P, et al. Prevalence of fragrance contact allergy in the general population of five European countries: a cross-sectional study. Br J Dermatol 2015;173:1411-1419

81   Klaschka U. Contact allergens for armpits - allergenic fragrances specified on deodorants. Int J Hyg Environ Health 2012;215:584-591

82   Schwensen JF, Johansen JD, Veien NK, Funding AT, Avnstorp C, Østerballe M, et al. Occupational contact dermatitis in hairdressers: an analysis of patch test data from the Danish Contact Dermatitis Group, 2002–2011. Contact Dermatitis 2014;70:233-237

83   Heydorn S, Menné T, Andersen KE, Bruze M, Svedman C, Basketter D, Johansen JD. The fragrance hand immersion study – an experimental model simulating real-life exposure for allergic contact dermatitis on the hands. Contact Dermatitis 2003;48:324-330

84   Jacob SE. Allergic contact dermatitis from Lyral in an aerosol deodorant. Dermatitis 2008;19:216-217

85   Hamann D, Hamann CR, Zimerson E, Bruze M. Hydroxyisohexyl 3-cyclohexene carboxaldehyde (Lyral) in patch test preparations under varied storage conditions. Dermatitis 2013;24:246-248

86   Engfeldt M, Hagvall L, Isaksson M, Matura M, Mowitz M, Ryberg K, et al. Patch testing with hydroxyisohexyl 3-cyclohexene carboxaldehyde (HICC) – a multicentre study of the Swedish Contact Dermatitis Research Group. Contact Dermatitis 2017;76:34-39

87   Isaksson M, Inerot A, Lidén C, Lindberg M, Matura M, Möller H, et al. Multicentre patch testing with fragrance mix II and hydroxyisohexyl 3-cyclohexene carboxaldehyde by the Swedish Contact Dermatitis Research Group. Contact Dermatitis 2014;70:187-189

88   Nardelli A, Carbonez A, Drieghe J, Goossens A. Results of patch testing with fragrance mix 1, fragrance mix 2, and their ingredients, and Myroxylon pereirae and colophonium, over a 21-year period. Contact Dermatitis 2013;68:307-313

89   Krautheim A, Uter W, Frosch P, Schnuch A, Geier J. Patch testing with fragrance mix II: results of the IVDK 2005–2008. Contact Dermatitis 2010;63:262-269

90   Carvalho R, Maio P, Amaro C, Santos R, Cardoso J. Hydroxyisohexyl 3-cyclohexene carboxaldehyde (Lyral(R)) as allergen: experience from a contact dermatitis unit. Cutan Ocul Toxicol 2011;30:249-250

91   Uter W, Geier J, Schnuch A, Gefeller O. Risk factors associated with sensitization to hydroxyisohexyl 3-cyclohexene carboxaldehyde. Contact Dermatitis 2013;69:72-77

92   Api AM, Vey M. A new IFRA Standard on the fragrance ingredient, hydroxyisohexyl 3-cyclohexene carboxalde-hyde. Contact Dermatitis 2010;62:254-255

93   Militello G, James W, Mowad CM. Lyral: a fragrance allergen. Dermatitis 2005;16:41-44

94   Basketter DA, Pons-Guiraud A, Van Asten A, Laverdet C, Marty J-P, Martin L, et al. Fragrance allergy: assessing the safety of washed fabrics. Contact Dermatitis 2010;62:349-354

95   Schnuch A, Uter W, Dickel H, Szliska C, Schliemann S, Eben R, et al. Quantitative patch and repeated open application testing in hydroxyisohexyl 3-cyclohexene carboxaldehyde sensitive-patients. Contact Dermatitis 2009;61:152-162

96   De Groot AC, Schmidt E. Essential oils: contact allergy and chemical composition. Boca Raton, Fl., USA: CRC Press, Taylor and Francis Group, 2016 (ISBN 9781482246407)

97   Assier H, Tetart F, Avenel-Audran M, Barbaud A, Ferrier-le Bouëdec MC, Giordano-Labadie F, et al. Is a specific eyelid patch test series useful? Results of a French prospective study. Contact Dermatitis 2018;79:157-161

98   Wieck S, Olsson O, Kümmerer K, Klaschka U. Fragrance allergens in household detergents. Regul Toxicol Pharmacol 2018;97:163-169

99   Directorate-General for Internal Market, Industry, Entrepreneurship and SMEs (European Commission). Commission Regulation (EU) 2017/1410 of 2 August 2017 amending Annexes II and III to Regulation (EC) No 1223/2009 of the European Parliament and of the Council on cosmetic products. Official J European Union 2017;L202:1-3

100 Ung CY, White JML, White IR, Banerjee P, McFadden JP. Patch testing with the European baseline series fragrance markers: a 2016 update. Br J Dermatol 2018;178:776-780

101 Nagtegaal MJC, Pentinga SE, Kuik J, Kezic S, Rustemeyer T. The role of the skin irritation response in polysensitization to fragrances. Contact Dermatitis 2012;67:28-35

102 Heisterberg MV, Andersen KE, Avnstorp C, Kristensen B, Kristensen O, Kaaber K, et al. Fragrance mix II in the baseline series contributes significantly to detection of fragrance allergy. Contact Dermatitis 2010;63:270-276

103 Schubert S, Bauer A, Molin S, Skudlik C, Geier J. Occupational contact sensitization in female geriatric nurses: Data of the Information Network of Departments of Dermatology (IVDK) 2005-2014. J Eur Acad Dermatol Venereol 2017;31:469-476

104 Geier J, Lessmann H, Uter W, Schnuch A. Experiences with the fragrance mix II – the German perspective. Contact Dermatitis 2006;55(suppl.1):12 (Abstract)

105 Claßen A, Buhl T, Schubert S, Worm M, Bauer A, Geier J, Molin S; Information Network of Departments of Dermatology (IVDK) study group. The frequency of specific contact allergies is reduced in patients with psoriasis. Br J Dermatol. 2018 Aug 12. doi: 10.1111/bjd.17080. [Epub ahead of print]

106 Girbig M, Hegewald J, Seidler A, Bauer A, Uter W, Schmitt J. Type IV sensitizations in physical therapists: patch test results of the Information Network of Departments of Dermatology (IVDK) 2007-2011. J Dtsch Dermatol Ges 2013;11:1185-1192

107 120 Dittmar D, Schuttelaar MLA. Contact sensitization to hydroperoxides of limonene and linalool: Results of consecutive patch testing and clinical relevance. Contact Dermatitis 2018 Oct 31. doi: 10.1111/cod.13137. [Epub ahead of print]

108 Silvestre JF, Mercader P, González-Pérez R, Hervella-Garcés M, Sanz-Sánchez T, Córdoba S, et al. Sensitization to fragrances in Spain: A 5-year multicentre study (2011-2015). Contact Dermatitis. 2018 Nov 14. doi: 10.1111/cod.13152. [Epub ahead of print]

Chapter 3.85   IONONE

IDENTIFICATION

Description/definition	: Ionone is the organic compound that conforms to the structural formulas shown below; it has an α- and a β-isomer; mixed isomers are either α- or β-ionone or a mixture
Chemical class(es)	: Ketones
INCI name USA	: Ionone; mixed ionones
Other names	: Cyclocitrylidenacetone, α- and β-isomers; irisone (alpha-)
RIFM monograph(s)	: Food Chem Toxicol 2007;45(suppl.1):S251-S257; Food Cosmet Toxicol 1975;13:549
Merck Index monograph	: 6369
Function(s) in cosmetics	: EU: adstringent; perfuming. USA: fragrance ingredients
Patch testing	: alpha- and beta-ionone 5% pet. (5); 10% pet., mixed isomers (1); based on RIFM data, alpha-ionone 8% pet. and mixed isomers 20% pet. are probably not irritant (6)
Molecular formula	: $C_{13}H_{20}O$

alpha-Ionone

Chemical/IUPAC name	: (E)-4-(2,6,6-Trimethyl-2-cyclohexen-1-yl)but-3-en-2-one
CAS registry number(s)	: 127-41-3
EC number(s)	: 204-841-6
RIFM monograph(s)	: Food Chem Toxicol 2016;97(suppl.):S1-S10; Food Chem Toxicol 2007;45(suppl.1):S235-S240
SCCS opinion(s)	: SCCNFP/0389/00, final (8)

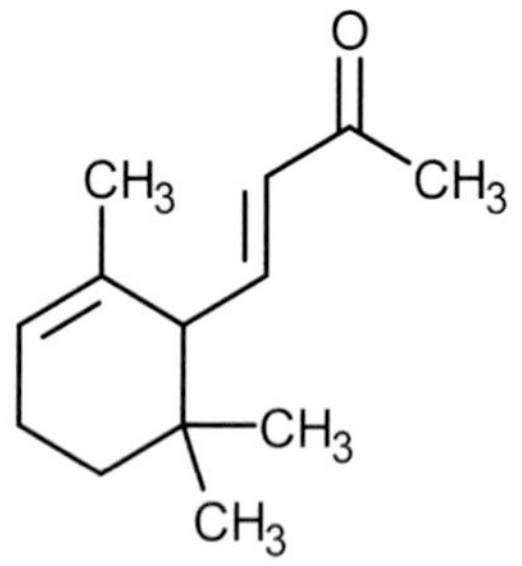

beta-Ionone

Chemical/IUPAC name	: (E)-4-(2,6,6-Trimethyl-1-cyclohexen-1-yl)but-3-en-2-one
CAS registry number(s)	: 8013-90-9; 79-77-6 (trans-β-)
EC number(s)	: 232-396-8; 201-224-3 (trans-β-)
RIFM monograph(s)	: Food Chem Toxicol 2007;45(suppl.1):S241-S247 and S248-S250 (trans-β-)
SCCS opinion(s)	: SCCNFP/0389/00, final (8)

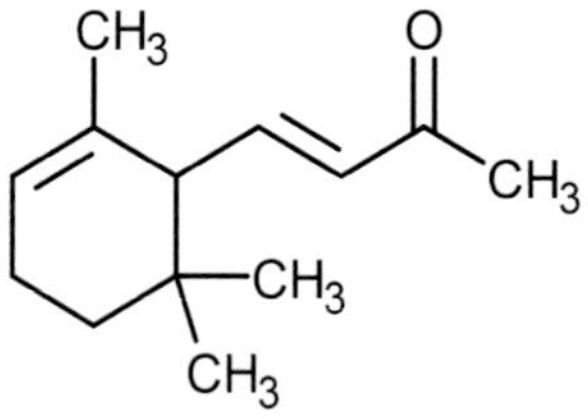

β-ionone 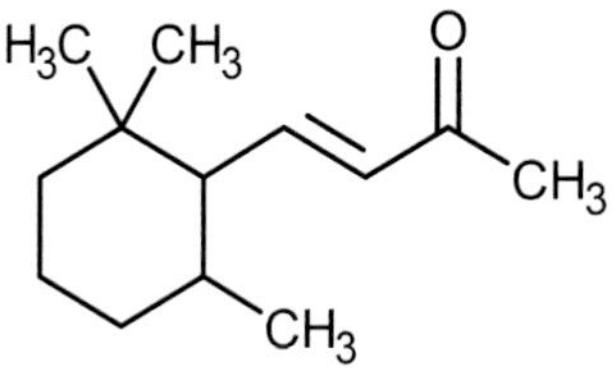   trans-β-ionone

GENERAL

Ionone is a pale yellow clear liquid; its odor type is floral and its odor at 10% in dipropylene glycol is described as 'violet sweet floral woody' (www.thegoodscentscompany.com). alpha-Ionone occurs naturally in plants including violets, blackberries and plums. It is also found in tobacco and tobacco smoke. alpha-Ionone is used as a fragrance in perfumes, cosmetics and personal care products, as well as in household cleaners and detergents. In addition, alpha-ionone is used as a food flavoring in beverages, ice cream, baked goods and candies. The chemical is present in bitter orange extract which is used widely in dietary supplements. alpha-Ionone is also used as an ingredient in cat and dog repellant applied on lawns, plants and outdoor furniture; conversely, it may be applied on roses to attract beetles (U.S. National Library of Medicine).

beta-Ionone is very widespread in nature and occurs in a wide variety of plants and plant oils. It is used to make vitamins A, E and K1, as a fragrance in perfumes, cosmetics and personal care products, and household cleaners and detergents and as a food flavoring in beverages, ice cream, baked goods and candies (U.S. National Library of Medicine).

See also Chapter 3.112 Methyl ionones.

Presence in essential oils

Ionone has been identified by chemical analysis in 12 (α-) and 21 (β-) of 91 essential oils, which have caused contact allergy / allergic contact dermatitis. In none of these oils, it belonged to the 'Top-10' of ingredients with the highest concentrations (7).

CONTACT ALLERGY

Patch testing in groups of patients

Patch testing in consecutive patients suspected of contact dermatitis: routine testing

In Germany, before 1995, alpha- and beta-ionone 5% and 1% in petrolatum were patch tested in 205 consecutive patients suspected of contact dermatitis. There was one reaction (0.5%) to alpha-ionone 5% and two (1.0%) to beta-ionone 5% pet., whereas no reactions were observed to the 1% test substances. The 'positive' reactions were either weakly positive (?+) or irritant (this was not specified). No mention was made of their relevance (5).

Patch testing in groups of selected patients

In 1984, in The Netherlands, 179 patients suspected of cosmetic allergy were patch tested with a test substance containing 10% ionone mixed isomers plus 10% γ-methylionone (alpha-isomethyl ionone) and there were two (1.1%) positive reactions. Their relevance was not mentioned (1).

Case reports and case series

Contact allergy to ionone and benzyl alcohol was described in an early German publication (4). One individual reacted to ionone and to benzyl alcohol, probably (as regards benzyl alcohol) from previous sensitization to Myroxylon pereirae resin. The patient had been in contact with flavoring agents for drinks. No data on the allergy to ionone are available.

Pigmented cosmetic dermatitis

While searching for causative ingredients of pigmented cosmetic dermatitis in Japan in the 1970s, both patients with ordinary (nonpigmented) cosmetic dermatitis and women with pigmented cosmetic dermatitis were tested with a large number of fragrance materials. In 1980 the accumulated data enabled the classification of fragrant materials into 4 groups: common sensitizers, rare sensitizers, virtually non-sensitizing fragrances and fragrances considered as non-sensitizers. alpha- and beta-Ionone were classified in the group of rare sensitizers, indicating that one or more cases of contact allergy / allergic contact dermatitis to them have been observed (3). More specific data are lacking, the results have largely or solely been published in Japanese journals only.

Presence in products and chemical analyses

In 2000, fifty-nine domestic and occupational products, purchased in retail outlets in Denmark, England, Germany and Italy were analyzed by GC-MS for the presence of fragrances. The product categories were liquid soap and soap bars (n=13), soft/hard surface cleaners (n=23), fabric conditioners/laundry detergents for hand wash (n=8), dish wash (n=10), furniture polish, car shampoo, stain remover (each n=1) and 2 products used in occupational environments. alpha- or beta-Ionone was present in 5 products (8%); quantification was not performed (2).

Cross-reactions, pseudo-cross-reactions and co-reactions

For general information on cross-/pseudo-cross-/co-reactivity of fragrance chemicals with other fragrances, fragrance markers (fragrance mix I, fragrance mix II, colophonium, Myroxylon pereirae resin [balsam of Peru]) and essential oils see Chapter 1.2 General information on cross-reactions, pseudo-cross-reactions and co-reactions.

A patient allergic to alpha-isomethylionone in 'methylionantheme' present in a cologne (Chapter 3.112) co-reacted to ionone (9).

LITERATURE

1   De Groot AC, Liem DH, Nater JP, van Ketel WG. Patch tests with fragrance materials and preservatives. Contact Dermatitis 1985;12:87-92

2   Rastogi SC, Heydorn S, Johansen JD, Basketter DA. Fragrance chemicals in domestic and occupational products. Contact Dermatitis 2001;45:221-225

3   Nakayama H. Fragrance hypersensitivity and its control. In: Frosch PJ, Johansen JD, White IR, Eds. Fragrances - beneficial and adverse effects. Berlin Heidelberg New York: Springer-Verlag, 1998:83-91

4   Schultheiss E. Überempfindlichkeit gegenüber Ionon und Benzylalkohol. Derm Monatsschr 1957;135:629. Data cited in: Shmunes E. Allergic dermatitis to benzyl alcohol in an injectable solution. Arch Dermatol1984;120:1200-1201

5   Frosch PJ, Pilz B, Andersen KE, Burrows D, Camarasa JG, Dooms-Goossens A, et al. Patch testing with fragrances: results of a multicenter study of the European Environmental and Contact Dermatitis Research Group with 48 frequently used constituents of perfumes. Contact Dermatitis 1995;33:333-342

6   De Groot AC. Patch Testing, 4th Edition. Wapserveen, The Netherlands: acdegroot publishing, 2018 (ISBN 978-90-813233-4-5)

7   De Groot AC, Schmidt E. Essential oils: contact allergy and chemical composition. Boca Raton, Fl., USA: CRC Press, Taylor and Francis Group, 2016 (ISBN 9781482246407)

8   Opinion of the Scientific Committee on Cosmetic Products and Non-Food Products Intended for Consumers concerning 'The 1st update of the inventory of ingredients employed in cosmetic products. Section II: Perfume and aromatic raw materials', 24 October 2000, SCCNFP/0389/00, final. Available at: http://ec.europa.eu/health/ph_risk/committees/sccp/documents/out131_en.pdf

9   Bernaola G, Escayol P, Fernandez E, Fernandez de Corrés L. Contact dermatitis from methylionone fragrance. Contact Dermatitis 1989;20:71-72

Chapter 3.86   ISOAMYL SALICYLATE

IDENTIFICATION

Description/definition   : Isoamyl salicylate is the amyl ester of salicylic acid that conform to the structural formula shown below

Chemical class(es)   : Aromatic compounds; esters; phenols

INCI name USA   : Not in the Personal Care Products Council Ingredient Database

Chemical/IUPAC name   : 3-Methylbutyl 2-hydroxybenzoate

Other names   : Isopentyl 2-hydroxybenzoate

CAS registry number(s)   : 87-20-7

EC number(s)   : 201-730-4

RIFM monograph(s)   : Food Chem Toxicol 2015;84(suppl.):S110-S121; Food Chem Toxicol 2007;45(suppl.1):S418-S423; Food Chem Toxicol 2007;45:S318-S361; Food Cosmet Toxicol 1973;11:859 (binder, page 87)

SCCS opinion(s)   : SCCS/1459/11 (1)

Merck Index monograph   : 6440

Function(s) in cosmetics   : EU: perfuming

Patch testing   : 5% pet. (7); 50% pet. (not irritant) (2); based on data from RIFM, 20% pet. is probably not irritant (6)

Molecular formula   : $C_{12}H_{16}O_3$

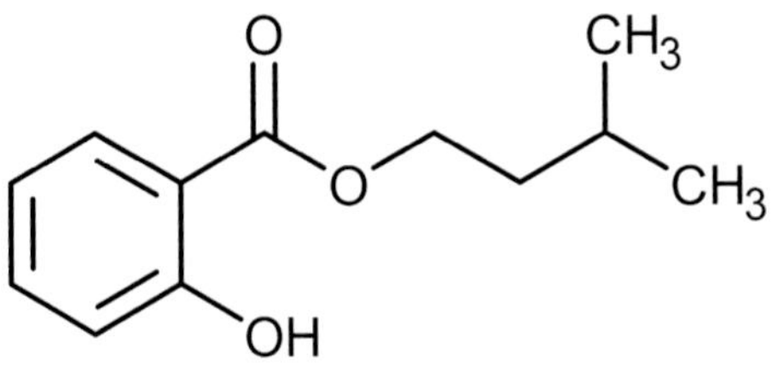

GENERAL

Isoamyl salicylate is a colorless clear oily liquid; its odor type is floral and its odor at 100% is described as 'floral herbal woody orchid metallic' (www.thegoodscentscompany.com).

Presence in essential oils

Isoamyl salicylate has been identified by chemical analysis in none of 91 essential oils, which have caused contact allergy / allergic contact dermatitis (8).

CONTACT ALLERGY

General

The SCCS (Scientific Committee on Consumer Safety), in a 2012 Opinion on Fragrance allergens in cosmetic products, has categorized isoamyl salicylate as 'likely fragrance contact allergen by combination of evidence' (1,5).

Patch testing in groups of patients

Patch testing in consecutive patients suspected of contact dermatitis: routine testing

In an early study from in Japan, 216 dermatitis patients where patch tested with 0.2% isoamyl salicylate in 99.9% ethanol or in a non-irritative cream base, applied for 24-48 hours to the upper inside arm; there were 8 (3.7%) positive reactions. More detailed information is not available (6).

Testing in groups of selected patients

In 1984, in The Netherlands, 179 patients suspected of cosmetic allergy were tested with isoamyl salicylate 50% in petrolatum and there was one (0.6%) positive reaction. Its relevance was not mentioned, but a false-positive reaction due to the excited skin syndrome could not be excluded (2).

Case reports and case series

Case reports of allergic contact dermatitis from isoamyl salicylate have not been found.

Presence in products and chemical analyses

In 2000, fifty-nine domestic and occupational products, purchased in retail outlets in Denmark, England, Germany and Italy were analyzed by GC-MS for the presence of fragrances. The product categories were liquid soap and soap bars (n=13), soft/hard surface cleaners (n=23), fabric conditioners/laundry detergents for hand wash (n=8), dish wash (n=10), furniture polish, car shampoo, stain remover (each n=1) and 2 products used in occupational environments. Isoamyl salicylate was present in 20 products (34%) with a mean concentration of 194 ppm and a range of 29-1157 ppm (3).

In 1997, 71 deodorants (22 vapo-spray, 22 aerosol spray and 27 roll-on products) were collected in Denmark, England, France, Germany and Sweden and analyzed by gas chromatography – mass spectrometry (GC-MS) for the presence of fragrances and other materials. Amyl / isoamyl salicylate was present in 21 (30%) of the products (4).

LITERATURE

1   SCCS (Scientific Committee on Consumer Safety). Opinion on Fragrance allergens in cosmetic products, 26-27 June 2012, SCCS/1459/11. Available at:
    https://ec.europa.eu/health/sites/health/files/scientific_committees/consumer_safety/docs/sccs_o_102.pdf
2   De Groot AC, Liem DH, Nater JP, van Ketel WG. Patch tests with fragrance materials and preservatives. Contact Dermatitis 1985;12:87-92
3   Rastogi SC, Heydorn S, Johansen JD, Basketter DA. Fragrance chemicals in domestic and occupational products. Contact Dermatitis 2001;45:221-225
4   Rastogi SC, Lepoittevin J-P, Johansen JD, Frosch PJ, Menné T, Bruze M, et al. Fragrances and other materials in deodorants: search for potentially sensitizing molecules using combined GC-MS and structure activity relationship (SAR) analysis. Contact Dermatitis 1998;39:293-303
5   Uter W, Johansen JD, Börje A, Karlberg A-T, Lidén C, Rastogi S, Roberts D, White IR. Categorization of fragrance contact allergens for prioritization of preventive measures: clinical and experimental data and consideration of structure–activity relationships. Contact Dermatitis 2013;69:196-230
6   Fujii T, Furukawa S, Suzuki S. Studies on compounded perfumes for toilet goods. On the non-irritative compounded perfumes for soaps. Yukugaku 1972;21:904-908 (article in Japanese). Data cited in: Lapczynski A, Jones L, McGinty D, Bhatia S, Letizia CS, Api AM. Fragrance material review on isoamyl salicylate. Food Chem Toxicol 2007;45(suppl.1):S418-S423
7   Frosch PJ, Pilz B, Andersen KE, Burrows D, Camarasa JG, Dooms-Goossens A, et al. Patch testing with fragrances: results of a multicenter study of the European Environmental and Contact Dermatitis Research Group with 48 frequently used constituents of perfumes. Contact Dermatitis 1995;33:333-342
8   De Groot AC, Schmidt E. Essential oils: contact allergy and chemical composition. Boca Raton, Fl., USA: CRC Press, Taylor and Francis Group, 2016 (ISBN 9781482246407)

Chapter 3.87   ISOEUGENOL

IDENTIFICATION

Description/definition	: Isoeugenol is the substituted phenol that conforms to the structural formula shown below
Chemical class(es)	: Ethers; phenols
Chemical/IUPAC name	: 2-Methoxy-4-(prop-1-enyl)phenol
CAS registry number(s)	: 97-54-1
EC number(s)	: 202-590-7
RIFM monograph(s)	: Food Chem Toxicol 2016;97(suppl.):S49-S56; Food Cosmet Toxicol 1975;13:815 (special issue II)
IFRA standard	: Restricted (www.ifraorg.org/en-us/standards-library) (table 3.87.1)
SCCS opinion(s)	: Various (9); SCCS/1459/11 (10); SCCNFP/0389/00, final (83); SCCNFP/0392/00, final (84)
Merck Index monograph	: 6486
Function(s) in cosmetics	: EU: flavouring; perfuming. USA: flavoring agents; fragrance ingredients
EU cosmetic restrictions	: Regulated in Annex III/73 of the Regulation (EC) No. 1223/2009, regulated by 2003/15/EC; Must be labeled on cosmetics and detergent products, if present at > 10 ppm (0.001%) in leave-on products and > 100 ppm (0.01%) in rinse-off products
Patch testing	: 1% Pet. (SmartPracticeEurope, SmartPracticeCanada); 2% pet. (Chemotechnique); also present in the fragrance mix I; TEST ADVICE: 2% pet.; some positive reactions to isoeugenol may be missed when the patient is not seen at D7 (13)
Molecular formula	: $C_{10}H_{12}O_2$

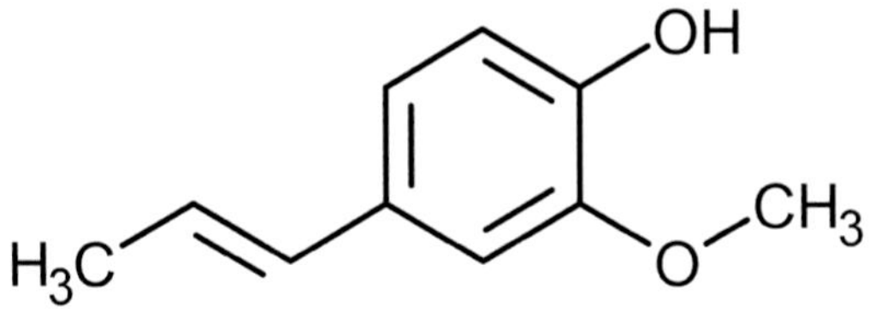

Table 3.87.1 IFRA restrictions for isoeugenol

Category [a]	Limits [b]	Category [a]	Limits [b]	Category [a]	Limits [b]
1	0.01%	5	0.02%	9	0.02%
2	0.01%	6	0.20%	10	0.02%
3	0.02%	7	0.02%	11	not restricted
4	0.02%	8	0.02%		

[a] For explanation of categories see pages 6-8
[b] Limits in the finished products

GENERAL

Isoeugenol is a colorless to yellow clear liquid; its odor type is spicy and its odor is described as 'sweet spicy, clove-like odor with a woody nuance' (www.thegoodscentscompany.com). Isoeugenol is used in perfumery in a large number of blossom compositions, mostly for clove and carnation types, but also in oriental perfumes. Small amounts are employed in aromas for foods and beverages and in reconstituted essential oils. Isoeugenol is used as a fragrance in household laundry and cleaning products including, most notably, laundry powders, laundry liquids, dish-washing liquids, hard surface cleaning products and toilet cleaning products. Other applications include or have included the manufacture of vanillin and as a fish anesthetic/sedative (U.S. National Library of Medicine).

Isoeugenol is one of the eight constituents of the fragrance mix I (Chapter 3.70 Fragrance mix I).

Presence in essential oils and Myroxylon pereirae resin (balsam of Peru)

Isoeugenol (any isomer) has been identified by chemical analysis in 24 of 91 essential oils, which have caused contact allergy / allergic contact dermatitis. In none of these oils, it belonged to the 'Top-10' of ingredients with the highest concentrations (80). Isoeugenol may also be present in Myroxylon pereirae resin (balsam of Peru) (0.85% in fraction BP3) (5).

CONTACT ALLERGY

General

The SCCS (Scientific Committee on Consumer Safety), in a 2012 Opinion on Fragrance allergens in cosmetic products, has marked isoeugenol as 'established contact allergen in humans' (10,52). The sensitizing potency of isoeugenol was classified as 'strong' based on an EC3 value of 0.54% in the LLNA (local lymph node assay) in animal experiments (10,47,52). The compound acts as a prohapten, which is a chemical that is itself non-sensitizing or low-sensitizing, but that is transformed into a hapten in the skin (bioactivation), usually via enzymatic catalysis (73).

Isoeugenol is a constituent of the fragrance mix I. In groups of patients reacting to the mix and tested with its 8 ingredients, isoeugenol scored 14.8-45.2% positive patch test reactions, median 19.6% and average 21.2%. It has rank number 2 in the list of most frequent reactors in the mix (Chapter 3.70 Fragrance mix I).

General population

In the period 2008-2011, in 5 European countries (Sweden, Germany, Netherlands, Portugal, Italy), a random sample of the general population of 3119 individuals aged 18-74 years were patch tested with the FM I, its 8 ingredients, the FM II, its 6 ingredients and Myroxylon pereirae resin. There were 21 reactions (0.7%) to isoeugenol, tested 2% in petrolatum. About half of all positive reactions to fragrances were considered to be relevant based on standardized criteria. Women were affected twice as often as men (68).

Patch testing in groups of patients

Results of studies testing isoeugenol in consecutive patients suspected of contact dermatitis (routine testing) are shown in table 3.87.2. Results of testing in groups of *selected* patients (e.g. patients with known or suspected fragrance or cosmetic dermatitis, individuals with eyelid dermatitis, nurses with occupational dermatitis) are shown in table 3.87.3.

Patch testing in consecutive patients suspected of contact dermatitis: routine testing

In sixteen studies in which routine testing with isoeugenol was performed, frequencies of sensitization have ranged from 1.0% to 4.5% (table 3.87.2). Test concentrations used were mostly 1% pet., more recently more often 2% pet. and in one older study 5%. An influence of the concentration on the frequency of sensitization is not readily apparent.

Table 3.87.2 Patch testing in groups of patients: Routine testing

Years and Country	Test conc. & vehicle	Number of patients tested	positive (%)	Selection of patients (S); Relevance (R); Comments (C)	Ref.
2015-7 Netherlands		821	21 (2.6%)	R: not stated	89
2015-2016 UK	2% pet.	2084	31 (1.5%)	R: not specified for individual fragrances; 25% of patients who reacted to any fragrance or fragrance marker had a positive fragrance intolerance history	86
2010-2015 Denmark	1% pet.	6004	(1.1%)	R: present relevance 39%, past relevance 31%	46
2009-2015 Sweden	2% pet.	4430	43 (1.0%)	R: not stated	53
2013-2014 Thailand		312	7 (2.2%)	R: 71%	49
2011-2012 UK	2% pet.	1951	40 (2.1%)	R: not stated	51
2010-2011 China	2% pet.	296	(3.4%)	R: 67% for all fragrances tested together (excluding FM I)	50
2008-2010 Denmark	1% pet.	1502	16 (1.1%)	S: mostly routine testing; R: 71%; 79% co-reactivity of FM I, 14% of FM II; C: of the relevant reactions to any of the 26 fragrances tested, 96% were caused by cosmetic products	1
2005-2008 IVDK	1% pet.	1214	(1.6%)	R: not stated	56
2001-2005 UK	1% pet.	3636	97 (2.7%)	R: not stated; C: increasing frequency in the study period	74
2003-2004 IVDK	1% pet.	2063	26 (1.3%)	R: not stated; C: 83% co-reactivity of FM I	3
2001-2 UK, Denmark, Belgium, Sweden	1% pet.	2261	40 (1.8%)	R: not stated; there were also 40 reactions to *trans-* (E)-isoeugenol (CAS 5932-68-3); in 36 of these cases (90%), there was a co-reaction to isoeugenol	75
1998 UK	1% pet.	155	7 (4.5%)	R: not stated; there were 5 (71%) co-reactions to isoeugenyl acetate	71
<1995 9 European countries + USA	1% pet.	1072	20 (1.9%)	R: not stated	30
1993 EECDRG	1% pet.	709	23 (3.3%)	R: not stated	62
1991 The Netherlands	5% pet.	677	15 (2.2%)	R: not stated	63

EECDRG: European Environmental and Contact Dermatitis Research Group; FM: Fragrance mix; IVDK: Informationsverbund Dermatologischer Kliniken (Germany, Switzerland, Austria)

In thirteen of the 16 investigations, no or no specific data on relevance were provided. In the studies that did address the issue, 71% (49), 71% (1) and 39% (present) resp. 31% (past) (46) of the reactions were considered to be relevant. In one study, of the relevant reactions to any of the 26 fragrances tested, 96% were caused by cosmetic products (1).

In two investigations in which patients allergic to Myroxylon pereirae (balsam of Peru) were patch tested with isoeugenol, high frequencies of positive reactions of 27.5% (5) and 61.6% (79) have been observed, although isoeugenol is not an important ingredient of the balsam. It has been suggested (79) that this is related to primary sensitization to possibly the most important allergen in balsam of Peru, coniferyl benzoate. The chemical structures of both chemicals have obvious similarities.

Results of testing isoeugenol in groups of patients reacting to the fragrance mix I are shown in Chapter 3.70 Fragrance mix I.

Table 3.87.3 Patch testing in groups of patients: Selected patient groups

Years and Country	Test conc. & vehicle	Number of patients tested | positive (%)		Selection of patients (S); Relevance (R); Comments (C)	Ref.
2011-2015 Spain	1% or 2% pet.	1013	138 (13.6%)	S: patients previously reacting to FM I, FM II, Myroxylon pereirae resin or hydroxyisohexyl 3-cyclohexene carboxaldehyde in the baseline series; R: not stated; C: the 2% test substances showed a higher rate of positive reactions than the 1% material	90
2003-2012 IVDK		621	32 (5.2%)	S: nurses with occupational contact dermatitis; R: not stated	45
2007-2011 IVDK	1% pet.	67	4 (6.0%)	S: physical therapists; R: not stated	88
2006-2010 USA	2% pet.	100	3 (3%)	S: patients with eyelid dermatitis; R: not stated	8
2005-10 Netherlands		100	12 (12%)	S: patients with known fragrance sensitivity based on a positive patch test to the FM I and/or the FM II; R: not stated	54
2000-2010 IVDK		1395	79 (2.3%)	S: patients with periorbital dermatitis; R: not stated; C: the frequency was lower than in a control group of routine testing	44
2004-2008 Spain	2% pet.	86	11 (13%)	S: patients previously reacting to the fragrance mix I or Myroxylon pereirae resin (n=54) or suspected of fragrance contact allergy (n=32); R: not stated	32
2005-7 Netherlands	2% pet.	320	4 (1.3%)	S: patients suspected of fragrance or cosmetic allergy; R: 61% relevance for all positive tested fragrances together	2
<2003 Israel		91	5 (5%)	S: patients with a positive or doubtful reaction to the fragrance mix and/or Myroxylon pereirae resin and/or to one or two commercial fine fragrances; R: not stated	31
1998-2002 IVDK	1% pet.	33	4 (12%)	S: patients who had a positive reaction to their own deodorant; R: not stated	35
1982-2001 UK		22	2 (9%)	S: patients with allergic contact cheilitis; R: the patients were selected on the basis of relevant positive reactions	66
1997-2000 Austria	1% pet.	747	40 (5.4%)	S: patients suspected of fragrance allergy; R: not stated	6
<1986 France	2.5% pet.	21	7 (33%)	S: patients with dermatitis caused by perfumes; R: not stated	82
<1985 Netherlands		242	36 (14.9%)	S: randomly selected patients with proven contact allergy of different origins; R: not stated	65
<1982 UK		50	6 (12%)	S: patients with photosensitivity dermatitis with actinic reticuloid syndrome (PD/AR); R: not specified for individual fragrances, but the authors concluded that in some subjects with PD/AR and persistent light reaction, a significant factor in the latter is likely to be exposure to substances such as fragrance materials; C: in a control group of 457 dermatitis patients, only 1.8% reacted positively to isoeugenol	42
1975 USA	2% pet.	20	5 (25%)	S: fragrance-allergic patients; R: not stated	11

Testing in groups of patients reacting to Myroxylon pereirae resin (balsam of Peru)

1995-1998 Germany	2% pet.	102	28 (27.5%)	S: patients allergic to balsam of Peru	5
1955-1960 Denmark	5% pet., later 2% pet.	133	82 (61.6%)	S: patients allergic to balsam of Peru	79

Testing in groups of patients reacting to the fragrance mix I

Results of testing isoeugenol in groups of patients reacting to the fragrance mix I are shown in Chapter 3.70 Fragrance mix I.

EECDRG: European Environmental and Contact Dermatitis Research Group. FM: Fragrance mix; IVDK: Informationsverbund Dermatologischer Kliniken (Germany, Switzerland, Austria)

Patch testing in groups of selected patients

Results of studies patch testing isoeugenol in groups of selected patients (e.g. patients with known or suspected fragrance or cosmetic dermatitis, individuals with eyelid dermatitis, nurses with occupational dermatitis) are shown in table 3.87.3. In 16 investigations, frequencies of sensitization to isoeugenol have ranged from 1.3% to 33%. Not unexpectedly, most high rates of positive reactions (12% [35,54], 13% [32], 13.6% [90], 25% [11] and 33% [82]) were observed in groups of patients with proven fragrance contact allergy, sometimes by positive reactions to the fragrance mix I, which contains isoeugenol as one of the most frequent allergenic ingredients. Relevance data were almost invariably lacking.

Case reports and case series

Case series

Isoeugenol was stated to be the (or an) allergen in 30 patients in a group of 603 individuals suffering from cosmetic dermatitis, seen in the period 2010-2015 in Leuven, Belgium (43).

In the period 1996-2013, in a tertiary referral center in Valencia, Spain, 5419 patients were patch tested. Of these, 628 individuals had allergic contact dermatitis to cosmetics. In this group, isoeugenol was the responsible allergen in 27 cases (27, overlap with ref. 28).

In the period 2000-2009, in Leuven, Belgium, an unspecified number of patients had positive patch tests or use tests to a total of 344 cosmetic products *and* positive patch tests to FM I, FM II, and/or to one or more of 28 selected specific fragrance ingredients. In two of 15 patients reacting to isoeugenol, the presence of this fragrance in the cosmetic product(s) was confirmed by reading the product label(s) (55).

In the period 2000-2007, 202 patients with allergic contact dermatitis caused by cosmetics were seen in Valencia, Spain. In this group, isoeugenol was the allergen in 4 individuals from its presence in gel/soap (n=2), cologne (n=1) and deodorant (n=1) (28, overlap with ref. 27).

In one center in Belgium, between 1985 and 1990, 3970 patients with dermatitis were patch tested. 462 of these reacted positively to patch tests with cosmetic allergens. The reactions were considered to be relevant in 68%, probably relevant in 25% and doubtfully relevant in 7% of the patients. In the list of 'most common allergens' isoeugenol had rank number 7 with 33 reactions. It should be appreciated that not all patients were patch tested with individual fragrances and that the presence of the allergen in cosmetic products causing dermatitis could not always be verified (at that time, ingredient labeling in the EU was not yet mandatory) (81).

In a group of 119 patients with allergic contact dermatitis from cosmetics, investigated in The Netherlands in 1986-1987, 2 cases were caused by isoeugenol in deodorant and perfume (24,25).

In Belgium, in the years before 1986, of 5202 consecutive patients with dermatitis patch tested, 156 were diagnosed with pure cosmetic allergy. Isoeugenol was the 'dermatitic ingredient' in 16 (10.3%) patients (frequency in the entire group: 1.0%). It should be realized, however, that only a very limited number of patients was tested with a fragrance series (64).

Isoeugenol was responsible for 10 out of 399 cases of cosmetic allergy where the causal allergen was identified in a study of the NACDG, USA, 1977-1983 (4).

Case reports

A woman had allergic contact dermatitis from isoeugenol and lanolin alcohol in eye cosmetics (26). A male patient developed allergic contact dermatitis from isoeugenol in his aftershave (76).

Cross-reactions, pseudo-cross-reactions and co-reactions

For general information on cross-/pseudo-cross-/co-reactivity of fragrance chemicals with other fragrances, fragrance markers (fragrance mix I, fragrance mix II, colophonium, Myroxylon pereirae resin [balsam of Peru]) and essential oils see Chapter 1.2 General information on cross-reactions, pseudo-cross-reactions and co-reactions.

Co-reactivity with the fragrance mix I can be expected, as the mix contains isoeugenol (pseudo-cross-reactions).

Eugenol

There is, according to some authors, limited cross-reactivity between isoeugenol and eugenol (29). Indeed, of 166 patients with positive reactions to eugenol, 41 (25%) were also allergic to isoeugenol. Conversely, of 219 patients with positive reactions to isoeugenol, 41 (19%) also reacted to eugenol, confirming 'limited' cross-reactivity (41). However, in an early study, a high degree of cross-reactivity between eugenol and isoeugenol was found (79). In the latter study, both eugenol and isoeugenol were tested at 5% pet.; whether this has influenced co-/cross-reactivity is unknown. Also, in a large study performed by the IVDK in the period 2005-2013, of 203 eugenol-positive patients, 137 (67%) also reacted to isoeugenol; conversely, of 523 individuals allergic to isoeugenol, 137 (26%) co-reacted to eugenol (67).

Isoeugenyl esters and ethers

In 40 patients allergic to isoeugenol, there were 36 (90%) co-reactions to *trans*-isoeugenol, 13 (33%) to isoeugenyl acetate, 3 (8%) to isoeugenyl benzoate, 15 (38%) to isoeugenyl phenyl acetate, and none to isoeugenyl methyl ether and isoeugenyl benzyl ether (75). Conversely, isoeugenol elicited concomitant positive reactions in 36/40 (90%) of those who reacted to *trans*-isoeugenol, 13/19 (68%) of those positive to isoeugenyl acetate, 3/4 (75%) of those positive to isoeugenyl benzoate and 15/16 (94%) of those who reacted to isoeugenyl phenylacetate; none of the 6 who reacted to isoeugenyl methyl ether or of the 2 reacting to isoeugenyl benzyl ether were positive to isoeugenol (75). Of 7 patients reacting to isoeugenol 1% pet., 5 (71%) co-reacted to isoeugenyl acetate 1.2% alc. (71).

Concomitant contact allergy to isoeugenol and its derivatives can occur either through multiple sensitization, direct chemical cross-reactivity or local skin metabolism to a common and/or cross-reactive derivative or derivatives. Isoeugenyl acetate and isoeugenyl benzoate are probably easily hydrolyzed in the skin to produce isoeugenol (75).

Myroxylon pereirae resin

Of 97 patients allergic to isoeugenol, 29 (30%) co-reacted to Myroxylon pereirae resin, which contains isoeugenol (74). In an early Danish study, in patients allergic to Myroxylon pereirae resin (MP) (balsam of Peru), reactions to isoeugenol occurred almost exclusively in those individuals who were also allergic to coniferyl benzoate. Isoeugenol therefore was regarded as a secondary allergen after primary sensitization with the coniferyl alcohol esters in the resin of MP (79).

Other co-reactions

In some studies, a significant association between positive reactions to the Fragrance mix I and to epoxy resin has been found (57,58). Supplementary testing with fragrance mix ingredients showed that the association was related to positive reactions to amyl cinnamal and isoeugenol (58). The clinical implications are not clarified, and the association, which was not found in several other studies, may have been coincidental.

Of 13 patients reacting to *p*-allylphenol 2% pet, 13 (87%) co-reacted to isoeugenol 2% in petrolatum (79).

Patch test sensitization

In 6 patients out of 230 with contact allergy to Myroxylon pereirae resin (balsam of Peru), there was a positive patch test to isoeugenol 5% pet. that developed 6 days or later after application. Whether these were simply 'delayed' reactions or indicative of patch test sensitization was not well investigated (79).

Presence in products and chemical analyses

In various studies, the presence of isoeugenol in cosmetic and sometimes other products has been investigated. Before 2006, most investigators used chemical analysis, usually GC-MS, for qualitative and quantitative determination. Since then, the presence of the target fragrances was usually investigated by screening the product labels for the 26 fragrances that must be labeled since 2005 on cosmetics and detergent products in the EU, if present at > 10 ppm (0.001%) in leave-on products and > 100 ppm (0.01%) in rinse-off products. This method, obviously, is less accurate and may result in underestimation of the frequency of the fragrances being present in the product. When they are in fact present, but the concentration is lower than mentioned above, labeling is not required and the fragrances' presence will be missed.

The results of the relevant studies for isoeugenol are summarized in table 3.87.4. More detailed information can be found in the corresponding text before and following the table. The percentage of products in which isoeugenol was found to be present shows wide variations, which can among other be explained by the selection procedure of the products, the method of investigation (false-negatives with information obtained from labels only) and changes in the use of individual fragrance materials over time (fashion). The use of isoeugenol appears to be decreasing in the last decade. Before that, it was most frequently used in fine fragrances.

In Denmark, in 2015-2016, 5588 fragranced cosmetic products were examined with a smartphone application for the 26 fragrances that need to be labeled in the EU. Isoeugenol was present in 2% of the products (rank number 18) (21).

In Germany, in 2015, fragrance allergens were evaluated based on lists of ingredients in 817 (unique) detergents (all-purpose cleaners, cleaning preparations for special purposes [e.g. bathroom, kitchen, dish-washing] and laundry detergents) present in 131 households. Isoeugenol was found to be present in 3 (0.4%) of the products (85).

Of 179 emollients available in online drugstores in 2014 in Poland, two (1.1%) contained isoeugenol, according to information available online (48).

In 2008, 2010 and 2011, 374 deodorants available in German retail shops were randomly selected and their labels checked for the presence of the 26 fragrances that need to be labeled. Isoeugenol was found to be present in 5 (1.3%) of the products (69).

Table 3.87.4 Presence of isoeugenol in products [a]

Year	Country	Product type	Nr. investigated	Nr. of products positive [b]	(%)	Method [c]	Ref.
2015-6	Denmark	Fragranced cosmetic products	5588		(2%)	Labeling	21
2015	Germany	Household detergents	817	3	(0.4%)	Labeling	85
2014	Poland	Emollients	179	2	(1%)	Online info	48
2008-11	Germany	Deodorants	374	5	(1%)	Labeling	69
2006-9	Germany	Cosmetic products	4991		(2%)	Labeling	20
2008	Sweden	Cosmetic products	204		(0.5%)	Labeling	12
		Detergents	97		(0%)	Labeling	
2006-7	Denmark	perfumes, aftershave lotions	29	16	(55%)	Analysis	70
2006	UK	Perfumed cosmetic and household products	300	27	(9%)	Labeling	19
2006	Denmark	Popular perfumed deodorants	88	8	(9%)	Labeling	23
			23	8	(35%)	Analysis	
2006	Netherlands	Laundry detergents	52	1	(2%)	Labeling + analysis	38
2006	Denmark	Rinse-off cosmetics for children	208	1	(0.5%)	Labeling + analysis	36
2006	Denmark	Perfume products	25	14	(56%)	Analysis	40
2002	Denmark	Home and car air fresheners	19	3	(16%)	Analysis	39
2001	Denmark	Women's fine fragrances	10	5	(50%)	Analysis	22
2001	Denmark	Non-cosmetic consumer products	43	3	(7%)	Analysis	37
2000	Denmark, UK, Germany, Italy	Domestic and occupational products	59	3	(5%)	Analysis	15
<2000	Sweden	Swedish cosmetic products	42	5	(12%)	Analysis	67
1997-8	Denmark, UK Germany, Sweden	Cosmetics and cosmetic toys for children	25	3	(12%)	Analysis	18
1996-7	Denmark	Deodorants that had caused allergic contact dermatitis	19	4	(21%)	Analysis	59
1996	Five European countries	Fragranced deodorants	70	20	(29%)	Analysis	14
1995-6	Denmark	Perfumes from lower-price range cosmetic products	17	2	(12%)	Analysis	60
1995	Denmark	Cosmetic products based on natural ingredients	42	3	(7%)	Analysis	16
1995	Denmark	The 10 most popular women's perfumes	10	7	(70%)	Analysis	17
1994	Denmark	Cosmetics that had given a positive patch or use test in FM I allergic patients	23	6	(23%)	Analysis	61

[a] See the corresponding text below for more details
[b] positive = containing the target fragrance
[c] Labeling: information from the ingredient labels on the product / packaging; Analysis: chemical analysis, most often GC-MS

In Germany, in the period 2006-2009, 4991 cosmetic products were randomly sampled for an official investigation of conformity of cosmetic products with legal provisions. The labels were inspected for the presence of the 26 fragrances that need to be labeled in the EU. Isoeugenol was present in 2% of the products (rank number 19) (20).

Isoeugenol was present (as indicated by labeling) in 0.5% of 204 cosmetic products (92 shampoos, 61 hair conditioners, 34 liquid soaps, 17 wet tissues) and in none of 97 detergents in Sweden, 2008 (12).

In Denmark, in 2006-2007, 29 hydroalcoholic products of international brands (2 aftershave lotions, 26 eaux de toilette/eaux de parfum [10 for men and 16 for women] and one parfum) were purchased from Danish retail outlets and investigated by GC-MS for the presence of isoeugenol, isoeugenyl acetate, methyl isoeugenol and benzyl isoeugenol. Isoeugenol was found to be present in 16 products (55%) in a concentration range of 26.6-202.8 ppm, mean of 70.5 ppm. Many of the products contained 2 or 3 of the fragrances (benzyl isoeugenol was not found in any sample) (70).

In 2006, of 88 popular perfume containing deodorants purchased in Denmark, 8 (9%) were labeled to contain isoeugenol. Analysis of 24 regulated fragrance substances in 23 selected deodorants (19 spray products, 2 deostick and 2 roll-on) was performed by GC-MS. Isoeugenol was identified in 8 of the products (35%) with a concentration range of 1–138 ppm (23).

In 2006, the labels of 208 cosmetics for children (especially shampoos, body shampoos and soaps) available in Denmark were checked for the presence of the 26 fragrances that need to be labeled in the EU. Isoeugenol was present in one product (0.5%), and ranked number 22 in the frequency list (36).

In January 2006, a study of perfumed cosmetic and household products available on the shelves of U.K. retailers was carried out. Products were included if 'parfum' or 'aroma' was listed among the ingredients. Three hundred products were surveyed and any of 26 mandatory labeling fragrances named on the label were recorded. Isoeugenol was present in 27 (9%) of the products (rank number 16) (19).

In 2006, in The Netherlands, 52 laundry detergents were investigated for the presence of allergenic fragrances by checking their labels and chemical analyses. Isoeugenol was found to be present in one of the products (2%) in a concentration 40 ppm. Isoeugenol had rank number 15 in the frequency list (38).

In Denmark, in 2006, 25 perfume products (13 eau de parfum, 8 eau de toilette, one parfum spray, one parfum, and 2 after-shave lotions) for both men and women were purchased from Danish retail outlets and investigated for the presence of isoeugenol, hydroxyisohexyl 3-cyclohexenecarboxaldehyde, atranol and chloroatranol. Isoeugenol was present in 14 products (56%) in a concentration range of 48-193 ppm (40).

In 2002, in Denmark, 19 air fresheners (6 for cars, 13 for homes) were analyzed for the presence of fragrances that need to be labeled on cosmetics. Isoeugenol was found to be present in 3 products (16%) in a concentration range of 23-120 ppm and ranked 18 in the frequency list (39).

In January 2001, in Denmark, ten women's fine fragrances were purchased; 5 of these had been launched years ago (1921–1990) and 5 were the latest launches by the same companies, introduced 2 months to 4 years before purchase. They were analyzed for the presence and quantity of the 7 well-identified fragrances present in the FM I (see Chapter 3.70 Fragrance mix I). The analysis revealed that the 5 old perfumes contained a mean of 5 of the 7 target allergens of the FM, while the new perfumes contained a mean of 2.8 of the allergens. The mean concentrations of the target allergens were 2.6 times higher in the old perfumes than in the new perfumes, range 2.2-337 ppm. Isoeugenol was present in 3 of the 5 old perfumes, in a concentration range of 0.0257-0.249% (m/m), mean 0.119%; in the new perfumes, it was identified in 2 of the 5 in a concentration range of 0.001-0.004% (m/m), mean 0.003% (22).

In 2001, in Denmark, 43 non-cosmetic consumer products (mainly dish-washing products, laundry detergents, and hard and soft surface cleaners) were analyzed for the 26 fragrances that are regulated for labeling in the EU. Isoeugenol was present in 3 products (7%) in a concentration range of 0.0048-0.0097% (m/m) and had rank number 17 in the frequency list (37).

In 2000, fifty-nine domestic and occupational products, purchased in retail outlets in Denmark, England, Germany and Italy were analyzed by GC-MS for the presence of fragrances. The product categories were liquid soap and soap bars (n=13), soft/hard surface cleaners (n=23), fabric conditioners/laundry detergents for hand wash (n=8), dish- wash (n=10), furniture polish, car shampoo, stain remover (each n=1) and 2 products used in occupational environments. Isoeugenol was present in 3 products (5%); quantification was not performed (15).

In Sweden, before 2000, 42 cosmetic products of a Swedish manufacturer were investigated for the presence of the ingredients of the FM I by chemical analysis. Isoeugenol was found to be present in 5 of the products (12%) in a concentration range of 3-30 ppm with a mean of 11 ppm. Data provided by the manufacturer on the qualitative and quantitative presence of the chemicals was quite different from chemical analyses for some of the fragrances (67).

Twenty-five cosmetics and cosmetic toys for children (5 shampoos and shower gels, 6 perfumes, 1 deodorant (roll-on), 4 baby lotions/creams, 1 baby wipes product, 1 baby oil, 2 lipcare products and 5 toy-cosmetic products: a cosmetic-toy set for blending perfumes and a makeup set) purchased in 1997-1998 in retail outlets in Denmark, Germany, England and Sweden were analyzed in 1998 for the presence of fragrances by GC-MS. Isoeugenol was found in 3 products (12%) in a concentration range of 0.019-0.074 % (w/w). For the analytical data in each product category, the original publication should be consulted (18).

In Denmark, in 1996-1997, nineteen deodorants that had caused axillary allergic contact dermatitis in 14 patients were analyzed for the presence of the 8 constituents of the FM I and isoeugenol was found to be present in 4 (21%) of the products in a concentration range of 0.0068-0.2183% (59).

Seventy fragranced deodorants, purchased at retail outlets in 5 European countries in 1996, were analyzed by gas chromatography - mass spectrometry (GC-MS) for the determination of the contents of 21 commonly used fragrance materials. Isoeugenol was identified in 20 products (29%) in a concentration range of 1–458 ppm (14).

In Denmark, in 1995-1996, nine perfumes from lower-price cosmetic wash-off products and 8 from stay-on products were analyzed for the presence of the ingredients of the FM I except oakmoss absolute. Isoeugenol was present in 2 of the 9 (22%) wash-off product perfumes in a concentration range of 0.1350-0.1702% w/v and in none of the 8 stay-on product perfumes (60).

In 1995, in Denmark, 42 cosmetic products based on natural ingredients from 12 European and US companies (of which 22 were perfumes and 20 various other cosmetics) were investigated by high-resolution gas chromatography-mass spectrometry (GC-MS) for the presence of 11 fragrances. Isoeugenol was present in 2 (9%) of the 22 perfumes in a concentration range of 0.027-0.139 w/w%; it was also identified in one of the other cosmetics (a body balm) in a concentration of 0.0127% (16).

In Denmark, in 1995, the 10 most popular women's perfumes were analyzed with gas chromatography-mass spectrometry for the presence of 7 ingredients of the Fragrance mix I (all except Evernia prunastri extract). Isoeugenol was identified in 7 of the perfumes (70%) with a mean concentration of 0.17% and in a concentration range of 0.05-0.34% (17).

In Denmark, in 1994, 23 cosmetic products, which had either given a positive patch and/or use test in a total of 11 fragrance-mix-positive patients, and which products completely or partly explained present or past episodes of dermatitis, were analyzed for the presence of the constituents of the Fragrance mix I (with the exception of oakmoss absolute) and a few other fragrances. Isoeugenol was found to be present in 6 of the 23 products (26%) in a concentration range of <0.001-0.03% v/v with a mean concentration of 0.009% v/v (61).

Serial dilution testing and Repeated Open Application Tests

To investigate whether patients allergic to isoeugenol could develop skin reactions from isoeugenol residues on fabrics deposited by washing powder and fabric softener, 19 isoeugenol-allergic individuals were patch tested with a dilution series of isoeugenol and with pieces of cotton containing isoeugenol (72). For the dose–response patch tests, the concentration of allergens used was between 0.00001 and 0.01% (v/v), equivalent to 0.00045–0.00049 to 0.45–0.49 $\mu g/cm^2$ which is for the latter more than 20-fold higher than the likely skin exposure levels associated with a fabric washed with washing powder and a fabric softener. The dose isoeugenol in the fabric for patch testing was 0.23 $\mu g/g$ cotton, representing a surface area dose of 0.0115 $\mu g/cm^2$, which is the highest exposure concentration measured in cotton washed with a washing powder and softener. The vehicle for isoeugenol in the dilution series and in the fabric (ethanol/diethyl phthalate 3:1 v/v) and an untreated piece of cotton served as controls (72). Two of the 19 panellists had a positive patch test to the highest concentration of isoeugenol 0.01%, the others were all negative, indicating that their lower threshold for elicitation is >0.01% (0.01% is 20-fold higher than the likely skin exposure levels associated with a fabric washed with washing powder and a fabric softener). Patch testing with the fabric containing isoeugenol at D4 showed 5 irritant reactions (also 5 in the control material without isoeugenol), 1 ?+ reaction (0 in controls) and one + reaction (also one in controls). In the patient with a + reaction, the vehicle control fabric also showed a + reaction. It was concluded that isoeugenol residues present on fabric do not appear to present a risk of the elicitation of contact allergic skin reactions on individuals already sensitized to isoeugenol (72).

Twenty-seven patients allergic to isoeugenol and 7 non-allergic controls participated in serial dilution patch tests with isoeugenol 2.0, 1.32, 1.0, 0.5, 0.25, 0.125, 0.063, 0.031, 0.016, 0.008, 0.004, 0.002, 0.001, 0.0005, 0.00025, 0.00012, and 0.00006% in alcohol. Three of the 27 previously isoeugenol-sensitive patients and all controls had negative patch tests. The threshold patch test concentration among the positive patients ranged from 0.0005 to 2% (not further specified) (7). The patients and controls also performed a double-blinded Repeated Open Application Test (ROAT) using two alcoholic solutions of 0.05% and 0.2% isoeugenol, applying them on the volar aspect of the right and left arm, respectively. The dosages applied were 9 $\mu g/cm^2$ for the 0.2% solution and 2.2 $\mu g/cm^2$ for the 0.05% solution, which amounts are compatible with a normal consumer use situation. For each test site, the applications continued until a reaction appeared or for a maximum of 28 days. All controls were negative, but 16/24 (67%) of the isoeugenol-sensitive subjects showed a positive ROAT to the 0.2% solution within the study period. Ten of the positive patients also reacted to the 0.05% solution. The median number of days until a positive reaction was 7 days for the 0.2% solution and 15 days for the solution containing 0.05% isoeugenol. There was a highly significant correlation between the patients' patch test threshold and the number of days until a positive ROAT: the lower the threshold, the faster the ROAT would become positive. None of the 3 patients with negative patch tests to isoeugenol and none of the controls had positive ROATs (7).

In 20 patients previously shown to be allergic to isoeugenol, serial dilution tests and ROATs were performed. For patch testing, 2%, 1%, 0.5%, 0.2%, 0.1%, 0.05%, 0.02% and 0.01% isoeugenol in petrolatum were used. One patient had a negative response. Ten had positive (+, ++ or +++) patch test reactions, the other 9 were doubtful (?+) positive. Four reacted to the lowest concentration of 0.01%, the threshold responses for the others were not well-specified. A repeated open application test (ROAT) was performed with 0.2% isoeugenol in alcohol as test solution and ethanol as vehicle control. An area of 5x5 cm on the outer aspect of the upper arm was used as test site for the first 14 days. In case of no reaction, the patients continued to apply the test solutions at the test site on the upper arm and at the base of the neck for the next 14 days. An area of 5 cm^2 at each side of the neck was used for applications. The isoeugenol solution was applied on one side and the vehicle ethanol as control on the other. Twelve of 19 (63%) patients developed eczema at the isoeugenol test area during the first 14 days of application. No reactions were observed at the ethanol test site and all control subjects had a negative ROAT. Of the 10 patients with a positive (+, ++ or +++) reaction to isoeugenol 2% pet, all had a positive ROAT; of the other nine, who had a doubtful (?+) reaction, only 2 (22%) had a positive ROAT. All patients with a positive ROAT to 0.2% isoeugenol also had a minimum patch test effect level at 0.2% or below (78).

In an early study, 12 patients allergic to isoeugenol performed a ROAT applying isoeugenol in petrolatum (3-5 mg) 2-3 times daily to the antecubital fossa for 2 weeks in concentrations of 0.008%, 0.08% (if no reaction to 0.008% occurred) and 0.8% (if no reaction occurred to 0.008% and 0.08%). There were 5 positive reactions: one to the 0.008% concentration, 3 to 0.08% and one to 0.8% as the lowest concentration. The author stated that the 'use test' had no added value over patch testing, because the test was positive in 5 individuals only and 'none of the volunteers in this study suffered from cosmetic dermatitis and applied a wide range of cosmetics without fear'. However, 6 of the patients had positive patch tests to isoeugenol 8% only and not to 0.8%, which may indicate either a very weak sensitivity or a false-positive reaction. Of the 5 individuals who had positive ROATs, 4 did react to both isoeugenol 8% and 0.8% patch tests (77).

OTHER SIDE EFFECTS

Irritant contact dermatitis
Isoeugenol and eugenol in carnation and spice-type perfumes in the past have apparently caused irritant cosmetic dermatitis which was enhanced by sunburn (photo-irritation) (33).

LITERATURE

1   Heisterberg MV, Menné T, Johansen JD. Contact allergy to the 26 specific fragrance ingredients to be declared on cosmetic products in accordance with the EU cosmetic directive. Contact Dermatitis 2011;65:266-275
2   Oosten EJ van, Schuttelaar ML, Coenraads PJ. Clinical relevance of positive patch test reactions to the 26 EU-labelled fragrances. Contact Dermatitis 2009;61:217-223
3   Schnuch A, Uter W, Geier J, Lessmann H, Frosch PJ. Sensitization to 26 fragrances to be labelled according to current European regulation: Results of the IVDK and review of the literature. Contact Dermatitis 2007;57:1-10
4   Adams RM, Maibach HI, for the North American Contact Dermatitis Group. A five-year study of cosmetic reactions. J Am Acad Dermatol 1985;13:1062-1069
5   Hausen BM. Contact allergy to Balsam of Peru. II. Patch test results in 102 patients with selected Balsam of Peru constituents. Am J Contact Derm 2001;12:93-102
6   Wöhrl S, Hemmer W, Focke M, Götz M, Jarisch R. The significance of fragrance mix, balsam of Peru, colophony and propolis as screening tools in the detection of fragrance allergy. Br J Dermatol 2001;145:268-273
7   Andersen KE, Johansen JD, Bruze M, Frosch PJ, Goossens A, Lepoittevin JP, et al. The time-dose-response relationship for elicitation of contact dermatitis in isoeugenol allergic individuals. Toxicol Appl Pharmacol 2001;170:166-171
8   Wenk KS, Ehrlich AE. Fragrance series testing in eyelid dermatitis. Dermatitis 2012;23:22-26
9   Various SCCS opinions on isoeugenol have been published and are available at: http://ec.europa.eu/growth/tools-databases/cosing/index.cfm?fuseaction=search.details_v2&id=91017
10 SCCS (Scientific Committee on Consumer Safety). Opinion on Fragrance allergens in cosmetic products, 26-27 June 2012, SCCS/1459/11. Available at: https://ec.europa.eu/health/sites/health/files/scientific_committees/consumer_safety/docs/sccs_o_102.pdf
11 Larsen WG. Perfume dermatitis. A study of 20 patients. Arch Dermatol 1977;113:623-626
12 Yazar K, Johnsson S, Lind M-L, Boman A, Lidén C. Preservatives and fragrances in selected consumer-available cosmetics and detergents. Contact Dermatitis 2011;64:265-272
13 Nagtegaal MJC, Pentinga SE, Kuik J, Kezic S, Rustemeyer T. The role of the skin irritation response in polysensitization to fragrances. Contact Dermatitis 2012;67:28-35
14 Rastogi SC, Johansen JD, Frosch P, Menné T, Bruze M, Lepoittevin JP, et al. Deodorants on the European market: quantitative chemical analysis of 21 fragrances. Contact Dermatitis 1998;38:29-35
15 Rastogi SC, Heydorn S, Johansen JD, Basketter DA. Fragrance chemicals in domestic and occupational products. Contact Dermatitis 2001;45:221-225
16 Rastogi SC, Johansen JD, Menné T. Natural ingredients based cosmetics. Content of selected fragrance sensitizers. Contact Dermatitis 1996;34:423-426
17 Johansen JD, Rastogi SC, Menné T. Contact allergy to popular perfumes: assessed by patch test, use test and chemical analyses. Br J Dermatol 1996;135:419-422
18 Rastogi SC, Johansen JD, Menné T, Frosch P, Bruze M, Andersen KE, et al. Content of fragrance allergens in children's cosmetics and cosmetic toys. Contact Dermatitis 1999;41:84-88
19 Buckley DA. Fragrance ingredient labelling in products on sale in the UK. Br J Dermatol 2007;157:295-300

20 Uter W, Yazar K, Kratz E-M, Mildau G, Lidén C. Coupled exposure to ingredients of cosmetic products: I. Fragrances. Contact Dermatitis 2013;69:335-341

21 Bennike NH, Oturai NB, Müller S, Kirkeby CS, Jørgensen C, Christensen AB, et al. Fragrance contact allergens in 5588 cosmetic products identified through a novel smartphone application. J Eur Acad Dermatol Venereol 2018;32:79-85

22 Rastogi SC, Menné T, Johansen JD. The composition of fine fragrances is changing. Contact Dermatitis 2003;48:130-132

23 Rastogi SC, Hellerup Jensen G, Johansen JD. Survey and risk assessment of chemical substances in deodorants. Survey of Chemical Substances in Consumer Products, No. 86 2007. Danish Ministry of the Environment, Environmental Protection Agency. Available at: https://www2.mst.dk/Udgiv/publications/2007/978-87-7052-625-8/pdf/978-87-7052-626-5.pdf

24 De Groot AC, Bruynzeel DP, Bos JD, van der Meeren HL, van Joost T, Jagtman BA, Weyland JW. The allergens in cosmetics. Arch Dermatol 1988;124:1525-1529

25 De Groot AC. Adverse reactions to cosmetics. PhD Thesis, University of Groningen, The Netherlands: 1988, chapter 3.4, pp.105-113

26 Schorr WF. Lip gloss and gloss type cosmetics. Contact Dermatitis Newsletter 1973;14:408-409

27 Zaragoza-Ninet V, Blasco Encinas R, Vilata-Corell JJ, Pérez-Ferriols A, Sierra-Talamantes C, Esteve-Martínez A, de la Cuadra-Oyanguren J. Allergic contact dermatitis due to cosmetics: A clinical and epidemiological study in a tertiary hospital. Actas Dermosifiliogr 2016;107:329-336

28 Laguna C, de la Cuadra J, Martín-González B, Zaragoza V, Martínez-Casimiro L, Alegre V. Allergic contact dermatitis to cosmetics. Actas Dermosifiliogr 2009;100:53-60

29 Buckley DA, Basketter DA, Smith Pease CK, Rycroft RJG, White IR, McFadden JP. Simultaneous sensitivity to fragrances. Br J Dermatol 2006;154:885-888

30 Frosch PJ, Pilz B, Andersen KE, Burrows D, Camarasa JG, Dooms-Goossens A, et al. Patch testing with fragrances: results of a multicenter study of the European Environmental and Contact Dermatitis Research Group with 48 frequently used constituents of perfumes. Contact Dermatitis 1995;33:333-342

31 Trattner A, David M. Patch testing with fine fragrances: comparison with fragrance mix, balsam of Peru and a fragrance series. Contact Dermatitis 2003:49:287-289

32 Cuesta L, Silvestre JF, Toledo F, Lucas A, Perez-Crespo M, Ballester I. Fragrance contact allergy: a 4-year retrospective study. Contact Dermatitis 2010;63:77-84

33 Klarmann EG. Perfume dermatitis. Annals of Allergy 1958;16:425-434. Data cited in ref. 34

34 Mitchell JC. Contact hypersensitivity to some perfume materials. Contact Dermatitis 1975;1:196-199

35 Uter W, Geier J, Schnuch A, Frosch PJ. Patch test results with patients' own perfumes, deodorants and shaving lotions: results of the IVDK 1998-2002. J Eur Acad Dermatol Venereol 2007;21:374-379

36 Poulsen PB, Schmidt A. A survey and health assessment of cosmetic products for children. Survey of chemical substances in consumer products, No. 88. Copenhagen: Danish Environmental Protection Agency, 2007. Available at: https://www2.mst.dk/udgiv/publications/2007/978-87-7052-638-8/pdf/978-87-7052-639-5.pdf

37 Rastogi SC. Survey of chemical compounds in consumer products. Contents of selected fragrance materials in cleaning products and other consumer products. Survey no. 8-2002. Copenhagen, Denmark, Danish Environmental Protection Agency. Available at: http://eng.mst.dk/media/mst/69131/8.pdf

38 Bouma K, Van Peursem AJJ. Marktonderzoek naleving detergenten verordening voor textielwasmiddelen. Dutch Food and Consumer Products Safety Authority (VWA) Report ND06K173, 2006 [in Dutch]. Available at: http://docplayer.nl/41524125-Marktonderzoek-naleving-detergenten-verordening-voor-textielwasmiddelen.html

39 Pors J, Fuhlendorff R. Mapping of chemical substances in air fresheners and other fragrance liberating products. Report Danish Ministry of the Environment, Environmental Protection Agency (EPA). Survey of Chemicals in Consumer Products, No 30, 2003. Available at: http://eng.mst.dk/media/mst/69113/30.pdf

40 Rastogi SC, Johansen JD, Bossi R. Selected important fragrance sensitizers in perfumes: current exposures. Contact Dermatitis 2007;56:201-204

41 Buckley DA, Wakelin SH, Seed PT, Holloway D, Rycroft RJ, White IR, et al. The frequency of fragrance allergy in a patch-test population over a 17-year period. Br J Dermatol 2000;142:279-283

42 Addo HA, Ferguson J, Johnson BF, Frain-Bell W. The relationship between exposure to fragrance materials and persistent light reaction in photosensitivity dermatitis with actinic reticuloid syndrome. Br J Dermatol 1982;107:261-274

43 Goossens A. Cosmetic contact allergens. Cosmetics 2016, 3, 5; doi:10.3390/cosmetics3010005

44 Landeck L, John SM, Geier J. Periorbital dermatitis in 4779 patients – patch test results during a 10-year period. Contact Dermatitis 2014;70:205-212

45 Molin S, Bauer A, Schnuch A, Geier J. Occupational contact allergy in nurses: results from the Information Network of Departments of Dermatology 2003–2012. Contact Dermatitis 2015;72:164-171

46 Bennike NH, Zachariae C, Johansen JD. Non-mix fragrances are top sensitizers in consecutive dermatitis patients – a cross-sectional study of the 26 EU-labelled fragrance allergens. Contact Dermatitis 2017;77:270-279

47 Lidén C, Yazar K, Johansen JD, Karlberg A-T, Uter W, White IR. Comparative sensitizing potencies of fragrances, preservatives, and hair dyes. Contact Dermatitis 2016;75:265-275

48 Osinka K, Karczmarz A, Krauze K, Feleszko W. Contact allergens in cosmetics used in atopic dermatitis: analysis of product composition. Contact Dermatitis 2016;75:241-243

49 Vejanurug P, Tresukosol P, Sajjachareonpong P, Puangpet P. Fragrance allergy could be missed without patch testing with 26 individual fragrance allergens. Contact Dermatitis 2016;74:230-235

50 Liu J, Li L-F. Contact sensitization to fragrances other than fragrance mix I in China. Contact Dermatitis 2015;73:252-253

51 Mann J, McFadden JP, White JML, White IR, Banerjee P. Baseline series fragrance markers fail to predict contact allergy. Contact Dermatitis 2014;70:276-281

52 Uter W, Johansen JD, Börje A, Karlberg A-T, Lidén C, Rastogi S, Roberts D, White IR. Categorization of fragrance contact allergens for prioritization of preventive measures: clinical and experimental data and consideration of structure–activity relationships. Contact Dermatitis 2013;69:196-230

53 Mowitz M, Svedman C, Zimerson E, Isaksson M, Pontén A, Bruze M. Simultaneous patch testing with fragrance mix I, fragrance mix II and their ingredients in southern Sweden between 2009 and 2015. Contact Dermatitis 2017;77:280-287

54 Nagtegaal MJC, Pentinga SE, Kuik J, Kezic S, Rustemeyer T. The role of the skin irritation response in polysensitization to fragrances. Contact Dermatitis 2012;67:28-35

55 Nardelli A, Drieghe J, Claes L, Boey L, Goossens A. Fragrance allergens in 'specific' cosmetic products. Contact Dermatitis 2011;64:212-219

56 Uter W, Geier J, Frosch P, Schnuch A. Contact allergy to fragrances: current patch test results (2005–2008) from the Information Network of Departments of Dermatology. Contact Dermatitis 2010;63:254-261

57 Pontén A, Björk J, Carstensen O, Gruvberger B, Isaksson M, Rasmussen K, Bruze M. Associations between contact allergy to epoxy resin and fragrance mix. Acta Derm Venereol 2004;84:151-152

58 Andersen KE, Porskjær Christensen L, Vølund A, Johansen JD, Paulsen E. Association between positive patch tests to epoxy resin and fragrance mix I ingredients. Contact Dermatitis 2009;60:155-157

59 Johansen JD, Rastogi SC, Bruze M, Andersen KE, Frosch P, Dreier B, et al. Deodorants: a clinical provocation study in fragrance-sensitive individuals. Contact Dermatitis 1998;39:161-165

60 Johansen JD, Rastogi SC, Andersen KE, Menné T. Content and reactivity to product perfumes in fragrance mix positive and negative eczema patients: A study of perfumes used in toiletries and skin-care products. Contact Dermatitis 1997;36:291-296

61 Johansen JD, Rastogi SC, Menné T. Exposure to selected fragrance materials: A case study of fragrance-mix-positive eczema patients. Contact Dermatitis 1996;34:106-110

62 Frosch PJ, Pilz B, Burrows D, Camarasa JG, Lachapelle J-M, Lahti A, et al. Testing with fragrance mix: Is the addition of sorbitan sesquioleate to the constituents useful? Contact Dermatitis 1995;32:266-272

63 De Groot AC, Van der Kley AMJ, Bruynzeel DP, Meinardi MMHM, Smeenk G, van Joost Th, Pavel S. Frequency of false-negative reactions to the fragrance mix. Contact Dermatitis 1993;28:139-140

64 Broeckx W, Blondeel A, Dooms-Goossens A, Achten G. Cosmetic intolerance. Contact Dermatitis 1987;16:189-194

65 Van Joost Th, Stolz E, Van Der Hoek JCS. Simultaneous allergy to perfume ingredients. Contact Dermatitis 1985;12:115-116

66 Strauss RM, Orton DI. Allergic contact cheilitis in the United Kingdom: a retrospective study. Dermatitis 2003;14:75-77

67 Bárány E, Lodén M. Content of fragrance mix ingredients and customer complaints of cosmetic products. Dermatitis 2000;11:74-79

68 Diepgen TL, Ofenloch R, Bruze M, Cazzaniga S, Coenraads PJ, Elsner P, et al. Prevalence of fragrance contact allergy in the general population of five European countries: a cross-sectional study. Br J Dermatol 2015;173:1411-1419

69 Klaschka U. Contact allergens for armpits - allergenic fragrances specified on deodorants. Int J Hyg Environ Health 2012;215:584-591

70 Rastogi SC, Johansen JD. Significant exposures to isoeugenol derivates in perfumes. Contact Dermatitis 2008;58:278-281

71 White IR, Johansen JD, Giménez-Arnau E, Lepoittevin JP, Rastogi S, Bruze M, et al. Isoeugenol is an important contact allergen: can it be safely replaced with isoeugenyl acetate? Contact Dermatitis 1999;41:272-275

72 Basketter DA, Pons-Guiraud A, Van Asten A, Laverdet C, Marty J-P, Martin L, et al. Fragrance allergy: assessing the safety of washed fabrics. Contact Dermatitis 2010;62:349-354

73 Karlberg A-T, Börje A, Johansen JD, Lidén C, Rastogi S, Roberts D, et al. Activation of non-sensitizing or low-sensitizing fragrance substances into potent sensitizers – prehaptens and prohaptens. Contact Dermatitis 2013;69:323-334

74 White JML, White IR, Glendinning A, Fleming J, Jefferies D, Basketter DA, McFadden JP, Buckley DA. Frequency of allergic contact dermatitis to isoeugenol is increasing: a review of 3636 patients tested from 2001 to 2005. Br J Dermatol 2007;157:580-582

75 Tanaka S, Royds C, Buckley D, Basketter DA, Goossens A, Bruze M, et al. Contact allergy to isoeugenol and its derivatives: problems with allergen substitution. Contact Dermatitis 2004;51:288-291

76 Hannuksela M, Kousa M, Pirilä V. Allergy to ingredients of vehicles. Contact Dermatitis 1976;2:105-110

77 Epstein WL. The use test for contact hypersensitivity. Arch Derm Res 1982;272:279-281

78 Johansen JD, Andersen KE, Menné T. Quantitative aspects of isoeugenol contact allergy assessed by use and patch tests. Contact Dermatitis 1996;34:414-418

79 Hjorth N. Eczematous allergy to balsams. Acta Derm Venereol 1961;41(suppl.46):1-216

80 De Groot AC, Schmidt E. Essential oils: contact allergy and chemical composition. Boca Raton, Fl., USA: CRC Press, Taylor and Francis Group, 2016 (ISBN 9781482246407)

81 Dooms-Goossens, A, Kerre S, Drieghe J, Bossuyt L, DeGreef H. Cosmetic products and their allergens. Eur J Dermatol 1992;2:465-468

82 Meynadier JM, Meynadier J, Peyron JL, Peyron L. Formes cliniques des manifestations cutanées d'allergie aux parfums. Ann Dermatol Venereol 1986;113:31-39

83 Opinion of the Scientific Committee on Cosmetic Products and Non-Food Products Intended for Consumers concerning 'The 1st update of the inventory of ingredients employed in cosmetic products. Section II: Perfume and aromatic raw materials', 24 October 2000, SCCNFP/0389/00, final. Available at: http://ec.europa.eu/health/ph_risk/committees/sccp/documents/out131_en.pdf

84 Opinion of the Scientific Committee on Cosmetic Products and Non-Food Products Intended for Consumers concerning 'An initial list of perfumery materials which must not form part of cosmetic products except subject to the Restrictions and Conditions laid down, 25 September 2001, SCCNFP/0392/00, final. Available at: http://ec.europa.eu/health/archive/ph_risk/committees/sccp/documents/out150_en.pdf

85 Wieck S, Olsson O, Kümmerer K, Klaschka U. Fragrance allergens in household detergents. Regul Toxicol Pharmacol 2018;97:163-169

86 Ung CY, White JML, White IR, Banerjee P, McFadden JP. Patch testing with the European baseline series fragrance markers: a 2016 update. Br J Dermatol 2018;178:776-780

87 Geier J, Uter W, Lessmann H, Schnuch A. Fragrance mix I and II: results of breakdown tests. Flavour Fragr J 2015;30:264-274

88 Girbig M, Hegewald J, Seidler A, Bauer A, Uter W, Schmitt J. Type IV sensitizations in physical therapists: patch test results of the Information Network of Departments of Dermatology (IVDK) 2007-2011. J Dtsch Dermatol Ges 2013;11:1185-1192

89 Dittmar D, Schuttelaar MLA. Contact sensitization to hydroperoxides of limonene and linalool: Results of consecutive patch testing and clinical relevance. Contact Dermatitis 2018 Oct 31. doi: 10.1111/cod.13137. [Epub ahead of print]

90 Silvestre JF, Mercader P, González-Pérez R, Hervella-Garcés M, Sanz-Sánchez T, Córdoba S, et al. Sensitization to fragrances in Spain: A 5-year multicentre study (2011-2015). Contact Dermatitis. 2018 Nov 14. doi: 10.1111/cod.13152. [Epub ahead of print]

Chapter 3.88   ISOEUGENYL ACETATE

IDENTIFICATION

Description/definition : Isoeugenyl acetate is the organic compound that conforms to the structural formula shown below
Chemical class(es) : Esters; ethers
Chemical/IUPAC name : (2-Methoxy-4-prop-1-enylphenyl) acetate
Other names : Acetyl isoeugenol
CAS registry number(s) : 93-29-8
EC number(s) : 202-236-1
RIFM monograph(s) : Food Cosmet Toxicol 1975;13:819 (special issue II)
Function(s) in cosmetics : EU: perfuming. USA: fragrance ingredients
Patch testing : 1.3% pet. (2); 1.2% alc. (5); it cannot be excluded that the latter concentration + vehicle is slightly irritant
Molecular formula : $C_{12}H_{14}O_3$

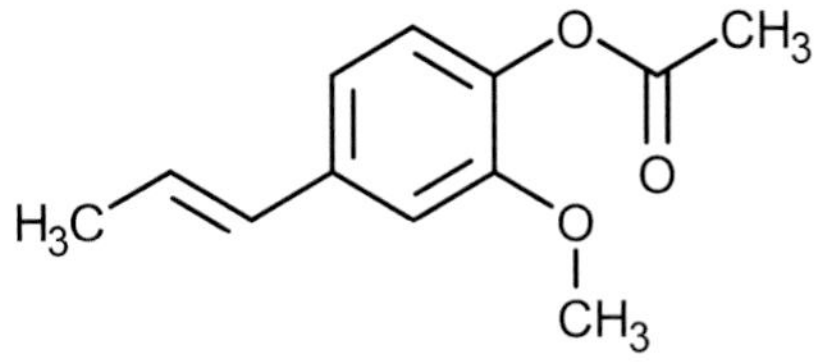

GENERAL

Isoeugenyl acetate is a white crystalline powder; its odor type is spicy and its odor at 100% is described as 'sweet spicy powdery floral carnation balsam' (www.thegoodscentscompany.com).

Presence in essential oils

Isoeugenyl acetate (any isomer) has been identified by chemical analysis in six of 91 essential oils, which have caused contact allergy / allergic contact dermatitis. In none of these oils, it belonged to the 'Top-10' of ingredients with the highest concentrations (6).

CONTACT ALLERGY

Patch testing in groups of patients

Patch testing in consecutive patients suspected of contact dermatitis: routine testing
The results of 2 studies in which isoeugenyl acetate was patch tested in consecutive patients suspected of contact dermatitis (routine testing) are shown in table 3.88.1. There were 0.8% positive reactions to isoeugenyl acetate 1.3% petrolatum in a group of 2261 patients tested in 2001-2002 in the United Kingdom, Belgium and Sweden (2) and an amazing 3.9% in 155 patients tested in the United Kingdom in 1998 with isoeugenyl acetate 1.2% in alcohol (5). Relevance was not mentioned in either study. The majority of allergic patients co-reacted to isoeugenol (2,5).

Table 3.88.1 Patch testing in groups of patients: Routine testing

Years and Country	Test conc. & vehicle	Number of patients tested	positive (%)	Selection of patients (S); Relevance (R); Comments (C)	Ref.
2001-2 UK, Denmark, Belgium, Sweden	1.3% pet.	2261	19 (0.8%)	R: not stated; C: there were 13 (68%) co-reactions to isoeugenol	2
1998 UK	1.2% alc.	155	6 (3.9%)	R: not stated; there were 5 (83%) co-reactions to isoeugenol and 6 (100%) co-reactions to the fragrance mix I	5

Testing in groups of selected patients
Studies in which isoeugenyl acetate was patch tested in groups of selected patients with positive results have not been found.

Case reports and case series
Case reports of allergic contact dermatitis from isoeugenyl acetate haven not been found.

Cross-reactions, pseudo-cross-reactions and co-reactions

For general information on cross-/pseudo-cross-/co-reactivity of fragrance chemicals with other fragrances, fragrance markers (fragrance mix I, fragrance mix II, colophonium, Myroxylon pereirae resin [balsam of Peru]) and essential oils see Chapter 1.2 General information on cross-reactions, pseudo-cross-reactions and co-reactions.

In a group of 19 patients with positive patch tests to isoeugenyl acetate, there were 13 (68%) co-reactions to isoeugenol (2). Of 6 patients reacting to isoeugenyl acetate 1.2% alc., 5 (83%) co-reacted to isoeugenol 1% pet. (5).

Concomitant contact allergy to isoeugenol and its derivatives can occur either through multiple sensitization, direct chemical cross-reactivity or local skin metabolism to one or more common and/or cross-reactive derivatives. Isoeugenyl acetate is probably easily hydrolyzed in the skin to produce isoeugenol (3).

Presence in products and chemical analyses

In Denmark, in 2006-2007, 29 hydroalcoholic products of international brands (2 aftershave lotions, 26 eaux de toilette/eaux de parfum [10 for men and 16 for women] and one parfum) were purchased from Danish retail outlets and investigated by GC-MS for the presence of isoeugenol, isoeugenyl acetate, methyl isoeugenol and benzyl isoeugenol. Isoeugenyl acetate was found to be present in 10 products (34%) in a concentration range of 20.1-4689.3 ppm, mean of 1569.5 ppm. Many of the products contained 2 or 3 of the fragrances, but benzyl isoeugenol was not found in any sample (4).

In 1997, 71 deodorants (22 vapo-spray, 22 aerosol spray and 27 roll-on products) were collected in Denmark, England, France, Germany and Sweden and analyzed by gas chromatography – mass spectrometry (GC-MS) for the presence of fragrances and other materials. Isoeugenyl acetate was present in 9 (13%) of the products (1).

LITERATURE

1   Rastogi SC, Lepoittevin J-P, Johansen JD, Frosch PJ, Menné T, Bruze M, et al. Fragrances and other materials in deodorants: search for potentially sensitizing molecules using combined GC-MS and structure activity relationship (SAR) analysis. Contact Dermatitis 1998;39:293-303

2   Tanaka S, Royds C, Buckley D, Basketter DA, Goossens A, Bruze M, et al. Contact allergy to isoeugenol and its derivatives: problems with allergen substitution. Contact Dermatitis 2004;51:288-291

3   Smith CK, Hotchkiss SAM. Allergic contact dermatitis: Chemical and metabolic mechanisms. London: Taylor & Francis, 2001

4   Rastogi SC, Johansen JD. Significant exposures to isoeugenol derivates in perfumes. Contact Dermatitis 2008;58:278-281

5   White IR, Johansen JD, Giménez-Arnau E, Lepoittevin J-P, Rastogi S, Bruze M, et al. Isoeugenol is an important contact allergen: can it be safely replaced with isoeugenyl acetate? Contact Dermatitis 1999;41:272-275

6   De Groot AC, Schmidt E. Essential oils: contact allergy and chemical composition. Boca Raton, Fl., USA: CRC Press, Taylor and Francis Group, 2016 (ISBN 9781482246407)

Chapter 3.89   ISOEUGENYL BENZOATE

IDENTIFICATION

Description/definition   : Isoeugenyl benzoate is the aromatic ester that conforms to the structural formula
                                shown below
Chemical class(es)   : Aromatic compounds; esters; unsaturated organic compounds
INCI name USA   : Not in the Personal Care Products Council Ingredient Database
Chemical/IUPAC name   : (2-Methoxy-4-prop-1-enylphenyl) benzoate
Other names   : Phenol, 2-methoxy-4-(1-propenyl)-, benzoate; propenylguaiacol benzoate
CAS registry number(s)   : 4194-00-7
EC number(s)   : 224-074-0
SCCS opinion(s)   : SCCNFP/0389/00, final (4)
Function(s) in cosmetics   : EU: perfuming
Patch testing   : 1.6% pet. (1)
Molecular formula   : $C_{17}H_{16}O_3$

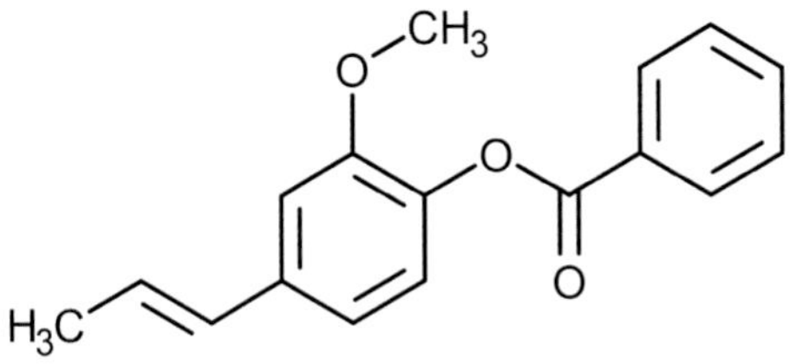

GENERAL

Isoeugenyl benzoate is a colorless to pale yellow clear liquid; its odor type and its odor description are not provided at www.thegoodscentscompany.com. Isoeugenyl benzoate is a synthetic chemical, not found in nature (and consequently not in essential oils (3)).

CONTACT ALLERGY

Patch testing in groups of patients: Routine testing

In the period 2001-2002, in the United Kingdom, Denmark, Belgium and Sweden, 2261 consecutive patients suspected of contact dermatitis (routine testing) were patch tested with isoeugenyl benzoate 1.6% pet. and there were four (0.2%) positive reactions. The relevance of these reactions was not mentioned (1).

Patch testing in groups of selected patients and Case reports

Studies in which isoeugenyl benzoate was patch tested in groups of selected patients with positive results have not been found. Case reports of allergic contact dermatitis from isoeugenyl benzoate have not been found.

Cross-reactions, pseudo-cross-reactions and co-reactions

In 4 patients with positive patch tests to isoeugenyl benzoate, there were 3 (75%) co-reactions to isoeugenol (1). Concomitant contact allergy to isoeugenol and its derivatives can occur either through multiple sensitization, direct chemical cross-reactivity or local skin metabolism to one or more common and/or cross-reactive derivatives. Isoeugenyl benzoate is probably easily hydrolyzed in the skin to produce isoeugenol (2).

LITERATURE

1   Tanaka S, Royds C, Buckley D, Basketter DA, Goossens A, Bruze M, et al. Contact allergy to isoeugenol and its
     derivatives: problems with allergen substitution. Contact Dermatitis 2004;51:288-291
2   Smith CK, Hotchkiss SAM. Allergic contact dermatitis: Chemical and metabolic mechanisms. London: Taylor &
     Francis, 2001
3   De Groot AC, Schmidt E. Essential oils: contact allergy and chemical composition. Boca Raton, Fl., USA: CRC Press,
     Taylor and Francis Group, 2016 (ISBN 9781482246407)
4   Opinion of the Scientific Committee on Cosmetic Products and Non-Food Products Intended for Consumers
     concerning 'The 1st update of the inventory of ingredients employed in cosmetic products. Section II: Perfume
     and aromatic raw materials', 24 October 2000, SCCNFP/0389/00, final. Available at:
     http://ec.europa.eu/health/ph_risk/committees/sccp/documents/out131_en.pdf

Chapter 3.90   ISOEUGENYL PHENYLACETATE

IDENTIFICATION

Description/definition	: Isoeugenyl phenylacetate is the aromatic ester that conforms to the structural formula shown below
Chemical class(es)	: Aromatic compounds; esters; unsaturated organic compounds
INCI name USA	: Not in the Personal Care Products Council Ingredient Database
Chemical/IUPAC name	: 2-Methoxy-4-prop-1-enylphenyl phenylacetate
Other names	: Propenylguaiacol phenylacetate; isoeugenyl α-toluate
CAS registry number(s)	: 120-24-1
EC number(s)	: 204-381-6
Function(s) in cosmetics	: EU: perfuming
Patch testing	: 1.7% pet. (1)
Molecular formula	: $C_{18}H_{18}O_3$

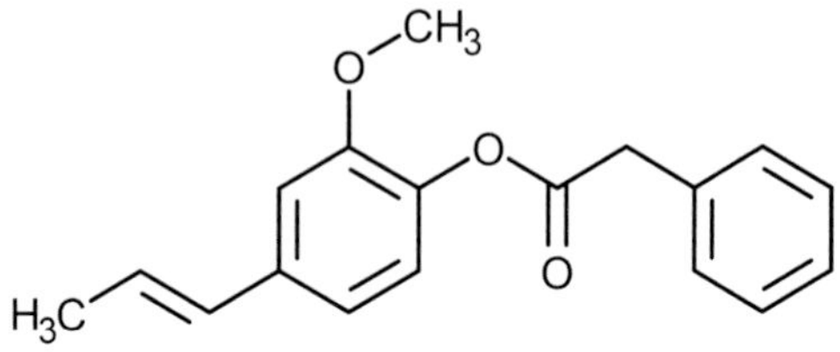

GENERAL

Isoeugenyl phenylacetate is a yellow clear viscous liquid; its odor type is spicy and its odor is described as 'sweet, spice, clove and cinnamon, floral and honey' (www.thegoodscentscompany.com). Isoeugenyl phenylacetate is a synthetic chemical, not found in nature (and consequently not in essential oils (2)).

CONTACT ALLERGY

Patch testing in consecutive patients suspected of contact dermatitis: routine testing

In the period 2001-2002, in the United Kingdom, Denmark, Belgium and Sweden, 2261 consecutive patients suspected of contact dermatitis (routine testing) were patch tested with isoeugenyl phenylacetate 1.7% pet. and there were sixteen (0.7%) positive reactions. The relevance of these reactions was not mentioned (1).

Patch testing in groups of selected patients

Studies in which isoeugenyl phenylacetate was patch tested in groups of selected patients with positive results have not been found.

Case reports and case series

Case reports of allergic contact dermatitis from isoeugenyl phenylacetate have not been found.

Cross-reactions, pseudo-cross-reactions and co-reactions

For general information on cross-/pseudo-cross-/co-reactivity of fragrance chemicals with other fragrances, fragrance markers (fragrance mix I, fragrance mix II, colophonium, Myroxylon pereirae resin [balsam of Peru]) and essential oils see Chapter 1.2 General information on cross-reactions, pseudo-cross-reactions and co-reactions.

In 16 patients with positive patch tests to isoeugenyl acetate, there were 15 (94%) co-reactions to isoeugenol (1). Concomitant contact allergy to isoeugenol and its derivatives can occur either through multiple sensitization, direct chemical cross-reactivity or local skin metabolism to one or more common and/or cross-reactive derivatives (1).

LITERATURE

1   Tanaka S, Royds C, Buckley D, Basketter DA, Goossens A, Bruze M, et al. Contact allergy to isoeugenol and its derivatives: problems with allergen substitution. Contact Dermatitis 2004;51:288-291
2   De Groot AC, Schmidt E. Essential oils: contact allergy and chemical composition. Boca Raton, Fl., USA: CRC Press, Taylor and Francis Group, 2016 (ISBN 9781482246407)

Chapter 3.91 ISOLONGIFOLANONE

IDENTIFICATION

Description/definition : Isolongifolanone is the tricyclic ketone that conforms to the structural formula shown below

Chemical class(es) : Ketones; tricyclic organic compounds

INCI name USA : Not in the Personal Care Products Council Ingredient Database

Chemical/IUPAC name : 2,2,8,8-Tetramethyl-octahydro-1H-2,4a-methanonapthalene-10-one

Other names : Isolongifolene ketone; 2,2,7,7-tetramethyltricyclo[6.2.1.0^{1,6}]undecan-5-one

CAS registry number(s) : 23787-90-8

EC number(s) : 245-890-3

RIFM monograph(s) : Food Chem Toxicol 2017;110(suppl.1):S59-S65; Food Chem Toxicol 2000;38(suppl.3): S129-S132; Food Chem Toxicol 1983;21:859

SCCS opinion(s) : SCCS/1459/11 (1)

Function(s) in cosmetics : EU: perfuming

Patch testing : 5% pet. (2)

Molecular formula : $C_{15}H_{24}O$

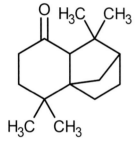

GENERAL

Isolongifolanone is a pale yellow clear liquid; its odor type is woody and its odor at 100% is described as 'dry woody patchouli cedar earthy tobacco incense' (www.thegoodscentscompany.com).

Presence in essential oils

(E)-Isolongifolanone has been identified by chemical analysis in two of 91 essential oils, which have caused contact allergy / allergic contact dermatitis: galbanum resin oil and sandalwood oil (4).

CONTACT ALLERGY

General

The SCCS (Scientific Committee on Consumer Safety), in a 2012 Opinion on Fragrance allergens in cosmetic products, has categorized isolongifolanone as 'likely fragrance contact allergen by combination of evidence' (1,3).

Patch testing in groups of patients

In 2000, in Japan, USA and several European countries, 178 patients with known fragrance sensitivity were tested with a series of fragrances and there was one (0.6%) positive patch test reaction to isolongifolanone 5% pet. The relevance of this reaction was not mentioned (2).

LITERATURE

1   SCCS (Scientific Committee on Consumer Safety). Opinion on Fragrance allergens in cosmetic products, 26-27 June 2012, SCCS/1459/11. Available at: https://ec.europa.eu/health/sites/health/files/scientific_committees/consumer_safety/docs/sccs_o_102.pdf

2   Larsen W, Nakayama H, Fischer T, Elsner P, Frosch P, Burrows D, et al. Fragrance contact dermatitis: A worldwide multicenter investigation (Part II). Contact Dermatitis 2001;44:344-346

3   Uter W, Johansen JD, Börje A, Karlberg A-T, Lidén C, Rastogi S, Roberts D, White IR. Categorization of fragrance contact allergens for prioritization of preventive measures: clinical and experimental data and consideration of structure–activity relationships. Contact Dermatitis 2013;69:196-230

4   De Groot AC, Schmidt E. Essential oils: contact allergy and chemical composition. Boca Raton, Fl., USA: CRC Press, Taylor and Francis Group, 2016 (ISBN 9781482246407)

Chapter 3.92   ALPHA-ISOMETHYL IONONE

IDENTIFICATION

Description/definition	: alpha-Isomethyl ionone is the organic compound that conforms to the structural formula shown below
Chemical class(es)	: Ketones
Chemical/IUPAC name	: 3-Methyl-4-(2,6,6-trimethylcyclohex-2-en-1-yl)but-3-en-2-one
Other names	: Methyl-γ-ionone; γ-methylionone
CAS registry number(s)	: 127-51-5
EC number(s)	: 204-846-3
RIFM monograph(s)	: Food Chem Toxicol 2007;45(suppl.1):S280-S289; Food Cosmetic Toxicol 1975;13:863 (isomer mixture) (special Issue II) (binder, page 559)
SCCS opinion(s)	: Various (5); SCCS/1459/11 (6); SCCNFP/0389/00, final (36)
Function(s) in cosmetics	: EU: perfuming; skin conditioning. USA: fragrance ingredients; skin-conditioning agents – miscellaneous
EU cosmetic restrictions	: Regulated in Annex III/90 of the Regulation (EC) No. 1223/2009, regulated by 2003/15/EC; Must be labeled on cosmetics and detergent products, if present at > 10 ppm (0.001%) in leave-on products and > 100 ppm (0.01%) in rinse-off products
Patch testing	: 10% Pet. (Chemotechnique); 1% pet. (SmartPracticeCanada); recommended test concentration: 10.0% wt./wt. pet. (1)
Molecular formula	: $C_{14}H_{22}O$

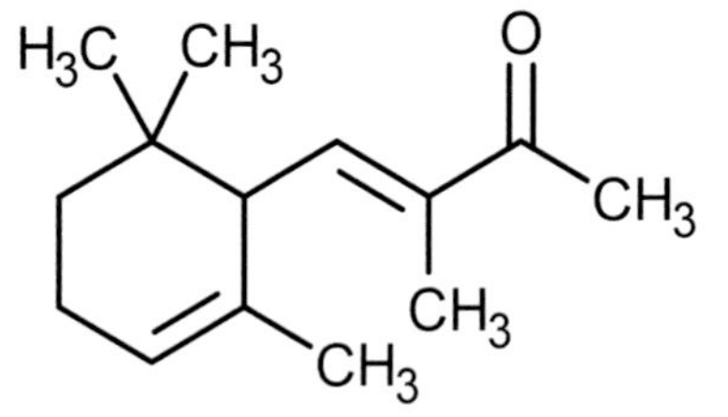

GENERAL

alpha-Isomethyl ionone is a colorless to yellow clear oily liquid; its odor type is floral and its odor at 10% in dipropylene glycol is described as 'violet sweet orris powdery floral woody' (www.thegoodscentscompany.com). alpha-Isomethyl ionone is a synthetic chemical, not found in nature (and consequently not in essential oils (35)).

See also Chapter 3.112 Methyl ionones.

CONTACT ALLERGY

General

The SCCS (Scientific Committee on Consumer Safety), in a 2012 Opinion on Fragrance allergens in cosmetic products, has marked alpha-isomethyl ionone as 'established contact allergen in humans' (6,31). The sensitizing potency of alpha-isomethyl ionone was classified as 'weak' based on an EC3 value of 21.8% in the LLNA (local lymph node assay) in animal experiments (6,31).

The literature on contact allergy to alpha-isomethyl ionone up to 2004 has been reviewed (8).

Patch testing in groups of patients

Results of studies testing alpha-isomethyl ionone in consecutive patients suspected of contact dermatitis (routine testing) and those of testing *selected* patients (patients with known or suspected fragrance or cosmetic dermatitis) are shown in table 3.92.1.

Patch testing in consecutive patients suspected of contact dermatitis: routine testing

In five studies in which consecutive patients suspected of contact dermatitis were patch tested with alpha-isomethyl ionone 1% pet., frequencies of sensitization were invariably low, ranging from 0.03% to 0.1% (2,29,30,38,41). In the one study where specific relevance data were provided, one of 2 positive reactions had current relevance, the other past relevance (29).

Patch testing in groups of selected patients

In five studies in which groups of selected patients (patients with known or suspected fragrance or cosmetic dermatitis) were patch tested with alpha-isomethyl ionone (1% pet., 5% pet. or 10% pet.), frequencies of sensitization were generally low, ranging from 0.4% to 2.1% (3,7,21,28,32). In four of the studies, no relevance data were provided (7,21,28,32), in the 4th relevance was not specified for individual fragrances (3).

Pigmented cosmetic dermatitis

While searching for causative ingredients of pigmented cosmetic dermatitis in Japan in the 1970s, both patients with ordinary (nonpigmented) cosmetic dermatitis and women with pigmented cosmetic dermatitis were tested with a large number of fragrance materials. In 1980 the accumulated data enabled the classification of fragrant materials into 4 groups: common sensitizers, rare sensitizers, virtually non-sensitizing fragrances and fragrances considered as non-sensitizers. alpha-Isomethyl ionone (γ-methylionone) was classified in the group of rare sensitizers, indicating that one or more cases of contact allergy / allergic contact dermatitis to it have been observed (27). More specific data are lacking, the results have largely or solely been published in Japanese journals only.

Table 3.92.1 Patch testing in groups of patients

Years and Country	Test conc. & vehicle	Number of patients tested | positive (%)		Selection of patients (S); Relevance (R); Comments (C)	Ref.
Routine testing					
2015-7 Netherlands		821	1 (0.1%)	R: not stated	41
2015-2016 UK	1% pet.	2084	1 (0.05%)	R: not specified for individual fragrances; 25% of patients who reacted to any fragrance or fragrance marker had a positive fragrance intolerance history	38
2010-2015 Denmark	1% pet.	6004	2 (0.03%)	R: present relevance 50%, past relevance 50%; current and/or past relevance: 100%	29
2011-2012 UK	1% pet.	1951	2 (0.1%)	R: not stated	30
2003-2004 IVDK	1% pet.	2004	1 (0.05%)	R: not stated	2
Testing in groups of selected patients					
2006-2011 IVDK	1% pet.	708	3 (0.4%)	S: patients with suspected cosmetic intolerance; R: not stated	28
2005-10 Netherlands		100	1 (1%)	S: patients with known fragrance sensitivity based on a positive patch test to the FM I and/or the FM II; R: not stated	32
2005-7 Netherlands	5% pet.	320	2 (0.6%)	S: patients suspected of fragrance or cosmetic allergy; R: 61% relevance for all positive tested fragrances together	3
2002-2003 Korea	5% pet.	422	9 (2.1%)	S: patients with suspected cosmetic dermatitis; R: not stated	21
1984 The Netherlands	10% pet.	179	2 (1.1%)	S: patients suspected of cosmetic allergy; R: not stated; C: the patch test material also contained 10% ionone (mixed isomers)	7

FM: Fragrance mix; IVDK: Informationsverbund Dermatologischer Kliniken (Germany, Switzerland, Austria)

Case reports and case series

In the period 2000-2009, in Leuven, Belgium, an unspecified number of patients had positive patch tests or use tests to a total of 344 cosmetic products *and* positive patch tests to FM I, FM II, and/or to one or more of 28 selected specific fragrance ingredients. In one of two patients reacting to alpha-isomethyl ionone, the presence of this fragrance in the cosmetic product(s) was confirmed by reading the product label(s) (33).

In a group of 119 patients with allergic contact dermatitis from cosmetics, investigated in The Netherlands in 1986-1987, one case was caused by alpha-isomethyl ionone in a skin care product (19,20).

A woman, with a previous history of dermatitis from adhesive tape, was hospitalized for an operation. Three days later, an itchy purpuric dermatitis appeared over the anterior trunk, its distribution suggesting production by a cologne profusely applied the previous day. The cologne had run over her breasts and abdomen, sparing the submammary folds, and had accumulated in her right groin due to her semi-lateral decubitus. The lesions became brownish and disappeared in 2 weeks. A series of 20 perfumes and cosmetic substances were patch tested with negative results. A patch test with the cologne (as is) gave a positive reaction at days 2 and 3. No purpura was seen. Two months later, 18 components of the cologne from the manufacturer were tested at the same concentration as in the cologne; 'methylionantheme' (0.0437% in alcohol) elicited a positive reaction. Other ionones were later tested and the patient now had positive patch test reactions to ionone and alpha-isomethyl ionone (test concentrations not specified) (39). alpha-Isomethyl ionone is part of Methylionantheme ®.

Presence in products and chemical analyses

In various studies, the presence of alpha-isomethyl ionone in cosmetic and sometimes other products has been investigated. Before 2006, most investigators used chemical analysis, usually GC-MS, for qualitative and quantitative determination. Since then, the presence of the target fragrances was usually investigated by screening the product labels for the 26 fragrances that must be labeled since 2005 on cosmetics and detergent products in the EU, if present at > 10 ppm (0.001%) in leave-on products and > 100 ppm (0.01%) in rinse-off products. This method, obviously, is less accurate and may result in underestimation of the frequency of the fragrances being present in the product. When they are in fact present, but the concentration is lower than mentioned above, labeling is not required and the fragrances' presence will be missed.

The results of the relevant studies for alpha-isomethyl ionone are summarized in table 3.92.2. More detailed information can be found in the corresponding text following the table. The percentage of products in which alpha-isomethyl ionone was found to be present shows wide variations, which can among other be explained by the selection procedure of the products, the method of investigation (false-negatives with information obtained from labels only) and changes in the use of individual fragrance materials over time (fashion). Generally speaking it can be stated that alpha-isomethyl ionone is one of the more frequently used fragrances in (cosmetic) products.

Table 3.92.2 Presence of alpha-isomethyl ionone in products [a]

Year	Country	Product type	Nr. investigated	Nr. of products positive [b]	(%)	Method [c]	Ref.
2015-6	Denmark	Fragranced cosmetic products	5588		(16%)	Labeling	17
2015	Germany	Household detergents	817	43	(5%)	Labeling	37
2008-11	Germany	Deodorants	374	115	(31%)	Labeling	34
2006-9	Germany	Cosmetic products	4991		(12%)	Labeling	16
2008	Sweden	Cosmetic products	204		(11%)	Labeling	4
		Detergents	97		(1%)	Labeling	
2007	Netherlands	Cosmetic products for children	23	10	(43%)	Analysis	23
2006	UK	Perfumed cosmetic and house-hold products	300	104	(35%)	Labeling	14
2006	Denmark	Popular perfumed deodorants	88	41	(47%)	Labeling	18
			23	15	(65%)	Analysis	
2006	Netherlands	Laundry detergents	52	21	(40%)	Labeling + analysis	25
2006	Denmark	Rinse-off cosmetics for children	208	12	(6%)	Labeling + analysis	22
2002	Denmark	Home and car air fresheners	19	10	(53%)	Analysis	26
2001	Denmark	Non-cosmetic consumer products	43	17	(40%)	Analysis	24
2000	Denmark, UK, Germany, Italy	Domestic and occupational products	59	5	(8.5%)	Analysis	10
1997-8	Denmark, UK Germany, Sweden	Cosmetics and cosmetic toys for children	25	9	(36%)	Analysis	11
1996	Five European countries	Fragranced deodorants	70	43	(61%)	Analysis	9
1992	Netherlands	Cosmetic products	300		(63%)	Analysis	15
1988	USA	Perfumes used in fine fragrances, household products and soap	400	50-64% (See text)		Analysis	13

[a] See the corresponding text below for more details
[b] positive = containing the target fragrance
[c] Labeling: information from the ingredient labels on the product / packaging; Analysis: chemical analysis, most often GC-MS

In Denmark, in 2015-2016, 5588 fragranced cosmetic products were examined with a smartphone application for the 26 fragrances that need to be labeled in the EU. alpha-Isomethyl ionone was present in 16% of the products (rank number 9) (17).

In Germany, in 2015, fragrance allergens were evaluated based on lists of ingredients in 817 (unique) detergents (all-purpose cleaners, cleaning preparations for special purposes [e.g. bathroom, kitchen, dish-washing] and laundry detergents) present in 131 households. Alpha-Isomethyl ionone was found to be present in 43 (5%) of the products (37).

In 2008, 2010 and 2011, 374 deodorants available in German retail shops were randomly selected and their labels checked for the presence of the 26 fragrances that need to be labeled. Alpha-Isomethyl ionone was found to be present in 115 (30.7%) of the products (34).

In Germany, in the period 2006-2009, 4991 cosmetic products were randomly sampled for an official investigation of conformity of cosmetic products with legal provisions. The labels were inspected for the presence of the 26 fragrances that need to be labeled in the EU. alpha-Isomethyl ionone was present in 12% of the products (rank number 7) (16).

alpha-Isomethyl ionone was present in 11% of 204 cosmetic products (92 shampoos, 61 hair conditioners, 34 liquid soaps, 17 wet tissues) and in 1% of 97 detergents in Sweden, 2008 (4).

In 2007, in The Netherlands, twenty-three cosmetic products for children were analyzed for the presence of fragrances that need to be labeled. alpha-Isomethyl ionone was identified in 10 of the products (43%) in a concentration range of 71-5395 ppm (23).

In 2006, of 88 popular perfume containing deodorants purchased in Denmark, 41 (47%) were labeled to contain alpha-isomethyl ionone. Analysis of 24 regulated fragrance substances in 23 selected deodorants (19 spray products, 2 deostick and 2 roll-on) was performed by GC-MS. alpha-Isomethyl iononewas identified in 15 of the products (65%) with a concentration range of 6–2588 ppm (18).

In 2006, the labels of 208 cosmetics for children (especially shampoos, body shampoos and soaps) available in Denmark were checked for the presence of the 26 fragrances that need to be labeled in the EU. alpha-Isomethyl ionone was present in 12 products (5.8%), and ranked number 15 in the frequency list. Seventeen products were analyzed quantitatively for the fragrances. The maximum concentration found for alpha-isomethyl ionone was 480 mg/kg (22).

In 2006, in The Netherlands, 52 laundry detergents were investigated for the presence of allergenic fragrances by checking their labels and chemical analyses. alpha-Isomethyl ionone was found to be present in 21 of the products (40%) in a concentration range of 10-160 ppm. The fragrance had rank number 3 (with limonene and linalool) in the frequency list (25).

In January 2006, a study of perfumed cosmetic and household products available on the shelves of U.K. retailers was carried out. Products were included if 'parfum' or 'aroma' was listed among the ingredients. Three hundred products were surveyed and any of 26 mandatory labeling fragrances named on the label were recorded. alpha-Isomethyl ionone was present in 104 (35%) of the products (rank number 8) (14).

In 2002, in Denmark, 19 air fresheners (6 for cars, 13 for homes) were analyzed for the presence of fragrances that need to be labeled on cosmetics. alpha-Isomethyl ionone was found to be present in 10 products (53%) in a concentration range of 220-11,000 ppm (26).

In 2001, in Denmark, 43 non-cosmetic consumer products (mainly dish-washing products, laundry detergents, and hard and soft surface cleaners) were analyzed for the 26 fragrances that are regulated for labeling in the EU. alpha-Isomethyl ionone was present in 17 products (40%) in a concentration range of 0.0073-0.1586% (m/m) and had rank number 5 in the frequency list (24).

In 2000, fifty-nine domestic and occupational products, purchased in retail outlets in Denmark, England, Germany and Italy were analyzed by GC-MS for the presence of fragrances. The product categories were liquid soap and soap bars (n=13), soft/hard surface cleaners (n=23), fabric conditioners/laundry detergents for hand wash (n=8), dish-wash (n=10), furniture polish, car shampoo, stain remover (each n=1) and 2 products used in occupational environments. alpha-Isomethyl ionone was present in 5 products; quantification was not performed (10).

Twenty-five cosmetics and cosmetic toys for children (5 shampoos and shower gels, 6 perfumes, 1 deodorant (roll-on), 4 baby lotions/creams, 1 baby wipes product, 1 baby oil, 2 lipcare products and 5 toy-cosmetic products: a cosmetic-toy set for blending perfumes and a makeup set) purchased in 1997-1998 in retail outlets in Denmark, Germany, England and Sweden were analyzed in 1998 for the presence of fragrances by GC-MS. alpha-Isomethyl ionone was found in 9 products (36%) in a concentration range of ≤0.001-0.231% (w/w). For the analytical data in each product category, the original publication should be consulted (11).

Seventy fragranced deodorants, purchased at retail outlets in 5 European countries in 1996, were analyzed by gas chromatography - mass spectrometry (GC-MS) for the determination of the contents of 21 commonly used fragrance materials. alpha-Isomethyl ionone was identified in 43 products (61%) in a concentration range of 1–2765 ppm (9).

In 1992, in The Netherlands, the presence of fragrances was analyzed in 300 cosmetic products. alpha-Isomethyl ionone was identified in 63% of the products (rank order 7) (15).

In 1988, in the USA, 400 perfumes used in fine fragrances, household products and soaps (number of products per category not mentioned) were analyzed for the presence of fragrance chemicals in a concentration of at least 1% and a list of the Top-25 (present in the highest number of products) presented. alpha-Isomethyl ionone was found to be present in 51% of the fine fragrances (rank number 10), 50% of the household product fragrances (rank number 9) and 64% of the fragrances used in soaps (rank number 8) (13).

OTHER SIDE EFFECTS

Immediate-type reactions

A female patient complained that application of her rouge, which she had used for many years without ill-effects, caused irritation and swelling of the face, starting after about one hour, the edema lasting for several hours. A closed patch test with rouge was negative, as was an open test in the antecubital fossa. However, when the rouge was applied to the face in the usual manner, a mild but definite swelling appeared after 40 minutes, lasting for up to 3 hours. A scratch test on the volar aspect of the lower arm with 0.9% NaCl solution, rubbed in with rouge, showed a wheal of 6 mm after 1 hour (control with saline only: 2 mm). Control tests in 2 persons showed a 1-2 mm wheal in both tests. Later, the ingredients of the rouge were patch tested separately: a strongly positive reaction was noted to alpha-isomethyl ionone 10% in petrolatum. However, an open test with this fragrance chemical on the face was negative; the other 18 ingredients of the rouge were not tested in this way, as the patient refused further investigations (40).

LITERATURE

1   Bruze M, Svedman C, Andersen KE, Bruynzeel D, Goossens A, Johansen JD, et al. Patch test concentrations (doses in mg/cm2) for the 12 non-mix fragrance substances regulated by European legislation. Contact Dermatitis 2012;66:131-136

2   Schnuch A, Uter W, Geier J, Lessmann H, Frosch PJ. Sensitization to 26 fragrances to be labelled according to current European regulation: Results of the IVDK and review of the literature. Contact Dermatitis 2007;57:1-10

3   Oosten EJ van, Schuttelaar ML, Coenraads PJ. Clinical relevance of positive patch test reactions to the 26 EU-labelled fragrances. Contact Dermatitis 2009;61:217-223

4   Yazar K, Johnsson S, Lind M-L, Boman A, Lidén C. Preservatives and fragrances in selected consumer-available cosmetics and detergents. Contact Dermatitis 2011;64:265-272

5   Various SCCS opinions on α-Isomethyl ionone have been published and are available at: http://ec.europa.eu/growth/tools-databases/cosing/index.cfm?fuseaction=search.details_v2&id=27939

6   SCCS (Scientific Committee on Consumer Safety). Opinion on Fragrance allergens in cosmetic products, 26-27 June 2012, SCCS/1459/11. Available at: https://ec.europa.eu/health/sites/health/files/scientific_committees/consumer_safety/docs/sccs_o_102.pdf

7   De Groot AC, Liem DH, Nater JP, van Ketel WG. Patch tests with fragrance materials and preservatives. Contact Dermatitis 1985;12:87-92

8   Hostýnek JJ, Maibach HI. Is there evidence that alpha-isomethylionone causes allergic contact dermatitis? Exog Dermatol 2004;3:121-125

9   Rastogi SC, Johansen JD, Frosch P, Menné T, Bruze M, Lepoittevin JP, et al. Deodorants on the European market: quantitative chemical analysis of 21 fragrances. Contact Dermatitis 1998;38:29-35

10   Rastogi SC, Heydorn S, Johansen JD, Basketter DA. Fragrance chemicals in domestic and occupational products. Contact Dermatitis 2001;45:221-225

11   Rastogi SC, Johansen JD, Menné T, Frosch P, Bruze M, Andersen KE, et al. Content of fragrance allergens in children's cosmetics and cosmetic toys. Contact Dermatitis 1999;41:84-88

12   De Groot AC. Contact allergy to cosmetics: causative ingredients. Contact Dermatitis 1987;17:26-34

13   Fenn RS. Aroma chemical usage trends in modern perfumery. Perfumer and Flavorist 1989;14:3-10

14   Buckley DA. Fragrance ingredient labelling in products on sale in the UK. Br J Dermatol 2007;157:295-300

15   Weyland JW. Personal Communication, 1992. Cited in: De Groot AC, Weyland JW, Nater JP. Unwanted effects of cosmetics and drugs used in dermatology, 3rd Ed. Amsterdam: Elsevier, 1994: 579

16   Uter W, Yazar K, Kratz E-M, Mildau G, Lidén C. Coupled exposure to ingredients of cosmetic products: I. Fragrances. Contact Dermatitis 2013;69:335-341

17   Bennike NH, Oturai NB, Müller S, Kirkeby CS, Jørgensen C, Christensen AB, et al. Fragrance contact allergens in 5588 cosmetic products identified through a novel smartphone application. J Eur Acad Dermatol Venereol 2018;32:79-85

18   Rastogi SC, Hellerup Jensen G, Johansen JD. Survey and risk assessment of chemical substances in deodorants. Survey of Chemical Substances in Consumer Products, No. 86 2007. Danish Ministry of the Environment, Environmental Protection Agency. Available at: https://www2.mst.dk/Udgiv/publications/2007/978-87-7052-625-8/pdf/978-87-7052-626-5.pdf

19   De Groot AC, Bruynzeel DP, Bos JD, van der Meeren HL, van Joost T, Jagtman BA, Weyland JW. The allergens in cosmetics. Arch Dermatol 1988;124:1525-1529

20 De Groot AC. Adverse reactions to cosmetics. PhD Thesis, University of Groningen, The Netherlands: 1988, chapter 3.4, pp.105-113

21 An S, Lee AY, Lee CH, Kim DW, Hahm JH, Kim KJ, et al. Fragrance contact dermatitis in Korea: a joint study. Contact Dermatitis 2005;53:320-323

22 Poulsen PB, Schmidt A. A survey and health assessment of cosmetic products for children. Survey of chemical substances in consumer products, No. 88. Copenhagen: Danish Environmental Protection Agency, 2007. Available at: https://www2.mst.dk/udgiv/publications/2007/978-87-7052-638-8/pdf/978-87-7052-639-5.pdf

23 VWA. Dutch Food and Consumer Product Safety Authority. Cosmetische producten voor kinderen: Inventarisatie van de markt en de veiligheidsborging door producenten en importeurs. Report ND04o065/ND05o170, 2007 (Report in Dutch), 2007. Available at: www.nvwa.nl/documenten/communicatie/inspectieresultaten/consument/2016m/cosmetische- producten-voor-kinderen

24 Rastogi SC. Survey of chemical compounds in consumer products. Contents of selected fragrance materials in cleaning products and other consumer products. Survey no. 8-2002. Copenhagen, Denmark, Danish Environmental Protection Agency. Available at: http://eng.mst.dk/media/mst/69131/8.pdf

25 Bouma K, Van Peursem AJJ. Marktonderzoek naleving detergenten verordening voor textielwasmiddelen. Dutch Food and Consumer Products Safety Authority (VWA) Report ND06K173, 2006 [in Dutch]. Available at: http://docplayer.nl/41524125-Marktonderzoek-naleving-detergenten-verordening-voor-textielwasmiddel-en.html

26 Pors J, Fuhlendorff R. Mapping of chemical substances in air fresheners and other fragrance liberating products. Report Danish Ministry of the Environment, Environmental Protection Agency (EPA). Survey of Chemicals in Consumer Products, No 30, 2003. Available at: http://eng.mst.dk/media/mst/69113/30.pdf

27 Nakayama H. Fragrance hypersensitivity and its control. In: Frosch PJ, Johansen JD, White IR, Eds. Fragrances - beneficial and adverse effects. Berlin Heidelberg New York: Springer-Verlag, 1998:83-91

28 Dinkloh A, Worm M, Geier J, Schnuch A, Wollenberg A. Contact sensitization in patients with suspected cosmetic intolerance: results of the IVDK 2006-2011. J Eur Acad Dermatol Venereol 2015;29:1071-1081

29 Bennike NH, Zachariae C, Johansen JD. Non-mix fragrances are top sensitizers in consecutive dermatitis patients – a cross-sectional study of the 26 EU-labelled fragrance allergens. Contact Dermatitis 2017;77:270-279

30 Mann J, McFadden JP, White JML, White IR, Banerjee P. Baseline series fragrance markers fail to predict contact allergy. Contact Dermatitis 2014;70:276-281

31 Uter W, Johansen JD, Börje A, Karlberg A-T, Lidén C, Rastogi S, Roberts D, White IR. Categorization of fragrance contact allergens for prioritization of preventive measures: clinical and experimental data and consideration of structure–activity relationships. Contact Dermatitis 2013;69:196-230

32 Nagtegaal MJC, Pentinga SE, Kuik J, Kezic S, Rustemeyer T. The role of the skin irritation response in polysensitization to fragrances. Contact Dermatitis 2012;67:28-35

33 Nardelli A, Drieghe J, Claes L, Boey L, Goossens A. Fragrance allergens in 'specific' cosmetic products. Contact Dermatitis 2011;64:212-219

34 Klaschka U. Contact allergens for armpits - allergenic fragrances specified on deodorants. Int J Hyg Environ Health 2012;215:584-591

35 De Groot AC, Schmidt E. Essential oils: contact allergy and chemical composition. Boca Raton, Fl., USA: CRC Press, Taylor and Francis Group, 2016 (ISBN 9781482246407)

36 Opinion of the Scientific Committee on Cosmetic Products and Non-Food Products Intended for Consumers concerning 'The 1st update of the inventory of ingredients employed in cosmetic products. Section II: Perfume and aromatic raw materials', 24 October 2000, SCCNFP/0389/00, final. Available at: http://ec.europa.eu/health/ph_risk/committees/sccp/documents/out131_en.pdf

37 Wieck S, Olsson O, Kümmerer K, Klaschka U. Fragrance allergens in household detergents. Regul Toxicol Pharmacol 2018;97:163-169

38 Ung CY, White JML, White IR, Banerjee P, McFadden JP. Patch testing with the European baseline series fragrance markers: a 2016 update. Br J Dermatol 2018;178:776-780

39 Bernaola G, Escayol P, Fernandez E, Fernandez de Corrés L. Contact dermatitis from methylionone fragrance. Contact Dermatitis 1989;20:71-72

40 De Groot AC, Liem DH. Contact urticaria to rouge. Contact Dermatitis 1983;9:322

41 Dittmar D, Schuttelaar MLA. Contact sensitization to hydroperoxides of limonene and linalool: Results of consecutive patch testing and clinical relevance. Contact Dermatitis 2018 Oct 31. doi: 10.1111/cod.13137. [Epub ahead of print]

Chapter 3.93   ISOPULEGOL

IDENTIFICATION

Description/definition : Isopulegol is the organic compound that conforms to the structural formula shown below
Chemical class(es) : Alcohols
Chemical/IUPAC name : 5-Methyl-2-prop-1-en-2-ylcyclohexan-1-ol
Other names : *p*-Menth-8-en-3-ol
CAS registry number(s) : 7786-67-6; 89-79-2
EC number(s) : 232-102-8; 201-940-6
RIFM monograph(s) : Food Chem Toxicol 2016;97(11)(suppl.):S129-S135; Food Chem Toxicol 2008;46(11)(suppl.):S185-S189; Food Chem Toxicol 2008;46(11)(suppl.):S1-S71; Food Cosmet Toxicol 1975;13:823 (special issue II)
Function(s) in cosmetics : EU: masking. USA: flavoring agents; fragrance ingredients
Patch testing : 5% pet. (1); based on RIFM data, 8% pet. is probably not irritant (2)
Molecular formula : $C_{10}H_{18}O$

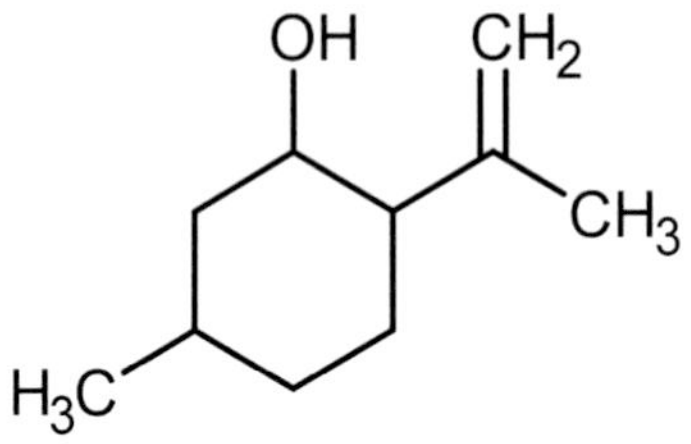

GENERAL

Isopulegol is a colorless clear liquid; its odor type is minty and its odor is described as 'minty, cooling, medicinal, woody with a green herbaceous undernote' (www.thegoodscentscompany.com).

Presence in essential oils

Isopulegol has been identified by chemical analysis in 27 of 91 essential oils, which have caused contact allergy / allergic contact dermatitis. In none of these oils, it belonged to the 'Top-10' of ingredients with the highest concentrations (3).

CONTACT ALLERGY

Patch testing in groups of patients

Patch testing in consecutive patients suspected of contact dermatitis: routine testing

Studies in which isopulegol was patch tested in consecutive patients suspected of contact dermatitis (routine testing) with positive results have not been found.

Testing in groups of selected patients

In a group of 20 patients allergic to fragrances and tested with a battery of fragrance materials, two (10%) reacted to isopulegol 5% pet. (1).

Case reports and case series

Case reports of allergic contact dermatitis from isopulegol have not been found.

LITERATURE

1   Larsen WG. Perfume dermatitis. A study of 20 patients. Arch Dermatol 1977;113:623-626
2   De Groot AC. Patch Testing, 4th Edition. Wapserveen, The Netherlands: acdegroot publishing, 2018 (ISBN 978-90-813233-4-5)
3   De Groot AC, Schmidt E. Essential oils: contact allergy and chemical composition. Boca Raton, Fl., USA: CRC Press, Taylor and Francis Group, 2016 (ISBN 9781482246407)

Chapter 3.94   ISOSAFROLE *
* Not officially an INCI name

IDENTIFICATION

Description/definition : Isosafrole is the bicyclic organic compound that conforms to the structural formula shown below

Chemical class(es) : Heterocyclic compounds; unsaturated compounds

INCI name USA : Neither in Cosing nor in the Personal Care Products Council Ingredient Database

Chemical/IUPAC name : 5-[(E or Z)-prop-1-enyl]-1,3-benzodioxole

CAS registry number(s) : 120-58-1; 4043-71-4 ((E)-isosafrole, beta-isosafrole); 17627-76-8 ((Z)-isosafrole, alpha-isosafrole)

EC number(s) : 204-410-2; 241-611-4 ((Z)-isosafrole, alpha-isosafrole)

RIFM monograph(s) : Food Cosmet Toxicol 1976;14:329 (binder, page 475)

IFRA standard : Restricted and prohibited; isosafrole as such should not be used as a fragrance ingredient; essential oils containing isosafrole should not be used at a level that the total concentration of isosafrole exceeds 0.01% in consumer products; the total concentration of isosafrole, safrole and dihydrosafrole should not exceed 0.01% in consumer products (www.ifraorg.org/en-us/standards-library)

Merck Index monograph : 6539

Patch testing : No patch test data available; based on RIFM data, 8% pet. is probably not irritant (1)

Molecular formula : $C_{10}H_{10}O_2$

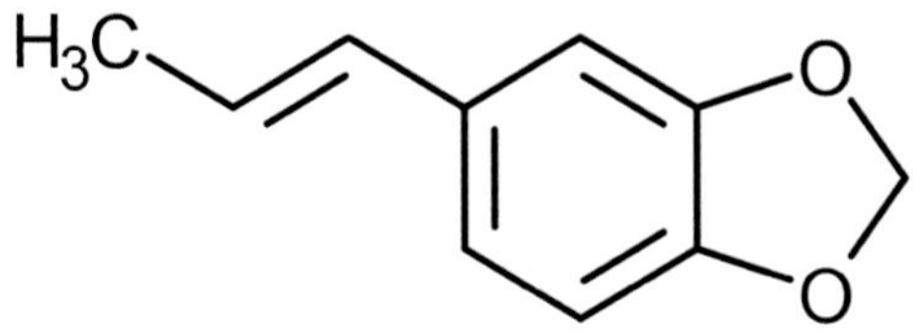

GENERAL

Isosafrole is a colorless to pale yellow clear liquid; its odor type is spicy and its odor at 10% in dipropylene glycol is described as 'sweet sassafrass spicy' (www.thegoodscentscompany.com). It is not used as fragrance ingredient because of carcinogenicity. Examples of essential oils with a high safrole content are Sassafras oil (*Sassafras officinale* Nees & Eberm.), Ocotea cymbarum oil (*Ocotea odorifera* (Vell.) Rohwer, synonym: *Ocotea pretiosa* Mez) and certain qualities of camphor oils.

Presence in essential oils

Isosafrole has been identified by chemical analysis in 3 of 91 essential oils, which have caused contact allergy / allergic contact dermatitis: laurel leaf oil, sweet orange oil and ylang-ylang oil. In none of these oils, isosafrole belonged to the 'Top-10' of ingredients with the highest concentrations which may be expected in commercial essential oils of this type (1). In fact, in all 3 oils, it was found in one publication each only and at very low concentrations, so the question may be raised whether the analytical identification has been correct.

CONTACT ALLERGY

Patch testing in groups of patients

Patch testing in consecutive patients suspected of contact dermatitis: routine testing
Studies in which isosafrole was patch tested in consecutive patients suspected of contact dermatitis (routine testing) with positive results have not been found.

Testing in groups of selected patients
In a group of 43 patients allergic to Myroxylon pereirae resin (balsam of Peru) and tested with isosafrole 5% pet., there was one positive reaction; this patient also reacted to safrole (8).

Case reports and case series

Case reports of allergic contact dermatitis from isosafrole have not been found.

Pigmented cosmetic dermatitis

In Japan, in the 1960s and 1970s, many female patients developed pigmentation of the face after having facial dermatitis (5). The skin manifestations of this so-called pigmented cosmetic dermatitis consisted of diffuse or patchy brown hyperpigmentation on the cheeks and/or forehead, sometimes the entire face was involved. In severe cases, the pigmentation was black, purple, or blue-black, and in mild cases, it was pale brown. Occasionally, erythematous macules or papules, suggesting a mild contact dermatitis, were observed and itching was also noted at varying times.

Pigmented cosmetic dermatitis was shown to be caused by contact allergy to components of cosmetic products, notably essential oils, other fragrance materials, antimicrobials, preservatives and coloring materials (4,5,6). In 1975, isosafrole was discovered to be one of the causative fragrance materials (3). The number of patients with pigmented cosmetic dermatitis decreased strongly after 1978, when major cosmetic companies began to eliminate strong contact sensitizers from their products (4). Since 1980, pigmented cosmetic dermatitis became a rare disease in Japan (7).

Cross-reactions, pseudo-cross-reactions and co-reactions

For general information on cross-/pseudo-cross-/co-reactivity of fragrance chemicals with other fragrances, fragrance markers (fragrance mix I, fragrance mix II, colophonium, Myroxylon pereirae resin [balsam of Peru]) and essential oils see Chapter 1.2 General information on cross-reactions, pseudo-cross-reactions and co-reactions.

Co-reactivity with safrole has been observed (8).

LITERATURE

1   De Groot AC, Schmidt E. Essential oils: contact allergy and chemical composition. Boca Raton, Fl., USA: CRC Press, Taylor and Francis Group, 2016 (ISBN 9781482246407)
2   De Groot AC. Patch Testing, 4th Edition. Wapserveen, The Netherlands: acdegroot publishing, 2018
3   Nakayama H. Fragrance hypersensitivity and its control. In: Frosch PJ, Johansen JD, White IR, Eds. Fragrances - beneficial and adverse effects. Berlin Heidelberg New York: Springer-Verlag, 1998:83-91
4   Nakayama H, Matsuo S, Hayakawa K, Takhashi K, Shigematsu T, Ota S. Pigmented cosmetic dermatitis. Int J Dermatol 1984;23:299-305
5   Nakayama H, Harada R, Toda M. Pigmented cosmetic dermatitis. Int J Dermatol 1976;15:673-675
6   Nakayama H, Hanaoka H, Ohshiro A. Allergen Controlled System. Tokyo: Kanehara Shuppan, 1974
7   Ebihara T, Nakayama H. Pigmented contact dermatitis. Clin Dermatol 1997;15:593-599
8   Hjorth N. Eczematous allergy to balsams. Acta Derm Venereol 1961;41(suppl.46):1-216

Chapter 3.95   LIMONENE

Limonene (INCI name EU, USA) has three forms: the isomers *D*-limonene ((*R*)-limonene, (+)-limonene) and *L*-limonene ((*S*)-limonene, (-)-limonene) and their racemic mixture *DL*-limonene (dipentene).

LIMONENE (general)

IDENTIFICATION

Chemical class(es)	: Hydrocarbons
SCCS opinion(s)	: SCCNFP/0392/00, final (18)
Merck Index monograph	: 6816
Function(s) in cosmetics	: EU: perfuming. USA: fragrance ingredients; solvents
IFRA standard	: Restricted; *D*-, *L*- and *DL*-limonene and natural products containing substantial amounts of it, should only be used when the level of peroxides is kept to the lowest practical level, for instance by adding antioxidants at the time of production; such products should have a peroxide value of less than 20 millimoles peroxides per liter, determined according to the FMA method (www.ifraorg.org/en-us/standards-library)
SCCS opinion(s)	: SCCS/1459/11 (19); SCCNFP/0389/00, final (110)
EU cosmetic restrictions	: Regulated in Annex III/88 of the Regulation (EC) No. 1223/2009, regulated by 2003/15/EC; Must be labeled on cosmetics and detergent products, if present at > 10 ppm (0.001%) in leave-on products and > 100 ppm (0.01%) in rinse-off products
Patch testing	: *D*-limonene 2% Pet. (SmartPracticeEurope); 2% and 3% pet. (SmartPracticeCanada); 10% pet. (Chemo); hydroperoxides 0.2% and 0.3% pet. (Chemotechnique); using the hydroperoxides is preferred; it has been recommended to add limonene hydroperoxides 0.3% pet. to the European (121) and British baseline series (115); most recently (November 2018); the European Environmental Contact Dermatitis Research Group (EECDRG) has recommended limonene hydroperoxides 0.2% and 0.3% as addition to the European baseline series (125); concentrations of limonene 5% (or higher) in alcohol may be (strongly) irritant in patch testing (12); 8% of allergies to limonene hydroperoxides are missed when the reaction is not read at day 7 (120)
Molecular formula	: $C_{10}H_{16}$

DL-LIMONENE *

* Not officially an INCI name but perfuming name

IDENTIFICATION

Description/definition	: *DL*-Limonene is the terpene that conforms to the structural formula shown below
Chemical/IUPAC name	: 1-Methyl-4-prop-1-en-2-ylcyclohexene
Other names	: 1,8(9)-*p*-Menthadiene; *p*-mentha-1,8-diene; 1-methyl-4-isopropenyl-1-cyclohexene; dipentene; cajeputene
CAS registry number(s)	: 138-86-3
EC number(s)	: 205-341-0
RIFM Monograph(s)	: Food Cosmet Toxicol 1974;12:703

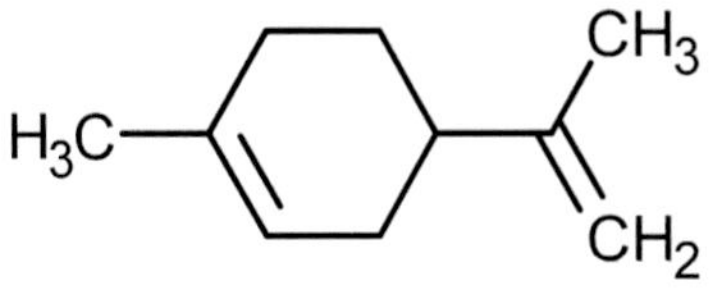

D-LIMONENE *

* Not officially an INCI name but perfuming name

IDENTIFICATION

Description/definition	: *D*-Limonene is the terpene that conforms to the structural formula shown below
Chemical/IUPAC name	: (4*R*)-1-Methyl-4-prop-1-en-2-ylcyclohexene

Other names   : (R)-p-Mentha-1,8-diene; (4R)-1-methyl-4-(1-methylethenyl)cyclohexene; (R)-limonene;
                           α-limonene; (+)-limonene
CAS registry number(s)   : 5989-27-5; 7705-13-7
EC number(s)   : 227-813-5
RIFM monograph(s)   : Food Cosmet Toxicol 1975;13:825 (special issue II)

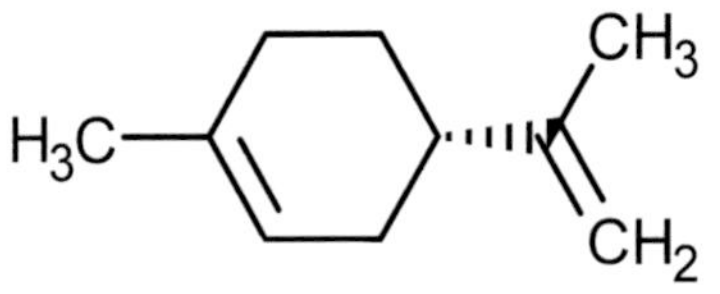

L-LIMONENE *
* Not officially an INCI name but perfuming name

IDENTIFICATION
Description/definition   : L-Limonene is the terpene that conforms to the structural formula shown below
Chemical/IUPAC name   : (4S)-1-Methyl-4-prop-1-en-2-ylcyclohexene
Other names   : (S)-p-Mentha-1,8-diene; (S)-limonene; β-limonene; (-)-limonene
CAS registry number(s)   : 5989-54-8
EC number(s)   : 227-815-6

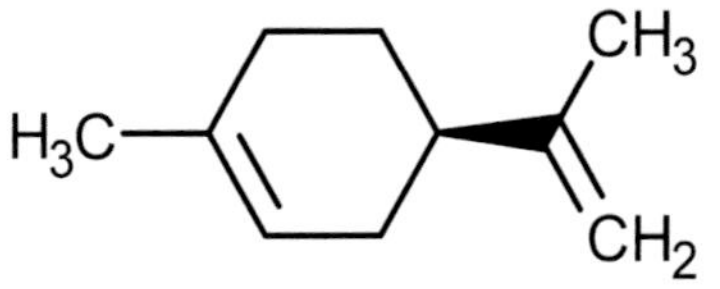

GENERAL
Limonene is a colorless clear liquid; its odor type is citrus and its odor at 100% is described as 'citrus herbal terpene camphor' (www.thegoodscentscompany.com). Limonene is found in many natural oils and fruits including orange, lemons and grapefruit (see below). Limonene is a natural emission of eucalyptus trees, needle-leaf trees, broad-leaf trees, shrubs, grasses and crops. It is present in wood smoke, tobacco, and tobacco smoke.

Limonene, often obtained as a by-product from the citrus juice industry, is an important commercial chemical that is used in many food products, soaps, perfumes and cleaning household products. Other uses include the synthesis of other chemicals, as a solvent, an industrial degreasing agent (often in a concentration up to 95%) before industrial painting and for cleaning assemblies, in therapeutic transdermal delivery systems as a penetration enhancer, in water-free hand cleansers, in chemicals used for histologic and cytologic specimen preparation, in tobacco substitute products and formerly as an ingredient in insect repellants, dog and cat repellants, and insecticides (U.S. National Library of Medicine, 5,10).

Presence in essential oils, Myroxylon pereirae resin (balsam of Peru) and propolis
D-Limonene is the main constituent of cold-pressed essential peel oils from citrus fruits, which contain 70-96% of this chemical. Limonene has been identified by chemical analysis in 88 of 91 essential oils, which have caused contact allergy / allergic contact dermatitis. In 49 oils, limonene belonged to the 'Top-10' of ingredients with the highest concentrations. These are shown in table 3.95.1 with the concentration range which may be expected in commercial essential oils of this type (23). Limonene may also be present in Myroxylon pereirae resin (balsam of Peru) (108) and in propolis (109).

CONTACT ALLERGY

General
The SCCS (Scientific Committee on Consumer Safety), in a 2012 Opinion on Fragrance allergens in cosmetic products, has marked DL-limonene (non-oxidized) as 'established contact allergen in humans' (19,70). The sensitizing potency of D-limonene (with low levels of oxidation) was classified as 'moderate' based on an EC3 value of <10% in the LLNA (local lymph node assay) in animal experiments, in another experiment as weak (EC3 30%); however, D-limonene oxidized for 10 weeks was a moderate sensitizer based on an EC3 value of 3.0% (19,70).

Limonene acts as a prehapten, which is a chemical that is itself non-sensitizing or low-sensitizing, but that is transformed into a hapten outside the skin by chemical transformation (air oxidation; photoactivation) and without the requirement for specific enzymatic systems (97). Indeed, limonene itself (pure) has a very low sensitizing capacity (8,10). However, both enantiomers, R-(+)- and S-(-)-limonene spontaneously autoxidize on air exposure to oxidation products such as limonene-1,2-oxide (a mixture of cis- and trans-isomers), limonene hydroperoxides, carvone and cis- and trans-carveol (9,10). Four main hydroperoxides are formed upon autoxidation of D-limonene: cis-p-mentha-2,8-diene-1-hydroperoxide, trans-p-mentha-2,8-diene-1-hydroperoxide (cis- and trans-limonene-1-hydroperoxide), cis-p-mentha-6,8-diene-2-hydroperoxide and trans-p-mentha-6,8-diene-2-hydroperoxide (cis- and trans-limonene-2-hydroperoxide); in addition, there are trace amounts of cis-p-mentha[1(7),8]-diene-2-hydroperoxide and trans-p-mentha[1(7),8]-diene-2-hydroperoxide (9,10,31).

The allergenicity of limonene is closely related to this oxidation process. The primary oxidation products formed, the hydroperoxides (limonene-1-hydroperoxide, limonene-2-hydroperoxide) are strong and clinically relevant contact allergens (5,9,10,25,26,27,104). Limonene-1-hydroperoxide is the stronger sensitizer (104) and clinically the most important allergen (105). Both hydroperoxides are unstable and readily degrade to secondary stable oxidation products such as carvone and carveol (5). R-(-)-Carvone is also a potent sensitizer in animal experiments, but cis- and trans-carveol have no or very little sensitizing capacity (10). If the oxidation process continues, polymers are created and the liquid will become viscous (3). The addition of an antioxidant such as BHT to limonene or limonene-containing products can prevent autoxidation for periods depending on the purity of the products and on the room temperature. Cold and dark storage of D-limonene in closed vessels can prevent autoxidation for one year without addition of anti-oxidant (16).

Oxidized d-limonene is more irritant than non-oxidized D-limonene; for the oxidized material when patch tested, irritation was found to start to increase at 5% pet. (44).

Table 3.95.1 Essential oils containing limonene in the 'Top-10' and concentration range in commercial oils (23)

Essential oil	Concentration range (min.-max.)	Essential oil	Concentration range (min.-max.)
Tangerine oil	81.8 - 97.8%	Cardamom oil	2.0 - 7.0%
Orange oil sweet	94.7 - 95.7%	Rosemary oil	0.7 - 6.7%
Orange oil bitter	92.2 - 95.6%	Sage oil Dalmatian	0.4 - 6.2%
Grapefruit oil	81.1 - 95.5%	Sage oil Spanish	2.0 - 6.0%
Mandarin oil	64.0 - 76.4%	Citronella oil Java	2.5 - 5.9%
Lemon oil	53.5 - 73.0%	Lemongrass oil East Indian	0.1 - 5.7%
Elemi oil	33.0 - 58.4%	Lemongrass oil West Indian	0.4 - 5.0%
Silver fir oil	6.1 - 54.7%	Turpentine oil	traces - 5.0%
Bergamot oil	31.4 - 45.1%	Nutmeg oil	3.8 - 4.5%
Pine needle oil	3.1 - 30.1%	Laurel leaf oil	1.0 - 4.0%
Black pepper oil	10.2 - 24.7%	Black cumin oil	0.08 - 3.7%
Dwarf pine oil	0.6 - 24.2%	Coriander fruit oil	1.0 - 3.6%
Spearmint oil	0.4 - 23.7%	Hyssop oil	1.0 - 3.5%
Neroli oil	10.1 - 20.3%	Aniseed oil	0.01 - 3.5%
Ravensara oil	0.08 - 19.4%	Star anise oil	0.2 - 3.3%
Olibanum oil	5.5 - 18.5%	Bay oil	2.4 - 3.2%
Peppermint oil	0.3 - 18.5%	Galbanum resin oil	0.4 - 3.2%
Litsea cubeba oil	6.4 - 15.6%	Spike lavender oil	0.2 - 3.0%
Angelica root oil	6.4 - 15.0%	Angelica fruit oil	2.3 - 2.9%
Eucalyptus globulus oil	4.5 - 12.9%	Thuja oil	1.1 - 2.7%
Cypress oil	0.1 - 10.8%	Petitgrain bigarade oil	0.3 - 2.6%
Citronella oil Sri Lanka	3.0 - 10.4%	Thyme oil Spanish	1.8 - 2.3%
Cajeput oil	1.8 - 10.2%	Palmarosa oil	0.1 - 1.4%
Niaouli oil	0.8 - 9.9%	Cassia oil	0.03 - 1.1%
Juniper berry oil	2.5 - 7.6%		

Patch testing in groups of patients

Results of patch testing limonene in consecutive patients suspected of contact dermatitis (routine testing) are shown in table 3.95.2 (non-oxidized limonene) and table 3.95.3 (oxidized limonene). Results of testing in groups of *selected* patients (e.g. patients with known or suspected fragrance or cosmetic dermatitis, individuals with eyelid dermatitis, patients with contact allergy to tea tree oil or turpentine oil [in which limonene is one of the sensitizers], car mechanics reporting hand eczema) are shown in table 3.95.4.

Testing in groups of patients: routine testing

Limonene non-oxidized

Limonene is a weak sensitizer (8,10) and results of patch testing with it are in accordance. In 10 studies in which limonene (non-oxidized) was routinely patch tested at 1%, 2%, 3% or 10% petrolatum, frequencies of sensitization have ranged from 0% to 1.6%, but 9 of 10 scored 0.7% or lower. The higher concentration of 1.6% was observed in an Australian population, which may have been selected (63). In the study with zero positives, the patients were also patch tested with oxidized limonene, which resulted in 2.8% positive reactions (5), testifying to the fact that patch testing with unoxidized limonene is highly unreliable. Few reactions were scored as relevant and culprit products were never mentioned (61,62,63,68).

Table 3.95.2 Patch testing in groups of patients: Routine testing (non-oxidized limonene)

Years and Country	Test conc. & vehicle	Number of patients tested	positive (%)		Selection of patients (S); Relevance (R); Comments (C)	Ref.
2015-7 Netherlands	2% pet.	821	1	(0.1%)	R: not stated	120
2013-2014 Thailand		312	2	(0.7%)	R: 50%	68
2011-12 NACDG	2% pet.	4230	9	(0.2%)	R: definite + probable relevance: 22%	61
2011-2012 UK	2% pet.	1951	1	(0.05%)	R: not stated	69
2011-2012 UK	10% pet.	4741	11	(0.2%)	R: not specified; 37% for linalool and limonene together positive to their hydroperoxides; the most important causative products for these reactions were fine fragrances, other cosmetics, detergents, essential oils and wet wipes; C: there were 6 (55%) co-reactions to limonene hydroperoxides	86
2009-10 NACDG	3% pet.	4304	4	(0.1%)	R: definite + probable relevance: 0%	62
2001-2010 Australia	1% pet.	3093	48	(1.6%)	R: 33%; C: possibly selected patients	63
2003-2004 IVDK	2% pet.	2396	3	(0.1%)	R: not stated	4
1998-2000 Six European countries	3% pet.	1606	9	(0.6%)	R: not stated	54
1977-1990 Belgium, Sweden, Spain, Portugal	10% pet. (?)	2273	0	(0%)	C: there were many reactions to *oxidized* limonene (see below)	5

IVDK: Informationsverbund Dermatologischer Kliniken (Germany, Switzerland, Austria)
NACDG: North American Contact Dermatitis Group (USA, Canada)

Limonene oxidized

Test preparations

Based on the increased sensitizing capacity of oxidized limonene and limonene hydroperoxides compared to pure limonene (9,10,19,70,104), higher frequencies of sensitization when testing with these materials could be anticipated. The results of such studies are shown in table 3.95.3. Test substances used have included oxidized limonene 2%, 3% and 5% and limonene hydroperoxides 0.1%, 0.2%, 0.3%, 0.5% and 1%, all in petrolatum. From 1991 to 2010, both oxidized limonene (containing limonene hydroperoxides) and limonene hydroperoxides, often in combination, were used for patch testing, sometimes in various concentrations to determine the optimal one (5,25,26,27,105,106). From 2011 on, all investigators, with one exception (75) have used limonene hydroperoxides, as this material had proven to be more suitable than oxidized limonene.

In two dose-finding investigations from Spain (37) and the United Kingdom (115), patients have been tested with three concentrations of limonene hydroperoxides (0.1%, 0.2% and 0.3%) and it was found that with rising concentrations, the percentages of positive patch test reactions also increased. In both studies, it was advised to use the 0.3% preparation for screening purposes and the authors of the UK study suggested to add limonene hydroperoxides 0.3% pet. to the British baseline series (115). Later, the EECDRG advised to add limonene hydroperoxides 0.3% pet., which by then had become commercially available, to the European baseline series (121).

Although it has convincingly been demonstrated that the 0.3% test material identifies a considerable number of allergic individuals not found by testing with the lower concentrations (37,115), it should be appreciated that the test material not infrequently causes irritant reactions and ?+ reactions (67,86,100,115,120), which are very hard to distinguish from each other and from true positive reactions. It is conceivable that, especially in the studies with the high frequencies of sensitization, a number of reactions judged to be 'allergic' have in fact been false-positive, irritant (117,120).

At this moment, the optimal test concentration for limonene hydroperoxides, which is now commercially available at 0.2% and 0.3% in petrolatum (www.chemotechnique.se), has not yet been established (125). When testing with 0.3% pet., the possibility of irritant reactions should always be kept in mind, also in case of ?+ reactions.

Table 3.95.3 Patch testing in groups of patients: Routine testing (oxidized limonene)

Years and Country	Test conc. & vehicle	Number of patients tested	positive (%)	Selection of patients (S); Relevance (R); Comments (C)	Ref.
2016-2018 UK	0.3% pet. hy-droperoxides	156	7 (4.5%)	R: 2/7 (29%)	114
2015-7 Netherlands	0.3% pet. hy-droperoxides	821	77 (9.4%)	R: certain 18%, probable 22%; C: there were 141 (17%) ?+ reactions and 7 (0.9%) irritant reactions	120
2015-2016 UK	3% pet.	2084	89 (4.3%)	R: not specified for individual fragrances; 25% of patients who reacted to any fragrance or fragrance marker had a positive fragrance history	75
2015-2016 Spain	0.1% pet.	3639	51 (1.4%)	R: 46% were currently relevant; most reactions to limonene and / or linalool were caused by cosmetics (including fine fragrances), a smaller number by detergents and wet wipes	37
	0.2% pet.	3639	124 (3.4%)		
	0.3% pet. all hydro-peroxides	3639	187 (5.1%)		
2012-2015 Denmark	0.3% pet. hy-droperoxides	4194	(2.5%)	R: present relevance 64%, past relevance 25%; current and/or past relevance: 76%; C: 13.7% doubtful positive reactions	100
2013-2014 UK	0.3% pet.	4563	241 (5.3%)	R: nearly 2/3 for all positives; C: 2.0% irritant reactions, 2.4% ?+ reactions	115
	0.2% pet.	4563	147 (3.2%)	C: 0.9% irritant reactions, 2.1% ?+ reactions	
	0.1% pet. all hydro-peroxides	4563	58 (1.3%)	C: 0.6% irritant reactions, 1.2% ?+ reactions	
2012-2014 UK	0.3% pet. hy-droperoxides	1292	65 (5.0%)	R: not stated; C: there were 4.3% ?+ and 9.8% irritant reactions	67
2011-2012 UK	0.3% pet. hy-droperoxides	4741	237 (5.0%)	R: 37% for linalool and limonene together; the most important causative products were fine fragrances, other cosmetics, detergents, essential oils and wet wipes; C: there were nearly 4% irritant reactions, but these included 'doubtful' reactions	86
2010-11 Denmark, Spain, Australia, UK, Sweden, Singapore	R-limonene, ox., 3% pet. with 0.33% hydroper-oxides	2900	152 (5.2%)	R: not stated; C: range of positive reactions: 2.3-12.1%; 7% (range: 0-24.5%) doubtful reactions, a number of which were probably weak positive patch test reactions, according to the authors; conversely, it may indicate that the test substance was marginal irritant and some positive reactions were false-positive	106
2007-2009 Sweden	R- 3% pet. [d]	763	9 (1.2%)	R: of 25 patients reacting to one or more of the limonene test substances, 11 (44%) had relevant reactions: 6 from cosmetics, 1 painter, one from a cleanser and 3 from occupational contact in the food industry	105
	1-OOH 0.5%	763	18 (2.4%)		
	2-OOH 0.5%, both in pet.	763	13 (1.7%)		
2000-2001 Belgium, Sweden, UK, Ger-many and Denmark	R- 3% pet. [d]	2411	41 (1.7%)	R: about 50% had a certain or probable history of adverse reactions to fragrances; C: 63 patients (2.6%) reacted to one of the two test materials; 28 reacted to both; 33% co-reactivity to fragrance mix I, 29% to Myroxylon pereirae resin	27
	S- 3% pet. [e]	2411	36 (1.5%)		
1997-1999 Belgium, Sweden, Spain, Portugal	see right column	2273	63 (2.8%)	R: 97% probable or certain relevance; C: the patients were patch tested with 4 materials: 3% oxidized D-limonene and 0.5% D-limonene hydroperoxide fraction in both stabilized and nonstabilized petrolatum; the 63 patients reacted to one or more of the 4 patch test materials; frequencies varied from 0.3% in Portugal to 6.5% in Spain; when retested, 18/30 patients (60%) again reacted positively; there were no reactions to pure (= non-oxidized) D-limonene; in Belgium, of 33 allergic patients, 19 (58%) co-reacted to the fragrance mix I	5,25
1991-1995 Sweden, Belgium	5% pet. [a]	277	14 (5.1%)	R: not stated; C: in Sweden, 2.4% of the patients reacted to any of the test substances versus 1.1% in Belgium; it was stated that a marginally irritant effect may be responsible for some of the 'positive' reactions	26
	3% pet. [a]	1366	22 (1.6%)		
	2% pet. [a]	154	2 (1.3%)		
	5% pet. [b]	426	4 (0.9%)		
	3% pet. [b]	369	6 (1.6%)		
	2% pet. [b]	208	0		
	1% pet. [c]	317	10 (3.2%)		
	0.5% pet. [c]	1237	13 (1.1%)		

[a] D-limonene oxidized for 10 weeks; [b] D-limonene oxidized for 20 weeks; [c] D-limonene hydroperoxides; [d] w/w oxidation mixture of R-(+)-limonene (D-limonene); [e] w/w oxidation mixture of S-(-)-limonene (L-limonene)

1-OOH: limonene-1-hydroperoxide in petrolatum; 2-OOH: limonene-2-hydroperoxide in petrolatum

In the case of such reactions or when otherwise in doubt, repeat testing, testing with a dilution series (or 0.2% pet., which has been recommended as an addition to the European baseline series in combination with 0.3% by the European Environmental Contact Dermatitis Research Group [125]) and studies with ROATs should be performed to reliably distinguish allergic from irritant reactions. Conversely, it has been suggested, in view of the large proportion of ?+ reactions, to increase the concentration, albeit the authors warned for the possibility of active sensitization (120).

Frequencies of sensitization

The results of routine patch testing with any limonene material in any concentration are shown in table 3.95.3 (previous page). In studies in which oxidized limonene 3% pet. was used, frequencies of sensitization – in order of decreasing rates – were 5.2% (106), 4.3% (75), 1.6% (26) and 1.2% (105). Patch testing with limonene hydroperoxides 0.3% pet. has shown – in order of decreasing frequencies – the following rates of sensitization: 9.4% (120), 5.3% (115), 5.1% (37), 5.0% (67,86), 4.5% (114), and 2.5% (100).

Relevance and causative products

In 7 of the 13 available studies, no (specific) relevance data were provided. In the investigations that did address this issue, percentages of the reactions to limonene considered to be relevant (sometimes definite + probable) ranged from 29 to 97% (5,25,37,100,105,114,120). Culprit products were mentioned in three investigations only. Most reactions were to fine fragrances and other cosmetics. Other causative products were detergents, essential oils, wet wipes, a cleanser and foods (37,86,105).

Table 3.95.4 Patch testing in groups of patients: Selected patient groups

Years and Country	Test conc. & vehicle	Number of patients tested	Number of patients positive (%)	Selection of patients (S); Relevance (R); Comments (C)	Ref.
2006-2011 IVDK	2% pet.	704	4 (0.6%)	S: patients with suspected cosmetic intolerance; R: not stated	64
2005-2008 IVDK	2% pet.	1241	(0.3%)	S: not specified; R: not stated	72
1999-2003 Germany	5% DEP	20	11 (55%)	S: patients with a positive patch test reaction to oxidized tea tree oil 5% DEP	15
2001-2 Denmark, Sweden	3% pet.	658	6 (0.9%)	S: consecutive patients with hand eczema; R: it was assumed that nearly all positive reactions were of present or past relevance; C: oxidized L-limonene was used for patch testing	13
	3% pet.	658	5 (0.8%)	S and R: see above; C: oxidized D-limonene was used for patch testing	
1999-2000 Germany, Austria	5% DEP	10	4 (40%)	S: patients with a positive patch test reaction to oxidized tea tree oil 5% DEP	11
<1999 Germany	5% vehicle?	16	1 (7%)	S: patients allergic to tea tree oil	14
1990-1992 Germany	1% and 5% alc.	7	6 (86%)	S: patients with a positive patch test reaction to tea tree oil 1% alc.; the test substances was D-limonene	12
1985 Spain	1% alc.	67	7 (10%)	S: patients allergic to turpentine oil; R: not specified; C: the test substance was L-limonene	81
	1% alc.	67	6 (9%)	S: patients allergic to turpentine oil; R: not specified; C: the test substance was D-limonene	
1984 The Netherlands	10% pet.	179	2 (1.1%)	S: patients suspected of cosmetic allergy; R: not stated; C: D-limonene was used for patch testing	20
1979-1983 Portugal	2% pet.	22	15 (68%)	S: patients allergic to turpentine oil; R: not stated	80
1976 Poland	1% pet.	15	3 (20%)	S: patients with positive patch tests to star anise oil 1% pet., negative to 0.5% but positive to one or more 'balsams' (Myroxylon pereirae resin, turpentine, wood tars, colophonium); C: limonene may be present in commercial star anise oils in a maximum concentration of 3.3% (23).	79
Oxidized limonene					
2014-2016 France		264	14 (5.3%)	S: patients suspected of eyelid allergic contact dermatitis; R: 6/14 (43%)	111
2014-2016 USA	0.3% pet. hy- Droperoxides	90	7 (8%)	S: patients suspected of fragrance allergy; R: probable relevance in 3/7 (42%) patients	98
1990 Sweden	D-, 5% pet., oxidized	105	2 (1.9%)	S: car mechanics reporting hand eczema; R: not mentioned, but it was stated that limonene '.. is used as a solvent and can be found in cleansing agents'	36

DEP: Diethyl phthalate
IVDK: Informationsverbund Dermatologischer Kliniken (Germany, Switzerland, Austria)

Patch testing in groups of selected patients

Results of testing in groups of selected patients (e.g. patients with known or suspected fragrance or cosmetic dermatitis, individuals with eyelid dermatitis, patients with contact allergy to tea tree oil or turpentine oil, car mechanics reporting hand eczema) are shown in table 3.95.4 (previous page). Limonene is a sensitizer in both tea tree oil (45) and turpentine oil. In groups of patients allergic to (oxidized) tea tree oil and patch tested with a number of its ingredients, 86% (12), 55% (15), 40% (11) and 7% (14) reacted to limonene (mean, adjusted for sample size: 40% [45]). In groups of patients previously reacting to turpentine oil, 10% (81) and 68% (80) reacted to limonene. In other groups of selected patients, generally low rates of sensitization to limonene have been observed, but in a 2014-2016 study from the USA, 7 of 90 (8%) patients suspected to be allergic to fragrances reacted to limonene hydroperoxides 0.3% pet. (98).

In most studies, no (specific) data on relevance were provided. In the investigations that did address the issue, 43% (111) and 42% (probable relevance) (98) were considered to be relevant, but causative products were not mentioned.

Case reports and case series

Case series

Limonene hydroperoxides was stated to be the (or an) allergen in 92 patients and limonene in one in a group of 603 individuals suffering from cosmetic dermatitis, seen in the period 2010-2015 in Leuven, Belgium (60).

In the period 1996-2013, in a tertiary referral center in Valencia, Spain, 5419 patients were patch tested. Of these, 628 individuals had allergic contact dermatitis to cosmetics. In this group, limonene was the responsible allergen in one case (51).

In the period 2000-2009, in Leuven, Belgium, an unspecified number of patients had positive patch tests or use tests to a total of 344 cosmetic products *and* positive patch tests to FM I, FM II, and/or to one or more of 28 selected specific fragrance ingredients. In 55 of 63 patients reacting to limonene, the presence of this fragrance in the cosmetic products was confirmed by reading the product labels (71).

In a perfume factory, three bottle fillers developed occupational allergic contact dermatitis from *DL*-limonene. Of twenty people working in the same factory who did *not* have dermatitis, none had positive reactions to it (17).

Three men working on a honing machine had occupational allergic contact dermatitis of the hands from dipentene (*DL*-limonene), added as an extreme pressure additive, in honing oil. On these machines, the metal workpiece has to be held in position around a rotating tool while being honed (finely ground). Honing oil is delivered to the interface between the workpiece and the honing tool by a pipe which is swung into position by the operator. As he holds the workpiece, the honing oil flows freely over his fingers and into his hands (33).

Case reports

<u>Occupational allergic contact dermatitis</u>

Cleaning and degreasing products, paint thinners, solvents and wax polish

A car mechanic reacted to oxidized *D*-limonene and to a degreasing agent used at work. Chemical analysis of this product revealed content of *D*-limonene and its oxidation products. Six more patients allergic to limonene had contact with cleaning products, in who 'contact allergy to oxidized limonene might be a contributing factor to their dermatitis' (26).

A painter and decorator had a 4-year history of work-exacerbated hand eczema. Patch tests showed a positive reaction to *D*-limonene 2% pet. It was found that the water-free hand cleansers het used at work contained *D*-limonene at concentrations of 7 and 1%, respectively (39).

A paint mixer at a car factory developed occupational allergic contact dermatitis of the hands and face from dipentene in a paint thinner (35). Allergy to dipentene in paint thinners has also been described in ref. 34.

A man working as painter and car mechanic developed occupational contact dermatitis from a wax polish. He reacted to the wax polish and its ingredients pine oil (5% and 10% in olive oil) and dipentene (*D,L*-limonene) and co-reacted to turpentine oil. This essential oil also contains limonene (up to 13%, depending on its origin) and is obtained from *Pinus* species, just as pine oil (92).

An installer of windows had a dyshidrotic and fissured, hyperkeratotic dermatitis of the fingers, which had existed for several months and correlated with his work where he came in contact with acrylic glues and several degreasers and detergents. Patch testing gave a positive reaction to the degreaser only. Because the label of this product indicated 'active component is a solvent obtained from the treatment of citrus fruits and has a lemon smell', further patch testing was done with oxidized *R*- and *S*-limonene 3% pet. and both showed a positive reaction. Avoiding this product has led to a clear improvement but not a complete resolution of his hand dermatitis, which was also partly irritant. The degreaser could not be analyzed for the presence of oxidized limonene (107).

A histopathology medical laboratory scientific officer had patchy dermatitis on the dorsum of his fingers and hands, which was caused by contact allergy to D-limonene in a solvent, which was being used as an alternative to xylene (38). Another histopathology technician had recalcitrant hand contact dermatitis apparently related to the use of a limonene-based solvent agent. Patch tests with the standard series, limonene-based solvent used by the patient and D- and L-limonene (both oxidized and non-oxidized form) and with Giemsa and methylene blue stains gave positive reactions to oxidized D- and L-limonene. The patient retired from work and promptly the hand dermatitis improved and healed. No oxidation products were identified in the limonene solvent by GC-MS, but it was assumed that oxidized limonene was produced during the handling of the solvent (40).

A man practicing competitive archery had linear allergic contact dermatitis of his left hand from limonene present in a paint stripper used on the bow before painting (122).

A mechanic had occupational hand dermatitis from contact allergy to limonene in a hand cleanser (101).

Other products

Four patients had allergic contact dermatitis from occupational exposure to limonene in fruits, flavors and vegetables (26).

A man presented with intensely itchy, erythematous, scaly, and fissured plaques localized to the back of both hands and several episodes of shortness of breath and swelling of the eyelids, occurring at work, which was picking and handling citrus fruits, particularly lemons. Spirometry showed a mild, mixed respiratory insufficiency, indicative of asthma. Patch tests were positive for DL-limonene 2% pet., citronellol 2% pet. and dichlorophene 1% pet. Prick tests with common aeroallergens and orange extract, lemon juice and lemon essence were negative, but RAST tests were positive for cow's milk, maize and orange/lemon. However, the patient reported that these foods had never caused any adverse reaction by ingestion. On stopping his work, there was complete remission of both dermatitis and asthma in about 6 weeks. Dermatitis as well as asthma reappeared when the patient resumed his work (43).

A porter became sensitized to oil of lemon, which he used occupationally. Patch tests were positive to oil of lemon, limonene, oil of citronella Java, oil of citronella Ceylon (= Sri Lanka), and turpentine oil (90). Limonene is the major ingredient in lemon oil and can also be present in high concentrations in commercial citronella and turpentine oils (23).

A male confectioner developed occupational contact dermatitis which was ascribed to working with cardamom powder. He reacted to cardamom powder, cardamom oil 2% in petrolatum, δ-carene, dipentene (DL-limonene), bergamot oil and turpentine peroxides (93). Limonene is the main component of bergamot oil, can be present in cardamom oil in concentrations up to 6%, has been found in commercial turpentine oils in concentrations up to 13.6% (23) and in its oxidized form can be the cause of sensitization to turpentine oils (94).

A car mechanic had occupational contact dermatitis of the hands and forearms for 3 years. Patch testing gave positive reactions to dipentene (D,L-limonene) and pine oil 5% pet. The patient usually washed his hands with a homemade hand-washing paste, prepared by the owner of the garage, at the end of the working day. This paste was obtained by mixing dish soap powder and fine sawdust from Swedish pine wood. On day 4, the patient showed a positive patch test reaction to the hand-washing paste (5% in water). Patch tests with this paste in 10 healthy volunteers gave negative results. The reaction was ascribed to pine oil and limonene present in the pine wood (123).

Non-occupational allergic contact dermatitis

A male patient who had an ileostomy secondary to underlying Crohn's disease developed allergic contact dermatitis inferior to the stoma bag from oakmoss extract and limonene in a deodorizer (76). It was shown that limonene and other fragrance components can permeate polythene. Citrus aroma could be detected by smell a few minutes after some deodorizer drops were placed in the stoma bag. It was postulated that exposure occurred via fragrance penetrating the stoma bag to affect the skin (76).

A man had developed contact allergy to and allergic contact dermatitis from turpentine oil from working in a laboratory. Many years later, he showed swelling of the tongue, lips, and gingival mucosa, and complained of a burning sensation in his mouth. Allergy to peppermint oil was suspected, which was present in an antiseptic spray, a mouthwash and candies he habitually sucked on. Patch tests were positive to colophonium, Myroxylon pereirae resin, turpentine peroxides, peppermint oil and its ingredients D-limonene, L-limonene (together dipentene) and alpha-pinene. The patient probably had primarily become sensitized to these substances in turpentine oil and later had allergic contact dermatitis from limonene and alpha-pinene in peppermint oil, which are important ingredients of this essential oil (limonene up to 18.5% and alpha-pinene up to 9.7% [23]) (52) .

A woman had allergic contact dermatitis from several fragrances in an eau de parfum, including limonene (74). Another female patient had dermatitis around a urostoma from contact allergy to D-limonene present in a stoma bag adhesive remover wipe (77).

A female patient was referred for patch testing because of vulval dermatitis. She reacted to limonene and linalool hydroperoxides only. On further questioning, it was revealed that she would regularly steam iron the gussets of her underwear with fragranced ironing water. A diagnosis of allergic contact dermatitis to limonene and linalool was made, further supported by a reduction of symptoms after stopping the use of ironing water. However, this diagnosis is premature and unsubstantiated, as apparently the presence of these fragrances in the ironing water was not confirmed and possibly not even looked for (87).

A woman with longstanding hand dermatitis reacted to limonene hydroperoxide, linalool, linalool hydroperoxide, lavender absolute (which contains high levels of linalool), Compositae mix and many other fragrances and fragrance markers. She had noticed exacerbations after peeling citrus fruit (limonene), gardening (Compositae mix) and using lavender sprigs to make furniture polish. Lavender oil on the pillow had caused a facial eruption (linalool). All her detergents contained limonene and/or linalool (89).

Another female patient had a widespread eczematous eruption with clear exacerbations after exposure to pine trees and after using an old bottle of perfume. Patch testing showed positive reactions to limonene hydroperoxide, linalool hydroperoxide and citral but colophonium (pine trees) was negative. Limonene and linalool were found in many of her cosmetics and detergents. On avoidance of these products and of pine trees, there was significant improvement (89).

A female patient had extensive lymphomatoid dermatitis of the lower abdomen and legs. Upon patch testing, she reacted to limonene hydroperoxides. She used several products labeled to contain limonene including a hair pack, a shower gel, a moisturizing cream, a shampoo, a washing-up liquid, and a floor mop. When stopping their use, the lesions disappeared after a few months. After the patient had strictly avoided contact with limonene and had been completely asymptomatic for 15 months, she used her former shampoo, shower gel and a moisturizing cream containing limonene for one month. A flare-up of lesions similar to the previous ones appeared over the same previously affected abdominal locations. The patient was patch tested a second time with limonene hydroperoxides 0.3% pet. and again had a positive test, but was negative to limonene 10% pet. (unoxidized) (112).

A woman became strongly sensitized after treating insect bites, herpes simplex, and other lesions of the skin with tea tree oil. When tested with its ingredients, she had positive patch test reactions to _D_-limonene (5%, vehicle unknown) and 6 other oil components (14). It should be noted that the reaction was weak and there were 6 other positive patch test reactions, of which 4 were extremely strong. Hence, a false-positive reaction to limonene cannot be excluded. However, limonene is an important allergen in tea tree oil. Of 73 patients allergic to tea tree oil and tested with a number of its ingredients, 29 (40%) reacted to (oxidized or unoxidized) _D_-limonene (45).

Cross-reactions, pseudo-cross-reactions and co-reactions

For general information on cross-/pseudo-cross-/co-reactivity of fragrance chemicals with other fragrances, fragrance markers (fragrance mix I, fragrance mix II, colophonium, Myroxylon pereirae resin [balsam of Peru]) and essential oils see Chapter 1.2 General information on cross-reactions, pseudo-cross-reactions and co-reactions.

Concomitant reactions to limonene hydroperoxides and linalool hydroperoxides are frequent. Of 281 patients reacting to either of these, 26% reacted to both. Of 200 patients allergic to linalool hydroperoxides, 71 (36%) co-reacted to limonene and of 152 patients reacting to limonene hydroperoxides, 71 (47%) also reacted to linalool hydroperoxides (99). In another study, 45% of the patients who reacted to oxidized _R_-limonene also reacted to oxidized linalool, whereas 38% of the patients who reacted to oxidized linalool also reacted to oxidized _R_-limonene (86). In yet another similar investigation, of 241 patient reacting to limonene hydroperoxides, 130 (54%) co-reacted to linalool hydroperoxides. Conversely, of 352 patients with a positive patch test to linalool hydroperoxides 1% pet., 130 (37%) co-reacted to limonene hydroperoxides 0.3% pet. (115). In a recent investigation from The Netherlands, 38/77 (49%) of patients allergic to limonene co-reacted to linalool and 38/96 (40%) of linalool-allergic individuals also reacted to limonene hydroperoxides (120). These frequent co-reactivities are explained by independent sensitizations from simultaneous exposure to both fragrances in everyday consumer products (99).

Limonene is an important ingredient of many essential oils and co-reactivity has been observed to bergamot oil (93), citronella oil (90), lemon oil (90), peppermint oil (52), sweet orange oil (91), tea tree oil (14,45,91,96,124), cardamom oil (93) and turpentine oil (23,52,90,92,93).

The hypothesis that patients sensitized to _p_-phenylenediamine are at increased risk of concomitant reactivity to limonene hydroperoxides, owing to a 'common pathway' of skin protein oxidation, has been rejected (65).

Presence in products and chemical analyses

In various studies, the presence of limonene in cosmetic and sometimes other products has been investigated. Before 2006, most investigators used chemical analysis, usually GC-MS, for qualitative and quantitative determination. Since then, the presence of the target fragrances was usually investigated by screening the product labels for the 26 fragrances that must be labeled since 2005 on cosmetics and detergent products in the EU, if present at > 10 ppm (0.001%) in leave-on products and > 100 ppm (0.01%) in rinse-off products. This method, obviously, is less accurate and may result in underestimation of the frequency of the fragrances being present in the product. When they are in fact present, but the concentration is lower than mentioned above, labeling is not required and the fragrances' presence will be missed.

The results of the relevant studies for limonene are summarized in table 3.95.5. More detailed information can be found in the corresponding text following the table. The percentage of products in which limonene was found to be present shows wide variations, which can among other be explained by the selection procedure of the products, the method of investigation (false-negatives with information obtained from labels only) and changes in the use of individual fragrance materials over time (fashion). Limonene is one of the most frequently used fragrances, both in cosmetic and in non-cosmetic products.

Table 3.95.5 Presence of limonene in products [a]

Year	Country	Product type	Nr. investigated	Nr. of products positive [b]	(%)	Method [c]	Ref.
2017	USA	Cosmetic products in hair-dye kits	539 products in 159 hair-dye kits	24	(4%)	Labeling	78
2016	Sweden	Toothpastes	66	34	(52%)	Labeling	82
2015-6	Denmark	Fragranced cosmetic products	5588		(49%)	Labeling	49
2015	Germany	Household detergents	817	182	(22%)	Labeling	113
2015	Sweden	Oxidative hair dye products	26	13	(50%)	Labeling	66
		Non-oxidative	35	9	(26%)	Labeling	
2013	USA	Pediatric cosmetics	187	12	(6%)	Labeling	53
2008-11	Germany	Deodorants	374	197	(53%)	Labeling	95
2009	Italy	Liquid household washing and cleaning products	291	127	(44%)	Labeling and website info	73
2006-9	Germany	Cosmetic products	4991		(30%)	Labeling	48
2008	Belgium	Fragranced topical pharmaceutical products	370	1	(0.3%)	Labeling	21
2008	Sweden	Cosmetic products	204		(28%)	Labeling	1
		Detergents	97		(25%)	Labeling	
2007	Netherlands	Cosmetic products for children	23	18	(78%)	Analysis	56
2006	UK	Perfumed cosmetic and household products	300	189	(63%)	Labeling	46
2006	Denmark	Popular perfumed deodorants	88	47	(54%)	Labeling	50
			23	16	(70%)	Analysis	
2006	Netherlands	Laundry detergents	52	21	(40%)	Labeling + analysis	58
2006	Denmark	Rinse-off cosmetics for children	208	48	(23%)	Labeling + analysis	55
2002	Denmark	Home and car air fresheners	19	15	(79%)	Analysis	59
2001	Denmark	Non-cosmetic consumer products	43	29	(67%)	Analysis	57
2000	Denmark, UK, Germany, Italy	Domestic and occupational products	59	46	(78%)	Analysis	2
1997	Denmark, UK, France, Germany, Sweden	Deodorants	71	48	(68%)	Analysis	24
1992	Netherlands	Cosmetic products	300		(71%)	Analysis	47

[a] See the corresponding text below for more details
[b] Positive = containing the target fragrance
[c] Labeling: information from the ingredient labels on the product / packaging; Analysis: chemical analysis, most often GC-MS

In 2017, in the USA, the ingredient labels 159 hair-dye kits containing 539 cosmetic products (e.g. colorants, conditioners, shampoos, toners) were screened for the most common sensitizers they contain. Limonene was found to be present in 24 (4%) of the products (78).

In 2016, in Sweden, 66 commercially available toothpastes obtained from local pharmacies and supermarkets in Malmö, Sweden were investigated for the presence of flavors by studying the packages and product labels. Limonene was found to be present in 34 (52%) of the products (82).

In Denmark, in 2015-2016, 5588 fragranced cosmetic products were examined with a smartphone application for the 26 fragrances that need to be labeled in the EU. Limonene was present in 49% of the products (rank number 2) (49).

In Germany, in 2015, fragrance allergens were evaluated based on lists of ingredients in 817 (unique) detergents (all-purpose cleaners, cleaning preparations for special purposes [e.g. bathroom, kitchen, dish-washing] and laundry detergents) present in 131 households. Limonene was found to be present in 182 (22%) of the products (113).

In Sweden, in 2015, contact allergens were identified on the ingredient labels of 26 oxidative hair dye products (from 4 different product series) and on the labels of 35 non-oxidative hair dye products (from 5 different product series, including so-called herbal hair colors). These products were selected on the basis of being advertised as 'organic', 'natural', or similar, or used in hairdressing salons branded with such attributes. Limonene was present in 13 (50%) of the 26 oxidative hair dyes and in nine (26%) of the 35 non-oxidative hair dye products (66).

In 2013, in the USA, the allergen content of 187 unique pediatric cosmetics from 6 different retailers marketed in the United States as hypoallergenic was evaluated on the basis of labeling. Inclusion criteria were products marketed as pediatric and 'hypoallergenic', 'dermatologist recommended/tested', 'fragrance free', or 'paraben free'. Limonene was found to be present in 12 (6.4%) of the products (53).

In 2008, 2010 and 2011, 374 deodorants available in German retail shops were randomly selected and their labels checked for the presence of the 26 fragrances that need to be labeled. Limonene was found to be present in 197 (52.7%) of the products (95).

In Italy, in 2009, the labels and website product information of 291 liquid household washing and cleaning products were studied for the presence of potential allergens. Limonene was found to be present in 127 (44%) of the products (73).

In 2008, 66 different fragrance components (including 39 essential oils) were identified in 370 (10% of the total) topical pharmaceutical products marketed in Belgium; one of these (0.3%) contained DL-limonene (21). Limonene was present (as indicated by labeling) in 28% of 204 cosmetic products (92 shampoos, 61 hair conditioners, 34 liquid soaps, 17 wet tissues) and in 25% of 97 detergents in Sweden, 2008 (1).

In Germany, in the period 2006-2009, 4991 cosmetic products were randomly sampled for an official investigation of conformity of cosmetic products with legal provisions. The labels were inspected for the presence of the 26 fragrances that need to be labeled in the EU. Limonene was present in 30% of the products (rank number 2) (48).

In 2007, in The Netherlands, twenty-three cosmetic products for children were analyzed for the presence of fragrances that need to be labeled. Limonene was identified in 18 of the products (78%) in a concentration range of 129-4096 ppm (56).

In 2006, in The Netherlands, 52 laundry detergents were investigated for the presence of allergenic fragrances by checking their labels and chemical analyses. Limonene was found to be present in 21 of the products (40%) in a concentration range of 13-689 ppm. Limonene had rank number 3 (with alpha-isomethyl ionone and linalool) in the frequency list (58).

In 2006, of 88 popular perfume containing deodorants purchased in Denmark, 47 (54%) were labeled to contain limonene. Analysis of 24 regulated fragrance substances in 23 selected deodorants (19 spray products, 2 deostick and 2 roll-on) was performed by GC-MS. Limonene was identified in 16 of the products (70%) with a concentration range of 1023–11387 ppm (50).

In 2006, the labels of 208 cosmetics for children (especially shampoos, body shampoos and soaps) available in Denmark were checked for the presence of the 26 fragrances that need to be labeled in the EU. Limonene was present in 48 products (23.1%), and ranked number one in the frequency list. Seventeen products were analyzed quantitatively for the fragrances. The maximum concentration found for limonene was 2200 mg/kg (55).

In January 2006, a study of perfumed cosmetic and household products available on the shelves of U.K. retailers was carried out. Products were included if 'parfum' or 'aroma' was listed among the ingredients. Three hundred products were surveyed and any of 26 mandatory labeling fragrances named on the label were recorded. Limonene was present in 189 (63%) of the products (rank number 2) (46).

In 2002, in Denmark, 19 air fresheners (6 for cars, 13 for homes) were analyzed for the presence of fragrances that need to be labeled on cosmetics. Limonene was found to be present in 15 products (79%) in a concentration range of 41-21,000 ppm and ranked first (with linalool) in the frequency list (59).

In 2001, in Denmark, 43 non-cosmetic consumer products (mainly dish-washing products, laundry detergents, and hard and soft surface cleaners) were analyzed for the 26 fragrances that are regulated for labeling in the EU. Limonene was present in 29 products (67%) in a concentration range of 0.0001-0.7693% (m/m) and had rank number 1 in the frequency list (57).

In 2000, fifty-nine domestic and occupational products, purchased in retail outlets in Denmark, England, Germany and Italy were analyzed by GC-MS for the presence of fragrances. The product categories were liquid soap and soap bars (n=13), soft/hard surface cleaners (n=23), fabric conditioners/laundry detergents for hand wash (n=8), dish- wash (n=10), furniture polish, car shampoo, stain remover (each n=1) and 2 products used in occupational environments. Limonene was present in 46 products (78%) with a mean concentration of 827 ppm and a range of 6-9443 ppm (2).

In 1997, 71 deodorants (22 vapo-spray, 22 aerosol spray and 27 roll-on products) were collected in Denmark, England, France, Germany and Sweden and analyzed by gas chromatography – mass spectrometry (GC-MS) for the presence of fragrances and other materials. Limonene was present in 48 (68%) of the products (24).

In 1992, in The Netherlands, the presence of fragrances was analyzed in 300 cosmetic products. Limonene was identified in 71% of the products (rank order 4) (47).

Limonene hydroperoxides in products

A sample of sweet orange oil showed contents of *D*-limonene in accordance with ISO standards. LC/MS/MS analyses detected 0.05% wt./wt. limonene-2-hydroperoxide in the essential oil. After 1 year of storage in darkness at 4^0C (refrigerator), the content of limonene-2-hydroperoxide in the essential oil had increased to 0.29% wt./wt. The authors concluded that 'Eliciting levels of terpene hydroperoxides, such as limonene-2-hydroperoxide, can be formed in the essential oils, regardless of handling and storage' (102).

In a study to quantify limonene-2-hydroperoxide in undiluted air-exposed sweet orange oil, a sample of the essential oil was air-exposed in Erlenmeyer flasks, and covered with aluminum foils in order to prevent contamination from the environment. The sample was stored at room temperature and stirred for 1 hour, 4 times a day for 63 days to mimic handling that can occur during production, storage and usage. Unexposed sweet orange oil contained 0.05% limonene-2-hydroperoxide. The concentration rose to 0.06% at D3, 0.07% at D7, 0.51% at D25 and 4.90% at D63 (103). A sample of the oil that had been stored in the refrigerator at+4^0C protected from daylight for a year before analysis was also examined. Limonene-2-hydroperoxide could be detected at a concentration of 0.35% w/w. Thus, storage in the refrigerator did not totally prevent hydroperoxide formation (103).

In a sample of sweet orange oil autoxidized for 2 months, 19 µg/mg (1.9%) limonene-2-hydroperoxides (isomers) was identified (88).

In a study by the fragrance industry, aged fine fragrances retrieved from consumers contained an average of 1990 µg/g limonene; however, limonene-2-hydroperoxide could be indirectly detected only up to 5 µg/g (ppm) in 14 of 39 aged fine fragrances (27).

A recently published method for selective analysis of hydroperoxides in perfumes investigated the content of limonene-2-hydroperoxide in 10 fine fragrances kept and used under normal conditions by consumers for one to five years after purchase. In four of these fine fragrances, limonene-2-hydroperoxide was detected at concentrations up to 56 ppm; the levels of the more sensitizing limonene-1-hydroperoxide were not determined (119).

Serial dilution testing and Repeated Open Application Tests

In 11 subjects previously reacting to limonene hydroperoxides 0.3% pet., a 3-week double-blinded vehicle-controlled repeated open application test study was performed with a simulated fine fragrance (hydro-alcoholic solution) containing limonene hydroperoxides at 0.13% (1260 ppm), 0.042% (420 ppm), and 0.014% (140 ppm). Of the eleven allergic subjects, 11 (100%), 7 (64%), and 3 (27%), respectively, reacted to the applied doses. In 17 healthy controls exposed to the highest dose, no reactions were observed. Among 13 subjects with a previous *doubtful* positive patch test to limonene hydroperoxides 0.3% pet., two (15%) had a positive ROAT to the highest dose applied. The authors estimated the dose, following repeated exposure in the ROAT, that will elicit allergic contact dermatitis in 10% of sensitized individuals to be 0.20 µg limonene hydroperoxides/cm^2, corresponding to a concentration in the simulated fragrance of 85 ppm. It was concluded that contact allergy to limonene hydroperoxides as shown by a positive patch test to 0.3% pet. is of clinical relevance in patients with a positive patch test. A doubtful patch test to the 0.3% pet. test substance can also be of clinical relevance (116).

The subjects were also patch tested with a serial dilution test of limonene hydroperoxides in alcohol in concentrations of 0.59%, 0.20%, 0.66%, 0.22%, 0.0073%, 0.0024% and the vehicle. Of the 11 subjects with a positive reaction to limonene hydroperoxides 0.3% pet., 11/11 (100%) reacted to the highest concentration, 10 (91%) to the 0.20% and 0.066% concentrations and 3 (27%) down to 0.0024% (24 ppm). Of the 13 subjects with a dubious positive patch test to limonene hydroperoxides 0.3% pet., 13/13 (100%) reacted to the highest concentration, 8/13 (62%) to the 0.20% test substance, 5 (38%) to 0.066%, one (8%) to 0.022% and one (8%) down to 0.0073% limonene hydroperoxides in alcohol. There were no reactions to the vehicle control. Thus, in allergic subjects the Minimal Eliciting Concentration (MEC) was 0.0024% (24 ppm) and in the doubtful allergic patients it was 0.0073% (73 ppm) limonene hydroperoxides (116).

Other information

Quenching

The term 'quenching' was employed to describe the complete abrogation of the sensitizing potential of 3 fragrance chemicals (cinnamal, citral and phenylacetaldehyde) by the presence of certain other fragrance chemicals (notably eugenol and limonene) (84). The conclusions were supported by a summary of human predictive test data. Unfortunately, the absence of any details (numbers tested, reproducibility, etc.) have tended to compromise the credibility of the report (83). Whilst there is some evidence in man for the occurrence of quenching during the induction of skin sensitization, a much more substantial body of work has failed to find supportive evidence in various animals models, at a chemical level or at elicitation in human subjects with existing allergy (83,85). In a thorough review of the subject in 2000, it was therefore concluded that the existence of quenching of these fragrance allergens by other specific fragrance components should be regarded as a hypothesis still lacking substantive proof (83).

OTHER SIDE EFFECTS

Irritant contact dermatitis

D-Limonene in high concentrations gives marked irritancy as shown experimentally in humans and animals (6,7). In a healthy volunteer, immersion of the hand for 2 hours in 98% *D*-limonene caused painful itching and burning, starting within a few minutes of exposure, and increasing throughout. Itching decreased after the end of exposure while burning continued to increase for at least 10 minutes post-exposure. After the exposure, the dorsal skin of the hand was moderately erythematous and swollen. The swelling was gone 100 minutes later. Six hours post-exposure, a severe purpuric eruption appeared, which was maximal after 1-2 days and remained for several weeks (7).

Irritant contact dermatitis caused by work in the citrus fruit canning industry has been described in older reports (28,29,30). However, such occupational exposure was complex, with many factors contributing to the dermatitis.

Immediate-type reactions

A man presented with a 6-month history of swelling of his lips within minutes of contact with toothpaste (22). After a further 5-10 minutes, he would also notice a swelling of his gingiva and shortness of breath. The patient had tried several brands of adult toothpaste, but experienced the same symptoms with all of them. The only exception was his children's fruit-flavored toothpaste. Open tests were positive to 2 brands of peppermint oil 2% pet. after 15 minutes, to (*R*)- and (*S*)-limonene 1% pet. after 15 minutes (limonene may be present in peppermint oil in a concentration range of 1-3% and in spearmint oil in a concentration range of 0-22%). There were also immediate reactions after two minutes to (*R*)- and (*S*)-carvone 5% pet.; carvone is the main ingredient of spearmint oil (57-84%) (23). Quite curiously, the authors did not comment on the composition of the toothpastes the patient had previously used, but they attributed the reaction to carvone, presumably because this was already positive in the open test after two minutes. Why menthol, the main ingredient of peppermint oil, was not tested, is unknown (22).

Other non-eczematous contact reactions

It has been shown that limonene is a non-specific airway irritant (41). There is a direct correlation between its concentration in indoor environments and bronchial hyperreactivity in people working in those environments (42).

A man presented with dermatitis of the hands and several episodes of shortness of breath, occurring at work, which was picking and handling citrus fruits, particularly lemons. Spirometry showed a mild, mixed respiratory insufficiency, indicative of asthma. Patch tests were positive for *DL*-limonene 2% pet. RAST tests were positive for orange/lemon, but the patient reported that orange or lemon had never caused any adverse reaction by ingestion. On stopping his work, there was complete remission of both dermatitis and asthma in about 6 weeks but the symptoms recurred when the patient resumed his work (43).

LITERATURE

1   Yazar K, Johnsson S, Lind M-L, Boman A, Lidén C. Preservatives and fragrances in selected consumer-available cosmetics and detergents. Contact Dermatitis 2011;64:265-272
2   Rastogi SC, Heydorn S, Johansen JD, Basketter DA. Fragrance chemicals in domestic and occupational products. Contact Dermatitis 2001;45:221-225
3   Nilsson U, Bergh M, Shao LP, Karlberg A-T. Analysis of contact allergenic compounds in oxidized *d*-limonene. Chromatographia 1996;42:199-205
4   Schnuch A, Uter W, Geier J, Lessmann H, Frosch PJ. Sensitization to 26 fragrances to be labelled according to current European regulation: Results of the IVDK and review of the literature. Contact Dermatitis 2007;57:1-10
5   Matura M, Goossens A, Bordalo O, Garcia-Bravo B, Magnusson K, Wrangsjö K, et al. Oxidized citrus oil (*R*-limonene): a frequent skin sensitizer in Europe. J Am Acad Dermatol 2002;47:709-714
6   Okabe H, Obata Y, Takayama K, Nagai T. Percutaneous absorption enhancing effect and skin irritation of monocyclic monoterpenes. Drug Des Deliv 1990;6:229-238
7   Falk A, Fischer T, Hagberg M. Purpuric rash caused by dermal exposure to *d*-limonene. Contact Dermatitis 1991;25:198-199

8 Karlberg A-T, Boman A, Melin B. Animal experiments on the allergenicity of *d*-limonene—the citrus solvent. Ann Occup Hyg 1991;35:419-426

9 Karlberg A-T, Shao L-P, Nilsson U, Gäfvert E, Nilsson J. Hydroperoxides in oxidized *d*-limonene identified as potent contact allergens. Arch Dermatol Res 1994;286:97-103

10 Karlberg A-T, Magnusson K, Nilsson U. Air oxidation of *d*-limonene (the citrus solvent) creates potent allergens. Contact Dermatitis 1992;26:332-340

11 Pirker C, Hausen BM, Uter W, Hillen U, Brasch J, Bayeret C, et al. Sensitization to tea tree oil in Germany and Austria. A multicenter Study of the German Contact Dermatitis group. J Dtsch Dermatol Ges 2003;1:629-634 (article in German)

12 Knight TE, Hausen BM. Melaleuca oil (tea tree oil) dermatitis. J Am Acad Dermatol 1994;30:423-427

13 Heydorn S, Johansen JD, Andersen KE, Bruze M, Svedman C, White IR, et al. Fragrance allergy in patients with hand eczema – a clinical study. Contact Dermatitis 2003;48:317-323

14 Hausen BM, Reichling J, Harkenthal M. Degradation products of monoterpenes are the sensitizing agents in tea tree oil. Am J Contact Dermat 1999;10:68-77

15 Hausen BM. Evaluation of the main contact allergens in oxidized tea tree oil. Dermatitis 2004;15:213-214

16 Karlberg AT, Magnusson K, Nilsson U. Influence of an antioxidant on the formation of allergenic compounds during autooxidation of *d*-limonene. Ann Occup Hyg 1994;38:199-207

17 Schubert HJ. Skin diseases in workers at a perfume factory. Contact Dermatitis 2006;55:81-83

18 SCCNFP (Scientific Committee on Cosmetic Products and Non-Food Products Intended for Consumers). Opinion of the Scientific Committee on Cosmetic Products and Non-Food Products Intended for Consumers concerning 'An initial list of perfumery materials which must not form part of cosmetic products except subject to the Restrictions and Conditions laid down, 25 September 2001, SCCNFP/0392/00, final. Available at: http://ec.europa.eu/health/archive/ph_risk/committees/sccp/documents/out150_en.pdf

19 SCCS (Scientific Committee on Consumer Safety). Opinion on Fragrance allergens in cosmetic products, 26-27 June 2012, SCCS/1459/11. Available at: https://ec.europa.eu/health/sites/health/files/scientific_committees/consumer_safety/docs/sccs_o_102.pdf

20 De Groot AC, Liem DH, Nater JP, van Ketel WG. Patch tests with fragrance materials and preservatives. Contact Dermatitis 1985;12:87-92

21 Nardelli A, D'Hooge E, Drieghe J, Dooms M, Goossens A. Allergic contact dermatitis from fragrance components in specific topical pharmaceutical products in Belgium. Contact Dermatitis 2009;60:303-313

22 Hansson C, Bergendorff O, Wallengren J. Contact urticaria caused by carvone in toothpaste. Contact Dermatitis 2011;65:362-364

23 De Groot AC, Schmidt E. Essential oils: contact allergy and chemical composition. Boca Raton, Fl., USA: CRC Press, Taylor and Francis Group, 2016 (ISBN 9781482246407)

24 Rastogi SC, Lepoittevin J-P, Johansen JD, Frosch PJ, Menné T, Bruze M, et al. Fragrances and other materials in deodorants: search for potentially sensitizing molecules using combined GC-MS and structure activity relationship (SAR) analysis. Contact Dermatitis 1998;39:293-303

25 Matura M, Goossens A, Bordalo O, Garcia-Bravo B, Magnusson K, Wrangsjö K, Karlberg AT. Patch testing with oxidized *R*-(+)-limonene and its hydroperoxide fraction. Contact Dermatitis 2003;49:15-21

26 Karlberg AT, Dooms-Goossens A. Contact allergy to oxidized *d*-limonene among dermatitis patients. Contact Dermatitis 1997;36:201-206

27 Matura M, Skold M, Börje A, Andersen KE, Bruze M, Frosch P, et al. Not only oxidized *R*-(+)- but also *S*-(-)-limonene is a common cause of contact allergy in dermatitis patients in Europe. Contact Dermatitis 2006;55:274-279

28 Beerman H, Fondé GH, Callaway JL. Citrus fruit dermatoses. Arch Derm Syph 1938;38:225-234

29 Schwartz L. Cutaneous hazards in the citrus fruit industry. Arch Dermatol 1938;37:631-649

30 Birmingham DJ, Campbell PC Jr, Doyle HN, McDonald JM. Investigation of occupational dermatoses in the citrus fruit canning industry. Arch Ind Hyg Occup Med 1951;3:57-63

31 Nilsson U, Magnusson K, Karlberg O, Karlberg A-T. Are contact allergens stable in patch test preparations? Investigation of the degradation of *D*-limonene hydroperoxides in petrolatum. Contact Dermatitis 1999;40:127-132

32 Bråred Christensson J, Matura M, Bäcktorp C, Börje A, Nilsson JLG, Karlberg A-T. Hydroperoxides form specific antigens in contact allergy. Contact Dermatitis 2006;55:230-237

33 Rycroft RJ. Allergic contact dermatitis from dipentene in honing oil. Contact Dermatitis 1980;6:325-329

34 Fregert S. Manual of Contact Dermatitis. Copenhagen: Munksgaard, 1974 (data cited in ref. 33)

35 Calnan CD. Allergy to dipentene in paint thinners. Contact Dermatitis 1979;5:123-124

36 Meding B, Barregard L, Marcus K. Hand eczema in car mechanics. Contact Dermatitis 1994;30:129-134

37 Deza G, García-Bravo B, Silvestre JF, Pastor-Nieto MA, González-Pérez R, Heras-Mendaza F, et al. Contact sensitization to limonene and linalool hydroperoxides in Spain: a GEIDAC* prospective study

Contact Dermatitis 2017;76:74-80

38 Wakelin SH, McFadden JP, Leonard JN, Rycroft RJ. Allergic contact dermatitis from *d*-limonene in a laboratory technician. Contact Dermatitis 1998;38:164-165

39 Topham EJ, Wakelin SH. *D*-Limonene contact dermatitis from hand cleansers. Contact Dermatitis 2003;49:108-109

40 Foti C, Zambonin CG, Conserva A, Casulli C, D'Accolti L, Angelini G. Occupational contact dermatitis to a limonene-based solvent in a histopathology technician. Contact Dermatitis 2007;56:109-112

41 Rohr AC, Wilkins CK, Clausen PA, Hammer M, Nielsen GD, Wolkoff P, et al. Upper airway and pulmonary effects of oxidation products of (+)-alpha-pinene, *d*-limonene, and isoprene in BALB/c mice. Inhal Toxicol 2002;14:663-684

42 Norback D, Bjornsson E, Janson C, Widstrom J, Boman G. Asthmatic symptoms and volatile organic compounds, formaldehyde, and carbon dioxide in dwellings. Occup Environ Med 1995;52:388-395

43 Guarneri F, Barbuzza O, Vaccaro M, Galtieri G. Allergic contact dermatitis and asthma caused by limonene in a labourer handling citrus fruits. Contact Dermatitis 2008;58:315-316

44 Bråred Christensson J, Forsström P, Wennberg A-M, Karlberg A-T, Matura M. Air oxidation increases skin irritation from fragrance terpenes. Contact Dermatitis 2009;60:32-40

45 De Groot AC, Schmidt E. Tea tree oil: contact allergy and chemical composition. Contact Dermatitis 2016;75:129-143

46 Buckley DA. Fragrance ingredient labelling in products on sale in the UK. Br J Dermatol 2007;157:295-300

47 Weyland JW. Personal Communication, 1992. Cited in: De Groot AC, Weyland JW, Nater JP. Unwanted effects of cosmetics and drugs used in dermatology, 3rd Ed. Amsterdam: Elsevier, 1994: 579

48 Uter W, Yazar K, Kratz E-M, Mildau G, Lidén C. Coupled exposure to ingredients of cosmetic products: I. Fragrances. Contact Dermatitis 2013;69:335-341

49 Bennike NH, Oturai NB, Müller S, Kirkeby CS, Jørgensen C, Christensen AB, et al. Fragrance contact allergens in 5588 cosmetic products identified through a novel smartphone application. J Eur Acad Dermatol Venereol 2018;32:79-85

50 Rastogi SC, Hellerup Jensen G, Johansen JD. Survey and risk assessment of chemical substances in deodorants. Survey of Chemical Substances in Consumer Products, No. 86 2007. Danish Ministry of the Environment, Environmental Protection Agency. Available at: https://www2.mst.dk/Udgiv/publications/2007/978-87-7052-625-8/pdf/978-87-7052-626-5.pdf

51 Zaragoza-Ninet V, Blasco Encinas R, Vilata-Corell JJ, Pérez-Ferriols A, Sierra-Talamantes C, Esteve-Martínez A, de la Cuadra-Oyanguren J. Allergic contact dermatitis due to cosmetics: A clinical and epidemiological study in a tertiary hospital. Actas Dermosifiliogr 2016;107:329-336

52 Dooms-Goossens A, Degreef H, Holvoet C, Maertens M. Turpentine-induced hypersensitivity to peppermint oil. Contact Dermatitis 1977;3:304-308

53 Hamann CR, Bernard S, Hamann D, Hansen R, Thyssen JP. Is there a risk using hypoallergenic cosmetic pediatric products in the United States? J Allergy Clin Immunol 2015;135:1070-1071

54 Frosch PJ, Johansen JD, Menné T, Pirker C, Rastogi SC, Andersen KE, et al. Further important sensitizers in patients sensitive to fragrances. II. Reactivity to essential oils. Contact Dermatitis 2002;47:279-287

55 Poulsen PB, Schmidt A. A survey and health assessment of cosmetic products for children. Survey of chemical substances in consumer products, No. 88. Copenhagen: Danish Environmental Protection Agency, 2007. Available at: https://www2.mst.dk/udgiv/publications/2007/978-87-7052-638-8/pdf/978-87-7052-639-5.pdf

56 VWA. Dutch Food and Consumer Product Safety Authority. Cosmetische producten voor kinderen: Inventarisatie van de markt en de veiligheidsborging door producenten en importeurs. Report ND04o065/ND05o170, 2007 (Report in Dutch), 2007. Available at: www.nvwa.nl/documenten/communicatie/inspectieresultaten/ consument/2016m/cosmetische- producten-voor-kinderen

57 Rastogi SC. Survey of chemical compounds in consumer products. Contents of selected fragrance materials in cleaning products and other consumer products. Survey no. 8-2002. Copenhagen, Denmark, Danish Environmental Protection Agency. Available at: http://eng.mst.dk/media/mst/69131/8.pdf

58 Bouma K, Van Peursem AJJ. Marktonderzoek naleving detergenten verordening voor textielwasmiddelen. Dutch Food and Consumer Products Safety Authority (VWA) Report ND06K173, 2006 [in Dutch]. Available at: http://docplayer.nl/41524125-Marktonderzoek-naleving-detergenten-verordening-voor-textielwasmiddelen.html

59 Pors J, Fuhlendorff R. Mapping of chemical substances in air fresheners and other fragrance liberating products. Report Danish Ministry of the Environment, Environmental Protection Agency (EPA). Survey of Chemicals in Consumer Products, No 30, 2003. Available at: http://eng.mst.dk/media/mst/69113/30.pdf

60 Goossens A. Cosmetic contact allergens. Cosmetics 2016, 3, 5; doi:10.3390/cosmetics3010005

61 Warshaw EM, Maibach HI, Taylor JS, Sasseville D, DeKoven JG, Zirwas MJ, et al. North American Contact Dermatitis Group patch test results: 2011-2012. Dermatitis 2015;26:49-59

62 Warshaw EM, Belsito DV, Taylor JS, Sasseville D, DeKoven JG, Zirwas MJ, et al. North American Contact Dermatitis Group patch test results: 2009 to 2010. Dermatitis 2013;24:50-59

63 Toholka R, Wang Y-S, Tate B, Tam M, Cahill J, Palmer A, Nixon R. The first Australian Baseline Series: Recommendations for patch testing in suspected contact dermatitis. Australas J Dermatol 2015;56:107-115

64 Dinkloh A, Worm M, Geier J, Schnuch A, Wollenberg A. Contact sensitization in patients with suspected cosmetic intolerance: results of the IVDK 2006-2011. J Eur Acad Dermatol Venereol 2015;29:1071-1081

65 Bennike NH, Lepoittevin J-P, Johansen JD. Can contact allergy to p-phenylenediamine explain the high rates of terpene hydroperoxide allergy? – An epidemiological study based on consecutive patch test results. Contact Dermatitis 2017;76:67-73

66 Thorén S, Yazar K. Contact allergens in 'natural' hair dyes. Contact Dermatitis 2016;74:302-304

67 Sabroe RA, Holden CR, Gawkrodger DJ. Contact allergy to essential oils cannot always be predicted from allergy to fragrance markers in the baseline series. Contact Dermatitis 2016;74:236-241

68 Vejanurug P, Tresukosol P, Sajjachareonpong P, Puangpet P. Fragrance allergy could be missed without patch testing with 26 individual fragrance allergens. Contact Dermatitis 2016;74:230-235

69 Mann J, McFadden JP, White JML, White IR, Banerjee P. Baseline series fragrance markers fail to predict contact allergy. Contact Dermatitis 2014;70:276-281

70 Uter W, Johansen JD, Börje A, Karlberg A-T, Lidén C, Rastogi S, Roberts D, White IR. Categorization of fragrance contact allergens for prioritization of preventive measures: clinical and experimental data and consideration of structure–activity relationships. Contact Dermatitis 2013;69:196-230

71 Nardelli A, Drieghe J, Claes L, Boey L, Goossens A. Fragrance allergens in 'specific' cosmetic products. Contact Dermatitis 2011;64:212-219

72 Uter W, Geier J, Frosch P, Schnuch A. Contact allergy to fragrances: current patch test results (2005–2008) from the Information Network of Departments of Dermatology. Contact Dermatitis 2010;63:254-261

73 Magnano M, Silvani S, Vincenzi C, Nino M, Tosti A. Contact allergens and irritants in household washing and cleaning products. Contact Dermatitis 2009;61:337-341

74 Nardelli A, Thijs L, Janssen K, Goossens A. Rosa centifolia in a 'non-scented' moisturizing body lotion as a cause of allergic contact dermatitis. Contact Dermatitis 2009;61:306-309

75 Ung CY, White JML, White IR, Banerjee P, McFadden JP. Patch testing with the European baseline series fragrance markers: a 2016 update. Br J Dermatol 2018;178:776-780

76 Elshimy N, Sheraz F, Lyon C. The secret sensitizer gets out of the bag. Contact Dermatitis 2018;79:54-55

77 Lazarov A, Trattner A. Allergic contact dermatitis from the adhesive remover wipe of stoma bags. Contact Dermatitis 1998;39:48-49

78 Hamann D, Kishi P, Hamann CR. Consumer hair dye kits frequently contain isothiazolinones, other common preservatives and fragrance allergens. Dermatitis 2018;29:48-49

79 Rudzki E, Grzywa Z. Sensitizing and irritating properties of star anise oil. Contact Dermatitis 1976;2:305-308

80 Cachao P, Menezes Brandao F, Carmo M, Frazao S, Silva M. Allergy to oil of turpentine in Portugal. Contact Dermatitis 1986;14:205-208

81 Romaguera C, Alomar A, Conde-Salazar L, Camarasa JMG, Grimalt F, Martin Pascual A, et al. Turpentine sensitization. Contact Dermatitis 1986;14:197

82 Kroona L, Warfvinge G, Isaksson M, Ahlgren C, Dahlin J, Sörensen Ö, Bruze M. Quantification of L-carvone in toothpastes available on the Swedish market. Contact Dermatitis 2017;77:224-230

83 Basketter D. Quenching: fact or fiction? Contact Dermatitis 2000;43:253-258

84 Opdyke DLJ. Inhibition of sensitization reactions induced by certain aldehydes. Fd Cosmet Toxicol 1976;14:197-198

85 Basketter D A, Allenby C F. Studies of the quenching phenomenon in delayed contact hypersensitivity reactions. Contact Dermatitis 1991;25:166-171

86 Audrain H, Kenward C, Lovell CR, Green C, Ormerod AD, Sansom J, et al. Allergy to oxidized limonene and linalool is frequent in the U.K. Br J Dermatol 2014;171:292-297

87 Duhovic C, Reckling C. Allergic contact dermatitis to limonene and linalool in ironing water. Contact Dermatitis 2016;75(suppl.1):76

88 Rudbäck J, Ramzy A, Karlberg A-T, Nilsson U. Determination of allergenic hydroperoxides in essential oils using gas chromatography with electron ionization mass spectrometry. J Sep Sci 2014;37:982-989

89 Whitley H, Lovell C, Buckley D. Oxidized terpene allergy has diverse clinical features. Br J Dermatol 2012;167(suppl.1):143

90 Keil H. Contact dermatitis due to oil of citronellal. J Invest Dermatol 1947;8:327-334

91 Kränke B. Allergisierende Potenz von Teebaumöl. Hautarzt 1997;48:203-204 (article in German)

92 Martins C, Gonçalo M, Gonçalo S. Allergic contact dermatitis from dipentene in wax polish. Contact Dermatitis 1995;33:126-127

93 Mobacken H, Fregert S. Allergic contact dermatitis from cardamom. Contact Dermatitis 1975;1:175-176

94 Hellerström S, Thyresson N, Widmark G. Chemical aspects on turpentine eczema. Dermatologica 1957;115:277-286

95 Klaschka U. Contact allergens for armpits - allergenic fragrances specified on deodorants. Int J Hyg Environ Health 2012;215:584-591

96 Santesteban R, Loidi L, Agulló A, Hervella M, Larrea M, Yanguas I. Allergic contact dermatitis to tea tree oil. Contact Dermatitis 2014:70(suppl.1):102

97 Karlberg A-T, Börje A, Johansen JD, Lidén C, Rastogi S, Roberts D, et al. Activation of non-sensitizing or low-sensitizing fragrance substances into potent sensitizers – prehaptens and prohaptens. Contact Dermatitis 2013;69:323-334

98 Nath NS, Liu B, Green C, Atwater AR. Contact allergy to hydroperoxides of linalool and *d*-limonene in a US population. Dermatitis 2017;28:313-316

99 Bråred Christensson J, Karlberg A-T, Andersen KE, Bruze M, Johansen JD, Garcia-Bravo B, et al. Oxidized limonene and oxidized linalool – concomitant contact allergy to common fragrance terpenes. Contact Dermatitis 2016;74:273-280

100 Bennike NH, Zachariae C, Johansen JD. Non-mix fragrances are top sensitizers in consecutive dermatitis patients – a cross-sectional study of the 26 EU-labelled fragrance allergens. Contact Dermatitis 2017;77:270-279

101 Chang Y-C, Karlberg A-T, Maibach HI. Allergic contact dermatitis from oxidized *d*-limonene. Contact Dermatitis 1997;37:308

102 Rudbäck J, Islam MN, Börje A, Nilsson U, Karlberg A-T. Essential oils can contain allergenic hydroperoxides at eliciting levels, regardless of handling and storage. Contact Dermatitis 2015;73:253-254

103 Rudbäck J, Islam N, Nilsson U, Karlberg AT. A sensitive method for determination of allergenic fragrance terpene hydroperoxides using liquid chromatography coupled with tandem mass spectrometry. J Sep Sci 2013;36:1370-1378

104 Bråred Christensson J, Johansson S, Hagvall L, Jonsson C, Börje A, Karlberg A-T. Limonene hydroperoxide analogues differ in allergenic activity. Contact Dermatitis 2008;59:344-352

105 Bråred Christensson J, Hellsén S, Börje A, Karlberg A-T. Limonene hydroperoxide analogues show specific patch test reactions. Contact Dermatitis 2014;70:291-299

106 Bråred Christensson J, Andersen KE, Bruze M, Johansen JD, Garcia-Bravo B, Giménez-Arnau A, et al. An international multicentre study on the allergenic activity of air-oxidized *R*-limonene. Contact Dermatitis 2013;68:214-223

107 Kerre S, Matura M, Goossens A. Allergic contact dermatitis from a degreaser. Contact Dermatitis 2006;55:117-118

108 Mammerler V. Contribution to the analysis and quality control of Peru Balsam. PhD Thesis, University of Vienna, Austria, 2007. Available at: http://othes.univie.ac.at/4056/1/2009-03-23_0201578.pdf

109 De Groot AC, Popova MP, Bankova VS. An update on the constituents of poplar-type propolis. Wapserveen, The Netherlands: acdegroot publishing, 2014, 11 pages. ISBN/EAN: 978-90-813233-0-7. Available at: https://www.researchgate.net/publication/262851225_AN_UPDATE_ON_THE_CONSTITUENTS_OF_POPLAR-TYPE_PROPOLIS

110 Opinion of the Scientific Committee on Cosmetic Products and Non-Food Products Intended for Consumers concerning 'The 1st update of the inventory of ingredients employed in cosmetic products. Section II: Perfume and aromatic raw materials', 24 October 2000, SCCNFP/0389/00, final. Available at: http://ec.europa.eu/health/ph_risk/committees/sccp/documents/out131_en.pdf

111 Assier H, Tetart F, Avenel-Audran M, Barbaud A, Ferrier-le Bouëdec MC, Giordano-Labadie F, et al. Is a specific eyelid patch test series useful? Results of a French prospective study. Contact Dermatitis 2018;79:157-161

112 Gatica-Ortega ME, Pastor-Nieto MA, Schoendorff-Ortega C, Mollejo-Villanueva M, Giménez-Arnau A. Lymphomatoid contact dermatitis caused by limonene hydroperoxides confirmed by an exposure provocation test with the involved personal hygiene products. Contact Dermatitis 2018;78:230-233

113 Wieck S, Olsson O, Kümmerer K, Klaschka U. Fragrance allergens in household detergents. Regul Toxicol Pharmacol 2018;97:163-169

114 Watts TJ, Watts S, Thursfield D, Haque R. A patch testing initiative for the investigation of allergic contact dermatitis in a UK allergy practice: a retrospective study. J Allergy Clin Immunol Pract. 2018 Sep 7. pii: S2213-2198(18)30567-1. doi: 10.1016/j.jaip.2018.08.030. (Epub ahead of print)

115 Wlodek C, Penfold CM, Bourke JF, Chowdhury MMU, Cooper SM, Ghaffar S, et al. Recommendation to test limonene hydroperoxides 0·3% and linalool hydroperoxides 1·0% in the British baseline patch test series. Br J Dermatol 2017;177:1708-1715

116 Bennike NH, Palangi L, Bråred Christensson J, Nilsson U, Zachariae C, Johansen JD, Hagvall L. Allergic contact dermatitis to hydroperoxides of limonene and dose-response relationship - a repeated open application test (ROAT) study. Contact Dermatitis. 2018 Oct 30. doi: 10.1111/cod.13168. [Epub ahead of print]

117 Uter W. Extended patch-test screening for fragrance contact allergy: findings and challenges. Br J Dermatol 2018;178:592-593

118 Kern S, Granier T, Dkhil H, Haupt T, Ellis G, Natsch A. Stability of limonene and monitoring of a hydroperoxide in fragranced products. Flavour Fragr J 2014;29:277-286

119 Ramzi A, Ahmadi H, Sadiktsis I, Nilsson U. A two-dimensional non-comprehensive reversed/normal phase high-performance liquid chromatography/tandem mass spectrometry system for determination of limonene and linalool hydroperoxides. J Chromatogr A 2018;1566:102-110

120 Dittmar D, Schuttelaar MLA. Contact sensitization to hydroperoxides of limonene and linalool: Results of consecutive patch testing and clinical relevance. Contact Dermatitis 2018 Oct 31. doi: 10.1111/cod.13137. [Epub ahead of print]

121 Wilkinson M, Gallo R, Goossens A, Johansen JD, Rustemeyer T, Sánchez-Pérez J, et al. A proposal to create an extension to the European baseline series. Contact Dermatitis 2018;78:101-108

122 Tammaro A, Cortesi G, Abruzzese C, Narcisi A, Ermini G, Parisella FR, Persechino S. Archer dermatitis: a new case of allergic contact dermatitis. Occup Environ Med 2013;70:750

123 D'Erme AM, Francalanci S, Milanesi N, Ricci L, Gola M. Contact dermatitis due to dipentene and pine oil in an automobile mechanic. Occup Environ Med 2012;69:452

124 Santesteban Muruzábal R, Hervella Garcés M, Larrea García M, Loidi Pascual L, Agulló Pérez A, Yanguas Bayona I. Secondary effects of topical application of an essential oil. Allergic contact dermatitis due to tea tree oil. An Sist Sanit Navar 2015;38:163-167 (article in Spanish).

125 Wilkinson M, Gonçalo M, Aerts O, Badulici S, Bennike NH, Bruynzeel D, et al. The European baseline series and recommended additions: 2019. Contact Dermatitis. 2018 Nov 12. doi: 10.1111/cod.13155. [Epub ahead of print]

Chapter 3.96   LINALOOL

IDENTIFICATION

Description/definition	: Linalool is the terpene that conforms to the structural formula shown below
Chemical class(es)	: Alcohols
Chemical/IUPAC name	: 3,7-Dimethylocta-1,6-dien-3-ol
Other names	: Linalyl alcohol
CAS registry number(s)	: 78-70-6
EC number(s)	: 201-134-4
RIFM monograph(s)	: Food Chem Toxicol 2016;97(suppl.):S11-S24 (*l*-Linalool); Food Chem Toxicol 2015;82(suppl.):S29-S38; Food Chem Toxicol 2008;46(11)(suppl.):S190-S192, S193-S194 (*d*-linalool) and S195-S196 (*l*-linalool); Food Chem Toxicol 2008;46(suppl.):S1-S71; Food Chem Toxicol 2003;41:943-964; Food Chem Toxicol 2003;41:919-942; Food Cosmet Toxicol 1975;13:827 (special issue II)
IFRA standard	: Restricted; linalool and natural products known to be rich in linalool, such as bois de rose, coriander or ho wood oil, should only be used when the level of peroxides is kept to the lowest practical level; it is recommended to add antioxidants at the time of production of the raw material, for example 0.1% BHT or alpha-tocopherol; the maximum peroxide level for products in use should be 20 millimoles per liter; the (hydro)peroxide content can be determined by using the FMA method (www.ifraorg.org/en-us/standards-library)
SCCS opinion(s)	: SCCNFP/0760/03 (14); SCCS/1459/11 (15)
Merck Index monograph	: 6820
Function(s) in cosmetics	: EU: deodorant; perfuming. USA: fragrance ingredients
EU cosmetic restrictions	: Regulated in Annex III/84 of the Regulation (EC) No. 1223/2009, regulated by 2003/15/EC; Must be labeled on cosmetics and detergent products, if present at > 10 ppm (0.001%) in leave-on products and > 100 ppm (0.01%) in rinse-off products
Patch testing	: Non-oxidized 10% Pet. (SmartPracticeEurope, Chemotechnique, SmartPracticeCanada); hydroperoxides 0.5% and 1% pet. (Chemotechnique); using the hydroperoxides is preferred; linalool hydroperoxides 1% pet. not infrequently causes irritant reactions and often dubiously positive reactions (46,62,63,80,85); it has been recommended to add linalool hydroperoxides 1% pet. to the British baseline series (80); most recently (November 2018), the European Environmental Contact Dermatitis Research Group (EECDRG) has recommended that linalool hydroperoxides 1% and 0.5% be added as an addition to the European baseline series (85); 4% of allergies to linalool hydroperoxides are missed when the reaction is not read at day 7 (81)
Molecular formula	: $C_{10}H_{18}O$

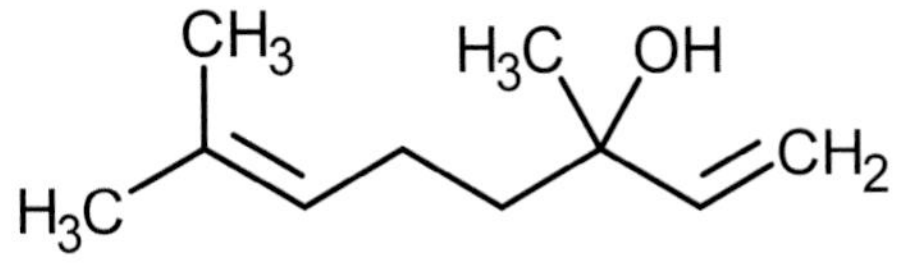

GENERAL

There are 2 forms of linalool: (*R*)-linalool (synonyms: licareol, (-)-linalool, *L*-linalool) and (*S*)-linalool (synonyms: coriandrol, (+)-linalool, *D*-linalool); the racemate of these 2 forms is referred to as linalool. Linalool is a colorless clear liquid; its odor type is floral and its odor is described as 'citrus, orange, floral, terpy, waxy and rose' (www.thegoodscentscompany.com). It is a naturally occurring terpene, present in large amounts in various plants, for example in lavender, rosewood, ylang-ylang, bergamot, geranium and jasmine (2). It is added to processed food and beverages, perfumes and fine fragrances, cosmetics and soaps. Linalool is also used in household detergents and waxes, and added to animal drugs, feeds and other products. Other applications include or have included its use as a pesticide in pet sprays, dips or shampoos, in carpet and surface treatments and as a pesticide fogger for indoor use (U.S. National Library of Medicine). Linalool is among the most commonly found fragrance ingredients in consumer products presently available (see 'Presence in products and chemical analyses' below).

The literature on contact allergy to linalool up to 2003 has been reviewed (16).

Presence in essential oils and propolis

Linalool has been identified by chemical analysis in 82 of 91 essential oils, which have caused contact allergy / allergic contact dermatitis. In 30 oils, linalool belonged to the 'Top-10' of ingredients with the highest concentrations. These are shown in table 3.96.1 with the concentration range which may be expected in commercial essential oils of this type (58). Linalool and cis-linalool oxide may also be present in propolis (74).

In rosewood oil, 'Top-10' concentrations have been found of cis-linalool oxide (0.9-2.1%), cis-linalool oxide, furanoid (0.03-2%), trans-linalool oxide (0.9-2.0%), and trans-linalool oxide, furanoid (0.06-1.7%).

Table 3.96.1 Essential oils containing linalool in the 'Top-10' and concentration range in commercial oils (58)

Essential oil	Concentration range (min.-max.)	Essential oil	Concentration range (min.-max.)
Rosewood oil	(73.0 - 88.4%)	Laurel leaf oil	(1.1 - 7.8%)
Coriander fruit oil	(55.0 - 81.2%)	Cinnamon bark oil Sri Lanka	(2.1 - 7.2%)
Thyme oil	(0.03 - 68.5%)	Cardamom oil	(3.0 - 7.0%)
Neroli oil	(31.9 - 57.7%)	Rose oil	(0.02 - 6.4%)
Lavandin oil	(26.0 - 56.2%)	Thyme oil Spanish	(3.2 - 5.2%)
Basil oil	(0.6 - 55.8%)	Palmarosa oil	(2.3 - 4.5%)
Lavender oil	(26.0 - 44.8%)	Lovage oil	(trace - 4.4%)
Spike lavender oil	(0.6 - 42.3%)	Sage oil Spanish	(0.3 - 4.0%)
Petitgrain bigarade oil	(19.8 - 34.0%)	Cananga oil	(1.2 - 2.8%)
Clary sage oil	(18.6 - 31.0%)	Cinnamon leaf oil Sri Lanka	(1.8 - 2.8%)
Ylang-ylang oil	(0.1 - 24.0%)	Bay oil	(0.5 - 2.7%)
Marjoram oil	(0.2 - 23.5%)	Litsea cubeba oil	(1.0 - 2.4%)
Bergamot oil	(4.7 - 16.7%)	Lemongrass oil West Indian	(0.6 - 1.4%)
Ravensara oil	(0.05 - 12.4%)	Star anise oil	(0.2 - 1.3%)
Geranium oil	(1.4 - 11.1%)	Orange oil bitter	(0.1 - 0.3%)

CONTACT ALLERGY

The SCCS (Scientific Committee on Consumer Safety), in a 2012 Opinion on Fragrance allergens in cosmetic products, has marked linalool (non-oxidized) as 'established contact allergen in humans' (15,48). The sensitizing potency of linalool (with low levels of oxidation) was classified as 'weak' based on EC3 values of 30% and 46.2% in the LLNA (local lymph node assay) in animal experiments. However, linalool oxidized for 10 weeks and linalool oxidized for 45 weeks were moderate sensitizers based on EC3 values of 9.4% and 4.8%, respectively (15,48).

Linalool itself is a very weak sensitizer (7) and as a pure compound it seldom causes positive patch test reactions (1,4). Purification of commercial linalool decreases its sensitizing potency even further (65). Linalool acts as a prehapten, which is a chemical that is itself non-sensitizing or low-sensitizing, but that is transformed into a hapten outside the skin by chemical transformation (air oxidation; photoactivation) and without the requirement for specific enzymatic systems (60). Indeed, on air exposure at room temperature linalool autoxidizes spontaneously forming different oxidation products. The major oxidation products are the linalool hydroperoxides, together with furan oxides and pyranoxides (table 3.96.2). Also, linalool alcohols and a minor amount of a linalyl aldehyde have been identified. The allergenicity of linalool is closely related to oxidation and the primary oxidation products, the hydroperoxides, are the main sensitizers (6). These hydroperoxides are potent sensitizers according to the murine local lymph node assay (LLNA), the aldehyde a moderate sensitizer, and the alcohols were non-sensitizing at the tested concentrations (6,7). The furan oxides and pyranoxides showed no significant sensitization potential when tested according to Freund's complete adjuvant test in guinea pigs (12).

Oxidized linalool is more irritant than non-oxidized linalool; for the oxidized material when patch tested, irritation starts to increase at 10% pet., and rises moderately at 20% pet. (11).

Table 3.96.2 Oxidation products formed by autoxidation of linalool (5,6,7)

2,6-Dimethylocta-1,7-diene-3,6-diol
2,6-Dimethylocta-2,7-diene-1,6-diol
2,6-Dimethylocta-3,7-diene-2,6-diol
6-Hydroxy-2,6-dimethylocta-2,7-dienal
6-Hydroperoxy-3,7-dimethylocta-1,7-diene-3-ol (minor hydroperoxide, 20% of the hydroperoxide fraction)
7-Hydroperoxy-3,7-dimethylocta-1,5-diene-3-ol (major hydroperoxide, 80% of the hydroperoxide fraction)
2-(5-Methyl-5-vinyltetrahydrofuran-2-yl)propan-2-ol
2,2,6-Trimethyl-6-vinyltetrahydro-2H-pyran-3-ol

Patch testing in groups of patients

Results of studies testing linalool in consecutive patients suspected of contact dermatitis (routine testing) are shown in table 3.96.3 (non-oxidized linalool) and table 3.96.4 (oxidized linalool). Results of testing linalool in groups of *selected* patients (e.g. patients with known or suspected fragrance or cosmetic dermatitis, individuals with eyelid dermatitis) are shown in table 3.96.5.

Testing in groups of patients: routine testing

Linalool non-oxidized

Linalool is a weak sensitizer (7) and results of patch testing with it are in accordance. In five studies in which linalool (non-oxidized) was routinely patch tested at 10% in petrolatum frequencies of sensitization were invariably low, ranging from 0.1% to 0.5% with an average (not adjusted for sample size) of 0.3% (2,4,24,47,62). Specific relevance data were provided in one study only (100%), but this concerned only one positive patch test (2). Culprit products were mainly fine fragrances, other cosmetics, detergents, essential oils and wet wipes (2,62).

Linalool oxidized

Test preparations

Based on the increased sensitizing capacity of oxidized linalool and linalool hydroperoxides compared to pure linalool (6,7,15,48), higher frequencies of sensitization when testing with these materials could be anticipated. The results of such studies are shown in table 3.96.4. Test substances used have included oxidized linalool 2%, 3%, 4%, 6% and 11%, and linalool hydroperoxides 0.25%, 0.5% and 1%, all in petrolatum.

From 2002 to 2011, mostly oxidized linalool was used for patch testing. In a dose-finding study, it was observed that with increasing concentrations of 2% to 11%, the percentages of positive patch tests also rose (22). Oxidized linalool 6% (containing about 1% linalool hydroperoxides) was considered most suitable for screening for linalool contact allergy (22) and the results of several studies performing routine patch testing with this test substance have since been published (5,56,73,77,78).

In the majority of the studies performed after 2010, however, linalool hydroperoxides was used for patch testing, as this material had proven to be more suitable than oxidized linalool. In two dose-finding investigations from Spain (61) and the United Kingdom (80), patients have been tested with three concentrations of linalool hydroperoxides (1%, 0.5% and 0.25%) and it was found that with rising concentrations, the percentages of positive patch test reactions also increased. In both studies, it was advised to use the 1% preparation for screening purposes and the authors of the UK study suggested to add linalool hydroperoxides 1% pet. to the British baseline series (80). Later, the EECDRG advised to add linalool hydroperoxides 1% pet., which by then had become commercially available, to the European baseline series (84).

Although it has convincingly been demonstrated that the 1% test material identifies a considerable number of allergic individuals not found by testing with the lower concentrations (61,80), it should be appreciated that the test material not infrequently causes irritant reactions and ?+ reactions (46,62,63,80,85), which are very hard to distinguish from each other and from true allergic reactions. It is conceivable that, especially in the studies with the high frequencies of sensitization, a number of reactions judged to be 'allergic' have in fact been false-positive, irritant (81,82).

At this moment, the optimal test concentration for linalool hydroperoxides, which is now commercially available at 0.5% and 1% in petrolatum (www.chemotechnique.se), has not yet been established (85). When testing with 1% pet., the possibility of irritant reactions should always be kept in mind, also in case of ?+ reactions. In the case of such reactions or when otherwise in doubt, repeat testing, testing with a dilution series (or 0.5% pet., which has been recommended by the EECDRG as an addition to the European baseline series in combination with 1% [85]) and studies with ROATs should be performed to reliably distinguish allergic from irritant reactions. Conversely, it has been suggested, in view of the large proportion of ?+ reactions, to increase the concentration, albeit the authors warned for the possibility of active sensitization (81).

Frequencies of sensitization

The results of routine patch testing with any linalool material in any concentration are shown in table 3.96.4. In studies in which oxidized linalool 6% pet. was used, frequencies of sensitization – in order of decreasing rates - were 7.4% (77), 6.9% (5), 5.3% (22), 3.9% (73), 3.4% (56) and 3.3% (78). Patch testing with linalool hydroperoxides 1% pet. has shown – in order of decreasing frequencies – the following rates of sensitization: 11.7% (81), 9.8% (46), 7.7% (80), 5.9% (62), 4.9% (61), 4.5% (79), and 3.9% (63). The highest rate was reported from The Netherlands (81), the following three all were in studies performed in the United Kingdom (46,62,80).

Relevance and causative products
In 9 of the 16 available studies, no (specific) relevance data were provided. In the investigations that did address this issue, percentages of the reactions to linalool considered to be relevant ranged from 20 to 66% (5,10,61,63,79,80,81). Culprit products were mentioned in two investigations only and most were fine fragrances, other cosmetics, detergents, essential oils and wet wipes (61,62).

Table 3.96.3 Patch testing in groups of patients: Routine testing (non-oxidized linalool)

Years and Country	Test conc. & vehicle	Number of patients tested | positive (%)		Selection of patients (S); Relevance (R); Comments (C)	Ref.
2011-2012 UK	10% pet.	1951	6 (0.3%)	R: not stated	47
2011-2012 UK	10% pet.	4741	12 (0.3%)	R: not specified; 37% for linalool and limonene together positive to their hydroperoxides; the most important causative products for these reactions were fine fragrances, other cosmetics, detergents, essential oils and wet wipes; C: there were 6 (50%) co-reactions to linalool hydroperoxide	62
2008-2010 Denmark	10% pet.	1503	1 (0.1%)	S: mostly routine testing; R: 100%; C: of the relevant reactions to any of the 26 fragrances tested, 96% were caused by cosmetic products	2
2003-2004 IVDK	10% pet.	2401	7 (0.3%)	R: not stated	4
1968 Denmark and Sweden	10% pet.	792	4 (0.5%)	R: not stated; C: routine testing was abandoned because of the low rate of sensitization	24

IVDK: Informationsverbund Dermatologischer Kliniken (Germany, Switzerland, Austria)

Table 3.96.4 Patch testing in groups of patients: Routine testing (oxidized linalool)

Years and Country	Test conc. & vehicle	Number of patients tested | positive (%)		Selection of patients (S); Relevance (R); Comments (C)	Ref.
2016-2018 UK	1% pet. hydroperoxides	156	7 (4.5%)	R: 4/7 (57%)	79
2015-7 Netherlands	1.0% pet. hydroperoxides	821	96 (11.7%)	R: certain 20%, probable 27%; C: there were 180 (22%) ?+ reactions and 16 (1.9%) irritant reactions	81
2015-2016 UK	6% pet. ox.	2084	154 (7.4%)	R: not specified for individual fragrances; 25% of patients who reacted to any fragrance or fragrance marker had a positive fragrance intolerance history	77
2015-2016 Spain	0.25% pet.	3639	46 (1.3%)	R: 47% were currently relevant; most reactions to linalool and/ or limonene were caused by cosmetics (including fine fragrances), a smaller number by detergents and wet wipes	61
	0.5% pet.	3639	106 (2.9%)		
	1.0% pet. all hydroperoxides	3639	179 (4.9%)		
2012-2015 Denmark	1% pet. hydroperoxides	4194	(3.9%)	R: present relevance 63%, past relevance 27%; current and/or past relevance: 76%; C: 21% doubtful positive reactions	63
2008-2014 UK	1% pet. hydroperoxides	1292	126 (9.8%)	R: not stated; C: there were 6.6% ?+ and 14% irritant reactions	46
2013-2014 UK	1% pet.	4563	352 (7.7%)	R: nearly 2/3 for all positives; C: 3.9% irritant reactions, 2.9% ?+ reactions	80
	0.5% pet.	4563	231 (5.1%)	C: 2% irritant reactions, 3.4% ?+ reactions	
	0.25% pet. all hydroperoxides	4563	115 (2.5%)	C: 1.1% irritant reactions, 2.9% ?+ reactions	
2011-2012 UK	1% pet. hydroperoxides	4741	281 (5.9%)	R: 37% for linalool and limonene together; the most important causative products were fine fragrances, other cosmetics, detergents, essential oils and wet wipes; C: there were nearly 6% irritant reactions, but these included 'doubtful' reactions	62
2010-11 Denmark, UK, Spain, Australia, Sweden, Singapore	6% pet., ox. with 1% hydroperoxides	2900	200 (6.9%)	R: 36% current relevance, 7% past; C: range: 3.3-14.3%; 9.2% doubtful reactions, a number of which were probably very weak positive patch test reactions, according to the authors; conversely, it may indicate that the test substance was a marginal irritant and some positive reactions were false-positive	5
2008-2011 Sweden	6% pet. ox.	1712	(3.4%)	R: not stated; probably the same data as in ref. 78 (below this entry)	56
2008-2010 Sweden	6% pet., oxidized	1674	56 (3.3%)	R: not stated; C: 55% co-reacted to oxidized lavender oil 6%, 39% to oxidized linalyl acetate 6% and 27% to both; probably the same data as in ref. 56 (above this entry)	78
2007-2010 UK	3% pet. ox.	483	11 (2.3%)	R: in 6 or 7 of the patients; C: 3 of 4 patients tested also	10

Table 3.96.4 Patch testing in groups of patients: Routine testing (oxidized linalool) (continued)

Years and Country	Test conc. & vehicle	Number of patients tested | positive (%)			Selection of patients (S); Relevance (R); Comments (C)	Ref.
					reacted to stabilized linalool 10% pet.	
2007-2009 Sweden	6% pet. ox.	1187	38	(3.9%)	R: not stated	73
2004-2007 Sweden	2% pet. ox.	1693	14	(0.8%)	R: ' the relevance of the findings in the present study was	22
	4% pet. ox.	2075	67	(3.2%)	supported by a high frequency of positive reactions to other	
	6% pet. ox.	1725	91	(5.3%)	fragrance markers and/or colophonium in patients showing	
	11% pet. ox.	1004	72	(7.2%)	positive patch test reactions to ox. linalool'; C: 5.1%-7.3%	
					doubtful reactions with increasing concentration; 6.0% was	
					suggested as patch test concentration for future screening of	
					patients with dermatitis	
2002-2003 Denmark,	2% pet. ox.	1511	20	(1.3%)	R: certain or probable history of fragrance allergy in 58% of	8
Sweden, Belgium,	0.5% hydro-	1511	16	(1.1%)	all terpenes tested (linalool, caryophyllene, caryophyllene	
Germany, UK	peroxides in				oxide and myrcene) together; C: 25 patients (1.7%) reacted	
	petrolatum				to either or both test substances; all 3 retests were positive	
2002-2003 Denmark	0.5% pet. hy-	262	5	(1.9%)	R: not stated	40
	droperoxides					
	2% pet. ox.	262	7	(2.7%)	R: not stated	

ox: oxidized

Patch testing in groups of selected patients

Results of testing linalool in groups of selected patients (e.g. patients with known or suspected fragrance or cosmetic dermatitis, individuals with eyelid dermatitis) are shown in table 3.96.5. Testing with unoxidized linalool 10% pet. yielded very low frequencies of sensitization, ranging from 0.2% to 1%. Adequate relevance data were not provided and causative products not mentioned (3,42,49,51,71).

In three investigations testing groups of patients, suspected of fragrance allergy or of allergic contact dermatitis of the eyelids, with oxidized linalool or linalool hydroperoxides, frequencies of sensitization were 4.5% (10), 6.8% (75) and 20% (71). The high percentage of 20 was found in the United States in a group of 96 patients suspected of fragrance allergy; they were also tested with pure linalool 10% pet., to which only one patient reacted (71).

Thirty-seven per cent (71), 39% (75) and 86% (10) of the positive patch tests were considered to be relevant, but causative products were not mentioned.

Table 3.96.5 Patch testing in groups of patients: Selected patient groups

Years and Country	Test conc. & vehicle	Number of patients tested | positive (%)			Selection of patients (S); Relevance (R); Comments (C)	Ref.
Linalool non-oxidized						
2014-2016 USA	10% pet.	96	1	(1%)	S: patients suspected of fragrance allergy; R: 'possible' relevance	71
2006-2011 IVDK	10% pet.	708	3	(0.4%)	S: patients with suspected cosmetic intolerance; R: not stated	42
2005-10 Netherlands		100	1	(1%)	S: patients with known fragrance sensitivity based on a positive patch test to the FM I and/or the FM II; R: not stated	49
2005-2008 IVDK	10% pet.	985	2	(0.2%)	S: not specified; R: not stated	51
2005-7 Netherlands	10% pet.	320	2	(0.6%)	S: patients suspected of fragrance or cosmetic allergy; R: 61% relevance for all positive tested fragrances together	3
Linalool oxidized						
2014-2016 France	0.5% pet. hy-droperoxides	264	18	(6.8%)	S: patients suspected of eyelid allergic contact dermatitis; R: 7/18 (39%)	75
2014-2016 USA	1.0% pet., oxidized	96	19	(20%)	S: patients suspected of fragrance allergy; R: definite + probable relevance: 37%	71
2007-2010 UK	3% pet. ox.	88	4	(4.5%)	S: patients suspected of fragrance allergy; R: 6/7 (86%) relevant; C: 3 of 4 patients tested also reacted to stabilized linalool 10% pet.	10

FM: Fragrance mix; IVDK: Informationsverbund Dermatologischer Kliniken (Germany, Switzerland, Austria); ox: oxidized

Case reports and case series

Case series

Linalool hydroperoxides was stated to be the (or an) allergen in 134 patients in a group of 603 individuals suffering from cosmetic dermatitis, seen in the period 2010-2015 in Leuven, Belgium (41). In the period 2000-2009, in Leuven, Belgium, an unspecified number of patients had positive patch tests or use tests to a total of 344 cosmetic products *and* positive patch tests to FM I, FM II, and/or to one or more of 28 selected specific fragrance ingredients. In all 10 patients reacting to linalool, the presence of this fragrance in the cosmetic product(s) was confirmed by reading the product label(s) (50).

In a perfume factory, three bottle fillers developed occupational allergic contact dermatitis from linalool (13).

Three individuals had allergic contact dermatitis from linalool in skin care products, and 3 others from this fragrance in 'dry shampoo', hair lotion and aftershave, respectively (20). In a group of 7 patients reacting to oxidized linalool with proven relevance, products giving positive patch test reactions and labeled as containing linalool were moisturizing creams (n=3), anti-aging creams (n=2), sunscreen (n=1), fine fragrance (n=1), wet wipes (n=1), tea tree oil (n=1), and citrus insect repellent (n=1) (10).

In a group of 119 patients with allergic contact dermatitis from cosmetics, investigated in The Netherlands in 1986-1987, one case was caused by linalool in dry shampoo (33,34).

Case reports

A young atopic girl had a 6-month history of a severely pruritic, burning, oozing eruption confined to her eyelids. The patient's mother had been assiduously protecting her daughter from all products known to contain fragrances or other common contact sensitizers. Examination revealed erythematous, eczematous lichenified plaques on both upper and lower eyelids, with extensive serous crusts. The patient underwent patch testing and she reacted only to hydroperoxides of linalool. As the patient was apparently already avoiding all fragrances, no specific recommendations could be given. One week later, the patient's mother told that her daughter's nanny washed her hair once a week with the shampoo of the child's father, which is fragranced. After removing the shampoo from the household, the patient's eyelid dermatitis had completely resolved 3 months later, without any other intervention. Headspace gas chromatography–mass spectrometry analysis showed easily detectable amounts of linalool and the major linalool oxide (the furan derivative: 2-(5-methyl-5-vinyltetrahydrofuran-2-yl)propan-2-ol). Later, liquid chromatography–mass spectrometry analysis showed the shampoo to contain 87 µg/g linalool, 0.8 µg/g linalool oxide (the furan derivative), and 0.2 µg/g linalool hydroperoxides. Although not conclusive, the authors stated that their results strongly suggest that hydroperoxides of linalool present in the shampoo was a critical factor contributing to this patient's eyelid dermatitis (64).

A man suffering from psoriasis developed allergic contact dermatitis from linalool and hydroxycitronellal in an aftershave, that evolved into facial psoriasis (Köbner-phenomenon) (23). Another male patient developed airborne contact dermatitis from contact allergy to lavender oil, jasmine absolute and rosewood oil from aromatherapy lamps, whereby the water vapor produced distributes the essential oils as an aerosol in the air; the patient also reacted to linalool 2% pet., which is an important constituent of all three products (25).

Two professional aromatherapists reacted upon patch testing to multiple essential oils. They were also patch tested with linalool (5% and 10% pet.), which was found to be present in many of the essential oils by GC-MS. One patient reacted to linalool at both concentrations (26). A woman had allergic contact dermatitis of the dorsa of both feet from linalool present in 'exfoliating socks', which she had worn for only one hour (44).

Another female patient had allergic contact dermatitis from several fragrances in an eau de parfum, including linalool (53). One individual developed contact allergy to linalool in a sunscreen cream (54). A woman was referred for patch testing because of vulval dermatitis. She reacted to limonene and linalool hydroperoxides only. On further questioning, it was revealed that she would regularly steam-iron the gussets of her underwear with fragranced ironing water. A diagnosis of allergic contact dermatitis to limonene and linalool was made, further supported by a reduction of symptoms after stopping the use of ironing water. However, this diagnosis is premature and unsubstantiated, as apparently the presence of these fragrances in the ironing water was not confirmed and possibly not even looked for (68).

A female individual with longstanding hand dermatitis reacted to linalool, linalool hydroperoxides, limonene hydroperoxides, lavender absolute (which contains high levels of linalool), Compositae mix and many other fragrances and fragrance markers. She had noticed exacerbations after gardening (Compositae mix), peeling citrus fruit (limonene) and using lavender sprigs to make furniture polish. Lavender oil on the pillow had caused a facial eruption (linalool). All her detergents contained linalool and/or limonene (69).

Another woman had a widespread eczematous eruption with clear exacerbations after exposure to pine trees and after using an old bottle of perfume. Patch testing showed positive reactions to linalool hydroperoxides, citral and to limonene hydroperoxides, but colophonium was negative. Linalool and limonene were found in many of her cosmetics and detergents. On avoidance of these products and of pine trees there was significant improvement (69).

Cross-reactions, pseudo-cross-reactions and co-reactions

For general information on cross-/pseudo-cross-/co-reactivity of fragrance chemicals with other fragrances, fragrance markers (fragrance mix I, fragrance mix II, colophonium, Myroxylon pereirae resin [balsam of Peru]) and essential oils see Chapter 1.2 General information on cross-reactions, pseudo-cross-reactions and co-reactions.

Linalool is an important ingredient in many essential oils and co-reactivity to lavender oil/absolute (25,69), jasmine absolute (25), rosewood oil (25) and various other essential oils containing linalool (26) has been observed.

Concomitant reactions to linalool hydroperoxides and limonene hydroperoxides are frequent. Of 200 patients allergic to linalool, 71 (36%) co-reacted to limonene and of 152 patients reacting to limonene hydroperoxides, 71 (47%) also reacted to linalool (67). This is explained by independent sensitization from the frequent simultaneous exposure to both fragrances in everyday consumer products (67). In another study, concomitant reactions between oxidized linalool and oxidized limonene were also frequent: 45% of the patients who reacted to oxidized (R)-limonene also reacted to oxidized linalool, whereas 38% of the patients who reacted to oxidized linalool also reacted to oxidized (R)-limonene (62). Of 352 patients with a positive patch test to linalool hydroperoxides 1% pet., 130 (37%) co-reacted to limonene hydroperoxides 0.3% pet. Conversely, of 241 patient reacting to limonene hydroperoxides, 130 (54%) co-reacted to linalool hydroperoxides (80).

Of 4 patients allergic to oxidized linalool, 3 co-reacted to oxidized linalyl acetate 4% pet. (57). Of 56 patients allergic to oxidized linalool, 21 (38%) co-reacted to oxidized linalyl acetate 6% pet. (78).

The hypothesis that patients sensitized to p-phenylenediamine are at increased risk of concomitant reactivity to linalool hydroperoxides, owing to a 'common pathway' of skin protein oxidation, has been rejected (43).

Testing with dilution series and Repeated Open Application Tests

Repeated open application tests (ROATs) were performed in 5 participants previously diagnosed with contact allergy to oxidized linalool and later confirmed to be allergic. Creams containing 3.0%, 1.0% and 0.30% oxidized linalool (corresponding to 0.56%, 0.19% and 0.056% linalool hydroperoxides, respectively) and 'fine fragrance' containing 1.0%, 0.30% and 0.10% oxidized linalool in alcohol (corresponding to 0.19%, 0.056% and 0.019% linalool hydroperoxides, respectively) were used twice daily for up to 3 weeks. All 5 participants reacted to the cream containing 3% oxidized linalool. With 1% oxidized linalool, a reaction was seen in 3 (cream) and 4 (fine fragrance) participants, respectively. With 0.3% oxidized linalool, 2 (cream) and 1 (fine fragrance) participants reacted.

Patch testing with a dilution series of oxidized linalool was also performed. All 5 reacted to a concentration of 5%, 4/5 to 2%, 4/5 to 0.7%, 2/5 to 0.2% and 1/5 to 0.07% oxidized linalool. It was concluded that 'Repeated exposure to low concentrations of oxidized linalool can elicit allergic contact dermatitis in previously sensitized individuals'. The authors admit, however, that 'The actual concentrations of linalool used in different consumer products are not well described' (70). However, they appear to be very low (66).

Presence in products and chemical analyses

In various studies, the presence of linalool in cosmetic and sometimes other products has been investigated. Before 2006, most investigators used chemical analysis, usually GC-MS, for qualitative and quantitative determination. Since then, the presence of the target fragrances was usually investigated by screening the product labels for the 26 fragrances that must be labeled since 2005 on cosmetics and detergent products in the EU, if present at > 10 ppm (0.001%) in leave-on products and > 100 ppm (0.01%) in rinse-off products. This method, obviously, is less accurate and may result in underestimation of the frequency of the fragrances being present in the product. When they are in fact present, but the concentration is lower than mentioned above, labeling is not required and the fragrances' presence will be missed.

The results of the relevant studies for linalool are summarized in table 3.96.6. More detailed information can be found in the corresponding text before and following the table. The percentage of products in which linalool was found to be present shows wide variations, which can among other be explained by the selection procedure of the products, the method of investigation (false-negatives with information obtained from labels only) and changes in the use of individual fragrance materials over time (fashion). Linalool is a very frequently used fragrance chemical in both cosmetic and non-cosmetic products, if not *the* most frequent fragrance material.

In Denmark, in 2015-2016, 5588 fragranced cosmetic products were examined with a smartphone application for the 26 fragrances that need to be labeled in the EU. Linalool was present in 50% of the products (rank number 1) (31).

In Germany, in 2015, fragrance allergens were evaluated based on lists of ingredients in 817 (unique) detergents (all-purpose cleaners, cleaning preparations for special purposes [e.g. bathroom, kitchen, dish-washing] and laundry detergents) present in 131 households. Linalool was found to be present in 154 (19%) of the products (76).

In Sweden, in 2015, contact allergens were identified on the ingredient labels of 26 oxidative hair dye products (from 4 different product series) and on the labels of 35 non-oxidative hair dye products (from 5 different product series, including so-called herbal hair colors). These products were selected on the basis of being advertised as 'organic', 'natural', or similar, or used in hairdressing salons branded with such attributes. Linalool was present in 13 (50%) of the 26 oxidative hair dyes and in 5 (14%) of the 35 non-oxidative hair dye products (45).

In a 2013 study from Switzerland and France, linalool content relative to the total fragrance oil content was assessed in 861 hydroalcoholic market formulations (fine fragrances, deodorants) by liquid chromatography–mass spectrometry with high mass resolution (LC-MS). Among these, 30% of the formulas contained linalool at 10,000–

30,000 µg/g (1-3%), 20% contained linalool at 30,000–50,000 µg/g (3-5%) and 21% contained linalool at more than 50,000 µg/g (5%) (expressed relative to the total fragrance content), with a median content of 23,000 µg/g (2.3%). Thus, at least 71% of these formulations contained linalool (66).

Table 3.96.6 Presence of linalool in products [a]

Year	Country	Product type	Nr. investigated	Nr. of products positive [b] (%)		Method [c]	Ref.
2015-6	Denmark	Fragranced cosmetic products	5588		(50%)	Labeling	31
2015	Germany	Household detergents	817	143	(19%)	Labeling	76
2015	Sweden	Oxidative hair dye products	26	13	(50%)	Labeling	45
		Non-oxidative	35	5	(14%)	Labeling	
2008-11	Germany	Deodorants	374	190	(51%)	Labeling	55
2009	Italy	Liquid household washing and cleaning products	291	74	(25%)	Labeling and website info	52
2006-9	Germany	Cosmetic products	4991		(31%)	Labeling	30
2008	Belgium	Fragranced topical pharmaceutical products	370	6	(2%)	Labeling	1
2008	Sweden	Cosmetic products	204		(38%)	Labeling	9
		Detergents	97		(10%)	Labeling	
2007	Netherlands	Cosmetic products for children	23	16	(70%)	Analysis	36
2006	UK	Perfumed cosmetic and household products	300	190	(63%)	Labeling	28
2006	Denmark	Popular perfumed deodorants	88	47	(53%)	Labeling	32
			23	22	(96%)	Analysis	
2006	Netherlands	Laundry detergents	52	21	(40%)	Labeling + analysis	38
2006	Denmark	Rinse-off cosmetics for children	208	45	(22%)	Labeling + analysis	35
2002	Denmark	Home and car air fresheners	19	15	(79%)	Analysis	39
2001	Denmark	Non-cosmetic consumer products	43	17	(40%)	Analysis	37
2000	Denmark, UK, Germany, Italy	Domestic and occupational products	59	36	(61%)	Analysis	18
1997-8	Denmark, UK, Germany, Sweden	Cosmetics and cosmetic toys for children	25	20	(80%)	Analysis	19
1996	Five European countries	Fragranced deodorants	70	68	(97%)	Analysis	17
1992	Netherlands	Cosmetic products	300		(91%)	Analysis	29
1988	USA	Perfumes used in fine fragrances, household products and soap	400	68-91% (see text)		Analysis	27

[a] See the corresponding text below for more details
[b] Positive = containing the target fragrance
[c] Labeling: information from the ingredient labels on the product / packaging; Analysis: chemical analysis, most often GC-MS

In 2008, 2010 and 2011, 374 deodorants available in German retail shops were randomly selected and their labels checked for the presence of the 26 fragrances that need to be labeled. Linalool was found to be present in 190 (50.9%) of the products (55).

In Italy, in 2009, the labels and website product information of 291 liquid household washing and cleaning products were studied for the presence of potential allergens. Linalool was found to be present in 74 (25%) of the products (52).

In 2008, 66 different fragrance components (including 39 essential oils) were identified in 370 (10% of the total) topical pharmaceutical products marketed in Belgium; 6 (1.6%) of these contained linalool (1).

Linalool was present (as indicated by labeling) in 38% of 204 cosmetic products (92 shampoos, 61 hair conditioners, 34 liquid soaps, 17 wet tissues) and in 10% of 97 detergents in Sweden, 2008 (9).

In Germany, in the period 2006-2009, 4991 cosmetic products were randomly sampled for an official investigation of conformity of cosmetic products with legal provisions. The labels were inspected for the presence of the 26 fragrances that need to be labeled in the EU. Linalool was present in 31% of the products (rank number 1) (30).

In 2007, in The Netherlands, twenty-three cosmetic products for children were analyzed for the presence of fragrances that need to be labeled. Linalool was identified in 16 of the products (70%) in a concentration range of 63-1534 ppm (36).

In 2006, in The Netherlands, 52 laundry detergents were investigated for the presence of allergenic fragrances by checking their labels and chemical analyses. Linalool was found to be present in 21 of the products (40%) in a concentration range of 6-335 ppm. Linalool had rank number 3 (with limonene and alpha-isomethyl ionone) in the frequency list (38).

In 2006, of 88 popular perfume containing deodorants purchased in Denmark, 47 (53%) were labeled to contain linalool. Analysis of 24 regulated fragrance substances in 23 selected deodorants (19 spray products, 2 deostick and 2 roll-on) was performed by GC-MS. Linalool was identified in 22 of the products (96%) with a concentration range of 8–3447 ppm (32).

In 2006, the labels of 208 cosmetics for children (especially shampoos, body shampoos and soaps) available in Denmark were checked for the presence of the 26 fragrances that need to be labeled in the EU. Linalool was present in 45 products (21.6%), and ranked number 2 in the frequency list. Seventeen products were analyzed quantitatively for the fragrances. The maximum concentration found for linalool was 1100 mg/kg (35).

In January 2006, a study of perfumed cosmetic and household products available on the shelves of U.K. retailers was carried out. Products were included if 'parfum' or 'aroma' was listed among the ingredients. Three hundred products were surveyed and any of 26 mandatory labeling fragrances named on the label were recorded. Linalool was present in 190 (63%) of the products (rank number 1) (28).

In 2002, in Denmark, 19 air fresheners (6 for cars, 13 for homes) were analyzed for the presence of fragrances that need to be labeled on cosmetics. Linalool was found to be present in 15 products (79%) in a concentration range of 970-39,000 ppm and ranked first (with limonene) in the frequency list (39).

In 2001, in Denmark, 43 non-cosmetic consumer products (mainly dish-washing products, laundry detergents, and hard and soft surface cleaners) were analyzed for the 26 fragrances that are regulated for labeling in the EU. Linalool was present in 17 products (40%) in a concentration range of 0.00002-0.0270% (m/m) and had rank number 4 in the frequency list (37).

In 2000, fifty-nine domestic and occupational products, purchased in retail outlets in Denmark, England, Germany and Italy were analyzed by GC-MS for the presence of fragrances. The product categories were liquid soap and soap bars (n=13), soft/hard surface cleaners (n=23), fabric conditioners/laundry detergents for hand wash (n=8), dish-wash (n=10), furniture polish, car shampoo, stain remover (each n=1) and 2 products used in occupational environments. Linalool was present in 36 products (61%) with a mean concentration of 148 ppm and a range of 3-439 ppm (18); linalool oxide was present in 2 of these products; quantification was not performed (18).

Twenty-five cosmetics and cosmetic toys for children (5 shampoos and shower gels, 6 perfumes, 1 deodorant (roll-on), 4 baby lotions/creams, 1 baby wipes product, 1 baby oil, 2 lipcare products and 5 toy-cosmetic products: a cosmetic-toy set for blending perfumes and a makeup set) purchased in 1997-1998 in retail outlets in Denmark, Germany, England and Sweden were analyzed in 1998 for the presence of fragrances by GC-MS. Linalool was found in 20 products (80%) in a concentration range of 0.005-0.343% (w/w). For the analytical data in each product category, the original publication should be consulted (19).

Seventy fragranced deodorants, purchased at retail outlets in 5 European countries in 1996, were analyzed by gas chromatography - mass spectrometry (GC-MS) for the determination of the contents of 21 commonly used fragrance materials. Linalool was identified in 68 products (97%) in a concentration range of 9–1927 ppm (17).

In 1992, in The Netherlands, the presence of fragrances was analyzed in 300 cosmetic products. Linalool was identified in 91% of the products (rank order 1) (29).

In 1988, in the USA, 400 perfumes used in fine fragrances, household products and soaps (number of products per category not mentioned) were analyzed for the presence of fragrance chemicals in a concentration of at least 1% and a list of the Top-25 (present in the highest number of products) presented. Linalool was found to be present in 90% of the fine fragrances (rank number 1), 68% of the household product fragrances (rank number 1) and 91% of the fragrances used in soaps (rank number 1) (27).

Linalool hydroperoxides in products

In lavender oil, the main ingredients are linalool (26-45%), linalyl acetate (26-43%), and caryophyllene (1.8-6%) (58). It has been shown that lavender oil lacks protection against autoxidation and that these three terpenes are oxidized in air-exposed lavender oil at the same rate as the pure compounds exposed to air, and that the same oxidation products are identified, thereby increasing the sensitizing potency of air-oxidized lavender oil (57).

In petitgrain bigarade oil, which may contain 10-32% linalool (58), linalool hydroperoxides were identified even after 1 year of storage in darkness at 4^0C (refrigerator) (59). Although their quantity was not mentioned, the authors concluded that 'Eliciting levels of terpene hydroperoxides, such as hydroperoxides of linalool, can be formed in the essential oils, regardless of handling and storage' (59).

In 2013, In a study performed by a Swiss manufacturer of fragrances, the amount of linalool hydroperoxides was investigated in some raw materials containing linalool. In essential oils, used by the fragrance industries as raw material for fine fragrances, levels of linalool hydroperoxides ranging from 88-220 µg/g were detected by liquid chromatography–mass spectrometry with high mass resolution (LC-MS). Samples of commercial synthetic linalool contained 276 µg/g and a natural linalool sample from *Cinnamomum camphora* contained 2986 µg/g (i.e. 0.3%); however, this sample was 1 year beyond its commercial expiration date. These data show that certain natural raw materials can be a source of linalool hydroperoxides (66). However, the amount was not elevated by storage in perfume formulations exposed to air. No indication of hydroperoxide formation in fine fragrances was found in stability studies. Aged fine fragrances recalled from consumers contained a geometric mean linalool concentration of 1888 µg/g and, corrected for matrix effects, linalool hydroperoxide at a concentration of around 14 µg/g. In antiperspirants, no oxidation products were detected. It was concluded that very low levels of linalool hydroperoxide in fragranced products may originate from raw materials, but no evidence for oxidation during storage of products was found. The levels detected were, according to the authors, orders of magnitude below the levels inducing sensitization in experimental animals (66).

In a study to quantify linalool hydroperoxides in undiluted light-exposed petitgrain oil, a sample of the essential oil was air-exposed in Erlenmeyer flasks and covered with aluminum foils in order to prevent contamination from the environment. The sample was stored at room temperature and stirred for 1 hour, 4 times a day for 63 days to mimic handling that can occur during production, storage and usage. In unexposed petitgrain oil, no linalool hydroperoxides were detected, which was also the case at D3 of exposure. At D7 of exposure, linalool hydroperoxides were detected, and quantified at day 25 as 0.07% and 0.37% at D63. A sample of the oil that had been stored in the refrigerator at +4^{0}C protected from daylight for a year before analysis was also examined, but no linalool hydroperoxides were detected (72).

A recently published method for selective analysis of hydroperoxides in perfumes investigated the content of linalool-6- and linalool-7-hydroperoxide in 10 fine fragrances kept and used under normal conditions by consumers for one to five years after purchase. The peroxides were found in all 10 products, in levels from 5-424 ppm for Lin-6-OOH, and 5 to 102 ppm for Lin-7-OOH. The highest detected level of total linalool hydroperoxides was 445 ± 23 ppm measured in an after-shave product (83).

LITERATURE

1   Nardelli A, D'Hooge E, Drieghe J, Dooms M, Goossens A. Allergic contact dermatitis from fragrance components in specific topical pharmaceutical products in Belgium. Contact Dermatitis 2009;60:303-313

2   Heisterberg MV, Menné T, Johansen JD. Contact allergy to the 26 specificc fragrance ingredients to be declared on cosmetic products in accordance with the EU cosmetic directive. Contact Dermatitis 2011;65:266-275

3   Oosten EJ van, Schuttelaar ML, Coenraads PJ. Clinical relevance of positive patch test reactions to the 26 EU-labelled fragrances. Contact Dermatitis 2009;61:217-223

4   Schnuch A, Uter W, Geier J, Lessmann H, Frosch PJ. Sensitization to 26 fragrances to be labelled according to current European regulation: Results of the IVDK and review of the literature. Contact Dermatitis 2007;57:1-10

5   Bråred Christensson J, Andersen KE, Bruze M, Johansen JD, Garcia-Bravo B, Gimenez Arnau A, et al. Air-oxidized linalool – a frequent cause of contact allergy. Contact Dermatitis 2012;67:247-259

6   Sköld M, Börje A, Harambasic E, Karlberg AT. Contact allergens formed on air exposure of linalool. Identification and quantification of primary and secondary oxidation products and the effect on skin sensitization. Chem Res Toxicol 2004;17:1697-1705

7   Sköld M, Börje A, Matura M, Karlberg AT. Studies on the autoxidation and sensitizing capacity of the fragrance chemical linalool, identifying a linalool hydroperoxide. Contact Dermatitis 2002;46:267-272

8   Matura M, Sköld M, Börje A, Andersen KE, Bruze M, Frosch P, et al. Selected oxidized fragrance terpenes are common contact allergens. Contact Dermatitis 2005;52:320-328

9   Yazar K, Johnsson S, Lind M-L, Boman A, Lidén C. Preservatives and fragrances in selected consumer-available cosmetics and detergents. Contact Dermatitis 2011;64:265-272

10 Buckley DA. Allergy to oxidized linalool in the UK. Contact Dermatitis 2011;64:240-241

11 Bråred Christensson J, Forsström P, Wennberg A-M, Karlberg A-T, Matura M. Air oxidation increases skin irritation from fragrance terpenes. Contact Dermatitis 2009;60:32-40

12 Bezard M, Karlberg A-T, Montelius J, Lepoittevin JP. Skin sensitization to linalyl hydroperoxide: support for radical intermediates. Chem Res Toxicol 1997;10:987-993

13 Schubert HJ. Skin diseases in workers at a perfume factory. Contact Dermatitis 2006;55:81-83

14 SCCFNP (Scientific Committee on Cosmetic Products and Non-Food Products Intended for Consumers). Opinion on linalool, 9 December 2003, SCCNFP/0760/03. Available at:
    http://ec.europa.eu/health/archive/ph_risk/committees/sccp/documents/out248_en.pdf

15 SCCS (Scientific Committee on Consumer Safety). Opinion on Fragrance allergens in cosmetic products, 26-27 June 2012, SCCS/1459/11. Available at: https://ec.europa.eu/health/sites/health/files/scientific_committees/consumer_safety/docs/sccs_o_102.pdf

16 Hostýnek JJ, Maibach HI. Is there evidence that linalool causes allergic contact dermatitis? Exog Dermatol 2003;2:223-229

17 Rastogi SC, Johansen JD, Frosch P, Menné T, Bruze M, Lepoittevin JP, et al. Deodorants on the European market: quantitative chemical analysis of 21 fragrances. Contact Dermatitis 1998;38:29-35

18 Rastogi SC, Heydorn S, Johansen JD, Basketter DA. Fragrance chemicals in domestic and occupational products. Contact Dermatitis 2001;45:221-225

19 Rastogi SC, Johansen JD, Menné T, Frosch P, Bruze M, Andersen KE, et al. Content of fragrance allergens in children's cosmetics and cosmetic toys. Contact Dermatitis 1999;41:84-88

20 De Groot AC. Contact allergy to cosmetics: causative ingredients. Contact Dermatitis 1987;17:26-34

21 Bråred Christensson J, Matura M, Bäcktorp C, Börje A, Nilsson JLG, Karlberg A-T. Hydroperoxides form specific antigens in contact allergy. Contact Dermatitis 2006;55:230-237

22 Christensson JB, Matura M, Gruvberger B, Bruze M, Karlberg A T. Linalool – a significant contact sensitizer after air exposure. Contact Dermatitis 2010;62:32-41

23 De Groot AC, Liem DH. Facial psoriasis caused by contact allergy to linalool and hydroxycitronellal in an aftershave. Contact Dermatitis 1983;9:230-232

24 Fregert S, Hjorth N. Results of standard patch tests with substances abandoned. Contact Dermatitis Newsletter 1969;5:85

25 Schaller M, Korting HC. Allergic airborne contact dermatitis from essential oils used in aromatherapy. Clin Exp Dermatol 1995;20:143-145

26 Dharmagunawardena B, Takwale A, Sanders KJ, Cannan S, Rodger A, Ilchyshyn A. Gas chromatography: an investigative tool in multiple allergies to essential oils. Contact Dermatitis 2002;47:288-292

27 Fenn RS. Aroma chemical usage trends in modern perfumery. Perfumer and Flavorist 1989;14:3-10

28 Buckley DA. Fragrance ingredient labelling in products on sale in the UK. Br J Dermatol 2007;157:295-300

29 Weyland JW. Personal Communication, 1992. Cited in: De Groot AC, Weyland JW, Nater JP. Unwanted effects of cosmetics and drugs used in dermatology, 3rd Ed. Amsterdam: Elsevier, 1994:579

30 Uter W, Yazar K, Kratz E-M, Mildau G, Lidén C. Coupled exposure to ingredients of cosmetic products: I. Fragrances. Contact Dermatitis 2013;69:335-341

31 Bennike NH, Oturai NB, Müller S, Kirkeby CS, Jørgensen C, Christensen AB, et al. Fragrance contact allergens in 5588 cosmetic products identified through a novel smartphone application. J Eur Acad Dermatol Venereol 2018;32:79-85

32 Rastogi SC, Hellerup Jensen G, Johansen JD. Survey and risk assessment of chemical substances in deodorants. Survey of Chemical Substances in Consumer Products, No. 86 2007. Danish Ministry of the Environment, Environmental Protection Agency. Available at: https://www2.mst.dk/Udgiv/publications/2007/978-87-7052-625-8/pdf/978-87-7052-626-5.pdf

33 De Groot AC, Bruynzeel DP, Bos JD, van der Meeren HL, van Joost T, Jagtman BA, Weyland JW. The allergens in cosmetics. Arch Dermatol 1988;124:1525-1529

34 De Groot AC. Adverse reactions to cosmetics. PhD Thesis, University of Groningen, The Netherlands: 1988, chapter 3.4, pp.105-113

35 Poulsen PB, Schmidt A. A survey and health assessment of cosmetic products for children. Survey of chemical substances in consumer products, No. 88. Copenhagen: Danish Environmental Protection Agency, 2007. Available at: https://www2.mst.dk/udgiv/publications/2007/978-87-7052-638-8/pdf/978-87-7052-639-5.pdf

36 VWA. Dutch Food and Consumer Product Safety Authority. Cosmetische producten voor kinderen: Inventarisatie van de markt en de veiligheidsborging door producenten en importeurs. Report ND04o065/ND05o170, 2007 (Report in Dutch), 2007. Available at: www.nvwa.nl/documenten/communicatie/inspectieresultaten/ consument/ 2016m/cosmetische- producten-voor-kinderen

37 Rastogi SC. Survey of chemical compounds in consumer products. Contents of selected fragrance materials in cleaning products and other consumer products. Survey no. 8-2002. Copenhagen, Denmark, Danish Environmental Protection Agency. Available at: http://eng.mst.dk/media/mst/69131/8.pdf

38 Bouma K, Van Peursem AJJ. Marktonderzoek naleving detergenten verordening voor textielwasmiddelen. Dutch Food and Consumer Products Safety Authority (VWA) Report ND06K173, 2006 [in Dutch]. Available at: http://docplayer.nl/41524125-Marktonderzoek-naleving-detergenten-verordening-voor-textielwasmiddelen.html

39 Pors J, Fuhlendorff R. Mapping of chemical substances in air fresheners and other fragrance liberating products. Report Danish Ministry of the Environment, Environmental Protection Agency (EPA). Survey of Chemicals in Consumer Products, No 30, 2003. Available at: http://eng.mst.dk/media/mst/69113/30.pdf

40 Paulsen E, Andersen KE. Colophonium and Compositae mix as markers of fragrance allergy: cross-reactivity between fragrance terpenes, colophonium and Compositae plant extracts. Contact Dermatitis 2005;53:285-291

41 Goossens A. Cosmetic contact allergens. Cosmetics 2016, 3, 5; doi:10.3390/cosmetics3010005

42 Dinkloh A, Worm M, Geier J, Schnuch A, Wollenberg A. Contact sensitization in patients with suspected cosmetic intolerance: results of the IVDK 2006-2011. J Eur Acad Dermatol Venereol 2015;29:1071-1081

43 Bennike NH, Lepoittevin J-P, Johansen JD. Can contact allergy to p-phenylenediamine explain the high rates of terpene hydroperoxide allergy? – An epidemiological study based on consecutive patch test results. Contact Dermatitis 2017;76:67-73

44 Millelid R, Isaksson M. Allergic contact dermatitis caused by exfoliating socks. Contact Dermatitis 2017;76:59-60

45 Thorén S, Yazar K. Contact allergens in 'natural' hair dyes. Contact Dermatitis 2016;74:302-304

46 Sabroe RA, Holden CR, Gawkrodger DJ. Contact allergy to essential oils cannot always be predicted from allergy to fragrance markers in the baseline series. Contact Dermatitis 2016;74:236-241

47 Mann J, McFadden JP, White JML, White IR, Banerjee P. Baseline series fragrance markers fail to predict contact allergy. Contact Dermatitis 2014;70:276-281

48 Uter W, Johansen JD, Börje A, Karlberg A-T, Lidén C, Rastogi S, Roberts D, White IR. Categorization of fragrance contact allergens for prioritization of preventive measures: clinical and experimental data and consideration of structure–activity relationships. Contact Dermatitis 2013;69:196-230

49 Nagtegaal MJC, Pentinga SE, Kuik J, Kezic S, Rustemeyer T. The role of the skin irritation response in polysensitization to fragrances. Contact Dermatitis 2012;67:28-35

50 Nardelli A, Drieghe J, Claes L, Boey L, Goossens A. Fragrance allergens in 'specific' cosmetic products. Contact Dermatitis 2011;64:212-219

51 Uter W, Geier J, Frosch P, Schnuch A. Contact allergy to fragrances: current patch test results (2005–2008) from the Information Network of Departments of Dermatology. Contact Dermatitis 2010;63:254-261

52 Magnano M, Silvani S, Vincenzi C, Nino M, Tosti A. Contact allergens and irritants in household washing and cleaning products. Contact Dermatitis 2009;61:337-341

53 Nardelli A, Thijs L, Janssen K, Goossens A. Rosa centifolia in a 'non-scented' moisturizing body lotion as a cause of allergic contact dermatitis. Contact Dermatitis 2009;61:306-309

54 De Groot AC, van der Walle HB, Jagtman BA, Weyland JW. Contact allergy to 4-isopropyl dibenzoylmethane and 3-(4'-methylbenzylidene) camphor in the sunscreen Eusolex 8021. Contact Dermatitis 1987;16:249-254

55 Klaschka U. Contact allergens for armpits - allergenic fragrances specified on deodorants. Int J Hyg Environ Health 2012;215:584-591

56 Hagvall L, Berglund V, Bråred Christensson J. Air-oxidized linalyl acetate – an emerging fragrance allergen? Contact Dermatitis 2015;72:216-223

57 Hagvall L, Sköld M, Bråred-Christensson J, Börje A, Karlberg AT. Lavender oil lacks natural protection against autoxidation, forming strong contact allergens on air exposure. Contact Dermatitis 2008;59:143-150

58 De Groot AC, Schmidt E. Essential oils: contact allergy and chemical composition. Boca Raton, Fl., USA: CRC Press, Taylor and Francis Group, 2016 (ISBN 9781482246407)

59 Rudbäck J, Islam MN, Börje A, Nilsson U, Karlberg A-T. Essential oils can contain allergenic hydroperoxides at eliciting levels, regardless of handling and storage. Contact Dermatitis 2015;73:253-254

60 Karlberg A-T, Börje A, Johansen JD, Lidén C, Rastogi S, Roberts D, et al. Activation of non-sensitizing or low-sensitizing fragrance substances into potent sensitizers – prehaptens and prohaptens. Contact Dermatitis 2013;69:323-334

61 Deza G, García-Bravo B, Silvestre JF, Pastor-Nieto MA, González-Pérez R, Heras-Mendaza F, et al. Contact sensitization to limonene and linalool hydroperoxides in Spain: a GEIDAC* prospective study. Contact Dermatitis 2017;76:74-80

62 Audrain H, Kenward C, Lovell CR, Green C, Ormerod AD, Sansom J, et al. Allergy to oxidized limonene and linalool is frequent in the U.K. Br J Dermatol 2014;171:292-297

63 Bennike NH, Zachariae C, Johansen JD. Non-mix fragrances are top sensitizers in consecutive dermatitis patients – a cross-sectional study of the 26 EU-labelled fragrance allergens. Contact Dermatitis 2017;77:270-279

64 Elliott JF, Ramzy A, Nilsson U, Moffat W, Suzuki K. Severe intractable eyelid dermatitis probably caused by exposure to hydroperoxides of linalool in a heavily fragranced shampoo. Contact Dermatitis 2017;76:114-115

65 Basketter DA, Wright ZM, Colson NR, Patlewicz GY, Smith Pease CK. Investigation of the skin sensitizing activity of linalool. Contact Dermatitis 2002;47:161-164

66 Kern S, Dkhil H, Hendarsa P, Ellis G, Natsch A. Detection of potentially skin sensitizing hydroperoxides of linalool in fragranced products. Anal Bioanal Chem 2014;406:6165-6178

67 Bråred Christensson J, Karlberg A-T, Andersen KE, Bruze M, Johansen JD, Garcia-Bravo B, et al. Oxidized limonene and oxidized linalool – concomitant contact allergy to common fragrance terpenes. Contact Dermatitis 2016;74:273-280

68 Duhovic C, Reckling C. Allergic contact dermatitis to limonene and linalool in ironing water. Contact Dermatitis 2016;75(suppl.1):76

69 Whitley H, Lovell C, Buckley D. Oxidized terpene allergy has diverse clinical features. Br J Dermatol 2012;167(suppl.1):143

70 Andersch Björkman Y, Hagvall L, Siwmark C, Niklasson B, Karlberg A-T, Bråred Christensson J. Air-oxidized linalool elicits eczema in allergic patients – a repeated open application test study. Contact Dermatitis 2014;70:129-138

71 Nath NS, Liu B, Green C, Atwater AR. Contact allergy to hydroperoxides of linalool and d-limonene in a US population. Dermatitis 2017;28:313-316

72 Rudbäck J, Islam N, Nilsson U, Karlberg AT. A sensitive method for determination of allergenic fragrance terpene hydroperoxides using liquid chromatography coupled with tandem mass spectrometry. J Sep Sci 2013;36:1370-1378

73 Bråred Christensson J, Hellsén S, Börje A, Karlberg A-T. Limonene hydroperoxide analogues show specific patch test reactions. Contact Dermatitis 2014;70:291-299

74 De Groot AC, Popova MP, Bankova VS. An update on the constituents of poplar-type propolis. Wapserveen, The Netherlands: acdegroot publishing, 2014, 11 pages. ISBN/EAN: 978-90-813233-0-7. Available at: https://www.researchgate.net/publication/262851225_AN_UPDATE_ON_THE_CONSTITUENTS_OF_POPLAR-TYPE_PROPOLIS

75 Assier H, Tetart F, Avenel-Audran M, Barbaud A, Ferrier-le Bouëdec MC, Giordano-Labadie F, et al. Is a specific eyelid patch test series useful? Results of a French prospective study. Contact Dermatitis 2018;79:157-161

76 Wieck S, Olsson O, Kümmerer K, Klaschka U. Fragrance allergens in household detergents. Regul Toxicol Pharmacol 2018;97:163-169

77 Ung CY, White JML, White IR, Banerjee P, McFadden JP. Patch testing with the European baseline series fragrance markers: a 2016 update. Br J Dermatol 2018;178:776-780

78 Hagvall L, Bråred Christensson J. Patch testing with main sensitizers does not detect all cases of contact allergy to oxidized lavender oil. Acta Derm Venereol 2016;96:679-683

79 Watts TJ, Watts S, Thursfield D, Haque R. A patch testing initiative for the investigation of allergic contact dermatitis in a UK allergy practice: a retrospective study. J Allergy Clin Immunol Pract. 2018 Sep 7. pii: S2213-2198(18)30567-1. doi: 10.1016/j.jaip.2018.08.030. (Epub ahead of print)

80 Wlodek C, Penfold CM, Bourke JF, Chowdhury MMU, Cooper SM, Ghaffar S, et al. Recommendation to test limonene hydroperoxides 0·3% and linalool hydroperoxides 1·0% in the British baseline patch test series. Br J Dermatol 2017;177:1708-1715

81 Dittmar D, Schuttelaar MLA. Contact sensitization to hydroperoxides of limonene and linalool: Results of consecutive patch testing and clinical relevance. Contact Dermatitis 2018 Oct 31. doi: 10.1111/cod.13137. [Epub ahead of print]

82 Uter W. Extended patch-test screening for fragrance contact allergy: findings and challenges. Br J Dermatol 2018;178:592-593

83 Ramzi A, Ahmadi H, Sadiktsis I, Nilsson U. A two-dimensional non-comprehensive reversed/normal phase high-performance liquid chromatography/tandem mass spectrometry system for determination of limonene and linalool hydroperoxides. J Chromatogr A 2018;1566:102-110

84 Wilkinson M, Gallo R, Goossens A, Johansen JD, Rustemeyer T, Sánchez-Pérez J, et al. A proposal to create an extension to the European baseline series. Contact Dermatitis 2018;78:101-108

85 Wilkinson M, Gonçalo M, Aerts O, Badulici S, Bennike NH, Bruynzeel D, et al. The European baseline series and recommended additions: 2019. Contact Dermatitis. 2018 Nov 12. doi: 10.1111/cod.13155. [Epub ahead of print]

Chapter 3.97   LINALYL ACETATE

IDENTIFICATION

Description/definition	: Linalyl acetate is the ester of linalool and acetic acid, that conforms to the structural formula shown below
Chemical class(es)	: Esters
Chemical/IUPAC name	: 3,7-Dimethylocta-1,6-dien-3-yl acetate
Other names	: Bergamol
CAS registry number(s)	: 115-95-7
EC number(s)	: 204-116-4
RIFM monograph(s)	: Food Chem Toxicol 2016;97(suppl.):S237-S241; Food Chem Toxicol 2015;82(suppl.):S39-S48; Food Chem Toxicol 2003;41:965-976; Food Chem Toxicol 2003;41:919-942
SCCS opinion(s)	: SCCS/1459/11 (1)
Merck Index monograph	: 6821
Function(s) in cosmetics	: EU: masking. USA: fragrance ingredients
Patch testing	: Oxidized linalyl acetate 4% pet. (15) or 6% pet. (17)
Molecular formula	: $C_{12}H_{20}O_2$

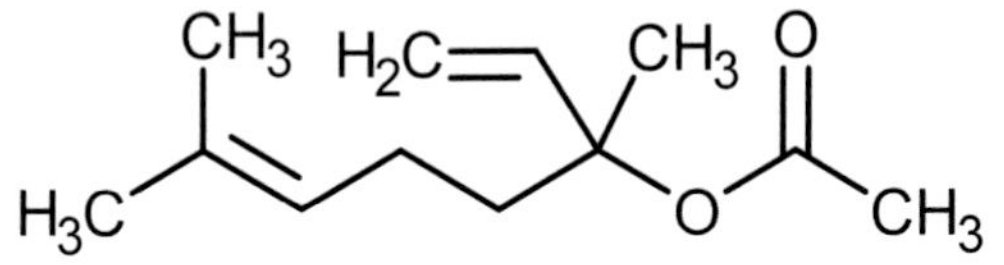

GENERAL

Linalyl acetate is a colorless clear liquid; its odor type is herbal and its odor is described as 'sweet, green, floral and spicy with a clean, woody, terpy and citrus nuance' (www.thegoodscentscompany.com). Linalyl acetate is an important commercial chemical. It is found in the oils of many plants (see below). It is used as a flavor additive in foods and in extracts, perfumes, personal and pet care products and oil-based paints (U.S. National Library of Medicine).

Presence in essential oils and propolis

Linalyl acetate has been identified by chemical analysis in 60 of 91 essential oils, which have caused contact allergy / allergic contact dermatitis. In 9 oils, linalyl acetate belonged to the 'Top-10' of ingredients with the highest concentrations which may be expected in commercial essential oils of this type: clary sage oil (31.2-64.2%), petitgrain bigarade oil (41.3-54.0%), lavender oil (26.1-43.3%), lavandin oil (14.9-36.0%), bergamot oil (20.3-35.6%), neroli oil (1.4-15.1%), cardamom oil (4.0-9.0%), sage oil Spanish (0.1-5.0%), and orange oil bitter (0.05-0.4%) (16).

Linalyl acetate may be also present in propolis (19).

CONTACT ALLERGY

The SCCS (Scientific Committee on Consumer Safety), in a 2012 Opinion on Fragrance allergens in cosmetic products, has marked linalyl acetate as 'established contact allergen in humans' (1,12). The sensitizing potency of linalyl acetate (pure) was classified as 'weak' based on an EC3 value of 25% in the LLNA (local lymph node assay) in animal experiments; however, linalyl acetate oxidized for 10 weeks was a moderate sensitizer based on an EC3 value of 3.6% (1,12).

Linalyl acetate acts as a prehapten, which is a chemical that is itself non-sensitizing or low-sensitizing, but that is transformed into a hapten outside the skin by chemical transformation (air oxidation; photoactivation) and without the requirement for specific enzymatic systems (13). Indeed, linalyl acetate autoxidizes spontaneously at air exposure. In samples taken from air-exposed linalyl acetate after 10, 16, 24, and 28 weeks, 74% of the linalyl acetate remained after 10 weeks, 55% after 16 weeks, 38% after 24 weeks, and 24% after 28 weeks (14). In autoxidized linalyl acetate samples, the following oxidation products were isolated and identified: 7-hydroperoxy-3,7-dimethylocta-1,5-dien-3-yl acetate, 6-hydroperoxy-3,7-dimethylocta-1,7-dien-3-yl acetate, 6,7-epoxy-3,7-dimethyl-1-octen-3-yl acetate and 7-hydroxy-3,7-dimethylocta-1,5-dien-3-yl acetate. In the murine local lymph node assay (LLNA), pure linalyl acetate was shown to be weak sensitizer, samples of linalyl acetate air-exposed for 10 weeks a moderate sensitizer and linalyl hydroperoxides also moderate sensitizers. Thus, autoxidation significantly increases the sensitizing capacity of linalyl acetate and the hydroperoxides are the sensitizers (14).

In lavender oil, the main ingredients are linalyl acetate (26-43%), linalool (26-45%) and caryophyllene (1.8-6%) (16). It has been shown that lavender oil lacks protection against autoxidation and that these three terpenes are oxidized in air-exposed lavender oil at the same rates as the pure compounds exposed to air, and that the same oxidation products are identified, thereby increasing the sensitizing potency of air oxidized lavender oil (15).

Patch testing in groups of patients

The results of two studies in which linalyl acetate has been tested in consecutive patients suspected of contact dermatitis are shown in table 3.97.1. In a European study with 1855 patients tested with linalyl acetate 10% pet., there were only 4 (0.2%) reactions (11). Testing with *oxidized* linalyl acetate 6% in petrolatum, however, resulted in a far higher frequency of sensitization of 2.2% in a group of 1717 patients tested in Sweden in the period 2008-2011 (17,20). The relevance of the observed positive patch tests was not mentioned in either study.

Studies in which linalyl acetate was tested in groups of *selected* patients or case reports of allergic contact dermatitis from the chemical have not been found.

Table 3.97.1 Patch testing in groups of patients: Routine testing

Years and Country	Test conc. & vehicle	Number of patients tested	positive (%)	Selection of patients (S); Relevance (R); Comments (C)	Ref.
2008-2011 Sweden	6% pet., oxidized	1717	37 (2.2%)	R: not stated; C: 41% co-reacted to oxidized linalool 6% pet.; despite this impressive percentage, the authors did not consider these co-reactivities to be cross-reactions but the result of con-comitant sensitization, 'as linalool and linalyl acetate are both present in lavender oil'; 47% co-reacted to oxidized lavender oil (in which linalyl acetate and linalool are the main ingredients) 28% to both linalool and lavender oil	17, 20
1997-8 Six European countries	10% pet.	1855	4 (0.2%)	R: not stated / specified	11

Case reports and case series

Two professional aromatherapists reacted upon patch testing to multiple essential oils. They were also patch tested with linalyl acetate (5% and 10% pet.), which was found to be present in many of the essential oils by GC-MS. One patient reacted to linalyl acetate at both concentrations (2).

Cross-reactions, pseudo-cross-reactions and co-reactions

For general information on cross-/pseudo-cross-/co-reactivity of fragrance chemicals with other fragrances, fragrance markers (fragrance mix I, fragrance mix II, colophonium, Myroxylon pereirae resin [balsam of Peru]) and essential oils see Chapter 1.2 General information on cross-reactions, pseudo-cross-reactions and co-reactions.

Linalyl acetate is an important ingredient of many essential oils and co-reactivity to several of them has been observed (2).

Of 37 patients allergic to oxidized linalyl acetate 6% pet., 15 (41%) co-reacted to oxidized linalool 6% pet. According to the authors, this does not support cross-reactivity between linalyl acetate hydroperoxides and linalool hydroperoxides, despite the possibility of hydrolysis of the ester function in linalyl acetate hydroperoxides resulting in the formation of linalool hydroperoxides. Instead, the authors suggested that concomitant exposure could explain the co-reactions, as linalool and linalyl acetate are both present in lavender oil (17). This statement is somewhat surprising, as if lavender oil were the only or a main source of sensitization to linalool and linalyl acetate.

Of 4 patients allergic to oxidized linalool, 4 (100%) co-reacted to oxidized lavender oil (in which linalool is one of the 2 main ingredients) 4% pet. and 3 to oxidized linalyl acetate 4% pet. (15).

Presence in products and chemical analyses

In 2008, 66 different fragrance components (including 39 essential oils) were identified in 370 (10% of the total) topical pharmaceutical products marketed in Belgium; 5 (1.4%) of these contained linalyl acetate (3).

In 2000, fifty-nine domestic and occupational products, purchased in retail outlets in Denmark, England, Germany and Italy were analyzed by GC-MS for the presence of fragrances. The product categories were liquid soap and soap bars (n=13), soft/hard surface cleaners (n=23), fabric conditioners/laundry detergents for hand wash (n=8), dish wash (n=10), furniture polish, car shampoo, stain remover (each n=1) and 2 products used in occupational environments. Linalyl acetate was present in 16 products (27%); quantification was not performed (5).

Twenty-five cosmetics and cosmetic toys for children (5 shampoos and shower gels, 6 perfumes, 1 deodorant (roll-on), 4 baby lotions/creams, 1 baby wipes product, 1 baby oil, 2 lipcare products and 5 toy-cosmetic products: a cosmetic-toy set for blending perfumes and a makeup set) purchased in 1997-1998 in retail outlets in Denmark, Germany, England and Sweden were analyzed in 1998 for the presence of fragrances by GC-MS. Linalyl acetate was found in 14 products (56%) in a concentration range of ≤0.001-1.872% (w/w). For the analytical data in each product category, the original publication should be consulted (6).

Seventy fragranced deodorants, purchased at retail outlets in 5 European countries in 1996, were analyzed by gas chromatography - mass spectrometry (GC-MS) for the determination of the contents of 21 commonly used fragrance materials. Linalyl acetate was identified in 51 products (73%) in a concentration range of 1–1810 ppm (4).

In 1992, in The Netherlands, the presence of fragrances was analyzed in 300 cosmetic products. Linalyl acetate was identified in 67% of the products (rank order 6) (8).

In 1988, in the USA, 400 perfumes used in fine fragrances, household products and soaps (number of products per category not mentioned) were analyzed for the presence of fragrance chemicals in a concentration of at least 1% and a list of the Top-25 (present in the highest number of products) presented. Linalyl acetate was found to be present in 78% of the fine fragrances (rank number 1), 44% of the household product fragrances (rank number 11) and 59% of the fragrances used in soaps (rank number 11) (7).

Linalyl acetate hydroperoxides in products

In a study to quantify linalyl acetate hydroperoxides in undiluted, air- and light exposed petitgrain oil, a sample of the essential oil was air-exposed in Erlenmeyer flasks and covered with aluminum foils in order to prevent contamination from the environment. The sample was stored at room temperature and stirred for 1 hour, 4 times a day for 63 days to mimic handling that can occur during production storage and usage. In air-exposed oil at D3 and D7, linalyl acetate hydroperoxides were detected, and were quantified at D25 as 0.09% and 0.55% at D63. A sample of the oil that had been stored in the refrigerator at $+4^0$C protected from daylight for a year before analysis was also examined. Linalyl acetate hydroperoxides were detected at a concentration of 0.03% w/w. Obviously, storage in the refrigerator did not totally prevent hydroperoxide formation (18).

LITERATURE

1   SCCS (Scientific Committee on Consumer Safety). Opinion on Fragrance allergens in cosmetic products, 26-27 June 2012, SCCS/1459/11. Available at:
    https://ec.europa.eu/health/sites/health/files/scientific_committees/consumer_safety/docs/sccs_o_102.pdf
2   Dharmagunawardena B, Takwale A, Sanders KJ, Cannan S, Rodger A, Ilchyshyn A. Gas chromatography: an investigative tool in multiple allergies to essential oils. Contact Dermatitis 2002;47:288-292
3   Nardelli A, D'Hooge E, Drieghe J, Dooms M, Goossens A. Allergic contact dermatitis from fragrance components in specific topical pharmaceutical products in Belgium. Contact Dermatitis 2009;60:303-313
4   Rastogi SC, Johansen JD, Frosch P, Menné T, Bruze M, Lepoittevin JP, et al. Deodorants on the European market: quantitative chemical analysis of 21 fragrances. Contact Dermatitis 1998;38:29-35
5   Rastogi SC, Heydorn S, Johansen JD, Basketter DA. Fragrance chemicals in domestic and occupational products. Contact Dermatitis 2001;45:221-225
6   Rastogi SC, Johansen JD, Menné T, Frosch P, Bruze M, Andersen KE, et al. Content of fragrance allergens in children's cosmetics and cosmetic toys. Contact Dermatitis 1999;41:84-88
7   Fenn RS. Aroma chemical usage trends in modern perfumery. Perfumer and Flavorist 1989;14:3-10
8   Weyland JW. Personal Communication, 1992. Cited in: De Groot AC, Weyland JW, Nater JP. Unwanted effects of cosmetics and drugs used in dermatology, 3rd Ed. Amsterdam: Elsevier, 1994: 579
9   De Groot AC, Bruynzeel DP, Bos JD, van der Meeren HL, van Joost T, Jagtman BA, Weyland JW. The allergens in cosmetics. Arch Dermatol 1988;124:1525-1529
10 De Groot AC. Adverse reactions to cosmetics. PhD Thesis, University of Groningen, The Netherlands: 1988, chapter 3.4, pp.105-113
11 Frosch PJ, Johansen JD, Menné T, Pirker C, Rastogi SC, Andersen KE, et al. Further important sensitizers in patients sensitive to fragrances. I. Reactivity to 14 frequently used chemicals. Contact Dermatitis 2002;47:78-85
12 Uter W, Johansen JD, Börje A, Karlberg A-T, Lidén C, Rastogi S, Roberts D, White IR. Categorization of fragrance contact allergens for prioritization of preventive measures: clinical and experimental data and consideration of structure–activity relationships. Contact Dermatitis 2013;69:196-230
13 Karlberg A-T, Börje A, Johansen JD, Lidén C, Rastogi S, Roberts D, et al. Activation of non-sensitizing or low-sensitizing fragrance substances into potent sensitizers – prehaptens and prohaptens. Contact Dermatitis 2013;69:323-334
14 Sköld M, Hagvall L, Karlberg AT. Autoxidation of linalyl acetate, the main component of lavender oil, creates potent contact allergens. Contact Dermatitis 2008;58:9-14
15 Hagvall L, Sköld M, Brared-Christensson J, Börje A, Karlberg AT. Lavender oil lacks natural protection against autoxidation, forming strong contact allergens on air exposure. Contact Dermatitis 2008;59:143-150
16 De Groot AC, Schmidt E. Essential oils: contact allergy and chemical composition. Boca Raton, Fl., USA: CRC Press, Taylor and Francis Group, 2016 (ISBN 9781482246407)

17 Hagvall L, Berglund V, Bråred Christensson J. Air-oxidized linalyl acetate – an emerging fragrance allergen? Contact Dermatitis 2015;72:216-223

18 Rudbäck J, Islam N, Nilsson U, Karlberg AT. A sensitive method for determination of allergenic fragrance terpene hydroperoxides using liquid chromatography coupled with tandem mass spectrometry. J Sep Sci 2013;36:1370-1378

19 De Groot AC, Popova MP, Bankova VS. An update on the constituents of poplar-type propolis. Wapserveen, The Netherlands: acdegroot publishing, 2014, 11 pages. ISBN/EAN: 978-90-813233-0-7. Available at: https://www.researchgate.net/publication/262851225_AN_UPDATE_ON_THE_CONSTITUENTS_OF_POPLAR-TYPE_PROPOLIS

20 Hagvall L, Christensson JB. Patch testing with main sensitizers does not detect all cases of contact allergy to oxidized lavender oil. Acta Derm Venereol 2016;96:679-683

Chapter 3.98   MALTOL

IDENTIFICATION

Description/definition   : Maltol is the organic compound that conforms to the formula shown below
Chemical class(es)   : Ethers; ketones; phenols
Chemical/IUPAC name   : 3-Hydroxy-2-methylpyran-4-one
Other names   : 2-Methyl-3-hydroxypyrone; larixinic acid
CAS registry number(s)   : 118-71-8
EC number(s)   : 204-271-8
RIFM monograph(s)   : Food Cosm Toxicol 1975;13:841 (special issue II) (binder, page 514)
Merck Index monograph : 7047
Function(s) in cosmetics   : EU: masking; tonic. USA: flavoring agents; fragrance ingredients
Patch testing   : 1% pet. (1)
Molecular formula   : $C_6H_6O_3$

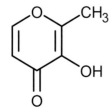

GENERAL

Maltol is a white powder; its odor type is caramellic and its odor is described as 'sweet, caramellic, cotton candy, jammy fruity, burnt with bready nuances' (www.thegoodscentscompany.com).

Presence in essential oils

Maltol has been identified by chemical analysis in one of 91 essential oils, which have caused contact allergy / allergic contact dermatitis: Dalmatian sage oil. However, it was only found in one study and in traces, so the validity of this report may be questioned (2).

CONTACT ALLERGY

Patch testing in groups of patients

Studies in which maltol was patch tested in either consecutive patients suspected of contact dermatitis (routine testing) or in groups of selected patients with positive results have not been found.

Case reports and case series

A woman presented with a 2-month history of perioral eczema mainly on the upper lip. The lips were edematous and erythematous, with peripheral scaling outside the vermilion border. Patch tests were carried out with the standard series, a dentist series, face and cosmetics series and one product used by the patient. Despite previous positive results, these were all negative. Biopsy of the oral mucosa of the upper lip showed histological features of contact dermatitis. At review, the patient mentioned her long-term use of a strawberry-flavored lip salve, with soothing extract of camomile. A patch test with this product was positive. Patch tests to the individual constituents of the lip salve were positive to the strawberry flavor 1% pet., but not to the others. Patch tests were subsequently carried out to the individual constituents of the flavor and a positive reaction was observed to maltol 1% pet.; 30 controls were negative to the same preparation. The use of the lip salve was stopped and the cheilitis resolved within a few days. It has not recurred in the following 12 months (1).

LITERATURE

1   Taylor AEM, Lever L, Lawrence CM. Allergic contact dermatitis from strawberry lipsalve. Contact Dermatitis 1996;34:142-143
2   De Groot AC, Schmidt E. Essential oils: contact allergy and chemical composition. Boca Raton, Fl., USA: CRC Press, Taylor and Francis Group, 2016 (ISBN 9781482246407)

Chapter 3.99   MENTHOL

IDENTIFICATION

Description/definition
: Menthol is a diterpene that conforms to the structural formula shown below; it has a *D*- and and *L*-isomer; *DL*-menthol, a mixture of the two isomers, is also called menthol, menthol racemic or racemic menthol

Chemical class(es)
: Alcohols

CAS registry number(s)
: 1490-04-6 (*DL*-); 89-78-1 (*DL*-); 15356-60-2 (*D*-); 2216-51-5 (*L*-)

EC number(s)
: 216-074-4 (*DL*-); 201-939-0 (*DL*-); 239-387-8 (*D*-); 218-690-9 (*L*-)

SCCS opinion(s)
: SCCS/1459/11 (7)

Merck Index monograph
: 5837

Function(s) in cosmetics
: EU: denaturant; masking; refreshing; soothing. USA: external analgesics; flavoring agents; fragrance ingredients; oral health care drugs

Patch testing
: 1% Pet. (SmartPracticeEurope, SmartPracticeCanada); 2% pet. (Chemotechnique)

Molecular formula
: $C_{10}H_{20}O$

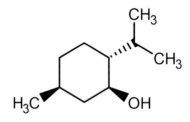

DL-Menthol

Chemical/IUPAC name
: 5-Methyl-2-propan-2-ylcyclohexan-1-ol

Other names
: Menthol; menthol racemic; combination of *D*- and *L*-menthol

CAS registry number(s)
: 89-78-1; 1490-04-6

EC number(s)
: 201-939-0; 216-074-4

RIFM monograph(s)
: Food Chem Toxicol 2008;46(11)(suppl.):S209-S214 (menthol); S224-S227 (*dl*-menthol) and S228-S233 (menthol racemic); Food Chem Toxicol 2008;46(11)(suppl.):S1-S71; Food Cosmet Toxicol 1976;14:473 (menthol racemic)

D-Menthol

Chemical/IUPAC name
: (1*S*,2*R*,5*S*)-5-Methyl-2-propan-2-ylcyclohexan-1-ol

Other names
: (+)-Menthol

CAS registry number(s)
: 15356-60-2

EC number(s)
: 239-387-8

RIFM monograph(s)
: Food Chem Toxicol 2008;46(suppl.):S215-S217

L-Menthol

Chemical/IUPAC name
: (1*R*,2*S*,5*R*)-5-Methyl-2-propan-2-ylcyclohexan-1-ol

Other names
: (-)-Menthol; levomenthol; (1*R*)-(-)-menthol

CAS registry number(s)
: 2216-51-5

EC number(s)
: 218-690-9

RIFM monograph(s)
: Food Chem Toxicol 2008;46(suppl.):S218-S223; Food Cosmet Toxicol 1976;14:471

GENERAL

Menthol appears as colorless crystalline fused; its odor type is mentholic and its odor at 10% in dipropylene glycol is described as 'peppermint cool woody' (www.thegoodscentscompany.com).

Presence in essential oils and propolis

Menthol has been identified by chemical analysis in 26 of 91 essential oils, which have caused contact allergy / allergic contact dermatitis. In two oils, menthol belonged to the 'Top-10' of ingredients with the highest concentrations which may be expected in commercial essential oils of this type: peppermint oil (23.0-47.9%) and spearmint oil (0.2-2.2%) (30). Menthol may be also present in propolis (40).

CONTACT ALLERGY

General

The SCCS (Scientific Committee on Consumer Safety), in a 2012 Opinion on Fragrance allergens in cosmetic products, has marked menthol as 'established contact allergen in humans' (7,10). The literature on contact allergy to menthol up to 2002 has been reviewed (4).

Patch testing in groups of patients

Results of studies testing menthol in consecutive patients suspected of contact dermatitis (routine testing) and those of testing in groups of *selected* patients (e.g. patients with suspected cosmetic intolerance, fragrance-allergic individuals, patients with intraoral symptoms) are shown in table 3.99.1. In one study in which menthol 5% pet. was routinely tested, there was only one positive reaction in 1200 patients with dermatitis (0.1%) (42).

In 8 studies in which groups of selected patients were patch tested with menthol 1%, 2% or 5% pet., frequencies of sensitization have ranged from 0.1% to 40% (table 3.99.1). The highest rate (40%) was observed in 10 patients allergic to peppermint oil (44), in which menthol is the main and probably the most frequent allergenic ingredient. A frequency of 5% was seen in a group of 20 patients known to be allergic to fragrances (only one positive reaction [8]) and 6.7% in a not well-defined group of patients in a 1975-1977 study from Belgium (20). Relevance was mentioned in one study only (all 12 positive reactions judged to be relevant), but it included 'questionable' and 'past' relevance (2). Culprit products were never mentioned.

Table 3.99.1 Patch testing in groups of patients

Years and Country	Test conc. & vehicle	Number of patients tested | positive (%)		Selection of patients (S); Relevance (R); Comments (C)	Ref.
Routine testing					
1983-1984 Italy	5% pet.	1200	1 (0.1%)	R: not stated	42
Testing in groups of selected patients					
2006-2011 IVDK	1% pet.	663	5 (0.8%)	S: patients with suspected cosmetic intolerance; R: not stated	6
2005-2008 IVDK	1% pet.	1147	(0.1%)	S: not specified; R: not stated	12
2000-2007 USA	2% pet.	870	12 (1.4%)	S: patients who were tested with a supplemental cosmetic screening series; R: 100%; C: weak study: a. high rate of macular erythema and weak reactions; b. relevance figures included 'questionable' and 'past' relevance	2
1989-1992 UK		512	12 (2.3%)	S: patients with intraoral symptoms; C: the 12 positive reactions were to menthol and/or peppermint oil; R: not specified	13
<1984 Japan		10	4 (40%)	S: patients allergic to peppermint oil, in which menthol is the main ingredient at 23-48% (30)	44
1975-1977 Belgium	1% pet.	330	20 (6.1%)	S: uncertain whether the patients were consecutive or selected; 88 (27%) had leg ulcers; R: not stated	20
1975 USA	5% pet.	20	1 (5%)	S: fragrance-allergic patients; R: not stated	8
1967-1970 Poland	5% pet.	877	9 (1.0%)	S: not stated; R: not stated	41

IVDK: Informationsverbund Dermatologischer Kliniken (Germany, Switzerland, Austria)

Case reports and case series

Toothpastes and other oral preparations

In one patient with a 3-year-history of burning mouth syndrome who was allergic to menthol, the symptoms cleared within 3 days of avoiding her menthol-containing toothpaste and mouthwash (which were not patch tested).

Another individual with menthol allergy reported cessation of an 8-year history of recurrent mouth ulcers on changing to a menthol-free toothpaste and avoiding a peppermint-flavored mouthwash (which were not patch tested) (13).

Two patients with cheilitis, who both reacted to peppermint oil and to menthol, have been presented; the causative products were not specified, but presumably toothpastes were implicated (21). One patient with oral burning and discomfort and a lichenoid reaction of the oral mucosa had positive patch test reactions to peppermint oil and menthol; the symptoms improved after avoiding mint-flavored mouthwashes and food (25).

One individual developed stomatitis and lip dermatitis from contact allergy to peppermint oil and menthol present in toothpastes (26). A man had cheilitis from contact allergy to menthol in toothpaste and throat spray (29). The patient also reacted to peppermint oil, commercial samples of which contain 23-48% menthol (30). One or more patients had stomatitis and perioral dermatitis from exposure to 'peppermint oil and/or menthol' in toothpastes (no details known, article not read) (46).

According to some sources (15,16 and 17), one or more cases of contact allergy to menthol in toothpastes were described in a Monograph on Myroxylon pereirae resin and other balsams (14), but the authors has not been able to verify this (menthol not mentioned in the Index).

Topical pharmaceutical preparations

In one clinic in Leuven, Belgium, in the period 1990-2016, two cases of dermatitis caused by contact allergy to menthol from its presence as active principle in 'topical botanical medicines' have been observed (47). In the same clinic, in the period 1978-2008, five patients were seen with allergic contact dermatitis from menthol in topical pharmaceutical preparations (3). A man had allergic contact dermatitis from a transcutaneous patch with flurbiprofen for lumbar pain; when patch tested, he reacted to the patch and its ingredients peppermint oil and menthol (5).

Another man had allergic contact dermatitis of his legs from applying a spray for topical treatment of musculoskeletal injuries. He reacted to FM I, Myroxylon pereirae resin, the spray and to the following ingredients of the spray: menthol (1% pet.), benzyl alcohol, essence of lilies (both fragrance materials) and dimethyl sulfoxide (DMSO) (22). However, there were 7 strong positive patch tests, and false-positive reactions to the excited skin syndrome cannot be excluded.

A male patient developed an eczematous reaction to a medicated tape. When patch and photopatch tested, he had a photocontact allergy to the ingredient ketoprofen and contact allergy to the ingredients menthol and the tackifying agent glyceryl hydrogenated rosinate (a colophonium-derivative) (27).

A woman had generalized erythema multiforme-like dermatitis from contact allergy to menthol, present in a concentration of 1.5% in two anti-inflammatory compresses to treat myalgia resulting from a car accident, applied to the back and arms. Patch tests were positive to 1.5% and 10% L-menthol. Generalization of the eruption was considered to be the result of hematogenic spread of the allergen (28).

Other products

In Leuven, Belgium, in the period 2000-2009, an unspecified number of patients had positive patch tests or use tests to a total of 344 cosmetic products *and* positive patch tests to FM I, FM II, and/or to one or more of 28 selected specific fragrance ingredients. In one patient reacting to menthol, the presence of this fragrance in the cosmetic product(s) was confirmed by reading the product label(s) (11). One patient had prolonged lip swelling, apparently from contact allergy to peppermint oil and menthol; another individual had oral ulcerations which was ascribed to menthol allergy (24).

A woman suffered from mild scaly erythema for 2 years affecting the upper lip, the perioral area and the dorsal aspect of the central fingers of both hands. She also often had intermittent outbreaks of erythema and intense facial itching. Patch testing did not reveal a cause. By chance, later contact allergy to menthol was discovered. When she stopped smoking menthol cigarettes, all symptoms disappeared (19).

A man had orofacial granulomatosis, mainly of the lower lip, and was allergic to peppermint oil and menthol. An exclusion diet resulted in reduction of the swelling; upon re-exposure to menthol, further episodes of lip swelling occurred (23). The same authors also presented a woman with recurrent mouth ulcerations for 12 months. She had a positive reaction to menthol 2% pet. on patch testing. Appropriate avoidance advice was given and her symptoms resolved rapidly (23).

Possibly, ref. 48 provides other information on menthol contact allergy not presented here (article not read).

Cross-reactions, pseudo-cross-reactions and co-reactions

For general information on cross-/pseudo-cross-/co-reactivity of fragrance chemicals with other fragrances, fragrance markers (fragrance mix I, fragrance mix II, colophonium, Myroxylon pereirae resin [balsam of Peru]) and essential oils see Chapter 1.2 General information on cross-reactions, pseudo-cross-reactions and co-reactions.

Menthol is the main ingredient of peppermint oil (23-48% [30]) and most likely also most important allergenic constituent. Co-reactivity between menthol and peppermint oil have been observed on numerous occasions (5,13,21,23,24,25,26,29,46). No cross-reaction of menthol to menthoxypropanediol contact allergy (1).

Presence in products and chemical analyses

In 2016, in Sweden, 66 commercially available toothpastes obtained from local pharmacies and supermarkets in Malmö, Sweden, were investigated for the presence of flavors by studying the packages and product labels. Menthol was found to be present in 2 (3%) of the products (18).

In 2008, 66 different fragrance components (including 39 essential oils) were identified in 370 (10% of the total) topical pharmaceutical products marketed in Belgium; 99 of these (27%) contained menthol (3).

In 1997, 71 deodorants (22 vapo-spray, 22 aerosol spray and 27 roll-on products) were collected in Denmark, England, France, Germany and Sweden and analyzed by gas chromatography – mass spectrometry (GC-MS) for the presence of fragrances and other materials. Menthol was present in one (1%) of the products (9).

OTHER SIDE EFFECTS

Irritant contact dermatitis
Local necrosis and interstitial nephritis have been attributed to topical methyl salicylate and menthol. Details are unknown (35, article not read).

At low concentrations, *L*-menthol (levomenthol) produces a cooling sensation when it comes into contact with the skin or mucous membranes. Other isomers of menthol do not exert this cooling effect. Menthol at higher concentrations (5-10% in mineral oil) causes a burning sensation when applied to the skin (45).

Immediate-type reactions
A woman had suffered from hot flashes for 3 years and generalized urticaria for 4 days. Menthol was suspected to be the cause, which she used in the form of peppermint-flavored toothpaste, eating peppermint candy throughout the day and smoking one pack of mentholated cigarettes daily. The patient was advised to avoid peppermint and all other sources of menthol, and the whealing and hot flashes promptly ceased. When a minute amount of peppermint oil was applied to the patient's volar wrist, within 40 minutes urticarial lesions developed at the sites of application, accompanied by a typical flushing reaction. An oral provocation test with 10 mg of menthol in 5 mL of 50% alcohol after 30 minutes resulted in a flushing reaction and at 40 minutes she complained of a pounding frontal headache. Three control patients showed no clinical response to an identical oral challenge. When subsequently 0.1 mL of menthol 75% in 50% alcohol was applied to the flexor forearm in a 3 cm circle under a plastic wrap, within 20 minutes the patient experienced a severe burning sensation, and a 9-cm fiery erythematous reaction formed about the treated area. Two control subjects felt only "cooling" and had slight erythema confined to the original 3-cm circle (32).

A female patient suffered from generalized urticaria. The cause was suspected to be menthol in cigarettes, mint candies, mentholated cough drops, a mentholated aerosol room spray, and liberal applications of a mentholated topical petrolatum product. She also regularly used a facial cream containing menthol, and brushed her teeth twice daily with a mint-flavored toothpaste. The patient was advised to avoid all sources of mint and menthol and the lesions disappeared within 2 days and she was completely free of hives. Two weeks later the patient experienced a single episode of hives which was subsequently traced to an "instant" iced tea preparation containing mint flavoring. A single attempt to reinstitute the use of a mint-flavored toothpaste resulted in an immediate flushing and a general burning sensation. An open test with peppermint oil gave some burning and erythema after 15 minutes, but also in controls. A skin prick test reaction was the same as in 2 controls. However, an oral provocation test with menthol in alcohol induced a warm flushed feeling, a mild frontal headache, a single urticarial wheal on her arm and mild general pruritus. Dermographism could be demonstrated. At two hours all symptoms had subsided. A positive basophil degranulation test to menthol showed, according to the authors, hypersensitivity to menthol with circulating antibodies (31).

See also the section 'Respiratory side effects' below for immediate-type respiratory effects of menthol.

Other non-eczematous contact reactions

Respiratory side effects
A case of rhinitis caused by various menthol-containing products, diagnostically proven by repeatedly positive urticarial reactions after application of 2% menthol in pet. or 5% peppermint oil in pet. and a positive provocation test with brushing of the teeth with menthol-flavored toothpaste, has been reported. The most likely explanation seemed to be – according to the authors – an IgE-mediated reaction (34).

Two patients had aspirin-induced and mint-flavor-sensitive asthma. In one patient, the challenge test with his flavored toothpaste was positive. A challenge was then performed with menthol, one of the components of the patient's toothpaste. He was instructed to rinse his mouth with 25 mg of menthol diluted in 50 ml of 5% alcohol for one minute and then spit it out. Five minutes later, FEV (Forced Expiratory Volume) was decreased from 4.49 liter to 4.08 liter. The patient complained of tightness of the chest (37).

A female nonsmoker had asthma and aspirin intolerance for 6 years. In spite of treatment, the patient required emergency care on 10 occasions because of acute asthma attacks. She reported a moderate increase in dyspnea after daily toothbrushing. Also, on one occasion she suffered an attack of bronchospasm after eating a menthol candy. A challenge was then performed with her toothpaste and a strong immediate response (36% decrease in FEV) was observed. The same test, performed with the same toothpaste but without any flavor, was completely negative. A challenge was then performed with each of the components of the patient's flavored toothpaste (anethole, spearmint oil, eucalyptol, peppermint oil, menthol) and an immediate and significant response was obtained with spearmint oil, peppermint oil, and menthol. The immediate bronchial reaction caused by menthol was completely inhibited by prior inhalation of sodium cromoglycate, even when the patient was challenged with the maximum dose of 100 mg. No specific IgE serum antibodies to these flavors was detected by ELISA (38).

A woman had suffered from dyspnea, wheezing and nasal symptoms for 2 years when exposed to mentholated products such as toothpaste and candies. The diagnosis of menthol-induced asthma was established by skin tests and bronchial challenge with menthol (39).

Systemic side effects
Local necrosis and interstitial nephritis have been attributed to topical methyl salicylate and menthol. Details are unknown (35, article not read).

An almost 2-month-old boy was referred to the intensive care unit 30 minutes after the mother instilled about 1 ml of a menthol solution into the nose instead of NaCl 0.9%. On examination the child was acutely dyspneic and unconscious. His breath smelled strongly of menthol. The pupils were deviated upwards to the left. The extremities were in hyperextension. There was an inspiratory stridor and an irregular respiration rate. Blood gas analysis showed a metabolic acidosis. Oxygen was administered. About 4 hours after admission the pulse, blood pressure and respiration rate returned to normal (36).

In France, two children aged 2 years and 3 months who received a cosmetic baby balm on the skin of their thorax containing eucalyptus, rosemary and lavender essential oils, developed convulsions. As there was no other explanation for this and the 'neurologic toxicity of terpene derivatives is well known' (referring to studies on camphor toxicity), the cosmetic was suspected to be the culprit product. Although no specific terpene ingredient was blamed, the authors discussed the possible role of camphor, menthol and eucalyptol (1,8-cineole). On the basis of these two hardly convincing cases, the product was withdrawn from the market (43).

Miscellaneous side effects
A case of nonthrombocytopenic purpura caused by mentholated cigarettes was reported in 1951. The generalized purpuric rash first appeared about two months after the patient began smoking one to two packs of mentholated cigarettes daily. The eruption disappeared when she discontinued smoking the cigarettes, and it was experimentally reproduced when she ingested 60 mg of menthol three times daily, and also on several occasions when she resumed smoking the mentholated cigarettes. The only consistent hematologic abnormality which paralleled the purpuric eruption was an increase in the blood coagulation time (33).

LITERATURE
1   Franken L, de Groot A, Laheij-de Boer A-M. Allergic contact dermatitis caused by menthoxypropanediol in a lip cosmetic. Contact Dermatitis 2013;69:377-378
2   Wetter DA, Yiannias JA, Prakash AV, Davis MDP, Farmer SA, el-Azhary RA. Results of patch testing to personal care product allergens in a standard series and a supplemental cosmetic series: an analysis of 945 patients from the Mayo Clinic Contact Dermatitis Group, 2000-2007. J Am Acad Dermatol 2010;63:789-798
3   Nardelli A, D'Hooge E, Drieghe J, Dooms M, Goossens A. Allergic contact dermatitis from fragrance components in specific topical pharmaceutical products in Belgium. Contact Dermatitis 2009;60:303-313
4   Ale SI, Hostynek JJ, Maibach HI. Menthol: a review of its sensitization potential. Exog Dermatol 2002;1:74–80
5   Foti C, Conserva A, Antelmi A, Lospalluti L, Angelini G. Contact dermatitis from peppermint and menthol in a local action transcutaneous patch. Contact Dermatitis 2003;49:312-313
6   Dinkloh A, Worm M, Geier J, Schnuch A, Wollenberg A. Contact sensitization in patients with suspected cosmetic intolerance: results of the IVDK 2006-2011. J Eur Acad Dermatol Venereol 2015;29:1071-1081
7   SCCS (Scientific Committee on Consumer Safety). Opinion on Fragrance allergens in cosmetic products, 26-27 June 2012, SCCS/1459/11. Available at:
    https://ec.europa.eu/health/sites/health/files/scientific_committees/consumer_safety/docs/sccs_o_102.pdf
8   Larsen WG. Perfume dermatitis. A study of 20 patients. Arch Dermatol 1977;113:623-626
9   Rastogi SC, Lepoittevin J-P, Johansen JD, Frosch PJ, Menné T, Bruze M, et al. Fragrances and other materials in deodorants: search for potentially sensitizing molecules using combined GC-MS and structure activity relationship (SAR) analysis. Contact Dermatitis 1998;39:293-303
10 Uter W, Johansen JD, Börje A, Karlberg A-T, Lidén C, Rastogi S, Roberts D, White IR. Categorization of fragrance contact allergens for prioritization of preventive measures: clinical and experimental data and consideration of structure–activity relationships. Contact Dermatitis 2013;69:196-230
11 Nardelli A, Drieghe J, Claes L, Boey L, Goossens A. Fragrance allergens in 'specific' cosmetic products. Contact Dermatitis 2011;64:212-219
12 Uter W, Geier J, Frosch P, Schnuch A. Contact allergy to fragrances: current patch test results (2005–2008) from the Information Network of Departments of Dermatology. Contact Dermatitis 2010;63:254-261
13 Morton CA, Garioch J, Todd P, Lamey PJ, Forsyth A. Contact sensitivity to menthol and peppermint in patients with intra-oral symptoms. Contact Dermatitis 1995;32:281-284
14 Hjorth N. Eczematous allergy to balsams. Acta Derm Venereol 1961;41(suppl.46):1-216

15 De Groot AC, Weyland JW, Nater JP. Unwanted effects of cosmetics and drugs used in dermatology. 3rd edition. Amsterdam: Elsevier Science BV; 1994:187-189

16 Hausen BM. Toothpaste allergy. Dtsch Med Wochenschr 1984;109:300-302 (article in German)

17 Sainio E-L, Kanerva L. Contact allergens in toothpastes and a review of their hypersensitivity. Contact Dermatitis 1995;33:100-105

18 Kroona L, Warfvinge G, Isaksson M, Ahlgren C, Dahlin J, Sörensen Ö, Bruze M. Quantification of L-carvone in toothpastes available on the Swedish market. Contact Dermatitis 2017;77:224-230

19 Camarasa G, Alomar A. Menthol dermatitis from cigarettes. Contact Dermatitis 1978;4:169-170

20 Blondeel A, Oleffe J, Achten G. Contact allergy in 330 dermatological patients. Contact Dermatitis 1978;4:270-276

21 Wilkinson SM, Beck MH. Allergic contact dermatitis from menthol in peppermint. Contact Dermatitis 1994;30:42-43

22 Aguirre A, Oleaga JM, Zabala R, Izu R, Díaz-Pérez JL. Allergic contact dermatitis from Reflex® spray. Contact Dermatitis 1994;30:52-53

23 Lewis FM, Shah M, Gawkrodger DJ. Contact sensitivity to food additives can cause oral and perioral symptoms. Contact Dermatitis 1995;33:429-430

24 Shah M, Lewis M, Gawkrodger DJ. Contact allergy in patients with oral symptoms: a study of 47 patients. Am J Cont Derm 1996;7:146-151

25 Fleming CJ, Forsyth A. D5 patch test reactions to menthol and peppermint. Contact Dermatitis 1998;38:337

26 Downs AMR, Lear JT, Sansom JE. Contact sensitivity in patients with oral symptoms. Contact Dermatitis 1998;39:258-259

27 Ota T, Oiso N, Iba Y, Narita T, Kawara S, Kawada A. Concomitant development of photoallergic contact dermatitis from ketoprofen and allergic contact dermatitis from menthol and rosin (colophony) in a compress. Contact Dermatitis 2007;56:47-48

28 Nakagawa S, Tagami H, Aiba S. Erythema multiforme-like generalized contact dermatitis to *l*-menthol contained in anti-inflammatory medical compresses as an ingredient. Contact Dermatitis 2009;61:178-179

29 Bourgeois P, Goossens A. Allergic contact cheilitis caused by menthol in toothpaste and throat medication: a case report. Contact Dermatitis 2016;75:113-115

30 De Groot AC, Schmidt E. Essential oils: contact allergy and chemical composition. Boca Raton, Fl., USA: CRC Press, Taylor and Francis Group, 2016 (ISBN 9781482246407)

31 McGowan EM. Menthol urticaria. Arch Dermatol 1966;94:62-63

32 Papa M, Shelley WB. Menthol hypersensitivity; diagnostic basophil response in a patient with chronic urticaria, flushing, and headaches. JAMA 1964;189:546-548

33 Highstein B, Zeligman I. Non-thrombocytopenic purpura caused by mentholated cigarettes. JAMA 1951;146:816

34 Andersson M, Hindsén M. Rhinitis because of toothpaste and other menthol-containing products. Allergy 2007;62:336-337

35 Heng MCY. Local necrosis and interstitial nephritis due to topical methyl salicylate and menthol. Cutis 1987;39:442-444

36 Melis K, Bochner A, Janssens G. Accidental nasal eucalyptol and menthol instillation. Eur J Pediatr 1989;148:786-787

37 Kawane H. Menthol and aspirin induced asthma. Respir Med 1996;90:247

38 Subiza J, Subiza JL, Valdivieso R, Escribano PM, Garcia R, Jerez M et al. Toothpaste flavour – induced asthma. J Allergy Clin Immunol 1992;90:1004-1006

39 Dos Santos MA, Santos Galvao CE, Morato Castro F. Menthol-induced asthma: a case report. J Investig Allergol Clin Immunol 2001;11:56-58

40 De Groot AC, Popova MP, Bankova VS. An update on the constituents of poplar-type propolis. Available at: https://www.researchgate.net/publication/262851225_AN_UPDATE_ON_THE_CONSTITUENTS_OF_POPLAR-TYPE_PROPOLIS

41 Rudzki E, Kleniewska D. The epidemiology of contact dermatitis in Poland. Br J Dermatol 1970;83:543-545

42 Santucci B, Cristaudo A, Cannistraci C, Picardo M. Contact dermatitis to fragrances. Contact Dermatitis 1987;16:93-95

43 Laribière A, Miremont-Salamé G, Bertrand S, François C, Haramburu F. Terpènes dans les cosmétiques: 2 cas d'épilepsie. Thérapie 2005;60: 607-609

44 Saito F, Miyazaki T, Matsuoka Y. Peppermint oil contact allergy. Skin Res 1984;26:636-643 (article in Japanese).

45 Eccles R. Menthol and related cooling compounds. J Pharm Pharmacol 1994;46:618-630

46 Baer PN. Toothpaste allergies. J Clin Pediatr Dent 1992;16:230-231. Data cited in ref. 47

47 Gilissen L, Huygens S, Goossens A. Allergic contact dermatitis caused by topical herbal remedies: importance of patch testing with the patients' own products. Contact Dermatitis 2018;78:177-184

48 Fisher AA. Reactions to menthol. Cutis 1986;38:17-18

Chapter 3.100 MENTHYL ACETATE

IDENTIFICATION

Description/definition : Menthyl acetate is the ester of menthol and acetic acid, that conforms to the structural formula shown below

Chemical class(es) : Esters

Chemical/IUPAC name : (5-Methyl-2-propan-2-ylcyclohexyl) acetate

Other names : Cyclohexanol, 5-methyl-2-(1-methylethyl)-, acetate; neomenthyl acetate

CAS registry number(s) : 89-48-5

EC number(s) : 201-911-8

RIFM monograph(s) : Food Chem Toxicol 2017;110(suppl.1):S619-S628 (isomer unspecified); Food Cosmet Toxicol 1976;14:477 & 479 (binder, pages 524-525)

Merck Index monograph : 7177

Function(s) in cosmetics : EU: masking; refreshing. USA: cosmetic astringents; flavoring agents; fragrance ingredients

Patch testing : No patch test data available; based on RIFM data, 8% pet. is probably not irritant (2)

Molecular formula : $C_{12}H_{22}O_2$

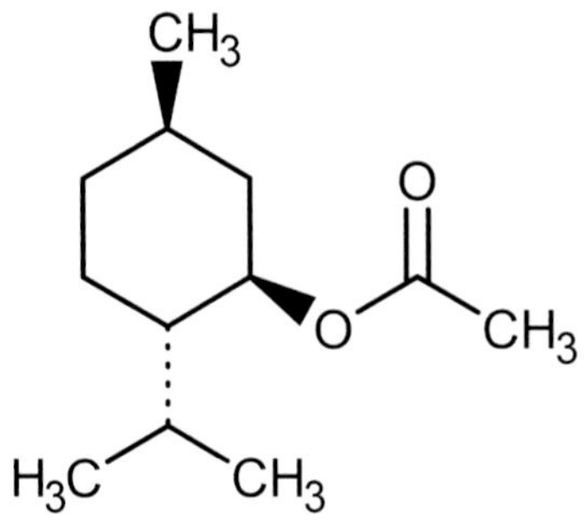

GENERAL

Menthyl acetate is a colorless clear liquid; its odor type is mentholic and its odor is described as 'tea-like, slightly cooling, minty and fruity' (www.thegoodscentscompany.com). In perfumery, menthyl acetate emphasizes floral notes, especially that of rose, used in toilet waters having a lavender odor. It is useful in mint, fruit, berry and caraway flavors (U.S. National Library of Medicine).

Presence in essential oils

Menthyl acetate has been identified by chemical analysis in 10 of 91 essential oils, which have caused contact allergy / allergic contact dermatitis. In one oil, menthyl acetate belonged to the 'Top-10' of ingredients with the highest concentrations which may be expected in commercial essential oils of this type: peppermint oil (0.5-7.7%) (3).

CONTACT ALLERGY

Patch testing in groups of patients

Ten patients allergic to peppermint oil (of who 4 co-reacted to spearmint oil) were patch tested with 24 ingredients. There was one positive reaction to menthyl acetate, 4 to menthol, 4 to piperitone, 3 to pulegone, 2 to tetrahydro-dimethylbenzofuran (menthofuran), and one to dihydrocarveol (1). Further details are lacking (article in Japanese).

LITERATURE

1   Saito F, Miyazaki T, Matsuoka Y. Peppermint oil contact allergy. Skin Research 1984;26:636-643 (article in Japanese)

2   De Groot AC. Patch Testing, 4th Edition. Wapserveen, The Netherlands: acdegroot publishing, 2018 (ISBN 978-90-813233-4-5)

3   De Groot AC, Schmidt E. Essential oils: contact allergy and chemical composition. Boca Raton, Fl., USA: CRC Press, Taylor and Francis Group, 2016 (ISBN 9781482246407)

Chapter 3.101 METHOXYCINNAMAL

IDENTIFICATION

Description/definition	: Methoxycinnamal is the organic compound that conforms to the structural formula shown below
Chemical class(es)	: Aldehydes
Chemical/IUPAC name	: 3-(2-Methoxyphenyl)prop-2-enal
Other names	: 2-(o-) or 4-(p)-Methoxycinnamaldehyde; o- or p-methoxycinnamic aldehyde
CAS registry number(s)	: 1504-74-1 (o-); 60125-24-8 (o-); 1963-36-6 (p-); 24680-50-0 (p-)
EC number(s)	: 216-131-3 (o-); 217-807-0 (p-)
RIFM monograph(s)	: Food Cosmet Toxicol 1975;13:845 (special issue II)
IFRA standard	: Restricted (www.ifraorg.org/en-us/standards-library) (table 3.101.1)
Function(s) in cosmetics	: EU: antioxidant; perfuming. USA: antioxidants; fragrance ingredients
Patch testing	: 4% pet. (1)
Molecular formula	: $C_{10}H_{10}O_2$

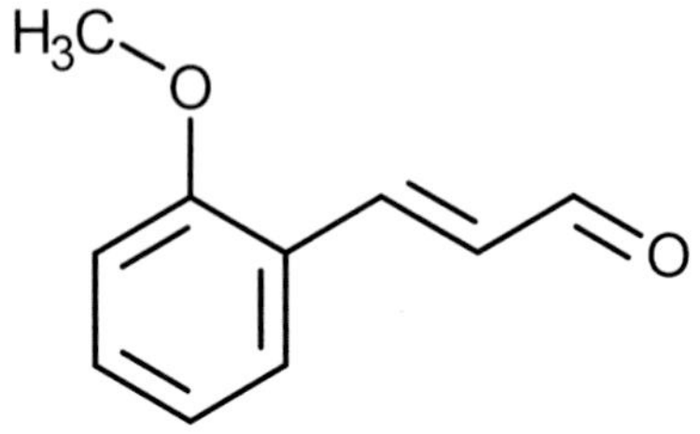

o-Methoxycinnamal 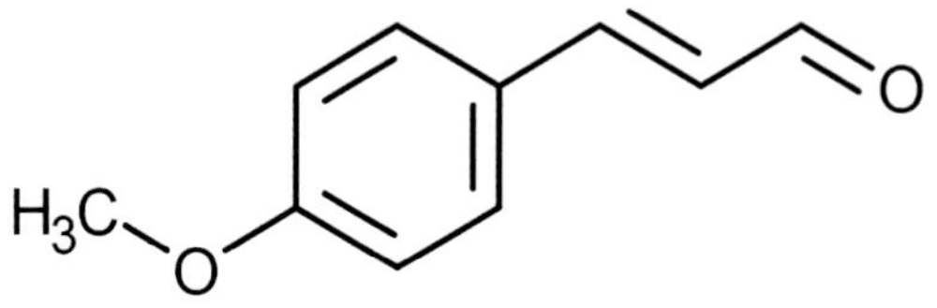   p-Methoxycinnamal

Table 3.101.1 IFRA restrictions for methoxycinnamal

Category [a]	Limits [b]	Category [a]	Limits [b]	Category [a]	Limits [b]
1	0.03%	5	0.24%	9	5.00%
2	0.04%	6	0.72%	10	2.50%
3	0.15%	7	0.08%	11	not restricted
4	0.45%	8	1.01%		

[a] For explanation of categories see pages 6-8

GENERAL

Methoxycinnamal appear as pale yellow crystals; its odor type is spicy and its odor at 100% is described as 'sweet cinnamon cassia oily woody paper' (www.thegoodscentscompany.com).

Presence in essential oils

Methoxycinnamal has been identified by chemical analysis in 4 of 91 essential oils, which have caused contact allergy / allergic contact dermatitis. In one oil, (E)-2-methoxycinnamal belonged to the 'Top-10' of ingredients with the highest concentrations which may be expected in commercial essential oils of this type: cassia oil (6.8-11.1%) (2).

CONTACT ALLERGY

Case reports and case series

A baker had recurrent dyshidrotic eczema of the hands. Routine patch testing was negative, but he reacted to the cinnamon powder he had brought from his work. When tested subsequently with a series of fragrances/flavors, he reacted to methoxycinnamal 4% and several other cinnamates. The author was 'inclined' to say that these reactions may have been relevant (1).

Cross-reactions, pseudo-cross-reactions and co-reactions

Co-reactions have been observed with other cinnamon-derivatives: cinnamyl alcohol, cinnamal, cinnamyl benzoate, cinnamyl cinnamate, and amyl cinnamate (1).

LITERATURE

1   Malten KE. Four bakers showing positive patch tests to a number of fragrance materials, which can also be used as flavors. Acta Derm Venereol 1979;59(suppl.85):117-121
2   De Groot AC, Schmidt E. Essential oils: contact allergy and chemical composition. Boca Raton, Fl., USA: CRC Press, Taylor and Francis Group, 2016 (ISBN 9781482246407)

Chapter 3.102 METHOXYCITRONELLAL

IDENTIFICATION

Description/definition   : Methoxycitronellal is the aldehyde that conforms to the structural formula shown
                            below
Chemical class(es)   : Organic compounds; aldehydes; ethers
INCI name USA   : Not in the Personal Care Products Council Ingredient Database
Chemical/IUPAC name   : 7-Methoxy-3,7-dimethyloctanal
CAS registry number(s)   : 3613-30-7
EC number(s)   : 222-784-5
RIFM monograph(s)   : Food Cosmet Toxicol 1976;14:807 (special issue III)
SCCS opinion(s)   : SCCS/1459/11 (1)
Function(s) in cosmetics : EU: perfuming
Patch testing   : 10% pet. (2)
Molecular formula   : $C_{11}H_{22}O_2$

GENERAL

Methoxycitronellal is a colorless clear liquid; its odor type is floral and its odor at 100% is described as 'fresh melon floral lily sweet' (www.thegoodscentscompany.com). Methoxycitronellal is a synthetic chemical, not found in nature (and consequently not in essential oils (7)).

CONTACT ALLERGY

General

The SCCS (Scientific Committee on Consumer Safety), in a 2012 Opinion on Fragrance allergens in cosmetic products, has categorized methoxycitronellal as 'likely fragrance contact allergen by combination of evidence' (1,6).

Patch testing in groups of patients

Studies in which methoxycitronellal was patch tested in either consecutive patients suspected of contact dermatitis (routine testing) or in groups of selected patients with positive results have not been found.

Pigmented cosmetic dermatitis

In Japan, in the 1960s and 1970s, many female patients developed pigmentation of the face after having facial dermatitis (3). The skin manifestations of this so-called pigmented cosmetic dermatitis consisted of diffuse or patchy brown hyperpigmentation on the cheeks and/or forehead, sometimes the entire face was involved. In severe cases, the pigmentation was black, purple, or blue-black, and in mild cases, it was pale brown. Occasionally, erythematous macules or papules, suggesting a mild contact dermatitis, were observed and itching was also noted at varying times.

Pigmented cosmetic dermatitis was shown to be caused by contact allergy to components of cosmetic products, notably essential oils, other fragrance materials, antimicrobials, preservatives and coloring materials (2,3,4). In a group of 137 Japanese patients with this condition investigated between 1971 and 1974, 9% had positive patch test reactions to methoxycitronellal 10% in petrolatum versus 1% in a control group of patients not suffering from pigmented cosmetic dermatitis (2).

The number of patients with pigmented cosmetic dermatitis decreased strongly after 1978, when major cosmetic companies began to eliminate strong contact sensitizers from their products (2). Since 1980, pigmented cosmetic dermatitis became a rare disease in Japan (5).

Case reports and case series

Case reports of allergic contact dermatitis from methoxycitronellal have not been found.

Cross-reactions, pseudo-cross-reactions and co-reactions

For general information on cross-/pseudo-cross-/co-reactivity of fragrance chemicals with other fragrances, fragrance markers (fragrance mix I, fragrance mix II, colophonium, Myroxylon pereirae resin [balsam of Peru]) and essential oils see Chapter 1.2 General information on cross-reactions, pseudo-cross-reactions and co-reactions.

Possibly cross-reactivity with hydroxycitronellal (4).

LITERATURE

1   SCCS (Scientific Committee on Consumer Safety). Opinion on Fragrance allergens in cosmetic products, 26-27 June 2012, SCCS/1459/11. Available at:
    https://ec.europa.eu/health/sites/health/files/scientific_committees/consumer_safety/docs/sccs_o_102.pdf
2   Nakayama H, Matsuo S, Hayakawa K, Takhashi K, Shigematsu T, Ota S. Pigmented cosmetic dermatitis. Int J Dermatol 1984;23:299-305
3   Nakayama H, Harada R, Toda M. Pigmented cosmetic dermatitis. Int J Dermatol 1976;15:673-675
4   Nakayama H, Hanaoka H, Ohshiro A. Allergen Controlled System. Tokyo: Kanehara Shuppan, 1974
5   Ebihara T, Nakayama H. Pigmented contact dermatitis. Clin Dermatol 1997;15:593-599
6   Uter W, Johansen JD, Börje A, Karlberg A-T, Lidén C, Rastogi S, Roberts D, White IR. Categorization of fragrance contact allergens for prioritization of preventive measures: clinical and experimental data and consideration of structure–activity relationships. Contact Dermatitis 2013;69:196-230
7   De Groot AC, Schmidt E. Essential oils: contact allergy and chemical composition. Boca Raton, Fl., USA: CRC Press, Taylor and Francis Group, 2016 (ISBN 9781482246407)

Chapter 3.103 2-METHOXYPHENOL/2,2-DIMETHYL-3-METHYLENEBICY-CLOHEPTANE HYDROGENATED

IDENTIFICATION

Description/definition	: 2-Methoxyphenol/2,2-dimethyl-3-methylenebicycloheptane hydrogenated is the bicyclic substituted cyclohexanol that conforms to the structural formula shown below
Chemical class(es)	: Bicyclic organic compounds; alcohols
INCI name USA	: Not in the Personal Care Products Council Ingredient Database
Chemical/IUPAC name	: (4R)-3,3-Dimethyl-2-methylidenebicyclo[2.2.1]heptane;2-methoxyphenol
Other names	: Phenol, 2-methoxy-, reaction products with 2,2-dimethyl-3-methylenebicyclo[2.2.1]heptane, hydrogenated; m-(isocamphyl-5)-cyclohexanol; sandela
CAS registry number(s)	: 70955-71-4
EC number(s)	: 275-062-7
Function(s) in cosmetics	: EU: perfuming
Patch testing	: 5% pet. (1); some irritant reactions cannot be excluded
Molecular formula	: $C_{16}H_{28}O$

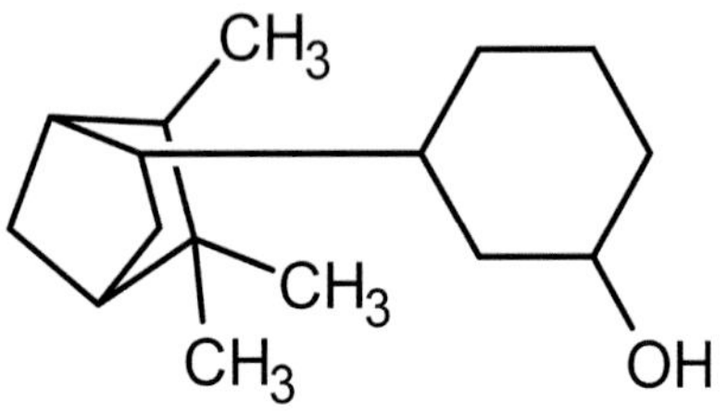

GENERAL

2-Methoxyphenol/2,2-dimethyl-3-methylenebicycloheptane hydrogenated is a colorless to pale yellow slightly viscous liquid; its odor type is woody and its odor at 100% is described as 'sandalwood clean sweet woody cashew' (www.thegoodscentscompany.com). 2-Methoxyphenol/2,2-dimethyl-3-methylenebicycloheptane is a synthetic chemical, not found in nature (and consequently not in essential oils (2)).

CONTACT ALLERGY

Patch testing in groups of patients

Patch testing in consecutive patients suspected of contact dermatitis: routine testing
Studies in which 2-methoxyphenol/2,2-dimethyl-3-methylenebicycloheptane hydrogenated was patch tested in consecutive patients suspected of contact dermatitis (routine testing) with positive results have not been found.

Testing in groups of selected patients
Before 1996, in Japan, some European countries and the USA, 167 patients known or suspected to be allergic to fragrances were patch tested with 2-methoxyphenol/2,2-dimethyl-3-methylenebicycloheptane hydrogenated 5% pet. and there were eleven (6.6%) positive reactions; their relevance was not mentioned (1). As the frequency is unexpectedly high, the possibility of (some) false-positive reactions due to irritancy of the test material should be considered.

Case reports and case series
Case reports of allergic contact dermatitis from 2-methoxyphenol/2,2-dimethyl-3-methylenebicycloheptane hydrogenated have not been found.

LITERATURE
1   Larsen W, Nakayama H, Fischer T, Elsner P, Burrows D, Jordan W, et al. Fragrance contact dermatitis: A worldwide multicenter investigation (Part I). Am J Cont Dermat 1996;7:77-83
2   De Groot AC, Schmidt E. Essential oils: contact allergy and chemical composition. Boca Raton, Fl., USA: CRC Press, Taylor and Francis Group, 2016 (ISBN 9781482246407)

Chapter 3.104 METHOXYTRIMETHYLHEPTANOL

IDENTIFICATION

Description/definition   : Methoxytrimethylheptanol is the organic compound that conforms to the structural
                              formula shown below
Chemical class(es)   : Alcohols; ethers
Chemical/IUPAC name   : 7-Methoxy-3,7-dimethyloctan-2-ol
Other names   : 3,7-Dimethyl-7-methoxyoctan-2-ol; osyrol; sandal octanol
CAS registry number (s)   : 41890-92-0
EC number(s)   : 225-574-7
RIFM monograph(s)   : Food Chem Toxicol 2010;48(suppl.4):S51-S54; Food Chem Toxicol 1992;30(suppl.1):S25
SCCS opinion(s)   : SCCS/1459/11 (1)
Function(s) in cosmetics   : EU: masking; perfuming. USA: fragrance ingredients
Patch testing   : 5% pet. (2) (uncertain)
Molecular formula   : $C_{11}H_{24}O_2$

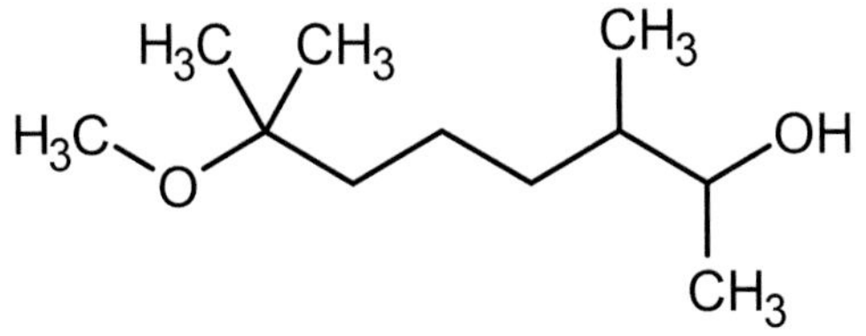

GENERAL

Methoxytrimethylheptanol is a colorless clear liquid; its odor type is woody and its odor at 100% is described as 'sweet sandalwood soapy floral woody' (www.thegoodscentscompany.com). Methoxytrimethylheptanol is a synthetic chemical, not found in nature (and consequently not in essential oils (4)).

CONTACT ALLERGY

General
The SCCS (Scientific Committee on Consumer Safety), in a 2012 Opinion on Fragrance allergens in cosmetic products, has categorized methoxytrimethylheptanol as 'possible fragrance contact allergen' (1,3).

Patch testing in consecutive patients suspected of contact dermatitis: routine testing
Studies in which methoxytrimethylheptanol was patch tested in consecutive patients suspected of contact dermatitis (routine testing) with positive results have not been found.

Testing in groups of selected patients
Before 2002, in Japan, European countries and the USA, 218 patients with known fragrance sensitivity were patch tested with methoxytrimethylheptanol (test concentration and vehicle unknown, probably 5% in petrolatum) and two positive reactions (0.9%) were observed; their relevance was not mentioned (2).

Case reports and case series
Case reports of allergic contact dermatitis from methoxytrimethylheptanol have not been found.

LITERATURE

1   SCCS (Scientific Committee on Consumer Safety). Opinion on Fragrance allergens in cosmetic products, 26-27 June 2012, SCCS/1459/11. Available at: https://ec.europa.eu/health/sites/health/files/scientific_committees/consumer_safety/docs/sccs_o_102.pdf
2   Larsen W, Nakayama H, Fischer T, Elsner P, Frosch P, Burrows D, et al. Fragrance contact dermatitis - a worldwide multicenter investigation (Part III). Contact Dermatitis 2002;46:141-144
3   Uter W, Johansen JD, Börje A, Karlberg A-T, Lidén C, Rastogi S, Roberts D, White IR. Categorization of fragrance contact allergens for prioritization of preventive measures: clinical and experimental data and consideration of structure–activity relationships. Contact Dermatitis 2013;69:196-230
4   De Groot AC, Schmidt E. Essential oils: contact allergy and chemical composition. Boca Raton, Fl., USA: CRC Press, Taylor and Francis Group, 2016 (ISBN 9781482246407)

Chapter 3.105 METHYL P-ANISATE

IDENTIFICATION

Description/definition	: Methyl p-anisate is the benzoic acid derivative that conforms to the structural formula shown below
Chemical class(es)	: Aromatic compounds; esters; ethers
INCI name USA	: Not in the Personal Care Products Council Ingredient Database
Chemical/IUPAC name	: Methyl 4-methoxybenzoate
Other names	: Methyl 4-anisate
CAS registry number(s)	: 121-98-2
EC number(s)	: 204-513-2
RIFM monograph(s)	: Food Cosmet Toxicol 1976;14:481
SCCS opinion(s)	: SCCS/1459/11 (1)
Function(s) in cosmetics	: EU: perfuming
Patch testing	: 4% pet. (2,4)
Molecular formula	: $C_9H_{10}O_3$

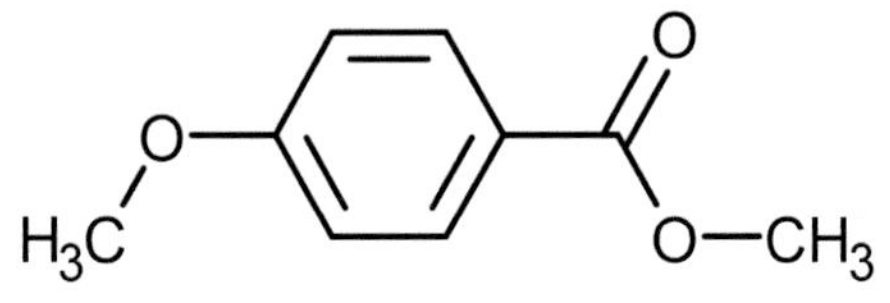

GENERAL

Methyl p-anisate is a white crystalline powder; its odor type is anisic and its odor at 100% is described as 'herbal anise sweet' (www.thegoodscentscompany.com).

Presence in essential oils

Methyl p-anisate has been identified by chemical analysis in four of 91 essential oils, which have caused contact allergy / allergic contact dermatitis: hyssop oil, star anise oil, ylang-ylang oil and zdravetz oil (5).

CONTACT ALLERGY

General

The SCCS (Scientific Committee on Consumer Safety), in a 2012 Opinion on Fragrance allergens in cosmetic products, has categorized methyl p-anisate as 'possible fragrance contact allergen' (1,3).

Patch testing in groups of patients

Patch testing in consecutive patients suspected of contact dermatitis: routine testing

Studies in which methyl p-anisate was patch tested in consecutive patients suspected of contact dermatitis (routine testing) with positive results have not been found.

Patch testing in groups of selected patients

In 1983, in The Netherlands, 182 patients suspected of cosmetic allergy were patch tested with methyl p-anisate 4% in petrolatum and there was one (0.5%) positive reaction; its relevance was not mentioned (2).

Case reports and case series

A metal grinder who previously suffered from posttraumatic thrombosis developed lower leg ulcers and later a weeping stasis dermatitis. When patch tested, the patient reacted to several allergens, including the paraben-mix, 3 topical pharmaceutical preparations containing parabens, to methyl p-anisate and ethyl anisate. The patient denied using perfumes, although – according to the author – perfumes may have been present in some cosmetics or therapeutics used by him. The author further suggested that the reaction to the perfume ingredients should be regarded as group specific reactions (cross-reactions) in a patient contact sensitized to parabens present in topically applied medicaments, because of the chemical similarities between the parabens and the anisates (4).

Cross-reactions, pseudo-cross-reactions and co-reactions

For general information on cross-/pseudo-cross-/co-reactivity of fragrance chemicals with other fragrances, fragrance markers (fragrance mix I, fragrance mix II, colophonium, Myroxylon pereirae resin [balsam of Peru]) and essential oils see Chapter 1.2 General information on cross-reactions, pseudo-cross-reactions and co-reactions.

Possibly cross-reactivity to or from ethyl anisate (4); possibly to or more likely from parabens (4).

LITERATURE

1   SCCS (Scientific Committee on Consumer Safety). Opinion on Fragrance allergens in cosmetic products, 26-27 June 2012, SCCS/1459/11. Available at:
     https://ec.europa.eu/health/sites/health/files/scientific_committees/consumer_safety/docs/sccs_o_102.pdf
2   Malten KE, van Ketel WG, Nater JP, Liem DH. Reactions in selected patients to 22 fragrance materials. Contact Dermatitis 1984;11:1-10
3   Uter W, Johansen JD, Börje A, Karlberg A-T, Lidén C, Rastogi S, Roberts D, White IR. Categorization of fragrance contact allergens for prioritization of preventive measures: clinical and experimental data and consideration of structure–activity relationships. Contact Dermatitis 2013;69:196-230
4   Malten KE. Sensitization to solcoseryl and methylanisate (fragrance ingredient). Contact Dermatitis 1977;3:219
5   De Groot AC, Schmidt E. Essential oils: contact allergy and chemical composition. Boca Raton, Fl., USA: CRC Press, Taylor and Francis Group, 2016 (ISBN 9781482246407)

Chapter 3.106 METHYL ANTHRANILATE

IDENTIFICATION

Description/definition   : Methyl anthranilate is the ester of methyl alcohol and 2-aminobenzoic acid, that
                             conforms to the structural formula shown below
Chemical class(es)   : Amines; esters
Chemical/IUPAC name   : Methyl 2-aminobenzoate
Other names   : Neroli oil, artificial
CAS registry number(s)   : 134-20-3
EC number(s)   : 205-132-4
RIFM monograph(s)   : Food Chem Toxicol 2017;110(suppl.1):S290-S298; Food Cosmet Toxicol 1974;12:935
                             (special issue I)
Merck Index monograph : 6020
Function(s) in cosmetics : EU: masking. USA: flavoring agents; fragrance ingredients
Patch testing   : 5% Pet. (Chemotechnique, SmartPracticeCanada)
Molecular formula   : $C_8H_9NO_2$

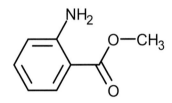

GENERAL

Methyl anthranilate is a pale yellow to dark yellow clear liquid to solid; its odor type is fruity and its odor is described as 'fruity, concord grape, musty with a floral powdery nuance' (www.thegoodscentscompany.com). Methyl anthranilate is used as a fragrance, flavor, pesticide, and in the manufacture of synthetic perfumes. The chemical is an effective, non-toxic and non-lethal bird repellant, with application potential for protecting crops, seeds, turf and fish stocks from bird damage (U.S. National Library of Medicine).

Presence in essential oils

Methyl anthranilate has been identified by chemical analysis in seven of 91 essential oils, which have caused contact allergy / allergic contact dermatitis. In none of these oils, it belonged to the 'Top-10' of ingredients with the highest concentrations (4).

CONTACT ALLERGY

Patch testing in groups of patients

Patch testing in consecutive patients suspected of contact dermatitis: routine testing
Studies in which methyl anthranilate was patch tested in consecutive patients suspected of contact dermatitis (routine testing) with positive results have not been found.

Patch testing in groups of selected patients
Results of studies patch testing methyl anthranilate in groups of selected patients (patients with eyelid dermatitis, patients with suspected photosensitivity or reactions to sunscreens) are shown in table 3.106.1. In two investigations, frequencies of sensitization were 1% in 100 patients with eyelid dermatitis (1) and 1.9% in a group of 160 patients with suspected photosensitivity or who developed pruritus or a rash after sunscreen application (2). In neither studies was the relevance of the positive patch test reactions mentioned (1,2).

Case reports and case series
Case reports of allergic contact dermatitis from methyl anthranilate have not been found.

Presence in products and chemical analyses
In 2000, fifty-nine domestic and occupational products, purchased in retail outlets in Denmark, England, Germany and Italy were analyzed by GC-MS for the presence of fragrances. The product categories were liquid soap and soap bars (n=13), soft/hard surface cleaners (n=23), fabric conditioners/laundry detergents for hand wash (n=8), dish

wash (n=10), furniture polish, car shampoo, stain remover (each n=1) and 2 products used in occupational environments. Methyl anthranilate was present in 7 products (12%); quantification was not performed (3).

Table 3.106.1 Patch testing in groups of patients: Selected patient groups

Years and Country	Test conc. & vehicle	Number of patients tested	positive (%)		Selection of patients (S); Relevance (R); Comments (C)	Ref.
2006-2010 USA	5% pet.	100	1	(1%)	S: patients with eyelid dermatitis; R: not stated	1
2001-2010 Canada	not stated	160	3	(1.9%)	S: patients with suspected photosensitivity and patients who developed pruritus or a rash after sunscreen application; R: not stated; C: inadequate reading of test results: erythema only was considered to represent a positive patch test reaction	2

OTHER SIDE EFFECTS

Photosensitivity

Photopatch testing in groups of patients

In the period 2001-2010, in Canada, 160 patients with suspected photosensitivity and patients who developed pruritus or a rash after sunscreen application were tested with methyl anthranilate (test concentration and vehicle not mentioned) and there were 2 (1.3%) positive photopatch tests; their relevance was not mentioned (2). It should be appreciated that erythema only was considered to represent a positive patch test, which is not conform internationally accepted criteria.

LITERATURE

1 Wenk KS, Ehrlich AE. Fragrance series testing in eyelid dermatitis. Dermatitis 2012;23:22-26
2 Greenspoon J, Ahluwalia R, Juma N, Rosen CF. Allergic and photoallergic contact dermatitis: A 10-year experience. Dermatitis 2013;24:29-32
3 Rastogi SC, Heydorn S, Johansen JD, Basketter DA. Fragrance chemicals in domestic and occupational products. Contact Dermatitis 2001;45:221-225
4 De Groot AC, Schmidt E. Essential oils: contact allergy and chemical composition. Boca Raton, Fl., USA: CRC Press, Taylor and Francis Group, 2016 (ISBN 9781482246407)

Chapter 3.107 METHYL CINNAMATE

IDENTIFICATION

Description/definition	: Methyl cinnamate is the methyl ester of cinnamic acid, that conforms to the structural formula shown below
Chemical class(es)	: Aromatic compounds; unsaturated compounds; esters
INCI name USA	: Not in the Personal Care Products Council Ingredient Database
Chemical/IUPAC name	: Methyl 3-phenylprop-2-enoate
Other names	: Methyl 3-phenylacrylate; cinnamic acid, methyl ester
CAS registry number(s)	: 103-26-4
EC number(s)	: 203-093-8
RIFM monograph(s)	: Food Chem Toxicol 2007;45(suppl.1):S113-S119; Food Chem Toxicol 2007;45(suppl.1):S1-S23; Food Cosmet Toxicol 1975;13:849 (special issue II)
SCCS opinion(s)	: SCCS/1459/11 (3)
Function(s) in cosmetics	: EU: perfuming
Patch testing	: 5% pet. (1);10% pet. (2); based on RIFM data, 8% pet. is probably not irritant (6)
Molecular formula	: $C_{10}H_{10}O_2$

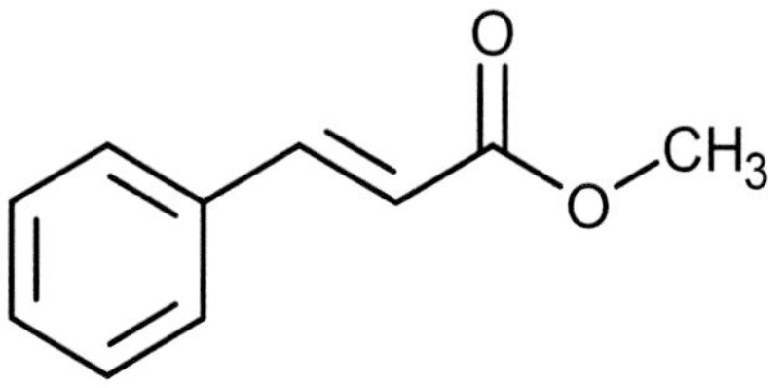

GENERAL

Methyl cinnamate appears as white crystalline fused; its odor type is balsamic and its odor at 100% is described as 'sweet balsam strawberry cherry cinnamon' (www.thegoodscentscompany.com).

Presence in essential oils, Myroxylon pereirae resin (balsam of Peru) and propolis

Methyl cinnamate (any isomer) has been identified by chemical analysis in 3 of 91 essential oils, which have caused contact allergy / allergic contact dermatitis. In one oil, (Z)-methyl cinnamate belonged to the 'Top-10' of ingredients with the highest concentrations which may be expected in commercial essential oils of this type: basil oil (0-23.6%) (8). Methyl cinnamate may also be present in Myroxylon pereirae resin (balsam of Peru) (2,9) and in propolis (1).

CONTACT ALLERGY

General

The SCCS (Scientific Committee on Consumer Safety), in a 2012 Opinion on Fragrance allergens in cosmetic products, has categorized methyl cinnamate as 'likely fragrance contact allergen by combination of evidence' (3,5).

Patch testing in groups of patients

Patch testing in consecutive patients suspected of contact dermatitis: routine testing

Studies in which methyl cinnamate was patch tested in consecutive patients suspected of contact dermatitis (routine testing) with positive results have not been found.

Patch testing in groups of selected patients

Results of studies patch testing methyl cinnamate in groups of selected patients (e.g. patients allergic to propolis, individuals with known contact allergy to Myroxylon pereirae resin [balsam of Peru]) are shown in table 3.107.1. In one study in which 27 patients allergic to propolis were tested with methyl cinnamate 5% pet., only one had a positive reaction (1). It appears that methyl cinnamate is a minor allergenic ingredient of propolis. The major sensitizers are caffeic acid esters.

Also in Myroxylon pereirae resin (balsam of Peru), methyl cinnamate is not an important allergenic constituent. In 3 groups of patients allergic to balsam of Peru and patch tested with a battery of its ingredients including methyl cinnamate, only 0%, 3% and 4.2% positive reactions to this chemical were observed (2,7,9).

The results of patch testing with all known allergenic ingredients of balsam of Peru are shown in Chapter 3.126 Myroxylon pereirae resin (balsam of Peru).

Table 3.107.1 Patch testing in groups of patients: Selected patient groups

Years and Country	Test conc. & vehicle	Number of patients tested	positive (%)		Selection of patients (S); Relevance (R); Comments (C)	Ref.
1995-2005 Germany	5% pet.	27	1	(4%)	S: patients allergic to propolis; C: minor allergenic ingredient in propolis cera; the major allergens are caffeic acid esters	1
Testing in patients allergic to Myroxylon pereirae resin (balsam of Peru)						
1995-1998 Germany	10% pet.	102	3	(3%)	S: patients allergic to balsam of Peru	2
<1990 Denmark	25% pet.	15	0	-	S: patients allergic to balsam of Peru	9
<1976 USA, Canada, Europe		142	6	(4.2%)	S: patients allergic to balsam of Peru	7

Case reports and case series
Case reports of allergic contact dermatitis from methyl cinnamate have not been found.

Presence in products and chemical analyses
In 1997, 71 deodorants (22 vapo-spray, 22 aerosol spray and 27 roll-on products) were collected in Denmark, England, France, Germany and Sweden and analyzed by gas chromatography – mass spectrometry (GC-MS) for the presence of fragrances and other materials. Methyl cinnamate was present in 2 (3%) of the products (4).

LITERATURE
1   Hausen BM. Evaluation of the main contact allergens in propolis (1995 to 2005). Dermatitis 2005;16:127-129
2   Hausen BM. Contact allergy to Balsam of Peru. II. Patch test results in 102 patients with selected Balsam of Peru constituents. Am J Contact Derm 2001;12:93-102
3   SCCS (Scientific Committee on Consumer Safety). Opinion on Fragrance allergens in cosmetic products, 26-27 June 2012, SCCS/1459/11. Available at: https://ec.europa.eu/health/sites/health/files/scientific_committees/consumer_safety/docs/sccs_o_102.pdf
4   Rastogi SC, Lepoittevin J-P, Johansen JD, Frosch PJ, Menné T, Bruze M, et al. Fragrances and other materials in deodorants: search for potentially sensitizing molecules using combined GC-MS and structure activity relationship (SAR) analysis. Contact Dermatitis 1998;39:293-303
5   Uter W, Johansen JD, Börje A, Karlberg A-T, Lidén C, Rastogi S, Roberts D, White IR. Categorization of fragrance contact allergens for prioritization of preventive measures: clinical and experimental data and consideration of structure–activity relationships. Contact Dermatitis 2013;69:196-230
6   De Groot AC. Patch Testing, 4th Edition. Wapserveen, The Netherlands: acdegroot publishing, 2018 (ISBN 978-90-813233-4-5)
7   Mitchell JC, Calnan CD, Clendenning WE, Cronin E, Hjorth N, Magnusson B, et al. Patch testing with some components of balsam of Peru. Contact Dermatitis 1976;2:57-58
8   De Groot AC, Schmidt E. Essential oils: contact allergy and chemical composition. Boca Raton, Fl., USA: CRC Press, Taylor and Francis Group, 2016 (ISBN 9781482246407)
9   Oxholm A, Heidenheim M, Larsen E, Batsberg W, Menné T. Extraction and patch testing of methylcinnamate, a newly recognized fraction of balsam of Peru. Dermatitis 1990;1:43-46

Chapter 3.108 6-METHYL COUMARIN

IDENTIFICATION

Description/definition   : 6-Methyl coumarin is the heterocyclic compound that conforms to the structural formula
                             shown below
Chemical class(es)   : Esters; heterocyclic compounds
Chemical/IUPAC name   : 6-Methylchromen-2-one
Other names   : Methyl coumarin; 6-methylcoumarin
CAS registry number(s)   : 92-48-8
EC number(s)   : 202-158-8
RIFM monograph(s)   : Food Cosmet Toxicol 1979;17:275; Food Cosmet Toxicol 1976;14:605
IFRA standard   : Prohibited (www.ifraorg.org/en-us/standards-library)
SCCS opinion(s)   : SCCNFP/0320/00, final (3); SCCS/1459/11 (4)
Function(s) in cosmetics   : EU: masking; oral care. USA: fragrance ingredients
EU cosmetic restrictions   : Regulated in Annex III/46 of the Regulation (EC) No. 1223/2009, regulated by
                             83/191/EEC
Patch testing   : 1% Pet. (Chemotechnique); 1% alc. (Chemotechnique)
Molecular formula   : $C_{10}H_8O_2$

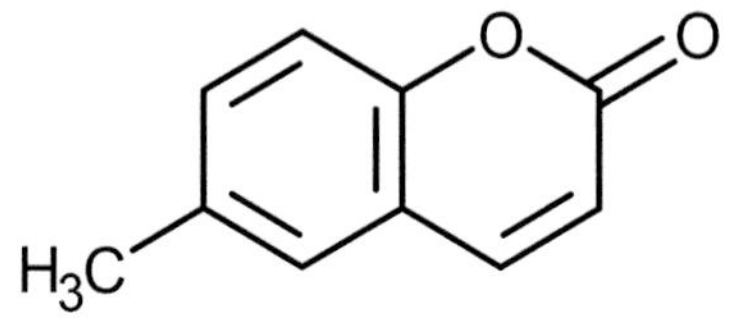

GENERAL

6-Methyl coumarin appears as white crystals; its odor type is coconut and its odor is described as 'sweet coconut, vanilla, creamy with a powdery floral nuance' (www.thegoodscentscompany.com). It is a synthetic chemical, not found in nature (and consequently not in essential oils (23)). 6-Methyl coumarin is prohibited by IFRA because of photoallergy (www.ifraorg.org) and is not used anymore in cosmetics.

General information on photosensitivity to 6-methyl coumarin can be found below in the section 'Photosensitivity, General'

CONTACT ALLERGY

General
The SCCS (Scientific Committee on Consumer Safety), in a 2012 Opinion on Fragrance allergens in cosmetic products, has marked 6-methyl coumarin as 'established **photo**contact allergen in humans' (4,9).

Patch testing in groups of patients

Patch testing in consecutive patients suspected of contact dermatitis: routine testing
Studies in which 6-methyl coumarin was patch tested in consecutive patients suspected of contact dermatitis (routine testing) with positive results have not been found.

Patch testing in groups of selected patients
Results of studies patch testing 6-methyl coumarin in groups of selected patients (patients with suspected photosensitivity) are shown in table 3.108.1. In three studies, rates of positive reactions were 0.3%, 1.7% and 11.9% (2,11,16). The latter study with 11.9% positive reactions, however, had certain flaws, notably that erythema only (?+ reaction) was regarded as 'positive', which is not according to internationally accepted criteria (2). In two of the investigations, no relevance data were provided, but in the third (16), 2 of 3 reactions were considered to be relevant. Culprit products were not mentioned, but it is unlikely that, given the well-known photosensitizing capacity of 6-methyl coumarin, it was still used in consumer products in the USA in the period 2000-2005.

Case reports and case series
Case reports of allergic contact dermatitis (*not* photoallergic) to 6-methyl coumarin have not been found.

Table 3.108.1 Patch testing in groups of patients: Selected patient groups

Years and Country	Test conc. & vehicle	Number of patients tested	positive (%)		Selection of patients (S); Relevance (R); Comments (C)	Ref.
2005-2014 China	1% pet.	2565	7	(0.3%)	S: patients suspected of photodermatoses; R: not stated	11
2001-2010 Canada	not stated	160	19	(11.9%)	S: patients with suspected photosensitivity and patients who developed pruritus or a rash after sunscreen application; R: not stated; C: weak study: inadequate reading of test results, erythema only was considered to represent a positive patch test reaction	2
2000-2005 USA	1% alc.	176	3	(1.7%)	S: patients photopatch tested for suspected photodermatitis; R: two of the three reactions were relevant	16

OTHER SIDE EFFECTS

Photosensitivity

General

6-Methyl coumarin (6-MC) is a synthetic compound, an organic lactone structurally related to the furocoumarins. 6-MC has been in use in the United States since 1920. It was employed as a fragrance in a great variety of cosmetics and toiletries including soaps, detergents, creams and perfumes. The usual concentration ranged from 0.001% to 0.4%. It was also used as an artificial flavoring substance in foods (22). In the late 1970s an epidemic of photodermatitis occurred in people using a popular sunscreen with an increased level of 6-methyl coumarin (17). The reactions occurred primarily in women and developed within several hours after they applied the suntan lotion and went into the sun. The reactions were particularly severe, requiring hospitalization in many cases. Most of the patients' eruptions took weeks to resolve and left (temporary) hyperpigmentation (17).

The fact that many patients had used the sunscreen lotion for the first time and the morphology of the reactions, beginning with burning and erythema often after a few hours already, suggested phototoxicity. However, photoallergy was thought to be the underlying mechanism, as sometimes the eruption would later spread beyond the areas of application with maculopapules and vesicles (17).

An early problem with the identification of this agent as etiologic occurred because of its apparent instability as a photoallergen once applied to skin. In routine photopatch testing, antigens are applied to skin 24-48 hours before UVA exposure. Such testing yielded negative results in one report in 4 of 5 patient (17). When 6-HC was applied shortly before exposure (30-60 minutes [17] to 6 hours [19]), strongly positive reactions were found in sensitized individuals (17). Photomaximization tests showed 6-methyl coumarin to be a potent photosensitizer (21,22).

The FDA received many consumer complaints of this particular sunscreen lotion containing 6-MC, and it initiated a shelf recall of all suntan products containing this ingredient (18); also, 6-HC was no longer recommended for use as a fragrance component (20).

6-Methyl coumarin has both been found to cause immediate and delayed positive photopatch tests, which were considered to be phototoxic in nature (8). Data from ref. 25 are not presented here (article not read).

Photopatch testing in groups of patients

Photopatch testing in consecutive patients suspected of contact dermatitis: routine testing
Studies in which 6-methyl coumarin was photopatch tested in consecutive patients suspected of contact dermatitis (routine testing) with positive results have not been found.

Photopatch testing in groups of selected patients
Results of studies photopatch testing 6-methyl coumarin in groups of selected patients (usually patients suspected of photosensitivity, photodermatoses or photoallergic contact dermatitis) are shown in table 3.108.2. In 12 investigations, frequencies of positive reactions have ranged from 0.1% to 7%; in ten, rates were 3% or lower and of these, 8 scored only 1% or even lower frequencies. The highest percentages positive reactions (5.6 and 7.0) were seen in studies with inadequate data or flaws and the issue of relevance of the observed reactions was addressed in neither of the two (1,2). In most of the other studies, relevance was also either not addressed or specified and only one reaction was considered to be relevant (14).

Case reports and case series
A woman applied a mixture of two popular sunscreens to her face, chest, and thighs. The active ingredient in one was amyl dimethyl PABA and in the other it was homosalate. Twenty-four hours later, the patient noted intense

erythema and pruritus, limited to the areas pre-treated with the sunscreens. By 48 hours, there was massive swelling and vesiculation, with oozing of the face, and she could not retract her eyelids. Edema, vesiculation, and erythema were also present over the chest and thighs. Photopatch testing showed positive reactions to the two sunscreens and to 6-MC. Unirradiated patch tests were negative, as were controls. Three patients known to be sensitive to 6-MC were also tested with the sunscreens and had strongly positive photopatch test reactions. High-pressure liquid chromatography analysis of the two sunscreens revealed 6-MC levels of 0.032% in one and 0.2% in the other (19).

Table 3.108.2 Photopatch testing in groups of patients: Selected patient groups

Years and Country	Test conc. & vehicle	Number of patients tested	positive (%)	Selection of patients (S); Relevance (R); Comments (C)	Ref.
2005-2014 China	1% pet.	2569	16 (0.6%)	S: patients suspected of photodermatoses; R: not stated	11
2001-2010 Canada		160	9 (5.6%)	S: patients with suspected photosensitivity and patients who developed pruritus or a rash after sunscreen application; R: not stated; C: weak study: inadequate reading of test results, erythema only was considered to represent a positive patch test reaction	2
2003-2007 Portugal	1% pet.	83	2 (2.4%)	S: patients with suspected photoaggravated facial dermatitis or systemic photosensitivity; R: not stated	12
1993-2006 USA	1% pet.	76	2 (3.0%)	S: not stated; R: not specified	6
2004-2006 Italy		1082	1 (0.1%)	S: patients with histories and clinical features suggestive of photoallergic contact dermatitis; R: not relevant	15
2000-2005 USA	1% alc.	176	1 (0.7%)	S: patients photopatch tested for suspected photodermatitis; R: not relevant	16
2001-2003 Colombia		82	1 (1%)	S: patients with a clinical diagnosis of photoallergic contact dermatitis; R: 65% of all reactions in the study were relevant	13
1985-1993 Italy		1050	6 (0.6%)	S: patients suspected of photoallergic contact dermatitis; R: not specified (78% for all photoallergens together)	5
1985-1990 USA	5% alc., later 1% alcohol	187	1 (0.5%)	S: patients with a history of photosensitivity; R: the reaction was considered to be relevant	14
1980-1985 USA	5% pet.	70	5 (7%)	S: not stated; R: not stated	1
1980-85 Germany, Austria, Switzerland	1% pet.	1129	2 (0.2%)	S: patients suspected of photoallergy, polymorphic light eruption, phototoxicity and skin problems with photo-distribution; R: not stated; C: there were 10 (0.9%) photo*toxic* reactions	7
1980-1 Denmark, Finland, Norway, Sweden	1% alc.	745	2 (0.3%)	S: patients with suspected photodermatoses; R: not specified; C: there was also one 'plain' contact allergic reaction	10

Two of 24 randomly selected volunteer college students were shown to be photosensitized to 6-MC. Neither had ever used the sunscreen that at that moment was implicated in many cases of photosensitivity in the USA. Also, neither was aware of having experienced a photosensitization reaction before. Both had positive photopatch tests to 6-MC 5% in alcohol, and one, who was tested with 3 other cosmetic products containing about 0.1% 6-MC, had photoallergic reactions to two of them.

Five patients developed severe erythema and edema with burning and pruritus following application of a suntan preparation containing 6-methylcoumarin and subsequent sunlight exposure. All were women who had never used this type of product before, although they had used other suntan agents without difficulty. All patients had severe reactions that required treatment with significant doses of systemic corticosteroids, and most of the patients' eruptions took weeks to resolve, leaving hyperpigmentation. Three patients had negative photopatch tests to the sunscreen and to 6-MC. In these tests, 6-methyl coumarin had been placed 48 hours before UVA exposure. A fourth individual had weak positive reactions, which were far stronger when the material was applied immediately before and 6 hours prior to UVA exposure. In the 5th patient, photopatch tests performed in the usual way (UVA exposure 48 hours after application) were entirely negative, whereas strong photopatch tests were observed when 6-MC was applied immediately before and 6 hours before application. The first 3 patients appear not to have been re-tested (17).

A woman from Thailand had the clinical picture of poikiloderma of Civatte on the anterior aspect and both sides of the neck; histopathology was consistent with this condition. She had a weak positive photopatch test to 6-methyl coumarin. This was apparently present in her perfume (which was negative on photopatch testing), but the authors also wrote that they found '**coumarin** listed in the ingredients on her perfume's package'. In addition, as it could not be ascertained that the poikiloderma disappeared or improved after avoidance of the product (she had laser treatment), the authors' proposition that photoallergy to 6-methyl coumarin may have played a role in producing poikiloderma of Civatte in this patient was insufficiently substantiated (24).

Photocross-reactions

Of four subjects photosensitized to 6-methyl coumarin, three photocross-reacted to 7-methylcoumarin, three to 7-methoxycoumarin, and two to coumarin (21).

LITERATURE

1   Menz J, Muller SA, Connnolly SM. Photopatch testing: A six year experience. J Am Acad Dermatol 1988;18:1044-1047

2   Greenspoon J, Ahluwalia R, Juma N, Rosen CF. Allergic and photoallergic contact dermatitis: A 10-year experience. Dermatitis 2013;24:29-32

3   SCCFNP (Scientific Committee on Cosmetic Products and Non-Food Products Intended for Consumers). Opinion of the Scientific Committee on Cosmetic Products and Non-Food Products Intended for Consumers concerning 'An initial list of perfumery materials which must not form part of fragrances compounds used in cosmetic products', 3 May 2000, SCCNFP/0320/00, final. Available at: http://ec.europa.eu/health/archive/ph_risk/committees/sccp/documents/out116_en.pdf

4   SCCS (Scientific Committee on Consumer Safety). Opinion on Fragrance allergens in cosmetic products, 26-27 June 2012, SCCS/1459/11. Available at: https://ec.europa.eu/health/sites/health/files/scientific_committees/consumer_safety/docs/sccs_o_102.pdf

5   Pigatto PD, Legori A, Bigardi AS,Guarrera M, Tosti A, Santucci B, et al. Gruppo Italiano recerca dermatiti da contatto ed ambientali Italian multicenter study of allergic contact photodermatitis: epidemiological aspects. Am J Contact Dermatitis 1996;7:158-163

6   Victor FC, Cohen DE, Soter NA. A 20-year analysis of previous and emerging allergens that elicit photoallergic contact dermatitis. J Am Acad Dermatol 2010;62:605-610

7   Hölzle E, Neumann N, Hausen B, Przybilla B, Schauder S, Hönigsmann H, et al. Photopatch testing: the 5-year experience of the German, Austrian and Swiss Photopatch Test Group. J Am Acad Dermatol 1991;25:59-68

8   Addo HA, Ferguson J, Johnson BF, Frain-Bell W. The relationship between exposure to fragrance materials and persistent light reaction in photosensitivity dermatitis with actinic reticuloid syndrome. Br J Dermatol 1982;107:261-274

9   Uter W, Johansen JD, Börje A, Karlberg A-T, Lidén C, Rastogi S, Roberts D, White IR. Categorization of fragrance contact allergens for prioritization of preventive measures: clinical and experimental data and consideration of structure–activity relationships. Contact Dermatitis 2013;69:196-230

10   Wennersten G, Thune P, Brodthagen H, Jansen C, Rystedt I, Crames M, et al. The Scandinavian multicenter photopatch study: Preliminary results. Contact Dermatitis 1984;10:305-309

11   Hu Y, Wang D, Shen Y, Tanh H. Photopatch testing in Chinese patients over 10 years. Dermatitis 2016;27:137-142

12   Cardoso JC, Canelas MM, Goncalo M, Figueiredo A. Photopatch testing with an extended series of photoallergens: a 5-year study. Contact Dermatitis 2009;60:325-329

13   Rodriguez E, Valbuena M, Rey M, Porras de Quintana L. Causal agents of photoallergic contact dermatitis diagnosed in the national institute of dermatology of Columbia. Photoderm Photoimmunol Photomed 2006;22:189-192

14   DeLeo VA, Suarez SM, Maso MJ. Photoallergic contact dermatitis. Results of photopatch testing in New York, 1985 to 1990. Arch Dermatol 1992;128:1513-1518

15   Pigatto PD, Guzzi G, Schena D, Guarrera M, Foti C, Francalanci S, et al. Photopatch tests: an Italian multicentre study from 2004 to 2006. Contact Dermatitis 2008;59:103-108

16   Scalf LA, Davis MDP, Rohlinger AL, Connolly SM. Photopatch testing of 182 patients: A 6-year experience at the Mayo Clinic. Dermatitis 2009;20:44-52

17   Jackson RT, Nesbitt LT, DeLeo VA. 6-Methylcoumarin photocontact dermatitis. J Am Acad Dermatol 1980;2:124-127

18   Eiermann HJ. Regulatory issues concerning AETT and 6-MC. Contact Dermatitis 1980;6:120-122

19   Kaidbey KH, Kligman AM. Contact photoallergy to 6-methylcoumarin in proprietary sunscreens. Arch Dermatol 1978;114:1709-1710

20   DeLeo VA. Photocontact dermatitis. Dermatol Ther 2004;17:279-288

21   Kaidbey KH, Kligman AM. Photosensitization by coumarin derivatives. Arch Dermatol 1981;117:258-263

22   Kaidbey KH, Kligman AM. Photocontact allergy to 6-methylcoumarin. Contact Dermatitis 1978;4:277-282

23   De Groot AC, Schmidt E. Essential oils: contact allergy and chemical composition. Boca Raton, Fl., USA: CRC Press, Taylor and Francis Group, 2016 (ISBN 9781482246407)

24   Vachiramon V, Wattanakrai P. Photoallergic contact sensitization to 6-methylcoumarin in poikiloderma of Civatte. Dermatitis 2005;16:136-138

25   Fisher AA. Perfume dermatitis. Part II. Photodermatitis to Musk Ambrette and 6-methylcoumarin. Cutis 1980;26:549, 552, 614

Chapter 3.109   METHYLDIHYDROJASMONATE

IDENTIFICATION

Description/definition	: Methyldihydrojasmonate is the organic compound that conforms to the structural formula shown below
Chemical class(es)	: Esters; ketones
Chemical/IUPAC name	: Methyl 2-(3-oxo-2-pentylcyclopentyl)acetate
Other names	: Cyclopentaneacetic acid, 3-oxo-2-pentyl-, methyl ester; Hedione ®
CAS registry number(s)	: 24851-98-7; 2630-39-9
EC number(s)	: 220-112-5; 246-495-9
RIFM monograph(s)	: Food Chem Toxicol 2015;82(suppl.):S114-S121; Food Chem Toxicol 1992;30(suppl.1): S85-S86
SCCS opinion(s)	: SCCS/1459/11 (1)
Function(s) in cosmetics	: EU: masking. USA: fragrance ingredients; skin-conditioning agents - miscellaneous
Patch testing	: 5% pet. (6); based on RIFM data, 20% pet. may not be irritant (8)
Molecular formula	: $C_{13}H_{22}O_3$

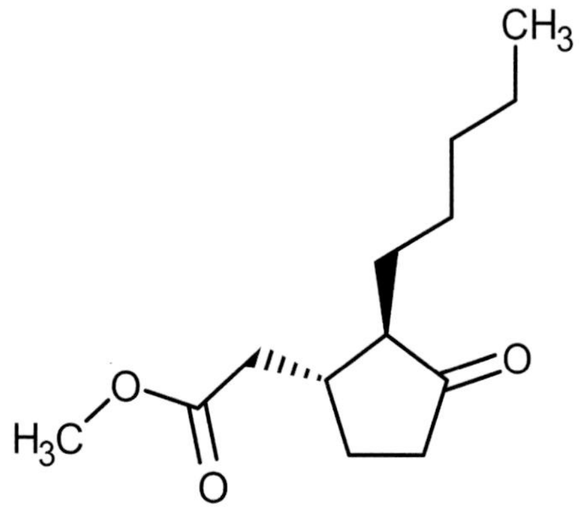

GENERAL

Methyldihydrojasmonate is a colorless to pale yellow clear oily liquid; its odor type is floral and its odor is described as 'sweet, fruity, floral, citrus lemon and grapefruit-like with woody jasmine and green nuances' (www.thegood scentscompany.com). It has repellent activities against the southern house mosquito, *Culex quinquefasciatus*, in laboratory assays (10).

Presence in essential oils

Methyldihydrojasmonate has been identified by chemical analysis in one of 91 essential oils, which have caused contact allergy / allergic contact dermatitis: Eucalyptus globulus oil (9). However, it was found in one study only, which may indicate misidentification.

CONTACT ALLERGY

General

The SCCS (Scientific Committee on Consumer Safety), in a 2012 Opinion on Fragrance allergens in cosmetic products, has categorized methyldihydrojasmonate as 'possible fragrance contact allergen' (1,7).

Patch testing in groups of patients

Patch testing in consecutive patients suspected of contact dermatitis: routine testing

In the period 1998-2000, in six European countries, 1606 consecutive patients with dermatitis were patch tested with methyldihydrojasmonate 5% pet. and there were three (0.2%) positive reactions. Their relevance was not mentioned (6).

Patch testing in groups of selected patients

Studies in which methyldihydrojasmonate was patch tested in groups of selected patients with positive results have not been found.

Case reports and case series

Case reports of allergic contact dermatitis from methyldihydrojasmonate have not been found.

Presence in products and chemical analyses

In 2018, methyldihydrojasmonate was found to be present in concentrations of 35 and 54 mg/ml in two eaux de parfum by GC-MS (10).

In 2000, fifty-nine domestic and occupational products, purchased in retail outlets in Denmark, England, Germany and Italy were analyzed by GC-MS for the presence of fragrances. The product categories were liquid soap and soap bars (n=13), soft/hard surface cleaners (n=23), fabric conditioners/laundry detergents for hand wash (n=8), dish wash (n=10), furniture polish, car shampoo, stain remover (each n=1) and 2 products used in occupational environments. Methyldihydrojasmonate was present in 14 products (24%); quantification was not performed (3).

Twenty-five cosmetics and cosmetic toys for children (5 shampoos and shower gels, 6 perfumes, 1 deodorant (roll-on), 4 baby lotions/creams, 1 baby wipes product, 1 baby oil, 2 lipcare products and 5 toy-cosmetic products: a cosmetic-toy set for blending perfumes and a makeup set) purchased in 1997-1998 in retail outlets in Denmark, Germany, England and Sweden were analyzed in 1998 for the presence of fragrances by GC-MS. Methyldihydrojasmonate (Hedione ®) was found in 12 products (48%) in a concentration range of ≤0.001-1.027% (w/w). For the analytical data in each product category, the original publication should be consulted (4).

Seventy fragranced deodorants, purchased at retail outlets in 5 European countries in 1996, were analyzed by gas chromatography - mass spectrometry (GC-MS) for the determination of the contents of 21 commonly used fragrance materials. Methyldihydrojasmonate (Hedione ®) was identified in 55 products (79%) in a concentration range of 1–17,587 ppm (2).

In 1988, in the USA, 400 perfumes used in fine fragrances, household products and soaps (number of products per category not mentioned) were analyzed for the presence of fragrance chemicals in a concentration of at least 1% and a list of the Top-25 (present in the highest number of products) presented. Methyldihydrojasmonate was found to be present in 56% of the fine fragrances (rank number 8), 17% of the household product fragrances (rank number 25) and an unknown percentage of the fragrances used in soaps (5).

LITERATURE

1 SCCS (Scientific Committee on Consumer Safety). Opinion on Fragrance allergens in cosmetic products, 26-27 June 2012, SCCS/1459/11. Available at:
https://ec.europa.eu/health/sites/health/files/scientific_committees/consumer_safety/docs/sccs_o_102.pdf

2 Rastogi SC, Johansen JD, Frosch P, Menné T, Bruze M, Lepoittevin JP, et al. Deodorants on the European market: quantitative chemical analysis of 21 fragrances. Contact Dermatitis 1998;38:29-35

3 Rastogi SC, Heydorn S, Johansen JD, Basketter DA. Fragrance chemicals in domestic and occupational products. Contact Dermatitis 2001;45:221-225

4 Rastogi SC, Johansen JD, Menné T, Frosch P, Bruze M, Andersen KE, et al. Content of fragrance allergens in children's cosmetics and cosmetic toys. Contact Dermatitis 1999;41:84-88

5 Fenn RS. Aroma chemical usage trends in modern perfumery. Perfumer and Flavorist 1989;14:3-10

6 Frosch PJ, Johansen JD, Menné T, Pirker C, Rastogi SC, Andersen KE, et al. Further important sensitizers in patients sensitive to fragrances. II. Reactivity to essential oils. Contact Dermatitis 2002;47:279-287

7 Uter W, Johansen JD, Börje A, Karlberg A-T, Lidén C, Rastogi S, Roberts D, White IR. Categorization of fragrance contact allergens for prioritization of preventive measures: clinical and experimental data and consideration of structure–activity relationships. Contact Dermatitis 2013;69:196-230

8 De Groot AC. Patch Testing, 4th Edition. Wapserveen, The Netherlands: acdegroot publishing, 2018 (ISBN 978-90-813233-4-5)

9 De Groot AC, Schmidt E. Essential oils: contact allergy and chemical composition. Boca Raton, Fl., USA: CRC Press, Taylor and Francis Group, 2016 (ISBN 9781482246407)

10 Zeng F, Xu P, Tan K, Zarbin PHG, Leal WS. Methyl dihydrojasmonate and lilial are the constituents with an "off-label" insect repellence in perfumes. PLoS One 2018;13(6):e0199386

Chapter 3.110 METHYLENEDIOXYPHENYL METHYLPROPANAL

DENTIFICATION

Description/definition	: Methylenedioxyphenyl methylpropanal is the organic compound that conforms to the structural formula shown below
Chemical class(es)	: Aldehydes; ethers
Chemical/IUPAC name	: 3-(1,3-Benzodioxol-5-yl)-2-methylpropanal
Other names	: α-Methyl-1,3-benzodioxole-5-propionaldehyde; Helional ®; tropional
CAS registry number(s)	: 1205-17-0
EC number(s)	: 214-881-6
IFRA standard	: Restricted (www.ifraorg.org/en-us/standards-library) (table 3.110.1)
Function(s) in cosmetics	: EU: perfuming. USA: fragrance ingredients; skin-conditioning agents - miscellaneous
Patch testing	: 5% pet. (1)
Molecular formula	: $C_{11}H_{12}O_3$

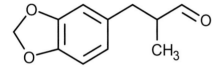

Table 3.110.1 IFRA restrictions for methylenedioxyphenyl methylpropanal

Category [a]	Limits [b]	Category [a]	Limits [b]	Category [a]	Limits [b]
1	0.34%	5	2.80%	9	5.00%
2	0.43%	6	8.60%	10	2.50%
3	1.78%	7	0.89%	11	not restricted
4	5.30%	8	2.00%		

[a] For explanation of categories see pages 6-8
[b] Limits in the finished products

GENERAL

Methylenedioxyphenyl methylpropanal is a pale yellow to yellow clear oily liquid; its odor type is floral and its odor at 100% is described as 'watery fresh green ozone cyclamen hay' (www.thegoodscentscompany.com). Methylene-dioxyphenyl methylpropanal is a synthetic chemical, not found in nature (and consequently not in essential oils (3)).

CONTACT ALLERGY

Patch testing in groups of patients

Before 1996, in Japan, some European countries and the USA, 167 patients known or suspected to be allergic to fragrances were patch tested with methylenedioxyphenyl methylpropanal and there were four (2.4%) positive reactions; their relevance was not mentioned (1).

Presence in products and chemical analyses

In 2000, fifty-nine domestic and occupational products, purchased in retail outlets in Denmark, England, Germany and Italy were analyzed by GC-MS for the presence of fragrances. The product categories were liquid soap and soap bars (n=13), soft/hard surface cleaners (n=23), fabric conditioners/laundry detergents for hand wash (n=8), dish wash (n=10), furniture polish, car shampoo, stain remover (each n=1) and 2 products used in occupational environments. Methylenedioxyphenyl methylpropanal (Helional ®) was present in one product (2%); quantification was not performed (2).

LITERATURE

1   Larsen W, Nakayama H, Fischer T, Elsner P, Burrows D, Jordan W, et al. Fragrance contact dermatitis: A worldwide multicenter investigation (Part I). Am J Cont Dermat 1996;7:77-83
2   Rastogi SC, Heydorn S, Johansen JD, Basketter DA. Fragrance chemicals in domestic and occupational products. Contact Dermatitis 2001;45:221-225
3   De Groot AC, Schmidt E. Essential oils: contact allergy and chemical composition. Boca Raton, Fl., USA: CRC Press, Taylor and Francis Group, 2016 (ISBN 9781482246407)

Chapter 3.111 METHYL EUGENOL *
Not an INCI name

IDENTIFICATION

Description/definition	: Methyl eugenol is the aromatic compound that conforms to the structural formula shown below
Chemical class(es)	: Ethers
Chemical/IUPAC name	: 1,2-Dimethoxy-4-prop-2-enylbenzene
Other names	: 4-Allylveratrole; eugenyl methyl ether
CAS registry number(s)	: 93-15-2
EC number(s)	: 202-223-0
RIFM monograph(s)	: Food Cosmet Toxicol 1975;13:857 (special issue II)
IFRA standard	: Restricted (www.ifraorg.org/en-us/standards-library) (table 3.111.1)
SCCS opinion(s)	: SCCNFP 0373/00 (1)
Function(s) in cosmetics	: EU: not mentioned. USA: fragrance ingredients
EU cosmetic restrictions	: Regulated in Annex III/102 of the Regulation (EC) No. 1223/2009
Patch testing	: 5% pet. (2); based on RIFM data, 8% pet. may not be irritant (3)
Molecular formula	: $C_{11}H_{14}O_2$

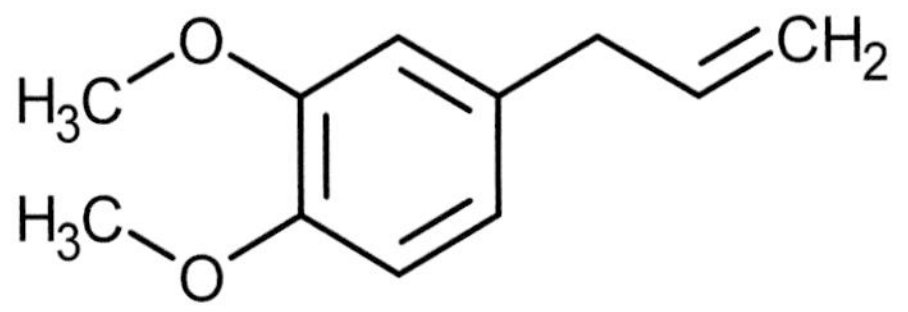

Table 3.111.1 IFRA restrictions for methyl eugenol

Fine fragrance:	0.02%
Eau de toilette:	0.008%
Fragrancing cream:	0.004%
Other leave-on products:	0.0004%
Rinse-off products:	0.001%
Non-skin, incidental skin contact:	0.01%

The limitations apply to methyl eugenol originating from all sources. Contributions from essential oils can be significant

GENERAL

Methyl eugenol is a colorless to pale yellow clear liquid; its odor type is spicy and its odor at 1% in dipropylene glycol is described as 'spicy, cinnamon, clove, musty, vegetative, waxy and peppery with phenolic nuances' (www.the good scentscompany.com). It is used as a fragrance, flavor, oriental fruit fly attractant and in veterinary medications (U.S. National Library of Medicine).

Presence in essential oils

Methyl eugenol has been identified by chemical analysis in 48 of 91 essential oils, which have caused contact allergy / allergic contact dermatitis. In 7 oils, methyl eugenol belonged to the 'Top-10' of ingredients with the highest concentrations which may be expected in commercial essential oils of this type: basil oil (0-24.7%), ravensara oil (trace-21.4%), citronella oil Sri Lanka (0.4-7.2%), calamus oil (0.03-6.5%), rose oil (0.06-4.3%), laurel leaf oil (1.0-3.0%), and clove bud/leaf/stem oil (0.04-0.2%) (4).

CONTACT ALLERGY

Patch testing in groups of patients

Patch testing in consecutive patients suspected of contact dermatitis: routine testing

Studies in which methyl eugenol was patch tested in consecutive patients suspected of contact dermatitis (routine testing) with positive results have not been found.

Testing in groups of selected patients

Before 2002, in Japan, European countries and the USA, 218 patients with known fragrance sensitivity were patch tested with methyl eugenol 5% in petrolatum and four positive reactions (1.8%) were observed; their relevance was not mentioned (2).

Case reports and case series

Case reports of allergic contact dermatitis from methyl eugenol have not been found.

LITERATURE

1   SCCFNP (Scientific Committee on Cosmetic Products and Non-Food Products Intended for Consumers). Opinion concerning Methyleugenol, 24 October 2000, SCCNFP 0373/00. Available at: http://ec.europa.eu/health/ scientificcommittees/consumersafety/opinions/sccnfp_opinions_97 _04/sccp_out126_en.htm
2   Larsen W, Nakayama H, Fischer T, Elsner P, Frosch P, Burrows D, et al. Fragrance contact dermatitis - a worldwide multicenter investigation (Part III). Contact Dermatitis 2002;46:141-144
3   De Groot AC. Patch Testing, 4th Edition. Wapserveen, The Netherlands: acdegroot publishing, 2018 (ISBN 978-90-813233-4-5)
4   De Groot AC, Schmidt E. Essential oils: contact allergy and chemical composition. Boca Raton, Fl., USA: CRC Press, Taylor and Francis Group, 2016 (ISBN 9781482246407)

Chapter 3.112 METHYL IONONES

IDENTIFICATION

Description/definition
: Methyl ionones is a mixture of isomers consisting of alpha-isomethyl ionone, beta-isomethylionone, alpha-methylionone, and beta-methylionone

Chemical class(es)
: Ketones

Chemical/IUPAC name
: α-isomethyl ionone: 3-Methyl-4-(2,6,6-trimethylcyclohex-2-en-1-yl)but-3-en-2-one
β-isomethyl ionone: 3-Methyl-4-(2,6,6-trimethylcyclohex-1-en-1-yl)but-3-en-2-one
α-methyl ionone: 1-(2,6,6-Trimethylcyclohex-2-en-1-yl)pent-1-en-3-one
β-methyl ionone: 1-(2,6,6-Trimethylcyclohex-1-en-1-yl)pent-1-en-3-one

Other names
: Methyl ionone, mixture of isomers; Methylionantheme ®; Iralia ®

CAS registry number (s)
: 79-89-0; 127-43-5; 127-51-5; 1335-46-2; 7779-30-8;127-42-4

EC number(s)
: 201-231-1;204-843-7; 204-846-3; 231-926-5

RIFM monograph(s)
: Food Chem Toxicol 2007;45(suppl.1):S300-S307 (mixture of isomers), S276-S279 (alpha-), 290-293 (beta-) and S297-S299 (beta-isomethyl-); Food Cosmet Toxicol 1975;13:863; see also Chapter 3.92 alpha-Isomethyl ionone

IFRA standard
: Restricted (www.ifraorg.org/en-us/standards-library) (table 3.112.1)

SCCS opinion(s)
: SCCS/1459/11 (1)

Function(s) in cosmetics
: EU: masking. USA: fragrance ingredients

Patch testing
: 0.0437% in alcohol (3), which seems too low for general use; based on RIFM data, 20% pet. is probably not irritant (4)

Molecular formula
: $C_{14}H_{22}O$

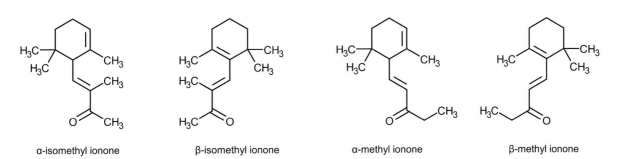

α-isomethyl ionone   β-isomethyl ionone   α-methyl ionone   β-methyl ionone

Table 3.112.1 IFRA restrictions for methyl ionone, mixed isomers

Category [a]	Limits [b]	Category [a]	Limits [b]	Category [a]	Limits [b]
1	2.00%	5	16.67%	9	5.00%
2	2.59%	6	50.72%	10	2.50%
3	10.56%	7	5.30%	11	not restricted
4	31.67%	8	2.00%		

[a] For explanation of categories see pages 6-8
[b] Limits in the finished products

GENERAL

Methyl ionones is a raw material for perfume composed of isomeric *n*-methyl ionones and isomethyl ionones (alpha-isomethyl ionone, beta-isomethylionone, alpha-methylionone, and beta-methylionone). It is prepared by condensing citral and methyl ethyl ketone with subsequent cyclization of pseudo-methyl ionone, and does not apparently occur in nature (and consequently, not in essential oils (5)).

alpha-Isomethyl ionone is a colorless to yellow clear oily liquid; its odor type is floral and its odor at 10% in dipropylene glycol is described as 'violet sweet orris powdery floral woody' (www.thegoodscentscompany.com).

beta-Isomethyl ionone has an unknown physical appearance; its odor type is floral and its odor at 10% in dipropylene glycol is described as 'woody ambergris waxy orris floral' (www.thegoodscentscompany.com).

alpha-Methyl ionone is a pale yellow clear liquid; its odor type is powdery and its odor at 10% in dipropylene glycol is described as 'sweet powdery fruity floral violet beeswax orris woody' (www.thegoodscentscompany.com).

beta-Methyl ionone is a pale yellow to yellow clear liquid; its odor type is woody and its odor at 10% in dipropylene glycol is described as 'woody orris tobacco powdery floral violet' (www.thegoodscentscompany.com).

See also Chapter 3.192 alpha-Isomethyl ionone and Chapter 3.85 Ionone .

CONTACT ALLERGY

The SCCS (Scientific Committee on Consumer Safety), in a 2012 Opinion on Fragrance allergens in cosmetic products, has categorized methyl ionones (methylionantheme) as 'likely fragrance contact allergen by combination of evidence' (1,2).

Patch testing in groups of patients

Studies in which methyl ionones was patch tested in either consecutive patients suspected of contact dermatitis (routine testing) or in groups of selected patients with positive results have not been found.

Case reports and case series

A woman, with a previous history of dermatitis from adhesive tape, was hospitalized for an operation. Three days later, an itchy purpuric dermatitis appeared over the anterior trunk, its distribution suggesting production by a cologne profusely applied the previous day. The cologne had run over her breasts and abdomen, sparing the submammary folds, and had accumulated in her right groin due to her semi-lateral decubitus. The lesions became brownish and disappeared in 2 weeks. A series of 20 perfumes and cosmetic substances were patch tested with negative results. A patch test with the cologne (as is) gave a ++ reaction at days 2 and 3. No purpura was seen. Two months later, 18 components of the cologne from the manufacturer were tested at the same concentration as in the cologne; 'methylionantheme' (0.0437% in alcohol) elicited a positive reaction. Other ionones were later tested and the patient now had positive patch test reactions to ionone and alpha-isomethyl ionone (test concentrations not specified) (3).

LITERATURE

1   SCCS (Scientific Committee on Consumer Safety). Opinion on Fragrance allergens in cosmetic products, 26-27 June 2012, SCCS/1459/11. Available at:
     https://ec.europa.eu/health/sites/health/files/scientific_committees/consumer_safety/docs/sccs_o_102.pdf
2   Uter W, Johansen JD, Börje A, Karlberg A-T, Lidén C, Rastogi S, Roberts D, White IR. Categorization of fragrance contact allergens for prioritization of preventive measures: clinical and experimental data and consideration of structure–activity relationships. Contact Dermatitis 2013;69:196-230
3   Bernaola G, Escayol P, Fernandez E, Fernandez de Corrés L. Contact dermatitis from methylionone fragrance. Contact Dermatitis 1989;20:71-72
4   De Groot AC. Patch Testing, 4th Edition. Wapserveen, The Netherlands: acdegroot publishing, 2018 (ISBN 978-90-813233-4-5)
5   De Groot AC, Schmidt E. Essential oils: contact allergy and chemical composition. Boca Raton, Fl., USA: CRC Press, Taylor and Francis Group, 2016 (ISBN 9781482246407)

Chapter 3.113 5-METHYL-ALPHA-IONONE

IDENTIFICATION

Description/definition	: 5-Methyl-alpha-ionone is the unsaturated cyclic ketone that conforms to the structural formula shown below
Chemical class(es)	: Unsaturated cyclic organic compounds; ketones
INCI name USA	: Not in the Personal Care Products Council Ingredient Database
Chemical/IUPAC name	: 4-(2,5,6,6-Tetramethylcyclohex-2-en-1-yl)but-3-en-2-one
Other names	: 6-Methylionone; 6-methyl-α-ionone; α-irone
CAS registry number(s)	: 79-69-6
EC number(s)	: 201-219-6
RIFM monograph(s)	: Food Chem Toxicol 2015;82(suppl.):S105-S113; Food Chem Toxicol 2007;45(suppl.1):S272-S275; Food Cosmet Toxicol 1975;13:551
SCCS opinion(s)	: SCCS/1459/11 (1)
Merck Index monograph	: 6410
Function(s) in cosmetics	: EU: perfuming
Patch testing	: 10% pet. (2)
Molecular formula	: $C_{14}H_{22}O$

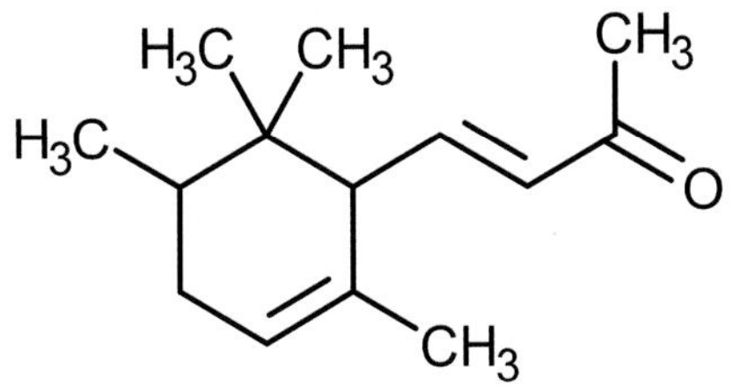

GENERAL

5-Methyl-alpha-ionone is a colorless to pale yellow clear liquid; its odor type is floral and its odor is described as 'sweet, orris, woody, raspberry and powdery' (www.thegoodscentscompany.com).

Presence in essential oils

5-Methyl-alpha-ionone has been identified by chemical analysis in 1 of 91 essential oils, which have caused contact allergy / allergic contact dermatitis: black cumin oil (5).

CONTACT ALLERGY

General

The SCCS (Scientific Committee on Consumer Safety), in a 2012 Opinion on Fragrance allergens in cosmetic products, has categorized 5-methyl-alpha-ionone as 'likely fragrance contact allergen by combination of evidence' (1,4).

Patch testing in groups of patients

Patch testing in consecutive patients suspected of contact dermatitis: routine testing

In the period 1998-2000, in six European countries, 1606 consecutive patients with dermatitis were patch tested with 5-methyl-alpha-ionone 10% in petrolatum and there were 5 (0.3%) positive reactions; their relevance was not mentioned (2).

Testing in groups of selected patients

While searching for causative ingredients of pigmented cosmetic dermatitis in Japan in the 1970s, both patients with ordinary (nonpigmented) cosmetic dermatitis and women with pigmented cosmetic dermatitis were tested with a large number of fragrance materials. In 1980 the accumulated data enabled the classification of fragrant materials into 4 groups: common sensitizers, rare sensitizers, virtually non-sensitizing fragrances and fragrances considered as non-sensitizers. 5-Methyl-alpha-ionone (alpha-methylionone) was classified in the group of rare sensitizers, indicating that one or more cases of contact allergy / allergic contact dermatitis to it have been observed (3). More specific data are lacking, the results have largely or solely been published in Japanese journals only.

Case reports and case series
Case reports of allergic contact dermatitis from 5-methyl-alpha-ionone have not been found.

LITERATURE

1   SCCS (Scientific Committee on Consumer Safety). Opinion on Fragrance allergens in cosmetic products, 26-27 June 2012, SCCS/1459/11. Available at: https://ec.europa.eu/health/sites/health/files/scientific_committees/consumer_safety/docs/sccs_o_102.pdf
2   Frosch PJ, Johansen JD, Menné T, Pirker C, Rastogi SC, Andersen KE, et al. Further important sensitizers in patients sensitive to fragrances. II. Reactivity to essential oils. Contact Dermatitis 2002;47:279-287
3   Nakayama H. Fragrance hypersensitivity and its control. In: Frosch PJ, Johansen JD, White IR, Eds. Fragrances - beneficial and adverse effects. Berlin Heidelberg New York: Springer-Verlag, 1998:83-91
4   Uter W, Johansen JD, Börje A, Karlberg A-T, Lidén C, Rastogi S, Roberts D, White IR. Categorization of fragrance contact allergens for prioritization of preventive measures: clinical and experimental data and consideration of structure–activity relationships. Contact Dermatitis 2013;69:196-230
5   De Groot AC, Schmidt E. Essential oils: contact allergy and chemical composition. Boca Raton, Fl., USA: CRC Press, Taylor and Francis Group, 2016 (ISBN 9781482246407)

Chapter 3.114   METHYL ISOEUGENOL

IDENTIFICATION

Description/definition	: Methyl isoeugenol is the aromatic compound that conforms to the structural formula shown below
Chemical class(es)	: Aromatic compounds; unsaturated organic compounds; ethers
INCI name USA	: Not in the Personal Care Products Council Ingredient Database
Chemical/IUPAC name	: 1,2-Dimethoxy-4-prop-1-enylbenzene
Other names	: 3,4-Dimethoxypropenylbenzene; isomethyleugenol; isoeugenyl methyl ether
CAS registry number (s)	: 93-16-3
EC number(s)	: 202-224-6
RIFM monograph(s)	: Food Cosmet Toxicol 1975;13:865 (special issue II)
Function(s) in cosmetics	: EU: perfuming
Patch testing	: 1.1% pet. (3); 5% pet. (1); based on RIFM data, 8% pet. is probably not irritant (5)
Molecular formula	: $C_{11}H_{14}O_2$

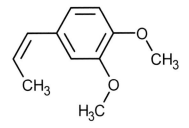

GENERAL
Methyl isoeugenol is a colorless to pale yellow clear liquid; its odor type is spicy and its odor at 100% is described as 'spicy clove blossom carnation woody' (www.thegoodscentscompany.com).

Presence in essential oils
Methyl isoeugenol (any isomer) has been identified by chemical analysis in 18 of 91 essential oils, which have caused contact allergy / allergic contact dermatitis. In one oil, methyl isoeugenol belonged to the 'Top-10' of ingredients with the highest concentrations which may be expected in commercial essential oils of this type: citronella oil Sri Lanka ((E)-, 6.7-10.7%; (Z)-, 0.4-9.9%) (6).

CONTACT ALLERGY

Patch testing in groups of patients

Patch testing in consecutive patients suspected of contact dermatitis: routine testing
In the period 2001-2002, in Denmark, Belgium and Sweden, 2261 consecutive dermatitis patients were patch tested with methyl isoeugenol and there were 6 (0.3%) positive reactions; their relevance was not mentioned. There were no co-reactions to isoeugenol (3).

Patch testing in groups of patients: Selected patient groups
Before 2002, in Japan, European countries and the USA, 218 patients with known fragrance sensitivity were patch tested with methyl isoeugenol 5% in petrolatum and 16 (7.3%) positive patch tests were observed; their relevance was not mentioned (1). Based on this unexpected high frequency, one may wonder whether the test concentration of 5% pet. may not be slightly irritant. However, RIFM data suggest that 8% pet. is probably not irritant (5).

While searching for causative ingredients of pigmented cosmetic dermatitis in Japan in the 1970s, both patients with ordinary (nonpigmented) cosmetic dermatitis and women with pigmented cosmetic dermatitis were tested with a large number of fragrance materials. In 1980 the accumulated data enabled the classification of fragrant materials into 4 groups: common sensitizers, rare sensitizers, virtually non-sensitizing fragrances and fragrances considered as non-sensitizers. Methyl isoeugenol was classified in the group of rare sensitizers, indicating that one or more cases of contact allergy / allergic contact dermatitis to it have been observed (2). More specific data are lacking, the results have largely or solely been published in Japanese journals only.

Case reports and case series
Case reports of allergic contact dermatitis from methyl isoeugenol have not been found.

Cross-reactions, pseudo-cross-reactions and co-reactions
For general information on cross-/pseudo-cross-/co-reactivity of fragrance chemicals with other fragrances, fragrance markers (fragrance mix I, fragrance mix II, colophonium, Myroxylon pereirae resin [balsam of Peru]) and essential oils see Chapter 1.2 General information on cross-reactions, pseudo-cross-reactions and co-reactions.

In 6 patients with positive patch tests to methyl isoeugenol, there were no co-reactions to isoeugenol (3).

Presence in products and chemical analyses
In Denmark, in 2006-2007, 29 hydroalcoholic products of international brands (2 aftershave lotions, 26 eaux de toilette/eaux de parfum [10 for men and 16 for women] and one parfum) were purchased from Danish retail outlets and investigated by GC-MS for the presence of isoeugenol, isoeugenyl acetate, methyl isoeugenol and benzyl isoeugenol. Methyl isoeugenol was present in 13 products (45%) in a concentration range of 64.9-1755.0 ppm, mean of 442.3 ppm. Many products contained 2 or 3 of the isoeugenol derivatives, but benzyl isoeugenol was not found in any sample (4).

LITERATURE

1   Larsen W, Nakayama H, Fischer T, Elsner P, Frosch P, Burrows D, et al. Fragrance contact dermatitis - a worldwide multicenter investigation (Part III). Contact Dermatitis 2002;46:141-144
2   Nakayama H. Fragrance hypersensitivity and its control. In: Frosch PJ, Johansen JD, White IR, Eds. Fragrances - beneficial and adverse effects. Berlin Heidelberg New York: Springer-Verlag, 1998:83-91
3   Tanaka S, Royds C, Buckley D, Basketter DA, Goossens A, Bruze M, et al. Contact allergy to isoeugenol and its derivatives: problems with allergen substitution. Contact Dermatitis 2004;51:288-291
4   Rastogi SC, Johansen JD. Significant exposures to isoeugenol derivates in perfumes. Contact Dermatitis 2008;58:278-281
5   De Groot AC. Patch Testing, 4th Edition. Wapserveen, The Netherlands: acdegroot publishing, 2018 (ISBN 978-90-813233-4-5)
6   De Groot AC, Schmidt E. Essential oils: contact allergy and chemical composition. Boca Raton, Fl., USA: CRC Press, Taylor and Francis Group, 2016 (ISBN 9781482246407)

Chapter 3.115 METHYL OCTINE CARBONATE *

* Not officially an INCI name but perfuming name

IDENTIFICATION

Description/definition	: Methyl octine carbonate is the nonynoic acid ester that conforms to the structural formula shown below
Chemical class(es)	: Unsaturated acid ester
INCI name USA	: Not in the Personal Care Products Council Ingredient Database
Chemical/IUPAC name	: Methyl non-2-ynoate
Other names	: Methyl 2-nonynoate
CAS registry number(s)	: 111-80-8
EC number(s)	: 203-909-2
RIFM monograph(s)	: Food Cosmet Toxicol 1975;13:871 (special issue II)
IFRA standard	: Restricted (www.ifraorg.org/en-us/standards-library) (table 3.115.1)
SCCS opinion(s)	: SCCP/1023/06 (1); SCCNFP/0392/00, final (2); SCCS/1459/11 (3); SCCNFP/0389/00, final (8)
Function(s) in cosmetics	: EU: perfuming
EU cosmetic restrictions	: Regulated in Annex III/173 of the Regulation (EC) No. 344/2013
Patch testing	: 1% Methyl ethyl ketone (5); based on RIFM data, 2% pet. is probably not irritant (7)
Molecular formula	: $C_{10}H_{16}O_2$

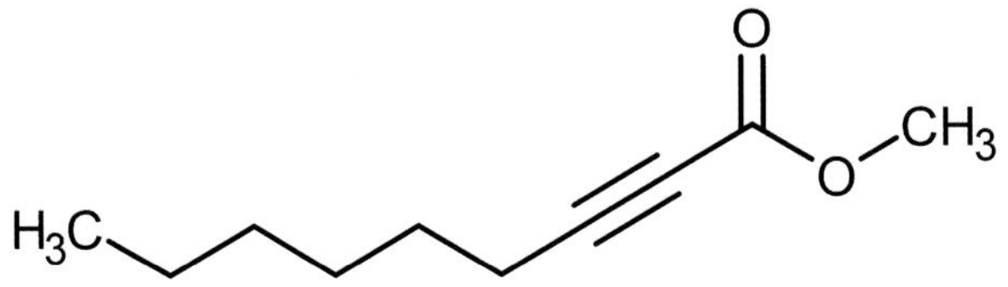

Table 3.115.1 IFRA restrictions for methyl octine carbonate

Category [a]	Limits [b]	Category [a]	Limits [b]	Category [a]	Limits [b]
1	0.00%	5	0.00%	9	0.00%
2	0.00%	6	0.00%	10	0.00%
3	0.00%	7	0.00%	11	not restricted
4	0.00%	8	0.00%		

[a] For explanation of categories see pages 6-8
[b] Limits in the finished products

GENERAL

Methyl octine carbonate is a colorless to pale yellow clear liquid; its odor type is green and its odor at 1% in dipropylene glycol is described as 'floral green violet leaf melon cucumber' (www.thegoodscentscompany.com). Methyl octine carbonate is a synthetic chemical, not found in nature (and consequently not in essential oils (6)).

CONTACT ALLERGY

General

The SCCS (Scientific Committee on Consumer Safety), in a 2012 Opinion on Fragrance allergens in cosmetic products, has marked methyl octine carbonate as 'Fragrance substance with positive human data, which are, however, not sufficient to categorize it as 'established contact allergen in humans' (3,4). The sensitizing potency of methyl octine carbonate was classified as 'moderate' based on an EC3 value of 2.5% in the LLNA (local lymph node assay) in animal experiments (3,4).

Patch testing in groups of patients

Studies in which methyl octine carbonate was patch tested in either consecutive patients suspected of contact dermatitis (routine testing) or in groups of selected patients with positive results have not been found.

Case reports and case series

A laboratory assistant developed a localized vesicular dermatitis on her wrist following direct skin contact with methyl heptine carbonate (MHC) (methyl 2-octynoate), which resolved within 2 weeks. Several months later, she developed hand dermatitis, which was relapsing and work-related. She had worked in a fragrance laboratory for 3 years, mixing fragrances, sunscreens and flavorings. She regularly worked with methyl octine carbonate (MOC) but only occasionally with MHC. Patch testing with the ICDRG standard series of allergens was negative, but both MHC (1% MEK) and MOC (1% MEK) produced very strong positive reactions at 2 and 4 days. The samples of MHC and MOC supplied were 96% pure (5).

Cross-reactions, pseudo-cross-reactions and co-reactions

For general information on cross-/pseudo-cross-/co-reactivity of fragrance chemicals with other fragrances, fragrance markers (fragrance mix I, fragrance mix II, colophonium, Myroxylon pereirae resin [balsam of Peru]) and essential oils see Chapter 1.2 General information on cross-reactions, pseudo-cross-reactions and co-reactions.

Possibly cross-reactivity to or from methyl heptine carbonate (methyl 2-octynoate), or possibly allergy to a common degradation product (5).

LITERATURE

1   SCCP (Scientific Committee on Consumer Products). Opinion on 'Clarifications to SCCNFP/0392/00 'An initial list of perfumery materials which must not form part of cosmetic products except subject to the Restrictions and Conditions laid down', 20 June 2006, SCCP/1023/06. Available at:
    http://ec.europa.eu/health/archive/ph_risk/committees/04_sccp/docs/sccp_o_062.pdf
2   SCCNFP (Scientific Committee on Cosmetic Products and Non-Food Products Intended for Consumers). Opinion of the Scientific Committee on Cosmetic Products and Non-Food Products Intended for Consumers concerning 'An initial list of perfumery materials which must not form part of cosmetic products except subject to the Restrictions and Conditions laid down, 25 September 2001, SCCNFP/0392/00, final. Available at:
    http://ec.europa.eu/health/archive/ph_risk/committees/sccp/documents/out150_en.pdf
3   SCCS (Scientific Committee on Consumer Safety). Opinion on Fragrance allergens in cosmetic products, 26-27 June 2012, SCCS/1459/11. Available at:
    https://ec.europa.eu/health/sites/health/files/scientific_committees/consumer_safety/docs/sccs_o_102.pdf
4   Uter W, Johansen JD, Börje A, Karlberg A-T, Lidén C, Rastogi S, Roberts D, White IR. Categorization of fragrance contact allergens for prioritization of preventive measures: clinical and experimental data and consideration of structure–activity relationships. Contact Dermatitis 2013;69:196-230
5   English JS, Rycroft RJ. Allergic contact dermatitis from methyl heptine and methyl octine carbonates. Contact Dermatitis 1988;18:174-175
6   De Groot AC, Schmidt E. Essential oils: contact allergy and chemical composition. Boca Raton, Fl., USA: CRC Press, Taylor and Francis Group, 2016 (ISBN 9781482246407)
7   De Groot AC. Patch Testing, 4th Edition. Wapserveen, The Netherlands: acdegroot publishing, 2018 (ISBN 978-90-813233-4-5)
8   Opinion of the Scientific Committee on Cosmetic Products and Non-Food Products Intended for Consumers concerning 'The 1st update of the inventory of ingredients employed in cosmetic products. Section II: Perfume and aromatic raw materials', 24 October 2000, SCCNFP/0389/00, final. Available at:
    http://ec.europa.eu/health/ph_risk/committees/sccp/documents/out131_en.pdf

Chapter 3.116 METHYL 2-OCTYNOATE

IDENTIFICATION

Description/definition : Methyl 2-octynoate is the organic compound that conforms to the structural formula shown below

Chemical class(es) : Esters

Chemical/IUPAC name : Methyl oct-2-ynoate

Other names : Methyl heptine carbonate; methyl pentylacetylenecarboxylate

CAS registry number(s) : 111-12-6

EC number(s) : 203-836-6

RIFM monograph(s) : Food Cosmet Toxicol 1979;17:375

IFRA standard : Restricted (www.ifraorg.org/en-us/standards-library) (table 3.116.1)

SCCS opinion(s) : SCCP/1023/06 (5); SCCNFP/0392/00, final (6); SCCS/1459/11 (7); SCCNFP/0389/00, final (33)

Function(s) in cosmetics : EU: perfuming. USA: fragrance ingredients

EU cosmetic restrictions : Regulated in Annex III/89 of the Regulation (EC) No. 1223/2009, regulated by 2003/15/EC; Must be labeled on cosmetics and detergent products, if present at > 10 ppm (0.001%) in leave-on products and > 100 ppm (0.01%) in rinse-off products

Patch testing : 0.2% Pet. (Chemotechnique); recommended test concentration: 0.2% wt./wt. pet. (1)

Molecular formula : $C_9H_{14}O_2$

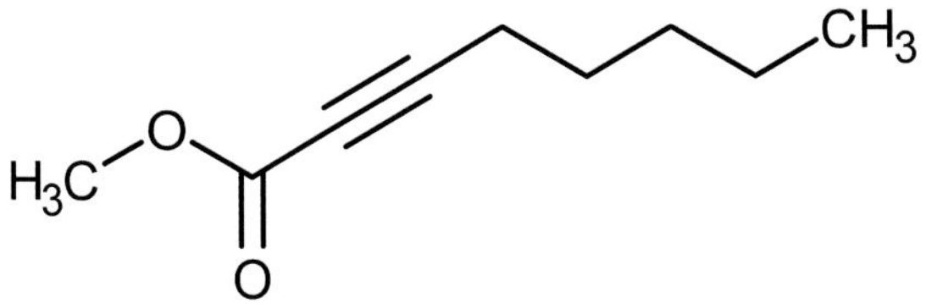

Table 3.116.1 IFRA restrictions for methyl 2-octynoate

Category [a]	Limits [b]	Category [a]	Limits [b]	Category [a]	Limits [b]
1	0.00%	5	0.01%	9	0.01%
2	0.00%	6	0.08%	10	0.01%
3	0.01%	7	0.01%	11	not restricted
4	0.01%	8	0.01%		

[a] For explanation of categories see pages 6-8
[b] Limits in the finished products

GENERAL

Methyl 2-octynoate is a colorless to pale yellow clear liquid; its odor type is green and its odor described as 'green, vegetative, fruity, fatty, waxy, cucumber, melon and violet leaf-like with floral nuances' (www.thegoodscents company.com). Methyl 2-octynoate is a synthetic chemical, not found in nature (and consequently not in essential oils (31)).

CONTACT ALLERGY

General

The SCCS (Scientific Committee on Consumer Safety), in a 2012 Opinion on Fragrance allergens in cosmetic products, has marked methyl 2-octynoate as 'established contact allergen in humans' (7,23).

Animal and human studies have shown methyl 2-octynoate to be a strong sensitizer (21,27,28,29,30). It was observed that this was not the case when freshly distilled preparations were tested. Only when a time-lapse had occurred did the test material appear to have a very powerful sensitizing capacity (27). It has been argued that a degradation product, not yet identified but not the result of autoxidation or peroxidation, is the allergen (27).

The literature on allergy to methyl 2-octynoate up to 2006 has been reviewed (30).

Patch testing in groups of patients

Results of studies testing methyl 2-octynoate in consecutive patients suspected of contact dermatitis (routine testing) and those of testing in groups of *selected* patients (e.g. patients with known or suspected fragrance or cosmetic dermatitis) are shown in table 3.116.2.

Patch testing in consecutive patients suspected of contact dermatitis: routine testing

In five studies in which consecutive patients with dermatitis have been tested with methyl 2-octynoate (in three tested at 1% pet., in the 4th 2% pet., the fifth not mentioned) rates of sensitization ranged from 0.1% to 0.9% (4,22,28,34), the latter percentage representing one positive reaction in a small group of 120 patients (28). Specific relevance data were not provided in any investigation.

Patch testing in groups of selected patients

The results of patch testing with methyl 2-octynoate in groups of selected patients are shown in table 3.116.2. In 5 studies, frequencies of sensitization have ranged from 0.1% to 5% (3,8,20,24,32), the latter representing one positive reaction in a very small group of 20 individuals who had dermatitis from perfumes (32). Specific relevance data were not provided in any investigation.

Table 3.116.2 Patch testing in groups of patients

Years and Country	Test conc. & vehicle	Number of patients tested	positive (%)	Selection of patients (S); Relevance (R); Comments (C)	Ref.
Routine testing					
2015-7 Netherlands		821	2 (0.2%)	R: not stated	35
2015-2016 UK	1% pet.	2084	2 (0.1%)	R: not specified for individual fragrances; 25% of patients who reacted to any fragrance or fragrance marker had a positive fragrance intolerance history	34
2011-2012 UK	1% pet.	1951	3 (0.2%)	R: not stated	22
2007-2008 France	2% pet.	120	1 (0.9%)	R: not stated; C: one other patient became sensitized by the test and one individual co-reacted to methyl octine carbonate	28
2003-2004 IVDK	1% pet.	2401	6 (0.2%)	R: not stated	4
Testing in groups of selected patients					
2006-2011 IVDK	1% pet.	708	6 (0.8%)	S: patients with suspected cosmetic intolerance; R: not stated	20
2005-2008 IVDK	1% pet.	988	(0.1%)	S: not specified; R: not stated	24
2005-7 Netherlands	0.5% pet.	320	1 (0.3%)	S: patients suspected of fragrance or cosmetic allergy; R: 61% relevance for all positive tested fragrances together	3
<1986 France	2% pet.	21	1 (5%)	S: patients with dermatitis caused by perfumes; R: not stated	32
1983 The Netherlands	0.5% pet.	182	2 (1.1%)	S: patients suspected of cosmetic allergy; R: not stated	8

IVDK: Informationsverbund Dermatologischer Kliniken (Germany, Switzerland, Austria)

Case reports and case series

A woman had severe dermatitis of the face and neck which was caused by methyl 2-octynoate in a face cream as shown by open application of 'the essential ingredients' of the product to the face (14). Another female patient had allergic contact cheilitis presumably caused by methyl 2-octynoate in a lipstick. The author mentions that the fragrance was 'the irritant', but its patch test concentration was probably too high (15).

A baker who later became cook had recurrent dermatitis of the hands, arms and face. He was known to react to his wife's perfumes and used fragranced cosmetic products himself. He had no reactions to any spice that he brought in himself, but when tested with a battery of fragrances, there were positive reactions to methyl 2-octynoate 0.5%, eugenol 8%, dihydrocoumarin 5%, phenylacetaldehyde 2% and cinnamyl benzoate 10%, all in petrolatum. The author was 'inclined' to say that these reactions may have been relevant (19).

A barber developed contact dermatitis localized to the dorsa of the fingers. All reactions to routine patch tests were negative. He was also tested with 10 cosmetics which he used frequently. Only one positive reaction to an aftershave was obtained. Further patch testing with its 22 perfume ingredients showed positive reactions to methyl 2-octynoate (0.5% pet.), hydroxycitronellal (10% pet.) and cinnamyl alcohol (5% pet.). By thin layer chromatography, column chromatography and gas chromatography all three fragrances were demonstrated in the aftershave. Whether this was the cause of the dermatitis of his hands was not stated (25).

A laboratory assistant developed a localized vesicular dermatitis on her wrist following direct skin contact with methyl heptine carbonate (MHC) (methyl 2-octynoate), which resolved within 2 weeks. Several months later, she developed hand dermatitis, which was relapsing and work-related. She had worked in a fragrance laboratory for 3 years, mixing fragrances, sunscreens and flavorings. She regularly worked with methyl octine carbonate (MOC) but only occasionally with MHC. Patch testing with the ICDRG standard series of allergens was negative, but both MHC (1% MEK) and MOC (1% MEK) produced very strong positive reactions at 2 and 4 days. The samples of MHC and MOC supplied were 96% pure (26).

Cross-reactions, pseudo-cross-reactions and co-reactions

For general information on cross-/pseudo-cross-/co-reactivity of fragrance chemicals with other fragrances, fragrance markers (fragrance mix I, fragrance mix II, colophonium, Myroxylon pereirae resin [balsam of Peru]) and essential oils see Chapter 1.2 General information on cross-reactions, pseudo-cross-reactions and co-reactions.

Methyl octine carbonate (26,28), possibly from a same degradation product (26).

Patch test sensitization

Two patients out of 230 tested with methyl 2-octynoate 1% in petrolatum and one out of 120 tested with 2% pet. were sensitized by the patch test (28). In testing methyl 2-octynoate in volunteers, 'primary sensitization' occurred (no further data known) (18).

Presence in products and chemical analyses

In various studies, the presence of methyl 2-octynoate in cosmetic and sometimes other products has been investigated. Before 2006, most investigators used chemical analysis, usually GC-MS, for qualitative and quantitative determination of target fragrances. Since then, the presence of the target fragrances was usually investigated by screening the product labels for the 26 fragrances that must be labeled since 2005 on cosmetics and detergent products in the EU, if present at > 10 ppm (0.001%) in leave-on products and > 100 ppm (0.01%) in rinse-off products. This method, obviously, is less accurate and may result in underestimation of the frequency of the fragrances being present in the product. When they are in fact present, but the concentration is lower than mentioned above, labeling is not required and the fragrances' presence will be missed.

The results of the relevant studies for methyl 2-octynoate are summarized in table 3.116.3. More detailed information can be found in the corresponding text following the table. Generally speaking, this fragrance appears to be little used or in concentrations lower than those that require labeling in the EU.

Table 3.116.3 Presence of methyl 2-octynoate in products [a]

Year	Country	Product type	Nr. investigated	Nr. of products positive [b]	(%)	Method [c]	Ref.
2015-6	Denmark	Fragranced cosmetic products	5588		(0.1%)	Labeling	12
2006-9	Germany	Cosmetic products	4991		(0.1%)	Labeling	11
2008	Sweden	Cosmetic products	204		(2%)	Labeling	9
		Detergents	97		(0%)	Labeling	
2007	Netherlands	Cosmetic products for children	23	1	(4%)	Analysis	16
2006	UK	Perfumed cosmetic and house-hold products	300	0	(0%)	Labeling	10
2006	Denmark	Popular perfumed deodorants	88	1	(1%)	Labeling	13
			23	0	(0%)	Analysis	
2002	Denmark	Home and car air fresheners	19	3	(16%)	Analysis	17

[a] See the corresponding text below for more details
[b] positive = containing the target fragrance
[c] Labeling: information from the ingredient labels on the product / packaging; Analysis: chemical analysis, most often GC-MS

In Denmark, in 2015-2016, 5588 fragranced cosmetic products were examined with a smartphone application for the 26 fragrances that need to be labeled in the EU. Methyl 2-octynoate was present in 0.1% of the products (rank number 25) (12).

In Germany, in the period 2006-2009, 4991 cosmetic products were randomly sampled for an official investigation of conformity of cosmetic products with legal provisions. The labels were inspected for the presence of the 26 fragrances that need to be labeled in the EU. Methyl 2-octynoate was present in 0.1% of the products (rank number 26) (11).

Methyl 2-octynoate was present in 2% of 204 cosmetic products (92 shampoos, 61 hair conditioners, 34 liquid soaps, 17 wet tissues) and in none of 97 detergents in Sweden, 2008 (9).

In 2007, in The Netherlands, twenty-three cosmetic products for children were analyzed for the presence of fragrances that need to be labelled. Methyl 2-octynoate was identified in one of the products (4%) in a concentration of 14 ppm (16).

In 2006, of 88 popular perfume containing deodorants purchased in Denmark, one (1%) were labeled to contain methyl 2-octynoate. Analysis of 24 regulated fragrance substances in 23 selected deodorants (19 spray products, 2 deostick and 2 roll-on) was performed by GC-MS. Methyl 2-octynoate was identified in none of the products (13).

In January 2006, a study of perfumed cosmetic and household products available on the shelves of U.K. retailers was carried out. Products were included if 'parfum' or 'aroma' was listed among the ingredients. Three hundred products were surveyed and any of 26 mandatory labeling fragrances named on the label were recorded. Methyl 2-oxtynoate was present in none of the products (rank number 26) (10).

In 2002, in Denmark, 19 air fresheners (6 for cars, 13 for homes) were analyzed for the presence of fragrances that need to be labelled on cosmetics. Methyl 2-octynoate was found to be present in 3 products (16%) in a concentration range of 3.5-270 ppm and ranked 19 in the frequency list (17).

LITERATURE

1   Bruze M, Svedman C, Andersen KE, Bruynzeel D, Goossens A, Johansen JD, et al. Patch test concentrations (doses in mg/cm2) for the 12 non-mix fragrance substances regulated by European legislation. Contact Dermatitis 2012;66:131-136

2   Heisterberg MV, Menné T, Johansen JD. Contact allergy to the 26 specific fragrance ingredients to be declared on cosmetic products in accordance with the EU cosmetic directive. Contact Dermatitis 2011;65:266-275

3   Oosten EJ van, Schuttelaar ML, Coenraads PJ. Clinical relevance of positive patch test reactions to the 26 EU-labelled fragrances. Contact Dermatitis 2009;61:217-223

4   Schnuch A, Uter W, Geier J, Lessmann H, Frosch PJ. Sensitization to 26 fragrances to be labelled according to current European regulation: Results of the IVDK and review of the literature. Contact Dermatitis 2007;57:1-10

5   SCCP (Scientific Committee on Consumer Products). Opinion on 'Clarifications to SCCNFP/0392/00 'An initial list of perfumery materials which must not form part of cosmetic products except subject to the Restrictions and Conditions laid down', 20 June 2006, SCCP/1023/06. Available at:
    http://ec.europa.eu/health/archive/ph_risk/committees/04_sccp/docs/sccp_o_062.pdf

6   SCCNFP (Scientific Committee on Cosmetic Products and Non-Food Products Intended for Consumers). Opinion of the Scientific Committee on Cosmetic Products and Non-Food Products Intended for Consumers concerning 'An initial list of perfumery materials which must not form part of cosmetic products except subject to the Restrictions and Conditions laid down, 25 September 2001, SCCNFP/0392/00, final. Available at:
    http://ec.europa.eu/health/archive/ph_risk/committees/sccp/documents/out150_en.pdf

7   SCCS (Scientific Committee on Consumer Safety). Opinion on Fragrance allergens in cosmetic products, 26-27 June 2012, SCCS/1459/11. Available at:
    https://ec.europa.eu/health/sites/health/files/scientific_committees/consumer_safety/docs/sccs_o_102.pdf

8   Malten KE, van Ketel WG, Nater JP, Liem DH. Reactions in selected patients to 22 fragrance materials. Contact Dermatitis 1984;11:1-10

9   Yazar K, Johnsson S, Lind M-L, Boman A, Lidén C. Preservatives and fragrances in selected consumer-available cosmetics and detergents. Contact Dermatitis 2011;64:265-272

10 Buckley DA. Fragrance ingredient labelling in products on sale in the UK. Br J Dermatol 2007;157:295-300

11 Uter W, Yazar K, Kratz E-M, Mildau G, Lidén C. Coupled exposure to ingredients of cosmetic products: I. Fragrances. Contact Dermatitis 2013;69:335-341

12 Bennike NH, Oturai NB, Müller S, Kirkeby CS, Jørgensen C, Christensen AB, et al. Fragrance contact allergens in 5588 cosmetic products identified through a novel smartphone application. J Eur Acad Dermatol Venereol 2018;32:79-85

13 Rastogi SC, Hellerup Jensen G, Johansen JD. Survey and risk assessment of chemical substances in deodorants. Survey of Chemical Substances in Consumer Products, No. 86 2007. Danish Ministry of the Environment, Environmental Protection Agency. Available at: https://www2.mst.dk/Udgiv/publications/2007/978-87-7052-625-8/pdf/978-87-7052-626-5.pdf

14 Hoffmann MJ, Peters J. Dermatitis due to facial cream, caused by methyl heptine carbonate. JAMA 1935;104:1072

15 Baer HL. Lipstick dermatitis. Arch Dermatol 1935;32:726-734

16 VWA. Dutch Food and Consumer Product Safety Authority. Cosmetische producten voor kinderen: Inventarisatie van de markt en de veiligheidsborging door producenten en importeurs. Report ND04o065/ND05o170, 2007 (Report in Dutch), 2007. Available at: www.nvwa.nl/documenten/communicatie/inspectieresultaten/consument/2016m/cosmetische- producten-voor-kinderen

17 Pors J, Fuhlendorff R. Mapping of chemical substances in air fresheners and other fragrance liberating products. Report Danish Ministry of the Environment, Environmental Protection Agency (EPA). Survey of Chemicals in Consumer Products, No 30, 2003. Available at: http://eng.mst.dk/media/mst/69113/30.pdf

18   Nakayama H. Fragrance hypersensitivity and its control. In: Frosch PJ, Johansen JD, White IR, Eds. Fragrances - beneficial and adverse effects. Berlin Heidelberg New York: Springer-Verlag, 1998:83-91

19   Malten KE. Four bakers showing positive patch tests to a number of fragrance materials, which can also be used as flavors. Acta Derm Venereol 1979;59(suppl.85):117-121

20   Dinkloh A, Worm M, Geier J, Schnuch A, Wollenberg A. Contact sensitization in patients with suspected cosmetic intolerance: results of the IVDK 2006-2011. J Eur Acad Dermatol Venereol 2015;29:1071-1081

21   Lidén C, Yazar K, Johansen JD, Karlberg A-T, Uter W, White IR. Comparative sensitizing potencies of fragrances, preservatives, and hair dyes. Contact Dermatitis 2016;75:265-275

22   Mann J, McFadden JP, White JML, White IR, Banerjee P. Baseline series fragrance markers fail to predict contact allergy. Contact Dermatitis 2014;70:276-281

23   Uter W, Johansen JD, Börje A, Karlberg A-T, Lidén C, Rastogi S, Roberts D, White IR. Categorization of fragrance contact allergens for prioritization of preventive measures: clinical and experimental data and consideration of structure–activity relationships. Contact Dermatitis 2013;69:196-230

24   Uter W, Geier J, Frosch P, Schnuch A. Contact allergy to fragrances: current patch test results (2005–2008) from the Information Network of Departments of Dermatology. Contact Dermatitis 2010;63:254-261

25   Van Ketel WG. Dermatitis from an aftershave. Contact Dermatitis 1978;4:117

26   English JS, Rycroft RJ. Allergic contact dermatitis from methyl heptine and methyl octine carbonates. Contact Dermatitis 1988;18:174-175

27   Opdyke DLJ. Fragrance raw materials monographs. Food Cosmet Toxicol 1979;17:375-376

28   Heisterberg MV, Vigan M, Johansen JD. Active sensitization and contact allergy to methyl 2-octynoate. Contact Dermatitis 2010;62:97-101

29   IFRA standard Methyl heptane carbonate. Available at: www.ifraorg.org/en-us/standards-library)

30   Hostynek JJ, Maibach HI. Is there evidence that methyl heptine carbonate causes allergic contact dermatitis? Cutan Ocul Toxicol 2006;25:259-271

31   De Groot AC, Schmidt E. Essential oils: contact allergy and chemical composition. Boca Raton, Fl., USA: CRC Press, Taylor and Francis Group, 2016 (ISBN 9781482246407)

32   Meynadier JM, Meynadier J, Peyron JL, Peyron L. Formes cliniques des manifestations cutanées d'allergie aux parfums. Ann Dermatol Venereol 1986;113:31-39

33   Opinion of the Scientific Committee on Cosmetic Products and Non-Food Products Intended for Consumers concerning 'The 1st update of the inventory of ingredients employed in cosmetic products. Section II: Perfume and aromatic raw materials', 24 October 2000, SCCNFP/0389/00, final. Available at: http://ec.europa.eu/health/ph_risk/committees/sccp/documents/out131_en.pdf

34   Ung CY, White JML, White IR, Banerjee P, McFadden JP. Patch testing with the European baseline series fragrance markers: a 2016 update. Br J Dermatol 2018;178:776-780

35   Dittmar D, Schuttelaar MLA. Contact sensitization to hydroperoxides of limonene and linalool: Results of consecutive patch testing and clinical relevance. Contact Dermatitis 2018 Oct 31. doi: 10.1111/cod.13137. [Epub ahead of print]

Chapter 3.117 METHYL SALICYLATE

IDENTIFICATION

Description/definition   : Methyl salicylate is the ester of methyl alcohol and salicylic acid that conforms to the structural formula shown below
Chemical class(es)   : Esters; phenols
Chemical/IUPAC name   : Methyl 2-hydroxybenzoate
Other names   : Synthetic wintergreen oil; synthetic sweet birch oil
CAS registry number(s)   : 119-36-8
EC number(s)   : 204-317-7
CIR review(s)   : Int J Toxicol 2003;22(suppl.3):S1-S108 (access: www.cir-safety.org/ingredients)
RIFM monograph(s)   : Food Chem Toxicol 2007;45(suppl.1):S428-S452; Food Chem Toxicol 2007;45(suppl.1): S318-S361; Food Cosmet Toxicol 1974;16:821 (special issue IV)
SCCS opinion(s)   : SCCS/1459/11 (2)
Merck Index monograph   : 7463
Function(s) in cosmetics   : EU: denaturant; perfuming; soothing. USA: denaturants; external analgesics; flavoring agents; fragrance ingredients; oral health care drugs
Patch testing   : 1% Pet. (SmartPracticeEurope, SmartPracticeCanada)
Molecular formula   : $C_8H_8O_3$

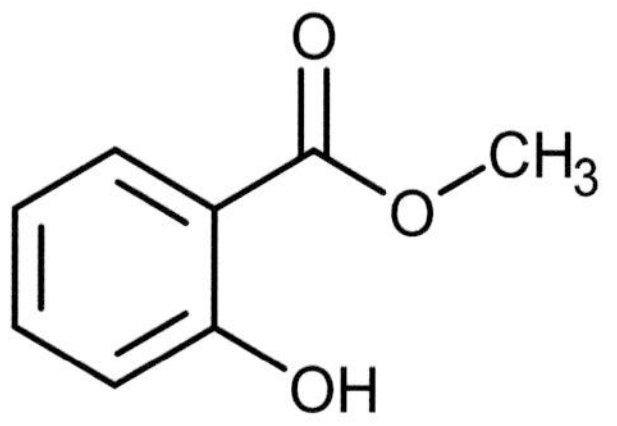

GENERAL

Methyl salicylate is a colorless to pink clear liquid; its odor type is minty and its odor is described as 'sweet, salicylate, root beer, wintergreen, aromatic, slightly phenolic and camphoreous' (www.thegoodscentscompany.com). It can be produced synthetically by esterification of salicylic acid with methyl alcohol or obtained from botanical sources, e.g. by maceration and subsequent distillation with steam from the leaves of *Gaultheria procumbrens* L. or from the bark of *Betula lenta* L. (18).

In perfumery, methyl salicylate is used as a modifier in blossom fragrances and as a mild antiseptic in oral hygiene products. Other uses include or have included (veterinary and human) medications, UV-absorber in sunburn lotions, flavor in foods and beverages, solvent for insecticides, polishes, and inks, and as chemical intermediate (U.S. National Library of Medicine). In many countries, it is available as an analgesic, anti-inflammatory agent, rubefacient and counterirritant in a wide range of over-the-counter liniments, ointments, lotions and medical oils for muscle pains (11,23). Cutaneous and non-cutaneous side effects of such preparations up to 1996 (12) and 2007 (26) have been reviewed (12).

Presence in essential oils and propolis

Methyl salicylate has been identified by chemical analysis in 16 of 91 essential oils, which have caused contact allergy / allergic contact dermatitis. In one oil, methyl salicylate belonged to the 'Top-10' of ingredients with the highest concentrations which may be expected in commercial essential oils of this type: clove bud/leaf/stem oil (0.02-0.3%) (20). Methyl salicylate may also be present in propolis (19).

CONTACT ALLERGY

General

The SCCS (Scientific Committee on Consumer Safety), in a 2012 Opinion on Fragrance allergens in cosmetic products, has marked methyl salicylate as 'established contact allergen in humans' (2,4). Few cases of contact allergy to methyl salicylate have been reported. Those that have were from topical pharmaceuticals rather than from cosmetics or other products containing methyl salicylate as a fragrance (8,9,11).

Patch testing in groups of patients

Results of studies testing methyl salicylate in consecutive patients suspected of contact dermatitis (routine testing) and those of testing in groups of *selected* patients (patients suspected of oral and lip contact allergy) are shown in table 3.117.1.

Patch testing in consecutive patients suspected of contact dermatitis: routine testing

In three studies in which methyl salicylate 2% pet. was tested in consecutive patients suspected of contact dermatitis, low frequencies of sensitization (0.1%, 0.4% and 0.5%) have been observed (1,10,16). The relevance of the positive patch test reactions was not mentioned.

Patch testing in groups of selected patients

In two studies in which methyl salicylate was tested in selected patient groups, low frequencies of sensitization of 1.3% and 1.6% have been observed (5,6). The relevance of the positive patch test reactions was not mentioned.

Table 3.117.1 Patch testing in groups of patients

Years and Country	Test conc. & vehicle	Number of patients tested	positive (%)		Selection of patients (S); Relevance (R); Comments (C)	Ref.
Routine testing						
1998-9 Netherlands	2% pet.	1825	7	(0.4%)	R: not stated	1
1978-1980 USA	2% pet.	585	3	(0.5%)	R: not stated; C: testing with it was abandoned	16
1973-1977 Spain	2% pet.	4600	6	(0.1%)	R: not stated	10
Testing in groups of selected patients						
2014-2015 USA		149	2	(1.3%)	S: patients suspected of oral and lip contact allergy; R: not stated	5
1975-1976 USA	2% pet.	183	3	(1.6%)	S: not stated; R: not stated	6

Case reports and case series

A man developed acute dermatitis of the neck, upper back, shoulders and dorsa of the hands. The patient had been applying an analgesic ointment to his neck and back containing menthol, camphor and 12% methyl salicylate. Patch testing to the constituents of the ointment gave a positive reaction to methyl salicylate 2% in olive oil. Three months later, the patient returned with a reappearance of his eczema at the previous sites. He denied using any topical applications but he had taken oral Aspirin (acetylsalicylic acid). Patch tests with acetylsalicylic acid 0.3% and 5% aqua were negative, but when he took 500 mg of Aspirin, the patient noticed pruritus and erythema again in the previously affected areas (8).

Two cases of contact allergy to methyl salicylate have been reported from a liniment containing 25% methyl salicylate in arachis oil (9).

A woman had a rectangular pruritic erythematous macule on the hip following the use of a compress. The manufacturer provided samples of the ingredients and patch testing showed a positive reaction to methyl salicylate 2% in olive oil (11).

Cross-reactions, pseudo-cross-reactions and co-reactions

For general information on cross-/pseudo-cross-/co-reactivity of fragrance chemicals with other fragrances, fragrance markers (fragrance mix I, fragrance mix II, colophonium, Myroxylon pereirae resin [balsam of Peru]) and essential oils see Chapter 1.2 General information on cross-reactions, pseudo-cross-reactions and co-reactions.

Cross-reactions (or pseudo-cross-reactions from the same allergenic moiety) have been observed to phenyl salicylate (5), benzyl salicylate (5) and sodium salicylate (8).

Presence in products and chemical analyses

In 1997, 71 deodorants (22 vapo-spray, 22 aerosol spray and 27 roll-on products) were collected in Denmark, England, France, Germany and Sweden and analyzed by gas chromatography – mass spectrometry (GC-MS) for the presence of fragrances and other materials. Methyl salicylate was present in 4 (6%) of the products (3).

OTHER SIDE EFFECTS

Irritant contact dermatitis

Methyl salicylate is said to be a strong irritant to the skin and can cause irritant dermatitis (12). One patient had applied a topical methyl salicylate- and menthol-containing ointment over his forearms, calves and thighs for the treatment of muscle aches and pains. He also applied heat to these areas periodically using a heating pad. The patient experienced full-thickness skin and muscle necrosis, in combination with systemic symptoms (14).

Immediate-type reactions

Methyl salicylate has been cited as having caused immediate contact reactions (contact urticaria) (27).

Other non-eczematous contact reactions

A woman may have developed bronchospasm from methyl salicylate ('wintergreen') in toothpaste. Alternatively, the culprit may have been peppermint flavor or methyl salicylate *and* peppermint flavor (7).

Severe urticaria and angioedema following the use of methyl salicylate-containing mints, toothpaste or liniments were seen in a young man with a past history of Aspirin (acetylsalicylic acid) hypersensitivity (15).

Systemic side effects

In many countries, methyl salicylate is available as an analgesic, anti-inflammatory agent, rubefacient and counterirritant in a wide range of over-the-counter liniments, ointments, lotions and medical oils for the self-treatment of muscle pains (11,23). Like other salicylates, methyl salicylate may be absorbed through the intact skin (22) and cause systemic side effects including salicylate intoxication ('salicylism'). A few examples are presented here, but detailed discussion of the subject is considered to fall outside the scope of this publication.

Systemic poisoning has been reported as a result of penetration of methyl and phenyl salicylate in a patient with psoriasis (13). Another patient had applied a topical methyl salicylate- and menthol-containing ointment over his forearms, calves and thighs for the treatment of muscle aches and pains. He also applied heat to these areas periodically using a heating pad. The patient experienced full-thickness skin and muscle necrosis, interstitial nephritis, hepatic dysfunction and metabolic acidosis. Some of his clinical presentations were attributed to toxicity of methyl salicylate (14).

A man developed the classical syndrome of salicylism with early tinnitus followed by hypernea, vomiting, diaphoresis, fever and central nervous system disturbance within an hour after full body application of a methyl salicylate-containing cream under a 'bodywrap' of plastic cling film for psoriasis. A salicylate level of 48.5mg/dL at time of presentation confirmed the diagnosis of salicylate intoxication (17).

Concomitant use of topical analgesic preparations containing methyl salicylate and oral warfarin (an anticoagulant) may result in prolonged international normalized ratio (INR) (a measure for clotting time of blood) with or without bleeding (12). Topical and oral administration of oil of wintergreen, containing 35% methyl salicylate, may have led to coma, seizures and death in an old man with end-stage renal disease (21).

Other case reports of toxicity from topical application of methyl salicylate-containing preparations include refs. 24 and 25. The literature on cutaneous and non-cutaneous side effects of preparations containing methyl salicylate up to 1996 (12) and 2007 (26) have been reviewed.

Side effects of oral administration

Accidental or deliberate ingestion of methyl salicylate (usually in the form of oil of wintergreen, which contains up to 98% methyl salicylate), poses the threat of severe, rapid-onset salicylate poisoning because of its liquid, concentrated form. The unusual number of deaths resulting from this agent in the past may be due to the ease of ingestion of many millilitres of this pleasantly smelling liquid. To put into perspective the danger of this compound: one teaspoon (5 ml) of oil of wintergreen (synthetic methyl salicylate) is equivalent to approximately 7000 mg of salicylate or 14 adult (500 mg) Aspirin tablets. Ingestions of as little as 4 ml in a child and 6 ml in an adult have been fatal (12).

Methyl salicylate is rapidly absorbed from the gastrointestinal tract. Much of the ester is hydrolyzed to free salicylate. The onset of symptoms is rapid, usually within 2 hours of ingestion. Clinical manifestations are similar to those observed with poisoning by other salicylates. However, in view of its lipid solubility, methyl salicylate is expected to be more toxic. The major toxic effects of salicylates may be grouped as gastrointestinal, central nervous system, hematological, and metabolic and acid-base disturbances. In adult patients with severe salicylate poisoning, delayed presentation, coma, hyperpyrexia, and pulmonary edema and acidemia appear to be more common among the fatal cases (12).

There is a vast amount of literature on toxicity from oral intake of methyl salicylate in various products (oil of wintergreen, herbal preparations); further discussion of this subject is considered to fall outside the scope of this publication.

LITERATURE

1   De Groot AC, Coenraads PJ, Bruynzeel DP, Jagtman BA, Van Ginkel CJW, Noz K, et al. Routine patch testing with fragrance chemicals in The Netherlands. Contact Dermatitis 2000;42:184-185
2   SCCS (Scientific Committee on Consumer Safety). Opinion on Fragrance allergens in cosmetic products, 26-27 June 2012, SCCS/1459/11. Available at:

https://ec.europa.eu/health/sites/health/files/scientific_committees/consumer_safety/docs/sccs_o_102.pdf

3   Rastogi SC, Lepoittevin J-P, Johansen JD, Frosch PJ, Menné T, Bruze M, et al. Fragrances and other materials in deodorants: search for potentially sensitizing molecules using combined GC-MS and structure activity relationship (SAR) analysis. Contact Dermatitis 1998;39:293-303

4   Uter W, Johansen JD, Börje A, Karlberg A-T, Lidén C, Rastogi S, Roberts D, White IR. Categorization of fragrance contact allergens for prioritization of preventive measures: clinical and experimental data and consideration of structure–activity relationships. Contact Dermatitis 2013;69:196-230

5   Scheman A, Te R. Contact allergy to salicylates and cross-reactions. Dermatitis 2017;28:291

6   Rudner EJ. North American group results. Contact Dermatitis 1977;3:208-209

7   Spurlock BW, Dailey TM. Shortness of (fresh) breath--toothpaste-induced bronchospasm. N Engl J Med 1990;323:1845-1846

8   Hindson C. Contact eczema from methyl salicylate reproduced by oral aspirin (acetyl salicylic acid). Contact Dermatitis 1977;3:348-349

9   Morgan JK. British Journal of Clinical Practice 1968;22:261. Data cited in ref. 8

10 Romaguera C, Grimalt F. Statistical and comparative study of 4600 patients tested in Barcelona (1973–1977). Contact Dermatitis 1980;6:309-315

11 Oiso N, Fukai K, Ishii M. Allergic contact dermatitis due to methyl salicylate in a compress. Contact Dermatitis 2004;51:34-35

12 Chan TY. Potential dangers from topical preparations containing methyl salicylate. Hum Exp Toxicol 1996;15:747-750

13 Von Weiss JF, Lever WF. Percutaneous salicylic acid intoxication in psoriasis. Arch Dermatol 1964;90:614-619

14 Heng MCY. Local necrosis and interstitial nephritis due to topical methyl salicylate and menthol. Cutis 1987;39:442-444

15 Speer F. Allergy to methyl salicylate. Ann Allergy 1979;43:36-37. Data cited in ref. 12

16 Mitchell JC, Adams RM, Glendenning WE, Fisher A, Kanof N, Larsen W, et al. Results of standard patch tests with substances abandoned. Contact Dermatitis 1982;8:336-337

17 Bell AJ, Duggin G. Acute methyl salicylate toxicity complicating herbal skin treatment for psoriasis. Emergency Medicine 2002;14:188-190

18 Cosmetic Ingredient Review Expert Panel. Safety assessment of salicylic acid, butyloctyl salicylate, calcium salicylate, C12-15 alkyl salicylate, capryloyl salicylic acid, hexyldodecyl salicylate, isocetyl salicylate, isodecyl salicylate, magnesium salicylate, MEA-salicylate, ethylhexyl salicylate, potassium salicylate, methyl salicylate, myristyl salicylate, sodium salicylate, tea-salicylate, and tridecyl salicylate. Int J Toxicol 2003;22(suppl.3):1-108

19 De Groot AC, Popova MP, Bankova VS. An update on the constituents of poplar-type propolis. Wapserveen, The Netherlands: acdegroot publishing, 2014, 11 pages. ISBN/EAN: 978-90-813233-0-7. Available at: https://www.researchgate.net/publication/262851225_AN_UPDATE_ON_THE_CONSTITUENTS_OF_POPLAR-TYPE_PROPOLIS

20 De Groot AC, Schmidt E. Essential oils: contact allergy and chemical composition. Boca Raton, Fl., USA: CRC Press, Taylor and Francis Group, 2016 (ISBN 9781482246407)

21 Chin R, Olson K, Dempsey D. Salicylate toxicity from ingestion and continued dermal absorption. Calif J Emerg Med 2007;8:23-25

22 Morra P, Bartle WR, Walker SE, Lee SN, Bowles SK, Reeves RA. Serum concentrations of salicylic acid following topically applied salicylate derivatives. Ann Pharmacother 1996;30:935-940

23 Anderson A, McConville A, Fanthorpe L, Davis J. Salicylate poisoning potential of topical pain relief agents: From age old remedies to engineered smart patches. Medicines (Basel) 2017 June 30;4(3). pii: E48. doi: 10.3390/medicines4030048

24 Thompson TM, Toerne T, Erickson TB. Salicylate toxicity from genital exposure to a methyl salicylate-containing rubefacient. West J Emerg Med 2016;17:181-183

25 Robinson K, Rauch A, Hannan L. Salicylate poisoning following topical administration of methylsalicylate. Emerg Med Australas 2015;27:374-375

26 Davis JE. Are one or two dangerous? Methyl salicylate exposure in toddlers. J Emerg Med 2007;32:63-69

27 De Groot AC. Patch Testing, 4th Edition. Wapserveen, The Netherlands: acdegroot publishing, 2018 (ISBN 978-90-813233-4-5)

Chapter 3.118   3-METHYL-5-(2,2,3-TRIMETHYL-3-CYCLOPENTENYL) PENT-4-EN-2-OL

IDENTIFICATION

Description/definition	: 3-Methyl-5-(2,2,3-trimethyl-3-cyclopentenyl)pent-4-en-2-ol is the unsaturated cyclic compound that conforms to the structural formula shown below
Chemical class(es)	: Unsaturated cyclic organic compounds; alcohols
INCI name USA	: Not in the Personal Care Products Council Ingredient Database
Chemical/IUPAC name	: 3-Methyl-5-(2,2,3-trimethylcyclopent-3-en-1-yl)pent-4-en-2-ol
Other names	: Sandal pentenol; Ebanol ®
CAS registry number(s)	: 67801-20-1
EC number(s)	: 267-140-4
RIFM monograph(s)	: Food Chem Toxicol 2018;115(suppl.1):S143-S152
SCCS opinion(s)	: SCCS/1459/11 (1)
Function(s) in cosmetics	: EU: perfuming
Patch testing	: 5% pet. (2,3)
Molecular formula	: $C_{14}H_{24}O$

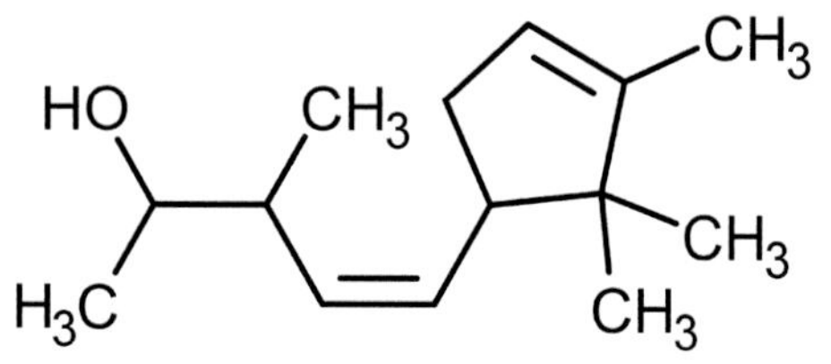

GENERAL

3-Methyl-5-(2,2,3-trimethyl-3-cyclopentenyl)pent-4-en-2-ol is a colorless to pale yellow clear liquid; its odor type is woody and its odor at 10% in dipropylene glycol is described as 'sandalwood woody musk' (www.thegoodscents company.com). 3-Methyl-5-(2,2,3-trimethyl-3-cyclopentenyl)pent-4-en-2-ol is a synthetic chemical, not found in nature (and consequently not in essential oils (5)).

CONTACT ALLERGY

General

The SCCS (Scientific Committee on Consumer Safety), in a 2012 Opinion on Fragrance allergens in cosmetic products, has marked 3-methyl-5-(2,2,3-trimethyl-3-cyclopentenyl)pent-4-en-2-ol as 'established contact allergen in humans' (1,4).

Patch testing in groups of patients

Patch testing in consecutive patients suspected of contact dermatitis: routine testing

Studies in which 3-methyl-5-(2,2,3-trimethyl-3-cyclopentenyl)pent-4-en-2-ol was patch tested in consecutive patients suspected of contact dermatitis (routine testing) with positive results have not been found.

Patch testing in groups of selected patients

Results of studies patch testing 3-methyl-5-(2,2,3-trimethyl-3-cyclopentenyl)pent-4-en-2-ol in groups of selected patients (patients with suspected cosmetic dermatitis, patients with known fragrance sensitivity) are shown in table 3.118.1. In 2002-2003, in Korea, 422 patients with suspected cosmetic dermatitis were patch tested and there were 12 (2.8%) positive reactions to 3-methyl-5-(2,2,3-trimethyl-3-cyclopentenyl)pent-4-en-2-ol (3). In 2000, in Japan, some European countries and the USA, a group of 178 patients with known fragrance sensitivity were patch tested with 3-methyl-5-(2,2,3-trimethyl-3-cyclopentenyl)pent-4-en-2-ol 5% pet. and only one (0.6%) positive reaction was observed (2). In neither study was the relevance of the positive reactions mentioned (2,3).

Table 3.118.1 Testing in groups of patients: Selected patient groups

Years and Country	Test conc. & vehicle	Number of patients tested | positive (%)		Selection of patients (S); Relevance (R); Comments (C)	Ref.
2002-2003 Korea	5% pet.	422	12 (2.8%)	S: patients with suspected cosmetic dermatitis; R: not stated	3
2000 Japan, Europe, USA	5% pet.	178	1 (0.6%)	S: patients with known fragrance sensitivity; R: not stated	2

Case reports and case series

Case reports of allergic contact dermatitis from 3-methyl-5-(2,2,3-trimethyl-3-cyclopentenyl)pent-4-en-2-ol have not been found.

LITERATURE

1 SCCS (Scientific Committee on Consumer Safety). Opinion on Fragrance allergens in cosmetic products, 26-27 June 2012, SCCS/1459/11. Available at: https://ec.europa.eu/health/sites/health/files/scientific_committees/consumer_safety/docs/sccs_o_102.pdf

2 Larsen W, Nakayama H, Fischer T, Elsner P, Frosch P, Burrows D, et al. Fragrance contact dermatitis: A worldwide multicenter investigation (Part II). Contact Dermatitis 2001;44:344-346

3 An S, Lee AY, Lee CH, Kim DW, Hahm JH, Kim KJ, et al. Fragrance contact dermatitis in Korea: a joint study. Contact Dermatitis 2005;53:320-323

4 Uter W, Johansen JD, Börje A, Karlberg A-T, Lidén C, Rastogi S, Roberts D, White IR. Categorization of fragrance contact allergens for prioritization of preventive measures: clinical and experimental data and consideration of structure–activity relationships. Contact Dermatitis 2013;69:196-230

5 De Groot AC, Schmidt E. Essential oils: contact allergy and chemical composition. Boca Raton, Fl., USA: CRC Press, Taylor and Francis Group, 2016 (ISBN 9781482246407)

Chapter 3.119 MUSK

IDENTIFICATION

Description/definition : Musk is the secretion from an abdominal gland of the musk deer, *Moschus moschiferus* L.
Chemical class(es) : Natural products and derivatives
INCI name USA : Neither in Cosing nor in the Personal Care Products Council Ingredient Database
Other names : Musk tonquin; Moschus moschiferus L. pod grain absolute; musk tonquin absolute
CAS registry number(s) : 68991-41-3; 8001-04-5; 90064-09-8
EC number(s) : 290-070-0
Merck Index monograph : 7669
Patch testing : unknown (1)

GENERAL

Musk is the secretion of an abdominal gland of the musk deer (*Moschus moschiferus*), a small, hornless deer species living in high plateaus of East Asia (Himalayas, Siberia). In the past, the animals were killed and the sac containing the secretion cut out. These sacs were dried and marketed. It contained a black brown, grainy mass with ammonia-animalic odor. The actual erogenic-animalic, dry woody musk odor develops on preparation of a tincture in 70-80% slightly alkaline ethanol. The musk tincture was used in the production of expensive luxury perfumes. Its major odor substance was muscone. Genuine musk is no longer used in Europe and the USA. It has been completely substituted by synthetic musk (2).

CONTACT ALLERGY

Patch testing in groups of patients

Studies in which musk was patch tested in either consecutive patients suspected of contact dermatitis (routine testing) or in groups of selected patients with positive results have not been found.

Case reports and case series

A woman had allergic contact dermatitis from the perfume in an eye cream. Subsequently, she was tested with 94 individual liquid fragrance materials from this perfume (test concentrations not stated). The patient at day 5 had 12 positive patch test reactions, including to musk (musk tonquin). Three controls were negative. She was not retested, so false-positive reactions due to the excited skin syndrome (there was an additional strong reaction to allyl cyclohexyl propionate which proved to be irritant) cannot be excluded (1).

Indeed, two years later, in a Letter to the Editor, the author mentioned that he had retested the patient with the 12 fragrances to which she had previously shown a positive patch test. Only hydroxycitronellal had again given a positive reaction (3). This means that, in fact, contact allergy to musk tonquin has not been demonstrated thus far beyond doubt.

LITERATURE

1   Larsen WG. Cosmetic dermatitis due to a perfume. Contact Dermatitis 1975;1:142-145
2   Steglich W Fugmann B, Lang-Fugmann S, , Eds. Römpp Encyclopedia Natural Products. Stuttgart – New York: Georg Thieme Verlag, 2000
3   Larsen WG. Perfume dermatitis revisited. Contact Dermatitis 1977;3:98

Chapter 3.120 MUSK AMBRETTE *

Not an INCI name

IDENTIFICATION

Description/definition : Musk ambrette is the dinitro aromatic compound that conforms to the structural formula shown below

Chemical class(es) : Aromatic organic compounds; ethers; nitro compounds

INCI name USA : Not in the Personal Care Products Council Ingredient Database

Chemical/IUPAC name : 1-*tert*-Butyl-2-methoxy-4-methyl-3,5-dinitrobenzene

CAS registry number(s) : 83-66-9

EC number(s) : 201-493-7

RIFM monograph(s) : Food Cosmet Toxicol 1975;13:875 (special issue II)

IFRA standard : Prohibited (www.ifraorg.org/en-us/standards-library)

SCCS opinion(s) : SCCNFP/0320/00, final (5)

Function(s) in cosmetics : Formerly used in perfuming

EU cosmetic restrictions : Regulated in Annex II/414 of the Regulation (EC) No. 1223/2009, regulated by 95/34/EC; Prohibited since 1995

Patch testing : 5% Pet. (SmartPracticeEurope, SmartPracticeCanada)

Molecular formula : $C_{12}H_{16}N_2O_5$

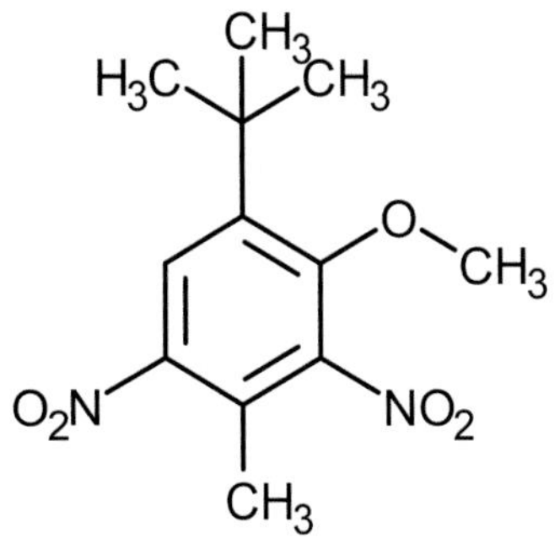

GENERAL

Musk ambrette is a pale yellow powder; its odor type is musk and its odor at 10% in benzyl benzoate is described as 'musty sweet ambrette seed' (www.thegoodscentscompany.com). It is a synthetic chemical, not found in nature (and consequently not in essential oils (57)). Musk ambrette is prohibited by the European Union and by IFRA because of photosensitization and neurotoxicity (www.ifraorg.org) and is not used anymore in cosmetics.

Musk ambrette is a synthetic nitro-musk fragrance that was formerly used in topical medications, detergents, food (37), women's perfumes, in shaving products, talcum powders, deodorants, hair creams and gels (49), hair sprays, shampoos, soaps (49) and baby products (31). However, musk ambrette's primary application was in men's shaving cosmetics (shaving cream, aftershave lotion), because of its fixative properties, animal-like musk scent, low price and solubility in most cosmetic vehicles (27,41). Musk ambrette-related chemicals extracted from the scent glands of animals and some plants had been used for years before as fixatives and enhancers in perfumes, but they were (too) expensive and difficult to purchase because of shortage of material.

In the 1970s and 1980s, huge quantities of musk ambrette were used in the United States and other countries in cosmetics, primarily men's after-shave lotions and colognes. Concentrations as high as 15% were used in such products (41). In the late 1970s, reports of photoallergy began to appear in the literature (14,27,28,29), and it was soon found out in guinea pig testing that musk ambrette is a photosensitizer, albeit not a very strong one (44). By the 1980s, this agent was the most frequently reported cause of photoallergic contact dermatitis (9,31,43,46). Many of the men sensitized to musk ambrette would develop persistent light reactions of the light-exposed skin (notably the face, neck and the back of the hands) despite avoiding the culprit products (usually an aftershave) and other cosmetics possibly containing musk ambrette (2,21,25,30,31,33,41,51,54,64). This not infrequently lead to chronic actinic dermatitis and in a single case, to erythroderma (2).

Perfume manufacturers in the early 1980s were already very aware of the problem and musk ambrette's concentrations in perfumes and toiletries was greatly reduced. Indeed, the International Fragrance Association (IFRA) had approved further restrictions in its use to a maximum of 0.1% for fragrance compounds intended for use in toilet waters, colognes, shaving products and sunscreen preparations (21). In the mid-nineties, the number of cases of photoallergic contact dermatitis dropped because IFRA had advised not to use musk ambrette in cosmetics anymore and its use was prohibited in the European Union by that time.

Further information on photocontact allergy to musk ambrette is discussed in the section 'Photosensitivity' below. Some additional data on (photo)contact allergy to musk ambrette not presented here can be found in refs. 34,35,40,42 and 47 (articles not read).

CONTACT ALLERGY

General
A number of 'plain' contact allergic reactions have been observed (sometimes with far stronger photopatch tests, 'photoaggravated contact allergy') (21,23,31,32,33,50,52,55) but the vast majority of reactions to musk ambrette consisted of photocontact allergy and photoallergic contact dermatitis.

Patch testing in groups of patients
Results of studies testing musk ambrette in consecutive patients suspected of contact dermatitis (routine testing) and those of testing in groups of selected patients (patients with suspected photosensitivity or photodermatoses, individuals known or suspected to be allergic to fragrances) are shown in table 3.120.1.

Patch testing in consecutive patients suspected of contact dermatitis: routine testing
In two studies in which musk ambrette was patch tested in consecutive patients, low frequencies of sensitization of 0.3% and 0.4% were observed. In one, the relevance was not mentioned (17), in the other investigation, two positive reactions were likely to be relevant, as the patients used cosmetic products known to contain musk ambrette (29).

Patch testing in groups of selected patients
Results of studies patch testing musk ambrette in groups of selected patients (patients with suspected photosensitivity or photodermatoses, individuals known or suspected to be allergic to fragrances) are shown in table 3.120.1. In seven investigations, frequencies of sensitization ranged from 0.15% to 10%, but were 1.6% or lower in 5/7 studies.

A high percentage 8 was observed in 1983-1984 in Singapore, where many cases of photocontact allergy to musk ambrette were diagnosed. The 4 patients with a positive patch test to musk ambrette in this study all had photo-aggravation (63). The highest percentage of 10 (five positive reactions) was in a group of 50 patients with photosensitivity dermatitis with actinic reticuloid syndrome. The relevance of the positive patch tests was not specified, but the authors suggested that fragrances may play a role in the etiology of this disease (16).

Table 3.120.1 Patch testing in groups of patients

Years and Country	Test conc. & vehicle	Number of patients tested	positive (%)	Selection of patients (S); Relevance (R); Comments (C)	Ref.
Routine testing					
1983-1984 Italy	5% pet.	1200	4 (0.3%)	R: not stated	17
1977-1978 Denmark	1% pet.	562	2 (0.4%)	R: both very likely relevant, the patients used cosmetics known to contain musk ambrette	29
Testing in groups of selected patients					
2005-2014 China	5% pet.	4930	15 (0.3%)	S: patients suspected of photodermatoses; R: not stated	19
1983-1998 UK	5% pet.	2715	4 (0.15%)	S: patients suspected of photosensitivity or with (a history of) dermatitis at exposed sites; R: not stated	45
<1996 Japan, Europe, USA	5% pet.	167	2 (1.2%)	S: patients known or suspected to be allergic to fragrances; R: not stated	6
1990-1994 France	5% pet.	370	6 (1.6%)	S: patients with suspected photodermatitis; R: not stated	10
1985-1990 USA	1% alc.	187	1 (0.5%)	S: patients with a history of photosensitivity; R: not relevant	46
1983-1984 Singapore	5% pet.	50	4 (8%)	S: not stated; R: not specified; C: all had photo-aggravation	63
<1982 UK		50	5 (10%)	S: patients with photosensitivity dermatitis with actinic reticuloid syndrome (PD/AR); R: not specified for individual fragrances, but the authors concluded that in some subjects with PD/AR and persistent light reaction, a significant factor in the latter is likely to be exposure to substances such as fragrance materials; C: in a control group of 457 dermatitis patients, only 1.5% reacted positively to musk ambrette	16

Case reports and case series
In the period 1996-2013, in a tertiary referral center in Valencia, Spain, 5419 patients were patch tested. Of these, 628 individuals had allergic contact dermatitis to cosmetics. In this group, musk ambrette was the responsible allergen in 3 cases (11, overlap with ref. 12).

In the period 2000-2007, 202 patients with allergic contact dermatitis caused by cosmetics were seen in Valencia, Spain. In this group, musk ambrette was stated to be the allergen in one individual from its presence in cologne (12, overlap with ref. 11), It may be doubtful whether this observation is correct, since musk ambrette has been prohibited in cosmetics since 1995.

Musk ambrette was responsible for 11 out of 399 cases of cosmetic (photo)allergy where the causal allergen was identified in a study of the NACDG, USA, 1977-1983 (1); most likely, these were all or virtually all photocontact reactions.

A man had allergic contact dermatitis related to his pre- and aftershave products (positive patch tests) and also had a positive patch test to musk ambrette. It was not investigated whether the cosmetic products contained musk ambrette. Another male patient presented with an acute eczema of the face, neck and chest on light-exposed surfaces. He used an aftershave lotion and a spray deodorant. The products themselves were not tested, the patient did react to musk ambrette. Contact allergy to the products was not proven nor was the presence of musk ambrette therein (29).

One patient suspected to be allergic to incense had positive patch tests to two brands of incense, sandalwood oil, musk ambrette and santalol; gas chromatography of pentane:ether extracts of the incense showed 9% and 34% musk ambrette and 8% santalol in both incenses (32).

A Japanese woman, who burnt incense every day, presented with itchy pigmentation of her face, suggestive of pigmented cosmetic dermatitis. Patch testing revealed contact allergy to musk ambrette 1%, 2% and 5% in petrolatum and to pentane:ether extracts of 2 incenses. The perfume components of the incenses were extracted and analyzed by gas chromatography, detecting 20 fragrance materials. All were patch tested but only musk ambrette reacted. The incenses which she used contained 33.7% and 15.3% musk ambrette in their perfume components. The use of the incenses was stopped and (with therapy) the pigmentation had disappeared two months later (23).

One patient had allergic contact dermatitis from allergy to musk ambrette in products used by the patient's partner. Details are lacking (42, article not read).

Cross-reactions, pseudo-cross-reactions and co-reactions

For general information on cross-/pseudo-cross-/co-reactivity of fragrance chemicals with other fragrances, fragrance markers (fragrance mix I, fragrance mix II, colophonium, Myroxylon pereirae resin [balsam of Peru]) and essential oils see Chapter 1.2 General information on cross-reactions, pseudo-cross-reactions and co-reactions.

Musk ketone
Of 21 patients with photocontact allergy to musk ambrette, one photo-co-reacted to musk ketone (31).
Musk moskene
Photo-co-reactions of musk moskene in patients photosensitive to musk ambrette have been observed in one of 2 individuals (27), in two of two (36), in 3 of 19 (21, overlap with ref. 31), in 8 of 21 (31, overlap with ref. 21) and in one of 8 patients with photocontact allergy to musk ambrette (58). In one individual, a contact allergic co-reaction to musk moskene was observed in a patient with 'plain' contact allergy to musk ambrette (31).
Musk tibetene
In 8 patients with photocontact allergy to musk ambrette, there was one photo-co-reaction to musk tibetene (58).
Musk xylene
Photo-co-reactions of musk xylene in patients photosensitive to musk ambrette have been observed in two of two patients (36), in three of 19 (21, overlap with ref. 31), in one of 21 (31, overlap with ref. 21) and in one of 13 patients with photocontact allergy to musk ambrette (58).
Although (some of) these reactions may have been actual cross-reactions, musk ketone and musk xylene have also been identified in men's colognes (20,60), so the reactions can also be explained by sensitization independent of musk ambrette photocontact allergy.

Presence in products and chemical analyses
In 2000, thirty 30 fragranced products were purchased in the USA and investigated by GC-MS for the presence of nitro-musks. Musk ambrette was not found in any of the products, but musk xlyene was found in 9 products at levels ranging from 0.001 to 0.22% and musk ketone was identified in 8 products at levels ranging from 0.023 to 0.45% (60).

In 1984, in Singapore, 32 different men's colognes were analysed with GC-MS for the presence of nitro-musks. Fourteen (44%) proved to contain musk ambrette in concentrations ranging from 0.02% w/v to 0.39% w/v (20).

In 1984, in Sweden, 21 perfumed commercial products, mainly aftershaves and eaux de toilette preparations, were examined by thin layer chromatography and high pressure liquid chromatography for the presence of nitro-musks. Musk ambrette was identified in 12 (57%) of the products in a concentration range of 0.014% to 7.049% (58).

OTHER SIDE EFFECTS

Photosensitivity
Musk ambrette in the past has been a very important cause of photocontact allergy from its use in men's aftershaves and colognes. See for additional information the section GENERAL, photosensitivity, above.

Clinical features of photoallergic contact dermatitis due to musk ambrette
The clinical features of patients with photoallergic contact dermatitis have been described in detail in 34 patients seen in London during the period 1979-1982 (31). The eruptions were eczematous. The initial stages were erythematous, and when acute often edematous, weeping and crusted. Secondary impetiginisation sometimes occurred. The chronic eruption was scaly and erythematous, the skin thickened and sometimes lichenified. In patients from Asian origin, post-inflammatory hyperpigmentation was prominent and persistent. The light-exposed areas, e.g. face, neck and backs of hands were chiefly affected. The pattern was not fixed and continued exposure or exposure to aerosols resulted in a change from a localized to a generalized facial dermatitis.

There were four main patterns of skin eruptions from photocontact allergy to musk ambrette: 1. plaques; 2. jaw-line (mandibular) dermatitis; 3. acute contact dermatitis; and 4. chronic actinic dermatitis (31).
1. In the first pattern, plaques of eczema were scattered over the cheeks, sides of the neck and occasionally the forehead. This was the most common pattern in the Asian men. This was initially often diagnosed as fixed drug eruption, discoid eczema or lupus erythematosus.
2. In the jaw-line pattern, a zone of eczema was present corresponding to the area of application of an after-shave, extending along the jaw-line and across the lower part of the ear, with an area of the neck both behind and below the ear. Initial diagnoses included seborrheic dermatitis, psoriasis and, in one very acute case, impetigo. This was the commonest pattern in the European men.
3. The third pattern was acute contact dermatitis of the face, with involvement of the whole face and marked swelling of the eyelids. These episodes were sometimes caused by exposure to aerosols of perfume or aftershave lotion.
4. The fourth pattern was a picture clinically indistinguishable from chronic actinic dermatitis present in 10/34 patients. The whole face apart from the periorbital area was involved with a chronic light-exacerbated dermatitis with lichenification in some cases. There was often extension behind the ears and below the chin. Some of these patients initially had a more localized form. These individuals all had abnormal monochromator tests (31).

These patterns varied from time to time within patients depending on degree of exposure, treatment and chronicity. Continued exposure often culminated in the picture of chronic actinic dermatitis. Involved sites other than the face were the hands (74%), particularly the backs of the hands and finger webs (probably because of aftershave trickling from the palms between the fingers during application and from light-exposure), the arms (42%), the trunk (31%), the legs (26%), and the axillae (20%), due to deodorant usage (31).

Unusual presentations of musk ambrette (photo)contact allergy
In rare cases, allergic reactions to musk ambrette presented as pigmented photoallergic contact dermatitis (22), airborne pigmented contact dermatitis (plain, not photocontact allergy) (23), airborne depigmented contact dermatitis (32) (plain, not photocontact allergy), or lichenoid photocontact dermatitis (25,26). Photodermatitis was sometimes acquired by 'connubial' (or 'consort') exposure (24,31).

Photopatch testing in groups of patients
In one study, a group of patients photopatch tested with musk ambrette consisted largely of consecutive patients suspected of contact dermatitis (53). Results of photopatch testing in groups of selected patients (patients suspected of photodermatoses / photosensitivity) are shown in table 3.120.2.

Photopatch testing in consecutive patients suspected of contact dermatitis: routine testing
In Denmark, in the period 1979-1980, a group of 495 individuals, mostly consecutive patients suspected of contact dermatitis, was photopatch tested with musk ambrette and there were four (0.8%) positive reactions, of which one had present and one past relevance (53).

Photopatch testing in groups of selected patients
Results of photopatch testing in groups of selected patients (patients suspected of photodermatoses / photosensitivity) are shown in table 3.120.2. In 16 studies, frequencies of photosensitization have ranged from 0.4% to 24%. The highest rates (13% and 24%) were both seen in Singapore (59,63). In the period 1983-1984, 12 of 50 patients (24%) who underwent photopatch testing were positive to musk ambrette with a high relevance rate of 75% from colognes shown to contain the fragrance (63). About a decade later, when the epidemic of photocontact allergy was on its

way back, the frequency of photocontact allergy in the same center in Singapore was still 13% (59). In the mid-nineties, the number of cases of photoallergic contact dermatitis dropped because IFRA had advised not to use musk ambrette in cosmetics anymore and its use was prohibited in the European Union by that time. Nevertheless, in the USA, in the period 1993-2006, still 6 of 76 (8.7%) patients photopatch tested reacted to musk ambrette. However, neither the selection criteria of the patients nor the relevance of the positive photopatch tests were mentioned and possibly, the reactions have been observed in the early years of that study (8). In most other studies, relevance was either not mentioned or not specified and culprit products not mentioned.

Table 3.120.2 Photopatch testing in groups of patients

Years and Country	Test conc. & vehicle	Number of patients tested | positive (%)		Selection of patients (S); Relevance (R); Comments (C)	Ref.
Routine testing					
1979-1980 Denmark	5% pet.	495	4 (0.8%)	S: **mostly** consecutive patients; R: one relevant, one reaction was of past relevance, 2 uncertain; C: the patients were also tested with musk ambrette 5% in dimethyl phthalate, but this had no advantages over petrolatum as vehicle	53
Testing in groups of selected patients					
2005-2014 China	5% pet.	4930	46 (0.9%)	S: patients suspected of photodermatoses; R: not stated	19
1993-2006 USA	1% pet. and 1% alc.	76	6 (8.7%)	S: not stated; R: not specified	8
2004-2005 Spain	5% pet.	224	1 (0.4%)	S: patients who were photopatch tested, indications not stated; R: the reaction was relevant	39
1994-9 Netherlands	5% pet.	55	1 (1.8%)	S: patients suspected of photosensitivity disorders; R: not stated; C: in this period, musk ambrette was hardly, if at all, used in The Netherlands (prohibited in cosmetics in the EU in 1995)	38
1983-1998 UK	5% pet.	2715	11 (0.4%)	S: patients suspected of photosensitivity or with (a history of) dermatitis at exposed sites; R: 37% for all photoallergens together	45
1991-97 Germany, Austria, Switzerland	5% pet.	1261	11 (0.9%)	S: patients suspected of photosensitivity; R: not stated; the reactions were considered to be phototoxic	4
1990-1994 France	5% pet.	370	4 (1.1%)	S: patients with suspected photodermatitis; R: not stated	10
1991-1993 Singapore	1% pet.	62	8 (13%)	S: patients suspected of photosensitivity; R: 100%; C: culprit products were cologne, toiletries, perfumes (each 2) and 'minyak atar', a fragrant oil used by Muslims before prayers	59
1985-1993 Italy		1050	36 (3.4%)	S: patients suspected of photoallergic contact dermatitis; R: not specified (78% for all photoallergens together)	7
1987-1992 UK	5% pet.	86	5 (6%)	S: patients with chronic actinic dermatitis; R: not stated	61
1985-1990 USA	1% alc.	187	9 (4.8%)	S: patients with a history of photosensitivity; R: all reactions were relevant	46
1980-1985 USA	5% alc.	70	9 (13%)	S: not stated; R: not stated	9
1980-85 Germany, Austria, Switzerland	5% pet.	1129	6 (0.5%)	S: patients suspected of photoallergy, polymorphic light eruption, phototoxicity and skin problems with photo-distribution; R: not stated; C: there were 9 (8%) photo*toxic* reactions	13
1983-1984 Singapore	5% pet.	50	12 (24%)	S: not stated; R: 9/12 (75%) from colognes; C: musk ambrette was identified in the products used by the patients	63
1980-1981 UK	5% pet.	49	4 (9%)	S: patients with chronic actinic dermatitis; R: unknown	56
1980-1 Denmark, Finland, Norway, Sweden	1% alc.	745	19 (2.6%)	S: patients with suspected photodermatoses; R: not specified; C: there were also 3 'plain' contact allergic reactions	18

Case reports and case series

Case series

In London, photopatch testing with musk ambrette was commenced at St. John's Hospital in 1979. It was performed routinely on all men with a facial dermatosis and all patients with a diagnosis of chronic actinic dermatitis. Thirty-four patients had positive patch and photopatch tests to musk ambrette during the period 1979-1982 (a number of the patients discussed in this study had previously been presented, with less detail, in ref. 21). Sixteen patients were studied in more detail using irradiated and covered patch tests to determine whether musk ambrette was a contact or a photocontact allergen. Eight patients manifested pure photocontact allergic dermatitis. The other 8 had ordinary allergic contact dermatitis, but in 6 of these, the reaction was much stronger when the patch test was exposed to UVA irradiation, so-called 'photo-aggravated contact allergy' (31).

All patients had initially used one or more aftershave lotions containing musk ambrette. The biggest selling brand in the U.K. was used by 21 patients. In many men the problem persisted despite abandoning the use of aftershave because they unknowingly continued to use products containing musk ambrette. In some patients, exposure to wives' or girlfriends' perfumes was a cause of both acute exacerbations and chronic dermatitis. In many individuals the scrupulous avoidance of all sources of musk ambrette has returned their skin to normal (31). A number of these patients had already been presented in less detail in ref. 21 (next paragraph).

In London, 19 patients with a positive photopatch test to musk ambrette were evaluated for clinical data, patch testing for 'plain' contact allergy and photocross-reactions to other nitro-musks (for the latter see the section 'Cross-reactions, pseudo-cross-reactions and co-reactions' above). Three patients had contact allergy to musk ambrette without photo-aggravation. Eight patients had normal tolerance to sunlight, six continued to be photosensitive, their sun intolerance dating from their reaction to an aftershave lotion. One had chronic actinic dermatitis with secondary photosensitization to musk ambrette and another one photosensitivity complicated by musk ambrette. In the latter 3, it was too soon after diagnosis to tell whether they would remain light intolerant (21). A number of these 19 patients would later be discussed again in more detail in ref. 31 (previous paragraph).

Musk ambrette was responsible for 11 out of 399 cases of cosmetic (photo)allergy where the causal allergen was identified in a study of the NACDG, USA, 1977-1983 (1); most likely, these were all or virtually all photocontact allergic reactions.

In one hospital in Portugal, during 1982, 7 male patients with photoallergy to musk ambrette were investigated. The clinical picture was similar in all of them: an erythematosquamous and pruriginous dermatitis of the beard area and neck, which became worse after sun exposure. All used colognes and lotions which were applied after shaving. All had positive photopatch tests to musk ambrette and one or more aftershaves or colognes (also to a number of commercial products sold in Portugal but not used by them). Two had plain contact allergy to the fragrance mix and their own aftershave/cologne and one had photoaggravated contact allergy to musk ambrette (52).

Of 5 patients with photocontact allergy to musk ambrette, mostly from shaving cosmetics, 4 developed persistent photosensitivity. Two of the five had a weak positive patch test reaction to musk ambrette, but a far stronger photopatch test, indicating photo-aggravation (33).

In a group of 50 patients suffering from photosensitivity dermatitis with actinic reticuloid syndrome (PD/AR) patch tested with a battery of fragrances, there were 5 reactions (10%) to musk ambrette versus 1.5% positive patch tests in a group of 457 routinely tested dermatitis patients. The frequency of reactions to various other fragrances was also elevated in the PD/AR group. In a subgroup of 35 patients (11 with PD/AR, 13 with chronic polymorphic light eruption, 11 with contact dermatitis) who were *photo*patch tested, there were 5 patients with positive reactions to musk ambrette, 3 of who also had an immediate-type reaction. These positive photopatch tests were tentatively interpreted as indicating a phototoxic reaction, although the possibility that this phototoxic response may merge subsequently with a delayed allergic type reaction could not be excluded. The authors concluded that in some subjects with PD/AR and persistent light reaction, a significant factor is likely to be exposure to fragrance materials such as musk ambrette which has the ability to produce dermatitis, not only from contact allergic sensitivity but also through photocontact reactions, involving either phototoxic or photoallergic mechanisms (16).

In Singapore, in the period 1983-1984, 12 patients were seen in one center with photosensitivity to musk ambrette. The majority of patients was in the older age group (>35 years of age) and most were men (n=1). The duration of presentation varied from four weeks to five years. All presented with dermatitis of the exposed parts of the face and neck and eight had dermatitis of the arms as well. All had positive photopatch tests to musk ambrette and five to the cologne that they were using. In three patients the source of musk ambrette photosensitivity was unknown. Two patients initially denied using any aftershaves or cologne, but later revealed that their barbers had used cologne during haircuts. Analysis of the colognes by GC-MS used by nine patients showed presence of musk ambrette in varying concentrations in all. Follow-up over a six months to one year period showed that three had persistent chronic dermatitis despite avoidance of perfumed preparations (63).

In one center in Australia, in an 18-month period (1983-1985), six cases of musk ambrette photoallergic contact dermatitis were seen and proven in a group of 210 patients evaluated for possible contact dermatitis. All were men with photoallergic contact dermatitis of the beard area from musk ambrette in the same brand of aftershave (62).

Three patients had photoallergic contact dermatitis from aftershave and cologne and positive photopatch tests to musk ambrette (27). The authors mention two more cases seen by other dermatologists with positive photopatch tests to musk ambrette and aftershaves. In one, the presence of musk ambrette in the cosmetic product was verified (27).

Three patients from France were presented as suffering from persistent light reaction to musk ambrette. They all had a positive photopatch test to musk ambrette, one also a plain contact allergic reaction. However, 2 of the patients also had positive patch tests to the fragrance mix and a number of individual fragrances and one of these also to colognes formerly used. Also, no products (formerly) used containing musk ambrette were mentioned, so the diagnosis was based merely on a positive photopatch test to musk ambrette, which is hardly convincing (50).

Case reports
The first case report of photocontact allergy to musk ambrette was reported in 1978. The patient used a well-known aftershave lotion containing musk ambrette and broke out with a severe dermatitis on the sun-exposed areas of the face and neck (14). Two patients had photoallergic contact dermatitis from musk ambrette (28, presented in more detail in ref. 27)

Two patients with longstanding photosensitivity were presented who had, according to the authors, photoallergic contact dermatitis from musk ambrette. However, no culprit products were identified (or even tested) and the patients also had many contact allergic reactions to other fragrances, so the causal relationship between persistent photosensitivity and photoallergy to musk ambrette was not proven (30).

In a similar case, a photoaggravated patch test with musk ambrette in a man with long-standing photosensitivity was enough for the author to conclude that 'the primary and major factor would seem to be a photosensitivity to musk ambrette'. The patient had not used perfumed goods for a long time since he was told earlier that he was allergic to an aftershave lotion. This product was not tested, but the aftershave with this product name was the culprit in several other publications, so it probably did contain musk ambrette (54).

Photoallergic contact dermatitis to musk ambrette in aftershave lotions in two male patients was reported from Germany (36). One patient had persistent light reaction leading to erythroderma from photocontact allergy to musk ambrette (2). Another man also suffered from persistent light reaction due to musk ambrette photosensitivity (3).

A male patient developed photoallergic contact dermatitis from musk ambrette in an aftershave followed by persistent light sensitivity on sun-exposed areas (48). Another male patient had photoallergic contact dermatitis of the face, neck and hands from musk ambrette in several aftershaves and other cosmetic products (53).

One patient had photocontact allergy to musk ambrette and an aftershave lotion. It could not be ascertained that the product contained musk ambrette. After removal of the product, the patient remained photosensitive and developed chronic actinic dermatitis. In these years, he had used some perfumed products, but they were negative on photopatch testing, so the authors concluded that the chronic actinic dermatitis was the result of musk ambrette photosensitivity (51).

A man developed acute exudative dermatitis of the face with temporary persisting light sensitivity from photocontact allergy to musk ambrette in a hair gel and toilet soap (49). Another male individual had the clinical picture of pigmented contact dermatitis of the face. He used an aftershave containing musk ambrette. Photopatch tests were positive to the aftershave and musk ambrette 5% pet. and both test sites later became pigmented (22).

Serial dilution tests
Two patients reacting in photopatch testing to musk ambrette 5% in DEP (diethyl phthalate) were tested with a serial dilution test of musk ambrette with concentrations of 0.01, 0.25, 0.5 and 1% using petrolatum and ethanol as the vehicles. Both patients experienced positive photopatch test reactions down to 0.25%, but were negative at 0.01% (27).

Immediate-type reactions
In a group of 35 patients (11 with photosensitivity dermatitis with actinic reticuloid syndrome, 13 with chronic polymorphic light eruption, 11 with contact dermatitis) who were photopatch tested, there were 5 patients with positive photopatch test reactions to musk ambrette, 3 of who also had an immediate-type reaction (16).

Other non-eczematous contact reactions
A man had violet-brown macules on the cheeks, chin, forehead and nose with lichenoid features in the histology. He had used aftershave containing musk ambrette. A photopatch test with musk ambrette was negative after 3 days, but, after a month, a bluish macule developed at the patch test site. A repeat test and photopatch test gave the same result, with a weaker reaction at the plain patch test site. Although de patient denied any dermatitis prior to the development of the pigmentation or itching, and the photopatch did not show any signs of dermatitis, clinically nor histologically, the authors chose to name their article 'Lichenoid photocontact dermatitis to musk ambrette' (26).

LITERATURE
1   Adams RM, Maibach HI, Clendenning WE, et al. A five-year study of cosmetic reactions. J Am Acad Dermatol 1985;13:1062-9
2   Lan LR, Lee JYY, Kao HF, et al. Persistent light reaction with erythroderma caused by musk ambrette. Cutis 1994;54:167-170
3   Giovinazzo VJ, Harber LC, Bickers DR, Armstrong RB, Silvers DN. Photoallergic contact dermatitis to musk ambrette. Histopathologic features of photobiologic reactions observed in a persistent light reactor. Arch Dermatol 1981;117:344-348
4   Neumann NJ, Hölzle E, Plewig G, Schwarz T, Panizzon RG, Breit R, et al. Photopatch testing: The 12-year experience of the German, Austrian and Swiss Photopatch Test Group. J Am Acad Dermatol 2000;42:183-192

5   SCCFNP (Scientific Committee on Cosmetic Products and Non-Food Products Intended for Consumers). Opinion of the Scientific Committee on Cosmetic Products and Non-Food Products Intended for Consumers concerning 'An initial list of perfumery materials which must not form part of fragrances compounds used in cosmetic products', 3 May 2000, SCCNFP/0320/00, final. Available at: http://ec.europa.eu/health/archive/ph_risk/committees/sccp/documents/out116_en.pdf

6   Larsen W, Nakayama H, Fischer T, Elsner P, Burrows D, Jordan W, et al. Fragrance contact dermatitis: A worldwide multicenter investigation (Part I). Am J Cont Dermat 1996;7:77-83

7   Pigatto PD, Legori A, Bigardi AS,Guarrera M, Tosti A, Santucci B, et al. Gruppo Italiano recerca dermatiti da contatto ed ambientali Italian multicenter study of allergic contact photodermatitis: epidemiological aspects. Am J Contact Dermatitis 1996;7:158-163

8   Victor FC, Cohen DE, Soter NA. A 20-year analysis of previous and emerging allergens that elicit photoallergic contact dermatitis. J Am Acad Dermatol 2010;62:605-610

9   Menz J, Muller SA, Connnolly SM. Photopatch testing: A six year experience. J Am Acad Dermatol 1988;18:1044-1047

10   Journe F, Marguery M-C, Rakotondrazafy J, El Sayed F, Bazex J. Sunscreen sensitization: a 5-year study. Acta Derm Venereol 1999;79:211-213

11   Zaragoza-Ninet V, Blasco Encinas R, Vilata-Corell JJ, Pérez-Ferriols A, Sierra-Talamantes C, Esteve-Martínez A, de la Cuadra-Oyanguren J. Allergic contact dermatitis due to cosmetics: A clinical and epidemiological study in a tertiary hospital. Actas Dermosifiliogr 2016;107:329-336

12   Laguna C, de la Cuadra J, Martín-González B, Zaragoza V, Martínez-Casimiro L, Alegre V. Allergic contact dermatitis to cosmetics. Actas Dermosifiliogr 2009;100:53-60

13   Hölzle E, Neumann N, Hausen B, Przybilla B, Schauder S, Hönigsmann H, et al. Photopatch testing: the 5-year experience of the German, Austrian and Swiss Photopatch Test Group. J Am Acad Dermatol 1991;25:59-68

14   Larsen WG. Photoallergy to musk ambrette found in an aftershave lotion. Presented at the Annual Meeting of the American Academy of Dermatology, San Francisco, CA, December, 1978. Data cited in ref. 15

15   Larsen W. Perfume dermatitis. J Am Acad Dermatol 1985;12:1-9

16   Addo HA, Ferguson J, Johnson BF, Frain-Bell W. The relationship between exposure to fragrance materials and persistent light reaction in photosensitivity dermatitis with actinic reticuloid syndrome. Br J Dermatol 1982;107:261-274

17   Santucci B, Cristaudo A, Cannistraci C, Picardo M. Contact dermatitis to fragrances. Contact Dermatitis 1987;16:93-95

18   Wennersten G, Thune P, Brodthagen H, Jansen C, Rystedt I, Crames M, et al. The Scandinavian multicenter photopatch study: Preliminary results. Contact Dermatitis 1984;10:305-309

19   Hu Y, Wang D, Shen Y, Tanh H. Photopatch testing in Chinese patients over 10 years. Dermatitis 2016;27:137-142

20   Goh CL, Kwok SF. A simple method of qualitative analysis for musk ambrette, musk ketone and musk xylene in cologne. Contact Dermatitis 1986;14:53-56

21   Cronin E. Photosensitivity to musk ambrette. Contact Dermatitis 1984;11:88-92

22   Gonçalo S, Gil J, Gonçalo M, Baptista AP. Pigmented photoallergic contact dermatitis from musk ambrette. Contact Dermatitis 1991;24:229-230

23   Hayakawa R, Matsunaga K, Arima Y. Airborne pigmented contact dermatitis due to musk ambrette in incense. Contact Dermatitis 1987;16:96-98

24   Leroy D, Dompmartin A. Connubial photosensitivity to musk ambrette. Photodermatol 1989;6:137-139

25   Megahed M, Holzle E, Plewig G. Persistent light reaction associated with photoallergic contact dermatitis to musk ambrette and allergic contact dermatitis to fragrance mix. Dermatologica 1991;182:199-202

26   Parodi G, Guerrera M, Rebora A. Lichenoid photocontact dermatitis to musk ambrette. Contact Dermatitis 1987;16:136-138

27   Raugi GJ, Storrs FJ, Larsen WG. Photoallergic contact dermatitis to men's perfumes. Contact Dermatitis 1979;5:251-260

28   Raugi GJ, Storrs FJ. Photosensitivity from men's colognes. Arch Dermatol 1979;115:106

29   Kroon S. Musk ambrette, a new cosmetic sensitizer and photosensitizer. Contact Dermatitis 1979;5:337-338

30   Giovinazzo VJ, Harber LC, Armstrong RB, Kochevar IE. Photoallergic contact dermatitis to musk ambrette: Clinical report of two patients with persistent light reactor patterns. J Am Acad Dermatol 1980;3:384-392

31   Wojnarowska F, Calnan CD. Contact and photocontact allergy to musk ambrette. Br J Dermatol 1986;114:667-675

32   Hayakawa R, Matsunaga K, Arima Y. Depigmented contact dermatitis due to incense. Contact Dermatitis 1987;16:272-274

33   Ramsay CA. Transient and persistent photosensitivity due to musk ambrette. Clinical and photobiological studies. Br J Dermatol 1984;111:423-429

34 Serrano G, Aliaga A, de la Cuadra J, Planells I, lorente M, Bonillo J. Photosensitivity to musk ambrette in Spain. Photodermatol 1986;3:186-188

35 Sánchez-Pedreño P, García-Bravo B, Rodriguez-Pichardo A, Camacho F. Different clinical presentations in photosensitivity to musk ambrette. Photodermatol 1989;6:103-105

36 Galosi A, Plewig G. Photoallergisches Ekzem durch Ambrette Moschus. Hautarzt 1982;33:589-594

37 Fisher AA. Perfume dermatitis (II). Photodermatitis to musk ambrette and 6-methyl coumarine. Cutis 1980;26:549-614 (page numbers incorrect, the article was probably spread over several individual, not successive, pages)

38 Bakkum RS, Heule F. Results of photopatch testing in Rotterdam during a 10-year period. Br J Dermatol 2002;146:275-279

39 De La Cuadra-Oyanguren J, Perez-Ferriols A, Lecha-Carrelero M, et al. Results and assessment of photopatch testing in Spain: towards a new standard set of photoallergens. Actas Dermosfiliogr 2007;98:96-101

40 Hosono K, Ishihara M, Ito M, Kantoh H, Nishimura M. Three solar dermatitis cases exhibiting positive reactions to musk ambrette in photopatch tests, Skin Research 1986;28:365-375 (article in Japanese)

41 DeLeo VA. Photocontact dermatitis. Dermatol Ther 2004;17:279-288

42 Fisher AA. Consort contact dermatitis due to musk ambrette. Cutis 1995;55:199-200

43 Thune P, Jansen C, Wennersten G, Rystedt I, Brodthagen H, McFadden N. The Scandinavian multicenter photopatch study 1980-1985: final report. Photodermatol 1988;5:261-269

44 Kochevar IE, Zalar GL, Einbinder J, Harber LC. Assay of contact photosensitivity to musk ambrette in guinea pigs. J Invest Dermatol 1979;73:144-146

45 Darvay A, White I, Rycroft R, Jones AB, Hawk JL, McFadden JP. Photoallergic contact dermatitis is uncommon. Br J Dermatol 2001;145:597-601

46 DeLeo VA, Suarez SM, Maso MJ. Photoallergic contact dermatitis. Results of photopatch testing in New York, 1985 to 1990. Arch Dermatol 1992;128:1513-1518

47 Lecha M, Romaguera C, Grimalt F, Vilaplana J, Mascaro JM. Photosensitivity to musk ambrette. Photodermatol 1984;1:313-315

48 Zugerman C. Persistent photosensitivity caused by musk ambrette. Arch Derm 1981;117:432-434

49 Shall L, Reynolds AJ, Holt PJA. Photosensitivity to musk ambrette in a toilet soap and hair gel. Contact Dermatitis 1986;14:324

50 Ducombs G, Abbauie D, Maleville J. Persistent light reaction from musk ambrette. Contact Dermatitis 1986;14:129-130

51 Cirne de Castro JL, Pereira MA, Prates Nunes F, Pereira dos Santos A. Musk ambrette and chronic actinic dermatitis. Contact Dermatitis 1985;13:302-306

52 Menezes Brandão F, Cirne De Castro J, Pecegueiro M. Photoallergy – musk ambrette. Contact Dermatitis 1983;9:332-333

53 Kroon S. Standard photopatch testing with musk ambrette. Contact Dermatitis 1983;9:1-4

54 Burry JN. Persistent light reaction associated with sensitivity to musk ambrette. Contact Dermatitis 1981;7:46-47

55 Thune P. Photosensitivity and allergy to cosmetics. Contact Dermatitis 1981;7:54-55

56 Barber K, Cronin E. Patch and photopatch testing in chronic actinic dermatitis. Contact Dermatitis 1984;10:69-73

57 De Groot AC, Schmidt E. Essential oils: contact allergy and chemical composition. Boca Raton, Fl., USA: CRC Press, Taylor and Francis Group, 2016 (ISBN 9781482246407)

58 Bruze M, Edman B, Niklasson B, Möller H. Thin layer chromatography and high pressure liquid chromatography of musk ambrette and other nitromusk compounds including photopatch studies. Photodermatol 1985;2:295-302

59 Leow YH, Wong WK, Ng SK, Goh CL. Two years' experience of photopatch testing in Singapore. Contact Dermatitis 1994;31:181-182

60 Wisneski HH. Determination of musk ambrette, musk xylol, and musk ketone in fragrance products by capillary gas chromatography with electron capture detection. J AOAC Int 2001;84:376-381

61 Menagé H, Ross JS, Norris PG, Hawk JL, White IR. Contact and photocontact sensitization in chronic actinic dermatitis: sesquiterpene lactone mix is an important allergen. Br J Dermatol 1995;132:543-547

62 O'Brien TJ. Contact photoallergy to musk ambrette. Australas J Dermatol 1986;27:134-137

63 Goh CL, Tham SN. Photosensitivity to musk ambrette. Australas J Dermatol 1985;26:133-136

64 Harber LC, Whitman GB, Armstrong RB, Deleo VA. Photosensitivity diseases related to interior lighting. Ann N Y Acad Sci 1985;453:317-327

Chapter 3.121 MUSK KETONE

IDENTIFICATION

Description/definition   : Musk ketone is the organic compound that conforms to the structural formula shown
                            below
Chemical class(es)   : Ketones
Chemical/IUPAC name   : 1-(4-*tert*-Butyl-2,6-dimethyl-3,5-dinitrophenyl)ethanone
CAS registry number(s)   : 81-14-1
EC number(s)   : 201-328-9
RIFM monograph(s)   : Food Cosmet Toxicol 1975;13:877 (special issue II)
IFRA standard   : Restricted; musk ketone should only be used if it contains less than 0.1% of musk xylene
                            (www.ifraorg.org/en-us/standards-library)
SCCS opinion(s)   : SCCNFP/0817/04 (3)
Function(s) in cosmetics : EU: masking; perfuming. USA: fragrance ingredients
EU cosmetic restrictions : Regulated in Annex III/97 of the Regulation (EC) No. 1223/2009, regulated by
                            2004/88/EC
Patch testing   : 1% Pet. (Chemotechnique)
Molecular formula   : $C_{14}H_{18}N_2O_5$

GENERAL

Musk ketone is a yellow powder; its odor type is musk and its odor at 10% in benzyl benzoate is described as 'fatty musk soapy dry powdery' (www.thegoodscentscompany.com). Musk ketone is widely used as a fixative in blossom and phantasy fragrance compositions (U.S. National Library of Medicine). Musk ketone is a synthetic chemical, not found in nature (and consequently not in essential oils (11)).

CONTACT ALLERGY

Patch testing in groups of patients

Results of studies testing musk ketone in consecutive patients suspected of contact dermatitis (routine testing) and those of testing in groups of *selected* patients (patients with eyelid dermatitis, patients with a positive or doubtful reaction to the fragrance mix and/or Myroxylon pereirae resin and/or to one or two commercial fine fragrances) are shown in table 3.121.1.

In one study from China, performed in 2010-2011, one of 296 routinely tested patients (0.3%) reacted to musk ketone 1% pet.; its relevance was not specified (9). In two studies performing patch testing with musk ketone in groups of selected patients, only 1% and 2% had positive reactions; relevance was not mentioned (1,8).

Table 3.121.1 Patch testing in groups of patients

Years and Country	Test conc. & vehicle	Number of patients tested	positive (%)	Selection of patients (S); Relevance (R); Comments (C)	Ref.
Routine testing					
2010-2011 China	1% pet.	296	1 (0.3%)	R: 67% for all fragrances tested together (excluding FM I)	9
Testing in groups of selected patients					
2006-2010 USA	1% pet.	100	2 (2%)	S: patients with eyelid dermatitis; R: not stated	1
<2003 Israel		91	1 (1%)	S: patients with a positive or doubtful reaction to the fragrance mix and/or Myroxylon pereirae resin and/or to one or two commercial fine fragrances; R: not stated	8

FM: Fragrance mix

Case reports and case series

Two patients had allergic contact dermatitis from musk ketone in topical pharmaceutical preparations (2).

Cross-reactions, pseudo-cross-reactions and co-reactions

For general information on cross-/pseudo-cross-/co-reactivity of fragrance chemicals with other fragrances, fragrance markers (fragrance mix I, fragrance mix II, colophonium, Myroxylon pereirae resin [balsam of Peru]) and essential oils see Chapter 1.2 General information on cross-reactions, pseudo-cross-reactions and co-reactions.

None of two (13), none of one or two (14) and none of 19 (15, overlap with ref. 16) patients photosensitive to musk ambrette photo-co-reacted to musk ketone. Of 21 patients with photocontact allergy to musk ambrette, one photo-co-reacted to musk ketone (16, overlap with ref. 15). Of 13 patients photoallergic to musk ambrette, one photo-co-reacted to musk ketone (17).

Presence in products and chemical analyses

In 2008, 66 different fragrance components (including 39 essential oils) were identified in 370 (10% of the total) topical pharmaceutical products marketed in Belgium; 6 of these (1.6%) contained musk ketone (2).

In 2000, thirty fragranced products were purchased in the USA and investigated by GC-MS for the presence of nitro-musks. Musk ketone was identified in 8 products (27%) at levels ranging from 0.023 to 0.45% (18).

In 2000, fifty-nine domestic and occupational products, purchased in retail outlets in Denmark, England, Germany and Italy were analyzed by GC-MS for the presence of fragrances. The product categories were liquid soap and soap bars (n=13), soft/hard surface cleaners (n=23), fabric conditioners/laundry detergents for hand wash (n=8), dish wash (n=10), furniture polish, car shampoo, stain remover (each n=1) and 2 products used in occupational environments. Musk ketone was present in one product (2%); quantification was not performed (4).

In 1997, 71 deodorants (22 vapo-spray, 22 aerosol spray and 27 roll-on products) were collected in Denmark, England, France, Germany and Sweden and analyzed by gas chromatography – mass spectrometry (GC-MS) for the presence of fragrances and other materials. Musk ketone was present in 18 (25%) of the of the products (5).

In 1992, in The Netherlands, the presence of fragrances was analyzed in 300 cosmetic products. Musk ketone was identified in 34% of the products (rank order 22) (7).

In 1988, in the USA, 400 perfumes used in fine fragrances, household products and soaps (number of products per category not mentioned) were analyzed for the presence of fragrance chemicals in a concentration of at least 1% and a list of the Top-25 (present in the highest number of products) presented. Musk ketone was found to be present in 38% of the fine fragrances (rank number 18), an unknown percentage of the household product fragrances and an unknown percentage of the fragrances used in soaps (6).

In 1984, in Singapore, 32 men's colognes were investigated for the presence of musk ambrette, musk ketone and musk xylene with the aid of thin-layer chromatography and GC-MS. Five products (16%) were found to contain musk ketone, the concentration varying from 0.04 to 0.60% w/v (10).

In 1984, in Sweden, 21 perfumed commercial products, mainly aftershave and eau de toilette preparations, were examined by thin layer chromatography and high pressure liquid chromatography for the presence of nitro-musks. Musk ketone was identified in 2 (10%) of the products in concentrations of 0.015% and 0.049% (17).

OTHER SIDE EFFECTS

Photosensitivity

Case reports and case series

A man with chronic actinic dermatitis (CAD) had positive photopatch tests to musk ketone, musk ambrette, and his aftershave lotion. The manufacturer confirmed the presence of musk ambrette (0.0007%) and musk ketone (0.0017%) in the cosmetic. The photosensitive eruption was ascribed to musk ketone in the aftershave, but the eruption only cleared after treatment with a combination of PUVA and cyclosporine, making it difficult to establish a causal relationship between the eruption and musk ketone photosensitivity (12).

LITERATURE

1   Wenk KS, Ehrlich AE. Fragrance series testing in eyelid dermatitis. Dermatitis 2012;23:22-26
2   Nardelli A, D'Hooge E, Drieghe J, Dooms M, Goossens A. Allergic contact dermatitis from fragrance components in specific topical pharmaceutical products in Belgium. Contact Dermatitis 2009;60:303-313
3   SCCFNP (Scientific Committee on Cosmetic Products and Non-Food Products Intended for Consumers). Opinion on Musk xylene and Musk ketone, 25 May 2004, SCCNFP/0817/04. Available at:
     http://ec.europa.eu/health/archive/ph_risk/committees/sccp/documents/out280_en.pdf

4   Rastogi SC, Heydorn S, Johansen JD, Basketter DA. Fragrance chemicals in domestic and occupational products. Contact Dermatitis 2001;45:221-225

5   Rastogi SC, Lepoittevin J-P, Johansen JD, Frosch PJ, Menné T, Bruze M, et al. Fragrances and other materials in deodorants: search for potentially sensitizing molecules using combined GC-MS and structure activity relationship (SAR) analysis. Contact Dermatitis 1998;39:293-303

6   Fenn RS. Aroma chemical usage trends in modern perfumery. Perfumer and Flavorist 1989;14:3-10

7   Weyland JW. Personal Communication, 1992. Cited in: De Groot AC, Weyland JW, Nater JP. Unwanted effects of cosmetics and drugs used in dermatology, 3rd Ed. Amsterdam: Elsevier, 1994:579

8   Trattner A, David M. Patch testing with fine fragrances: comparison with fragrance mix, balsam of Peru and a fragrance series. Contact Dermatitis 2003:49:287-289

9   Liu J, Li L-F. Contact sensitization to fragrances other than fragrance mix I in China. Contact Dermatitis 2015;73:252-253

10   Goh CL, Kwok SF. A simple method of qualitative analysis for musk ambrette, musk ketone and musk xylene in cologne. Contact Dermatitis 1986;14:53-56

11   De Groot AC, Schmidt E. Essential oils: contact allergy and chemical composition. Boca Raton, Fl., USA: CRC Press, Taylor and Francis Group, 2016 (ISBN 9781482246407)

12   Gardeazábal J, Arregui MA, Gil N, Landa N, Ratón JA, Diáz-Pérez JL. Successful treatment of musk ketone-induced chronic actinic dermatitis with cyclosporine and PUVA. J Am Acad Dermatol 1992;27(5 Pt. 2):838-842

13   Raugi GJ, Storrs FJ, Larsen WG. Photoallergic contact dermatitis to men's perfumes. Contact Dermatitis 1979;5:251-260

14   Galosi A, Plewig G. Photoallergisches Ekzem durch Ambrette Moschus. Hautarzt 1982;33:589-594

15   Cronin E. Photosensitivity to musk ambrette. Contact Dermatitis 1984;11:88-92

16   Wojnarowska F, Calnan CD. Contact and photocontact allergy to musk ambrette. Br J Dermatol 1986;114:667-675

17   Bruze M, Edman B, Niklasson B, Möller H. Thin layer chromatography and high pressure liquid chromatography of musk ambrette and other nitromusk compounds including photopatch studies. Photodermatol 1985;2:295-302

18   Wisneski HH. Determination of musk ambrette, musk xylol, and musk ketone in fragrance products by capillary gas chromatography with electron capture detection. J AOAC Int 2001;84:376-381

Chapter 3.122 MUSK MOSKENE *

Not an INCI name

IDENTIFICATION

Description/definition	: Musk moskene is the bicyclic dinitro compound that conforms to the structural formula shown below
Chemical class(es)	: Bicyclic organic compounds; aromatic compounds; nitro compounds
INCI name USA	: Not in the Personal Care Products Council Ingredient Database
Chemical/IUPAC name	: 1,1,3,3,5-Pentamethyl-4,6-dinitro-2H-indene
Other names	: Moskene
CAS registry number(s)	: 116-66-5
EC number(s)	: 204-149-4
SCCS opinion(s)	: SCCFNP/1431/96 (11)
RIFM monograph(s)	: Food Cosmet Toxicol 1979;17:885 (special issue V)
IFRA standard	: Prohibited (www.ifraorg.org/en-us/standards-library)
EU cosmetic restrictions	: Regulated in Annex II/421 of the Regulation (EC) No. 1223/2009, regulated by 98/62/EC; (Prohibited since 1999)
Patch testing	: 1% Pet. (Chemotechnique); 5% pet. (7)
Molecular formula	: $C_{14}H_{18}N_2O_4$

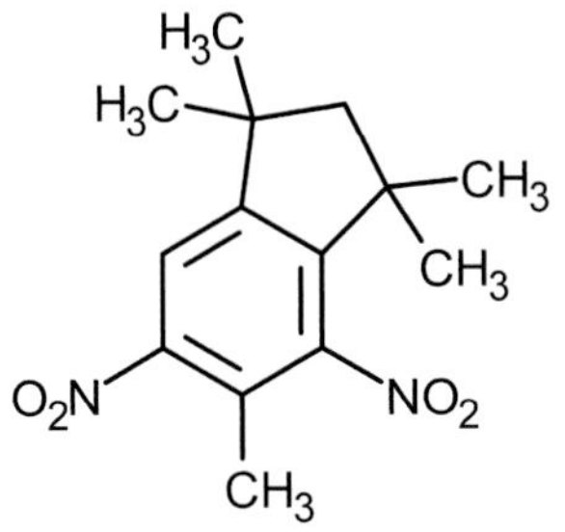

GENERAL

Musk moskene is a yellow powder; its odor type is musk and its odor at 10% in benzyl benzoate is described as 'sweet musk ambrette ketone powdery dry' (www.thegoodscentscompany.com). It is a synthetic chemical, not found in nature (and consequently not in essential oils (8)). Musk moskene is prohibited by IFRA because of photosensitization (www.ifraorg.org) and is not used anymore in cosmetics.

CONTACT ALLERGY

Patch testing in groups of patients

Musk moskene 1% in petrolatum was patch tested in 2010-2011 in China in 296 consecutive patients suspected of contact dermatitis and there were 4 (1.4%) positive reactions; their relevance was not specified (1).

Case reports and case series

A female patient had suffered from itchy hyperpigmentation of the face for 3 years. Despite daily application of a topical corticosteroid, her itching had not subsided. Every day she used skin care cosmetics and makeup. Histology showed liquefaction degeneration of basal cells, incontinence of pigment, and inflammatory round cell infiltration into the dermis. A diagnosis of pigmented contact dermatitis was made. Patch tests were positive for three cheek rouges of the same brand, which reactions continued for 2 weeks and resulted in hyperpigmentation. Testing with their ingredients yielded a positive reaction to the perfume only, which was present in all 3 products. In a third session, the patient was patch tested with the components of the perfume, provided by the manufacturer; there now were strongly positive reactions to musk moskene 5% and 25% in petrolatum. Hyperpigmentation developed in all three positive reactions after subsidence of the inflammation. Control patch tests on 11 patients with contact dermatitis were negative (2).

Another patient from Japan had pigmented cosmetic dermatitis from musk moskene in a hair tonic (6). A third woman presented with acute facial eczema within a few weeks of using a new moisturizer. Patch testing gave positive reactions to musk ambrette in the face series, oakmoss in the fragrance series, the facial moisturizer as is, and the perfume in the moisturizer tested 5% and 10% pet. Further patch testing to the individual ingredients of the perfume revealed positive reactions to oakmoss 2% pet. and musk moskene 5% pet. Photopatch tests were not performed (7).

Cross-reactions, pseudo-cross-reactions and co-reactions
For general information on cross-/pseudo-cross-/co-reactivity of fragrance chemicals with other fragrances, fragrance markers (fragrance mix I, fragrance mix II, colophonium, Myroxylon pereirae resin [balsam of Peru]) and essential oils see Chapter 1.2 General information on cross-reactions, pseudo-cross-reactions and co-reactions.

Contact allergy
Co-reaction to musk ambrette (2). Of 8 patients with contact allergy to musk ambrette, one (13%) co-reacted to musk moskene (9, overlap with ref. 5).

Photocontact allergy
Photo-co-reaction to musk ambrette (3). One of two patients photosensitive to musk ambrette photo-co-reacted to musk moskene 0.5% pet. (4). In one or two patients with photocontact allergy to musk ambrette, there were co-reactions to musk moskene (12). Of 8 patients photoallergic to musk ambrette, one photo-co-reacted to musk moskene (13).

Of 16 individuals with photocontact allergy to musk ambrette, 8 (50%) co-reacted to musk moskene (9, overlap with ref. 5). Of 19 patients photoallergic to musk ambrette and tested with 4 related nitro-musks, 3 photo-co-reacted to musk moskene (5, overlap with ref. 9).

LITERATURE

1   Liu J, Li L-F. Contact sensitization to fragrances other than fragrance mix I in China. Contact Dermatitis 2015;73:252-253
2   Hayakawa R, Hirose O, Arima Y. Pigmented contact dermatitis due to musk moskene. J Dermatol 1991;18:420-424
3   Hosono K, Ishihara M, Ito M, Kantoh H. Three solar dermatitis cases exhibiting positive reactions to musk ambrette in photopatch tests. Skin Research 1986;28:365-375 (article in Japanese). Data cited in ref. 2
4   Raugi GI, Storrs FJ, Larsen WG. Photoallergic contact dermatitis to men's perfume. Contact Dermatitis 1979;5:251-260
5   Cronin E. Photosensitivity to musk ambrette. Contact Dermatitis 1984;11:88-92
6   Ito M, Kurosaka R, Kantoh H, Hosono K. Pigmented contact dermatitis due to musk moskene in a hair tonic. Hifubyo Rinsho 1990;12:243-246 (article in Japanese). Data cited in ref. 2
7   Parry EJ, Beck MH. Contact allergy to musk moskene in a perfumed moisturizing cream. Contact Dermatitis 1997;37:236
8   De Groot AC, Schmidt E. Essential oils: contact allergy and chemical composition. Boca Raton, Fl., USA: CRC Press, Taylor and Francis Group, 2016 (ISBN 9781482246407)
9   Wojnarowska F, Calnan CD. Contact and photocontact allergy to musk ambrette. Br J Dermatol 1986;114:667-675
10 Bruze M, Edman B, Niklasson B, Möller H. Thin layer chromatography and high pressure liquid chromatography of musk ambrette and other nitromusk compounds including photopatch studies. Photodermatol 1985;2:295-302
11 SCCFNP (Scientific Committee on Cosmetic Products and Non-Food Products Intended for Consumers). Opinion on 4,6-dinitro-1,1,3,3,5-pentamethylindane 24 June 1997, SCCFNP/1431/96. Available at: http://ec.europa.eu/health/scientific_committees/consumer_safety/opinions/sccnfp_opinions_97_04/sccp_out08_en.htm
12 Galosi A, Plewig G. Photoallergisches Ekzem durch Ambrette Moschus. Hautarzt 1982;33:589-594
13 Bruze M, Edman B, Niklasson B, Möller H. Thin layer chromatography and high pressure liquid chromatography of musk ambrette and other nitromusk compounds including photopatch studies. Photodermatol 1985;2:295-302

Chapter 3.123 MUSK TIBETENE *
Not an INCI name

IDENTIFICATION

Description/definition   : Musk tibetene is the dinitro aromatic compound that conforms to the structural
                            formula shown below
Chemical class(es)   : Aromatic compounds; nitro compounds
INCI name USA   : Not in the Personal Care Products Council Ingredient Database
Chemical/IUPAC name   : 1-*tert*-Butyl-3,4,5-trimethyl-2,6-dinitrobenzene
Other name(s)   : 1,2,3-Trimethyl-5-(2-methyl-2-propanyl)-4,6-dinitrobenzene; 5-*tert*-butyl-1,2,3-trimethyl-
                            4,6-dinitrobenzene
CAS registry number(s)   : 145-39-1
EC number(s)   : 205-651-6
SCCS opinion(s)   : SCCFNP/1430/96 (7)
RIFM monograph(s)   : Food Cosmet Toxicol 1975;13:879 (special issue II)
IFRA standard   : Prohibited (www.ifraorg.org/en-us/standards-library)
Function(s) in cosmetics : Formerly used for perfuming
EU cosmetic restrictions : Regulated in Annex II/422 of the Regulation (EC) No. 1223/2009, regulated by 98/62/EC;
                            (Prohibited since 1998)
Patch testing   : 2-5% pet. (5)
Molecular formula   : $C_{13}H_{18}N_2O_4$

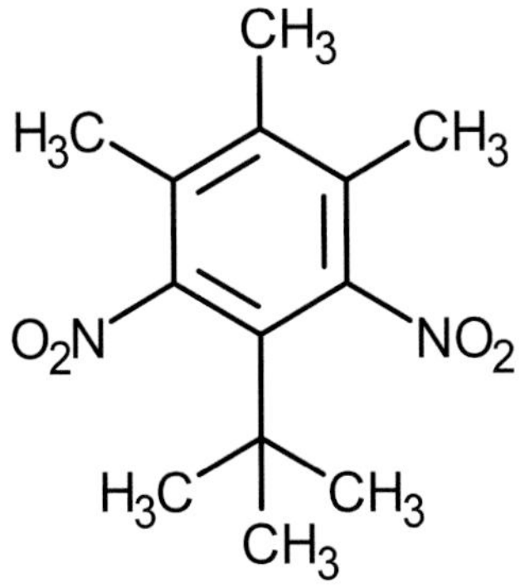

GENERAL

Musk tibetene appears as pale yellow crystals; its odor type is musk and its odor at 10% in benzyl benzoate is described as 'musk ketone sweet powdery fatty' (www.thegoodscentscompany.com). It is a synthetic chemical, not found in nature (and consequently not in essential oils (1)). Musk tibetene is prohibited by IFRA because of photosensitization (www.ifraorg.org) and is not used anymore.

Allergic or photoallergic contact dermatitis from musk tibetene appears not to have been reported, one positive photopatch test reaction observed was interpreted as a photocross-reaction to musk ambrette (6).

CONTACT ALLERGY

Patch testing in groups of patients
Studies in which musk tibetene was patch tested or photopatch tested in either consecutive patients suspected of contact dermatitis (routine testing) or in groups of selected patients with positive results have not been found.

Case reports and case series
Case reports of (photo)allergic contact dermatitis from musk tibetene have not been found.

Cross-reactions, pseudo-cross-reactions and co-reactions
For general information on cross-/pseudo-cross-/co-reactivity of fragrance chemicals with other fragrances, fragrance markers (fragrance mix I, fragrance mix II, colophonium, Myroxylon pereirae resin [balsam of Peru]) and essential oils see Chapter 1.2 General information on cross-reactions, pseudo-cross-reactions and co-reactions.

Of twenty-two patients with photocontact allergy to musk ambrette, there were no photo-co-reactions to musk tibetene (2,3,4). Of 8 patients photoallergic to musk ambrette, one photo-co-reacted to musk tibetene (6).

LITERATURE

1   De Groot AC, Schmidt E. Essential oils: contact allergy and chemical composition. Boca Raton, Fl., USA: CRC Press, Taylor and Francis Group, 2016 (ISBN 9781482246407)

2   Cronin E. Photosensitivity to musk ambrette. Contact Dermatitis 1984;11:88-92

3   Raugi GJ, Storrs FJ, Larsen WG. Photoallergic contact dermatitis to men's perfumes. Contact Dermatitis 1979;5:251-260

4   Galosi A, Plewig G. Photoallergisches Ekzem durch Ambrette Moschus. Hautarzt 1982;33:589-594

5   De Groot AC. Patch Testing, 4th Edition. Wapserveen, The Netherlands: acdegroot publishing, 2018 (ISBN 978-90-813233-4-5)

6   Bruze M, Edman B, Niklasson B, Möller H. Thin layer chromatography and high pressure liquid chromatography of musk ambrette and other nitromusk compounds including photopatch studies. Photodermatol 1985;2:295-302

7   SCCFNP (Scientific Committee on Cosmetic Products and Non-Food Products Intended for Consumers). Opinion on 5-tert-Butyl-1,2,3-trimethyl-4,6-dinitrobenzene, 24 June 1997, SCCFNP/1430/96. Available at: http://ec.europa.eu/health/scientific_committees/consumer_safety/opinions/sccnfp_opinions_97_04/sccp_out 07_en.htm

Chapter 3.124 MUSK XYLENE

IDENTIFICATION

Description/definition	: Musk xylene is the trinitro aromatic compound that conforms to the structural formula shown below
Chemical class(es)	: Aromatic compounds; nitro compounds
INCI name USA	: Not in the Personal Care Products Council Ingredient Database
Chemical/IUPAC name	: 1-*tert*-Butyl-3,5-dimethyl-2,4,6-trinitrobenzene
Other names	: 1-(1,1-Dimethylethyl)-3,5-dimethyl-2,4,6-trinitrobenzene; musk xylol
CAS registry number(s)	: 81-15-2
EC number(s)	: 201-329-4
RIFM monograph(s)	: Food Cosmet Toxicol 1975;13:881 (special issue II) (binder page 577)
SCCS opinion(s)	: SCCNFP/0817/04 (2)
IFRA standard	: Prohibited (www.ifraorg.org/en-us/standards-library)
Function(s) in cosmetics	: EU: masking; perfuming
EU cosmetic restrictions	: Regulated in Annex III/96 Annex of the Regulation (EC) No. 1223/2009 (Regulated by 2004/88/EC)
Patch testing	: 1% Pet. (Chemotechnique)
Molecular formula	: $C_{12}H_{15}N_3O_6$

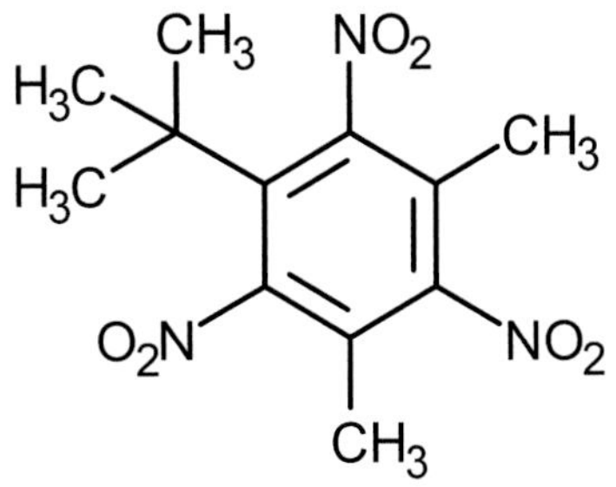

GENERAL

Musk xylene appears as pale yellow crystals; its odor type is musk and its odor at 10% in benzyl benzoate is described as 'fatty dry sweet soapy musk' (www.thegoodscentscompany.com). It is a synthetic chemical, not found in nature (and consequently not in essential oils (8)). Musk xylene is prohibited by IFRA, because it fulfils the criteria for being classified vPvB (very Persistent and very Bioaccumulative; Environmental half-life >180 days; BCF>5000) (www.ifraorg.org/en-us/standards-library) and is not used anymore.

CONTACT ALLERGY

Patch testing in groups of patients

Patch testing in consecutive patients suspected of contact dermatitis: routine testing
In China, in the period 2010-2011, 296 consecutive patients suspected of contact dermatitis (routine testing) were patch tested with musk xylene 1% in petrolatum and there were 2 (0.7%) positive reactions; their relevance was not specified (5).

Patch testing in groups of selected patients
In the USA, in the period 2006-2010, 100 patients with eyelid dermatitis were patch tested with musk xylene 1% in petrolatum and there were 2 (2%) positive reactions; their relevance was not mentioned (1).

Case reports and case series
In the period 2000-2007, 202 patients with allergic contact dermatitis caused by cosmetics were seen in Valencia, Spain. In this group, musk xylene was stated to be the allergen in one individual from its presence in cologne (4).

Cross-reactions, pseudo-cross-reactions and co-reactions
For general information on cross-/pseudo-cross-/co-reactivity of fragrance chemicals with other fragrances, fragrance markers (fragrance mix I, fragrance mix II, colophonium, Myroxylon pereirae resin [balsam of Peru]) and essential oils see Chapter 1.2 General information on cross-reactions, pseudo-cross-reactions and co-reactions.

Of 18 patients photoallergic to musk ambrette and tested with 4 related nitro-musks, 3 photo-co-reacted to musk xylene; one reaction was weak (7). Of 13 other individuals photoallergic to musk ambrette, one photo-co-reacted to musk xylene (9). In one or 2 patients with photocontact allergy to musk ambrette, there were co-reactions to musk xylene (10).

Presence in products and chemical analyses
In 2000, thirty fragranced products were purchased in the USA and investigated by GC-MS for the presence of nitro-musks. Musk xylene was found in 9 (30%) products at levels ranging from 0.001 to 0.22% (11).

In 1988, in the USA, 400 perfumes used in fine fragrances, household products and soaps (number of products per category not mentioned) were analyzed for the presence of fragrance chemicals in a concentration of at least 1% and a list of the Top-25 (present in the highest number of products) presented. Musk xylene was found to be present in an unknown percentage of the fine fragrances, an unknown percentage of the household product fragrances and 28% of the fragrances used in soaps (rank number 25) (3).

In 1984, in Singapore, 32 different men's colognes were analysed with GC-MS for the presence of nitro-musks. Eleven (34%) proved to contain musk xylene in concentrations ranging from 0.02% w/v to 0.78% w/v (6).

LITERATURE

1   Wenk KS, Ehrlich AE. Fragrance series testing in eyelid dermatitis. Dermatitis 2012;23:22-26
2   SCCFNP (Scientific Committee on Cosmetic Products and Non-Food Products Intended for Consumers). Opinion on Musk xylene and Musk ketone, 25 May 2004, SCCNFP/0817/04. Available at: http://ec.europa.eu/health/archive/ph_risk/committees/sccp/documents/out280_en.pdf
3   Fenn RS. Aroma chemical usage trends in modern perfumery. Perfumer and Flavorist 1989;14:3-10
4   Laguna C, de la Cuadra J, Martín-González B, Zaragoza V, Martínez-Casimiro L, Alegre V. Allergic contact dermatitis to cosmetics. Actas Dermosifiliogr 2009;100:53-60
5   Liu J, Li L-F. Contact sensitization to fragrances other than fragrance mix I in China. Contact Dermatitis 2015;73:252-253
6   Goh CL, Kwok SF. A simple method of qualitative analysis for musk ambrette, musk ketone and musk xylene in cologne. Contact Dermatitis 1986;14:53-56
7   Cronin E. Photosensitivity to musk ambrette. Contact Dermatitis 1984;11:88-92
8   De Groot AC, Schmidt E. Essential oils: contact allergy and chemical composition. Boca Raton, Fl., USA: CRC Press, Taylor and Francis Group, 2016 (ISBN 9781482246407)
9   Bruze M, Edman B, Niklasson B, Möller H. Thin layer chromatography and high pressure liquid chromatography of musk ambrette and other nitromusk compounds including photopatch studies. Photodermatol 1985;2:295-302
10 Galosi A, Plewig G. Photoallergisches Ekzem durch Ambrette Moschus. Hautarzt 1982;33:589-594 (article in German)
11 Wisneski HH. Determination of musk ambrette, musk xylol, and musk ketone in fragrance products by capillary gas chromatography with electron capture detection. J AOAC Int 2001;84:376-381

Chapter 3.125 MYRCENE

IDENTIFICATION

Description/definition	: Myrcene is the unsaturated compound that conforms to the structural formula shown below
Chemical class(es)	: Unsaturated organic compounds
INCI name USA	: Not in the Personal Care Products Council Ingredient Database
Chemical/IUPAC name	: 7-Methyl-3-methylideneocta-1,6-diene
Other names	: β-Myrcene
CAS registry number(s)	: 123-35-3
EC number(s)	: 204-622-5
RIFM monograph(s)	: Food Cosmet Toxicol 1976;14:615
SCCS opinion(s)	: SCCS/1459/11 (4)
Merck Index monograph	: 7686
Function(s) in cosmetics	: EU: perfuming
Patch testing	: Oxidized myrcene, 3% pet. (7); 5% diethyl phthalate (1,3)
Molecular formula	: $C_{10}H_{16}$

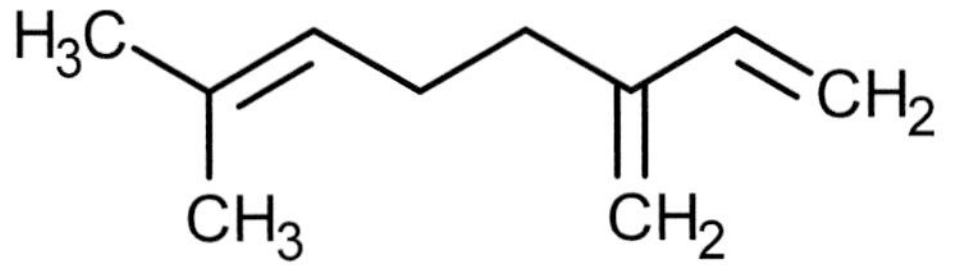

GENERAL

Myrcene is a colorless clear liquid; its odor type is spicy and its odor at 5% in dipropylene glycol is described as 'peppery terpene spicy balsam plastic' (www.thegoodscentscompany.com). Myrcene is the starting material for a range of industrially important chemicals, e.g. geraniol, nerol, linalool, and isophytol. Besides its main use as an intermediate for the production of terpene alcohols, myrcene is used in the production of terpene polymers, terpene-phenol resins, and terpene-maleate resins. It can also be used as a solvent or diluting agent for dyes and varnishes and is added to foods and beverages as flavor (U.S. National Library of Medicine).

Presence in essential oils

Myrcene has been identified by chemical analysis in 81 of 91 essential oils, which have caused contact allergy / allergic contact dermatitis. In 26 oils, myrcene belonged to the 'Top-10' of ingredients with the highest concentrations. These are shown in table 3.125.1 with the concentration range which may be expected in commercial essential oils of this type (8).

Table 3.125.1 Essential oils containing myrcene in the 'Top-10' and concentration range in commercial oils (8)

Essential oil	Concentration range (min.-max.)	Essential oil	Concentration range (min.-max.)
Rosemary oil	0.2 - 46.0%	Petitgrain bigarade oil	0.4 - 3.6%
Bay oil	20.5 - 32.0%	Grapefruit oil	1.3 - 3.5%
Dwarf pine oil	1.6 - 30.2%	Orange oil sweet	1.4 - 3.5%
Juniper berry oil	11.6 - 21.6%	Cypress oil	1.0 - 2.9%
Pine needle oil	0.4 - 13.5%	Spearmint oil	0.01 - 2.6%
Nutmeg oil	2.3 - 10.5%	Orange oil bitter	1.5 - 2.5%
Olibanum oil	1.8 - 10.4%	Silver fir oil	0.7 - 2.5%
Galbanum resin oil	0.1 - 6.6%	Cardamom oil	trace - 2.5%
Black pepper oil	1.5 - 6.3%	Lemon oil	1.2 - 2.2%
Angelica root oil	1.4 - 5.4%	Tangerine oil	0.1 - 2.2%
Angelica fruit oil	0.6 - 5.0%	Mandarin oil	0.08 - 2.2%
Lemongrass oil East Indian	0.07 - 5.0%	Bergamot oil	0.7 - 1.8%
Niaouli oil	0.3 - 3.8%	Turpentine oil	trace - 1.0%

CONTACT ALLERGY

The SCCS (Scientific Committee on Consumer Safety), in a 2012 Opinion on Fragrance allergens in cosmetic products, has categorized myrcene as 'likely fragrance contact allergen by combination of evidence' (4,6).

Experimental studies have shown that myrcene easily autoxidizes on air exposure. The pure compound myrcene was found to be a non-sensitizer in animal experiments, but its oxidation mixture was sensitizing (unpublished data, cited in ref. 7). Myrcene is a minor allergen in tea tree oil. Of 61 patients allergic to tea tree oil and tested with a number of its ingredients in various studies, 10 (16%) reacted to myrcene (5).

Patch testing in groups of patients
Results of studies testing myrcene in consecutive patients suspected of contact dermatitis (routine testing) and those of testing in groups of *selected* patients (patients allergic to (oxidized) tea tree oil) are shown in table 3.125.2.

Patch testing in consecutive patients suspected of contact dermatitis: routine testing
In one study in which routine testing with myrcene was performed, only one of 1511 patients with dermatitis (0.1%) reacted to oxidized myrcene, tested 3% in petrolatum (7). Relevance was not specified.

Patch testing in groups of selected patients
In three studies in which small groups of patients allergic to tea tree oil were patch tested with myrcene 5% in diethyl phthalate, 10-35% reacted positively (1,2,3). In some other studies, no reactions to myrcene were observed, and of all 61 patients tested, 10 (16%) reacted to myrcene, making it a minor allergenic ingredient of tea tree oil (5).

Table 3.125.2 Patch testing in groups of patients

Years and Country	Test conc. & vehicle	Number of patients tested	positive (%)		Selection of patients (S); Relevance (R); Comments (C)	Ref.
Routine testing						
2002-2003 Denmark, Sweden, Belgium, Germany, UK	3% pet., oxidized	1511	1	(0.1%)	R: certain or probable history of fragrance allergy in 58% of all terpenes tested (linalool, caryophyllene, caryophyllene oxide and myrcene) together	7
Testing in groups of selected patients						
1999-2003 Germany	5% DEP	20	7	(35%)	S: patients with a positive patch test reaction to oxidized tea tree oil 5% DEP	3
1999-2000 Germany, Austria	5% DEP	10	1	(10%)	S: patients with a positive patch test reaction to oxidized tea tree oil 5% DEP	1
<1999 Germany	5% vehicle?	16	2	(13%)	S: patients allergic to tea tree oil	2

DEP: Diethyl phthalate

Case reports and case series
A man used to wash his hair with a shampoo to which his wife had added tea tree oil. Another male patient used herbal extracts for hygiene and cosmetic purposes, including several tea tree oil bottles. Both developed allergic contact dermatitis. When patch tested, they reacted to tea tree oil, its ingredient myrcene (5%, vehicle unknown) and 3 resp. 5 other oil components (2).

LITERATURE
1   Pirker C, Hausen BM, Uter W, Hillen U, Brasch J, Bayeret C, et al. Sensitization to tea tree oil in Germany and Austria. A multicenter Study of the German Contact Dermatitis group. J Dtsch Dermatol Ges 2003;1:629-634 (article in German)
2   Hausen BM, Reichling J, Harkenthal M. Degradation products of monoterpenes are the sensitizing agents in tea tree oil. Am J Contact Dermat 1999;10:68-77
3   Hausen BM. Evaluation of the main contact allergens in oxidized tea tree oil. Dermatitis 2004;15:213-214
4   SCCS (Scientific Committee on Consumer Safety). Opinion on Fragrance allergens in cosmetic products, 26-27 June 2012, SCCS/1459/11. Available at:
    https://ec.europa.eu/health/sites/health/files/scientific_committees/consumer_safety/docs/sccs_o_102.pdf
5   De Groot AC, Schmidt E. Tea tree oil: contact allergy and chemical composition. Contact Dermatitis 2016;75:129-143
6   Uter W, Johansen JD, Börje A, Karlberg A-T, Lidén C, Rastogi S, Roberts D, White IR. Categorization of fragrance contact allergens for prioritization of preventive measures: clinical and experimental data and consideration of structure–activity relationships. Contact Dermatitis 2013;69:196-230
7   Matura M, Sköld M, Börje A, Andersen KE, Bruze M, Frosch P, et al. Selected oxidized fragrance terpenes are common contact allergens. Contact Dermatitis 2005;52:320-328
8   De Groot AC, Schmidt E. Essential oils: contact allergy and chemical composition. Boca Raton, Fl., USA: CRC Press, Taylor and Francis Group, 2016 (ISBN 9781482246407)

Chapter 3.126 MYROXYLON PEREIRAE RESIN (BALSAM OF PERU)

IDENTIFICATION

Description/definition	: Myroxylon pereirae resin is an oleoresin obtained from the bark exudate of the balsam Peru tree, *Myroxylon pereirae*, Leguminosae
Chemical class(es)	: Botanical products and botanical derivatives
INCI name USA	: Myroxylon pereirae (Balsam Peru) resin
Other names	: Balsam Peru; Balsam fir oleoresin (*Abies balsamea* (L.) Mill.)
CAS registry number(s)	: 8007-00-9; 8016-42-0
EC number(s)	: 232-352-8
RIFM monograph(s)	: Food Cosmet Toxicol 1974;12:953 (special issue 1)
IFRA standard	: Prohibited as crude material; extracts and distillates are restricted (www.ifraorg.org/en-us/standards-library) (table 3.126.1)
SCCS opinion(s)	: SCCP/0988/06 (22); SCCNFP/0771/03 (23); SCCNFP/0389/00, final (oil and extract) (133); SCCNFP/0392/00, final (oil and extract) (205)
Merck Index monograph	: 2212
Function(s) in cosmetics	: EU: film forming; hair conditioning; masking. USA: film formers; fragrance ingredients
EU cosmetic restrictions	: Regulated in Annex II/1136 of the Regulation (EC) No. 1223/2009; Prohibited, when used as a fragrance ingredient
Patch testing	: 25% Pet. (SmartPracticeEurope, Chemotechnique, SmartPracticeCanada); the TRUE test is less sensitive in detecting contact allergy to MP (101)

Table 3.126.1 IFRA restrictions for Peru balsam extracts and distillates

Category [a]	Limits [b]	Category [a]	Limits [b]	Category [a]	Limits [b]
1	0.03%	5	0.20%	9	0.40%
2	0.04%	6	0.70%	10	0.40%
3	0.10%	7	0.07%	11	not restricted
4	0.40%	8	0.40%		

[a] For explanation of categories see pages 6-8
[b] Limits in the finished products

GENERAL

General

Balsam of Peru (Peru balsam; INCI name: Myroxylon pereirae resin, in this chapter often abbreviated as MP) is the balsam obtained from the scorched and wounded bark of *Myroxylon balsamum* (L.) Harms var. *pereirae* (Royle) Baillon of the Leguminosae family, a tree that reaches a height of 30-35 meter and grows between 300 and 700 meter above the sea in the coastal regions of El Salvador (14,167) and apparently also in Honduras, Guatemala, Cuba, Mexico, Costa Rica and Panama, but not in Peru (197). The correct botanical name according to the database www.theplantlist.org is *Myroxylon balsamum* var. *pereirae* (Royle) Harms.

Crude MP is a dark brown, viscous liquid which is transparent and yellowish-brown when viewed in a thin layer; the liquid is not sticky, it is non-drying and does not form threads. MP is practically insoluble in water, freely soluble in alcohol, and not miscible with fatty oils, except for castor oil (197). It has an aromatic smell of cinnamon and vanilla, and a bitter taste. To remove it from the tree, the bark is alternately scorched and beaten. The balsam in the bark is obtained by boiling. Following removal of strips of bark from the tree, the exposed wood also secretes balsam. The material is absorbed into rags wrapped around the tree, which are then boiled in water. The balsam sinks to the bottom and is then collected (197).

MP is an oleoresin which is said to contain some 250 ingredients with a resin content of 20-40% (12,14); the rest is a volatile oil (often incorrectly called 'essential oil') named cinnamein. The quantitatively most important chemicals appear to be benzyl cinnamate, benzyl benzoate, cinnamic acid, benzoic acid, coniferyl benzoate (only in fresh MP), nerolidol, benzyl alcohol, and vanillin (13,14). According to the European Pharmacopoeia, Balsamum Peruvianum contains not less than 45.0% w/w and not more than 70.0% w/w of esters, mainly benzyl benzoate and benzyl cinnamate (197). Further information on its chemical composition is provided below in the section 'Constituents of Myroxylon pereirae resin'.

The name Balsam of Peru is misleading. Most MP in worldwide circulation comes from El Salvador, none from Peru (where the source tree does not grow). The misnomer does not originate, as is often stated, from El Salvador belonging to the Viceroyalty of Peru in the 16th century, but from the fact that, at that time, this balsam was originally packed and shipped by the Spanish to Europe from the port of Callao in Lima, Peru, one of the main ports of the time in the New World. MP was extremely valued for religious ceremonies in Spain and thus was an attraction to robbers in the New World. To distract merchants and pirates from its true origin, the Spanish authorities exported MP from Peru around Cape Horn, rather than directly from El Salvador (171).

MP has a long history of medicinal use. In the 17th century the 'drug' appeared in German pharmacies and it was included in the U.S.P. from 1820. MP has also been described in many other national pharmacopoeias, for example in those of Argentina, Austria, Belgium, Brazil, Chile, France, Germany, Italy, Japan, Mexico, Netherlands and Spain. Applied externally, MP has been described as an antiseptic and vulnerary (wound healing), either alone, in alcoholic solution, or in the form of an ointment. Internally it has been used as a stimulating expectorant, but the internal use is rather rare, also because it is irritating. Indications for its topical use have included chronic ulcers, poorly healing wounds, decubitus, eczema, pruritus, hemorrhoids and anal pruritus (in the form of rectal suppositories), scabies (later replaced with its ingredient benzyl benzoate), frostbite, diaper rash, and intertrigo. It has also been an ingredient of preparations designed to be inhaled after dispersion in hot water. However, in 2016 the European Medicines Agency concluded that 'There is no documentation available for Peru balsam to support a well-established use indication' (216).

The main buyers of pure MP are pharmaceutical companies, perfume manufacturers, the food industry, and stores selling natural or herbal products. MP as a complete mixture has been substituted more and more by single constituents or fractions of MP now used in foods, sweets, bakery goods, chocolate, pastries, toothpaste, suntan products and medicinal ointments (13). MP or its ingredients may also be added to tobacco. Crude MP, as such, has not been used in perfumery (and consequently not in cosmetics) since 1982, when the International Fragrance Association IFRA banned its use in fragrances (36,113). Extracts or distillates are allowed (it has been stated that MP-sensitized subjects react even more strongly to these extracts [176], but evidence was not provided), and the current IFRA Standard restricts the use of these products to a level of 0.03%-0.7% in consumer products, depending on the product category (83) (table 3.126.1). MP used in perfumery is prepared either by vacuum distillation (Peru Balsam oil) or by solvent extraction (Peru Balsam absolute). Neither material is used at high volumes in fragrances, but of the two, the oil is the more important. In 2000, the worldwide volume of use of the oil was less than 10 metric tons and the worldwide volume of use of the absolute was less than 1 metric ton (IFRA Volume of Use Survey, 2000, cited in ref. 113).

The first observation of a skin lesion was described as an urticarial reaction to an MP-containing ointment in 1880 (12,14). Since then, case reports increased steadily and, up to 1995, over 500 articles on MP concerning constituents, case reports and patch test results have been published up to 1990. Most often, positive patch tests results were found in women with leg ulcers. In those days, MP was used extensively in topical medicinal wound and healing preparations (14). However, apparently, in the USA, topical pharmaceutical preparations containing MP are readily available even now (200).

MP has been used as a marker for fragrance sensitivity since Hjorth in 1961 (12) found that half of his patients with a positive reaction to MP were also sensitive to one or more toilet soap perfumes and half of the reactions to toilet soap perfumes in a standard patch test series coincided with a reaction to balsam of Peru (167). The reason for this may be that many scent allergens either happen to be ingredients of MP or are closely related to them (208).

Currently, in most patients reacting to MP, fragrance allergy is already detected by reactions to other fragrance indicators such as the fragrance mixes, and it has been suggested by some that MP may be of limited value in detecting cases of clinically relevant fragrance allergy and that consideration should be given to the replacement of MP with more well-defined markers of fragrance allergy in order to detect cases not identified by the FM (15,190). Nevertheless, now, 20 years later, MP is still part of most baseline series and, when discussing fragrance markers in recent literature, MP is always mentioned.

The literature up to 1961 has been reviewed by Hjorth in his famous PhD Thesis 'Eczematous allergy to balsams' (12).

Chemical composition of Myroxylon pereirae resin

Surprisingly little qualitative and quantitative information is available on the chemical composition of MP resin and its extracts (oil, essential oil, absolute) (12,13,14,113,197,198). The quantitatively most important chemicals in MP appear to be benzyl cinnamate (up to 40%), benzyl benzoate (up to 30%), cinnamic acid (3-30%), benzoic acid (1.5-11%), coniferyl benzoate (only in fresh MP up to 8.5% [possibly a mistake, should be 1.5%, see legends under table 3.126.2]), nerolidol (2-7%), benzyl alcohol (1-2%), vanillin (0.2-1.3%), cinnamyl cinnamate (0.5%), cinnamyl alcohol (0.4%), ferulic acid (0.1-0.4%), benzyl isoferulate (0.2%) and coniferyl alcohol (0.2%) (13,14). These and other ingredients identified by gas chromatography - mass spectrometry (GC-MS) analyses are shown in Table 3.126.2 (12,13,14,113, 197,198). Concentrations for most are not mentioned, as they have been presented as percentages of various fractions of MP or as MP derivatives and therefore cannot be compared. Contrary to what is often stated, cinnamal has not been identified in MP products.

The flavor of MP can be divided into four major ingredient aromatic groups: 1. vanilla (vanillic acid and its derivatives vanillin, benzyl vanillate, acetovanillone); 2. rose oil (benzoates); 3. cinnamon (cinnamic acid, cinnamyl alcohol, benzyl cinnamate, cinnamyl cinnamate, methyl cinnamate, other cinnamates); 4. (to a lesser degree) clove (eugenol, isoeugenol).

Table 3.126.2 Ingredients identified in Myroxylon pereirae resin, extracts and essential oils (12,13,14,113,197, 198, 215)

Constituent	
Acetic acid [a]	Ferulic acid (0.1-0.4%) [d]
Acetophenone [a]	Formic acid [a]
Acetovanillone [c]	Geranyl acetone [a]
α-Amorphene [a]	Guaiacol [a]
Amyrin [c]	Heptadecanoic acid (margaric acid) [c]
Aristolene [a]	Hexacosanoic acid (cerotic acid) [c]
Benzaldehyde [a]	1-Hexacosanol [c]
Benzoic acid [c]	Hexadecanoic acid (palmitic acid) [c]
Benzyl alcohol (1-2%) [d]	Hydroconiferyl benzoate [c]
Benzyl benzoate (up to 30%) [d]	Hydroconiferyl cinnamate [c]
Benzyl cinnamate (up to 40%) [d]	Hydroxycinnamic acid (148)
Benzyl p- coumarate [c]	4-Hydroxy-3-methoxyacetophenone (acetovanillone) [c]
Benzyl ferulate [c]	4-Hydroxy-3-methoxybenzoic acid (vanillic acid) [c]
Benzyl formate [a]	2-Hydroxypropanoic acid (lactic acid) [c]
Benzyl-trans-4-hydroxycinnamate (benzyl p-coumarate) [c]	Isoeugenol (0.85% in fraction BP3) [d]
Benzyl 4-hydroxy-3-methoxybenzoate (benzyl vanillate) [c]	Isoferulic acid (traces) [d]
	Limonene [a]
Benzyl isoferulate (cis- and trans) (0.2%) [d]	Methoxyeugenol [c]
Benzyl vanillate	Methyl benzoate
cis-α-, β- and cis- and trans-γ-Bisabolene [a]	Methyl cinnamate [d]
β-Caryophyllene [a]	Methyl vanillyl ketone (215)
1,8-Cineole [a]	α-Muurolene [a]
Cinnamic acid (cis- and trans-) (3-30%) [d]	Naphthalene
Cinnamyl alcohol (0.4%) [d]	Nerolidol (2-7%) [d]
Cinnamyl cinnamate (0.5%) [d]	allo-, cis- and trans-β-Ocimene [a]
Coniferyl alcohol (0.2%) [d]	1-Octacosanol [c]
Coniferyl benzoate (cis- and trans-) (up to 8.5% in fresh MP) [b,c,d]	Octadecanoic acid (stearic acid) [c]
	Patchoulene [a]
Coniferyl cinnamate [c]	α- and β-Phellandrene [a]
α-Copaene [a]	1-Phenylethanol (α-methylbenzyl alcohol) [c]
α-Curcumene [a]	3-Phenylpropanol [c]
Cycloisosativene [a]	α- and β-Pinene [a]
p- and trans-beta-Cymene [a]	β-Sesquiphellandrene [a]
Docosanoic acid [c]	Styrene [a]
Dodecanoic acid [c]	α-and γ-Terpinene [a]
Eicosanoic acid (arachidic acid) [c]	Terpinen-4-ol [a]
Ethylbenzene [a]	α-Terpineol [a]
Ethyl benzoate	1-Tetracosanol (lignoceryl alcohol) [c]
Ethyl cinnamate [a]	Tetradecanoic acid (myristic acid) [c]
Ethylhexanoic acid (tentatively identified) [c]	1-Undecanol [c]
Eugenol (0.2% in fraction BP3) [d]	Vanillic acid [c]
α-and β-Farnesene [a]	Vanillin (0.2-1.3%) [d]
Farnesol (traces) [d]	p-Vinylguaiacol (215)

[a] Ref. 197 (volatile fraction); [b] according to ref. 13. It is uncertain whether this is correct; the data are derived from the author's previous investigation (14), where he found up to a maximum of 8.5% coniferyl benzoate in fraction MP2, which constitutes 2.6% of total MP content; in fraction MP3, which constitutes 8-15% of total BP, 6.61% coniferyl benzoate was found; for the total amount of MP, the calculated maximum concentration of coniferyl benzoate would then be 1.5%; [c] Ref. 14; [d] Ref. 13

Chemical composition of Myroxylon pereirae *extracts* and *essential oil*

MP used in perfumery is prepared either by vacuum distillation (Peru balsam oil) or by solvent extraction (Peru balsam absolute); it can also be hydrodistilled to obtain Peru balsam essential oil. In all materials, the most important chemicals are benzyl benzoate (at least half of the composition), benzyl cinnamate, cinnamic acid, benzoic acid, E-nerolidol, benzyl alcohol and vanillin (198, 214,215). In one investigation, nerolidol was the major constituent in a hydrodistilled essential oil sample and in an oil obtained by solid phase micro extraction (197). It is well known that botanical products may have very different compositions and that the method of preparation heavily influences the analytical results (218).

In studies for an Austrian PhD Thesis, the volatile fraction of MP was investigated by the following extracting methods: supercritical fluid extraction (SFE-CO2 with CO2), solid phase micro extraction (SPME) and hydrodistillation (197). The major constituents identified by hydrodistillation were the sesquiterpene nerolidol with 46,1% and benzyl benzoate with 44,6%. Eighteen components of MP were identified all together. Major constituents in the volatile fraction extracted by SPME were nerolidol with 38.0%, benzyl benzoate with 31.1%, as well as benzyl alcohol, benzaldehyde, benzoic acid and trans-beta-cymene. The major constituents in SFE´s extracts were benzyl benzoate with around 60%, followed by benzyl cinnamate showing the highest value of 33% in vial4 and nerolidol with approximately 16% in vial2 (197).

One sample of MP essential oil (it should be realized that this can also mean an extract obtained by other methods than hydrodistillation) from an American company was investigated by gas chromatography – mass spectrometry (GC-MS) which gave the following results (% w/w): benzyl benzoate 66.24%, benzyl cinnamate 15.92%, benzoic acid 8.91%, (E)-nerolidol 3.41%, cinnamic acid 3.01%, vanillin 0.93%, (+)-α-pinene 0.87%, benzyl alcohol 0.62%, terpin-4-ol 0.32%, (+)-limonene 0.36% and (−)-limonene 0.08% (198).

Another sample of MP essential oil (steam-distilled, ergo indeed an essential oil) had the following composition: benzyl benzoate 70.49%, benzyl cinnamate 21.96%, trans-nerolidol 4.75%, vanillin 1.14%, benzyl alcohol 0.99% and cinnamein 0.67% (214). Yet another batch of Peru balsam essential oil from El Salvador was shown by GC-MS to contain benzyl benzoate 93.34%, benzyl cinnamate 3.26%, E-cinnamic acid 1.05%, benzoic acid 0.89%, E-nerolidol 0.38%, benzyl alcohol 0.28%, vanillin 0.10%, methyl vanillyl ketone 0.09%, and p-vinylguaiacol 0.05% (215).

CONTACT ALLERGY

General
The SCCS (Scientific Committee on Consumer Safety), in a 2012 Opinion on Fragrance allergens in cosmetic products, has marked Myroxylon pereirae extract as 'established contact allergen in humans' (211,212). The sensitizing potency of Peru balsam absolute was classified as 'moderate' based on an EC3 value of 2.5% in the LLNA (local lymph node assay) in animal experiments and Peru balsam oil had also a moderate sensitizing potency based on an EC3 value of 4% (211,212).

Contact allergy in the general population
There have been several investigations, especially in Europe, in which random samples of the population of certain age groups were patch tested with Myroxylon pereirae resin (MP). In a 2018 meta-analysis of 12 studies covering 8002 patch tested individuals from the general population, the pooled prevalence of sensitization to MP was 1.8% (women 1.7%, men 1.6%) (28). Ten years earlier, based on data from a systematic literature review up to 2008, the median prevalence of MP sensitization among adults was found to be 1.1% (women 1.4%; men 0%). The weighted average prevalence of MP sensitization among adults was 1.6% (173).

Estimates of the 10-year prevalence of contact allergy to MP in the general population of Denmark based on the CE-DUR method ranged from 0.57% to 0.77% (45). In a similar study from Germany, the estimated prevalence in the general population in the period 1992-2000 ranged from 1.3% to 3.0% (46).

Patch testing in groups of patients
Results of patch testing MP I in consecutive patients suspected of contact dermatitis (routine testing) back to 2000 are shown in table 3.126.3. Results of testing in groups of selected patients (e.g. physical therapists, individuals with eyelid / periorbital dermatitis, patients with allergic contact cheilitis, individuals with stasis dermatitis / leg ulcers, patients suspected of cosmetic intolerance or fragrance allergy, patients with hand dermatitis) are shown in table 3.126.4.

Patch testing in consecutive patients suspected of contact dermatitis: routine testing
As MP is present in most, if not all, baseline / routine / screening / standard series tested worldwide, data on testing MP in consecutive patients (routine testing) is abundant. The results of nearly 55 such published investigations back to 2000 are shown in table 3.126.3.

USA
In 14 studies from the USA, 10 of which were performed by the North American Contact Dermatitis Group (NACDG), frequencies of sensitization have ranged from 6.6% to 13.7% (10,16,17,18,29,47,57,58,63,66,71,74,125,161). Generally speaking, the rates appear to have decreased somewhat in the last decade, ranging in all NACDG studies

between 7 and 8%. In the studies from the NACDG, 'definite' + 'probable' relevance was usually 30-35%. In two non-NACDG centers, relevance was scored in 57% (71) and 65% (10) of the positive patch test reactions.

Europe, multicenter studies
In seven multinational multicenter studies performed in Europe (European Surveillance System on Contact Allergy network, European Environmental and Contact Dermatitis Research Group, other parties) frequencies of sensitization have ranged in a very narrow band of 5.3% to 6.4% (1,11,62,69,72,75,101). In most studies, there was a significant variability in the results per center or country: 3.6-12.8% (101), 1.6-10.6% (1), 1.4-14.6% (11), 2.3-12.9% (62) and 2.8-10.9% (69). Relevance data were not provided in any of the 7 investigations.

IVDK (Informationsverbund Dermatologischer Kliniken: Germany, Switzerland, Austria)
The results of testing large groups of patients with MP by the IVDK have been reported in 5 publications (25,38,60, 103 ,161). Rates of sensitization have ranged from 6.8% to 9.2%. Relevance data were not provided.

Other European countries
Prevalence rates of sensitization in various European countries published after 2000 are shown in table 3.126.3. In 4 Danish studies with overlapping study periods and populations, frequencies of sensitization ranged from 2.8% to 4.4% and in 2 of those, relevance was 50% and 58%, resp. (7,61,106,174). In 4 investigations from the UK, frequencies of sensitization ranged from 2.9% to 6.4%, with lower rates in recent periods; relevance data were not provided or specified (26,98,102,172). In Spain, positivity rates were 2.4%, 6.4% and 5.8% (48,35,168). In two, 66% (35) and 75% (168) of the positive reactions were considered to be relevant. Culprit products were mainly topical pharmaceuticals and cosmetics (168).
In Sweden, 4.8% to 6.5% of routine patients reacted to MP; relevance data were not provided (65,70,134). The results of investigations performed in other European countries (The Netherlands, Finland, Belgium, Switzerland, Czech Republic) can be found in table 3.126.3.

Non-European countries
Prevalence rates of sensitization in various non-European countries published after 2000 are shown in table 3.126.3. These were 6.8% in Thailand (99, 67% relevance), 4.2% in Singapore (95, present + past relevance 38%), 5.1% in China (100), a high 8.7% and 8.9% in Australia (73,210, relevance rates 28% and 30%), 2.8% in Iran (20), 3.6% and 6.1% in Israel (34,59), and 2.1% in Turkey (67). Culprit products were not mentioned in any investigation.

Table 3.126.3 Patch testing in groups of patients: Routine testing

Years and Country	Test conc. & vehicle	Number of patients tested | positive (%)		Selection of patients (S); Relevance (R); Comments (C)	Ref.
2015-2017 NACDG	25% pet.	5595	392 (7.0%)	R: definite + probable relevance: 27%	47
2015-7 Netherlands		821	237 (2.8%)	R: not stated; low rate can partly be explained by the use of the TRUE test, which has a lower sensitivity for detecting contact allergy to MP	49
2015-2016 UK	25% pet.	2084	61 (2.9%)	R: not specified for individual fragrances; 25% of patients who reacted to any fragrance or fragrance marker had a positive fragrance history	172
2011-2015 Spain	25% pet.	19,588	481 (2.4%)	R: not stated	48
2011-2015 USA	25% pet.	2573	236 (9.2%)	R: not stated	29
2013-2014 NACDG	25% pet.	4859	348 (7.2%)	R: definite + probable relevance: 34%	74
2013-2014 Twelve European countries, 46 departments [a]	25% pet.	27,274	(5.7%)	R: not stated; C: results of 6 occupational dermatology clinics and one pediatric clinic not included in these figures; range of positive reactions: 0.7%-13.3%	75
2013-2014 Thailand		312	21 (6.8%)	R: 67%	99
2010-2014 IVDK	25% pet.	48,956	3944 (8.1%)	R: not stated	161
2009-2014 NACDG	25% pet.	13,398	991 (7.4%)	R: not stated	161
2008-2014 UK	25% pet.	3502	130 (3.7%)	R: not stated; C: there were 1.9% ?+ and 1.7% irritant reactions	98
2009-2013 Singapore	25% pet.	2598	(4.2%)	R: present + past relevance: 38%; C: range of positive reactions per year 2.5-6.2%	95
2011-2012 NACDG	25% pet.	4234	333 (7.9%)	R: definite + probable relevance: 38%	57
2011-2012 UK	25% pet.	1951	68 (3.5%)	R: not stated	102
2009-2012 Twelve European countries [a]	25% pet.	57,027	(5.9%)	R: not stated; C: range per country: 3.6-12.8%; the TRUE ® test system is less sensitive for detecting sensitivity to MP than the pet.-based chamber systems	101
1999-2012 IVDK	25% pet.	130,258	(8.4%)	R: not stated	38
2010-2011 China	25% pet.	296	(5.1%)	R: 67% for all fragrances tested together (excluding FM I)	100

Table 3.126.3 Patch testing in groups of patients: Routine testing (continued)

Years and Country	Test conc. & vehicle	Number of patients tested	positive (%)		Selection of patients (S); Relevance (R); Comments (C)	Ref.
2009-2010 NACDG	25% pet.	4308		(7.2%)	R: definite + probable relevance: 35%	58
2008-2010 Denmark	25% pet.	1503	53	(3.5%)	R: 58% present clinical relevance	7
2006-2010 USA	25% pet.	3082		(12.6%)	R: 57%	71
2001-2010 Australia	25% pet.	5198	461	(8.7%)	R: 30%	73
1993-2010 Australia	25% pet.	5646	500	(8.9%)	R: 142/500 (28%)	210
2009 Sweden	25% pet.	3112		(4.8%)	R: not stated	70
2007-2009 Sweden	25% pet.	1180	68	(5.8%)	R: not stated	134
2007-2008 Eleven European countries [a]	25% pet.	25,181	1338	(5.3%)	R: not stated; C: prevalences ranged from 1.6% (Italy) to 10.6% (Austria)	1
2007-2008 NACDG	25% pet.	5083		(11.0%)	R: definite + probable relevance: 34%	17
2005-2008 Denmark	25% pet.	12,302	347	(2.8%)	R: 50%	174
2005-2008 IVDK	25% pet.	36,919		(6.8%)	R: not stated	103
2004-2008 Spain	25% pet.	1253	80	(6.4%)	R: 66%	35
2004-2008 Iran	25% pet.	1135	32	(2.8%)	R: 82% of all reactions to FM I, FM II, Myroxylon pereirae resin, hydroxyisohexyl 3-cyclohexene carboxaldehyde and/or turpentine were clinically relevant	20
1985-2007 Denmark	25% pet.	16,173		(4.0%)	R: not stated; C: significant decline of positive reactions to BP from 1997 to 2007 in women but not in men	106
2005-2006 Ten European countries [a]	25% pet.	18,533	1156	(6.4%)	R: not stated; C: prevalences were 6.8% in Central Europe, 5.4% in West, 6.2% in Northeast and 5.4% in South Europe	72
2005-2006 NACDG	25% pet.	4449		(11.9%)	R: definite + probable relevance: 34%	16
2001-2005 USA	25% pet.	3837		(13.7%)	R: 65%	10
1990-2005 Belgium	25% pet.	10,128	617	(6.1%)	R: not stated	108
1985-2005 Denmark	25% pet.	14,998		(4.4%)	R: not stated	61
2004, Eleven European countries [a]	25% pet.	9978	607	(5.7%)	R: not stated; C: range positives per center: 1.4%-14.6%	11
2003-2004 NACDG	25% pet.	5140	545	(10.6%)	R: not stated	18
2001-2004 IVDK	25% pet.	30,999		(9.2%)	R: not stated	60
2001-2004 Spain	25% pet.	863	50	(5.8%)	R: 75% from topical medication (n=19) and from cosmetics (n=13)	168
2000-4 Switzerland	25% pet.	4094	318	(7.8%)	R: not stated	104
1998-2004 Israel	25% pet.	2156	78	(3.6%)	R: not stated	59
1992-2004 Turkey	25% pet.	1038	22	(2.1%)	R: not stated; C: prevalence in women 1.5%, in men 3.3%	67
2003 NACDG	25% pet.	1603	105	(6.6%)	R: definite + probable relevance: 26%	125
2002-2003 Europe [a]	25% pet.	9672		(6.1%)	R: not stated; C: 17 centers in 9 European countries; range per center: 2.3-12.9%	62
<2003 Israel	25% pet.	641	39	(6.1%)	R: not stated	34
2001-2002 NACDG	25% pet.	4910		(11.6%)	R: definite + probable relevance: 13%	63
2000-2002 Finland	25% pet.	11,806		(6.2%)	R: not stated	64
2001-2002 UK	25% pet.	766	49	(6.4%)	R: not stated	26
1996-2002 IVDK	25% pet.	59,334			R: not stated; C: range per year: 7.3-11.5%; significant increase in the frequency between 1996 and 1998, and a significant decline from 1999 to 2002	25
1999-2001 Sweden	25% pet.	3790		(6.5%)	R: not stated; C: prevalence in women 9.0%, in men 5.7% (standardized prevalences)	65
1997-2001 Czech Rep.	25% pet.	12,058	878	(7.3%)	R: not stated; C: prevalence in men 6.3%, in women 7.8%	68
2000 Sweden	25% pet.	3825		(6.5%)	R: not stated	70
1998-2000 USA	25% pet.	1322		(11.3%)	R: not stated	66
1996-2000 Europe	25% pet.	26,210		(6.0%)	R: not stated; C: prevalence in women 6.7%, in men 5.1%; C: ten centers, seven countries, EECDRG study; range per center 2.8-10.9%	69

[a] study of the ESSCA (European Surveillance System on Contact Allergies)
EECDRG: European Environmental and Contact Dermatitis Research Group; FM: Fragrance mix; IVDK: Information Network of Departments of Dermatology, Germany, Austria, Switzerland; NACDG: North American Contact Dermatitis Group (USA, Canada)

Patch testing in groups of selected patients

Results of testing in groups of selected patients (e.g. physical therapists, individuals with eyelid / periorbital dermatitis, patients with allergic contact cheilitis, individuals with stasis dermatitis / leg ulcers, patients suspected of cosmetic intolerance or fragrance allergy, patients with hand dermatitis) are shown in table 3.126.4. The studies shown are selected, and the table does not provide a full literature review. Hairdressers are not included, as the prevalence of MP sensitization in most studies is not or only slightly elevated (87,88,89,90,94), which also applies to health care professionals / nurses (77,96,97). However, adequate controls groups are largely lacking.

Patients with eyelid dermatitis / periorbital dermatitis
In 7 studies, in which patients with eyelid dermatitis / periorbital dermatitis were patch tested with MP, frequencies of sensitization have ranged from 1.7% to 17%, but 5/7 scored lower than 7% (21,53,78,79,82,92,124). In 3 investigations where relevance was addressed, rates of relevant reactions were 43% (124), 58% (53) and 75% (79), but culprit products were not mentioned. In 4 studies with a control group, the frequency of sensitization to MP was significantly lower than in routine testing (53,78,79,82).

Patients with stasis dermatitis / leg ulcers
In 8 studies testing patients with stasis dermatitis / leg ulcers, frequencies of sensitization to MP have ranged from 14.8% to 50%; most scored 30-40% positive reactions (55,85,105,109,110,130,170,206). Relevance was mentioned in one study only: 'definite' zero per cent, 'probable' 6% (55). It is clear that in all studies, the frequencies of sensitization to MP were higher than in routinely tested patients (85,109,206) or than expected.

In a meta-analysis, 26 studies investigating sensitization in leg ulcer / stasis dermatitis patients published between 1975 and 2003 were analyzed (130). In the period 1975-1990, the average percentage of positive reactions (unadjusted for sample size) in 15 studies to MP was 16.0% (range2.6-37.5%) and in the period 1991-2003 in 11 investigations was 25.4% (range 5.9-40.0%). In three French studies, extremely high percentages of sensitization (up to 40%) were found. It was assumed that this was mainly due to the presence of MP (for unproven healing properties) in topical treatments, including over-the-counter products widely used on leg ulcers or stasis dermatitis in France. The overall rate of sensitization to MP during the period 1991-2003 (25.4%) dropped to 14.6% when the French studies were removed from the calculation (130). The older studies (<2004) mentioned above may have been part of the meta-analysis (130).

Patients suspected of fragrance or cosmetic allergy
In 6 studies in groups of patients suspected of cosmetic or fragrance allergy (8,19,32,76,86,91) frequencies of sensitization have ranged from 9.4% to 19.6%. Relevance was mentioned in one study only (95%), but this investigation had certain weaknesses (8). There was a control group in only one study; the frequency of sensitization in the group suspected of cosmetic / fragrance allergy (7.9%) was significantly higher than in a control group of routine testing (86).

Patients with cosmetic allergy including allergic contact cheilitis
In 6 studies in groups of patients with cosmetic allergy (allergic contact cheilitis, patients known to be allergic to cosmetics or fragrances, patients with previous positive patch tests to deodorant, perfume, eau de toilette, aftershave, bath or shower products, skin creams), frequencies of sensitization to MP ranged from 14% to 45%, mostly between 17 and 24% (24,37,52,80,111,126). These high frequencies are hardly surprizing considering the selection criteria. Relevance in 3 studies addressing this issue were 100% (52,80,126[the latter selected on the basis of relevant reactions]), but causative products were not mentioned.

Miscellaneous indications for patch testing
For information on testing patients with psoriasis (53), individuals suspected of photodermatoses (123), children (84; there are many such studies not mentioned here), physical therapists (50), patients with pure allergic hand dermatitis (54), with poikiloderma of Civatte (131) and with facial allergic contact dermatitis (79) please consult table 3.126.4. In the studies in patients with poikiloderma of Civatte (131), with pure allergic hand dermatitis (54) and with facial allergic contact dermatitis (81) the frequency of sensitization may have been elevated, but in the latter two, the patients were selected on the basis of relevant reactions (54,81).

Case reports and case series

General
In many reports, MP was stated to be the responsible allergen in patients with allergic contact dermatitis, notably when caused by cosmetics (see the sections 'Case series' and 'Case reports' below). As MP *per se* is not used in cosmetics, this statement is not quite correct. What is probably meant in these studies is that one or more of MP's ingredients or its extracts (oil or absolute) were the allergens or were *supposed to be* the allergens, without verification by patch testing and ascertaining their presence in causative products. It is plausible, though, that in a number of these patients, individual ingredients have been patch tested and were positive, but that MP was *also*

counted as allergen. Another possibility is that MP was considered to be a marker for fragrance allergy, and that, when the patient reacted to other fragrances or fragranced products, the reaction to MP was scored as relevant.

Table 3.126.4 Patch testing in groups of patients: Selected patient groups

Years and Country	Test conc. & vehicle	Number of patients		Selection of patients (S); Relevance (R); Comments (C)	Ref.
		tested	positive (%)		
2014-2016 France		264	14 (5.3%)	S: patients suspected of eyelid allergic contact dermatitis; R: 6/14 (43%)	124
1996-2015 IVDK	25% pet.	2239	102 (3.8%)	S: patients with psoriasis; R: not stated; C: the percentage of positive reactions was significantly lower than in the control group of consecutive dermatitis patients (7.6%)	51
<2015 Turkey	25% pet.	40	20 (50%)	S: patients with leg ulcers and dermatitis of the surrounding skin; R: not stated; C: the percentage was significantly higher than in a control group of patients with dermatitis of the foot or lower legs but without ulcers (20%)	206
2005-2014 China	25% pet.	1292	43 (3.3%)	S: patients suspected of photodermatoses; R: not stated	123
2003-2014 IVDK	25% pet.	5202	(14.8%)	S: patients with stasis dermatitis / chronic leg ulcers; R: not stated; C: percentage of reactions significantly higher than in a control group of routine testing	85
1996-2013 Nether-Lands	25% pet.	1004	38 (3.8%)	S: children aged 0-17 years; R: not stated; significantly more reactions in children with atopic dermatitis (5.6%) than in those without atopic dermatitis (2.0%)	84
2007-2011 IVDK	25% pet.	116	9 (7.8%)	S: physical therapists; R: not stated; C: the rate was probably not higher than in routine testing	50
2006-2011 IVDK	25% pet.	10,124	755 (7.9%)	S: patients with suspected cosmetic intolerance; R: not stated; C: the prevalence was significantly higher than in a control group matched for sex and age	86
2001-2011 USA	25% pet.	41	10 (24%)	S: patients with allergic contact cheilitis; R: 100%	52
2006-2010 USA	25% pet.	100	17 (17%)	S: patients with eyelid dermatitis; R: not stated	21
2000-2010 IVDK		4384	281 (5.3%)	S: patients with periorbital dermatitis; R: not stated; C: the frequency was lower than in a control group of routine testing	78
2005-2008 France	25% pet.	423	172 (40%)	S: patients with leg ulcers; R: not stated, but is was mentioned that, at that time, wound dressing with Myroxylon pereirae resin were still used in France for leg ulcers	105
2000-2007 USA	25% pet.	936	116 (12.4%)	S: patients who were tested with a supplemental cosmetic screening series; R: 95%; C: weak study: a. high rate of macular erythema and weak reactions; b. relevance figures included 'questionable' and 'past' relevance	8
1990-2006 USA	25% pet.	266	19 (7.1%)	S: patients with periorbital dermatitis; R: 11/19 (58%); C: the frequency was lower than in controls (12.7%)	53
<2005 Poland	25% pet.	50	19 (38%)	S: patients with chronic venous leg ulcers; R: not stated	110
<2004 USA, Canada	25% pet.	54	16 (30%)	S: patients with past or present leg ulcers with or without dermatitis; R: definite zero, probable 6%	55
<2004 Poland		300	90 (30.0%)	S: patients with stasis dermatitis; R: unknown, but topical medications were probably important	170
2001-2004 NACDG	25% pet.	60	14 (23%)	S: patients with allergic contact cheilitis and relevant contact allergies to allergens in the NACDG series; R: these reactions were probably all relevant, but the causative products were not mentioned	80
1999-2004 Germany	25% pet.	88	12 (14%)	S: patients with periorbital eczema; R: in 48 patients with allergic contact dermatitis, 5 reactions to MP (10%) were considered to be relevant; cosmetics were the most frequent causative products	92
1994-2004 NACDG	25% pet.	959	(9.6%)	S: patients with pure allergic contact dermatitis of the hands; R: the patients were selected on the basis of relevant reactions	54
2002-2003 Korea	25% pet.	422	31 (7.3%)	S: patients with suspected cosmetic dermatitis; R: not stated	32
1993-2003 IVDK	25% pet.	1233	92 (7.5%)	S: patients patch tested to confirm of rule out (secondary) allergic contact dermatitis of the scalp; R: not stated; C: the frequency was lower than in the total IVDK test population	91
2001-2002 NACDG	25% pet.	2193	431 (19.6%)	S: patients with (presumed) cosmetic allergy; R: not stated	76
2001-2002 France	25% pet.	106	42 (39.6%)	S: patients admitted to hospital for leg ulcers; R: not stated; C: this study was included in the meta-analysis discussed in the text in the section 'Patch testing in groups of selected patients'	130
2000-2002 Serbia	25% pet.	75	16 (21.3%)	S: patients with venous leg ulcers and documented dermatitis	109

Table 3.126.4 Patch testing in groups of patients: Selected patient groups (continued)

Years and Country	Test conc. & vehicle	Number of patients tested | positive (%)		Selection of patients (S); Relevance (R); Comments (C)	Ref.
				around the ulcers; R: not stated; C: the frequency was significantly higher than in a control group of patients suspected of allergic contact dermatitis but without venous insufficiency	
1998-2002 IVDK	25% pet.	60	17 (23%)	S: patients who had a positive reaction to their own deodorant; R: not stated; C: there was a significant difference in percentage positive reactions compared with a control group of dermatitis patients who had *not* reacted to their own deodorant	37
		56	13 (23%)	S: patients who had a positive reaction to their own perfume, eau de toilette or shaving product; R: not stated; C: there was a significant difference in percentage positive reactions compared with a control group of dermatitis patients who had *not* reacted to their own cosmetic products of this type	
1998-2002 IVDK	25% pet.	70	13 (17%)	S: patients with a positive patch test to one or more bath and shower products; R: not stated; C: the frequency was significantly higher than in a control group of patients not reacting to bath and shower products (8%)	111
1998-2002 IVDK	25% pet.	304	64 (21.2%)	S: patients with a positive patch test to one or more skin care cream products; R: not stated; C: the frequency was significantly higher than in a control group of patients not reacting to skin care cream products (9.1%)	
1982-2001 UK	25% pet.	22	3 (14%)	S: patients with allergic contact cheilitis; R: the patients were selected on the basis of relevant positive reactions	126
1997-2000 Austria	25% pet.	747	70 (9.4%)	S: patients suspected of fragrance allergy; R: not stated	19
1995-1999 IVDK	25% pet.	972	(6.5%)	S: patients with allergic periorbital contact dermatitis; R: not stated; rate was significantly lower than in a control group of routine testing	82
1995-1998 Greece	25% pet.	32	4 (13%)	S: patients with Poikiloderma of Civatte; R: it was suggested that fragrances play an etiological role; C: the frequency of sensitization to *all* fragrances together was significantly higher than in a control group of patients suspected of contact dermatitis	131
1994-1998 UK	25% pet.	232	4 (1.7%)	S: patients with eyelid dermatitis; R: 3/4 were currently relevant, but the causative products were not mentioned; C: the frequency was lower than in a controls group of routine testing	79
1995-1997 USA	25% pet.	57	12 (21%)	S: patients with facial allergic contact dermatitis; R: only relevant reactions were mentioned, causative products were not indicated	81
<1977	25% pet.	20	9 (45%)	S: patients allergic to fragrances; R: not stated	24

IVDK: Informationsverbund Dermatologischer Kliniken (Germany, Switzerland, Austria)
NACDG: North American Contact Dermatitis Group (USA, Canada)

Case series

In the period 1990-2016, in a clinic in Belgium, 125 patients were investigated for allergic contact dermatitis from a medicinal herbal preparation. In 30 (24%), MP was the active principle in these preparations. MP was formerly often present in dermatological preparations, especially hand and lip balms, as well as in preparations for the treatment of hemorrhoids, because of its (alleged) wound-healing and antimicrobial effects. Currently, these preparations are only rarely used in Belgium and the majority of the positive reactions were observed before the year 2000 (203).

MP was stated to be the (or an) allergen in 71 patients in a group of 603 individuals suffering from cosmetic dermatitis, seen in the period 2010-2015 in Leuven, Belgium (41).

In the period 1996-2013, in a tertiary referral center in Valencia, Spain, 5419 patients were patch tested. Of these, 628 individuals had allergic contact dermatitis to cosmetics. In this group, MP was stated to be the responsible allergen in 17 cases (42, overlap with ref. 43). In the period 2000-2007, 202 patients with allergic contact dermatitis caused by cosmetics were seen in Valencia, Spain. In this group, Myroxylon pereirae resin was the allergen in 4 individuals from its presence in moisturizing cream (n=2), deodorant (n=1) and perfume (n=1) (43, overlap with ref. 42).

Twenty-five case reports of contact allergy to MP mentioning the patients' sex, age, profession, site of skin lesions, co-reactions, reactions to constituents, individual habits, possible etiologies and comments/remarks were reported in the mid-1990's in Germany (13). The most important (possible) etiologies were plastics (in patients reacting to resorcinol monobenzoate, an ultraviolet stabilizer in cellulose acetate and other plastic materials; this chemical has not been identified in MP but frequently reacts for unknown reasons in MP-positive individuals), consumption of sweets, smoking (in those days, MP, Tolu balsam, vanilla, as well benzoic and cinnamic acid, benzyl alcohol, benzyl cinnamate, cinnamyl alcohol, farnesol, and nerolidol were added to tobacco in the manufacturing of cigarettes), and wound healing / herbal ointments. MP or its ingredients added to cigarettes resulted in hand eczema in smokers (13). Patients presented who reacted to foods and drinks are discussed in the section 'Case reports / Foods and drinks' below.

In one center in Belgium, between 1985 and 1990, 3970 patients with dermatitis were patch tested. 462 of these reacted positively to patch tests with cosmetic allergens. The reactions were considered to be relevant in 68%, probably relevant in 25% and doubtfully relevant in 7% of the patients. In the list of 'most common allergens' MP had rank number 2 with 114 reactions. It should be realized that, in those days, MP was already not used any more in cosmetics.

In Belgium, in the years before 1986, of 5202 consecutive patients with dermatitis patch tested, 156 were diagnosed with pure cosmetic allergy. MP was the 'dermatitic ingredient' in 52 (33.3%) patients (frequency in the entire group: 7.0%) (118). Balsam of Peru was responsible for 3 out of 399 cases of cosmetic allergy where the causal allergen was identified in a study of the NACDG, USA, 1977-1983 (9).

In Hjorth's investigations, published in his 1961 PhD Thesis (12), of a group of 230 patients with positive reactions to MP, seen in the second half of the 1950s in Denmark, data on previous use of MP was available for 182. There had been previous contact with MP in 126 (69%) of the cases. Forty-eight (of the 230) were referred for eczema caused by MP preparations. Among the 126 patients who had reported having used preparations containing MP, 111 had used the official 10% pet. Balsamum Peruvianum of the Danish pharmacopoeia, about half of them for burns. Apart from perfumes in soap, other perfumes and cosmetics were the contributory or the sole cause in 35 cases (12).

In Chapter 18 of the thesis, 21 case histories 'to serve as illustration of the potential causes of eczema in patients allergic to balsam of Peru' were described in some detail (12). Most reactions were caused by pure MP or MP in topical pharmaceutical preparations including ointments, gauzes and suppositories. There were also reactions to Arning's tincture and compound tincture of benzoin, which have similar ingredients as MP and therefore show pseudo-cross-reactions. Other causative products were perfumed soaps, perfumes, fragranced cosmetics (including a toothpaste containing oil of cinnamon and a hair lacquer with benzoin), and orange peel in 3 patients. There were also some descriptions of patients with exacerbations of dermatitis after eating sweets and ice cream (12).

Sixteen patients had allergic contact dermatitis from Myroxylon pereirae resin in topical pharmaceutical preparations (2). Eight patients had allergic contact cheilitis from MP in 'Dermophil Indien', a lip balm (40).

Case reports

Pharmaceuticals and cosmetics

Two patients presented with cheilitis and perioral dermatitis. Patch testing revealed positive reactions to MP and to an ointment used as lip balm, for minor burns, cuts, nappy rash, sunburn, rash and scalds. MP was not listed as an ingredient in this ointment, but the manufacturer confirmed that a small amount of MP was present in the product (210).

A man presented with a 12-week history of nonhealing peri-anal erosions. The patient experienced a blistering reaction 10 days after daily self-treatment of his chronic perianal pruritus with an analgesic cream that contained menthol, eugenol and methyl salicylate. He had used the cream intermittently in the past. Sores developed in the area. His primary care provider prescribed a healing spray containing trypsin, MP and castor oil and the sores progressed to ulcerations. The spray was discontinued, and the patient was patch tested, which revealed positive reactions to MP, eugenol, and the spray. During the patch test, the perianal area became indurated. The authors suggest that this patient became sensitized to the eugenol in the initial analgesic cream and then propagated the reaction with the MP-containing spray aimed at healing the area. The presentation of a nonhealing wound as contact dermatitis may suggest, according to the authors, an aberrant T-cell response in the chronic wound (200).

A woman developed severe weeping dermatitis of the face from the application of an MP-containing ointment. This was followed by dissemination to the legs, where the ointment had not been applied. The eruption on the legs resembled vasculitis with diffuse redness and numerous partly purpuric papules and some slightly hemorrhagic bullae. Patch testing showed her to be allergic to MP, FM I, colophonium, wood tars, eugenol,, isoeugenol, oil of cloves and lavender oil. Although the authors suggested that a systemic spread of the allergen was plausible, they did not, quite curiously, consider the possibility of systemic contact dermatitis from food or drinks (192). One other patient apparently also had purpuric vasculitis-like lesions due to allergy to MP (specific data unknown, article not read) (193).

A veterinarian had occupational allergic contact dermatitis of the hands from MP-containing ointments he used for treating animals (13).

Sixteen patients had allergic contact dermatitis from Myroxylon pereirae resin in topical pharmaceutical preparations (2). Eight patients had allergic contact cheilitis from MP in 'Dermophil Indien', a lip balm (40).

Foods and drinks

General

There are many case reports of patients allergic to MP, who improved when following a diet in which foods and drinks containing MP or specific ingredients of the material were avoided. These are presented below. It should be realized that most assessments of improvement were made by the patients themselves, that no prospective studies to support advice for dietary restriction have been published in the last 25 years, that the placebo effect of following such a diet may probably be considerable and that provocation and elimination experiments after initial improvement on a diet have rarely been performed or at least rarely been published. This topic is discussed further in the section 'Myroxylon pereirae resin and restrictive diets' below.

Foods and drinks Case reports

A female patient presented with a 10-year history of painful ulcerations on her tongue. She reported that she drank large quantities of diet cola and that she used cinnamon-flavored toothpaste and mouthwash nightly. Patch testing elicited positive reactions to MP and cinnamal, the main ingredient of cinnamon oil used for flavoring. The patient was put on a restricted diet and a fragrance-free regimen, and her condition resolved (189).

One individual allergic to Myroxylon pereirae resin was sensitized to cinnamon in a toothpaste; his dermatitis flared after drinking vermouth that contained cinnamon (127, cited in ref. 128). Another patient allergic to MP experienced a flare of dermatitis after drinking vermouth with cinnamon (181) and yet another one from eating half a teaspoon of vanilla sugar (182).

A man had contact dermatitis of the face, presumably caused by an after-shave. Upon patch testing, he reacted to MP. Later, he had recurrences that improved during the week, but would flare up on Mondays. It was found that that the patient consumed large quantities of sweets, mostly with a chocolate base, on Sundays. Oral administration of 20 mg/day MP provoked the dermatitis on the 3rd day (total intake 40 mg) (158) .

A woman known to be allergic to MP had suffered from dyshidrotic hand eczema for 9 years. After eating chocolate, an acute rash with vesicles and some pustules developed on her neck, trunk and thighs with some fever. In addition to topical and systemic corticosteroid therapy, an MP-reduced diet was initiated, resulting in complete clearance of the patient's symptoms. Patch tests showed multiple contact allergic reactions, including to MP, fragrance mix, propolis, cinnamyl alcohol, eugenol and isoeugenol. Oral MP challenge resulted in the development of eczema on the face, neck, chest and upper back after one day (188). Another patient in the same report had dyshidrotic eczema of the hands and dermatitis of the groins (classic for systemic contact dermatitis). She proved to be allergic to MP. Following an MP-reduced diet and treatment with topical steroids she had complete clearing of the inflamed skin changes. Oral MP challenge led to pruritic erythema on the trunk, and this continued to spread to the head and extremities. A third patient, a woman, had experienced new episodes of eczema on her face, trunk and extremities which often appeared after handling conifer branches, applying different cosmetics or eating cinnamon cakes. Patch testing showed contact allergic reactions to a variety of substances but not to MP. Because of the reactions to group allergens of MP (colophonium, fragrance mix), an oral MP challenge was performed, leading to severe pruritus and heat flush after 6 hours, and eczema on the hands, arms, neck and upper chest (188).

Four children with widespread dermatitis (atopic in three) were contact allergic to MP, 2 also reacted to cinnamyl alcohol. When they avoided intake of tomato ketchup and some other triggering foods, the dermatitis improved some 80% in all four. Both MP and tomatoes contain cinnamyl alcohol (201).

Three other children with dermatitis (2 atopic) and reacting to MP improved upon avoidance of fragranced products but improved more, and in one the dermatitis resolved, when a low MP diet was administered (202). A man with chronic intermittent dermatitis for 10 years and contact allergy to MP much improved on a low MP diet (204).

A brewer with chronic eczema of the hands showed positive patch test reactions to MP and fragrance mix I. A low MP diet resulted in clear improvement. Oral challenge with MP 2x0.5 gram with a 2-hour interval (or every two hours?) led to exacerbation of the eczema after 5 days. In a second provocation test, the dermatitis worsened after 2 days already (56).

Eating or sucking of wine gums, licorice, marzipan, caramels, cream toffees and other sweets/candies produced or maintained skin lesions in several MP-reactive patients, which disappeared after stopping these particular habits. Some patients had glossodynia which resolved by avoiding such sweets and candies (13).

Miscellaneous products

A factory worker preparing copper mirrors for carbon anhydride lasers developed dermatitis of the fingers of his right hand. He had positive patch tests to MP and a cutting fluid. The manufacturer did not provide data on the composition of the fluid, but other patients allergic to MP also reacted to the fluid; additionally, neither the patient nor other MP-allergic individuals had positive tests to the non-perfumed variety of the same brand of cutting fluid (152).

In the late 1980s, when Myroxylon pereirae resin was already recommended by IFRA to be banned because of its sensitizing potential, it was still present in several popular over-the-counter diaper products and may have caused fragrance dermatitis in children (162).

The sensitizers in Myroxylon pereirae

In 1948, it was reported that balsam of Peru was a common allergen; cinnamal was found to be an important allergenic ingredient (175). However, MP contains no cinnamal, but may be formed in the skin from cinnamyl alcohol and act as a sensitizer (see Chapter 3.34 Cinnamal and Chapter 3.36 Cinnamyl alcohol). Since Hjorth's classic study on balsam of Peru in 1961 (12), in which he found that 80% of his patients allergic to MP reacted to coniferyl benzoate, this was considered to be the most important allergen in the product. However, coniferyl benzoate was first identified in MP in 1995, 34 years later (14)! It was the strongest sensitizer of all MP ingredients tested in guinea pigs (12,14). However, it can only be found when fresh samples of MP are investigated, as it is a very unstable and is degrades in MP and syringes very quickly (14).

In several studies, patients known to be allergic to MP have been tested with selected ingredients; their results are shown in table 3.126.5 (12,13,148,150,156). The results have varied widely. There were differences in the methodology of patch testing, the size of the populations tested, in the number and nature of ingredients tested, in the test concentrations and sometimes the vehicles used and, of course, different samples of MP were used with different compositions. Therefore, reliably identifying the main sensitizers in MP based on the available data is not possible. The highest percentages positive reactions were scored by coniferyl benzoate, isoeugenol, eugenol, cinnamyl alcohol, cinnamic acid and cinnamyl cinnamate. Coniferyl benzoate is a potent sensitizer and MP may contain up to 30% cinnamic acid. However, the other substances appear to be present in MP in low concentrations. Whether these are high enough in MP to induce contact allergy and / or elicit allergic contact dermatitis has not been investigated. Possibly, there may be cross-reactivity between eugenol and isoeugenol and between cinnamic acid, cinnamyl alcohol and cinnamyl cinnamate. Also, some patients may well have become sensitized to these substances from their presence in other products.

Table 3.126.5 Results of patch tests with components of Myroxylon pereirae resin in patients allergic to MP

Compound	Germany (13)			Denmark (12)			Denmark (148)			Canada, USA, Europe (150)			Poland (156)			R
	N	C	% Pos.	N	C	% Pos.	N	C	% Pos.	N	C	% Pos.	N	C	% Pos.	
Benzaldehyde				100	5	10%										10
Benzoic acid	102	5	20%	139	5	8%										8-20
Benzyl alcohol	102	5	8%	95	5 c	20%										8-20
Benzyl benzoate	102	5	4%	115	5	12%				142	?	7%	12	5	0%	0-12
Benzyl cinnamate	102	5	3%	110	5	19%				142	?	8%	12	5	9%	3-19
Benzyl isoferulate	102	1	2%													2
Benzyl salicylate										142	?	4%				4
Cinnamal e				71	2	21%				142	?	10%				10-21
Cinnamic acid	102	5	32%	128	5	25%	15	5	13%	142	?	18%				13-32
Cinnamyl alcohol	102	5	37%	93	5	25%				142	?	20%	12	10	0%	0-37
Cinnamyl cinnamate	102	5	20%										12	5	25%	20-25
Coniferyl alcohol	102	1	14%													14
Coniferyl benzoate a	102	1	28%	82	2 h	81%										28-81
Eugenol	102	5	19%	127	5	62%				142	?	14%	12	2	0%	0-62
Farnesol	102	5	4%	53	50 i	2%										2-4
Ferulic acid	102	5	0													0
Isoeugenol	102	2	27%	133	5 f	62%										27-62
Isoferulic acid	102	5	1%													1
Methyl cinnamate	102	10	3%				15	25	0%	142	?	4%				0-4
Nerolidol	102	1	3%	51	3 i	6%										3-6
Resorcinol monobenzoate b	102	2	16%													16
Vanillin	102	5	0	164	10 d	13%				142	?	6%	12	10	17%	0-17

a coniferyl benzoate is an unstable chemical, which is swiftly degraded in MP and in commercial test syringes; b resorcinol monobenzoate has not been identified in MP; however, patients sensitized to resorcinol monobenzoate almost (146,147) invariably react to MP (13,135,145); conversely, only 0-16% of patients sensitized to MP co-react to resorcinol monobenzoate (13,142); c 5% pet. or 10% alcohol; d 10% pet. or as is; e not a constituent of MP, may be a sensitizer after conversion in the skin of cinnamyl alcohol into cinnamal; f first 5% pet., later 2% pet.; g 5% pet., 2% or 0.5% pet.; h 2% pet., later 0.5% pet. (because of patch test sensitization); i in olive oil

C: test concentration (petrolatum unless otherwise indicated); N: number of patients allergic to MP tested; R: range of percentage positive reactions; % Pos.: percentage of patients with a positive patch test reaction

Patch testing with *fractions* of MP has given contradictory results (12,199) or results that were incomparable because of the use of different methods for fractionation (148).

Cross-reactions, pseudo-cross-reactions and co-reactions

General
For general information on cross-/pseudo-cross-/co-reactivity of fragrance chemicals with other fragrances, fragrance markers (fragrance mix I, fragrance mix II, colophonium, Myroxylon pereirae resin [balsam of Peru]) and essential oils see Chapter 1.2 General information on cross-reactions, pseudo-cross-reactions and co-reactions.

Co-reactivity of many fragrant chemicals with Myroxylon pereirae resin (MP) can be expected, when these are present in MP in concentrations adequate for elicitation of a positive patch test reaction (pseudo-cross-reactions). The chemicals that have been identified in MP are summarized in table 3.126.2.

Fragrance mix I
In a group of 102 patients allergic to MP, 49 (48%) co-reacted to the fragrance mix I (13). A high degree of co-reactivity between MP and FM I and *vice versa* has been observed in numerous studies. These two substances share common components, that is, eugenol, isoeugenol, and cinnamyl alcohol. FM I also contains cinnamal; MP does not, but cinnamyl alcohol in MP may be converted in the skin into cinnamal, which then acts as a sensitizer. Indeed, cinnamal reacts in 10-20% of the patients allergic to MP (12,150).

Propolis
Of 21 patients allergic to propolis, 19 (90%) co-reacted to MP 25% pet. (156). Conversely, of 11 patients positive to MP who had never come into contact with propolis, 5 (45%) also reacted to propolis (156). Of 7 patients reacting to propolis, 6 (86%) co-reacted to MP (164). Of 102 patients allergic to MP, 9 co-reacted to propolis (13). Chemicals present in both propolis and Myroxylon pereirae include benzoic acid, benzyl alcohol, benzyl benzoate, benzyl caffeate, benzyl cinnamate, benzyl ferulate, benzyl isoferulate, caffeic acid, cinnamic acid, cinnamyl alcohol, coniferyl benzoate, farnesol, nerolidol and vanillin (119).

Essential oils
Of 31 patients allergic to MP, 18 (58%) had positive patch test reactions to one (n=12), 2 (n=3), 5 (n=1), 6 (n=1) or 9 (n=1) of 35 essential oils. Most positive reactions were observed to cassia oil (cinnamon-derivatives) and to clove oil (eugenol) (151).

Resins and balsams
In patients allergic to MP, frequent co-reactions were observed to balsam of Tolu (INCI name: Myroxylon balsamum resin) (47%), Styrax / storax (INCI name: Liquidambar orientalis resin) (43%), Siam benzoin (INCI name: Styrax tonkinensis resin, contains 75% coniferyl benzoate and 10% benzoic acid) (80%), Sumatra benzoin (INCI name: Styrax benzoin gum) (43%) and Compound tincture of benzoin U.S.P (contains styrax, benzoin and balsam of Tolu) (90%) (12,14). In a group of 21 patients allergic to tincture of benzoin, 13 (62%) co-reacted to MP (203).

A series of resins and balsams was tested 10% in alcohol in a small series of patients allergic to MP. Six of eleven (55%) reacted to Opoponax (Commiphora erythrea glabrescens gum), 7 of 13 (54%) to Copaiba balsam (Copaifera reticulata balsam) and 3 to Galbanum (Ferula galbaniflua gum) (12). In addition, 3 of 14 MP-allergic patients (21%) reacted to an extract of poplar buds (the source material for propolis, which often co-reacts with MP), 7/20 (35%) to ginger resinoid 10% pet., and all 5 tested with Tiger Balm ® (12).

Other co-reactions
Positive patch test reactions to Myroxylon pereirae (and to the fragrance mix I) are very frequently observed in patients photoallergic to ketoprofen; this may be due to cross-reactivity, as there is a strong similarity between the standard structure of cinnamyl alcohol (which is present in both the fragrance mix I and Myroxylon pereirae) and the UVA–excited ketoprofen structure (6). This topic is further discussed in Chapter 3.36 Cinnamyl alcohol.

Patients sensitized to resorcinol monobenzoate almost (146,147) invariably react to MP (13,135,145); conversely, only 0-16% of patients sensitized to MP co-react to resorcinol monobenzoate (13,142). Resorcinol monobenzoate has not been identified in MP and the mechanism behind the co-reactivity is unknown, but may be related to benzoate / benzoic acid.

Of 11 patients with contact allergy to oranges (peel), 5 (45%) co-reacted to MP. Eight patients known to be sensitive to MP were patch tested with an ether extract of orange peel 10% pet. and 5 (63%) had strong reactions to the extract (12).

In 73 patients sensitive to MP, 34 (47%) co-reacted to vanilla. This is not – entirely - due to vanillin in both products, as vanilla has only a low concentration of vanillin and reactions to vanillin 10% pet. and vanillin pure were *less* frequent than reactions to vanilla (12).

A statistically significant overrepresentation has been found of simultaneous patch test reactions to MP and phenol-formaldehyde resins (PFR) (166). About 20% of those allergic to MP co-react to PFR. It was suggested that this was due to the presence of low-molecular weight phenols in both substances (165). Indeed, IN at least one patient, a non-relevant reaction to MP proved to be an indication of contact allergy to phenol-formaldehyde resins (165).

Other information on co-reactivity

Patients with a positive patch test reaction to Myroxylon pereirae resin have an increased risk of being polysensitized, i.e. having two or more additional contact allergies (107). In patients with polysensitization (defined as at least 3 positive patch test reactions), the following allergens were particularly associated with the MP: FM II (odds ratio [OR] 34.2), FM I (OR 17.3), propolis (OR 38.9), nickel sulfate (OR 23.8), colophonium (OR 46.2) and lanolin alcohols (OR 42.8) (93).

Patch test sensitization

A man was sensitized by a patch test with MP 25% pet. (149). Patch testing with fresh samples of MP may actively sensitize (14). Patch testing with MP 25% in lanoline occasionally showed delayed patch test reactions appearing after 7-14 days; whether these were simply 'delayed' reactions or were indicative of patch test sensitization was not investigated (12).

Presence in products

In 2013, in the USA, the allergen content of 187 unique pediatric cosmetics from 6 different retailers marketed in the United States as hypoallergenic was evaluated on the basis of labeling. Inclusion criteria were products marketed as pediatric and 'hypoallergenic', 'dermatologist recommended/tested', 'fragrance free', or 'paraben free'. Myroxylon pereirae resin was found to be present in three (1.6%) of the products (31).

In 2008, 66 different fragrance components (including 39 essential oils) were identified in 370 (10% of the total) topical pharmaceutical products marketed in Belgium; 13 of these (3.5%) contained Myroxylon pereirae resin (2).

Myroxylon pereirae resin and restrictive diets

Already in the 1939 and 1961, it was noted that the oral intake of MP or individual components of BP such as cinnamic acid, vanillin or eugenol, which are used as aromas in food and drink items, can cause a flare of dermatitis in some patients allergic to MP (12,200). Later, several such case reports were published (see the section 'Case reports / Foods and drinks / Foods and drinks Case reports' above).

In the 1980s, Danish investigators observed that the eczema of several patients with *negative* patch tests to MP could also flare following ingestion of food items containing balsams. In a preliminary open study, 42 individuals with eczema, in who neither history nor standard patch tests had revealed the cause of the dermatitis (9 with perianal dermatitis, 17 with bilateral hand eczema and 16 with eczema at other sites) were challenged with 900 mg MP orally once a day taken as capsules. Nine patients (21%) had unequivocal flares 1-3 days after the challenge with (sometimes generalized) pruritus and aggravation at the usual sites of the eczema. These 9 patients with a positive challenge were instructed to avoid food items suspected of containing balsams for at least one month. At the end of this period, five (56%) patients showed cessation of all symptoms and signs of eczema (177).

In a second study from the same investigators, during 1982-1984, placebo-controlled, double-blind, oral challenges with MP 1 gram once a day in 210 patients with various types of dermatitis were performed. Forty-five of them (21%) experienced a flare of their symptoms within 4 days after challenge with MP but not after placebo. Of 17 patients with a positive patch test to MP, 10 (59%) had a positive challenge, including all 4 patients with vesicular hand dermatitis. In MP-*negative* patients, the symptoms of 12/58 (21%) patients with vesicular hand eczema flared, as was the case in of 5/18 (28%) individuals with anogenital dermatitis, and of 3/8 (38%) with axillary eczema; of other patients, only 6 (9%) had a positive oral challenge. Patients with a positive reaction to MP but negative to placebo were instructed to avoid food items suspected to contain balsams including products containing the peel of citrus fruits, products flavored with essences, perfumed products, various types of cough medicines and lozenges, eugenol (used by dentists), ice cream, cola and other spiced soft drinks, spices such as cinnamon, cloves, vanilla, and curry and products made with these spices. Dietary restriction of the intake of balsams was followed by marked improvement or clearance of the dermatitis in approximately half of the patients who adhered to the diet for at least one month; only one of these patients had a positive patch test reaction to MP (178).

In a subsequent publication by this group of authors, the results of long-term dietary restrictions were reported (179). 64 patients participated in this study. 24 were patients who had positive patch tests to MP and in 40 individuals, the dermatitis had previously flared after oral challenge with MP. All 64 patients were asked to avoid food items suspected of containing balsams for 1 to 2 months and the dermatitis of 37 (58%) cleared or improved markedly. If an improvement had taken place, the patient was asked to continue to diet moderately; 6 months to 3 years later, 30 (47%) felt there was a long-term effect and 27 still followed the diet instructions to some degree. In the subgroup of the 24 patients with a positive patch test to MP, 15 (63%) reported benefit from the diet. Food items most commonly mentioned by patients as causes of flare of dermatitis were spices, cinnamon, curry, vanilla, liver paste, pickled herring, fruit, citrus fruit, cake, ice cream, vegetables, candy and wine (179).

In yet another study by the same group, the long term effect of dietary restrictions were investigated in 15 patients positive to MP and/or FM, 13 of who had a positive oral challenge test. Most had vesicular hand dermatitis. Nine of 15 (60%) reported long-term improvement from dietary restrictions. However, in a group of 12 patients with a *negative* patch test to MP, but a positive challenge, a higher percentage (67%, 6/9) reported long-term improvement. Food items most commonly mentioned as aggravating factors were citrus fruits, spices (unspecified), curry, cinnamon, bitters, wine and pickled herring (180).

In a final study from this group, in 1996, it was investigated whether the results of oral challenge with MP can predict possible benefit from a low-balsam diet (183). 46 patients with positive patch tests to MP and/or the fragrance mix I and a chronic dermatitis of a morphology consistent with endogenous (systemic) dermatitis, had experienced improvement of a low-balsam diet for 1-2 months and continued it. Twenty-eight of these (71%) stated in a questionnaire mailed after 1-3 years that they had long-term benefits from the diet treatment. In the group of 22 with a positive oral provocation test, 16 (73%) reported benefit; 3/10 (30%) who had a negative challenge, and 9/14 (64%) of the patients in who no oral challenge had been performed reported benefit. This indicated that the oral challenge procedure offers only limited assistance in selecting patients who are likely to benefit from diet treatment. Food items that caused flares of dermatitis in 31 patients included wine (n=14), candy (n=8), chocolate (n=7), cinnamon, curry, flavorings (all n=7), citrus fruit, cake, drinks with citrus / lemon (all n=6), jam, tomatoes (both n=5) and ketchup and bitters (both n=4) (183). It should be appreciated that in all these Danish studies, the symptoms were interpreted largely by the patients themselves, no objective signs have been observed by the investigators.

In a study from Finland, a group of 118 patients allergic to MP was patch tested with a series of (powdered) spices. There were positive reactions in 48 (41%) individuals: clove (46%), Jamaica pepper (21%), cinnamon (15%), ginger (6%), curry (6%), cardamom (4%), white pepper (3%), vanilla (3%) and paprika (3%). In a control group of MP-*negative* patients, only a few reactions were seen. 71 patients with MP allergy had peroral challenge tests with spices and 7 (10%) had reactions, notably a vesicular reaction of the hands but also 2 urticarial reactions; in 3, the patch test with spices had been negative. The author suggested that spices are potential but rare causes of contact dermatitis and that they may also cause skin symptoms, most frequently a pompholyx reaction, as a consequence of internal exposure in patients with contact allergy to MP (184).

Ten years later, the same author performed double-blind placebo-controlled peroral challenges with MP and spices in patients with delayed-type allergy to MP (185). 29 patients previously reacting to MP 25% pet. were tested with MP and spices. The 2nd patch test with MP was positive in 17 (59%) of the 29 re-tested patients. Positive reactions to one or more spices were seen in 5 patients (17%), all of who reacted to clove and Jamaica pepper and 2 to cinnamon. One of the patients with positive patch tests to the spices was negative to balsam of Peru in the 2nd patch test. Twenty-two patients were challenged perorally with 1 gram BP and a spice mixture with equal parts of cinnamon, Jamaica pepper, clove and vanilla sugar, in 2 capsules of 200 mg each, and glucose as placebo. Eight of the 22 patients (36%) reacted to the active substances, but not to placebo (of who 4 were MP-positive and 4 MP-negative). The 8 patients with positive oral challenges exhibited an increase of at least 30% in the number of palmar vesicles from ingested balsam of Peru or spices. It was concluded that it seems possible that ingested MP and related spices cause systemic contact reactions in patients with delayed contact allergy to MP (185).

In a retrospective study from the USA, published in 2001, of 45 patients allergic to MP and/or FM I in who balsam dietary avoidance was recommended, 21 (47%) reported complete or significant improvement primarily related to dietary modification. Nine of 45 did not follow the recommended diet, and of these, only 1 (11%) had significant improvement. Food items most commonly mentioned as causes of flare-up of dermatitis were tomatoes (which contain coniferyl alcohol and cinnamyl alcohol [196,209]), citrus, spices, cola/soda, chocolate, chili, cinnamon, beer/wine and vinegar (186). This study entirely relied on subjective patients' opinions (186).

From these studies, it may be concluded that some patients with dermatitis, especially those with forms suggestive of systemic contact dermatitis (vesicular hand dermatitis, other types of symmetrical dermatitis of the hands or feet, anogenital dermatitis, symmetrical dermatitis in the large skin folds such as the axillae and the groins [207]) may benefit from a diet restricting foods with balsams, and certain spices like cinnamon, cloves, and vanilla. Especially patients with a positive patch test to MP (and probably also some patients negative to MP but reacting to the fragrance mix I) but also patients with a negative patch test (177,178) may benefit. An oral provocation test is not very helpful in predicting which patients may benefit from a diet. As restrictive diets are difficult to adhere to and often disrupt normal social life, it is recommended that dietary treatment be restricted to those with severe, long-standing dermatitis which responds poorly to conventional treatment (179). Initially, the patients can be placed on a balsam-restricted diet for at least 4 weeks and, if the dermatitis significantly improves, long-term compliance can be recommended. Subsequently, one food group can be reintroduced into the diet every several weeks to ascertain whether this particular substance exacerbates the dermatitis. Those foods worsening the eruption would then be permanently have to be avoided (187).

A recently provided possibly useful suggestion is to divide the food allergens in MP into the following groups: eugenol, cinnamate, vanillin, benzoate, ferulic acid, and coniferin. By establishing to which of these the MP-allergic patient reacts, it is possible to give more specific instructions which foods, drinks and spices best be avoided. The authors suggested the following screening allergens for this: eugenol and isoeugenol (eugenol group), vanillin (vanillin group), cinnamal, cinnamyl alcohol and benzyl cinnamate (cinnamate group), benzoic acid and sodium benzoate (benzoate group), ferulic acid (ferulic acid group) and coniferyl alcohol (coniferin group). The authors in this article also provide a table with a large number of foods, drinks and spices, indicating which of the food allergens groups are present in them (and therefore need to be avoided in allergic patients) (195). Studies into the efficacy of such measures appear not to have been published thus far.

Detailed lists of high risk processed foods (foods and drinks that frequently contain ingredients high in MP) and of primary ingredients (vanillin, eugenol, cinnamon, etc.) can be found at https://www.dermatitisacademy.com/bop-diet/#toggle-id-6. However, one might start with avoiding citrus peels, spices (cinnamon, cloves, vanilla, curry) and products containing them, ice cream, flavored beverages and colas, and tomatoes.

It should be realized that no prospective studies to support advice for dietary restriction have been published in the last 25 years, that most of the work on this subject is practically oriented rather than scientific (208), that the placebo effect of following such a diet may probably be considerable and that provocation and elimination experiments after initial improvement on a diet have rarely been performed or at least rarely been published. In addition, there is a lack of validated evidence with regard to the balsam content of various foods and, consequently, there is no objective scientific measure to quantify dietary balsam exposure. Therefore, to the question 'What, if any, is the value of a low-balsam diet?', there is at this moment no convincing clear-cut answer (208).

Serial dilution testing
Seventeen patients allergic to MP were tested with a dilution series and 12 of them (63%) reacted to 10%, 9 (53%) to 5%, 1 (6%) to 1% and 0 to 0.5% MP in petrolatum (186).

OTHER SIDE EFFECTS

Photosensitivity

Photopatch testing in groups of patients

Photocontact allergy
The results of photopatch testing with MP in groups of patients suspected of photosensitivity disorders are shown in table 3.126.6. In six studies performed between 1980 and 2014, frequencies of sensitization were low, ranging from 0.1% to 2.4%. Some of the reactions were considered to be phototoxic rather than photoallergic (3,5). In 4 of the investigations, no (specific) relevance data were provided, in the fifth, the 4 observed positive photopatch tests had no clinical relevance (5). In other photopatch test studies, MP caused positive reactions in 0.7% and 3 % of two groups of 1129 and 1993 patients, respectively (217; no specific data available, article not read).

Phototoxicity
When MP is photopatch tested, occasional phototoxic reactions (1.4%) have been observed (30). Myroxylon pereirae resin has been found to cause delayed positive photopatch tests which were considered to be phototoxic in nature (39). Of 161 patients photopatch tested in 1979-1980 in Denmark with a mixture of various samples of MP, tested pure, 2 had a phototoxic reaction (157). In two other studies too, some positive photopatch tests were considered to be phototoxic (3,5).

Immediate-type photocontact reactions
Photocontact urticaria has been observed within 20 minutes after photopatch testing with MP in 3 patients (122). Myroxylon pereirae resin has been found to cause immediate positive photopatch tests, which were considered to be phototoxic in nature (39).

Table 3.126.6 Photopatch testing in groups of patients

Years and Country	Test conc. & vehicle	Number of patients tested	positive (%)		Selection of patients (S); Relevance (R); Comments (C)	Ref.
2010-2014 India	25% pet.	86	2	(2%)	S: patients with dermatitis of photo-exposed areas suspected of chronic actinic dermatitis; R: not stated	129
2005-2014 China	25% pet.	1292	31	(2.4%)	S: patients suspected of photodermatoses; R: not stated	123
1991-97 Germany, Austria, Switzerland	25% pet.	1261	4	(0.3%)	S: patients suspected of photosensitivity; R: not stated; there were also 21 (1.7%) phototoxic reactions	3
1993-1994 France		370	4	(1.1%)	S: patients with suspected photodermatitis; R: no relevance; C: (some of) the reactions were considered to be phototoxic by the authors	5
1985-1993 Italy		1050	10	(0.1%)	S: patients suspected of photoallergic contact dermatitis; R: not specified (78% for all photoallergens together)	4
1980-1 Denmark, Finland, Norway, Sweden	25% pet.	745	6	(0.8%)	S: patients with suspected photodermatoses; R: not specified; C: there were also 30 'plain' contact allergic reactions	121

Immediate-type reactions

General

Myroxylon pereirae resin can provoke an immediate-type reaction within 20-30 minutes, mostly consisting of erythema, less often also of wheals, in the majority of patients and healthy subjects. The frequency of such reactions is dose-dependent, higher concentrations having higher scores. Symptoms usually disappear within 1-3 hours. The causative ingredients have not clearly been identified. In some studies, patients with positive immediate reactions to MP co-reacted to benzoic acid (153,155), cinnamon / cinnamon oil (153,159), benzaldehyde (155), cinnamic acid (155), vanillin (153) or oil of cloves (high concentration of eugenol [159]). Benzoic acid is a well-known cause of non-immune immediate contact reactions. Other culprit ingredients probably are cinnamon-derivatives such as cinnamic acid (155,159), but cinnamal, also a well-known cause of non-immune immediate contact reactions, is not a constituent of MP. Another possible causative ingredient is eugenol (120).

Anaphylactic symptoms from patch testing with MP have been recorded in one study (163).

Routine testing

In a group of 60 patients with a positive patch test reaction to FM I and/or MP, 34 (57%) had immediate contact reactions to MP 25% pet. In a control group of 50 non-allergic patients, the percentage of immediate reactions was 58, which was not significantly different. It was concluded that these results underline the non-immunological nature of the immediate contact reactions (112).

In Greece, however, in the period 1996-1998, of 664 patients patch tested with MP, in who reactions were read after 30 minutes, 113 (17%) had positive immediate-type reactions. Of these, 10 (9%) later also proved to have delayed-type allergy to MP. The percentage was significantly higher than in patients with negative immediate reactions and also than in the entire group. It was suggested that allergen-specific immune responses may in fact be involved in immediate contact reactions (33,115,132). However, most other studies clearly point at an non-immune related pathogenesis.

In a group of 401 patients suffering from periorbital dermatitis, 9 (2.2%) had immediate contact reactions to the patch test with MP (44). Sixteen patients with atopic dermatitis were patch tested with MP and the reactions were read at 30 minutes; 3 (19%) showed erythema, termed 'immediate positive reactions' by the authors (117). Of 50 individuals who had open tests with MP 25% pet. on the forearm, 32 (64%) showed local macular erythema after 45 minutes, termed 'contact urticaria' by the authors (120). In a group of 246 patients reacting to the FM I, 16 (6.5%) had immediate contact reactions to MP (114).

Testing MP in various concentrations

Fifty-seven patients were tested with MP in 4 different concentrations for immediate contact reactions after 30 minutes. The percentage positive reactions at 1.25% was 19, at 2.5% 32, at 5% 39 and 56% reacted to MP 10% in petrolatum. Only 8% of all reactions was erythema plus edema, the rest erythema only. The higher concentrations more often induced whealing. Reactions could persist for up to three hours. The authors suggested that the reaction might be due to histamine-releasing effect of the substance (160).

In a study in the mid-1970's in Sweden, closed patch tests with BP in concentrations ranging from 1.56% to 50% and 11 of its components (benzoic acid 5%, benzaldehyde 5%, cinnamal 2% [not an ingredient of MP], cinnamyl alcohol 2%, cinnamic acid 5%, methyl cinnamate 0.5%, benzyl benzoate 5%, benzyl salicylate 2%, benzyl cinnamate 5%, eugenol 5%, vanillin 10%) were applied to the upper part of the back for a period of 30 minutes. The result was read immediately after removal and after every hour until the reaction disappeared. The tests were performed on

121 patients with different dermatoses and on 57 patients with chronic urticaria, the components only in 5 patients (not specified). MP gave rise to 9/121 (7.4%) and 16/57 (28%) patients, respectively. Most reactions were caused by the higher concentrations, with 12.5% < 25% < 50% pet. The reaction appeared earliest 10 minutes after application of MP and normally after 20 minutes and would fade within 2 hours. Conventional patch tests were negative.

Among the components of MP tested in 5 individuals, cinnamal caused 4 urticarial reactions, cinnamic acid 3, benzoic acid 3 and benzaldehyde 1. In seven patients repeat testing was performed. In five cases the urticarial reaction could be reproduced after a duration of 3-12 months. Oral provocation with 25 mg MP and 25 mg cinnamic acid failed to precipitate urticaria or other skin changes in four patients with urticaria and in one with allergic contact dermatitis. Passive transfer with serum from two patients to eight normal volunteers was negative. The urticarial reactions were diminished but not always inhibited by pre-treatment with oral antihistamines (clemastine 2 mg) (155).

Testing in patients with (contact) urticaria

In 1976, in Hungary, 6 patients were seen who had contact urticaria from deodorants, perfumed soaps or detergents, or urticaria, sometimes accompanied by angio-edema or anaphylaxis and gastro-intestinal symptoms (nausea, vomiting) from certain foods and drinks, notably cola, vermouth, chocolate, or foods flavored with vanilla or cinnamon. They all had positive immediate patch tests to MP, 2 to vanillin, 3 to cinnamon (oil), and one to benzoic acid (153).

In the UK, before 1981, 56 patients with 'ordinary chronic urticaria' were patch tested with MP 25% pet. The materials were removed and reactions read after 1 hour. There were 35 positive reactions, associated with 17 reactions to cinnamon oil 0.5% in and 4 to oil of cloves 0.2%. Thirteen of these 35 had a large weal after one hour, and of these, 10 also to cinnamon oil. There were only 2 delayed patch tests to MP (159).

In an associated survey in London, 8 out of 12 patients with chronic urticaria had positive immediate patch tests (IPTs) to MP and 7 of these were also positive to cinnamon. In 23 normal controls, positive IPTs were found with balsam of Peru in 4 subjects and with cinnamon in 12 subjects (including the 4 positive to balsam of Peru) (159). The authors stated 'It would seem that a positive IPT to balsam of Peru and cinnamon occurs in the majority of normal subjects as a nonspecific phenomenon due to direct release of vaso-active substances'. They did not speculate on an etiological role of MP in chronic urticaria (159).

In a study in the mid-1970's in Sweden, closed patch tests with BP on 57 patients with chronic urticaria gave rise to positive reactions in 16 (28%) of the patients. Oral provocation with 25 mg MP and 25 cinnamic acid failed to precipitate urticaria or other skin changes in four patients with urticaria (155).

A female patient had recurrent episodes of widespread urticaria. When patch tested, she showed a local response to MP and fragrance mix at both 30 and 60 minutes. Moreover, at 60 minutes, the patient developed widespread urticaria, unassociated with respiratory or other systemic symptoms, which lasted for about 6 hours before spontaneously disappearing. When the patient was instructed to strictly avoid further contact with such substances, this resulted in rapid and complete remission of symptoms, which lasted for 6 months of follow-up (116).

Another woman developed contact urticaria from a popular Polish eau de cologne. A patch test with BP was strongly positive after 20 minutes. She also had immediate positive reactions to ethyl vanillin, with which she had contact at work from its presence in toffee mass (154).

Other non-eczematous contact reactions

A consistent and significant association has been found between perfume contact allergy diagnosed by positive patch tests to the fragrance mix I and/or Myroxylon pereirae resin and symptoms elicited by fragrance products from the eyes and airways. The symptoms are mostly reported as occurring within seconds or minutes after airborne exposure to fragrance products. However, contact dermatitis in sensitized individuals usually develops hours to days after exposure to an allergen and immediate responses are not in agreement with a type IV immunological reaction. As yet, the mechanism remains undetermined (27).

In 3 pediatric patients with atopic eczema, including the scalp and leading to circumscribed alopecia, therapeutic exposure to balm-containing remedies (including a fluocinolone ointment) had apparently induced contact allergy to Myroxylon pereirae resin (balsam of Peru), and avoidance of these products led to resolution of scalp inflammation and alopecia (219).

LITERATURE

1   Uter W, Aberer W, Armario-Hita JC, Fernandez-Vozmediano JM, Ayala F, Balato A, et al. Current patch test
     results with the European baseline series and extensions to it from the 'European Surveillance System on
     Contact Allergy' network, 2007-2008. Contact Dermatitis 2012;67:9-19
2   Nardelli A, D'Hooge E, Drieghe J, Dooms M, Goossens A. Allergic contact dermatitis from fragrance components
     in specific topical pharmaceutical products in Belgium. Contact Dermatitis 2009;60:303-313

3   Neumann NJ, Hölzle E, Plewig G, Schwarz T, Panizzon RG, Breit R, et al. Photopatch testing: The 12-year experience of the German, Austrian and Swiss Photopatch Test Group. J Am Acad Dermatol 2000;42:183-192

4   Pigatto PD, Legori A, Bigardi AS,Guarrera M, Tosti A, Santucci B, et al. Gruppo Italiano recerca dermatiti da contatto ed ambientali Italian multicenter study of allergic contact photodermatitis: epidemiological aspects. Am J Contact Dermatitis 1996;7:158-163

5   Journe F, Marguery M-C, Rakotondrazafy J, El Sayed F, Bazex J. Sunscreen sensitization: a 5-year study. Acta Derm Venereol (Stockh) 1999;79:211-213

6   Foti C, Bonamonte D, Conserva A, , Stingeni L, Lisi P, Lionetti N, et al. Allergic and photoallergic contact dermatitis from ketoprofen: evaluation of cross-reactivities by a combination of photopatch testing and computerized conformational analysis. Curr Pharm Des 2008;14:2833-2839

7   Heisterberg MV, Menné T, Johansen JD. Contact allergy to the 26 specific fragrance ingredients to be declared on cosmetic products in accordance with the EU cosmetic directive. Contact Dermatitis 2011;65:266-275

8   Wetter DA, Yiannias JA, Prakash AV, Davis MDP, Farmer SA, el-Azhary RA. Results of patch testing to personal care product allergens in a standard series and a supplemental cosmetic series: an analysis of 945 patients from the Mayo Clinic Contact Dermatitis Group, 2000-2007. J Am Acad Dermatol 2010;63:789-798

9   Adams RM, Maibach HI, for the North American Contact Dermatitis Group. A five-year study of cosmetic reactions. J Am Acad Dermatol 1985;13:1062-1069

10 Davis MDP, Scalf LA, Yiannias JA, Cheng JF, El-Azhary RA, Rohlinger AL, et al. Changing trends and allergens in the patch test standard series. Arch Dermatol 2008;144:67-72

11 ESSCA Writing Group. The European Surveillance System of Contact Allergies (ESSCA): results of patch testing the standard series, 2004. J Eur Acad Dermatol Venereol 2008;22:174-181

12 Hjorth N. Eczematous allergy to balsams. Acta Derm Venereol 1961;41(suppl.46):1-216

13 Hausen BM. Contact allergy to Balsam of Peru. II. Patch test results in 102 patients with selected balsam of Peru constituents. Am J Cont Derm 2001;12:93-102

14 Hausen BM, Simatupang T, Bruhn G, Evers P, Koenig WA. Identification of new allergenic constituents and proof of evidence for coniferyl benzoate in Balsam of Peru. Am J Cont Derm 1995;6:199-208

15 Johansen JD, Anderson TF, Veien N, Avnstorp C, Andersen KE, Menné T. Patch testing with markers of fragrance contact allergy. Do clinical tests correspond to patients' self-reported problems? Acta Derm Venereol 1997;77:149-153

16 Zug KA, Warshaw EM, Fowler JF jr, Maibach HI, Belsito DL, Pratt MD, et al. Patch-test results of the North American Contact Dermatitis Group 2005-2006. Dermatitis 2009;20:149-160

17 Fransway AF, Zug KA, Belsito DV, et al. North American Contact Dermatitis Group patch test results for 2007-2008. Dermatitis 2013;24:10-21

18 Warshaw EM, Belsito DV, DeLeo VA, et al. North American Contact Dermatitis Group patch-test results, 2003-2004 study period. Dermatitis 2008;19:129-36

19 Wöhrl S, Hemmer W, Focke M, Götz M, Jarisch R. The significance of fragrance mix, balsam of Peru, colophony and propolis as screening tools in the detection of fragrance allergy. Br J Dermatol 2001;145:268-273

20 Firooz A, Nassiri-Kashani M, Khatami A, Gorouhi F, Babakoohi S, Montaser-Kouhsari L, et al. Fragrance contact allergy in Iran. J Eur Acad Dermatol Venereol 2010;24:1437-1441

21 Wenk KS, Ehrlich AE. Fragrance series testing in eyelid dermatitis. Dermatitis 2012;23:22-26

22 SCCP (Scientific Committee on Consumer Products). Opinion on Peru Balsam, 28 March 2006, SCCP/0988/06. Available at: http://ec.europa.eu/health/ph_risk/committees/04_sccp/docs/sccp_o_055.pdf

23 SCCFNP (Scientific Committee on Cosmetic Products and Non-Food Products Intended for Consumers). Opinion concerning An update of the initial list of perfumery materials which must not form part of fragrance compounds used in cosmetic products, 9 December 2003, SCCNFP/0771/03.
    Available at: http://ec.europa.eu/health/ph_risk/committees/sccp/documents/out251_en.pdf

24 Larsen WG. Perfume dermatitis. A study of 20 patients. Arch Dermatol 1977;113:623-626

25 Schnuch A, Lessmann H, Geier J, Frosch PJ, Uter W. Contact allergy to fragrances: frequencies of sensitization from 1996 to 2002. Results of the IVDK. Contact Dermatitis 2004;50:65-76

26 Baxter KF, Wilkinson SM, Kirk SJ. Hydroxymethyl pentylcyclohexene-carboxaldehyde (Lyral) as a fragrance allergen in the UK. Contact Dermatitis 2003;48:117-118

27 Elberling J, Linneberg A, Mosbech H, Dirksen A, Frolund L, Madsen F, et al. A link between skin and airways regarding sensitivity to fragrance products? Br J Dermatol 2004;151:1197-1203

28 Alinaghi F, Bennike NH, Egeberg A, Thyssen JP, Johansen JD. Prevalence of contact allergy in the general population: A systematic review and meta-analysis. Contact Dermatitis 2018 Oct 29. doi: 10.1111/cod.13119. [Epub ahead of print]

29 Veverka KK, Hall MR, Yiannias JA, Drage LA, El-Azhary RA, Killian JM, et al. Trends in patch testing with the Mayo Clinic standard series, 2011-2015. Dermatitis 2018;29:310-315

30   Hölzle E, Neumann N, Hausen B, Przybilla B, Schauder S, Hönigsmann H, et al. Photopatch testing: the 5-year experience of the German, Austrian and Swiss Photopatch Test Group. J Am Acad Dermatol 1991;25:59-68

31   Hamann CR, Bernard S, Hamann D, Hansen R, Thyssen JP. Is there a risk using hypoallergenic cosmetic pediatric products in the United States? J Allergy Clin Immunol 2015;135:1070-1071

32   An S, Lee AY, Lee CH, Kim DW, Hahm JH, Kim KJ, et al. Fragrance contact dermatitis in Korea: a joint study. Contact Dermatitis 2005;53:320-323

33   Katsarou A, Armenaka M, Kalogeromitros D, Koufou V, Georgala S. Contact reactions to fragrances. Ann Allergy Asthma Immunol 1999;82:449-455

34   Trattner A, David M. Patch testing with fine fragrances: comparison with fragrance mix, balsam of Peru and a fragrance series. Contact Dermatitis 2003:49:287-289

35   Cuesta L, Silvestre JF, Toledo F, Lucas A, Perez-Crespo M, Ballester I. Fragrance contact allergy: a 4-year retrospective study. Contact Dermatitis 2010;63:77-84

36   IFRA. Standard Peru balsam crude, 2007 (www.ifraorg.org/en-us/standards-library)

37   Uter W, Geier J, Schnuch A, Frosch PJ. Patch test results with patients' own perfumes, deodorants and shaving lotions: results of the IVDK 1998-2002. J Eur Acad Dermatol Venereol 2007;21:374-379

38   Uter W, Fießler C, Gefeller O, Geier J, Schnuch A. Contact sensitization to fragrance mix I and II, to *Myroxylon pereirae* resin and oil of tupentine: multifactorial analysis of risk factors based on data of the IVDK network. Flav Fragr J 2015;30:255-263

39   Addo HA, Ferguson J, Johnson BF, Frain-Bell W. The relationship between exposure to fragrance materials and persistent light reaction in photosensitivity dermatitis with actinic reticuloid syndrome. Br J Dermatol 1982;107:261-274

40   Foussereau J. Allergy to Dermophil Indien. Contact Dermatitis 1975;1:257

41   Goossens A. Cosmetic contact allergens. Cosmetics 2016, 3, 5; doi:10.3390/cosmetics3010005

42   Zaragoza-Ninet V, Blasco Encinas R, Vilata-Corell JJ, Pérez-Ferriols A, Sierra-Talamantes C, Esteve-Martínez A, de la Cuadra-Oyanguren J. Allergic contact dermatitis due to cosmetics: A clinical and epidemiological study in a tertiary hospital. Actas Dermosifiliogr 2016;107:329-336

43   Laguna C, de la Cuadra J, Martín-González B, Zaragoza V, Martínez-Casimiro L, Alegre V. Allergic contact dermatitis to cosmetics. Actas Dermosifiliogr 2009;100:53-60

44   Temesvári E, Pónyai G, Németh I, Hidvégi B, Sas S, Kárpáti S. Periocular dermatitis: a report of 401 patients. JEADV 2009;23:124-128

45   Thyssen JP, Uter W, Schnuch A, Linneberg A, Johansen JD. 10-year prevalence of contact allergy in the general population in Denmark estimated through the CE-DUR method. Contact Dermatitis 2007;57:265-272

46   Schnuch A, Uter W, Geier J, Gefeller O (for the IVDK study group). Epidemiology of contact allergy: an estimation of morbidity employing the clinical epidemiology and drug-utilization research (CE-DUR) approach. Contact Dermatitis 2002;47:32-39

47   DeKoven JG, Warshaw EM, Zug KA, Maibach HI, Belsito DV, Sasseville D, et al. North American Contact Dermatitis Group patch test results: 2015-2016. Dermatitis 2018;29:297-309

48   Silvestre JF, Mercader P, González-Pérez R, Hervella-Garcés M, Sanz-Sánchez T, Córdoba S, et al. Sensitization to fragrances in Spain: A 5-year multicentre study (2011-2015). Contact Dermatitis. 2018 Nov 14. doi: 10.1111/cod.13152. [Epub ahead of print]

49   Dittmar D, Schuttelaar MLA. Contact sensitization to hydroperoxides of limonene and linalool: Results of consecutive patch testing and clinical relevance. Contact Dermatitis 2018 Oct 31. doi: 10.1111/cod.13137. [Epub ahead of print]

50   Girbig M, Hegewald J, Seidler A, Bauer A, Uter W, Schmitt J. Type IV sensitizations in physical therapists: patch test results of the Information Network of Departments of Dermatology (IVDK) 2007-2011. J Dtsch Dermatol Ges 2013;11:1185-1192

51   Claßen A, Buhl T, Schubert S, Worm M, Bauer A, Geier J, Molin S; Information Network of Departments of Dermatology (IVDK) study group. The frequency of specific contact allergies is reduced in patients with psoriasis. Br J Dermatol. 2018 Aug 12. doi: 10.1111/bjd.17080. [Epub ahead of print]

52   O'Gorman SM, Torgerson RR. Contact allergy in cheilitis. Int J Dermatol 2016;55:e386-e391

53   Landeck L, Schalock PC, Baden LA, Gonzalez E. Periorbital contact sensitization. Am J Ophthalmol 2010;150:366-370

54   Warshaw EM, Ahmed RL, Belsito DV, DeLeo VA, Fowler JF Jr, Maibach HI, et al. Contact dermatitis of the hands: cross-sectional analyses of North American Contact Dermatitis Group Data, 1994-2004. J Am Acad Dermatol 2007;57:301-314

55   Saap L, Fahim S, Arsenault E, Pratt M, Pierscianowski T, Falanga V, Pedvis-Leftick A. Contact sensitivity in patients with leg ulcerations: a North American study. Arch Dermatol 2004;140:1241-1246

56   Pfützner W, Niedermeier A, Thomas P, Przybilla B. Hämatogen-allergisches Kontaktekzem auf Perubalsam (Systemic contact eczema against Balsam of Peru). J Dtsch Dermatol Ges 2003;1:719-721 (Article in German)

57 Warshaw EM, Maibach HI, Taylor JS, Sasseville D, DeKoven JG, Zirwas MJ, et al. North American Contact Dermatitis Group patch test results: 2011-2012. Dermatitis 2015;26:49-59

58 Warshaw EM, Belsito DV, Taylor JS, Sasseville D, DeKoven JG, Zirwas MJ, et al. North American Contact Dermatitis Group patch test results: 2009 to 2010. Dermatitis 2013;24:50-59

59 Lazarov A. European Standard Series patch test results from a contact dermatitis clinic in Israel during the 7-year period from 1998 to 2004. Contact Dermatitis 2006;55:73-76

60 Worm M, Brasch J, Geier J, Uter W, Schnuch A. Epikutantestung mit der DKG-Standardreihe 2001-2004. Hautarzt 2005;56:1114-1124

61 Carlsen BC, Menné T, Johansen JD. 20 Years of standard patch testing in an eczema population with focus on patients with multiple contact allergies. Contact Dermatitis 2007;57:76-83

62 Uter W, Hegewald J, Aberer W, Ayala F, Bircher AJ, Brasch J, et al. The European standard series in 9 European countries, 2002/2003 – First results of the European Surveillance System on Contact Allergies. Contact Dermatitis 2005;53:136-145

63 Pratt MD, Belsito DV, DeLeo VA, Fowler JF Jr, Fransway AF, Maibach HI, et al. North American Contact Dermatitis Group patch-test results, 2001-2002 study period. Dermatitis 2004;15:176-183

64 Hasan T, Rantanen T, Alanko K, Harvima RJ, Jolanki R, Kalimo K, et al. Patch test reactions to cosmetic allergens in 1995-1997 and 2000-2002 in Finland – a multicentre study. Contact Dermatitis 2005;53:40-45

65 Lindberg M, Edman B, Fischer T, Stenberg B. Time trends in Swedish patch test data from 1992 to 2000. A multi-centre study based on age- and sex-adjusted results of the Swedish standard series. Contact Dermatitis 2007;56:205-210

66 Wetter DA, Davis MDP, Yiannias JA, Cheng JF, Connolly SM, el-Azhary RA, et al. Patch test results from the Mayo Contact Dermatitis Group, 1998–2000. J Am Acad Dermatol 2005;53:416-421

67 Akyol A, Boyvat A, Peksari Y, Gurgey E. Contact sensitivity to standard series allergens in 1038 patients with contact dermatitis in Turkey. Contact Dermatitis 2005;52:333-337

68 Machovcova A, Dastychova E, Kostalova D, , Vojtechovska A, Reslova J, Smejkalova D, et al. Common contact sensitizers in the Czech Republic. Patch test results in 12,058 patients with suspected contact dermatitis. Contact Dermatitis 2005;53:162-166

69 Bruynzeel DP, Diepgen TL, Andersen KE, Brandão FM, Bruze M, Frosch PJ, et al (EECDRG). Monitoring the European Standard Series in 10 centres 1996–2000. Contact Dermatitis 2005;53:146-152

70 Fall S, Bruze M, Isaksson M, Lidén C, Matura M, Stenberg B, Lindberg M. Contact allergy trends in Sweden – a retrospective comparison of patch test data from 1992, 2000, and 2009. Contact Dermatitis 2015;72:297-304

71 Wentworth AB, Yiannias JA, Keeling JH, Hall MR, Camilleri MJ, Drage LA, et al. Trends in patch-test results and allergen changes in the standard series: a Mayo Clinic 5-year retrospective review (January 1, 2006, to December 31, 2010). J Am Acad Dermatol 2014;70:269-275

72 Uter W, Rämsch C, Aberer W, Ayala F, Balato A, Beliauskiene A, et al. The European baseline series in 10 European Countries, 2005/2006 – Results of the European Surveillance System on Contact Allergies (ESSCA). Contact Dermatitis 2009;61:31-38

73 Toholka R, Wang Y-S, Tate B, Tam M, Cahill J, Palmer A, Nixon R. The first Australian Baseline Series: Recommendations for patch testing in suspected contact dermatitis. Australas J Dermatol 2015;56:107-115

74 DeKoven JG, Warshaw EM, Belsito DV, Sasseville D, Maibach HI, Taylor JS, et al. North American Contact Dermatitis Group Patch Test Results: 2013-2014. Dermatitis 2017;28:33-46

75 Uter W, Amario-Hita JC, Balato A, Ballmer-Weber B, Bauer A, Belloni Fortina A, et al. European Surveillance System on Contact Allergies (ESSCA): results with the European baseline series, 2013/14 J Eur Acad Dermatol Venereol 2017;31:1516-1525

76 Warshaw EM, Buchholz HJ, Belsito DV et al. Allergic patch test reactions associated with cosmetics: Retrospective analysis of cross-sectional data from the North American Contact Dermatitis Group, 2001-2004. J Am Acad Dermatol 2009;60:23-38

77 Molin S, Bauer A, Schnuch A, Geier J. Occupational contact allergy in nurses: results from the Information Network of Departments of Dermatology 2003–2012. Contact Dermatitis 2015;72:164-171

78 Landeck L, John SM, Geier J. Periorbital dermatitis in 4779 patients – patch test results during a 10-year period. Contact Dermatitis 2014;70:205-212

79 Cooper SM, Shaw S. Eyelid dermatitis: an evaluation of 232 patch test patients over 5 years. Contact Dermatitis 2000;42:291-293

80 Zug KA, Kornik R, Belsito DV, DeLeo VA, Fowler JF Jr, Maibach HI, et al. Patch-testing North American lip dermatitis patients: Data from the North American Contact Dermatitis Group, 2001 to 2004. Dermatitis 2008;19:202-208

81 Katz AS, Sherertz EF. Facial dermatitis: Patch test results and final diagnoses. Am J Cont Dermat 1999;10:153-156

82   Herbst RA, Uter W, Pirker C, Geier J, Frosch PJ. Allergic and non-allergic periorbital dermatitis: patch test results of the Information Network of the Departments of Dermatology during a 5-year period. Contact Dermatitis 2004;51:13-19

83   IFRA. Standard Peru balsam extracts and distillates, 2008 (www.ifraorg.org/en-us/standards-library)

84   Lubbes S, Rustemeyer T, Sillevis Smitt JH, Schuttelaar ML, Middelkamp-Hup MA. Contact sensitization in Dutch children and adolescents with and without atopic dermatitis - a retrospective analysis. Contact Dermatitis 2017;76:151-159

85   Erfurt-Berge C, Geier J, Mahler V. The current spectrum of contact sensitization in patients with chronic leg ulcers or stasis dermatitis - new data from the Information Network of Departments of Dermatology (IVDK). Contact Contact Dermatitis 2017;77:151-158

86   Dinkloh A, Worm M, Geier J, Schnuch A, Wollenberg A. Contact sensitization in patients with suspected cosmetic intolerance: results of the IVDK 2006-2011. J Eur Acad Dermatol Venereol 2015;29:1071-1081

87   Schwensen JF, Johansen JD, Veien NK, Funding AT, Avnstorp C, Østerballe M, et al. Occupational contact dermatitis in hairdressers: an analysis of patch test data from the Danish Contact Dermatitis Group, 2002–2011. Contact Dermatitis 2014;70:233-237

88   Uter W, Lessmann H, Geier J, Schnuch A. Contact allergy to ingredients of hair cosmetics in female hairdressers and clients: an 8-year analysis of IVDK data. Contact Dermatitis 2003;49:236-240

89   Uter W, Lessmann H, Geier J, Schnuch A. Contact allergy to hairdressing allergens in female hairdressers and clients – current data from the IVDK 2003–2006. J Dtsch Dermatol Ges 2007;5:993-1001

90   Uter W, Gefeller O, John SM, Schnuch A, Geier J. Contact allergy to ingredients of hair cosmetics – a comparison of female hairdressers and clients based on IVDK 2007–2012 data. Contact Dermatitis 2014;71:13-20

91   Hillen U, Grabbe S, Uter W. Patch test results in patients with scalp dermatitis: analysis of data of the Information Network of Departments of Dermatology. Contact Dermatitis 2007;56:87-93

92   Feser A, Plaza T, Vogelgsang L, Mahler V. Periorbital dermatitis – a recalcitrant disease: causes and differential diagnoses. Brit J Dermatol 2008;159:858-863

93   Adler W, Gefeller O, Uter W. Positive reactions to pairs of allergens associated with polysensitization: analysis of IVDK data with machine-learning techniques. Contact Dermatitis 2017;76:247-251

94   Carøe TK, Ebbehøj NE, Tove Agner. Occupational dermatitis in hairdressers – influence of individual and environmental factors. Contact Dermatitis 2017;76:146-150

95   Ochi H, Cheng SWN, Leow YH, Goon ATJ. Contact allergy trends in Singapore – a retrospective study of patch test data from 2009 to 2013. Contact Dermatitis 2017;76:49-50

96   Higgins CL, Palmer AM, Cahill JL, Nixon RL. Occupational skin disease among Australian healthcare workers: a retrospective analysis from an occupational dermatology clinic, 1993–2014. Contact Dermatitis 2016;75:213-222

97   Ibler KS, Jemec GBE, Garvey LH, Agner T. Prevalence of delayed-type and immediate-type hypersensitivity in healthcare workers with hand eczema. Contact Dermatitis 2016;75:223-229

98   Sabroe RA, Holden CR, Gawkrodger DJ. Contact allergy to essential oils cannot always be predicted from allergy to fragrance markers in the baseline series. Contact Dermatitis 2016;74:236-241

99   Vejanurug P, Tresukosol P, Sajjachareonpong P, Puangpet P. Fragrance allergy could be missed without patch testing with 26 individual fragrance allergens. Contact Dermatitis 2016;74:230-235

100 Liu J, Li L-F. Contact sensitization to fragrances other than fragrance mix I in China. Contact Dermatitis 2015;73:252-253

101 Frosch PJ, Johansen JD, Schuttelaar M-LA, Silvestre JF, Sánchez-Pérez J, Weisshaar E, et al. (on behalf of the ESSCA network). Patch test results with fragrance markers of the baseline series – analysis of the European Surveillance System on Contact Allergies (ESSCA) network 2009–2012. Contact Dermatitis 2015;73:163-171

102 Mann J, McFadden JP, White JML, White IR, Banerjee P. Baseline series fragrance markers fail to predict contact allergy. Contact Dermatitis 2014;70:276-281

103 Uter W, Geier J, Frosch P, Schnuch A. Contact allergy to fragrances: current patch test results (2005–2008) from the Information Network of Departments of Dermatology. Contact Dermatitis 2010;63:254-261

104 Janach M, Kühne A, Seifert B, French FE, Ballmer-Weber B, Hofbauer GFL. Changing delayed-type sensitizations to the baseline series allergens over a decade at the Zurich University Hospital. Contact Dermatitis 2010;63:42-48

105 Barbaud A, Collet E, Le Coz CJ, Meaume S, Gillois P. Contact allergy in chronic leg ulcers: results of a multicentre study carried out in 423 patients and proposal for an updated series of patch tests. Contact Dermatitis 2009;60:279-287

106 Thyssen JP, Carlsen BC, Menné T, Johansen JD. Trends of contact allergy to fragrance mix I and Myroxylon pereirae among Danish eczema patients tested between 1985 and 2007. Contact Dermatitis 2008;59:238-244

107 Carlsen BC, Menné T, Johansen JD. Associations between baseline allergens and polysensitization. Contact Dermatitis 2008;59:96-102

108 Nardelli A, Carbonez A, Ottoy W, Drieghe J, Goossens A. Frequency of and trends in fragrance allergy over a 15-year period. Contact Dermatitis 2008;58:134-141

109 Jankićević J, Vesić S, Vukićević J, Gajić M, Adamič M, Pavlović MD. Contact sensitivity in patients with venous leg ulcers in Serbia: comparison with contact dermatitis patients and relationship to ulcer duration. Contact Dermatitis 2008;58:32-36

110 Zmudzinska M, Czarnecka-Operacz M, Silny W, Kramer L. Contact allergy in patients with chronic venous leg ulcers – possible role of chronic venous insufficiency. Contact Dermatitis 2006;54:100-105

111 Uter W, Balzer C, Geier J, Frosch PJ, Schnuch A. Patch testing with patients' own cosmetics and toiletries – results of the IVDK, 1998–2002. Contact Dermatitis 2005;53:226-233

112 Tanaka S, Matsumoto Y, Dlova N, Ostlere LS, Goldsmith PC, Rycroft RJG, et al. Immediate contact reactions to fragrance mix constituents and Myroxylon pereirae resin. Contact Dermatitis 2004;51:20-21

113 Api AM. Only Peru balsam extracts or distillates are used in perfumery. Contact Dermatitis 2006;54:179

114 Temesvári E, Németh I, Baló-Banga MJ, Husz S, Kohánka V, Somos Z, et al. Multicentre study of fragrance allergy in Hungary: Immediate and late type reactions. Contact Dermatitis 2002;46:325-330

115 Katsarou A, Armenaka M, Ale I, Koufou V, Kalogeromitros D. Frequency of immediate reactions to the European standard series. Contact Dermatitis 1999;41:276-279

116 Cancian M, Belloni Fortini A, Peserico A. Contact urticaria syndrome from constituents of balsam of Peru and fragrance mix in a patient with chronic urticaria. Contact Dermatitis 1999;41:300

117 Abifadel R, Mortureux P, Perromat M, Ducombs G, Taier A. Contact sensitivity to flavourings and perfumes in atopic dermatitis. Contact Dermatitis 1992;27:43-46

118 Broeckx W, Blondeel A, Dooms-Goossens A, Achten G. Cosmetic intolerance. Contact Dermatitis 1987;16:189-194

119 De Groot AC, Popova MP, Bankova VS. An update on the constituents of poplar-type propolis. Wapserveen, The Netherlands: acdegroot publishing, 2014, 11 pages. ISBN/EAN: 978-90-813233-0-7. Available at: https://www.researchgate.net/publication/262851225_AN_UPDATE_ON_THE_CONSTITUENTS_OF_POPLAR-TYPE_PROPOLIS

120 Emmons WW, Marks JG Jr. Immediate and delayed reactions to cosmetic ingredients. Contact Dermatitis 1985;13:258-265

121 Wennersten G, Thune P, Brodthagen H, Jansen C, Rystedt I, Crames M, et al. The Scandinavian multicenter photopatch study: Preliminary results. Contact Dermatitis 1984;10:305-309

122 Thune P. Photosensitivity and allergy to cosmetics. Contact Dermatitis 1981;7:54-55

123 Hu Y, Wang D, Shen Y, Tanh, H. Photopatch testing in Chinese patients over 10 years. Dermatitis 2016;27:137-142

124 Assier H, Tetart F, Avenel-Audran M, Barbaud A, Ferrier-le Bouëdec MC, Giordano-Labadie F, et al. Is a specific eyelid patch test series useful? Results of a French prospective study. Contact Dermatitis 2018;79:157-161

125 Belsito DV, Fowler JF Jr, Sasseville D, Marks JG Jr, De Leo VA, Storrs FJ. Delayed-type hypersensitivity to fragrance materials in a select North American population. Dermatitis 2006;17:23-28

126 Strauss RM, Orton DI. Allergic contact cheilitis in the United Kingdom: a retrospective study. Dermatitis 2003;14:75-77

127 Fisher AA. The clinical significance of patch test reactions to balsam of Peru. Cutis 1976;13:910-913

128 Rietschel RL, Fowler JF, Jr, Eds. Fisher's Contact Dermatitis, 6th edition. Hamilton BC Decker Inc. 2008: 418,702,703

129 Sharma VK, Bhari N, Wadhwani AR, Bhatia R. Photo-patch and patch tests in patients with dermatitis over the photo-exposed areas: A study of 101 cases from a tertiary care centre in India. Australas J Dermatol 2018;59:e1-e5

130 Machet L, Couhe C, Perrinaud A, Hoarau C, Lorette G, Vaillant L. A high prevalence of sensitization still persists in leg ulcer patients: a retrospective series of 106 patients tested between 2001 and 2002 and a meta-analysis of 1975-2003. Br J Dermatol 2004;150:929-935

131 Katoulis AC, Stavrianeas NG, Katsarou A, Antoniou C, Georgala S, Rigopoulos D, et al. Evaluation of the role of contact sensitization and photosensitivity in the pathogenesis of poikiloderma of Civatte. Br J Dermatol 2002;147:493-497

132 Katsarou A, Armenaka M, Kalogeromitros D, Koufou V, Georgala S. Contact reactions to fragrances. Ann Allergy Asthma Immunol 1999;82:1-7

133 Opinion of the Scientific Committee on Cosmetic Products and Non-Food Products Intended for Consumers concerning 'The 1st update of the inventory of ingredients employed in cosmetic products. Section II: Perfume and aromatic raw materials', 24 October 2000, SCCNFP/0389/00, final. Available at: http://ec.europa.eu/health/ph_risk/committees/sccp/documents/out131_en.pdf

134 Bråred Christensson J, Hellsén S, Börje A, Karlberg A-T. Limonene hydroperoxide analogues show specific patch test reactions. Contact Dermatitis 2014;70:291-299

135 Jordan WP. Clothing and shoe dermatitis. Postgrad Med 1972;52:143-148

136 Spirig W, Elsner P. Hörstückekzem auf die Weichplastikzusätze Resorcin-Monobenzoat und Triphenylphosphat. Akt Dermatol 1995;21:51-53

137 Kanerva L, Tarvainen K, Jolanki R, Henriks-Eckerman ML, Estlander T. Airborne occupational allergic contact dermatitis to trimethylolpropane triacrylate (TMPTA) used in the manufacture of printed circuit boards. Contact Dermatitis 1998;38:292-294

138 Ongenae K, Matthieu L, Constandt L, Van Hecke E. Contact allergy to resorcinol monobenzoate. Dermatology 1998;196:470-473

139 Jordan WP. Resorcinol monobenzoate, steering wheels, peruvian balsam. Arch Derm 1973;108:278

140 Calnan CD. Resorcinol monobenzoate. Contact Dermatitis 1975;1:59-60

141 Jordan WP, Dahl MV. Contact dermatitis from cellulose ester plastics. Arch Dermatol 1972;105:880-885

142 Ljunggren B. Contact dermatitis to estradiol benzoate. Contact Dermatitis 1981;7:141-144

143 Sonnex TS, Rycroft RJG. Dermatitis from phenyl salicylate in safety spectacle frames. Contact Dermatitis 1986;14:268-270

144 Telang GH, Brod BA. Allergic contact dermatitis to eyeglass frame nose pieces. J Am Acad Dermatol 1994;31:114-115

145 Goossens A, Blondeel S, Zimerson E. Resorcinol monobenzoate: a potential sensitizer in a computer mouse. Contact Dermatitis 2002;47:235

146 Tung RC, Taylor JS. Contact dermatitis from polyvinyl chloride identification bands. Am J Contact Dermat 1998;9:234-236

147 Nakagawa M, Kawai K, Kawai K. Cross-sensitivity between resorcinol, resorcinol monobenzoate and phenyl salicylate. Contact Dermatitis 1992;27:199-200

148 Øxholm A, Heidenheim M, Larsen E, Batsberg W, Menné T. Extraction and patch testing of methylcinnamate, a newly recognized fraction of balsam of Peru. Am J Cont Dermat 1990;1:43-46

149 Calnan CD. Active sensitization to para and balsam of Peru. Contact Dermatitis 1975;1:126-127

150 Mitchell JC, Calnan CD, Clendenning WE, Cronin E, Hjorth N, Magnusson B, et al. Patch testing with some components of balsam of Peru. Contact Dermatitis 1976;2:57-58

151 Rudzki E, Grzywa Z, Bruo WS. Sensitivity to 35 essential oils. Contact Dermatitis 1976;2:196-200

152 Panconesi E, Sertoli A, Spallazani P, Giorgini S. Balsam of Peru sensitivity from a perfumed cutting fluid in a laser factory. Contact Dermatitis 1980;6:297

153 Temesvári E, Soos G, Podányi B, Kovács I, Nemeth I. Contact urticaria provoked by balsam of Peru. Contact Dermatitis 1978;4:65-68

154 Rudzki E, Grzywa Z. Immediate reactions to balsam of Peru, cassia oil and ethyl vanillin. Contact Dermatitis 1976;2:360-361

155 Forsbeck M, Skog E. Immediate reactions to patch tests with balsam of Peru. Contact Dermatitis 1977;3:201-205

156 Rudzki E, Grzywa Z. Dermatitis from propolis. Contact Dermatitis 1983;9:40-45

157 Kroon S. Standard photopatch testing with Waxtar®, para-aminobenzoic acid, potassium dichromate and balsam of Peru. Contact Dermatitis 1983;9:5-9

158 Bedello PG, Goitre M, Cane D. Contact dermatitis and flare from food flavouring agents. Contact Dermatitis 1982;8:143-144

159 Warin RP, Smith RJ. Chronic urticaria investigations with patch and challenge tests. Contact Dermatitis 1982;8:117-121

160 Friis B, Hjorth N. Immediate reactions to patch tests with balsam of Peru. Contact Dermatitis Newsletter 1973;13:389

161 Warshaw EM, Zug KA, Belsito DV, Fowler JF Jr, DeKoven JG, Sasseville D, et al. Positive patch-test reactions to essential oils in consecutive patients: Results from North America and Central Europe. Dermatitis 2017;28:246-252

162 Fisher AA. Perfume dermatitis in children sensitized to balsam of Peru in topical agents. Cutis 1990;45:21-23

163 Lahti A, Maibach HI. Immediate contact reactions. In: Menné T, Maibach HI, Eds. Exogenous dermatoses, Environmental contact dermatitis. Boca Raton, Fl., USA: CRC Press, 1990:21-35. Data cited in: De Groot AC, Weyland JW, Nater JP. Unwanted effects of cosmetics and drugs used in dermatology, 3rd Edition. Amsterdam – London – New York – Tokyo: Elsevier, 1994

164 Hausen BM, Evers P, Stüwe H-T, König WA, Wollenweber E. Propolis allergy (IV) Studies with further sensitizers from propolis and constituents common to propolis, poplar buds and balsam of Peru. Contact Dermatitis 1992;26:34-44

165 Bruze M. A nonrelevant contact allergy to balsam of Peru as an indication of a relevant contact allergy to phenol-formaldehyde resin. Am J Cont Dermat 1994;5:162-164

166 Bruze M. Simultaneous reactions to phenol-formaldehyde resins colophony/hydrpabietyl alcohol and balsam of peru/perfume mixture. Contact Dermatitis 1986;14:119-120

167 Hjorth N. The Prosser-White oration 1980. Skin reactions to balsams and perfumes. Clin Exp Dermatol 1982;7:1-9

168 Avalos-Peralta P, García-Bravo B, Camacho FM. Sensitivity to Myroxylon pereirae resin (balsam of Peru). A study of 50 cases. Contact Dermatitis 2005;52:304-306

169 Rudzki E, Rebandel P. 100 patients positive to balsam of Peru observed in Warsaw (Poland). Contact Dermatitis 2006;55:255

170 Rudzki E, Rebandel P, Parapura K. Alergeny w wyprysku podudzi (Allergens of stasis dermatitis). Przegl Dermatol (Warszawa, Poland) 2004;91:127-130 (article in Polish)

171 Amado A, Taylor JS. Balsam of Peru or Balsam of El Salvador? Contact Dermatitis 2006;55:119

172 Ung CY, White JML, White IR, Banerjee P, McFadden JP. Patch testing with the European baseline series fragrance markers: a 2016 update. Br J Dermatol 2018;178:776-780

173 Thyssen J P, Menné T, Linneberg A, Johansen JD. Contact sensitization to fragrances in the general population: a Koch's approach may reveal the burden of disease. Br J Dermatol 2009;160:729-735

174 Heisterberg MV, Andersen KE, Avnstorp C, Kristensen B, Kristensen O, Kaaber K, et al. Fragrance mix II in the baseline series contributes significantly to detection of fragrance allergy. Contact Dermatitis 2010;63:270-276

175 Bonnevie P. Some experiences of war-time industrial dermatoses. Acta Derm Venereol 1948;28:231-237

176 Nardelli A, Carbonez A, Drieghe J, Goossens A. Results of patch testing with fragrance mix 1, fragrance mix 2, and their ingredients, and Myroxylon pereirae and colophonium, over a 21-year period. Contact Dermatitis 2013;68:307-313

177 Veien NK, Hattel T, Justesen O, Nørholm A. Oral challenge with balsam of Peru in patients with eczema: a preliminary study. Contact Dermatitis 1983;9:75-76

178 Veien NK, Hattel T, Justesen O, Nørholm N. Oral challenge with balsam of Peru. Contact Dermatitis 1985;12:104-107

179 Veien NK, Hattel T, Justesen O, Nørholm A. Reduction of intake of balsams in patients sensitive to balsam of Peru. Contact Dermatitis 1985;12:270-273

180 Veien NK, Hattel T, Justesen O, Nørholm A. Dietary restrictions in the treatment of adult patients with eczema. Contact Dermatitis 1987;17:223-227

181 Fisher AA. The clinical significance of positive patch test reactions to balsam of Peru. Cutis 1974;13:909-913

182 Pirilä V. Endogenic contact eczema. Allergie und Asthma 1970;16:15-19

183 Veien NK, Hattel T, Laurberg G. Can oral challenge with balsam of Peru predict possible benefit from a low-balsam diet? Am J Cont Dermat Dermatitis 1996;7:84-87

184 Niinimäki A. Delayed-type allergy to spices: Contact Dermatitis 1984;11:34-40

185 Niinimäki A. Double-blind placebo-controlled peroral challenges in patients with delayed-type allergy to balsam of Peru. Contact Dermatitis 1995;33:78-83

186 Salam TN, Fowler JF Jr. Balsam-related systemic contact dermatitis. J Am Acad Dermatol 2001;45:377-381

187 Belsito DV. Surviving on a balsam-restricted diet: cruel and unusual punishment or medically necessary therapy? J Am Acad Dermatol 2001;45:470-472

188 Pfutzner W, Thomas P, Niedermeier A, Pfeiffer C, Sander C, Przybilla B. Systemic contact dermatitis elicited by oral intake of balsam of Peru. Acta Derm Venereol 2003;83:294-295

189 Jacob SE, Steele T. Tongue erosions and diet cola. Ear Nose Throat J 2007;86:232-233

190 Johansen JD. Contact allergy to fragrances: clinical and experimental investigations of the fragrance mix and its ingredients. Contact Dermatitis 2002;46(suppl.3):1-31

191 Fabbro SK, Zirwas MJ. Systemic contact dermatitis to foods: nickel, BOP, and more. Curr Allergy Asthma Rep 2014;14:463 (7 pages)

192 Bruynzeel D, van den Hoogenband H, Koedijk F. Purpuric vasculitis-like eruption in a patient sensitive to balsam of Peru. Contact Dermatitis 1984;11:207-209

193 Meneghini C L, Angelini G. Secondary polymorphic eruptions in allergic contact dermatitis. Dermatologica 1981;163:63-70 (data cited in ref. 192)

194 Bonnevie P. Aetiologie und pathogenese der Ekzemkrankheiten. Copenhagen: Busck, 1939

195 Scheman A, Rakowski EM, Chou V, Chhatriwala A, Ross J, Jacob SE. Balsam of Peru: past and future. Dermatitis 2013;24:153-160

196 Srivastava D, Cohen D. Identification of the constituents of balsam of Peru in tomatoes. Dermatitis 2009;20:99-105

197 Mammerler V. Contribution to the analysis and quality control of Peru Balsam. PhD Thesis, University of Vienna, Austria, 2007. Available at: http://othes.univie.ac.at/4056/1/2009-03-23_0201578.pdf

198 Seo SM, Park HM, Park IK. Larvicidal activity of ajowan (Trachyspermum ammi) and Peru balsam (Myroxylon pereira) oils and blends of their constituents against mosquito, Aedes aegypti, acute toxicity on water flea, Daphnia magna, and aqueous residue. J Agric Food Chem 2012;60:5909-5914

199 Matthies C, Dooms-Goossens A, Lachapelle J-M, Lahti A, Menné T, White IR, et al. Patch testing with fractionated balsam of Peru. Contact Dermatitis 1988;19:384-385

200 Hill H, Jacob SE. Peri-anal ulcerations in a patient with essential pruritus. Dermatitis 2015;26:292-293

201 Herro EM, Jacob SE. Systemic contact dermatitis – Kids and ketchup. Pediatr Dermatol 2013;30:e32–e33

202 Matiz C, Jacob SE. Systemic contact dermatitis in children: How an avoidance diet can make a difference. Pediatr Dermatol 2011;28:368-374

203 Gilissen L, Huygens S, Goossens A. Allergic contact dermatitis caused by topical herbal remedies: importance of patch testing with the patients' own products. Contact Dermatitis 2018;78:177-184

204 Nanda A, Wasan A. Allergic contact dermatitis to balsam of Peru. Ann Allergy Asthma Immunol 2016;117:208-209

205 Opinion of the Scientific Committee on Cosmetic Products and Non-Food Products Intended for Consumers concerning ' An initial list of perfumery materials which must not form part of cosmetic products except subject to the Restrictions and Conditions laid down, 25 September 2001, SCCNFP/0392/00, final. Available at: http://ec.europa.eu/health/archive/ph_risk/committees/sccp/documents/out150_en.pdf

206 Artüz F, Yılmaz E, Külcü Çakmak S, Polat Düzgün A. Contact sensitisation in patients with chronic leg ulcers. Int Wound J 2016;13:1190-1192

207 Kulberg A, Schliemann S, Elsner P. Contact dermatitis as a systemic disease. Clin Dermatol 2014;32:414-419

208 Wolf R, Orion E, Ruocco E, Baroni A, Ruocco V. Contact dermatitis: facts and controversies. Clin Dermatol 2013;31:467-478

209 Paulsen E, Christensen LP, Andersen KE. Tomato contact dermatitis. Contact Dermatitis 2012;67:321-327

210 Tan S, Tam MM, Nixon RL. Allergic contact dermatitis to Myroxylon pereirae (Balsam of Peru) in papaw ointment causing cheilitis. Australas J Dermatol 2011;52:222-223

211 Uter W, Johansen JD, Börje A, Karlberg A-T, Lidén C, Rastogi S, Roberts D, White IR. Categorization of fragrance contact allergens for prioritization of preventive measures: clinical and experimental data and consideration of structure–activity relationships. Contact Dermatitis 2013;69:196-230

212 SCCS (Scientific Committee on Consumer Safety). Opinion on Fragrance allergens in cosmetic products, 26-27 June 2012, SCCS/1459/11. Available at: https://ec.europa.eu/health/sites/health/files/scientific_committees/consumer_safety/docs/sccs_o_102.pdf

213 Dooms-Goossens, A, Kerre S, Drieghe J, Bossuyt L, DeGreef H. Cosmetic products and their allergens. Eur J Dermatol 1992;2:465-468

214 Ananda Apothecary, Boulder, Colorado, USA. Available at: https://www.anandaapothecary.com/media/catalog/product/p/e/peru_balsam_lia105bp.pdf.

215 Plant therapy. Available at: https://www.planttherapy.com/test_reports/Peru%20Balsam%20PN0100.pdf

216 European Medicines Agency. Committee on Herbal Medicinal Products (HMPC). Assessment report on Myroxylon balsamum (L.) Harms var. pereirae (Royle) Harms, balsamum. 31 May 2016, EMA/HMPC/712648/2014. Available at: www.ema.europa.eu/documents/herbal-report/final-assessment-report-myroxylon-balsamum-l-harms-var-pereirae-royle-harms-balsamum_en.pdf217

217 Hänsel R, Keller K, Rimpler H, Schneider G, Eds. Hagers Handbuch der Pharmazeutischen Praxis. Drogen E-O. Vol 5, 4th Edition. Berlin, Germany: Springer-Verlag, 1993: 894-902 (data cited in ref. 216)

218 De Groot AC, Schmidt E. Essential oils: contact allergy and chemical composition. Boca Raton, Fl., USA: CRC Press, Taylor and Francis Group, 2016 (ISBN 9781482246407)

219 Admani S, Goldenberg A, Jacob SE. Contact alopecia: Improvement of alopecia with discontinuation of fluocinolone oil in individuals allergic to balsam fragrance. Pediatr Dermatol 2017;34:e57-e60

Chapter 3.127 NARCISSUS POETICUS FLOWER EXTRACT

IDENTIFICATION

Description/definition : Narcissus poeticus flower extract is an extract of the flowers of *Narcissus poeticus* L.,
Agavaceae

Chemical class(es) : Botanical products and botanical derivatives

Other names : Narcissus absolute

CAS registry number(s) : 90064-26-9

EC number(s) : 290-087-3

RIFM monograph(s) : Food Cosmet Toxicol 1978;16:827 (special issue IV)

Function(s) in cosmetics : EU: perfuming; tonic. USA: fragrance ingredients

Patch testing : Narcissus poeticus absolute 2% pet. (Chemotechnique, SmartPracticeEurope,
SmartPracticeCanada)

GENERAL

Narcissus poeticus flower extract is very scarce and, partly for that reason, very rarely used perfume ingredient. The raw material for this product is made from a solvent extraction of the flowers of *Narcissus poeticus*. The material is a viscous, dark brown or dark orange to olive brown liquid of heavy, honey-like, deep sweet floral odor with a strong green back note and a somewhat bitter, very tenacious dry out note (www.chemotechnique.se).

The most important ingredients of Narcissus absolute (odoriferous part 20%) are cited to be alpha-terpineol (23.7%), *trans*-isoeugenyl methyl ether (20.0%), benzyl benzoate (19.4%), coumarin (6.9%), benzyl alcohol (5.0%), 3-carene (3.4%), phenethyl alcohol (2.2%), ethyl palmitate (2.2%), cinnamyl alcohol (2.2%), phenylpropyl acetate (1.7%), 1,8-cineole (1.5%), caryophyllene (1.0%), and benzyl acetate (0.7%) (3). Of course these concentrations are merely an indication, as the compositions of botanical extracts often differ considerably.

CONTACT ALLERGY

General

The SCCS (Scientific Committee on Consumer Safety), in a 2012 Opinion on Fragrance allergens in cosmetic products, has marked *Narcissus* species extracts as 'established contact allergen in humans' (10,11).

Patch testing in groups of patients

Results of studies testing Narcissus absolute in consecutive patients suspected of contact dermatitis (routine testing) are shown in table 3.127.1. Results of testing in groups of *selected* patients (e.g. patients with known or suspected fragrance or cosmetic dermatitis, individuals with eyelid dermatitis) are shown in table 3.127.2.

Patch testing in consecutive patients suspected of contact dermatitis: routine testing

In three studies in which routine testing with Narcissus absolute 2% in petrolatum was performed, frequencies of sensitization were 0.5%, 0.7% and 1.3% (4,5,9). In two of these investigations, the relevance of the positive patch test reactions was not mentioned (4,5), in the third not specified for Narcissus absolute (9).

Table 3.127.1 Patch testing in groups of patients: Routine testing

Years and Country	Test conc. & vehicle [b]	Number of patients tested	positive (%)	Selection of patients (S); Relevance (R); Comments (C)	Ref.
2010-2011 China	2% pet.	296	2 (0.7%)	R: 67% for all fragrances tested together (excluding FM I)	9
2000-2008 IVDK	2% pet.	2446	12 (0.5%) [a]	R: not stated	5
1998-2000 Six European countries	2% pet.	1606	21 (1.3%)	R: not stated	4

FM: Fragrance mix

Patch testing in groups of selected patients

In six studies in which groups of selected patients were patch tested with Narcissus absolute 2% pet., frequencies of sensitization ranged from 0.6% to 6.6% (1,2,5,7,8,12, Table 3.127.2). In four out of six, the frequency was 1% or lower. The high rate of 6.6% positive reactions was observed in an international study in a group of 167 patients with known or suspected fragrance sensitivity, but the relevance of the reactions was not mentioned (1). In only one study was the issue of relevance addressed. In this study from the USA, all 8 positive reactions were considered to be relevant (2). However, this study had certain flaws: there was a high rate of macular erythema (which was scored as positive) and weak reactions and relevance figures included 'questionable' and 'past' relevance (2).

Table 3.127.2 Patch testing in groups of patients: Selected patient groups

Years and Country	Test conc. & vehicle [a]	Number of patients tested	positive (%)		Selection of patients (S); Relevance (R); Comments (C)	Ref.
2011-2015 Spain	2% pet.	607	13	(2.1%)	S: patients previously reacting to FM I, FM II, Myroxylon pereirae resin or hydroxyisohexyl 3-cyclohexene carboxaldehyde in the baseline series and subsequently tested with a fragrance series; R: not stated	12
2006-2011 IVDK	2% pet.	513	4	(0.8%)	S: patients with suspected cosmetic intolerance; R: not stated	8
2006-2010 USA		100	1	(1.0%)	S: patients with eyelid dermatitis; R: not stated	7
2000-2008 IVDK	2% pet.	809	5	(0.6%)	S: patients with dermatitis suspected of causal exposure to fragrances; R: not stated	5
2000-2007 USA	2% pet.	863	8	(0.9%)	S: patients who were tested with a supplemental cosmetic screening series; R: 100%; C: weak study: a. high rate of macular erythema and weak reactions; b. relevance figures included 'questionable' and 'past' relevance	2
<1996 Japan, Europe, USA	2% pet.	167	11	(6.6%)	S: patients with known or suspected fragrance sensitivity; R: not stated	1

[a] mostly Narcissus (poeticus) absolute

IVDK: Information Network of Departments of Dermatology, Germany, Switzerland, Austria (www.ivdk.org)

Case reports and case series

Case reports of allergic contact dermatitis from Narcissus poeticus flower extract have not been found.

Cross-reactions, pseudo-cross-reactions and co-reactions

For general information on cross-/pseudo-cross-/co-reactivity of fragrance chemicals with other fragrances, fragrance markers (fragrance mix I, fragrance mix II, colophonium, Myroxylon pereirae resin [balsam of Peru]) and essential oils see Chapter 1.2 General information on cross-reactions, pseudo-cross-reactions and co-reactions.

Co-reactivity between Narcissus absolute and the Compositae mix has been observed (6).

LITERATURE

1   Larsen W, Nakayama H, Fischer T, Elsner P, Burrows D, Jordan W, et al. Fragrance contact dermatitis: A worldwide multicenter investigation (Part I). Am J Cont Dermat 1996;7:77-83

2   Wetter DA, Yiannias JA, Prakash AV, Davis MDP, Farmer SA, el-Azhary RA. Results of patch testing to personal care product allergens in a standard series and a supplemental cosmetic series: an analysis of 945 patients from the Mayo Clinic Contact Dermatitis Group, 2000-2007. J Am Acad Dermatol 2010;63:789-798

3   Petrzilka M, Ehret C. Natural products. In: Müller PM, Lamparsky D, Eds. Perfumes. Art, Science and Technology. London: Blackie, 1994:499-531

4   Frosch PJ, Johansen JD, Menné T, Pirker C, Rastogi SC, Andersen KE, et al. Further important sensitizers in patients sensitive to fragrances. II. Reactivity to essential oils. Contact Dermatitis 2002;47:279-287

5   Uter W, Schmidt E, Geier J, Lessmann H, Schnuch A, Frosch PJ. Contact allergy to essential oils: current patch test results (2000-2008) from the IVDK network. Contact Dermatitis 2010;63:277-283

6   Paulsen E, Andersen KE. Colophonium and Compositae mix as markers of fragrance allergy: cross-reactivity between fragrance terpenes, colophonium and Compositae plant extracts. Contact Dermatitis 2005;53:285-291

7   Wenk KS, Ehrlich AE. Fragrance series testing in eyelid dermatitis. Dermatitis 2012;23:22-26

8   Dinkloh A, Worm M, Geier J, Schnuch A, Wollenberg A. Contact sensitization in patients with suspected cosmetic intolerance: results of the IVDK 2006-2011. J Eur Acad Dermatol Venereol 2015;29:1071-1081

9   Liu J, Li L-F. Contact sensitization to fragrances other than fragrance mix I in China. Contact Dermatitis 2015;73:252-255

10 SCCS (Scientific Committee on Consumer Safety). Opinion on Fragrance allergens in cosmetic products, 26-27 June 2012, SCCS/1459/11. Available at: https://ec.europa.eu/health/sites/health/files/scientific_committees/consumer_safety/docs/sccs_o_102.pdf

11 Uter W, Johansen JD, Börje A, Karlberg A-T, Lidén C, Rastogi S, Roberts D, White IR. Categorization of fragrance contact allergens for prioritization of preventive measures: clinical and experimental data and consideration of structure–activity relationships. Contact Dermatitis 2013;69:196-230

12 Silvestre JF, Mercader P, González-Pérez R, Hervella-Garcés M, Sanz-Sánchez T, Córdoba S, et al. Sensitization to fragrances in Spain: A 5-year multicentre study (2011-2015). Contact Dermatitis. 2018 Nov 14. doi: 10.1111/cod.13152. [Epub ahead of print]

Chapter 3.128 NERAL

IDENTIFICATION

Description/definition : Neral is the aldehyde that conforms to the structural formula shown below; it is the *cis*-isomer of citral

Chemical class(es) : Aldehydes

INCI name USA : Not in the Personal Care Products Council Ingredient Database

Chemical/IUPAC name : (2*Z*)-3,7-Dimethylocta-2,6-dienal

Other names : *cis*-Citral; β-citral; citral B

CAS registry number(s) : 106-26-3

EC number(s) : 203-379-2

RIFM monograph(s) : Food Cosmet Toxicol 1979;17:259 (citral)

SCCS opinion(s) : SCCNFP/0389/00, final (7)

Merck Index monograph : 3591 (Citral)

Function(s) in cosmetics : EU: perfuming

Patch testing : 3.5% pet. (5)

Molecular formula : $C_{10}H_{16}O$

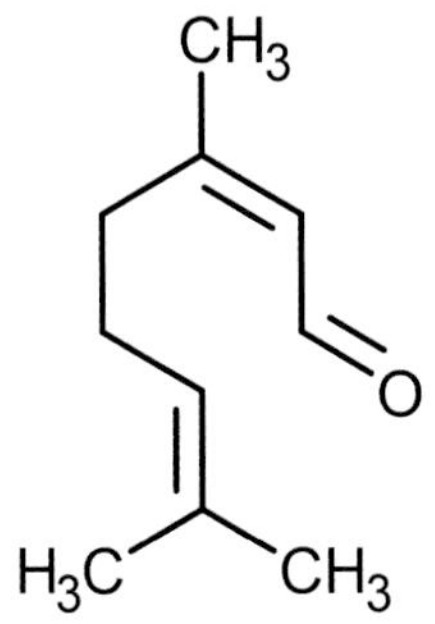

GENERAL

Neral is a pale yellow to yellow clear liquid; its odor type is citrus and its odor at 100% is described as 'sweet citral lemon peel' (www.thegoodscentscompany.com). Neral (*cis*-citral) in a 1:2 isomeric mixture with geranial (*trans*-citral) = citral. For more information on neral see Chapter 3.39 Citral.

Neral has – as has geranial - been identified as secondary oxidation product when geraniol autoxidizes (3). Both fragrances have also been identified as metabolites of geraniol (4).

Presence in essential oils

Neral has been identified by chemical analysis in 44 of 91 essential oils, which have caused contact allergy / allergic contact dermatitis. In 7 oils, neral belonged to the 'Top-10' of ingredients with the highest concentrations which may be expected in commercial essential oils of this type: lemongrass oil East Indian (27.5-35.5%), litsea cubeba oil (28.7-34.5%), lemongrass oil West Indian (30.3-33.3%), melissa oil (0.5-31.0%), ginger oil (0.3-10.2%), lemon oil (0.3-1.4%), and grapefruit oil (0.01-0.4%) (6).

CONTACT ALLERGY

Patch testing in groups of patients

Results of studies testing neral in consecutive patients suspected of contact dermatitis (routine testing) and those of testing *selected* patients (patients with suspected cosmetic allergy) are shown in table 3.128.1.

Patch testing in consecutive patients suspected of contact dermatitis: routine testing

In two studies performed in Sweden in groups of consecutive patients, rates of sensitization ranged from 0.1% to 0.9%, depending on the concentration (1,5). The higher test concentration of 3.5% may be preferable (5). In one study, relevance was not specified for individual fragrances (5) and in the other, no certain relevance for the positive patch test reactions to neral was found (1).

Patch testing in groups of selected patients

In 1983, in The Netherlands, 182 patients suspected of cosmetic allergy were patch tested with neral 1% in petrolatum and 5 positive reactions (2.7%) were observed (2). No relevance data were provided (2).

Case reports and case series
Case reports of allergic contact dermatitis from neral have not been found.

Table 3.128.1 Patch testing in groups of patients

Years and Country	Test conc. & vehicle	Number of patients tested	positive (%)		Selection of patients (S); Relevance (R); Comments (C)	Ref.
Routine testing						
2010-2011 Sweden	3.5% pet.	655	6	(0.9%)	R: not specified for individual fragrances	5
2006-2010 Sweden	1.5% pet.	680	1	(0.1%)	R: no certain relevance found	1
	1.0% pet.	946	4	(0.4%)		
Testing in groups of selected patients						
1983 The Netherlands	1% pet.	182	5	(2.6%)	S: patients suspected of cosmetic allergy; R: not stated	2

Cross-reactions, pseudo-cross-reactions and co-reactions
For general information on cross-/pseudo-cross-/co-reactivity of fragrance chemicals with other fragrances, fragrance markers (fragrance mix I, fragrance mix II, colophonium, Myroxylon pereirae resin [balsam of Peru]) and essential oils see Chapter 1.2 General information on cross-reactions, pseudo-cross-reactions and co-reactions.

Co-reactivity to oxidized geraniol (neral and geranial have been identified as secondary oxidation products when geraniol autoxidizes [3]), citral (= geranial + neral), and geranial (isomer of neral) have been observed (1).

Most patients with positive patch tests to geranial do not react to neral, indicating that there is no general cross-reactivity between neral and geranial. Although the only difference between the two molecules is the *cis/trans*-conformation of the α,β-double bond, this is most likely enough to induce separate immunological responses (5).

LITERATURE

1   Hagvall L, Karlberg A-T, Christensson JB. Contact allergy to air-exposed geraniol: clinical observations and report of 14 cases. Contact Dermatitis 2012;67:20-27
2   Malten KE, van Ketel WG, Nater JP, Liem DH. Reactions in selected patients to 22 fragrance materials. Contact Dermatitis 1984;11:1-10
3   Hagvall L, Backtorp C, Svensson S, Nyman G, Börje A, Karlberg AT. Fragrance compound geraniol forms contact allergens on air exposure. Identification and quantification of oxidation products and effect on skin sensitization. Chem Res Toxicol 2007;20:807-814
4   Hagvall L, Baron J M, Börje A, Weidolf L, Merk H, Karlberg AT. Cytochrome P450-mediated activation of the fragrance compound geraniol forms potent contact allergens. Toxicol Appl Pharmacol 2008;233:308-313
5   Hagvall L, Bråred Christensson J. Cross-reactivity between citral and geraniol – can it be attributed to oxidized geraniol? Contact Dermatitis 2014;71:280-288
6   De Groot AC, Schmidt E. Essential oils: contact allergy and chemical composition. Boca Raton, Fl., USA: CRC Press, Taylor and Francis Group, 2016 (ISBN 9781482246407)
7   Opinion of the Scientific Committee on Cosmetic Products and Non-Food Products Intended for Consumers concerning 'The 1st update of the inventory of ingredients employed in cosmetic products. Section II: Perfume and aromatic raw materials', 24 October 2000, SCCNFP/0389/00, final. Available at: http://ec.europa.eu/health/ph_risk/committees/sccp/documents/out131_en.pdf

Chapter 3.129 NEROL

IDENTIFICATION

Description/definition   : Nerol is the unsaturated alcohol that conforms to the structural formula shown below
Chemical class(es)   : Unsaturated organic compounds; alcohols
INCI name USA   : Not in the Personal Care Products Council Ingredient Database
Chemical/IUPAC name   : (2Z)-3,7-Dimethylocta-2,6-dien-1-ol
Other names   : Neryl alcohol; (Z)-geraniol
CAS registry number(s)   : 106-25-2
EC number(s)   : 203-378-7
RIFM monograph(s)   : Food Chem Toxicol 2008;46(11)(suppl.):S1-S71; Food Chem Toxicol 2008;46(11)(suppl.): S241-S244; Food Cosmet Toxicol 1976;14:623
SCCS opinion(s)   : SCCS/1459/11 (1)
Merck Index monograph   : 7830
Function(s) in cosmetics : EU: perfuming
Patch testing   : 5% pet. (2)
Molecular formula   : $C_{10}H_{18}O$

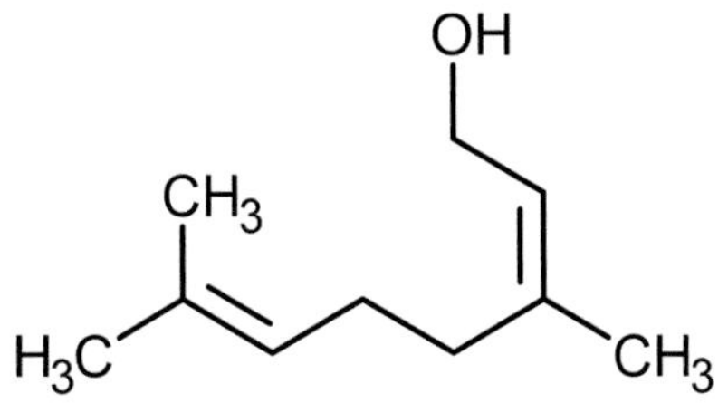

GENERAL

Nerol is a colorless clear liquid; its odor type is floral and its odor is described as 'fresh, citrus, floral, green, sweet, lemon/lime and waxy with a spicy depth' (www.thegoodscentscompany.com). Nerol occurs in many plants (see 'Presence in essential oils' below). It is a component of tobacco and tobacco smoke. Nerol is an important commercial chemical. It is used as a fragrance ingredient (e.g. in household products), an intermediate to make other terpene products (particularly citral, ionones, methyl ionones, citronellol, citronellal, hydroxycitronellal, menthol, and carotenoids) and as a flavoring compound in foods (U.S. National Library of Medicine).

Presence in essential oils

Nerol has been identified by chemical analysis in 58 of 91 essential oils, which have caused contact allergy / allergic contact dermatitis. In two oils, nerol belonged to the 'Top-10' of ingredients with the highest concentrations which may be expected in commercial essential oils of this type: melissa oil (0.1-16.2%) and rose oil (0.6-11.0%) (5).

CONTACT ALLERGY

General

The SCCS (Scientific Committee on Consumer Safety), in a 2012 Opinion on Fragrance allergens in cosmetic products, has categorized nerol as 'likely fragrance contact allergen by combination of evidence' (1,4).

Patch testing in groups of patients

Patch testing in consecutive patients suspected of contact dermatitis: routine testing

Studies in which nerol was patch tested in consecutive patients suspected of contact dermatitis (routine testing) with positive results have not been found.

Patch testing in groups of selected patients

Before 2002, in Japan, European countries and the USA, 218 patients with known fragrance sensitivity were patch tested with nerol 5% in petrolatum and 13 positive reactions (6.0%) were observed; their relevance was not mentioned (2).

Case reports and case series

Case reports of allergic contact dermatitis from nerol have not been found.

Presence in products and chemical analyses

In 2000, fifty-nine domestic and occupational products, purchased in retail outlets in Denmark, England, Germany and Italy were analyzed by GC-MS for the presence of fragrances. The product categories were liquid soap and soap bars (n=13), soft/hard surface cleaners (n=23), fabric conditioners/laundry detergents for hand wash (n=8), dish wash (n=10), furniture polish, car shampoo, stain remover (each n=1) and 2 products used in occupational environments. Nerol was present in 17 (29%) products; quantification was not performed (3).

LITERATURE

1   SCCS (Scientific Committee on Consumer Safety). Opinion on Fragrance allergens in cosmetic products, 26-27 June 2012, SCCS/1459/11. Available at:
    https://ec.europa.eu/health/sites/health/files/scientific_committees/consumer_safety/docs/sccs_o_102.pdf
2   Larsen W, Nakayama H, Fischer T, Elsner P, Frosch P, Burrows D, et al. Fragrance contact dermatitis - a worldwide multicenter investigation (Part III). Contact Dermatitis 2002;46:141-144
3   Rastogi SC, Heydorn S, Johansen JD, Basketter DA. Fragrance chemicals in domestic and occupational products. Contact Dermatitis 2001;45:221-225
4   Uter W, Johansen JD, Börje A, Karlberg A-T, Lidén C, Rastogi S, Roberts D, White IR. Categorization of fragrance contact allergens for prioritization of preventive measures: clinical and experimental data and consideration of structure–activity relationships. Contact Dermatitis 2013;69:196-230
5   De Groot AC, Schmidt E. Essential oils: contact allergy and chemical composition. Boca Raton, Fl., USA: CRC Press, Taylor and Francis Group, 2016 (ISBN 9781482246407)

Chapter 3.130 NEROLIDOL

IDENTIFICATION

Description/definition   : Nerolidol is the organic compound that conforms to the structural formula shown below
Chemical class(es)   : Alcohols
Chemical/IUPAC name   : 3,7,11-Trimethyldodeca-1,6,10-trien-3-ol
Other names   : Peruviol; melaleucol
CAS registry number(s)   : 142-50-7; 7212-44-4; 40716-66-3 (trans-); 3790-78-1 (cis-)
EC number(s)   : 205-540-2; 230-597-5; 255-053-4 (trans-); 223-263-5 (cis-)
RIFM monograph(s)   : Food Chem Toxicol 2010;48(suppl.3):S43-S45; Food Chem Toxicol 2008;46(suppl.11):S245-
                                          S246 (cis-nerolidol) and S247-S250 (isomer unspecified); Food Chem Toxicol
                                          2008;46(suppl.):S1-S71; Food Cosmet Toxicol 1975;13:887 (special issue II)
SCCS opinion(s)   : SCCS/1459/11 (2)
Merck Index monograph : 7831
Function(s) in cosmetics : EU: perfuming. USA: denaturants; flavoring agents; fragrance ingredients
Patch testing   : 3% olive oil (5); 1% pet. (1); according to RIFM data, 4% pet. is probably not irritant (7)
Molecular formula   : $C_{15}H_{26}O$

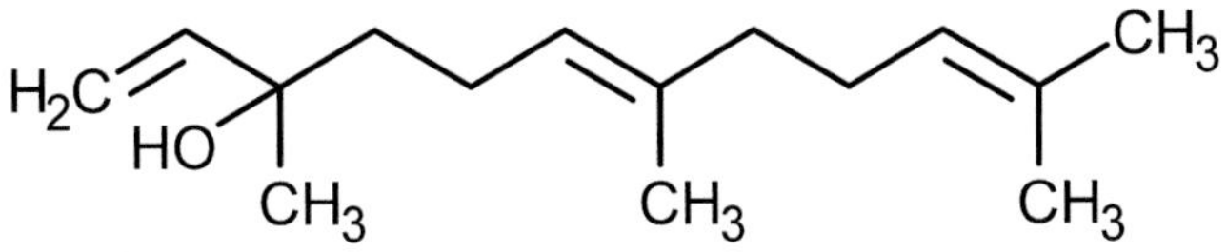

GENERAL

Nerolidol is a colorless to pale yellow clear oily liquid; its odor type is floral and its odor at 100% is described as 'floral, green and citrus like, with woody waxy nuances' (www.thegoodscentscompany.com).

Presence in essential oils and in Myroxylon pereirae resin (balsam of Peru)

Nerolidol (any isomer) has been identified by chemical analysis in 65 of 91 essential oils, which have caused contact allergy / allergic contact dermatitis. In three oils, (E)-nerolidol belonged to the 'Top-10' of ingredients with the highest concentrations which may be expected in commercial essential oils of this type: niaouli oil (0.3-80.3%), neroli oil (1.7-4.9%) and cardamom oil (0.5-2.0%) (4). Nerolidol may also be present in Myroxylon pereirae resin (balsam of Peru) (2-7%) (1).

CONTACT ALLERGY

General

The SCCS (Scientific Committee on Consumer Safety), in a 2012 Opinion on Fragrance allergens in cosmetic products, has categorized nerolidol as 'likely fragrance contact allergen by combination of evidence' (2,3).

Patch testing in groups of patients

Results of studies testing nerolidol in consecutive patients suspected of contact dermatitis (routine testing) and those of testing in groups of selected patients (patients allergic to balsam of Peru) are shown in table 3.130.1.

Patch testing in consecutive patients suspected of contact dermatitis: routine testing

In an early study from Poland 200 consecutive patients were patch tested with nerolidol 50% pet. and there were seven (3.5%) positive reactions (6). Their relevance was not mentioned and considering the unexpectedly high rate of positive reactions, some may have been irritant from the high (50%) nerolidol concentration.

Patch testing in groups of selected patients

In a group of 102 patients from Germany allergic to balsam of Peru tested with a battery of its ingredients, 3 (3%) positive reactions to nerolidol were observed (1). In an early Danish investigation, of 51 individuals previously reacting to balsam of Peru, 3 (6%) had positive patch tests to nerolidol 3% in olive oil (5). This seems to indicate that nerolidol in not an important allergenic ingredient of this material. The results of testing with all allergenic components of balsam of Peru are discussed in Chapter 3.126 Myroxylon pereirae resin.

Table 3.130.1 Patch testing in groups of patients

Years and Country	Test conc. & vehicle	Number of patients tested | positive (%)			Selection of patients (S); Relevance (R); Comments (C)	Ref.
Routine testing						
<1973 Poland	50% pet.	200	7	(3.5%)	R: not stated; C: probably some irritant reactions	6
Testing in groups of selected patients						
1995-1998 Germany	1% pet.	102	3	(3%)	S: patients allergic to Myroxylon pereirae resin (balsam of Peru)	1
1955-1960 Denmark	3% o.o.	51	3	(6%)	S: patients allergic to Myroxylon pereirae resin (balsam of Peru)	5

o.o.: Olive oil

Case reports and case series
Case reports of allergic contact dermatitis from nerolidol have not been found.

Cross-reactions, pseudo-cross-reactions and co-reactions
For general information on cross-/pseudo-cross-/co-reactivity of fragrance chemicals with other fragrances, fragrance markers (fragrance mix I, fragrance mix II, colophonium, Myroxylon pereirae resin [balsam of Peru]) and essential oils see Chapter 1.2 General information on cross-reactions, pseudo-cross-reactions and co-reactions.

Co-reactivity with Myroxylon pereirae resin (MP) may be explained by the presence of nerolidol (2-7%) in MP (pseudo-cross-reactions).

LITERATURE
1   Hausen BM. Contact allergy to Balsam of Peru. II. Patch test results in 102 patients with selected Balsam of Peru constituents. Am J Contact Derm 2001;12:93-102
2   SCCS (Scientific Committee on Consumer Safety). Opinion on Fragrance allergens in cosmetic products, 26-27 June 2012, SCCS/1459/11. Available at:
     https://ec.europa.eu/health/sites/health/files/scientific_committees/consumer_safety/docs/sccs_o_102.pdf
3   Uter W, Johansen JD, Börje A, Karlberg A-T, Lidén C, Rastogi S, Roberts D, White IR. Categorization of fragrance contact allergens for prioritization of preventive measures: clinical and experimental data and consideration of structure–activity relationships. Contact Dermatitis 2013;69:196-230
4   De Groot AC, Schmidt E. Essential oils: contact allergy and chemical composition. Boca Raton, Fl., USA: CRC Press, Taylor and Francis Group, 2016 (ISBN 9781482246407)
5   Hjorth N. Eczematous allergy to balsams. Acta Derm Venereol 1961;41(suppl.46):1-216
6   Rudzki E, Kielak D. Sensitivity to some compounds related to Balsam of Peru. Contact Dermatitis Newsletter 1972;nr.13:335-336
7   De Groot AC. Patch Testing, 4th Edition. Wapserveen, The Netherlands: acdegroot publishing, 2018 (ISBN 978-90-813233-4-5)

Chapter 3.131 NONANAL

IDENTIFICATION

Description/definition	: Nonanal is the aliphatic aldehyde that conforms to the structural formula shown below
Chemical class(es)	: Aliphatic organic compounds; aldehydes
INCI name USA	: Not in the Personal Care Products Council Ingredient Database
Chemical/IUPAC name	: Nonanal
Other names	: Pelargonaldehyde; aldehyde C-9
CAS registry number(s)	: 124-19-6
EC number(s)	: 204-688-5
RIFM monograph(s)	: Food Cosmet Toxicol 1973;11:115; Food Cosmet Toxicol 1973;11:1080
Function(s) in cosmetics	: EU: perfuming
Patch testing	: No patch test data available; based on RIFM data, 1% pet. is probably not irritant (3)
Molecular formula	: $C_9H_{18}O$

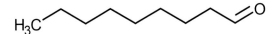

GENERAL

Nonanal is a colorless to pale yellow clear liquid; its odor type is aldehydic and its odor at 1% is described as 'waxy, aldehydic, citrus, with a fresh slightly green lemon peel like nuance, and a cucumber fattiness' (www.thegoodscents company.com). Nonanal occurs naturally in many citrus fruits, spices and some trees. It is an important commercial chemical that is used in perfumery and as a flavoring agent in food and cigarettes (National Library of Medicine).

Presence in essential oils

Nonanal has been identified by chemical analysis in 40 of 91 essential oils, which have caused contact allergy / allergic contact dermatitis. In none of these oils, it belonged to the 'Top-10' of ingredients with the highest concentrations (4).

CONTACT ALLERGY

Patch testing in groups of patients

Studies in which nonanal was patch tested in either consecutive patients suspected of contact dermatitis (routine testing) or in groups of selected patients with positive results have not been found.

Case reports and case series

A woman had allergic contact dermatitis from the perfume in an eye cream. Subsequently, she was tested with 94 individual liquid fragrance materials from this perfume (test concentrations not stated). The patient at day 5 had 12 positive patch test reactions, including to nonanal (aldehyde C-9). Three controls were negative. She was not retested, so false-positive reactions due to the excited skin syndrome (there was an additional strong reaction to allyl cyclohexyl propionate which proved to be irritant) cannot be excluded (1).

Indeed, two years later, in a Letter to the Editor, the author mentioned that he had retested the patient with the 12 fragrances to which she had previously shown a positive patch test. Only hydroxycitronellal had again given a positive reaction (2). This means that, in fact, contact allergy to nonanal has not been demonstrated thus far beyond doubt.

LITERATURE

1 Larsen WG. Cosmetic dermatitis due to a perfume. Contact Dermatitis 1975;1:142-145
2 Larsen WG. Perfume dermatitis revisited. Contact Dermatitis 1977;3:98
3 De Groot AC. Patch Testing, 4th Edition. Wapserveen, The Netherlands: acdegroot publishing, 2018 (ISBN 978-90-813233-4-5)
4 De Groot AC, Schmidt E. Essential oils: contact allergy and chemical composition. Boca Raton, Fl., USA: CRC Press, Taylor and Francis Group, 2016 (ISBN 9781482246407)

Chapter 3.132 NONYL ALCOHOL

IDENTIFICATION

Description/definition	: Nonyl alcohol is the aliphatic alcohol that conforms to the structural formula shown below
Chemical class(es)	: Aliphatic organic compounds; alcohols
INCI name USA	: Not in the Personal Care Products Council Ingredient Database
Chemical/IUPAC name	: Nonan-1-ol
Other names	: 1-Nonanol; alcohol C-9; N-nonyl alcohol
CAS registry number(s)	: 143-08-8; 28473-21-4
EC number(s)	: 205-583-7; 249-048-6
RIFM monograph(s)	: Food Cosmet Toxicol 1973;11:103; Food Cosmet Toxicol 1973;11:1079 (binder, page 41)
Merck Index monograph	: 8036
Function(s) in cosmetics	: EU: perfuming
Patch testing	: No patch test data available; based on RIFM data, 2% pet. is probably not irritant (3)
Molecular formula	: $C_9H_{20}O$

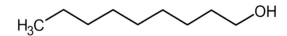

GENERAL

Nonyl alcohol is a colorless to pale yellow clear liquid; its odor type is floral and its odor at 100% is described as 'fresh clean fatty floral rose orange dusty wet oily' (www.thegoodscentscompany.com). The alcohol is used in perfumery and flavoring (manufacture of artificial lemon oil). Other uses include or have included the rubber and dyestuff industry, and as chemical intermediate in the production of plasticizers and surfactants (as alcohol mixture) (National Library of Medicine).

Presence in essential oils

Nonyl alcohol has been identified by chemical analysis in 10 of 91 essential oils, which have caused contact allergy / allergic contact dermatitis. In none of these oils, it belonged to the 'Top-10' of ingredients with the highest concentrations (4).

CONTACT ALLERGY

Patch testing in groups of patients

Studies in which nonyl alcohol was patch tested in either consecutive patients suspected of contact dermatitis (routine testing) or in groups of selected patients with positive results have not been found.

Case reports and case series

A woman had allergic contact dermatitis from the perfume in an eye cream. Subsequently, she was tested with 94 individual liquid fragrance materials from this perfume (test concentrations not stated). The patient at day 5 had 12 positive patch test reactions, including to nonyl alcohol (alcohol C-9). Three controls were negative. She was not retested, so false-positive reactions due to the excited skin syndrome (there was an additional strong reaction to allyl cyclohexyl propionate which proved to be irritant) cannot be excluded (1).

   Indeed, two years later, in a Letter to the Editor, the author mentioned that he had retested the patient with the 12 fragrances to which she had previously shown a positive patch test. Only hydroxycitronellal had again given a positive reaction (2). This means that, in fact, contact allergy to nonyl alcohol has not been demonstrated thus far beyond doubt.

LITERATURE

1   Larsen WG. Cosmetic dermatitis due to a perfume. Contact Dermatitis 1975;1:142-145
2   Larsen WG. Perfume dermatitis revisited. Contact Dermatitis 1977;3:98
3   De Groot AC. Patch Testing, 4th Edition. Wapserveen, The Netherlands: acdegroot publishing, 2018 (ISBN 978-90-813233-4-5)
4   De Groot AC, Schmidt E. Essential oils: contact allergy and chemical composition. Boca Raton, Fl., USA: CRC Press, Taylor and Francis Group, 2016 (ISBN 9781482246407)

Chapter 3.133 NOPYL ACETATE

IDENTIFICATION

Description/definition : Nopyl acetate is the organic compound that conforms to the structural formula shown below

Chemical class(es) : Esters

Chemical/IUPAC name : 2-(6,6-Dimethyl-4-bicyclo[3.1.1]hept-3-enyl)ethyl acetate

Other names : Lignyl acetate; nopol acetate

CAS registry number (s) : 128-51-8

EC number(s) : 204-891-9

RIFM monograph(s) : Food Cosmet Toxicol 1974;12:943 (special issue I)

SCCS opinion(s) : SCCS/1459/11 (1)

Function(s) in cosmetics : EU: masking. USA: fragrance ingredients

Patch testing : 25% pet. (2); based on RIFM data, 10% pet. is probably not irritant (6)

Molecular formula : $C_{13}H_{20}O_2$

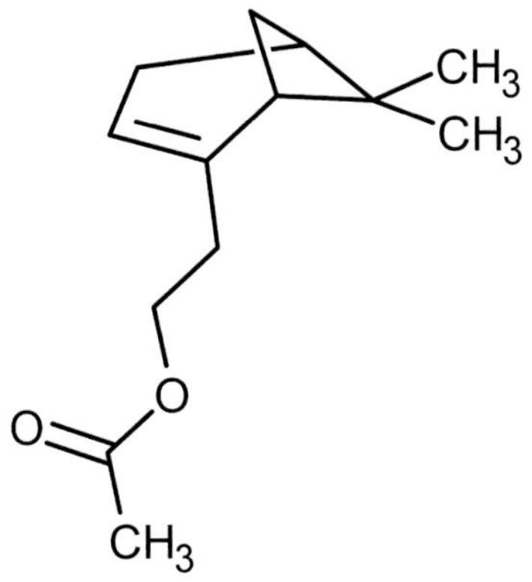

GENERAL

Nopyl acetate is a colorless clear liquid; its odor type is herbal and its odor at 100% is described as 'herbal linalyl acetate woody pine lavender' (www.thegoodscentscompany.com).

Presence in essential oils

Nopyl acetate has been identified by chemical analysis in 1 of 91 essential oils, which have caused contact allergy / allergic contact dermatitis: lavender oil (5). However, nopyl acetate is according to various sources not found in nature and therefore, the analytical identification of this chemical may have been erroneous.

CONTACT ALLERGY

General

The SCCS (Scientific Committee on Consumer Safety), in a 2012 Opinion on Fragrance allergens in cosmetic products, has categorized nopyl acetate as 'likely fragrance contact allergen by combination of evidence' (1,4).

Patch testing in groups of patients

Patch testing in consecutive patients suspected of contact dermatitis: routine testing

Studies in which nopyl acetate was patch tested in consecutive patients suspected of contact dermatitis (routine testing) with positive results have not been found.

Patch testing in groups of selected patients

In 1984, in The Netherlands, 179 patients suspected of cosmetic allergy were patch tested with nopyl acetate 25% pet. and there were 2 (1.1%) positive reactions. Their relevance was not mentioned, but false-positive reactions due to the excited skin syndrome could not be excluded (2).

Case reports and case series

Case reports of allergic contact dermatitis from nopyl acetate have not been found.

Presence in products and chemical analyses

In 2000, fifty-nine domestic and occupational products, purchased in retail outlets in Denmark, England, Germany and Italy were analyzed by GC-MS for the presence of fragrances. The product categories were liquid soap and soap bars (n=13), soft/hard surface cleaners (n=23), fabric conditioners/laundry detergents for hand wash (n=8), dish wash (n=10), furniture polish, car shampoo, stain remover (each n=1) and 2 products used in occupational environments. Nopyl acetate was present in one product (2%); quantification was not performed (3).

LITERATURE

1   SCCS (Scientific Committee on Consumer Safety). Opinion on Fragrance allergens in cosmetic products, 26-27 June 2012, SCCS/1459/11. Available at:
    https://ec.europa.eu/health/sites/health/files/scientific_committees/consumer_safety/docs/sccs_o_102.pdf
2   De Groot AC, Liem DH, Nater JP, van Ketel WG. Patch tests with fragrance materials and preservatives. Contact Dermatitis 1985;12:87-92
3   Rastogi SC, Heydorn S, Johansen JD, Basketter DA. Fragrance chemicals in domestic and occupational products. Contact Dermatitis 2001;45:221-225
4   Uter W, Johansen JD, Börje A, Karlberg A-T, Lidén C, Rastogi S, Roberts D, White IR. Categorization of fragrance contact allergens for prioritization of preventive measures: clinical and experimental data and consideration of structure–activity relationships. Contact Dermatitis 2013;69:196-230
5   De Groot AC, Schmidt E. Essential oils: contact allergy and chemical composition. Boca Raton, Fl., USA: CRC Press, Taylor and Francis Group, 2016 (ISBN 9781482246407)
6   De Groot AC. Patch Testing, 4th Edition. Wapserveen, The Netherlands: acdegroot publishing, 2018 (ISBN 978-90-813233-4-5)

Chapter 3.134 PENTAMETHYLCYCLOPENT-3-ENE-BUTANOL

IDENTIFICATION

Description/definition : Pentamethylcyclopent-3-ene-butanol is the cyclic alcohol that conforms to the structural formula shown below
Chemical class(es) : Unsaturated cyclic organic compounds; alcohols
INCI name USA : Not in the Personal Care Products Council Ingredient Database
Chemical/IUPAC name : 3-Methyl-5-(2,2,3-trimethylcyclopent-3-en-1-yl)pentan-2-ol
Other names : α,β,2,2,3-Pentamethylcyclopent-3-ene-1-butanol; sandal pentanol; Sandalore ®
CAS registry number(s) : 65113-99-7
EC number(s) : 265-453-0
Function(s) in cosmetics : EU: perfuming
Patch testing : 5% pet. (1)
Molecular formula : $C_{14}H_{26}O$

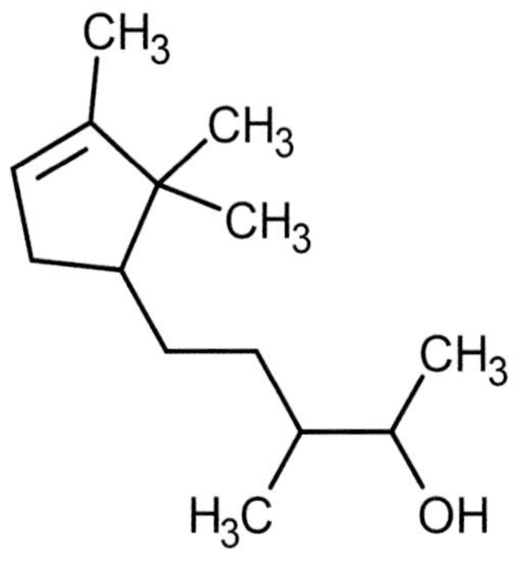

GENERAL

Pentamethylcyclopent-3-ene-butanol is a pale yellow clear viscous liquid; its odor type is woody and its odor at 100% is described as 'sweet sandalwood amyris woody' (www.thegoodscentscompany.com). Pentamethylcyclopent-3-ene-butanol is a synthetic chemical, not found in nature (and consequently not in essential oils (2)).

CONTACT ALLERGY

Patch testing in groups of patients

Patch testing in consecutive patients suspected of contact dermatitis: routine testing
Studies in which pentamethylcyclopent-3-ene-butanol was patch tested in consecutive patients suspected of contact dermatitis (routine testing) with positive results have not been found.

Patch testing in groups of selected patients
Before 1996, in Japan, some European countries and the USA, 167 patients known or suspected to be allergic to fragrances were patch tested with pentamethylcyclopent-3-ene-butanol and there were five (3.0%) positive reactions; their relevance was not mentioned (1).

Case reports and case series
Case reports of allergic contact dermatitis from pentamethylcyclopent-3-ene-butanol have not been found.

LITERATURE

1 Larsen W, Nakayama H, Fischer T, Elsner P, Burrows D, Jordan W, et al. Fragrance contact dermatitis: A worldwide multicenter investigation (Part I). Am J Cont Dermat 1996;7:77-83
2 De Groot AC, Schmidt E. Essential oils: contact allergy and chemical composition. Boca Raton, Fl., USA: CRC Press, Taylor and Francis Group, 2016 (ISBN 9781482246407)

Chapter 3.135 ALPHA-PHELLANDRENE

IDENTIFICATION

Description/definition : alpha-Phellandrene is the cyclic organic compound that conforms to the structural formula shown below
Chemical class(es) : Unsaturated cyclic organic compounds
INCI name USA : Not in the Personal Care Products Council Ingredient Database
Chemical/IUPAC name : 2-Methyl-5-propan-2-ylcyclohexa-1,3-diene
Other names : Dihydro-p-cymene; p-mentha-1,5-diene
CAS registry number(s) : 99-83-2
EC number(s) : 202-792-5
RIFM monograph(s) : Food Cosmet Toxicol 1978;16:843 (special issue IV)
Merck Index monograph : 8585
Function(s) in cosmetics : EU: perfuming
Patch testing : 5% pet.; concentrations of 5% (or higher) *in alcohol* may be (strongly) irritant (3)
Molecular formula : $C_{10}H_{16}$

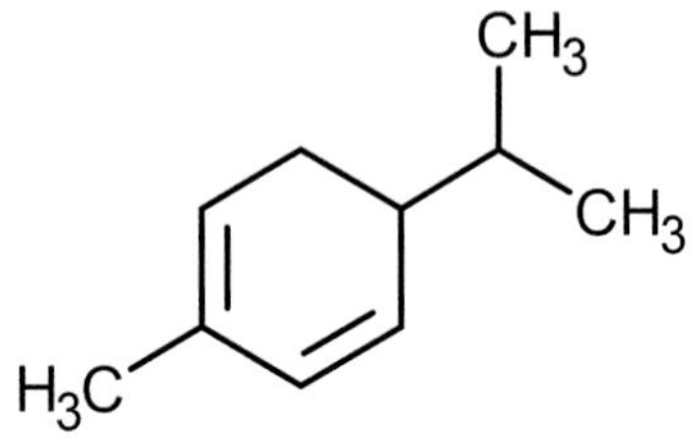

GENERAL

alpha-Phellandrene is a colorless to pale yellow clear liquid; its odor type is terpenic and its odor is described as 'citrus, terpenic, slightly green, black pepper-like' (www.thegoodscentscompany.com).

Presence in essential oils and Myroxylon pereirae resin (balsam of Peru)

alpha-Phellandrene has been identified by chemical analysis in 78 of 91 essential oils, which have caused contact allergy / allergic contact dermatitis. In 10 oils, alpha-phellandrene belonged to the 'Top-10' of ingredients with the highest concentrations. These are shown in table 3.135.1. with the concentration range which may be expected in commercial essential oils of this type (11). α-Phellandrene may also be present in Myroxylon pereirae resin (balsam of Peru) (10).

Table 3.135.1 Essential oils containing alpha-phellandrene in the 'Top-10' and concentration range in commercial oils

Essential oil	Concentration range (min.-max.)	Essential oil	Concentration range (min.-max.)
Elemi oil	10.3-23.9%	Angelica fruit oil	0.7-3.7%
Angelica root oil	4.5-22.0%	Galbanum resin oil	0.2-3.6%
Black pepper oil	0.8-17.4%	Cinnamon bark oil Sri Lanka	0.5-3.2%
Ravensara oil	0.04-11.8%	Cinnamon leaf oil Sri Lanka	0.5-1.5%
Pine needle oil	0.04-5.3%	Star anise oil	0.2-0.6%

CONTACT ALLERGY

General

alpha-Phellandrene has been shown to be a prohapten (9), which is a chemical that is itself non-sensitizing or low-sensitizing, but that is transformed into a hapten in the skin (bioactivation), usually via enzymatic catalysis. It is an important allergen in tea tree oil. Of 61 patients allergic to tea tree oil and tested with a number of its ingredients in various studies, 24 (39%) reacted to α-phellandrene (1,2,3,4,5,6). It is also one of the allergenic ingredients of Bulgarian turpentine oil (7).

Patch testing in consecutive patients suspected of contact dermatitis: routine testing

Studies in which alpha-phellandrene was patch tested in consecutive patients suspected of contact dermatitis (routine testing) with positive results have not been found.

Patch testing in groups of selected patients

Results of studies patch testing alpha-phellandrene in groups of selected patients (in all studies patients with known contact allergy to (oxidized) tea tree oil) are shown in table 3.135.2. In five investigations, in the period 1990-2003, small groups of 7-20 patients allergic to (oxidized) tea tree oil (which contains alpha-phellandrene) were patch tested with a number of its ingredients including alpha-phellandrene 5% in various vehicles and there were 14% - 63% positive reactions with an average (unadjusted for sample size) of 39% (1,2,3,4,5,6). This seems to indicate that alpha-phellandrene is an important allergenic ingredient of (oxidized) tea tree oil.

Table 3.135.2 Patch testing in groups of patients: Selected patient groups

Years and Country	Test conc. & vehicle	Number of patients tested	positive (%)		Selection of patients (S); Relevance (R); Comments (C)	Ref.
1999-2003 Germany	5% DEP	20	7	(35%)	S: patients with a positive patch test reaction to oxidized tea tree oil 5% DEP	5
1999-2000 Germany, Austria	5% DEP	10	6	(60%)	S: patients with a positive patch test reaction to oxidized tea tree oil 5% DEP	1
1999 Germany	5% water	8	5	(63%)	S: patients with a positive patch test reaction to oxidized tea tree oil 20% in olive oil	2
<1999 Germany	5% vehicle?	16	5	(31%)	S: patients allergic to tea tree oil	4
1990-1992 Germany	1% and 5% alc.	7	1	(14%)	S: patients with a positive patch test reaction to tea tree oil 1% alc.	3

DEP: Diethyl phthalate

Case reports and case series

A woman treated irritant reactions on her breast caused by a plaster applied to the skin after an operation and insect bites with tea tree oil, to which she became sensitized. When patch tested, she reacted to the oil, its ingredient alpha-phellandrene (5%, vehicle unknown) and three other components of tea tree oil (4).

A male patient used to wash his hair with a shampoo to which his wife had added tea tree oil and developed dermatitis. He showed positive patch tests to the oil, alpha-phellandrene and four other components of tea tree oil (4).

Two more patients were presented by the same authors, who had used tea tree oil for various reasons and indications, who developed allergic contact dermatitis from it and reacted on ingredient patch testing to alpha-phellandrene and 5 resp. 6 other oil components (4).

LITERATURE

1   Pirker C, Hausen BM, Uter W, Hillen U, Brasch J, Bayeret C, et al. Sensitization to tea tree oil in Germany and Austria. A multicenter Study of the German Contact Dermatitis group. J Dtsch Dermatol Ges 2003;1:629-634 (article in German)
2   Lippert U, Walter A, Hausen BM, Fuchs Th. Increasing incidence of contact dermatitis to tea tree oil. J Allergy Clin Immunol 2000;105;S43 (abstract 127)
3   Knight TE, Hausen BM. Melaleuca oil (tea tree oil) dermatitis. J Am Acad Dermatol 1994;30:423-427
4   Hausen BM, Reichling J, Harkenthal M. Degradation products of monoterpenes are the sensitizing agents in tea tree oil. Am J Contact Dermat 1999;10:68-77
5   Hausen BM. Evaluation of the main contact allergens in oxidized tea tree oil. Dermatitis 2004;15:213-214
6   De Groot AC, Schmidt E. Tea tree oil: contact allergy and chemical composition. Contact Dermatitis 2016;75:129-143
7   Michailov P, Berowa N, Zuzulowa A. Klinische und biochemische Untersuchungen über die berufsbedingten allergischen und toxischen Erscheinungen durch Terpentin. Allergie und Asthma 1970;16:201-205. Data cited in ref. 8
8   Dooms-Goossens A, Degreef H, Holvoet C, Maertens M. Turpentine-induced hypersensitivity to peppermint oil. Contact Dermatitis 1977;3:304-308
9   Bergström MA, Luthman K, Nilsson JL, Karlberg AT. Conjugated dienes as prohaptens in contact allergy: in *vivo* and in *vitro* studies of structure-activity relationships, sensitizing capacity, and metabolic activation. Chem Res Toxicol 2006;19:760-769
10 Mammerler V. Contribution to the analysis and quality control of Peru Balsam. PhD Thesis, University of Vienna, Austria, 2007. Available at: http://othes.univie.ac.at/4056/1/2009-03-23_0201578.pdf
11 De Groot AC, Schmidt E. Essential oils: contact allergy and chemical composition. Boca Raton, Fl., USA: CRC Press, Taylor and Francis Group, 2016 (ISBN 9781482246407)

Chapter 3.136 PHENETHYL ALCOHOL

IDENTIFICATION

Description/definition   : Phenethyl alcohol is the aromatic alcohol that conforms to the structural formula shown
                              below
Chemical class(es)   : Alcohols
Chemical/IUPAC name   : 2-Phenylethanol
Other names   : Phenylethyl alcohol; benzeneethanol
CAS registry number(s)   : 60-12-8
EC number(s)   : 200-456-2
CIR review(s)   : J Am Coll Toxicol 1990;9:165-183 (access: www.cir-safety.org/ingredients)
RIFM monograph(s)   : Food Chem Toxicol 2012;50(suppl.2):S224-S239; Food Cosmet Toxicol 1975;13:903
                              (special issue II)
SCCS opinion(s)   : SCCS/1459/11 (2)
Merck Index monograph   : 8608
Function(s) in cosmetics   : EU: masking. USA: fragrance ingredients; preservatives
Patch testing   : 25% pet. (3); 5% pet.(8); based on RIFM data, 8% pet. is probably not irritant (8)
Molecular formula   : $C_8H_{10}O$

GENERAL

Phenethyl alcohol is a colorless clear oily liquid; its odor type is floral and its odor at 100% is described as 'sweet, floral, fresh and bready with a rosey honey nuance' (www.thegoodscentscompany.com). Phenethyl alcohol occurs naturally in the environment. It is produced by microorganisms, plants, and animals. It has been found as the free alcohol or esterified in a number of natural essential oils, and in food, beers, wines, whiskeys, spices, and tobacco. Commercial quantities of phenethyl alcohol are produced synthetically (9).

Phenethyl alcohol is used in small quantities in fragrances for cosmetics and detergents and in larger amounts for the production of its esters, which are more important fragrance compounds. Phenethyl alcohol may also be added as a flavor to foods and beverages. Other uses include or have included the synthesis of artificial rose oil, as an antibacterial agent or preservative, e.g. in eye drops, and as an intermediate in the preparation of dyestuffs and photographic materials (9, National Library of Medicine).

Presence in essential oils

Phenethyl alcohol has been identified by chemical analysis in 18 of 91 essential oils, which have caused contact allergy / allergic contact dermatitis. In one oil, phenethyl alcohol belonged to the 'Top-10' of ingredients with the highest concentrations which may be expected in commercial essential oils of this type: cassia oil (0.2-0.7%) (10).

CONTACT ALLERGY

General

The SCCS (Scientific Committee on Consumer Safety), in a 2012 Opinion on Fragrance allergens in cosmetic products, has categorized phenethyl alcohol as 'possible fragrance contact allergen' (2,7).

Patch testing in groups of patients

Patch testing in consecutive patients suspected of contact dermatitis: routine testing

Studies in which phenethyl alcohol was patch tested in consecutive patients suspected of contact dermatitis (routine testing) with positive results have not been found.

Patch testing in groups of selected patients

In 1984, in The Netherlands, 179 patients suspected of cosmetic allergy were patch tested with a battery of fragrances and there were 2 positive reactions (1.1%) to phenethyl alcohol 25% pet. (3). In a group of 20 patients allergic to fragrances and tested with a battery of fragrance materials before 1977 in the USA, one (5%) reacted to phenethyl alcohol 5% pet. (1). In neither investigation was the relevance of the observed positive patch test reactions mentioned.

Case reports and case series

Case reports of allergic contact dermatitis from phenethyl alcohol have not been found.

Presence in products and chemical analyses

In 1997, 71 deodorants (22 vapo-spray, 22 aerosol spray and 27 roll-on products) were collected in Denmark, England, France, Germany and Sweden and analyzed by gas chromatography – mass spectrometry (GC-MS) for the presence of fragrances and other materials. Phenethyl alcohol was present in 58 (82%) of the products (4).

In 1992, in The Netherlands, the presence of fragrances was analyzed in 300 cosmetic products. Phenethyl alcohol was identified in 79% of the products (rank order 2) (6).

In 1988, in the USA, 400 perfumes used in fine fragrances, household products and soaps (number of products per category not mentioned) were analyzed for the presence of fragrance chemicals in a concentration of at least 1% and a list of the Top-25 (present in the highest number of products) presented. Phenethyl alcohol was found to be present in 82% of the fine fragrances (rank number 3), 63% of the household product fragrances (rank number 3) and 87% of the fragrances used in soaps (rank number 2) (5).

LITERATURE

1   Larsen WG. Perfume dermatitis. A study of 20 patients. Arch Dermatol 1977;113:623-626
2   SCCS (Scientific Committee on Consumer Safety). Opinion on Fragrance allergens in cosmetic products, 26-27 June 2012, SCCS/1459/11. Available at: https://ec.europa.eu/health/sites/health/files/scientific_committees/consumer_safety/docs/sccs_o_102.pdf
3   De Groot AC, Liem DH, Nater JP, van Ketel WG. Patch tests with fragrance materials and preservatives. Contact Dermatitis 1985;12:87-92
4   Rastogi SC, Lepoittevin J-P, Johansen JD, Frosch PJ, Menné T, Bruze M, et al. Fragrances and other materials in deodorants: search for potentially sensitizing molecules using combined GC-MS and structure activity relationship (SAR) analysis. Contact Dermatitis 1998;39:293-303
5   Fenn RS. Aroma chemical usage trends in modern perfumery. Perfumer and Flavorist 1989;14:3-10
6   Weyland JW. Personal Communication, 1992. Cited in: De Groot AC, Weyland JW, Nater JP. Unwanted effects of cosmetics and drugs used in dermatology, 3rd Ed. Amsterdam: Elsevier, 1994: 579
7   Uter W, Johansen JD, Börje A, Karlberg A-T, Lidén C, Rastogi S, Roberts D, White IR. Categorization of fragrance contact allergens for prioritization of preventive measures: clinical and experimental data and consideration of structure–activity relationships. Contact Dermatitis 2013;69:196-230
8   De Groot AC. Patch Testing, 4th Edition. Wapserveen, The Netherlands: acdegroot publishing, 2018 (ISBN 978-90-813233-4-5)
9   Cosmetic Ingredient Review Expert Panel. Final report on the safety assessment of phenethyl alcohol. J Am Coll Toxicol 1990;9:165-183
10   De Groot AC, Schmidt E. Essential oils: contact allergy and chemical composition. Boca Raton, Fl., USA: CRC Press, Taylor and Francis Group, 2016 (ISBN 9781482246407)

Chapter 3.137 PHENYLACETALDEHYDE

IDENTIFICATION

Description/definition	: Phenylacetaldehyde is the aromatic aldehyde that conforms to the structural formula shown below
Chemical class(es)	: Aromatic compounds; aldehydes
INCI name USA	: Not in the Personal Care Products Council Ingredient Database
Chemical/IUPAC name	: 2-Phenylacetaldehyde
Other names	: α-Tolualdehyde; hyacinthin
CAS registry number(s)	: 122-78-1
EC number(s)	: 204-574-5
RIFM monograph(s)	: Food Cosmet Toxicol 1979;17:377
IFRA standard	: Restricted (www.ifraorg.org/en-us/standards-library) (table 3.137.1)
SCCS opinion(s)	: SCCP/1153/08 (1); SCCS/1459/11 (2); SCCNFP/0389/00, final (6)
Merck Index monograph	: 8647
Function(s) in cosmetics	: EU: perfuming
Patch testing	: 0.5% pet. (9); risk of patch test sensitization with 0.5% in alcohol (8)
Molecular formula	: C_8H_8O

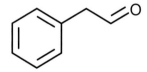

Table 3.137.1 IFRA restrictions for phenylacetaldehyde

Category [a]	Limits [b]	Category [a]	Limits [b]	Category [a]	Limits [b]
1	0.02%	5	0.10%	9	3.00%
2	0.02%	6	0.40%	10	2.50%
3	0.09%	7	0.04%	11	not restricted
4	0.30%	8	0.60%		

[a] For explanation of categories see pages 6-8
[b] Limits in the finished products

GENERAL

Phenylacetaldehyde is a colorless to pale yellow clear oily liquid; its odor type is green and its odor at 2% is described as 'honey, floral rose, sweet, powdery, fermented, chocolate with a slight earthy nuance' (www.thegoodscentscompany.com).

Presence in essential oils

Phenylacetaldehyde has been identified by chemical analysis in 27 of 91 essential oils, which have caused contact allergy / allergic contact dermatitis. In none of these oils, it belonged to the 'Top-10' of ingredients with the highest concentrations (5).

CONTACT ALLERGY

General

The SCCS (Scientific Committee on Consumer Safety), in a 2012 Opinion on Fragrance allergens in cosmetic products, has marked phenylacetaldehyde as 'Fragrance substance with positive human data, which are, however, not sufficient to categorize it as 'established contact allergen in humans' (2,4). The sensitizing potency of phenylacetaldehyde was classified as 'moderate' based on an EC3 value of 3% in the LLNA (local lymph node assay) in animal experiments (2,4).

Patch testing in groups of patients

Patch testing in consecutive patients suspected of contact dermatitis: routine testing
Before 1970, in Sweden, 275 consecutive patients with dermatitis were patch tested with phenylacetaldehyde 0.5% in alcohol and there were 4 (1.5%) positive patch test reactions. Their relevance was not mentioned (8). Three of the 4 co-reacted to Myroxylon pereirae resin (balsam of Peru) and two of the four were sensitized by the patch test (8).

Patch testing in groups of selected patients
In 1983, in The Netherlands, 182 patients suspected of cosmetic allergy were patch tested with phenylacetaldehyde 2% pet. and there were 2 (1.1%) positive reactions; their relevance was not mentioned (7).

Case reports and case series
A man, working as a joiner in a perfume factory, received pure phenylacetaldehyde on his face, trunk and arms, during the manipulation of a defected join. The substance absorbed by his clothes came in contact with the skin. Very quickly the worker took off his clothes and had a long shower of pure water. The same day he attended the emergency room with a discrete erythema of the chin, trunk and arms, without any systemic involvement. The day after, papular erythematous and vesicular pruriginous plaques appeared on the arms and trunk. The patient was patch tested 3 months after the work accident and reacted to phenylacetaldehyde 2%, 1% and 0.5% pet. Ten controls were negative. The authors were not sure whether this was is a primary sensitization reaction or if the patient was already sensitized to phenylacetaldehyde (10). The swift reaction after 2 days seems to favour previous sensitization.

A baker who later became cook had recurrent dermatitis of the hands, arms and face. He was known to react to his wife's perfumes and used fragranced cosmetic products himself. He had no reactions to any spice that he brought in himself, but when tested with a battery of fragrances, there were positive reactions to phenylacetaldehyde 2%, eugenol 8%, dihydrocoumarin 5%, methyl 2-octynoate 0.5% and cinnamyl benzoate 10%, all in petrolatum. The author was 'inclined' to say that these reactions may have been relevant (3).

Cross-reactions, pseudo-cross-reactions and co-reactions
For general information on cross-/pseudo-cross-/co-reactivity of fragrance chemicals with other fragrances, fragrance markers (fragrance mix I, fragrance mix II, colophonium, Myroxylon pereirae resin [balsam of Peru]) and essential oils see Chapter 1.2 General information on cross-reactions, pseudo-cross-reactions and co-reactions.

Of 4 patients with positive reactions to phenylacetaldehyde 0.5% alc., 3 (75%) co-reacted to Myroxylon pereirae resin (8).

Patch test sensitization
Of 275 patients patch tested with phenylacetaldehyde 0.5% alcohol, 2 (0.7%) were sensitized by the patch test; the author of this study was sensitized himself by a patch test with phenylacetaldehyde 10% in alcohol (8).

Quenching
The term 'quenching' was employed to describe the complete abrogation of the sensitizing potential of 3 fragrance chemicals (cinnamal, citral and phenylacetaldehyde) by the presence of certain other fragrance chemicals (notably eugenol and limonene) (12). The conclusions were supported by a summary of human predictive test data. Unfortunately, the absence of any details (numbers tested, reproducibility, etc.) have tended to compromise the credibility of the report (11). Whilst there is some evidence in man for the occurrence of quenching during the induction of skin sensitization, a much more substantial body of work has failed to find supportive evidence in various animal models, at a chemical level or at elicitation in human subjects with existing allergy (11,13). In a thorough review of the subject in 2000, it was therefore concluded that the existence of quenching of these fragrance allergens by other specific fragrance components should be regarded as a hypothesis still lacking substantive proof (11).

Other information
A patch test with phenylacetaldehyde 10% alc. caused irritant erythema after 2 days (8).

LITERATURE

1   SCCP (Scientific Committee on Consumer Products). Opinion on Dermal sensitisation quantitative risk assessment (Citral, Farnesol and Phenylacetaldehyde), 24 June 2008, SCCP/1153/08. Available at: http://ec.europa.eu/health/archive/ph_risk/committees/04_sccp/docs/sccp_o_135.pdf

2   SCCS (Scientific Committee on Consumer Safety). Opinion on Fragrance allergens in cosmetic products, 26-27 June 2012, SCCS/1459/11. Available at: https://ec.europa.eu/health/sites/health/files/scientific_committees/consumer_safety/docs/sccs_o_102.pdf

3   Malten KE. Four bakers showing positive patch tests to a number of fragrance materials, which can also be used as flavors. Acta Derm Venereol 1979;59(suppl.85):117-121

4   Uter W, Johansen JD, Börje A, Karlberg A-T, Lidén C, Rastogi S, Roberts D, White IR. Categorization of fragrance contact allergens for prioritization of preventive measures: clinical and experimental data and consideration of structure–activity relationships. Contact Dermatitis 2013;69:196-230

5   De Groot AC, Schmidt E. Essential oils: contact allergy and chemical composition. Boca Raton, Fl., USA: CRC Press, Taylor and Francis Group, 2016 (ISBN 9781482246407)

6   Opinion of the Scientific Committee on Cosmetic Products and Non-Food Products Intended for Consumers concerning 'The 1st update of the inventory of ingredients employed in cosmetic products. Section II: Perfume and aromatic raw materials', 24 October 2000, SCCNFP/0389/00, final. Available at: http://ec.europa.eu/health/ph_risk/committees/sccp/documents/out131_en.pdf

7   Malten KE, van Ketel WG, Nater JP, Liem DH. Reactions in selected patients to 22 fragrance materials. Contact Dermatitis 1984;11:1-10

8   Fregert S. Sensitization to phenylacetaldehyde. Dermatologica 1970;141:11-14

9   De Groot AC. Patch Testing, 4th Edition. Wapserveen, The Netherlands: acdegroot publishing, 2018 (ISBN 978-90-813233-4-5)

10   Sanchez-Politta S, Campanelli A, Pashe-Koo F, Saurat JH, Piletta P. Allergic contact dermatitis to phenylacetaldehyde: a forgotten allergen? Contact Dermatitis 2007;56:171-172

11   Basketter D. Quenching: fact or fiction? Contact Dermatitis 2000;43:253-258

12   Opdyke DLJ. Inhibition of sensitization reactions induced by certain aldehydes. Fd Cosmet Toxicol 1976;14:197-198

13   Basketter D A, Allenby C F. Studies of the quenching phenomenon in delayed contact hypersensitivity reactions. Contact Dermatitis 1991;25:166-171

Chapter 3.138 PHENYLPROPANOL

IDENTIFICATION

Description/definition : Phenylpropanol is the organic compound that conforms to the structural formula shown below
Chemical class(es) : Alcohols
Chemical/IUPAC name : 3-Phenylpropan-1-ol
Other names : Benzenepropanol; hydrocinnamic alcohol; hydrocinnamyl alcohol; phenethyl carbinol
CAS registry number(s) : 122-97-4
EC number(s) : 204-587-6
RIFM monograph(s) : Food Chem Toxicol 2011;49(suppl.2):S246-S251; Food Cosmet Toxicol 1979;17:893 (special issue V)
SCCS opinion(s) : SCCS/1459/11 (1)
Function(s) in cosmetics : EU: masking; perfuming; solvent. USA: fragrance ingredients; solvents
Patch testing : 5% pet. (2)
Molecular formula : $C_9H_{12}O$

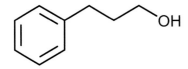

GENERAL

Phenylpropanol (3-phenyl propyl alcohol) is a colorless clear oily liquid; its odor type is balsamic and its odor at 100% is described as 'sweet spicy cinnamyl mignonette hyacinth balsam' (www.thegoodscentscompany.com). Phenylpropanol occurs in many fruits and berries, cinnamon and some types of balsam. It is also present in tobacco smoke. Phenylpropanol is used as a food flavoring, a cosmetic preservative, and as a fragrance in perfumes, personal care products, detergents, fabric softeners, candles, and incense (National Library of Medicine).

Presence in essential oils

Phenylpropanol (hydrocinnamyl alcohol) has been identified by chemical analysis in four of 91 essential oils, which have caused contact allergy / allergic contact dermatitis: cassia bark oil, cassia leaf oil, cinnamon bark oil Sri Lanka and cinnamon leaf oil Sri Lanka (4).

CONTACT ALLERGY

The SCCS (Scientific Committee on Consumer Safety), in a 2012 Opinion on Fragrance allergens in cosmetic products, has categorized phenylpropanol as 'possible fragrance contact allergen' (1,3).

Patch testing in groups of patients

Patch testing in groups of patients with phenylpropanol with positive results has been performed in one international study only (2). Before 2002, in Japan, European countries and the USA, 218 patients with known fragrance sensitivity were patch tested with phenylpropanol 5% in petrolatum and two positive reactions (0.9%) were observed; their relevance was not mentioned (2).

Case reports and case series

Case reports of allergic contact dermatitis from phenylpropanol have not been found.

LITERATURE

1 SCCS (Scientific Committee on Consumer Safety). Opinion on Fragrance allergens in cosmetic products, 26-27 June 2012, SCCS/1459/11. Available at: https://ec.europa.eu/health/sites/health/files/scientific_committees/consumer_safety/docs/sccs_o_102.pdf
2 Larsen W, Nakayama H, Fischer T, Elsner P, Frosch P, Burrows D, et al. Fragrance contact dermatitis - a worldwide multicenter investigation (Part III). Contact Dermatitis 2002;46:141-144
3 Uter W, Johansen JD, Börje A, Karlberg A-T, Lidén C, Rastogi S, Roberts D, White IR. Categorization of fragrance contact allergens for prioritization of preventive measures: clinical and experimental data and consideration of structure–activity relationships. Contact Dermatitis 2013;69:196-230
4 De Groot AC, Schmidt E. Essential oils: contact allergy and chemical composition. Boca Raton, Fl., USA: CRC Press, Taylor and Francis Group, 2016 (ISBN 9781482246407)

Chapter 3.139 ALPHA-PINENE *

Not an INCI name

IDENTIFICATION

Description/definition   : alpha-Pinene is the bicyclic organic compound that conforms to the structural formula shown below
Chemical class(es)   : Bicyclic organic compounds; unsaturated organic compounds
INCI name USA   : Pinene
Chemical/IUPAC name   : 4,6,6-Trimethylbicyclo[3.1.1]hept-3-ene
Other names   : 2-Pinene
CAS registry number(s)   : 80-56-8
EC number(s)   : 201-291-9
RIFM monograph(s)   : Food Cosmet Toxicol 1978;16:853 (special issue IV)
SCCS opinion(s)   : SCCS/1459/11 (2); SCCNFP/0389/00, final (10)
Merck Index monograph   : 8826
Function(s) in cosmetics   : EU: perfuming. USA: antifungal agents; fragrance ingredients
EU cosmetic restrictions   : Regulated in Annex III/130 of the Regulation (EC) No. 344/2013
Patch testing   : 15% Pet. (SmartPracticeEurope, SmartPracticeCanada); 10% pet. (15); concentrations of alpha-pinene 5% (or higher) *in alcohol* may be (strongly) irritant (1)
Molecular formula   : $C_{10}H_{16}$

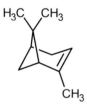

GENERAL

alpha-Pinene is a colorless to pale yellow clear liquid; its odor type is herbal and its odor at 10% is described as 'woody, piney and turpentine-like, with a slight cooling camphoraceous nuance and a fresh herbal lift' (www.thegoodscentscompany.com). alpha-Pinene is used to improve the odor of industrial products such as lubricating oils. It may also be employed in cosmetics and is added as flavor to foods and beverages. Other uses include or have included as solvent for protective coatings, polishes, and waxes, in the synthesis of camphene, camphor, geraniol, esters and ethers, synthetic pine oil, and terpene synthetic resins (U.S. National Library of Medicine).

Presence in essential oils, Myroxylon pereirae resin (balsam of Peru) and propolis

alpha-Pinene has been identified by chemical analysis in 88 of 91 essential oils, which have caused contact allergy / allergic contact dermatitis. In 45 oils, alpha-pinene belonged to the 'Top-10' of ingredients with the highest concentrations. These are shown in table 3.139.1 with the concentration range which may be expected in commercial essential oils of this type (7). alpha-Pinene may also be present in Myroxylon pereirae resin (balsam of Peru) (16) and in propolis (17).

CONTACT ALLERGY

General

The SCCS (Scientific Committee on Consumer Safety), in a 2012 Opinion on Fragrance allergens in cosmetic products, has marked alpha-pinene as 'established contact allergen in humans' (2,8).

alpha-Pinene has not been described as causing allergic contact dermatitis from its presence in fragrances or fragranced products. However, it used to be an important allergen in turpentine oil (1,3,11,12,13, Chapter 6.75 Turpentine oil) and may occasionally (potentially) be a sensitizer or one of the sensitizers in other essential oils (14,15).

Patch testing in groups of patients

Patch testing in consecutive patients suspected of contact dermatitis: routine testing

Studies in which alpha-pinene was patch tested in consecutive patients suspected of contact dermatitis (routine testing) with positive results have not been found.

Table 3.139.1 Essential oils containing alpha-pinene in the 'Top-10' and concentration range in commercial oils (7)

Essential oil	Concentration range (min.-max.)	Essential oil	Concentration range (min.-max.)
Turpentine oil	65.0 - 90.0%	Cajeput oil	0.6 - 7.6%
Juniper berry oil	18.1 - 66.6%	Laurel leaf oil	4.4 - 7.5%
Cypress oil	43.2 - 68.0%	Sage oil Dalmatian	1.1 - 6.5%
Olibanum oil	14.8 - 46.5%	Black cumin oil	0.7 - 4.1%
Rosemary oil	1.9 - 46.0%	Litsea cubeba oil	0.6 - 3.7%
Dwarf pine oil	0.3 - 38.8%	Thuja oil	1.4 - 3.6%
Black pepper oil	5.1 - 29.5%	Spike lavender oil	0.6 - 3.6%
Angelica root oil	11.4 - 27.0%	Eucalyptus citriodora oil	0.2 - 3.5%
Nutmeg oil	12.6 - 25.3%	Mandarin oil	1.2 - 3.1%
Pine needle oil	13.3 - 20.4%	Lovage oil	0.2 - 3.1%
Myrrh oil	0.3 - 15.8%	Silver fir oil	0.5 - 2.8%
Niaouli oil	4.7 - 15.0%	Lemon oil	1.5 - 2.4%
Angelica fruit oil	2.3 - 13.3%	Rosewood oil	0.2 - 2.2%
Carrot seed oil	1.9 - 12.5%	Zdravetz oil	0.05 - 2.1%
Calamus oil	0.02 - 12.4%	Cardamom oil	1.0 - 2.0%
Chamomile oil Roman	2.2 - 11.5%	Tangerine oil	0.08 - 1.9%
Sage oil Spanish	4.0 - 11.0%	Star anise oil	0.3 - 1.8%
Galbanum resin oil	2.3 - 10.1%	Bergamot oil	0.6 - 1.7%
Peppermint oil	0.06 - 9.7%	Cinnamon leaf oil Sri Lanka	0.4 - 1.4%
Tea tree oil	1.8 - 9.2%	Grapefruit oil	0.2 - 1.0%
Coriander fruit oil	0.9 - 8.7%	Orange oil sweet	0.2 - 1.0%
Ravensara oil	0.3 - 8.3%	Orange oil bitter	0.4 - 0.7%
Eucalyptus globulus oil	0.3 - 8.2%		

Patch testing in groups of selected patients

Results of studies patch testing alpha-pinene in groups of selected patients (e.g. patients allergic to turpentine oil, individuals allergic to tea tree oil) are shown in table 3.139.2. In five investigations, high frequencies of sensitization to alpha-pinene were observed, ranging from 50% to 77% (1,9,11,12,13). This is the result of selection of patients allergic to turpentine oil, in which alpha-pinene is one of the main allergens, and in some types the most frequent one (Chapter 6.75 Turpentine oil). The fact that 4 out of 7 (57%) of patients allergic to tea tree oil in a German study also reacted to alpha-pinene (1) is more difficult to explain, as this chemical is not an important allergen in tea tree oil (Chapter 6.71 Tea tree oil). Possibly, these tea tree oil-allergic patients had previously also become sensitized to turpentine oil, an allergy which is very common in Germany.

Table 3.139.2 Patch testing in groups of patients: Selected patient groups

Years and Country	Test conc. & vehicle	Number of patients tested | positive (%)		Selection of patients (S); Relevance (R); Comments (C)	Ref.
<1996 UK	10% pet.	14	7 (50%)	S: patients with occupational hand dermatitis working in the pottery industry and sensitized to Indonesian turpentine oil with high 3-carene content	13
1990-1992 Germany	10% alc.	7	4 (57%)	S: patients with a positive patch test reaction to tea tree oil 1% alc.	1
1985 Spain	15% o.o	67	36 (54%)	S: patients allergic to turpentine oil; R: not specified	12
1979-1983 Portugal	15% o.o.	22	17 (77%)	S: patients allergic to turpentine oil; R: not stated	11
<1976 Poland		15	8 (53%)	S: patients with positive patch tests to star anise oil 1% pet., negative to 0.5% but positive to one or more 'balsams' (Myroxylon pereirae resin, turpentine, wood tars, colophonium); all 8 patients co-reacted to turpentine, in which α-pinene is a very important allergen; alpha-pinene is not an important ingredient of star anise oil and the high percentage of positive reactions to alpha-pinene is the result of selecting patients for sensitivity to turpentine oil and other 'balsams'	9

o.o.: Olive oil

Case reports and case series

Fourteen pottery workers developed occupational contact dermatitis from sensitization to Indonesian turpentine oil with high 3-carene content. Seven (50%) co-reacted to α-pinene (13).

Two professional aromatherapists reacted upon patch testing to multiple essential oils. They were also patch tested with alpha-pinene (2%, 5% and 10% pet.), which was found to be present in many of the essential oils by GC-MS. One reacted to the 5% and 10% pet. test substances, the other only to 10% pet. There were no reactions to beta-pinene (15).

A man had developed contact allergy to and allergic contact dermatitis from turpentine oil from working in a laboratory. Many years later, he showed swelling of the tongue, lips, and gingival mucosa, and complained of a burning sensation in his mouth. Allergy to peppermint oil was suspected, which was present in an antiseptic spray, a mouthwash and candies he habitually sucked on. Patch tests were positive to colophonium, Myroxylon pereirae resin, turpentine peroxides, peppermint oil and its ingredients alpha-pinene, d-limonene and l-limonene (together dipentene). The patient probably had primarily become sensitized to these substances in turpentine oil and later had allergic contact dermatitis from alpha-pinene and limonene in peppermint oil, which are important ingredients of this essential oil (limonene up to 18.5% and alpha-pinene up to 9.7% [7]) (6) .

Bergamot oil sensitized one worker in the fragrance industry; she also reacted to α-pinene and β-pinene; commercial bergamot oils were investigated for the presence of these chemicals and they were identified in maximum concentrations of 1.7% (α-pinene) resp. 9.3% (β-pinene) (14).

Cross-reactions, pseudo-cross-reactions and co-reactions

For general information on cross-/pseudo-cross-/co-reactivity of fragrance chemicals with other fragrances, fragrance markers (fragrance mix I, fragrance mix II, colophonium, Myroxylon pereirae resin [balsam of Peru]) and essential oils see Chapter 1.2 General information on cross-reactions, pseudo-cross-reactions and co-reactions.

alpha-Pinene is an important ingredient of many essential oils (table 3.139.1) and co-reactivity has been observed especially with turpentine oil (6,9,11,12,13), but also with peppermint oil (6), tea tree oil (1) and various other essential oils (15).

Presence in products and chemical analyses

In 2000, fifty-nine domestic and occupational products, purchased in retail outlets in Denmark, England, Germany and Italy were analyzed by GC-MS for the presence of fragrances. The product categories were liquid soap and soap bars (n=13), soft/hard surface cleaners (n=23), fabric conditioners/laundry detergents for hand wash (n=8), dish wash (n=10), furniture polish, car shampoo, stain remover (each n=1) and 2 products used in occupational environments. alpha-Pinene was present in 23 products (39%) with a mean concentration of 41 ppm and a range of 5-157 ppm (4).

In 1992, in The Netherlands, the presence of fragrances was analyzed in 300 cosmetic products. alpha-Pinene was identified in 35% of the products (rank number 19) (5).

LITERATURE

1   Knight TE, Hausen BM. Melaleuca oil (tea tree oil) dermatitis. J Am Acad Dermatol 1994;30:423-427
2   SCCS (Scientific Committee on Consumer Safety). Opinion on Fragrance allergens in cosmetic products, 26-27 June 2012, SCCS/1459/11. Available at: https://ec.europa.eu/health/sites/health/files/scientific_committees/consumer_safety/docs/sccs_o_102.pdf
3   Michailov P, Berowa N, Zuzulowa A. Klinische und biochemische Untersuchungen über die berufsbedingten allergischen und toxischen Erscheinungen durch Terpentin. Allergie und Asthma 1970;16:201-205
4   Rastogi SC, Heydorn S, Johansen JD, Basketter DA. Fragrance chemicals in domestic and occupational products. Contact Dermatitis 2001;45:221-225
5   Weyland JW. Personal Communication, 1992. Cited in: De Groot AC, Weyland JW, Nater JP. Unwanted effects of cosmetics and drugs used in dermatology, 3rd Ed. Amsterdam: Elsevier, 1994:579
6   Dooms-Goossens A, Degreef H, Holvoet C, Maertens M. Turpentine-induced hypersensitivity to peppermint oil. Contact Dermatitis 1977;3:304-308
7   De Groot AC, Schmidt E. Essential oils: contact allergy and chemical composition. Boca Raton, Fl., USA: CRC Press, Taylor and Francis Group, 2016 (ISBN 9781482246407
8   Uter W, Johansen JD, Börje A, Karlberg A-T, Lidén C, Rastogi S, Roberts D, White IR. Categorization of fragrance contact allergens for prioritization of preventive measures: clinical and experimental data and consideration of structure–activity relationships. Contact Dermatitis 2013;69:196-230
9   Rudzki E, Grzywa Z. Sensitizing and irritating properties of star anise oil. Contact Dermatitis 1976;2:305-306

10 Opinion of the Scientific Committee on Cosmetic Products and Non-Food Products Intended for Consumers concerning 'The 1st update of the inventory of ingredients employed in cosmetic products. Section II: Perfume and aromatic raw materials', 24 October 2000, SCCNFP/0389/00, final. Available at: http://ec.europa.eu/health/ph_risk/committees/sccp/documents/out131_en.pdf

11 Cachao P, Menezes Brandao F, Carmo M, Frazao S, Silva M. Allergy to oil of turpentine in Portugal. Contact Dermatitis 1986;14:205-208

12 Romaguera C, Alomar A, Conde-Salazar L, Camarasa JMG, Grimalt F, Martin Pascual A, et al. Turpentine sensitization. Contact Dermatitis 1986;14:197

13 Lear JT, Heagerty AH, Tan BB, Smith AG, English JS. Transient re-emergence of oil of turpentine allergy in the pottery industry. Contact Dermatitis 1996;35:169-172

14 Zacher KD, Ippen H. Kontaktekzem durch Bergamottöl. Derm Beruf Umwelt 1984;32:95-97

15 Dharmagunawardena B, Takwale A, Sanders KJ, Cannan S, Roger A, Ilchyshyn A. Gas chromatography: an investigative tool in multiple allergies to essential oils. Contact Dermatitis 2002;47:288-292

16 Mammerler V. Contribution to the analysis and quality control of Peru Balsam. PhD Thesis, University of Vienna, Austria, 2007. Available at: http://othes.univie.ac.at/4056/1/2009-03-23_0201578.pdf

17 De Groot AC, Popova MP, Bankova VS. An update on the constituents of poplar-type propolis. Wapserveen, The Netherlands: acdegroot publishing, 2014, 11 pages. ISBN/EAN: 978-90-813233-0-7. Available at: https://www.researchgate.net/publication/262851225_AN_UPDATE_ON_THE_CONSTITUENTS_OF_POPLAR-TYPE_PROPOLIS

Chapter 3.140 BETA-PINENES *
* Not officially an INCI name but perfuming name

IDENTIFICATION

Description/definition   : beta-Pinene is the bicyclic organic compound that conforms to the structural formula
                                shown below
Chemical class(es)   : Bicyclic organic compounds; unsaturated organic compounds
INCI name USA   : Not in the Personal Care Products Council Ingredient Database
Chemical/IUPAC name   : 6,6-Dimethyl-4-methylidenebicyclo[3.1.1]heptane
Other names   : Nopinene; pseudopinene
CAS registry number(s)   : 127-91-3
EC number(s)   : 204-872-5
RIFM monograph(s)   : Food Cosmet Toxicol 1978;16:859 (special issue IV)
SCCS opinion(s)   : SCCS/1459/11 (1); SCCNFP/0389/00, final (12)
Merck Index monograph   : 8827
Function(s) in cosmetics   : EU: perfuming
EU cosmetic restrictions   : Regulated in Annex III/130 of the Regulation (EC) No. 344/2013
Patch testing   : 15% olive oil (5,6); 1% pet. (4); according to data from RIFM, 12% pet. is probably not
                                irritant (10)
Molecular formula   : $C_{10}H_{16}$

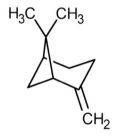

GENERAL

beta-Pinene is a colorless clear liquid; its odor type is herbal and its odor at 10% is described as 'cooling, woody, piney and turpentine-like with a fresh minty, eucalyptus and camphoraceous note with a spicy peppery and nutmeg nuance' (www.thegoodscentscompany.com). It is used as a chemical intermediate for the production of other fragrances such as myrcene (the starting material for acyclic terpenes), geraniol and linalool. Other uses include or have included as monomer for polyterpene resins, the production of hot melt adhesives, substitute for alpha-pinene, and flavoring agent for ice cream, candy and baked goods (U.S. National Library of Medicine).

Presence in essential oils and Myroxylon pereirae resin (balsam of Peru)
beta-Pinene has been identified by chemical analysis in 78 of 91 essential oils, which have caused contact allergy / allergic contact dermatitis. In 32 oils, beta-pinene belonged to the 'Top-10' of ingredients with the highest concentrations. These are shown in table 3.140.1 with the concentration range which may be expected in commercial essential oils of this type (9). β-Pinene may also be present in Myroxylon pereirae resin (balsam of Peru) (11).

CONTACT ALLERGY

General
The SCCS (Scientific Committee on Consumer Safety), in a 2012 Opinion on Fragrance allergens in cosmetic products, has marked β-pinene as 'established contact allergen in humans' (1,3).

There are no reports of allergic contact dermatitis caused by β-pinene from its presence in a fragrance or fragranced product. However, it used to be an important allergen in certain turpentine oils (5,6). Possibly, it was the allergen or one of the allergens in single patients who became sensitized to bergamot oil (7) and lemon oil (8).

Patch testing in groups of patients
Results of studies testing beta-pinene in consecutive patients suspected of contact dermatitis (routine testing) and those of testing in groups of *selected* patients (patients allergic to turpentine oil) are shown in table 3.140.2.

Patch testing in consecutive patients suspected of contact dermatitis: routine testing

In Italy, in the period 1983-1984, beta-pinene 1% pet. was tested in 1200 consecutive patients with dermatitis and there were 2 (0.2%) positive reactions; their relevance was not mentioned (4).

Table 3.140.1 Essential oils containing beta-pinene in the 'Top-10' and concentration range in commercial oils (9)

Essential oil	Concentration range (min.-max.)	Essential oil	Concentration range (min.-max.)
Galbanum resin oil	51.0 - 81.2%	Lovage oil	trace - 12.3%
Silver fir oil	7.4 - 31.7%	Rosemary oil	0.3 - 10.3%
Dwarf pine oil	0.01 - 29.0%	Bergamot oil	4.8 - 9.3%
Black pepper oil	6.7 - 20.3%	Sage oil Dalmatian	1.0 - 9.2%
Turpentine oil	3.0 - 18.0%	Juniper berry oil	1.8 - 7.8%
Lemon oil	7.4 - 17.8%	Pine needle oil	0.9 - 7.1%
Hyssop oil	8.2 - 17.2%	Peppermint oil	0.2 - 6.5%
Neroli oil	3.8 - 16.9%	Eucalyptus globulus oil	0.3 - 5.8%
Nutmeg oil	2.6 - 16.5%	Laurel leaf oil	3.2 - 5.0%
Ravensara oil	0.1 - 15.7%	Valerian oil	0.3 - 4.9%
Black cumin oil	0.7 - 4.4%	Petitgrain bigarade oil	0.09 - 1.9%
Cajeput oil	0.7 - 4.4%	Bay oil	0.05 - 1.8%
Carrot seed oil	0.4 - 4.4%	Eucalyptus citriodora oil	0.4 - 1.3%
Spike lavender oil	0.4 - 2.6%	Tangerine oil	trace - 0.9%
Mandarin oil	0.5 - 2.2%	Orange oil bitter	0.2 - 0.8%
Lavandin oil	0.5 - 1.9%	Orange oil sweet	0.01 - 0.5%

Patch testing in groups of selected patients

In two studies from Spain, groups of patients known to be allergic to oil of turpentine were patch tested with a number of its ingredients and 25 of 67 patients (37%) (6) resp. 2 of 22 (9%) (5) had positive reactions to beta-pinene 15% in olive oil.

Table 3.140.2 Patch testing in groups of patients

Years and Country	Test conc. & vehicle	Number of patients tested	positive (%)		Selection of patients (S); Relevance (R); Comments (C)	Ref.
Routine testing						
1983-1984 Italy	1% pet.	1200	2	(0.2%)	R: not stated	4
Testing in groups of selected patients						
1985 Spain	15% o.o	67	25	(37%)	S: patients allergic to turpentine oil	6
1979-1983 Portugal	15% o.o.	22	2	(9%)	S: patients allergic to turpentine oil	5

o.o.: Olive oil

Case reports and case series

One worker in the fragrance industry was sensitized by bergamot oil. She also reacted to beta-pinene and alpha-pinene. Commercial bergamot oils were investigated for the presence of these chemicals and they were identified in maximum concentrations of 9.3% (beta-pinene) and of 1.7% (alpha-pinene) (7).

A porter became sensitized to oil of lemon, which he used occupationally. Patch tests were positive to oil of lemon, limonene, oil of citronella Java, oil of citronella Ceylon (= Sri Lanka), turpentine and its component beta-pinene (8). Limonene is the major ingredient in lemon oil and beta-pinene has also been found in commercial lemon oils in concentrations up to 17.8% (9).

Cross-reactions, pseudo-cross-reactions and co-reactions

For general information on cross-/pseudo-cross-/co-reactivity of fragrance chemicals with other fragrances, fragrance markers (fragrance mix I, fragrance mix II, colophonium, Myroxylon pereirae resin [balsam of Peru]) and essential oils see Chapter 1.2 General information on cross-reactions, pseudo-cross-reactions and co-reactions.

beta-Pinene is an important ingredient of many essential oils and co-reactions have been observed with turpentine oil (5,6,8) and bergamot oil (7).

Presence in products and chemical analyses

In 1992, in The Netherlands, the presence of fragrances was analyzed in 300 cosmetic products. beta-Pinene was identified in 51% of the products (rank order 9) (2).

LITERATURE

1　SCCS (Scientific Committee on Consumer Safety). Opinion on Fragrance allergens in cosmetic products, 26-27 June 2012, SCCS/1459/11. Available at: https://ec.europa.eu/health/sites/health/files/scientific_committees/consumer_safety/docs/sccs_o_102.pdf

2　Weyland JW. Personal Communication, 1992. Cited in: De Groot AC, Weyland JW, Nater JP. Unwanted effects of cosmetics and drugs used in dermatology, 3rd Ed. Amsterdam: Elsevier, 1994:579

3　Uter W, Johansen JD, Börje A, Karlberg A-T, Lidén C, Rastogi S, Roberts D, White IR. Categorization of fragrance contact allergens for prioritization of preventive measures: clinical and experimental data and consideration of structure–activity relationships. Contact Dermatitis 2013;69:196-230

4　Santucci B, Cristaudo A, Cannistraci C, Picardo M. Contact dermatitis to fragrances. Contact Dermatitis 1987;16:93-95

5　Cachao P, Menezes Brandao F, Carmo M, Frazao S, Silva M. Allergy to oil of turpentine in Portugal. Contact Dermatitis 1986;14:205-208

6　Romaguera C, Alomar A, Conde-Salazar L, Camarasa JMG, Grimalt F, Martin Pascual A, et al. Turpentine sensitization. Contact Dermatitis 1986;14:197

7　Zacher KD, Ippen H. Kontaktekzem durch Bergamottöl. Derm Beruf Umwelt 1984;32:95-97

8　Keil H. Contact dermatitis due to oil of citronellal. J Invest Dermatol 1947;8:327-334

9　De Groot AC, Schmidt E. Essential oils: contact allergy and chemical composition. Boca Raton, Fl., USA: CRC Press, Taylor and Francis Group, 2016 (ISBN 9781482246407)

10　De Groot AC. Patch Testing, 4th Edition. Wapserveen, The Netherlands: acdegroot publishing, 2018 (ISBN 978-90-813233-4-5)

11　Mammerler V. Contribution to the analysis and quality control of Peru Balsam. PhD Thesis, University of Vienna, Austria, 2007. Available at: http://othes.univie.ac.at/4056/1/2009-03-23_0201578.pdf

12　Opinion of the Scientific Committee on Cosmetic Products and Non-Food Products Intended for Consumers concerning 'The 1st update of the inventory of ingredients employed in cosmetic products. Section II: Perfume and aromatic raw materials', 24 October 2000, SCCNFP/0389/00, final. Available at: http://ec.europa.eu/health/ph_risk/committees/sccp/documents/out131_en.pdf

Chapter 3.141 PIPERITONE

IDENTIFICATION

Description/definition : Piperitone is the cyclohexene derivative that conforms to the structural formula shown below
Chemical class(es) : Cyclic organic compounds; ketones
INCI name USA : Not in the Personal Care Products Council Ingredient Database
Chemical/IUPAC name : 3-Methyl-6-propan-2-ylcyclohex-2-en-1-one
Other names : 3-Carvomenthenone; *p*-menth-1-en-3-one
CAS registry number(s) : 89-81-6
EC number(s) : 201-942-7
RIFM monograph(s) : Food Cosmet Toxicol 1978;16:863 (special issue IV)
Merck Index monograph : 8855
Function(s) in cosmetics : EU: perfuming
Patch testing : No patch test data available; based on RIFM data, 10% pet. is probably not irritant (4)
Molecular formula : $C_{10}H_{16}O$

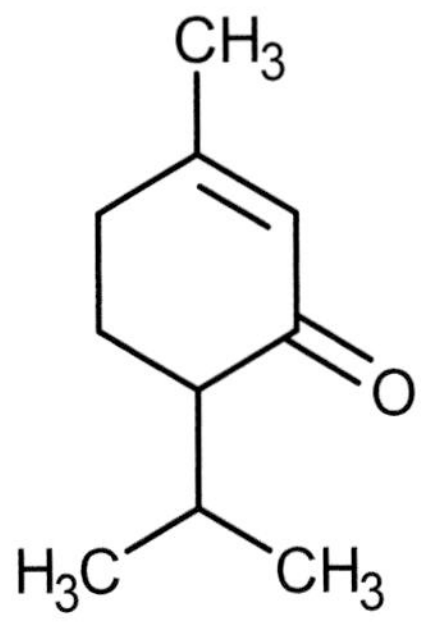

GENERAL

Piperitone is a colorless to pale yellow clear liquid; its odor type is herbal and its odor at 10% in dipropylene glycol is described as 'herbal minty camphor medicinal' (www.thegoodscentscompany.com).

Presence in essential oils

Piperitone has been identified by chemical analysis in 40 of 91 essential oils, which have caused contact allergy / allergic contact dermatitis. In none of these oils, it belonged to the 'Top-10' of ingredients with the highest concentrations (3).

CONTACT ALLERGY

Patch testing in groups of patients

Patch testing in consecutive patients suspected of contact dermatitis: routine testing
Studies in which piperitone was patch tested in consecutive patients suspected of contact dermatitis (routine testing) with positive results have not been found.

Patch testing in groups of selected patients
In Japan, three patients with allergic contact dermatitis from peppermint oil were patch tested with individual ingredients of the oil. It was established that the allergens were piperitone, menthol or pulegone (no further details known, article in Japanese) (1). Piperitone has been found in a maximum concentration of 5.4% in commercial peppermint oils (3).

Ten more patients allergic to peppermint oil (of who 4 co-reacted to spearmint oil) were patch tested with 24 ingredients. There were 4 positive reactions to piperitone, 4 to menthol, 3 to pulegone, 2 to tetrahydrodimethylbenzofuran (menthofuran), one to menthyl acetate and one to dihydrocarveol (2). Further details are lacking (article in Japanese).

Case reports and case series
Case reports of allergic contact dermatitis from dihydrocarveol have not been found.

OTHER SIDE EFFECTS

Other non-eczematous contact reactions
One patient with orofacial granulomatosis had a positive patch test to piperitone, which was apparently present in a toothpaste. After stopping the use of this product, partial improvement of the swelling was noted (5).

LITERATURE
1   Saito F, Oka K. Allergic contact dermatitis due to peppermint oil. Skin Res 1990;32:161-167 (article in Japanese). THIS REFERENCE IS INCORRECT. Cited in: Cosmetic Ingredient Review Expert Panel. Final report on the safety assessment of Mentha piperita (peppermint) oil, Mentha piperita (peppermint) leaf extract, Mentha piperita (peppermint) leaf, and Mentha piperita (peppermint) leaf water. Int J Toxicol 2001;20(suppl.3):61-73
2   Saito F, Miyazaki T, Matsuoka Y. Peppermint oil (title incomplete, partly in Japanese). Skin Research 1984;26:636-643 (article in Japanese)
3   De Groot AC, Schmidt E. Essential oils: contact allergy and chemical composition. Boca Raton, Fl., USA: CRC Press, Taylor and Francis Group, 2016 (ISBN 9781482246407)
4   De Groot AC. Patch Testing, 4th Edition. Wapserveen, The Netherlands: acdegroot publishing, 2018 (ISBN 978-90-813233-4-5)
5   Patton DW, Ferguson MM, Forsyth A, James J. Oro-facial granulomatosis: a possible allergic basis. Br J Oral Maxillofac Surg 1985;23:235-242

Chapter 3.142 PROPYLIDENE PHTHALIDE *
* Not officially an INCI name but perfuming name

IDENTIFICATION

Description/definition	: Propylidene phthalide is the bicyclic organic compound that conforms to the structural formula shown below
Chemical class(es)	: Aromatic compounds; heterocyclic compounds; lactones
INCI name USA	: Not in the Personal Care Products Council Ingredient Database
Chemical/IUPAC name	: 3-Propylidene-2-benzofuran-1-one
CAS registry number (s)	: 17369-59-4
EC number(s)	: 241-402-8
RIFM monograph(s)	: Food Cosmet Toxicol 1978;16:865 (special issue IV)
IFRA standard	: Restricted (www.ifraorg.org/en-us/standards-library) (table 3.142.1)
SCCS opinion(s)	: SCCNFP/0392/00, final (1); SCCS/1459/11 (2); SCCNFP/0389/00, final (7)
Function(s) in cosmetics	: EU: perfuming
EU cosmetic restrictions	: Regulated in Annex III/175 of the Regulation (EC) No. 344/2013
Patch testing	: 2% pet. (4); based on RIFM data, 4% pet. may not be irritant (5)
Molecular formula	: $C_{11}H_{10}O_2$

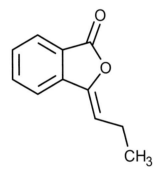

Table 3.142.1 IFRA restrictions for propylidene phthalide

Category [a]	Limits [b]	Category [a]	Limits [b]	Category [a]	Limits [b]
1	0.01%	5	0.01%	9	0.01%
2	0.01%	6	0.70%	10	0.01%
3	0.01%	7	0.01%	11	not restricted
4	0.01%	8	0.01%		

[a] For explanation of categories see pages 6-8
[b] Limits in the finished products

GENERAL

Propylidene phthalide is a colorless to pale yellow clear liquid; its odor type is herbal and its odor is described as 'celery, sweet, lovage and maple-like with herbal, brown, vegetative nuances' (www.thegoodscentscompany.com).

Presence in essential oils

(Z)-3-Propylidene phthalide has been identified by chemical analysis in one of 91 essential oils, which have caused contact allergy / allergic contact dermatitis: lovage oil (6).

CONTACT ALLERGY

General

The SCCS (Scientific Committee on Consumer Safety), in a 2012 Opinion on Fragrance allergens in cosmetic products, has marked propylidene phthalide as 'established contact allergen in humans' (2,3).

Patch testing in groups of patients

Patch testing in consecutive patients suspected of contact dermatitis: routine testing

Studies in which propylidene phthalide was patch tested in consecutive patients suspected of contact dermatitis (routine testing) with positive results have not been found.

Patch testing in groups of selected patients
In 1983, in The Netherlands, 182 patients suspected of cosmetic allergy were patch tested with propylidene phthalide and there were 5 (2.7%) positive reactions; their relevance was not mentioned (4).

Case reports and case series
Case reports of allergic contact dermatitis from propylidene phthalide have not been found.

LITERATURE

1   SCCNFP (Scientific Committee on Cosmetic Products and Non-Food Products Intended for Consumers). Opinion of the Scientific Committee on Cosmetic Products and Non-Food Products Intended for Consumers concerning 'An initial list of perfumery materials which must not form part of cosmetic products except subject to the Restrictions and Conditions laid down, 25 September 2001, SCCNFP/0392/00, final. Available at: http://ec.europa.eu/health/archive/ph_risk/committees/sccp/documents/out150_en.pdf
2   SCCS (Scientific Committee on Consumer Safety). Opinion on Fragrance allergens in cosmetic products, 26-27 June 2012, SCCS/1459/11. Available at: https://ec.europa.eu/health/sites/health/files/scientific_committees/consumer_safety/docs/sccs_o_102.pdf
3   Uter W, Johansen JD, Börje A, Karlberg A-T, Lidén C, Rastogi S, Roberts D, White IR. Categorization of fragrance contact allergens for prioritization of preventive measures: clinical and experimental data and consideration of structure–activity relationships. Contact Dermatitis 2013;69:196-230
4   Malten KE, van Ketel WG, Nater JP, Liem DH. Reactions in selected patients to 22 fragrance materials. Contact Dermatitis 1984;11:1-10
5   De Groot AC. Patch Testing, 4th Edition. Wapserveen, The Netherlands: acdegroot publishing, 2018 (ISBN 978-90-813233-4-5)
6   De Groot AC, Schmidt E. Essential oils: contact allergy and chemical composition. Boca Raton, Fl., USA: CRC Press, 7 Taylor and Francis Group, 2016 (ISBN 9781482246407)
7   Opinion of the Scientific Committee on Cosmetic Products and Non-Food Products Intended for Consumers concerning 'The 1st update of the inventory of ingredients employed in cosmetic products. Section II: Perfume and aromatic raw materials', 24 October 2000, SCCNFP/0389/00, final. Available at: http://ec.europa.eu/health/ph_risk/committees/sccp/documents/out131_en.pdf

Chapter 3.143 D-PULEGONE

IDENTIFICATION

Description/definition : *D*-Pulegone is the cyclohexane derivative that conforms to the structural formula shown below
Chemical class(es) : Cyclic organic compounds; unsaturated compounds; ketones
INCI name USA : Not in the Personal Care Products Council Ingredient Database
Chemical/IUPAC name : (5*R*)-5-Methyl-2-propan-2-ylidenecyclohexan-1-one
Other names : (+)-Pulegone; pulegone; (*R*)-pulegone; (1*R*)-(+)-*p*-menth-4(8)-en-3-one
CAS registry number(s) : 89-82-7
EC number(s) : 201-943-2
RIFM monograph(s) : Food Cosmet Toxicol 1978;16:867 (special issue IV)
Merck Index monograph : 9316
Function(s) in cosmetics : EU: perfuming
Patch testing : No patch test data available; based on RIFM data, 10% pet. is probably not irritant (4)
Molecular formula : $C_{10}H_{16}O$

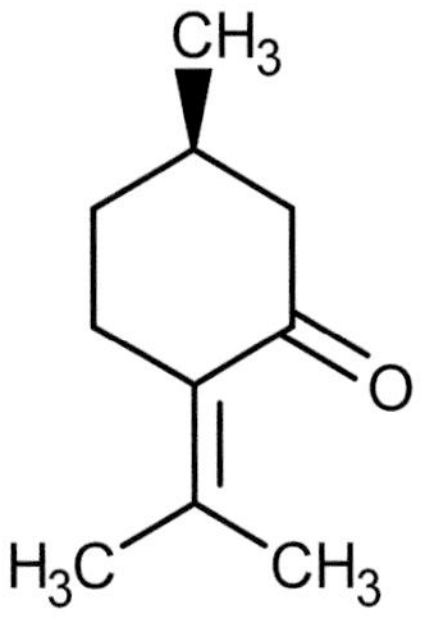

GENERAL

D-Pulegone is a colorless clear oily liquid; its odor type is minty and its odor is described as 'minty, sulfuraceous, sweet with metallic buchu nuances' (www.thegoodscentscompany.com). Pulegone is used as chemical intermediate and for flavoring. Pennyroyal oil contains 60%-90% pulegone and may be used for flavoring foods, drinks, and dental products. This oil has also been used as a herbal medicine proposed to induce menstruation and abortion (U.S. National Library of Medicine).

Presence in essential oils

Pulegone has been identified by chemical analysis in 24 of 91 essential oils, which have caused contact allergy / allergic contact dermatitis. In none of these oils, it belonged to the 'Top-10' of ingredients with the highest concentrations (3).

CONTACT ALLERGY

Patch testing in groups of patients

Patch testing in consecutive patients suspected of contact dermatitis: routine testing

Studies in which pulegone was patch tested in consecutive patients suspected of contact dermatitis (routine testing) with positive results have not been found.

Patch testing in groups of selected patients

In Japan, three patients with allergic contact dermatitis from peppermint oil were patch tested with individual ingredients of the oil. It was established that the allergens were pulegone, menthol or piperitone (no further details known, article in Japanese) (1). Pulegone has been found in a maximum concentration of 5.4% in commercial peppermint oils (3).

Ten more patients allergic to peppermint oil (of who 4 co-reacted to spearmint oil) were patch tested with 24 ingredients. There were 3 positive reactions to pulegone, 4 to menthol, 4 to piperitone, 2 to tetrahydrodimethyl-benzofuran (menthofuran), one to menthyl acetate and one to dihydrocarveol (2). Further details are lacking (article in Japanese).

Case reports and case series

Case reports of allergic contact dermatitis from pulegone have not been found.

LITERATURE

1   Saito F, Oka K. Allergic contact dermatitis due to peppermint oil. Skin Res 1990;32:161-167 (article in Japanese). THIS REFERENCE IS INCORRECT. cited in: Cosmetic Ingredient Review Expert Panel. Final report on the safety assessment of Mentha piperita (peppermint) oil, Mentha piperita (peppermint) leaf extract, Mentha piperita (peppermint) leaf, and Mentha piperita (peppermint) leaf water. Int J Toxicol 2001;20(suppl.3):61-73
2   Saito F, Miyazaki T, Matsuoka Y. Peppermint oil (title incomplete, partly in Japanese). Skin Research 1984;26:636-643 (article in Japanese)
3   De Groot AC, Schmidt E. Essential oils: contact allergy and chemical composition. Boca Raton, Fl., USA: CRC Press, Taylor and Francis Group, 2016 (ISBN 9781482246407)
4   De Groot AC. Patch Testing, 4th Edition. Wapserveen, The Netherlands: acdegroot publishing, 2018 (ISBN 978-90-813233-4-5)

Chapter 3.144 RHODINOL

IDENTIFICATION

Description/definition : Rhodinol is the unsaturated alcohol that conforms to the structural formula shown below
Chemical class(es) : Unsaturated organic compounds; alcohols
INCI name USA : Not in the Personal Care Products Council Ingredient Database
Chemical/IUPAC name : (3S)-3,7-Dimethyloct-7-en-1-ol
Other names : α-Citronellol
CAS registry number(s) : 6812-78-8
EC number(s) : 229-887-4
RIFM monograph(s) : Food Chem Toxicol 2008;46(11)(suppl.):S1-S71; Food Chem Toxicol 2008;46(11)(suppl.): S259-S262; Food Chem Toxicol 1992;30(suppl.1):S113-S114
IFRA standard : Restricted (www.ifraorg.org/en-us/standards-library) (table 3.144.1)
SCCS opinion(s) : SCCS/1459/11 (1)
Merck Index monograph : 9579
Function(s) in cosmetics : EU: perfuming
Patch testing : 'Citronellol' 1% pet. (SmartPracticeEurope, Chemotechnique, SmartPracticeCanada); 'citronellol' is also part of the fragrance mix II; it is unknown whether contact allergy to rhodinol (α-citronellol) will be shown by a positive patch test to 'citronellol' (β-citronellol); rhodinol itself may be tested 3-5% in petrolatum (3,4,7)
Molecular formula : $C_{10}H_{20}O$

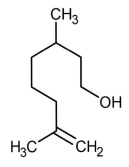

Table 3.144.1 IFRA restrictions for citronellol (CAS 6812-78-8)

Category [a]	Limits [b]	Category [a]	Limits [b]	Category [a]	Limits [b]
1	0.80%	5	7.00%	9	5.00%
2	1.10%	6	21.40%	10	2.50%
3	4.40%	7	2.20%	11	not restricted
4	13.30%	8	2.00%		

[a] For explanation of categories see pages 6-8
[b] Limits in the finished products

GENERAL

Rhodinol is a colorless to pale yellow clear liquid; its odor type is floral and its odor at 100% is described as 'floral red rose' (www.thegoodscentscompany.com).

See also Chapter 3.42 Citronellol (an isomer of rhodinol) and Chapter 3.71 Fragrance mix II.

Presence in essential oils

Rhodinol has been identified by chemical analysis in none of 91 essential oils, which have caused contact allergy / allergic contact dermatitis (6).

CONTACT ALLERGY

General

The SCCS (Scientific Committee on Consumer Safety), in a 2012 Opinion on Fragrance allergens in cosmetic products, has categorized rhodinol as 'likely fragrance contact allergen by combination of evidence' (1,2).

Patch testing in groups of patients

Patch testing in consecutive patients suspected of contact dermatitis: routine testing
Studies in which rhodinol was patch tested in consecutive patients suspected of contact dermatitis (routine testing) with positive results have not been found.

Patch testing in groups of selected patients
Before 1986, in France, 21 patients with allergic contact dermatitis caused by perfumes were patch tested with rhodinol 3% pet. and there was one (5%) positive reaction; its relevance was not mentioned (7).

In a series of patch tests conducted from 1978 to 1985 in Japan with cosmetic ingredients on 96 cosmetic dermatitis patients, two facial melanosis patients and 104 'non-cosmetic dermatitis and eczema patients', rhodinol 5% (vehicle not reported) produced reactions in one of the 104 (1.0%) non-cosmetic dermatitis and eczema patients. Further details are lacking (3,4).

Case reports and case series
Case reports of allergic contact dermatitis from rhodinol have not been found.

LITERATURE
1   SCCS (Scientific Committee on Consumer Safety). Opinion on Fragrance allergens in cosmetic products, 26-27 June 2012, SCCS/1459/11. Available at: https://ec.europa.eu/health/sites/health/files/scientific_committees/consumer_safety/docs/sccs_o_102.pdf
2   Uter W, Johansen JD, Börje A, Karlberg A-T, Lidén C, Rastogi S, Roberts D, White IR. Categorization of fragrance contact allergens for prioritization of preventive measures: clinical and experimental data and consideration of structure–activity relationships. Contact Dermatitis 2013;69:196-230
3   Itoh M, Ishihara M, Hosono K, Kantoh H, Kinoshita M, Yamada K, Nishimura M. Results of patch tests conducted between 1978 and 1985 using cosmetic ingredients. Skin Research 1986;28(suppl.2):110-119 (article in Japanese). Data cited in ref. 5
4   Itoh M, Hosono K, Kantoh H, Kinoshita M, Yamada K, Kurosaka R, Nishimura M. Patch test results with cosmetic ingredients conducted between 1978 and 1986. J Soc Cosm Science 1988;12:27-41 (article in Japanese). Data cited in ref. 5
5   Lapczynski A, Bhatia SP, Letizia CS, Api AM. Fragrance material review on rhodinol. Food Chem Toxicol 2008;46:S259-S262
6   De Groot AC, Schmidt E. Essential oils: contact allergy and chemical composition. Boca Raton, Fl., USA: CRC Press, Taylor and Francis Group, 2016 (ISBN 9781482246407)
7   Meynadier JM, Meynadier J, Peyron JL, Peyron L. Formes cliniques des manifestations cutanées d'allergie aux parfums. Ann Dermatol Venereol 1986;113:31-39

Chapter 3.145 ROSE KETONE-4 *

Not officially an INCI name but perfuming name

IDENTIFICATION

Description/definition : Rose ketone-4 is the cyclohexadiene derivative that conforms to the structural formula shown below

Chemical class(es) : Unsaturated organic compounds; ketones

INCI name USA : Not in the Personal Care Products Council Ingredient Database

Chemical/IUPAC name : 1-(2,6,6-Trimethyl-1,3-cyclohexadien-1-yl)-2-buten-1-one

Other names : Damascenone

CAS registry number.(s) : 23696-85-7

EC number(s) : 245-833-2

RIFM monograph(s) : Food Chem Toxicol 2007;45(suppl.1):S172-S178

IFRA standard : Restricted (www.ifraorg.org/en-us/standards-library) (table 3.145.1)

SCCS opinion(s) : SCCNFP/0392/00, final (2); SCCS/1459/11 (1); SCCNFP/0389/00, final (7)

Function(s) in cosmetics : EU: perfuming

EU cosmetic restrictions : Regulated in Annex III/160 of the Regulation (EC) No. 344/2013

Patch testing : No patch test data available; based on RIFM data, 3% in triacetin (glyceryl triacetate) and 0.5% alc. are probably not irritant (8)

Molecular formula : $C_{13}H_{18}O$

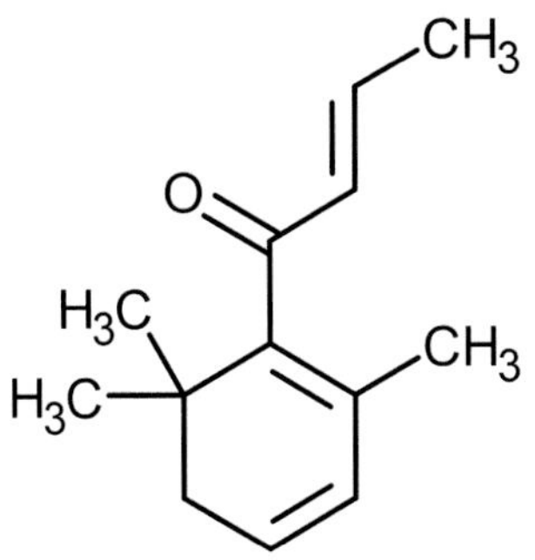

Table 3.145.1 IFRA restrictions for rose ketone-4

Category [a]	Limits [b]	Category [a]	Limits [b]	Category [a]	Limits [b]
1	0.00%	5	0.02%	9	0.02%
2	0.00%	6	0.07%	10	0.02%
3	0.02%	7	0.01%	11	not restricted
4	0.02%	8	0.02%		

[a] For explanation of categories see pages 6-8
[b] Limits in the finished products

GENERAL

Rose ketone-4 is a yellow clear liquid; its odor type is floral and its odor is described as 'woody, sweet, fruity, earthy with green floral nuances' (www.thegoodscentscompany.com).

Presence in essential oils

Rose ketone-4 (damascenone: alpha-, beta-, any isomer) has been identified by chemical analysis in 11 of 91 essential oils, which have caused contact allergy / allergic contact dermatitis. In none of these oils, it belonged to the 'Top-10' of ingredients with the highest concentrations (6).

CONTACT ALLERGY

General

The SCCS (Scientific Committee on Consumer Safety), in a 2012 Opinion on Fragrance allergens in cosmetic products, has marked rose ketone-4 as 'established contact allergen in humans' (1,5). The sensitizing potency of rose ketone-4 may be classified as 'moderate' based on EC3 values of 1.22% and 1.24% in the LLNA (local lymph node assay) in animal experiments (1).

Patch testing in groups of patients

Patch testing in consecutive patients suspected of contact dermatitis: routine testing
Studies in which rose ketone-4 was patch tested in consecutive patients suspected of contact dermatitis (routine testing) with positive results have not been found.

Patch testing in groups of selected patients: Pigmented cosmetic dermatitis
While searching for causative ingredients of pigmented cosmetic dermatitis in Japan in the 1970s, both patients with ordinary (nonpigmented) cosmetic dermatitis and women with pigmented cosmetic dermatitis were tested with a large number of fragrance materials. In 1980 the accumulated data enabled the classification of fragrant materials into 4 groups: common sensitizers, rare sensitizers, virtually non-sensitizing fragrances and fragrances considered as non-sensitizers. Rose ketone-4 (beta-damascenone) was classified in the group of rare sensitizers, indicating that one or more cases of contact allergy / allergic contact dermatitis to it have been observed (4). More specific data are lacking, the results have largely or solely been published in Japanese journals only.

Case reports and case series
Case reports of allergic contact dermatitis from rose ketone-4 have not been found.

Patch test sensitization
Rose ketone-4 (damascenone) was found to sensitize volunteers by patch testing (test concentration and vehicle unknown) (4).

Presence in products and chemical analyses
In 1997, 71 deodorants (22 vapo-spray, 22 aerosol spray and 27 roll-on products) were collected in Denmark, England, France, Germany and Sweden and analyzed by gas chromatography – mass spectrometry (GC-MS) for the presence of fragrances and other materials. beta-Damascenone (synonym for rose ketone-4) was present in one (1%) of the products (3).

LITERATURE
1   SCCS (Scientific Committee on Consumer Safety). Opinion on Fragrance allergens in cosmetic products, 26-27 June 2012, SCCS/1459/11. Available at:
    https://ec.europa.eu/health/sites/health/files/scientific_committees/consumer_safety/docs/sccs_o_102.pdf
2   SCCP (Scientific Committee on Consumer Products). Opinion on 'Clarifications to SCCNFP/0392/00 'An initial list of perfumery materials which must not form part of cosmetic products except subject to the Restrictions and Conditions laid down', 20 June 2006, SCCP/1023/06. Available at:
    http://ec.europa.eu/health/archive/ph_risk/committees/04_sccp/docs/sccp_o_062.pdf
3   Rastogi SC, Lepoittevin J-P, Johansen JD, Frosch PJ, Menné T, Bruze M, et al. Fragrances and other materials in deodorants: search for potentially sensitizing molecules using combined GC-MS and structure activity relationship (SAR) analysis. Contact Dermatitis 1998;39:293-303
4   Nakayama H. Fragrance hypersensitivity and its control. In: Frosch PJ, Johansen JD, White IR, Eds. Fragrances - beneficial and adverse effects. Berlin Heidelberg New York: Springer-Verlag, 1998:83-91
5   Uter W, Johansen JD, Börje A, Karlberg A-T, Lidén C, Rastogi S, Roberts D, White IR. Categorization of fragrance contact allergens for prioritization of preventive measures: clinical and experimental data and consideration of structure–activity relationships. Contact Dermatitis 2013;69:196-230
6   De Groot AC, Schmidt E. Essential oils: contact allergy and chemical composition. Boca Raton, Fl., USA: CRC Press, Taylor and Francis Group, 2016 (ISBN 9781482246407)
7   Opinion of the Scientific Committee on Cosmetic Products and Non-Food Products Intended for Consumers concerning 'The 1st update of the inventory of ingredients employed in cosmetic products. Section II: Perfume and aromatic raw materials', 24 October 2000, SCCNFP/0389/00, final. Available at:
    http://ec.europa.eu/health/ph_risk/committees/sccp/documents/out131_en.pdf
8   De Groot AC. Patch Testing, 4th Edition. Wapserveen, The Netherlands: acdegroot publishing, 2018 (ISBN 978-90-813233-4-5)

Chapter 3.146 SABINENE

IDENTIFICATION

Description/definition : Sabinene is the bicyclic organic compound that conforms to the structural formula shown below
Chemical class(es) : Bicyclic organic compounds; unsaturated compounds
INCI name USA : Neither in Cosing nor in the Personal Care Products Council Ingredient Database
Chemical/IUPAC name : 4-Methylidene-1-propan-2-ylbicyclo[3.1.0]hexane
Other names : 4(10)-Thujene; 1-isopropyl-4-methylenebicyclo[3.1.0]hexane
CAS registry number(s) : 3387-41-5
EC number(s) : 222-212-4
Patch testing : 5% in diethyl phthalate (1)
Molecular formula : $C_{10}H_{16}$

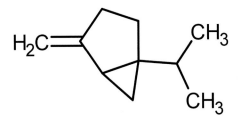

GENERAL

Sabinene is a colorless to pale yellow clear liquid; its odor type is woody and its odor at 10% in dipropylene glycol is described as 'woody terpene citrus pine spice' (www.thegoodscentscompany.com).

Presence in essential oils

Sabinene has been identified by chemical analysis in 80 of 91 essential oils, which have caused contact allergy / allergic contact dermatitis. In 21 oils, sabinene belonged to the 'Top-10' of ingredients with the highest concentrations. These are shown in table 3.146.1 with the concentration range which may be expected in commercial essential oils of this type (3).

Table 3.146.1 Essential oils containing sabinene in the 'Top-10' and concentration range in commercial oils (3)

Essential oil	Concentration range (min.-max.)	Essential oil	Concentration range (min.-max.)
Nutmeg oil	16.5 - 36.7%	Marjoram oil	1.0 - 9.4%
Ravensara oil	0.1 - 25.5%	Olibanum oil	0.5 - 7.2%
Juniper berry oil	1.0 - 17.7%	Elemi oil	2.5 - 6.6%
Black pepper oil	0.1 - 15.4%	Litsea cubeba oil	0.2 - 5.1%
Carrot seed oil	0.2 - 12.2%	Cardamom oil	2.0 - 5.0%
Laurel leaf oil	7.3 - 11.8%	Cajeput oil	0.01 - 4.5%
Angelica root oil	0.6 - 11.3%	Thuja oil	1.7 - 4.4%
Sage oil Spanish	0.1 - 3.5%	Grapefruit oil	0.2 - 0.8%
Lemon oil	1.1 - 2.9%	Orange oil sweet	0.02 - 0.7%
Cypress oil	0.5 - 2.2%	Tangerine oil	0.1 - 0.6%
Bergamot oil	0.03 - 1.3%		

CONTACT ALLERGY

Sabinene is a minor allergen in tea tree oil. Of 38 patients allergic to tea tree oil and tested with a number of its ingredients in various studies, 2 (5%) reacted to sabinene (2).

Patch testing in groups of patients

Patch testing in consecutive patients suspected of contact dermatitis: routine testing
Studies in which sabinene was patch tested in consecutive patients suspected of contact dermatitis (routine testing) with positive results have not been found.

Patch testing in groups of selected patients
In Germany, in the period 1999-2003, 20 patients who had previously shown a positive patch test reaction to oxidized tea tree oil 5% in DEP (diethyl phthalate) were patch tested with sabinene (5% in DEP) and 2 (10%) had a positive reaction to this ingredient of tea tree oil (1).

Case reports and case series
Case reports of allergic contact dermatitis from sabinene have not been found.

LITERATURE
1   Hausen BM. Evaluation of the main contact allergens in oxidized tea tree oil. Dermatitis 2004;15:213-214
2   De Groot AC, Schmidt E. Tea tree oil: contact allergy and chemical composition. Contact Dermatitis 2016;75:129-143
3   De Groot AC, Schmidt E. Essential oils: contact allergy and chemical composition. Boca Raton, Fl., USA: CRC Press, Taylor and Francis Group, 2016 (ISBN 9781482246407)

Chapter 3.147 SAFROLE *
* Not officially an INCI name but perfuming name

IDENTIFICATION

Description/definition : Safrole is the bicyclic organic compound that conforms to the structural formula shown below

Chemical class(es) : Heterocyclic aromatic compounds; unsaturated compounds

INCI name USA : Not in the Personal Care Products Council Ingredient Database

Chemical/IUPAC name : 5-Prop-2-enyl-1,3-benzodioxole

Other names : 5-Allyl-1,3-benzodioxole; shikimole

CAS registry number(s) : 94-59-7

EC number(s) : 202-345-4

RIFM monograph(s) : Food Cosmet Toxicol 1976;14:329 (binder, page 475)

IFRA standard : Restricted and prohibited; safrole as such should not be used as a fragrance ingredient; essential oils containing safrole should not be used at a level that the total concentration of safrole exceeds 0.01% in consumer products; the total concentration of safrole, isosafrole and dihydrosafrole should not exceed 0.01% in consumer products (www.ifraorg.org/en-us/standards-library)

Merck Index monograph : 9723

EU cosmetic restrictions : Regulated by (EC) No. 1223/2009, Annex II/360 (Prohibited, except for normal content in natural essences used with a maximum amount of 50-100 ppm, depending on the product category)

Patch testing : 1% pet. (2)

Molecular formula : $C_{10}H_{10}O_2$

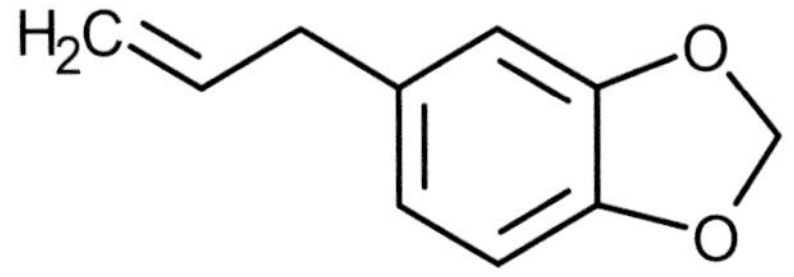

GENERAL

Safrole is a colorless to pale yellow clear liquid; its odor type is spicy and its odor at 10% in dipropylene glycol is described as 'sweet warm spicy woody floral sassafrass anise' (www.thegoodscentscompany.com). It is not used as fragrance ingredient because of carcinogenicity (4). Examples of essential oils with a high safrole content are Sassafras oil (*Sassafras officinale* Nees & Eberm.), Ocotea cymbarum oil (*Ocotea odorifera* (Vell.) Rohwer, synonym: *Ocotea pretiosa* Mez), nutmeg oil (Myristica fragrans kernel oil, Chapter 6.50), and certain qualities of camphor oils.

Presence in essential oils

Safrole has been identified by chemical analysis in 13 of 91 essential oils, which have caused contact allergy / allergic contact dermatitis. In none of the oils, safrole belonged to the 'Top-10' of ingredients with the highest concentrations which may be expected in commercial essential oils of this type. In fact, in most oils (with the notable exception of nutmeg oil where it may be present in a concentration range of 1.0-2.5% according to the ISO standard), it was found in rare publications only, at very low concentrations and sometimes the question was raised whether the identification was correct (3).

CONTACT ALLERGY

Patch testing in groups of patients

Patch testing in consecutive patients suspected of contact dermatitis: routine testing

Studies in which safrole was patch tested in consecutive patients suspected of contact dermatitis (routine testing) with positive results have not been found.

Testing in groups of selected patients

Fifteen patients with positive patch tests to star anise oil 1% in petrolatum, negative to 0.5% but positive to one or more 'balsams' (Myroxylon pereirae resin, turpentine, wood tars, colophonium) were tested with 9 components of star anise oil with the following results: one reaction to safrole, 8 to α-pinene, 5 to anethole (the main component of star anise oil), and 3 to limonene (2).

In a group of 46 patients allergic to Myroxylon pereirae resin (balsam of Peru) and tested with safrole 5% pet., there was one positive reaction; this patient also reacted to isosafrole (1).

One patient who was sensitized by patch testing with 0.5%, 1% and 2% in petrolatum was tested with 9 components of star anise oil and this individual reacted to safrole, anethole (the main ingredient of star anise oil), α-pinene, and methylchavicol, all tested 1% in petrolatum (2).

Case reports and case series
Case reports of allergic contact dermatitis from safrole have not been found.

Cross-reactions, pseudo-cross-reactions and co-reactions
For general information on cross-/pseudo-cross-/co-reactivity of fragrance chemicals with other fragrances, fragrance markers (fragrance mix I, fragrance mix II, colophonium, Myroxylon pereirae resin [balsam of Peru]) and essential oils see Chapter 1.2 General information on cross-reactions, pseudo-cross-reactions and co-reactions.

Co-reactivity to Isosafrole has been observed (1).

Patch test sensitization
One hundred consecutive patients with dermatitis were tested with star anise oil 0.5%, 1% and 2% in petrolatum and in five, patch test sensitization occurred, with flare-up of the 1% and 2% concentrations (2).

LITERATURE
1   Hjorth N. Eczematous allergy to balsams. Acta Derm Venereol 1961;41(suppl.46):1-216
2   Rudzki E, Grzywa Z. Sensitizing and irritating properties of star anise oil. Contact Dermatitis 1976;2:305-306
3   De Groot AC, Schmidt E. Essential oils: contact allergy and chemical composition. Boca Raton, Fl., USA: CRC Press, Taylor and Francis Group, 2016 (ISBN 9781482246407)
4   No authors listed. Safrole. Rep Carcinog 2004;11:III229-230

Chapter 3.148 SALICYLALDEHYDE

IDENTIFICATION

Description/definition : Salicylaldehyde is the aldehyde that conforms to the structural formula shown below
Chemical class(es) : Aldehydes
INCI name USA : Not in the Personal Care Products Council Ingredient Database
Chemical/IUPAC name : 2-Hydroxybenzaldehyde
CAS registry number (s) : 90-02-8
EC number(s) : 201-961-0
Merck Index monograph : 9732
RIFM monograph(s) : Food Cosmet Toxicol 1979;17:903 (special issue V)
SCCS opinion(s) : SCCS/1459/11 (2)
Function(s) in cosmetics : EU: perfuming
Patch testing : 2% Pet. (SmartPracticeEurope, SmartPracticeCanada)
Molecular formula : $C_7H_6O_2$

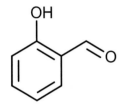

GENERAL
Salicylaldehyde is a colorless to pale yellow clear liquid; its odor type is medicinal and its odor at 10% in dipropylene glycol is described as 'medical spicy cinnamon wintergreen cooling' (www.thegoodscentscompany.com). It is or has been used as flavor ingredient in foods and beverages, perfume fragrance, chemical intermediate for the production of coumarin, medicinal chemicals and chelates to stabilize cracked gasoline, as auxiliary fumigant and as reagent in analytical chemistry (U.S. National Library of Medicine).

Presence in essential oils
Salicylaldehyde has been identified by chemical analysis in 7 of 91 essential oils, which have caused contact allergy / allergic contact dermatitis. In none of these oils, it belonged to the 'Top-10' of ingredients with the highest concentrations (10).

CONTACT ALLERGY

General
The SCCS (Scientific Committee on Consumer Safety), in a 2012 Opinion on Fragrance allergens in cosmetic products, has marked salicylaldehyde as 'established contact allergen in humans' (2,4).

Patch testing in groups of patients

Patch testing in consecutive patients suspected of contact dermatitis: routine testing
Studies in which salicylaldehyde was patch tested in consecutive patients suspected of contact dermatitis (routine testing) with positive results have not been found.

Patch testing in groups of selected patients
Results of studies patch testing salicylaldehyde in groups of selected patients (e.g. patients with known or suspected fragrance or cosmetic dermatitis) are shown in table 3.148.1. In four investigations, frequencies of sensitization ranged from 0.1% to 2.5% (1,3,5,6). The latter concentration was observed in a small group of 40 patients (only one positive reaction to salicylaldehyde = 2.5%) with known fragrance sensitivity (6). The relevance of the positive reactions was not mentioned in any study (1,3,5,6).

Case reports and case series
An elk researcher developed occupational allergic contact dermatitis from exposure to salicylaldehyde and salicyl alcohol by their presence in the barks of aspen (the main food of elks), rowan and willows (9).

Table 3.148.1 Patch testing in groups of patients: Selected patient groups

Years and Country	Test conc. & vehicle	Number of patients tested | positive (%)			Selection of patients (S); Relevance (R); Comments (C)	Ref.
2006-2011 IVDK	2% pet.	665	4	(0.6%)	S: patients with suspected cosmetic intolerance; R: not stated	3
2005-2008 IVDK	2% pet.	2729		(0.5%)	S: not specified; R: not stated	5
1997-2000 Austria	2% pet.	747	1	(0.1%)	S: patients suspected of fragrance allergy; R: not stated	1
1994-1995 UK	2% pet.	40	1	(2.5%)	S: patients reacting to the FM I and tested with an extended fragrance series; R: not stated	6

FM: Fragrance mix; IVDK: Informationsverbund Dermatologischer Kliniken (Germany, Switzerland, Austria)

Cross-reactions, pseudo-cross-reactions and co-reactions

For general information on cross-/pseudo-cross-/co-reactivity of fragrance chemicals with other fragrances, fragrance markers (fragrance mix I, fragrance mix II, colophonium, Myroxylon pereirae resin [balsam of Peru]) and essential oils see Chapter 1.2 General information on cross-reactions, pseudo-cross-reactions and co-reactions.

Of 8 patients with contact allergy to methylol phenols present in phenolformaldehyde resins, 4 (50%) co-reacted to salicylaldehyde (7). Among 17 patients sensitised to resorcinol by application of a wart remover, 2 positive reactions to salicylaldehyde were observed (8).

A possible cross-reaction with salicyl alcohol has been observed, but this may also have been caused by simultaneous sensitization, as the causative allergenic material in this case, aspen bark, contained both chemicals (9).

No co-reactions in case of primary sensitization to N,N'-disalicylidene-1,2-diaminopropane, a copper inhibitor present in some adhesive plasters, rubber products and gasoline, although this material upon contact with water is hydrolyzed to salicylaldehyde and 1,2-diaminopropane (11).

LITERATURE

1　Wöhrl S, Hemmer W, Focke M et al. The significance of fragrance mix, balsam of Peru, colophonium and propolis as screening tools in the detection of fragrance allergy. Br J Dermatol 2001;145:268-73

2　SCCS (Scientific Committee on Consumer Safety). Opinion on Fragrance allergens in cosmetic products, 26-27 June 2012, SCCS/1459/11. Available at: https://ec.europa.eu/health/sites/health/files/scientific_committees/consumer_safety/docs/sccs_o_102.pdf

3　Dinkloh A, Worm M, Geier J, Schnuch A, Wollenberg A. Contact sensitization in patients with suspected cosmetic intolerance: results of the IVDK 2006-2011. J Eur Acad Dermatol Venereol 2015;29:1071-1081

4　Uter W, Johansen JD, Börje A, Karlberg A-T, Lidén C, Rastogi S, Roberts D, White IR. Categorization of fragrance contact allergens for prioritization of preventive measures: clinical and experimental data and consideration of structure–activity relationships. Contact Dermatitis 2013;69:196-230

5　Uter W, Geier J, Frosch P, Schnuch A. Contact allergy to fragrances: current patch test results (2005–2008) from the Information Network of Departments of Dermatology. Contact Dermatitis 2010;63:254-261

6　Katsarma G, Gawkrodger DJ. Suspected fragrance allergy requires extended patch testing to individual fragrance allergens. Contact Dermatitis 1999;41:193-197

7　Bruze M, Zimerson E. Cross-reaction patterns in patients with contact allergy to simple methylol phenols. Contact Dermatitis 1997;37:82-86

8　Barbaud A, Reichert-Penetrat S, Trechot P, Granel F, Schmutz JL. Sensitization to resorcinol in a prescription verrucide preparation: unusual systemic clinical features and prevalence. Ann Dermatol Venereol 2001;128:615-618 (article in French)

9　Aalto-Korte K, Valimaa J, Henriks-Eckerman ML, Jolanki R. Allergic contact dermatitis from salicyl alcohol and salicylaldehyde in aspen bark (*Populus tremula*). Contact Dermatitis 2005;52:93-95

10　De Groot AC, Schmidt E. Essential oils: contact allergy and chemical composition. Boca Raton, Fl., USA: CRC Press, Taylor and Francis Group, 2016 (ISBN 9781482246407)

11　Bergendorff O, Hansson C. Activation and cross-reactivity pattern of a new allergen in adhesive plaster. Contact Dermatitis 2000;42:11-17

Chapter 3.149 SANTALOL

IDENTIFICATION

Description/definition : Santalol is the polycyclic organic compound that conforms to the structural formula shown below; it has 2 isomers, alpha- and beta-santalol; the α-isomer is tricyclic and the β-isomer is bicyclic; natural santalol is a mixture of both

Chemical class(es) : Polycyclic organic compounds; unsaturated compounds; alcohols

INCI name USA : Not in the Personal Care Products Council Ingredient Database

RIFM monograph(s) : Food Chem Toxicol 2008;46(11)(suppl.):S1-S71; Food Chem Toxicol 2008;46(11) (suppl.):S263-S266 and S267-S269 (α-santalol); Food Cosmet Toxicol 1974;12:991 (special issue I)

SCCS opinion(s) : SCCS/1459/11 (1)

Function(s) in cosmetics : EU: perfuming

Patch testing : 5% pet. (2); 10% pet. (mixed isomers) may be preferable; based on RIFM data, 20% pet. is probably not irritant (8)

Molecular formula : $C_{15}H_{24}O$

Natural santalol

Chemical/IUPAC name : See alpha- and beta-santalol below

Other names : Santalol; santalol, alpha- and beta-; santalol (natural)

CAS registry number(s) : 11031-45-1

EC number(s) : 234-262-4

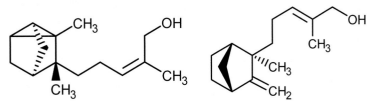

| alpha-Santalol | beta-Santalol |

alpha-Santalol

Chemical/IUPAC name : 5-(2,3-Dimethyl-4,5,6,7-tetrahydro-1H-tricyclo[2.2.1.0^{2,6}]heptan-3-yl)-2-methylpent-2-en-1-ol

CAS registry number(s) : 115-71-9

EC number(s) : 204-102-8

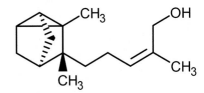

beta-Santalol

Chemical/IUPAC name : 2-Methyl-5-(3-methyl-2-methylidene-3-bicyclo[2.2.1]heptanyl)pent-2-en-1-ol

CAS registry number(s) : 77-42-9

EC number(s) : 201-027-2

GENERAL

Santalol is a colorless to pale yellow clear viscous liquid; its odor type is woody and its odor at 100% is described as 'deep sweet sandalwood woody' (www.thegoodscentscompany.com). It may be used in perfumes, soaps and detergents and as synthetic flavor (U.S. National Library of Medicine). alpha-Santalol is also used for its (alleged) medicinal properties (11).

Presence in essential oils

Santalol (all isomers) has been identified by chemical analysis in 17 of 91 essential oils, which have caused contact allergy / allergic contact dermatitis. In one oil, santalol belonged to the 'Top-10' of ingredients with the highest concentrations which may be expected in commercial essential oils of this type: sandalwood oil ((Z)-α- 17.0-53.3%; (Z)-β- 13.2-23.6%; (E)-β- 0.5-2.0%) (6).

CONTACT ALLERGY

General

The SCCS (Scientific Committee on Consumer Safety), in a 2012 Opinion on Fragrance allergens in cosmetic products, has marked alpha-santalol and beta-santalol as 'established contact allergens in humans' (1,4).

Patch testing in groups of patients

Patch testing in consecutive patients suspected of contact dermatitis: routine testing

In Japan, in the period between 1973 and 1994, studies testing santalol in consecutive patients suspected of contact dermatitis (routine testing) seem to have been performed, but details are lacking (results published in Japanese journals only). See the following section 'Patch testing in groups of selected patients'.

Patch testing in groups of selected patients

The results of 2 studies performing patch tests with santalol in groups of selected patients (patients with known fragrance sensitivity, patients with facial dermatoses) are shown in table 3.149.1. In one study in patients with known fragrance sensitivity, 1.1% reacted to santalol 5%, a mixture of alpha- and beta-santalol (2). In a Japanese study, 327 patients with facial dermatoses were tested with santalol mixed isomers 10%, 2% and 0.5% in petrolatum, and there were 1.5%, 0.6% and 0.6% positive reactions to these test concentrations, respectively. Quite curiously, 2% was chosen as the preferred concentration, although 10% showed more reactions and this concentration was apparently not irritant (9). In neither study, data on relevance of the positive reactions were provided (2,9).

Between 1973 and 1994, at least 10 studies have been performed in Japan testing unselected and selected groups of patients with santalol, all of which have been published in Japanese journals only. The numbers of patients tested ranged from 106 to 3123. Some were studies in consecutive patients, others in patients with cosmetic dermatitis and most probably also series of women with pigmented cosmetic dermatitis. Patch test concentrations were 1%, 2%, 5% or 10% in petrolatum or 0.05%-0.5% in cream base or alcohol. The frequencies of sensitization ranged from 0.3% to 5.7%. Summaries of these studies (albeit with incomplete data) can be found in ref. 7.

Table 3.149.1 Patch testing in groups of patients: Selected patient groups

Years and Country	Test conc. & vehicle	Number of patients tested | positive (%)		Selection of patients (S); Relevance (R); Comments (C)	Ref.
2000 Japan, Europe, USA	5% pet.	178	2 (1.1%)	S: patients with known fragrance sensitivity; R: not stated; C: the test substance was a mixture of (Z)-alpha- and (Z)-beta-santalol	2
1979 Japan	10% pet.	327	5 (1.5%)	S: patients with facial dermatoses; R: not stated; C: the test substance contained a mixture of alpha- and beta-santalol; 2% pet. was chosen to be the proper patch test concentration, although 10% yielded more positive reactions and no irritant reactions were observed	9
	2% pet.	327	2 (0.6%)		
	0.5% pet.	327	2 (0.6%)		

Case reports and case series

A patient suspected to be allergic to incense had positive patch tests to two brands of incense, sandalwood oil, musk ambrette and santalol. Gas chromatography of pentane:ether extracts of the incense showed 9% and 34% musk ambrette and 8% santalol in both incenses (5). The sandalwood oil extract contained 73% santalol (5), which is the dominant component of sandalwood oil (6).

Cross-reactions, pseudo-cross-reactions and co-reactions

For general information on cross-/pseudo-cross-/co-reactivity of fragrance chemicals with other fragrances, fragrance markers (fragrance mix I, fragrance mix II, colophonium, Myroxylon pereirae resin [balsam of Peru]) and essential oils see Chapter 1.2 General information on cross-reactions, pseudo-cross-reactions and co-reactions.

Santalol is the dominant ingredient of sandalwood oil and co-reactivity between them has been observed (5). Of 5 patients reacting to santalol 10% pet., all co-reacted to farnesol and fragrance mix I, 4 to Myroxylon pereirae resin, colophonium, jasmine absolute, cananga oil, lavender oil and sandalwood oil and 3 to various other essential oils and fragrances (10). It should be realized that the presented group of 8 patients had been selected on the basis of a positive patch test to farnesol. Had the search criterium been a positive patch test to santalol, the data may well have been different.

Presence in products and chemical analyses

In 1997, 71 deodorants (22 vapo-spray, 22 aerosol spray and 27 roll-on products) were collected in Denmark, England, France, Germany and Sweden and analyzed by gas chromatography – mass spectrometry (GC-MS) for the presence of fragrances and other materials. Santalol / alpha-santalol was present in 11 (15%) of the products (3).

LITERATURE

1 SCCS (Scientific Committee on Consumer Safety). Opinion on Fragrance allergens in cosmetic products, 26-27 June 2012, SCCS/1459/11. Available at:
   https://ec.europa.eu/health/sites/health/files/scientific_committees/consumer_safety/docs/sccs_o_102.pdf

2 Larsen W, Nakayama H, Fischer T, Elsner P, Frosch P, Burrows D, et al. Fragrance contact dermatitis: A worldwide multicenter investigation (Part II). Contact Dermatitis 2001;44:344-346

3 Rastogi SC, Lepoittevin J-P, Johansen JD, Frosch PJ, Menné T, Bruze M, et al. Fragrances and other materials in deodorants: search for potentially sensitizing molecules using combined GC-MS and structure activity relationship (SAR) analysis. Contact Dermatitis 1998;39:293-303

4 Uter W, Johansen JD, Börje A, Karlberg A-T, Lidén C, Rastogi S, Roberts D, White IR. Categorization of fragrance contact allergens for prioritization of preventive measures: clinical and experimental data and consideration of structure–activity relationships. Contact Dermatitis 2013;69:196-230

5 Hayakawa R, Matsunaga K, Arima Y. Depigmented contact dermatitis due to incense. Contact Dermatitis 1987;16:272-274

6 De Groot AC, Schmidt E. Essential oils: contact allergy and chemical composition. Boca Raton, Fl., USA: CRC Press, Taylor and Francis Group, 2016 (ISBN 9781482246407).

7 Bhatia SP, McGinty D, Letizia CS, Api AM. Fragrance material review on alpha-santalol. Food Chem Toxicol 2008;46(11)(suppl.):S267-S269

8 De Groot AC. Patch Testing, 4th Edition. Wapserveen, The Netherlands: acdegroot publishing, 2018 (ISBN 978-90-813233-4-5)

9 Mid-Japan Contact Dermatitis Research Group. Determination of suitable concentrations for patch testing of various fragrance materials. A summary of group study conducted over a 6-year period. J Dermatol 1984;11:31-35

10 Goossens A, Merckx L. Allergic contact dermatitis from farnesol in a deodorant. Contact Dermatitis 1997;37:179-180

11 Bommareddy A, Brozena S, Steigerwalt J, Landis T, Hughes S, Mabry E, et al. Medicinal properties of alpha-santalol, a naturally occurring constituent of sandalwood oil: review. Nat Prod Res 2017;Nov 13:1-17. https://doi-org.proxy-ub.rug.nl/10.1080/14786419.2017.1399387

Chapter 3.150 STYRYL ACETATE

IDENTIFICATION

Description/definition	: Styryl acetate is the aromatic ester that conforms to the structural formula shown below
Chemical class(es)	: Aromatic compounds; unsaturated compounds; esters
INCI name USA	: Not in the Personal Care Products Council Ingredient Database
Chemical/IUPAC name	: 2-Phenylethenyl acetate
Other names	: Ethenol, 2-phenyl-, 1-acetate
CAS registry number(s)	: 10521-96-7
EC number(s)	: 234-065-3
Function(s) in cosmetics	: EU: perfuming
Patch testing	: 1% pet. (1)
Molecular formula	: $C_{10}H_{10}O_2$

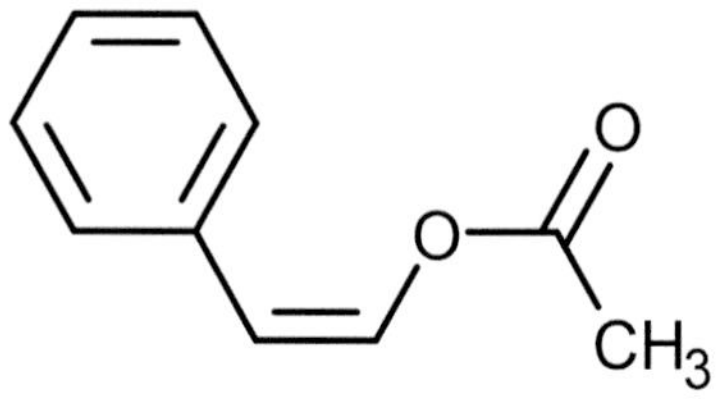

GENERAL

Styryl acetate is a colorless clear liquid; its odor type is fruity and its odor at 10% in dipropylene glycol is described as 'sweet fruity rum' (www.thegoodscentscompany.com).

Presence in essential oils

Styryl acetate has been identified by chemical analysis in none of 91 essential oils, which have caused contact allergy / allergic contact dermatitis (2).

CONTACT ALLERGY

Patch testing in groups of patients

Patch testing in consecutive patients suspected of contact dermatitis: routine testing

Studies in which styryl acetate was patch tested in consecutive patients suspected of contact dermatitis (routine testing) with positive results have not been found.

Patch testing in groups of selected patients

In a perfume factory, where several bottle fillers developed occupational allergic contact dermatitis from one or more fragrances, two of twenty people working in the same factory who did *not* have dermatitis had positive patch test reactions to styryl acetate 1% pet. (1).

Case reports and case series

Case reports of allergic contact dermatitis from styryl acetate have not been found.

LITERATURE

1   Schubert HJ. Skin diseases in workers at a perfume factory. Contact Dermatitis 2006;55:81-83
2   De Groot AC, Schmidt E. Essential oils: contact allergy and chemical composition. Boca Raton, Fl., USA: CRC Press, Taylor and Francis Group, 2016 (ISBN 9781482246407)

Chapter 3.151 ALPHA-TERPINENE *

Not officially an INCI name but perfuming name

IDENTIFICATION

Description/definition	: alpha-Terpinene is the unsaturated cyclic compound that conforms to the structural formula shown below
Chemical class(es)	: Cyclic organic compounds; unsaturated compounds
INCI name USA	: Not in the Personal Care Products Council Ingredient Database
Chemical/IUPAC name	: 1-Methyl-4-propan-2-ylcyclohexa-1,3-diene
Other names	: *p*-Mentha-1,3-diene; 1-methyl-4-isopropyl-1,3-cyclohexadiene
CAS registry number(s)	: 99-86-5
EC number(s)	: 202-795-1
RIFM monograph(s)	: Food Cosmet Toxicol 1976;14:873 (special issue III)
SCCS opinion(s)	: SCCNFP/0389/00, final (9)
Merck Index monograph	: 10582 (Terpinene)
Function(s) in cosmetics	: EU: perfuming
EU cosmetic restrictions	: Regulated in Annex III/131 of the Regulation (EC) No. 344/2013
Patch testing	: 5% in Diethyl phthalate (1,6); based on RIFM data, 5% pet. is probably not irritant (13), but concentrations of 5% (or higher) *in alcohol* may be (strongly) irritant (3).
Molecular formula	: $C_{10}H_{16}$

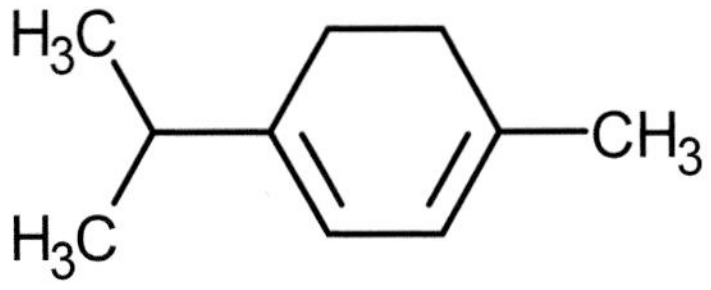

GENERAL

alpha-Terpinene is a colorless to pale yellow clear oily liquid; its odor type is woody and its odor at 10% is described as 'citrusy, woody, terpy with camphoraceous and thymol notes. It has spicy and juicy citrus nuances' (www.thegoodscentscompany.com). alpha-Terpinene is a naturally occurring cyclic monoterpene produced in the secondary metabolism of plants. It has been identified in numerous plant extracts and is a constituent of several commonly used essential oils, especially tea tree oil (see 'Presence in essential oils' below and Chapter 6.71 Tea tree oil). α-Terpinene is sometimes present in fragrances at low levels as part of natural oils that are used in the actual fragrances. The chemical has antioxidant activity and it is one of the most important constituents responsible for the antioxidant activity of tea tree oil.

Presence in essential oils and Myroxylon pereirae resin (balsam of Peru)

alpha-Terpinene has been identified by chemical analysis in 77 of 91 essential oils, which have caused contact allergy / allergic contact dermatitis. In 7 oils, alpha-terpinene belonged to the 'Top-10' of ingredients with the highest concentrations which may be expected in commercial essential oils of this type: tea tree oil (2.3-11.7%), marjoram oil (0.07-10.3%), nutmeg oil (2.4-4.6%), dwarf pine oil (0.07-4.2%), thyme oil Spanish (0.7-3.3%), cinnamon bark oil Sri Lanka (0.3-2.6%), and lemongrass oil East Indian (0.02-2.3%) (15). α-Terpinene may also be present in Myroxylon pereirae resin (balsam of Peru) (14).

CONTACT ALLERGY

General

alpha-Terpinene acts both as a prohapten (a chemical that is itself non-sensitizing or low-sensitizing, but that is transformed into a hapten in the skin (bioactivation), usually via enzymatic catalysis) and as a prehapten (a chemical that is itself non-sensitizing or low-sensitizing, but that is transformed into a hapten outside the skin by chemical transformation (air oxidation; photoactivation) and without the requirement for specific enzymatic systems) (12).

It has been shown that α-terpinene is a moderate sensitizer in the murine local lymph node assay (LLNA) (8). In fact, the sensitizing potency of pure α-terpinene is rather high as compared with that of other pure terpenes. This may be attributed to bioactivation in the skin, which gives highly sensitizing conjugated epoxides (alpha-terpinene as a prohapten) (8). However, autoxidation further increases its sensitizing potency (alpha-terpinene as a prehapten (12).

On air exposure, it undergoes rapid autoxidation and forms oxidation products including α-terpinene-1,2-epoxide, alpha-terpinene-3,4-epoxide, alpha-terpinenediol, ascaridole (16) and p-cymene; (E)-3-isopropyl-6-oxohept-2-enal (an α,β-unsaturated aldehyde) is another chemical in autoxidized alpha-terpinene as are several non-identified compounds. These oxidation products are strong sensitizers in the murine LLNA. The sensitization potency of autoxidized alpha-terpinene is approximately 9 times higher compared to that of pure α-terpinene (7,12).

Both alpha-terpinene and its oxidation products can be identified in tea tree oil samples (7). Indeed, alpha-terpinene is one of the most important components responsible for contact allergy to tea tree oil (1,2,3,5,6,11; see Chapter 6.71Tea tree oil). Of 64 patients allergic to tea tree oil and tested with a number of its ingredients in various studies, 49 (77%) reacted to alpha-terpinene (11).

Patch testing in groups of patients

Patch testing in consecutive patients suspected of contact dermatitis: routine testing
Studies in which alpha-terpinene was patch tested in consecutive patients suspected of contact dermatitis (routine testing) with positive results have not been found.

Patch testing in groups of selected patients
Results of studies patch testing alpha-terpinene in groups of selected patients (in all studies: patients previously shown to be allergic to (oxidized) tea tree oil) are shown in table 3.151.1. In the period 1990-2003, five small series of 7-20 patients allergic to (oxidized) tea tree oil have been tested with a battery of its ingredients, including alpha-terpinene 5% in various vehicles (1,2,3,5,6). Frequencies of sensitization have ranged from 69 to 100%, attesting to the fact that alpha-terpinene is an important allergenic ingredient of tea tree oil. On average, 77% of patients allergic to tea tree oil have reacted to alpha-terpinene (11).

Table 3.151.1 Patch testing in groups of patients: Selected patient groups

Years and Country	Test conc. & vehicle	Number of patients tested | positive (%)		Selection of patients (S); Relevance (R); Comments (C)	Ref.
1999-2003 Germany	5% DEP	20	16 (80%)	S: patients with a positive patch test reaction to oxidized tea tree oil 5% DEP	6
1999-2000 Germany, Austria	5% DEP	10	10 (100%)	S: patients with a positive patch test reaction to oxidized tea tree oil 5% DEP	1
1999 Germany	5% water	8	6 (75%)	S: patients with a positive patch test reaction to oxidized tea tree oil 20% in olive oil	2
<1999 Germany	5% vehicle?	16	11 (69%)	S: patients allergic to tea tree oil	5
1990-1992 Germany	1% and 5% alc.	7	5 (71%)	S: patients with a positive patch test reaction to tea tree oil 1% alc.	3

DEP: Diethyl phthalate

Case reports and case series
In 1995, in Australia, 25 volunteers without a history of dermatitis from tea tree oil were tested with 8 samples of the oil. Quite unexpectedly, 3 had positive reactions. They were subsequently patch tested with a number of its ingredients and one had a positive reaction to alpha-terpinene tested 5.90% in petrolatum (4).

A man became sensitized after using tea tree oil in his shampoo and for blisters on his face. When patch tested, he reacted to tea tree oil; in a second session, he was tested with its ingredients and now had positive reactions to alpha-terpinene (5%, vehicle unknown), terpinolene (10%, vehicle unknown) and ascaridole (5%, vehicle unknown) (5,10).

Another patient had treated warts on his hands with tea tree oil and became sensitized within three weeks. When patch tested, he reacted to tea tree oil and its ingredients alpha-terpinene (5%, vehicle unknown), terpinolene (10%, vehicle unknown) and ascaridole (5%, vehicle unknown) (5). A woman, who treated her atopic dermatitis with tea tree oil, also became sensitized to the essential oil from contact allergy to the same ingredients (5).

Four more patients are presented by the same authors, who had used tea tree oil for various reasons and indications, who developed allergic contact dermatitis from it and reacted on ingredient patch testing to alpha-terpinene and 3-5 other oil components (5).

LITERATURE

1   Pirker C, Hausen BM, Uter W, Hillen U, Brasch J, Bayeret C, et al. Sensitization to tea tree oil in Germany and Austria. A multicenter Study of the German Contact Dermatitis group. J Dtsch Dermatol Ges 2003;1:629-634 (article in German)

2   Lippert U, Walter A, Hausen BM, Fuchs Th. Increasing incidence of contact dermatitis to tea tree oil. J Allergy Clin Immunol 2000;105;S43 (abstract 127)

3   Knight TE, Hausen BM. Melaleuca oil (tea tree oil) dermatitis. J Am Acad Dermatol 1994;30:423-427

4   Rubel DM, Freeman S, Southwell I. Tea tree oil allergy: what is the offending agent? Report of three cases of tea tree oil allergy and review of the literature. Australas J Dermatol 1998;39:244-247

5   Hausen BM, Reichling J, Harkenthal M. Degradation products of monoterpenes are the sensitizing agents in tea tree oil. Am J Contact Dermat 1999;10:68-77

6   Hausen BM. Evaluation of the main contact allergens in oxidized tea tree oil. Dermatitis 2004;15:213-214

7   Rudbäck J, Andresen Bergström M, Börje A, Nilsson U, Karlberg AT. α-Terpinene, an antioxidant in tea tree oil, autoxidizes rapidly to skin allergens on air exposure. Chem Res Toxicol 2012;25:713-721

8   Bergström MA, Luthman K, Nilsson JLG, Karlberg AT. Conjugated dienes as prohaptens in contact allergy: *In vivo* and *in vitro* studies of structure - activity relationships, sensitizing capacity, and metabolic activation. Chem Res Toxicol 2006;19:760-769

9   Opinion of the Scientific Committee on Cosmetic Products and Non-Food Products Intended for Consumers concerning 'The 1st update of the inventory of ingredients employed in cosmetic products. Section II: Perfume and aromatic raw materials', 24 October 2000, SCCNFP/0389/00, final. Available at: http://ec.europa.eu/health/ph_risk/committees/sccp/documents/out131_en.pdf

10 Hausen BM. Kontaktallergie auf Teebaumöl und Ascaridol. Akt Derm 1998;24:60-62

11 De Groot AC, Schmidt E. Tea tree oil: contact allergy and chemical composition. Contact Dermatitis 2016;75:129-143

12 Karlberg A-T, Börje A, Johansen JD, Lidén C, Rastogi S, Roberts D, et al. Activation of non-sensitizing or low-sensitizing fragrance substances into potent sensitizers – prehaptens and prohaptens. Contact Dermatitis 2013;69:323-334

13 De Groot AC. Patch Testing, 4th Edition. Wapserveen, The Netherlands: acdegroot publishing, 2018 (ISBN 978-90-813233-4-5)

14 Mammerler V. Contribution to the analysis and quality control of Peru Balsam. PhD Thesis, University of Vienna, Austria, 2007. Available at: http://othes.univie.ac.at/4056/1/2009-03-23_0201578.pdf

15 De Groot AC, Schmidt E. Essential oils: contact allergy and chemical composition. Boca Raton, Fl., USA: CRC Press, Taylor and Francis Group, 2016 (ISBN 9781482246407)

16 Chittiboyina AG, Avonto C, Khan IA. What happens after activation of ascaridole? Reactive compounds and their implications for skin sensitization. Chem Res Toxicol 2016;29:1488-1492

Chapter 3.152 4-TERPINEOL

IDENTIFICATION

Description/definition	: 4-Terpineol is the organic compound that conforms to the structural formula shown below
Chemical class(es)	: Alcohols
Chemical/IUPAC name	: 4-Methyl-1-propan-2-ylcyclohex-3-en-1-ol
Other names	: Terpen-4-ol; terpinen-4-ol; 1-*p*-menthen-4-ol; 4-carvomenthenol; 4-terpinenol; 4-methyl-1-(1-methylethyl)-3-cyclohexen-1-ol
CAS registry number(s)	: 562-74-3
EINECS number(s)	: 209-235-5
RIFM monograph(s)	: Food Chem Toxicol 2008;46(11)(suppl.):S91-S94 (4-Carvomenthenol);Food Chem Toxicol 1982;20:833 (special issue VI)
Function(s) in cosmetics	: EU: masking. USA: fragrance ingredients
Patch testing	: 5% diethyl phthalate (DEP) (3); according to RIFM data, 5% pet. is probably not irritant (10)
Molecular formula	: $C_{10}H_{18}O$

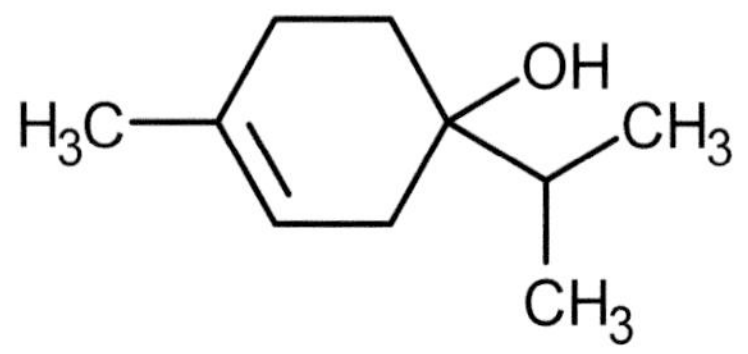

GENERAL

4-Terpineol is a pale yellow clear liquid; its odor type is spicy and its odor at 100% is described as 'pepper woody earth musty sweet' (www.thegoodscentscompany.com). It is used in artificial geranium and pepper oils and in perfumery for creating herbaceous and lavender notes and also as food and non-alcoholic beverages flavor (U.S. National Library of Medicine).

Presence in essential oils and propolis

4-Terpineol has been identified by chemical analysis in 82 of 91 essential oils, which have caused contact allergy / allergic contact dermatitis. In 10 oils, 4-terpineol belonged to the 'Top-10' of ingredients with the highest concentrations. These are shown in table 3.152.1 with the concentration range which may be expected in commercial essential oils of this type (9). 4-Terpineol may also be present in propolis (8).

Table 3.152.1 Essential oils containing 4-terpineol the 'Top-10' and concentration range in commercial oils (9)

Essential oil	Concentration range (min.-max.)	Essential oil	Concentration range (min.-max.)
Tea tree oil	6.2 - 44.9%	Cardamom oil	0.8 - 3.0%
Marjoram oil	0.5 - 29.7%	Lavandin oil	2.0 - 5.5%
Nutmeg oil	0.2 - 8.4%	Juniper berry oil	1.9 - 5.4%
Lavender oil	0.07 - 5.9%	Laurel leaf oil	1.7 - 3.4%
Olibanum oil	0.2 - 5.8%	Thuja oil	1.5 - 3.4%

CONTACT ALLERGY

4-Terpineol is a minor allergen in tea tree oil. Of patients allergic to tea tree oil and tested with a number of its ingredients in various studies, 4 (6%) reacted to 4-terpineol (4).

Patch testing in groups of patients

Patch testing in consecutive patients suspected of contact dermatitis: routine testing

Studies in which 4-terpineol was patch tested in consecutive patients suspected of contact dermatitis (routine testing) with positive results have not been found.

Patch testing in groups of selected patients

Results of studies patch testing 4-terpineol in groups of selected patients (in all 3 investigations: patients allergic to (oxidized) tea tree oil) are shown in table 3.152.2.

In Germany, in the period 1990-2003, three small groups of 7-20 patients allergic to tea tree oil were patch tested with a battery of its ingredients including 4-terpineol. Frequencies of sensitization ranged from 5-29% (1,2,3) with an average of 5% (4). 4-Terpineol is therefore a minor allergenic ingredient of tea tree oil.

Table 3.152.2 Patch testing in groups of patients: Selected patient groups

Years and Country	Test conc. & vehicle	Number of patients tested | positive (%)			Selection of patients (S); Relevance (R); Comments (C)	Ref.
1999-2003 Germany	5% DEP	20	1	(5%)	S: patients with a positive patch test reaction to tea tree oil 5% DEP	3
1999 Germany	10% water	8	1	(13%)	S: patients with a positive patch test reaction to oxidized tea tree oil 20% in olive oil	1
1990-1992 Germany	1% and 10% alc.	7	2	(29%)	S: patients with a positive patch test reaction to tea tree oil 1% alc.	2

DEP: Diethyl phthalate

Case reports and case series

Six patients had allergic contact dermatitis from 'terpineol' in topical pharmaceutical preparations (5); see also Chapter 3.153 alpha-Terpineol.

Presence in products and chemical analyses

In 2008, 66 different fragrance components (including 39 essential oils) were identified in 370 (10% of the total) topical pharmaceutical products marketed in Belgium; 7 of these (1.9%) contained 'terpineol' (5).

In 1992, in The Netherlands, the presence of fragrances was analyzed in 300 cosmetic products. 'Terpineol' was identified in 52% of the products (rank number 8) (7).

In 1988, in the USA, 400 perfumes used in fine fragrances, household products and soaps (number of products per category not mentioned) were analyzed for the presence of fragrance chemicals in a concentration of at least 1% and a list of the Top-25 (present in the highest number of products) presented. 'Terpineol' was found to be present in 66% of the fine fragrances (rank number 7), 66% of the household product fragrances (rank number 2) and 62% of the fragrances used in soaps (rank number 9) (6).

LITERATURE

1   Lippert U, Walter A, Hausen BM, Fuchs Th. Increasing incidence of contact dermatitis to tea tree oil. J Allergy Clin Immunol 2000;105;S43 (abstract 127)
2   Knight TE, Hausen BM. Melaleuca oil (tea tree oil) dermatitis. J Am Acad Dermatol 1994;30:423-427
3   Hausen BM. Evaluation of the main contact allergens in oxidized tea tree oil. Dermatitis 2004;15:213-214
4   De Groot AC, Schmidt E. Tea tree oil: contact allergy and chemical composition. Contact Dermatitis 2016;75:129-143
5   Nardelli A, D'Hooge E, Drieghe J, Dooms M, Goossens A. Allergic contact dermatitis from fragrance components in specific topical pharmaceutical products in Belgium. Contact Dermatitis 2009;60:303-313
6   Fenn RS. Aroma chemical usage trends in modern perfumery. Perfumer and Flavorist 1989;14:3-10
7   Weyland JW. Personal Communication, 1992. Cited in: De Groot AC, Weyland JW, Nater JP. Unwanted effects of cosmetics and drugs used in dermatology, 3rd Ed. Amsterdam: Elsevier, 1994:579
8   De Groot AC, Popova MP, Bankova VS. An update on the constituents of poplar-type propolis. Wapserveen, The Netherlands: acdegroot publishing, 2014, 11 pages. ISBN/EAN: 978-90-813233-0-7. Available at: https://www.researchgate.net/publication/262851225_AN_UPDATE_ON_THE_CONSTITUENTS_OF_POPLAR-TYPE_PROPOLIS
9   De Groot AC, Schmidt E. Essential oils: contact allergy and chemical composition. Boca Raton, Fl., USA: CRC Press, Taylor and Francis Group, 2016 (ISBN 9781482246407)
10 De Groot AC. Patch Testing, 4th Edition. Wapserveen, The Netherlands: acdegroot publishing, 2018 (ISBN 978-90-813233-4-5)

Chapter 3.153 ALPHA-TERPINEOL

IDENTIFICATION

Description/definition   : alpha-Terpineol is the cyclic unsaturated alcohol that conforms to the structural formula
                            shown below
Chemical class(es)   : Cyclic organic compounds; unsaturated compounds; alcohols
INCI name USA   : Not in the Personal Care Products Council Ingredient Database
Chemical/IUPAC name   : 2-(4-Methylcyclohex-3-en-1-yl)propan-2-ol
Other names   : Terpenol; p-menth-1-en-8-ol
CAS registry number(s)   : 10482-56-1; 98-55-5
EC number(s)   : 233-986-8; 202-680-6
RIFM monograph(s)   : Food Chem Toxicol 2017;110(suppl.1):S392-S402; Food Chem Toxicol 2008;46(11)(suppl.)
                            : S1-S71; Food Chem Toxicol 2008;46(11)(suppl.):S204-S205, S275-S279 (mixed isomers)
                            and S280-S285 (alpha-); Food Cosmet Toxicol 1974;12:997 (special issue I) (mixed isomers)
SCCS opinion(s)   : SCCS/1459/11 (4)
Merck Index monograph   : 10583
Function(s) in cosmetics : EU: perfuming
Patch testing   : 5% pet.
Molecular formula   : $C_{10}H_{18}O$

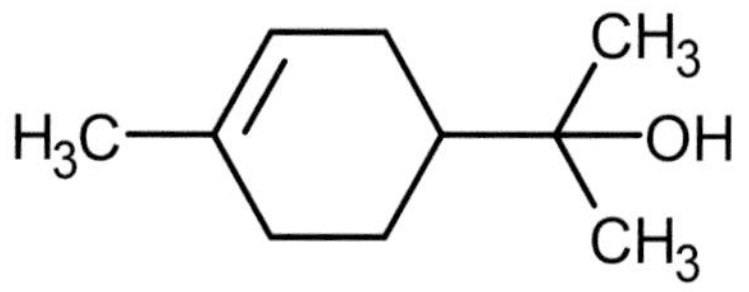

GENERAL

alpha-Terpineol is a colorless viscous liquid to solid; its odor type is terpenic and its odor at 100% is described as 'pine terpene lilac citrus woody floral' (www.thegoodscentscompany.com). alpha-Terpineol is an important commercial chemical. It is one of the most frequently used fragrances in soaps, perfumes and cosmetics. It is also used as a flavoring agent, disinfectant, antioxidant, and solvent (U.S. National Library of Medicine). alpha-Terpineol is one of the three isomers of terpineol (alpha-, beta-, and gamma-terpineol), the last two differing only by the location of the double bond. Terpineol is usually a mixture of these isomers with alpha-terpineol as the major constituent.

Presence in essential oils and Myroxylon pereirae resin (balsam of Peru)

alpha-Terpineol has been identified by chemical analysis in 85 of 91 essential oils, which have caused contact allergy / allergic contact dermatitis. In 16 oils, alpha-terpineol belonged to the 'Top-10' of ingredients with the highest concentrations. These are shown in table 3.153.1 with the concentration range which may be expected in commercial essential oils of this type (14). α-Terpineol may also be present in Myroxylon pereirae resin (balsam of Peru) (11).

Table 3.153.1 Essential oils containing alpha-terpineol in the 'Top-10' and concentration range in commercial oils [a]

Essential oil	Concentration range (min.-max.)	Essential oil	Concentration range (min.-max.)
Ravensara oil	0.2 - 14.7%	Cedarwood oil Atlas	0 - 6.0%
Cajeput oil	2.5 - 11.6%	Clary sage oil	0.6 - 5.1%
Niaouli oil	2.1 - 9.2%	Tea tree oil	1.9 - 4.2%
Rosewood oil	1.9 - 8.8%	Elemi oil	0.4 - 3.1%
Neroli oil	3.2 - 7.6%	Silver fir oil	0.07 - 2.3%
Petitgrain bigarade oil	4.6 - 7.5%	Eucalyptus globulus oil	0.02 - 1.9%
Rose oil	0.06 - 7.5%	Lavandin oil	0.3 - 1.7%
Cardamom oil	trace - 7.0%	Mandarin oil	0.07 - 1.1%

[a] Ref. 14

CONTACT ALLERGY

General
The SCCS (Scientific Committee on Consumer Safety), in a 2012 Opinion on Fragrance allergens in cosmetic products, has marked terpineol (mixed isomers and alpha-terpineol) as 'established contact allergen in humans' (4,8).

Patch testing in groups of patients
Results of studies testing alpha-terpineol in consecutive patients suspected of contact dermatitis (routine testing) and those of testing in groups of *selected* patients (e.g. fragrance-allergic patients, individuals allergic to turpentine oil) are shown in table 3.153.2.

Patch testing in consecutive patients suspected of contact dermatitis: routine testing
In two studies from six European countries (7) and an older one from Italy (9), very low frequencies of sensitization of 0.1% resp. 0.2% were observed to alpha-terpineol 5% in petrolatum. In neither study were relevance data provided (7,9)

Patch testing in groups of selected patients
Patch testing with alpha-terpineol in groups of selected patients (including 2 small groups of patients of 22 and 20 who were allergic to turpentine oil (10) resp. fragrances (1)) has been performed only in studies at least 30 years old. The rates of sensitization ranged from 1.3% to 14%. The latter one was in patients allergic to turpentine oil, in which alpha-terpineol may be present and is a minor allergenic ingredient (10, Chapter 3.75 Turpentine oil). Relevance data were not provided in any study.

Table 3.153.2 Patch testing in groups of patients

Years and Country	Test conc. & vehicle	Number of patients tested | positive (%)		Selection of patients (S); Relevance (R); Comments (C)	Ref.
Routine testing					
1998-2000 6 European countries	5% pet.	1606	1 (0.1%)	R: not stated	7
1983-1984 Italy	5% pet.	1200	2 (0.2%)	R: not stated	9
Testing in groups of selected patients					
<1986 Japan		312	4 (1.3%)	S: unknown; R: unknown; C: the patients were tested with 0.05-0.5% terpineol in a base cream or in 99% alcohol	12
1979-1983 Portugal	10% o.o.	22	3 (14%)	S: patients allergic to turpentine oil; R: not stated	10
1975 USA	5% pet.	20	1 (5%)	S: fragrance-allergic patients; R: not stated	1

o.o.: Olive oil

Case reports and case series
Six patients had allergic contact dermatitis from 'terpineol' in topical pharmaceutical preparations (3); see also Chapter 3.152 4-terpineol.

Presence in products and chemical analyses
In 2008, 66 different fragrance components (including 39 essential oils) were identified in 370 (10% of the total) topical pharmaceutical products marketed in Belgium; 7 (2%) of these contained 'terpineol' (3).

In 1997, 71 deodorants (22 vapo-spray, 22 aerosol spray and 27 roll-on products) were collected in Denmark, England, France, Germany and Sweden and analyzed by gas chromatography – mass spectrometry (GC-MS) for the presence of fragrances and other materials. alpha-Terpineol / terpinyl acetate was present in 53 (75%) of the products (5).

In 1992, in The Netherlands, the presence of fragrances was analyzed in 300 cosmetic products. 'Terpineol' was identified in 52% of the products (rank order 8) (6).

In 1988, in the USA, 400 perfumes used in fine fragrances, household products and soaps (number of products per category not mentioned) were analyzed for the presence of fragrance chemicals in a concentration of at least 1% and a list of the Top-25 (present in the highest number of products) presented. 'Terpineol' was found to be present in 66% of the fine fragrances (rank number 7), 66% of the household product fragrances (rank number 2) and 62% of the fragrances used in soaps (rank number 9) (2).

LITERATURE

1   Larsen WG. Perfume dermatitis. A study of 20 patients. Arch Dermatol 1977;113:623-626

2   Fenn RS. Aroma chemical usage trends in modern perfumery. Perfumer and Flavorist 1989;14:3-10

3   Nardelli A, D'Hooge E, Drieghe J, Dooms M, Goossens A. Allergic contact dermatitis from fragrance components in specific topical pharmaceutical products in Belgium. Contact Dermatitis 2009;60:303-313

4   SCCS (Scientific Committee on Consumer Safety). Opinion on Fragrance allergens in cosmetic products, 26-27 June 2012, SCCS/1459/11. Available at: https://ec.europa.eu/health/sites/health/files/scientific_committees/consumer_safety/docs/sccs_o_102.pdf

5   Rastogi SC, Lepoittevin J-P, Johansen JD, Frosch PJ, Menné T, Bruze M, et al. Fragrances and other materials in deodorants: search for potentially sensitizing molecules using combined GC-MS and structure activity relationship (SAR) analysis. Contact Dermatitis 1998;39:293-303

6   Weyland JW. Personal Communication, 1992. Cited in: De Groot AC, Weyland JW, Nater JP. Unwanted effects of cosmetics and drugs used in dermatology, 3rd Ed. Amsterdam: Elsevier, 1994:579

7   Frosch PJ, Johansen JD, Menné T, Pirker C, Rastogi SC, Andersen KE, et al. Further important sensitizers in patients sensitive to fragrances. II. Reactivity to essential oils. Contact Dermatitis 2002;47:279-287

8   Uter W, Johansen JD, Börje A, Karlberg A-T, Lidén C, Rastogi S, Roberts D, White IR. Categorization of fragrance contact allergens for prioritization of preventive measures: clinical and experimental data and consideration of structure–activity relationships. Contact Dermatitis 2013;69:196-230

9   Santucci B, Cristaudo A, Cannistraci C, Picardo M. Contact dermatitis to fragrances. Contact Dermatitis 1987;16:93-95

10 Cachao P, Menezes Brandao F, Carmo M, Frazao S, Silva M. Allergy to oil of turpentine in Portugal. Contact Dermatitis 1986;14:205-208

11 Mammerler V. Contribution to the analysis and quality control of Peru Balsam. PhD Thesis, University of Vienna, Austria, 2007. Available at: http://othes.univie.ac.at/4056/1/2009-03-23_0201578.pdf

12 Takenaka T, Hasegawa E, Takenaka U, Saito F, Odaka T. Fundamental studies of safe compound perfumes for cosmetics. Part 1. The primary irritation of compound materials to the skin. Unknown Source, 1986;?: 313-329 (article in Japanese). Data cited in ref 13

13 Bhatia SP, McGinty D, Foxenberg RJ, Letizia CS, Api AM. Fragrance material review on terpineol. Food Chem Toxicol 2008;46(11)(suppl.):S275-S279

14 De Groot AC, Schmidt E. Essential oils: contact allergy and chemical composition. Boca Raton, Fl., USA: CRC Press, Taylor and Francis Group, 2016 (ISBN 9781482246407)

Chapter 3.154 TERPINOLENE *
* Not officially an INCI name but perfuming name

IDENTIFICATION

Description/definition : Terpinolene is the cyclic unsaturated compound that conforms to the structural formula shown below
Chemical class(es) : Cyclic organic compounds; unsaturated compounds
INCI name USA : Not in the Personal Care Products Council Ingredient Database
Chemical/IUPAC name : 1-Methyl-4-propan-2-ylidenecyclohexene
Other names : *p*-Mentha-1,4(8)-diene; isoterpinene; 4-isopropylidene-1-methylcyclohexene
CAS registry number(s) : 586-62-9
EC number(s) : 209-578-0
RIFM monograph(s) : Food Cosmet Toxicol 1976;14:877 (special issue III)
SCCS opinion(s) : SCCS/1459/11 (8); SCCNFP/0389/00, final (7)
Function(s) in cosmetics : EU: perfuming
EU cosmetic restrictions : Regulated in Annex III/133 of the Regulation (EC) No. 344/2013
Patch testing : 5-10% pet.; according to RIFM data, 20% pet. is probably not irritant (14); concentrations of terpinolene 5% (or higher) *in alcohol* may be (strongly) irritant (3)
Molecular formula : $C_{10}H_{16}$

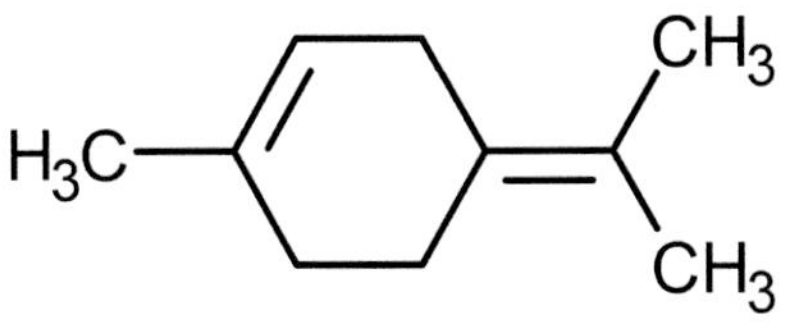

GENERAL

Terpinolene is a colorless clear liquid; its odor type is herbal and its odor at 10% in dipropylene glycol is described as 'fresh woody sweet pine citrus' (www.thegoodscentscompany.com). Terpinolene is given off naturally from tissues of many plants, especially trees. It is a component of many types of oranges as well as several oils, notably tea tree oil (see 'Presence in essential oils' below). Terpinolene is an important commercial chemical that is used as a solvent, as a flavoring ingredient in foods, and to make other chemicals including synthetic resins and flavors. It is also used as a fragrance in industrial and household cleaners, soaps, lotions, and perfumes (U.S. National Library of Medicine).

Presence in essential oils

Terpinolene has been identified by chemical analysis in 76 of 91 essential oils, which have caused contact allergy / allergic contact dermatitis. In 10 oils, terpinolene belonged to the 'Top-10' of ingredients with the highest concentrations. These are shown in table 3.154.1 with the concentration range which may be expected in commercial essential oils of this type (13).

Table 3.154.1 Essential oils containing terpinolene in the 'Top-10' and concentration range in commercial oils (13)

Essential oil	Concentration range (min.-max.)	Essential oil	Concentration range (min.-max.)
Tea tree oil	0.04 - 45.7%	Eucalyptus globulus oil	0.02 - 3.6%
Dwarf pine oil	0.4 - 8.3%	Cypress oil	0.8 - 3.5%
Marjoram oil	0.2 - 6.8%	Elemi oil	0.7 - 3.1%
Cajeput oil	0.4 - 5.3%	Tangerine oil	0.2 - 2.9%
Mandarin oil	0.06 - 4.2%	Bay oil	0.1 - 2.1%

CONTACT ALLERGY

General

The SCCS (Scientific Committee on Consumer Safety), in a 2012 Opinion on Fragrance allergens in cosmetic products, has marked terpinolene as 'established contact allergen in humans' (8,11).

Terpinolene is an important hapten in tea tree oil. Of 64 patients allergic to tea tree oil and tested with a number of its ingredients in various studies, 50 (78%) reacted to terpinolene (6).

Patch testing in groups of patients

Patch testing in consecutive patients suspected of contact dermatitis: routine testing
Studies in which terpinolene was patch tested in consecutive patients suspected of contact dermatitis (routine testing) with positive results have not been found.

Patch testing in groups of selected patients
Results of studies patch testing terpinolene in groups of selected patients (in all studies: patients previously shown to be allergic to (oxidized) tea tree oil) are shown in table 3.154.2. In the period 1990-2003, five small series of 7-20 patients allergic to (oxidized) tea tree oil have been tested with a battery of its ingredients, including terpinolene 5% or 10% in various vehicles (1,2,4,5,9). Frequencies of sensitization have ranged from 85 to 100%, attesting to the fact that terpinolene is an important allergenic ingredient of tea tree oil (6).

Table 3.154.2 Patch testing in groups of patients: Selected patient groups

Years and Country	Test conc. & vehicle	Number of patients tested	positive (%)	Selection of patients (S); Relevance (R); Comments (C)	Ref.
1999-2003 Germany	5% DEP	20	17 (85%)	S: patients with a positive patch test reaction to oxidized tea tree oil 5% DEP	5
1999-2000 Germany, Austria	10% DEP	10	10 (100%)	S: patients with a positive patch test reaction to oxidized tea tree oil 5% DEP	1
1999 Germany	10% water	8	7 (88%)	S: patients with a positive patch test reaction to oxidized tea tree oil 20% in olive oil	2
<1999 Germany	10% vehicle?	16	16 (100%)	S: patients allergic to tea tree oil	4
1990-1992 Germany	10% alc.	7	6 (86%)	S: patients with a positive patch test reaction to tea tree oil 1% alc.	9

DEP: diethyl phthalate

Case reports and case series
A man became sensitized after using tea tree oil in his shampoo and for blisters on his face. When patch tested, he reacted to tea tree oil; in a second session, the patient was tested with a number of its ingredients and now had positive reactions to terpinolene (10%, vehicle unknown), ascaridole (5%, vehicle unknown), and alpha-terpinene (5%, vehicle unknown) (4,10).

Another patient had treated warts on his hands with tea tree oil and became sensitized within three weeks. When patch tested, he reacted to tea tree oil and the same 3 ingredients (4). A woman, who treated her atopic dermatitis with tea tree oil, also became sensitized to the essential oil from contact allergy to these three tea tree oil components (4).

Eight more patients are presented by the same authors, who had used tea tree oil for various reasons and indications, who developed allergic contact dermatitis from it and reacted on ingredient patch testing to terpinolene and 1-6 other oil components (4).

A woman developed occupational allergic contact dermatitis from terpinolene and 3-carene in a cleanser for the machine she worked with. Patch tests were positive to both substances at 5% pet. and 1% in water; 10 controls were negative (12).

LITERATURE
1   Pirker C, Hausen BM, Uter W, Hillen U, Brasch J, Bayeret C, et al. Sensitization to tea tree oil in Germany and Austria. A multicenter Study of the German Contact Dermatitis group. J Dtsch Dermatol Ges 2003;1:629-634 (article in German)
2   Lippert U, Walter A, Hausen BM, Fuchs Th. Increasing incidence of contact dermatitis to tea tree oil. J Allergy Clin Immunol 2000;105;S43 (abstract 127)
3   Knight TE, Hausen BM. Melaleuca oil (tea tree oil) dermatitis. J Am Acad Dermatol 1994;30:423-427
4   Hausen BM, Reichling J, Harkenthal M. Degradation products of monoterpenes are the sensitizing agents in tea tree oil. Am J Contact Dermat 1999;10:68-77

5   Hausen BM. Evaluation of the main contact allergens in oxidized tea tree oil. Dermatitis 2004;15:213-214

6   De Groot AC, Schmidt E. Tea tree oil: contact allergy and chemical composition. Contact Dermatitis 2016;75:129-143

7   Opinion of the Scientific Committee on Cosmetic Products and Non-Food Products Intended for Consumers concerning 'The 1st update of the inventory of ingredients employed in cosmetic products. Section II: Perfume and aromatic raw materials', 24 October 2000, SCCNFP/0389/00, final. Available at: http://ec.europa.eu/health/ph_risk/committees/sccp/documents/out131_en.pdf

8   SCCS (Scientific Committee on Consumer Safety). Opinion on Fragrance allergens in cosmetic products, 26-27 June 2012, SCCS/1459/11. Available at: https://ec.europa.eu/health/sites/health/files/scientific_committees/consumer_safety/docs/sccs_o_102.pdf

9   Knight TE, Hausen BM. Melaleuca oil (tea tree oil) dermatitis. J Am Acad Dermatol 1994;30:423-427

10 Hausen BM. Kontaktallergie auf Teebaumöl und Ascaridol. Akt Derm 1998;24:60-62

11 Uter W, Johansen JD, Börje A, Karlberg A-T, Lidén C, Rastogi S, Roberts D, White IR. Categorization of fragrance contact allergens for prioritization of preventive measures: clinical and experimental data and consideration of structure–activity relationships. Contact Dermatitis 2013;69:196-230

12 Castelain PY, Camoin JP, Jouglard J. Contact dermatitis to terpene derivatives in a machine cleaner. Contact Dermatitis 1980;6:358-360

13 De Groot AC, Schmidt E. Essential oils: contact allergy and chemical composition. Boca Raton, Fl., USA: CRC Press, Taylor and Francis Group, 2016 (ISBN 9781482246407)

14 De Groot AC. Patch Testing, 4th Edition. Wapserveen, The Netherlands: acdegroot publishing, 2018 (ISBN 978-90-813233-4-5)

Chapter 3.155 TERPINYL ACETATE

Terpinyl acetate is the ester of acetic acid and terpineol. CosIng distinguishes terpineol acetate (CAS 8007-35-0; EINECS 232-357-5) from α-terpinyl acetate (CAS 80-26-2; EINECS 201-265-7); according to the PubChem project database (https://pubchem.ncbi.nlm.nih.gov) they are identical. Between the various chemical databases there are many discrepancies.

TERPINEOL ACETATE

IDENTIFICATION
Description/definition   : Terpineol acetate is the ester of acetic acid and terpineol
Chemical class(es)   : Esters
Chemical/IUPAC name   : 2-(4-Methylcyclohex-3-en-1-yl)propan-2-yl acetate (PubChem)
CAS registry number(s)   : 8007-35-0
EC number(s)   : 232-357-5

α-TERPINYL ACETATE

IDENTIFICATION
Description/definition   : α-Terpinyl acetate is the ester of acetic acid and terpineol
Chemical class(es)   : Esters
INCI name USA   : Not in the Personal Care Products Council Ingredient Database
Chemical/IUPAC name   : 1-Methyl-1-(4-methylcyclohex-3-enyl)ethyl ethanoate (CosIng)
Other names   : p-Menth-1-en-8-yl acetate (CosIng)
CAS registry number(s)   : 80-26-2
EC number(s)   : 201-265-7

Terpineol acetate and α-Terpinyl acetate

RIFM monograph(s)   : Food Chem Toxicol 2018 Sep 20. pii: S0278-6915(18)30675-6. doi: 10.1016/
                           j.fct.2018.09.031; Food Cosmet Toxicol 1974;12:999 (special issue I) (mixed isomers)
Function(s) in cosmetics : EU: masking; fragrance. USA: fragrance ingredients (Terpineol acetate)
Patch testing   : 5% Pet. (1)
Molecular formula   : $C_{12}H_{20}O_2$

GENERAL
Terpineol / terpinyl acetate is a colorless to pale yellow clear liquid; its odor type is herbal and its odor at 100% is described as 'sweet herbal bergamot pine lavender floral' (www.thegoodscentscompany.com).

Presence in essential oils
Terpinyl acetate (terpinyl acetate, alfa-, beta-, gamma-, delta-) has been identified by chemical analysis in 55 of 91 essential oils, which have caused contact allergy / allergic contact dermatitis. In four oils, terpinyl acetate belonged to the 'Top-10' of ingredients with the highest concentrations which may be expected in commercial essential oils of this type: cardamom oil (32.0-45.0%), laurel leaf oil (6.3-12.0%), sage oil Spanish (0.5-9.0%) and cypress oil (1.2-3.2%) (5).

CONTACT ALLERGY

Patch testing in groups of patients

Patch testing in consecutive patients suspected of contact dermatitis: routine testing
Studies in which terpinyl acetate was patch tested in consecutive patients suspected of contact dermatitis (routine testing) with positive results have not been found.

Patch testing in groups of selected patients
In a group of 20 patients allergic to fragrances and tested with a battery of fragrance materials, one reacted to terpinyl acetate 5% pet. The relevance of this reaction was not mentioned (1).

Case reports and case series
Case reports of allergic contact dermatitis from terpinyl acetate have not been found.

Presence in products and chemical analyses
In 1997, 71 deodorants (22 vapo-spray, 22 aerosol spray and 27 roll-on products) were collected in Denmark, England, France, Germany and Sweden and analyzed by gas chromatography – mass spectrometry (GC-MS) for the presence of fragrances and other materials. alpha-Terpineol / terpinyl acetate was present in 53 (75%) products (2).

In 1988, in the USA, 400 perfumes used in fine fragrances, household products and soaps (number of products per category not mentioned) were analyzed for the presence of fragrance chemicals in a concentration of at least 1% and a list of the Top-25 (present in the highest number of products) presented. Terpinyl acetate was found to be present in 50% of the fine fragrances (rank number 11), 51% of the household product fragrances (rank number 8) and an unknown percentage of the fragrances used in soaps (3).

OTHER SIDE EFFECTS

Immediate-type reactions
A woman developed contact urticaria within minutes after wearing spray-starched clothes. Contact with the spray starch reproduced the symptoms. When tested with its ingredients, there were positive reactions to the perfume (undiluted) and formaldehyde. Ingredient testing with the 44 fragrance compounds in the perfume showed terpinyl acetate (tested undiluted), which was present in the perfume in a concentration of 0.25%, to be the culprit. Twelve controls had negative open tests to undiluted terpinyl acetate (4).

LITERATURE
1   Larsen WG. Perfume dermatitis. A study of 20 patients. Arch Dermatol 1977;113:623-626
2   Rastogi SC, Lepoittevin J-P, Johansen JD, Frosch PJ, Menné T, Bruze M, et al. Fragrances and other materials in deodorants: search for potentially sensitizing molecules using combined GC-MS and structure activity relationship (SAR) analysis. Contact Dermatitis 1998;39:293-303
3   Fenn RS. Aroma chemical usage trends in modern perfumery. Perfumer and Flavorist 1989;14:3-10
4   McDaniel WH, Marks JG Jr. Contact urticaria due to sensitivity to spray starch. Arch Dermatol 1979;115:628
5   De Groot AC, Schmidt E. Essential oils: contact allergy and chemical composition. Boca Raton, Fl., USA: CRC Press, Taylor and Francis Group, 2016 (ISBN 9781482246407)

Chapter 3.156 TETRAHYDRO-DIMETHYLBENZOFURAN

IDENTIFICATION

Description/definition   : Tetrahydro-dimethylbenzofuran is the bicyclic organic compound that conforms to the
                             structural formula shown below
Chemical class(es)   : Heterocyclic organic compounds; unsaturated compounds
INCI name USA   : Not in the Personal Care Products Council Ingredient Database
Chemical/IUPAC name   : 3,6-Dimethyl-4,5,6,7-tetrahydro-1-benzofuran
Other names   : Menthofuran; 4,5,6,7-tetrahydro-3,6-dimethylbenzofuran
CAS registry number(s)   : 494-90-6
EC number(s)   : 207-795-5
Function(s) in cosmetics   : EU: perfuming
Patch testing   : No data available
Molecular formula   : $C_{10}H_{14}O$

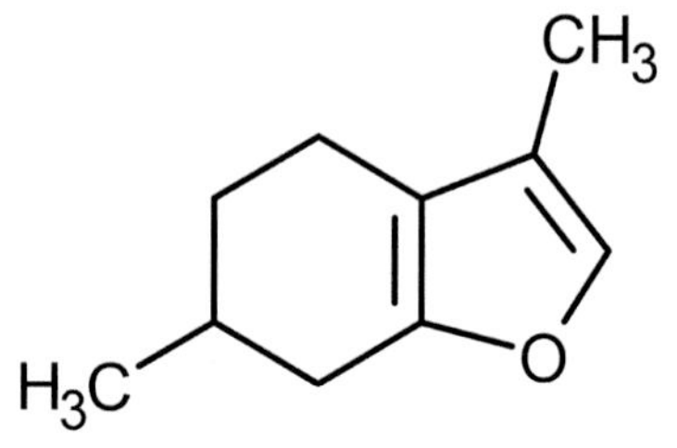

GENERAL

Tetrahydro-dimethylbenzofuran is a bluish clear liquid; its odor type is musty and its odor is described as 'diffusive, pungent, musty, nutty, pyrazine like, nutty, earthy and coffee' (www.thegoodscentscompany.com).

Presence in essential oils

Tetrahydro-dimethylbenzofuran has been identified by chemical analysis in 5 of 91 essential oils, which have caused contact allergy / allergic contact dermatitis: basil oil (sweet), laurel leaf oil, marjoram oil (sweet), peppermint oil and spearmint oil. In one oil, tetrahydro-dimethylbenzofuran belonged to the 'Top-10' of ingredients with the highest concentrations which may be expected in commercial essential oils of this type: peppermint oil (0.07%-7%) (2).

CONTACT ALLERGY

Patch testing in groups of patients

Patch testing in groups of patients: Selected patient groups

Ten patients allergic to peppermint oil (of who 4 co-reacted to spearmint oil) were patch tested with 24 ingredients. There were 2 positive reactions to tetrahydro-dimethylbenzofuran (menthofuran), 4 to menthol, 4 to piperitone, 3 to pulegone, one to menthyl acetate and one to dihydrocarveol (1). Further details are lacking (article in Japanese).

Case reports and case series

Case reports of allergic contact dermatitis from tetrahydro-dimethylbenzofuran have not been found.

LITERATURE

1   Saito F, Miyazaki T, Matsuoka Y. Peppermint oil (title incomplete, partly in Japanese). Skin Research
    1984;26:636-643 (article in Japanese)
2   De Groot AC, Schmidt E. Essential oils: contact allergy and chemical composition. Boca Raton, Fl., USA: CRC Press,
    Taylor and Francis Group, 2016 (ISBN 9781482246407)

Chapter 3.157 TETRAMETHYL ACETYLOCTAHYDRONAPHTHALENE

IDENTIFICATION

Description/definition : Tetramethyl acetyloctahydronaphthalene is the bicyclic unsaturated organic compound that conforms to the structural formula shown below

Chemical class(es) : Bicyclic organic compounds; unsaturated compounds; ketones

Chemical/IUPAC name : 1-(1,2,3,4,5,6,7,8-Octahydro-2,3,8,8-tetramethyl-2-naphthyl)ethan-1-one

Other names : Patchouli ethanone; Iso E super ®; isocyclemone E; 1-(2,3,8,8-tetramethyl-1,2,3,4,5,6,7,8-octahydronaphthalen-2-yl)ethanone

CAS registry number(s) : 54464-57-2; The actual INCI name is tetramethyl acetyloctahydronaphthaleneS, which includes isomers with CAS numbers 54464-59-4, 68155-66-8 and 68155-67-9

EC number(s) : 259-174-3

RIFM monograph(s) : Food Chem Toxicol 2013;62(suppl.1)S120-S132

IFRA standard : Restricted (www.ifraorg.org/en-us/standards-library) (table 3.157.1)

SCCS opinion(s) : SCCS/1459/11 (1)

Function(s) in cosmetics : EU: perfuming. USA: fragrance ingredients; skin-conditioning agents - miscellaneous

Patch testing : 5% pet.

Molecular formula : $C_{16}H_{26}O$

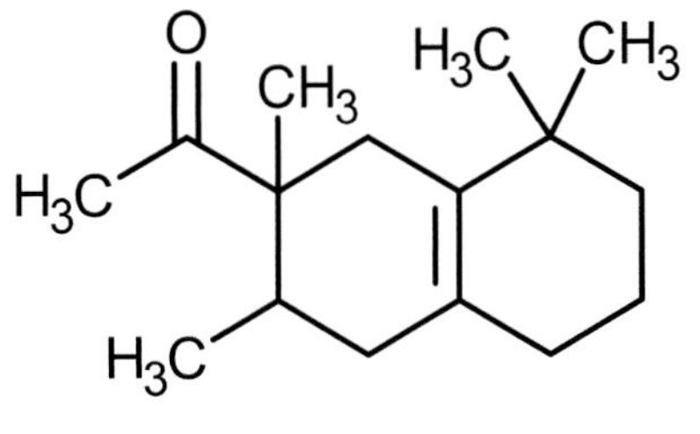

Table 3.157.1 IFRA restrictions for tetramethyl acetyloctahydronaphthalene

Category [a]	Limits [b]	Category [a]	Limits [b]	Category [a]	Limits [b]
1	1.34%	5	11.20%	9	5.00%
2	1.73%	6	34.20%	10	2.50%
3	7.10%	7	3.60%	11	not restricted
4	21.40%	8	2.00%		

[a] For explanation of categories see pages 6-8
[b] Limits in the finished products

GENERAL

Tetramethyl acetyloctahydronaphthalene is a colorless to pale yellow clear liquid; its odor type is floral and its odor at 100% is described as 'woody dry ambergris cedar old wood ketonic phenolic' (www.thegoodscentscompany.com). Tetramethyl acetyloctahydronaphthalene is a synthetic chemical, not found in nature (and consequently not in essential oils (8)).

CONTACT ALLERGY

General

The SCCS (Scientific Committee on Consumer Safety), in a 2012 Opinion on Fragrance allergens in cosmetic products, has marked tetramethyl acetyloctahydronaphthalene as 'established contact allergen in humans' (1,7).

Patch testing in groups of patients

Results of studies testing tetramethyl acetyloctahydronaphthalene in consecutive patients suspected of contact dermatitis (routine testing) and those of testing in groups of *selected* patients (patients with known fragrance sensitivity) are shown in table 3.157.2.

Patch testing in consecutive patients suspected of contact dermatitis: routine testing

In two investigations in which routine testing was performed with tetramethyl acetyloctahydronaphthalene, very low frequencies of sensitization of 0.2% and 0.3% were observed (4,5). In one study, the relevance was not specified, in the other, the one positive reaction was considered not to be relevant and a ROAT with the material was negative (4).

Patch testing in groups of selected patients

In a selected group of 178 patients with known fragrance sensitivity, 3 individuals (1.7%) reacted to tetramethyl acetyloctahydronaphthalene 5% in petrolatum. The relevance of the positive patch tests was not mentioned (2).

While searching for causative ingredients of pigmented cosmetic dermatitis in Japan in the 1970s, both patients with ordinary (nonpigmented) cosmetic dermatitis and women with pigmented cosmetic dermatitis were tested with a large number of fragrance materials. In 1980 the accumulated data enabled the classification of fragrant materials into 4 groups: common sensitizers, rare sensitizers, virtually non-sensitizing fragrances and fragrances considered as non-sensitizers. Tetramethyl acetyloctahydronaphthalene (Iso E super) was classified in the group of rare sensitizers, indicating that one or more cases of contact allergy / allergic contact dermatitis to it have been observed (6). More specific data are lacking, the results have largely or solely been published in Japanese journals only.

Table 3.157.2 Patch testing in groups of patients

Years and Country	Test conc. & vehicle	Number of patients tested	positive (%)		Selection of patients (S); Relevance (R); Comments (C)	Ref.
Routine testing						
1997-8 six European countries	5% pet.	1855	3	(0.2%)	R: not stated / specified	5
<1995 France and UK	1% pet.	313	1	(0.3%)	R: not relevant; C: unknown whether the reactions were in one	4
	5% pet.	313	1	(0.3%)	patient; a ROAT was negative	
Testing in groups of selected patients						
2000 Japan, Europe, USA	5% pet.	178	3	(1.7%)	S: patients with known fragrance sensitivity; R: not stated	2

Case reports and case series

Case reports of allergic contact dermatitis from tetramethyl acetyloctahydronaphthalene have not been found.

Presence in products and chemical analyses

In 1988, in the USA, 400 perfumes used in fine fragrances, household products and soaps (number of products per category not mentioned) were analyzed for the presence of fragrance chemicals in a concentration of at least 1% and a list of the Top-25 (present in the highest number of products) presented. Tetramethyl acetyloctahydronaphthalene was found to be present in an unknown percentage of the fine fragrances, 17% of the household product fragrances (rank number 24) and an unknown percentage of the fragrances used in soaps (3).

LITERATURE

1   SCCS (Scientific Committee on Consumer Safety). Opinion on Fragrance allergens in cosmetic products, 26-27 June 2012, SCCS/1459/11. Available at:
     https://ec.europa.eu/health/sites/health/files/scientific_committees/consumer_safety/docs/sccs_o_102.pdf
2   Larsen W, Nakayama H, Fischer T, Elsner P, Frosch P, Burrows D, et al. Fragrance contact dermatitis: A worldwide multicenter investigation (Part II). Contact Dermatitis 2001;44:344-346
3   Fenn RS. Aroma chemical usage trends in modern perfumery. Perfumer and Flavorist 1989;14:3-10
4   Frosch PJ, Pilz B, Andersen KE, Burrows D, Camarasa JG, Dooms-Goossens A, et al. Patch testing with fragrances: results of a multicenter study of the European Environmental and Contact Dermatitis Research Group with 48 frequently used constituents of perfumes. Contact Dermatitis 1995;33:333-342
5   Frosch PJ, Johansen JD, Menné T, Pirker C, Rastogi SC, Andersen KE, et al. Further important sensitizers in patients sensitive to fragrances. I. Reactivity to 14 frequently used chemicals. Contact Dermatitis 2002;47:78-85
6   Nakayama H. Fragrance hypersensitivity and its control. In: Frosch PJ, Johansen JD, White IR, Eds. Fragrances - beneficial and adverse effects. Berlin Heidelberg New York: Springer-Verlag, 1998:83-91
7   Uter W, Johansen JD, Börje A, Karlberg A-T, Lidén C, Rastogi S, Roberts D, White IR. Categorization of fragrance contact allergens for prioritization of preventive measures: clinical and experimental data and consideration of structure–activity relationships. Contact Dermatitis 2013;69:196-230
8   De Groot AC, Schmidt E. Essential oils: contact allergy and chemical composition. Boca Raton, Fl., USA: CRC Press, Taylor and Francis Group, 2016 (ISBN 9781482246407)

Chapter 3.158 THYMOL

IDENTIFICATION

Description/definition : Thymol is the substituted phenol that conforms to the structural formula shown below
Chemical class(es) : Phenols
Chemical/IUPAC name : 5-Methyl-2-propan-2-ylphenol
Other names : Isopropyl-*m*-cresol; 5-methyl-2-(1-methylethyl)phenol; *p*-cymen-3-ol
CAS registry number(s) : 89-83-8
EC number(s) : 201-944-8
CIR review(s) : Int J Toxicol 2006;25(suppl.1):S29-S127 (access: www.cir-safety.org/ingredients)
Merck Index monograph : 10824
Function(s) in cosmetics : EU: denaturant; hair dyeing; masking. USA: denaturants; fragrance ingredients; oral health care drugs
Patch testing : 1% Pet. (SmartPracticeEurope, SmartPracticeCanada)
Molecular formula : $C_{10}H_{14}O$

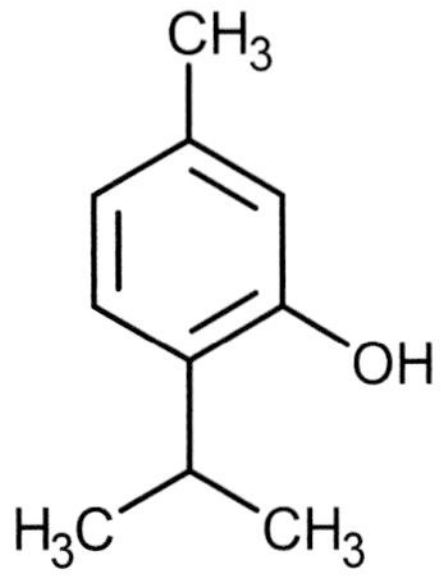

GENERAL

Thymol is a white crystalline solid; its odor type is herbal and its odor is described as 'spicy, phenolic and thymol with a chemical, medicinal, camphoreous nuance' (www.thegoodscentscompany.com). Thymol is a major constituent of oil of thyme (see 'Presence in essential oils' below). It also occurs naturally in food stuffs such as lime honey and cooking herbs and thymol is used as a synthetic flavoring for foods. In addition it is used in lavender compositions, in men's fragrances, and as a disinfectant in oral hygiene products. It is an ingredient in topical over-the-counter cold and cough preparations. Thymol is used as a preservative for documents, art objects and urine. The chemical is also used to make other compounds, notably racemic menthol, and has applications as a laboratory reagent. In addition, thymol is employed in products applied to beehives to control the varroa mite and in animal repellant products (U.S. National Library of Medicine).

Thymol is produced synthetically from *m*-cresol and isopropyl chloride and can also be derived from thyme, savory, marjoram, cumin and oregano (6). Health aspects and potential uses of thymol and its source plant *Thymus vulgaris* have been reviewed in 2018 (11).

Presence in essential oils and propolis

Thymol has been identified by chemical analysis in 43 of 91 essential oils, which have caused contact allergy / allergic contact dermatitis. In two oils, this chemical belonged to the 'Top-10' of ingredients with the highest concentrations which may be expected in commercial essential oils of this type: thyme oil Spanish (39.2-56.2%) and thyme oil ex *Thymus vulgaris* (0.2-47.8%) (10). Thymol may also be present in propolis (9).

CONTACT ALLERGY

General

Only a few cases of contact allergy to thymol have been reported (2,3,4,5), but never as a component of a fragrance.

Patch testing in groups of patients

Patch testing in consecutive patients suspected of contact dermatitis: routine testing

Studies in which thymol was patch tested in consecutive patients suspected of contact dermatitis (routine testing) with positive results have not been found.

Patch testing in groups of selected patients

Results of studies patch testing thymol in groups of selected patients (staff of stomatology departments, fragrance-allergic patients) are shown in table 3.158.1. In 2 studies, frequencies of positive reactions were 1.2% and 5%, but in both investigations, there was only one case of contact allergy (1,8). The relevance of the positive patch tests was either unknown or not mentioned.

Table 3.158.1 Patch testing in groups of patients: Selected patient groups

Years and Country	Test conc. & vehicle	Number of patients tested | positive (%)		Selection of patients (S); Relevance (R); Comments (C)	Ref.
<1990 country?	1% pet.	84	1 (1.2%)	S: staff of stomatology departments; R: unknown; C: thymol was tested as it is used in dental antiseptics	8
1975 USA	1% pet.	20	1 (5%)	S: fragrance-allergic patients; R: not stated	1

Case reports and case series

A woman was prescribed a solution of 4% thymol in chloroform for the treatment of chronic paronychia of the middle and ring fingers of the right hand. Six weeks after starting treatment, she developed severe erythema and edema, with intense itching, in the treated areas. The thymol solution was discontinued and a topical corticosteroid prescribed. After a few weeks, she had clinical resolution. One month later, the patient was patch tested with the GIRDCA standard series and her solution of 4% thymol in chloroform; the latter gave a positive test. Further testing with thymol 1% pet. and chloroform 40% in olive oil confirmed contact allergy to thymol. Control patch tests with thymol 1% pet. in 20 volunteers were negative (3).

A similar case of contact allergy to thymol from an antiseptic solution applied for chronic paronychia under occlusion had previously been reported from the USA (4).

Three patients had allergic contact dermatitis from thymol in topical pharmaceutical preparations (2). In an early study, one patient had cheilitis and glossitis from a toothpaste. Ingredient patch testing indicated thymol (patch test concentration and vehicle not mentioned) to be the offending allergen (5).

Presence in products and chemical analyses

In 2008, 66 different fragrance components (including 39 essential oils) were identified in 370 (10% of the total) topical pharmaceutical products marketed in Belgium; 9 of these (2.4%) contained thymol (2).

Other information

Twenty-three patients had allergic contact dermatitis from a topical pharmaceutical preparation. The patients had positive patch test reactions to the cream base, but not to its individual ingredients, including the preservatives thymol and 1,3,5-trihydroxyethylhexahydrotriazine. It was found that thymol and a degradation product of the triazine formed a new contact allergen ('compound allergy'). This chemical was identified by nuclear magnetic resonance spectroscopy and infrared spectroscopy as 3-(hydroxyethyl)-5-methyl-8-(2-methylethyl)-3,4-dihydro-2H-1,3-benzoxazine (7).

OTHER SIDE EFFECTS

Systemic side effects

Three patients were reported to have developed thyroid intoxication from the use of a mouthwash containing thymol for 6 months to 3 years. Two of the patients had lost weight, the third exhibited tremors, restlessness, sleeplessness, languidness, palpitations, perspirations and diarrhea. All recovered after stopping the use of the mouthwash (6).

LITERATURE

1   Larsen WG. Perfume dermatitis. A study of 20 patients. Arch Dermatol 1977;113:623-626
2   Nardelli A, D'Hooge E, Drieghe J, Dooms M, Goossens A. Allergic contact dermatitis from fragrance components in specific topical pharmaceutical products in Belgium. Contact Dermatitis 2009;60:303-313
3   Lorenzi S, Placucci F, Vincenzi C, Bardazzi F, Tosti A. Allergic contact dermatitis due to thymol. Contact Dermatitis 1995;33:439-440
4   Fisher AA. Allergic contact dermatitis due to thymol in Listerine® for treatment of paronychia. Cutis 1989;43:531-532

5   Beinhauer LG. Cheilitis and glossitis from toothpaste. Arch Dermatol Syphilol 1940;41:892-894

6   Andersen A. Final report on the safety assessment of sodium *p*-chloro-*m*-cresol, *p*-chloro-*m*-cresol, chlorothymol, mixed cresols, *m*-cresol, *o*-cresol, *p*-cresol, isopropyl cresols, thymol, *o*-cymen-5-ol, and carvacrol. Int J Toxicol 2006;25(suppl.1):S29-S127

7   Smeenk G, Kerckhoffs HP, Schreurs PH. Contact allergy to a reaction product in Hirudoid cream: an example of compound allergy. Br J Dermatol 1987;116:223-231

8   Berova N. Studies on contact dermatitis in stomatological staff. Dermatol Monstsschr 1990;176:15-18 (article in German). Data cited in ref. 6

9   De Groot AC, Popova MP, Bankova VS. An update on the constituents of poplar-type propolis. Wapserveen, The Netherlands: acdegroot publishing, 2014, 11 pages. ISBN/EAN: 978-90-813233-0-7. Available at: https://www.researchgate.net/publication/262851225_AN_UPDATE_ON_THE_CONSTITUENTS_OF_POPLAR-TYPE_PROPOLIS

10 De Groot AC, Schmidt E. Essential oils: contact allergy and chemical composition. Boca Raton, Fl., USA: CRC Press, Taylor and Francis Group, 2016 (ISBN 9781482246407)

11 Salehi B, Mishra AP, Shukla I, Sharifi-Rad M, Contreras MDM, Segura-Carretero A, et al. Thymol, thyme, and other plant sources: Health and potential uses. Phytother Res 2018;32:1688-1706

Chapter 3.159 TRIMETHYLBENZENEPROPANOL

IDENTIFICATION

Description/definition	: Trimethylbenzenepropanol is the organic compound that conforms to the structural formula shown below
Chemical class(es)	: Alcohols
Chemical/IUPAC name	: 2,2-Dimethyl-3-(3-methylphenyl)propan-1-ol
Other names	: β,β,3-Trimethylbenzenepropanol; lily propanol; 2,2-dimethyl-3-(3-tolyl)propan-1-ol; Majantol ®
CAS registry number(s)	: 103694-68-4
EC number(s)	: 403-140-4
IFRA standard	: Restricted (www.ifraorg.org/en-us/standards-library) (table 3.159.1)
RIFM monograph(s)	: Food Chem Toxicol 2012;50(suppl.2):S263-S268
SCCS opinion(s)	: SCCS/1459/11 (2)
Function(s) in cosmetics	: EU: masking; perfuming. USA: fragrance ingredients
Patch testing	: 5% Pet. (SmartPracticeCanada, Chemotechnique, SmartPracticeEurope)
Molecular formula	: $C_{12}H_{18}O$

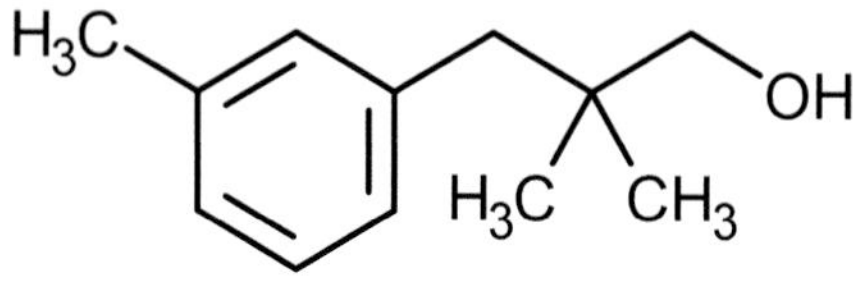

Table 3.159.1 IFRA restrictions for trimethylbenzenepropanol

Category [a]	Limits [b]	Category [a]	Limits [b]	Category [a]	Limits [b]
1	0.28%	5	2.40%	9	5.00%
2	0.36%	6	7.20%	10	2.50%
3	1.50%	7	0.80%	11	not restricted
4	4.50%	8	2.00%		

Trimethylbenzenepropanol should only be used as a fragrance ingredient if traces of organochlorine compounds are restricted. Total chlorine, which can be measured by Atomic Absorption Spectroscopy, must not exceed 25 ppm in the raw material

[a] For explanation of categories see pages 6-8
[b] Limits in the finished products

GENERAL

Trimethylbenzenepropanol is a colorless to pale yellow clear oily liquid; its odor type is floral and its odor at 100% is described as 'floral lily of the valley green tropical' (www.thegoodscentscompany.com). Trimethylbenzenepropanol is a synthetic chemical (16), not found in nature (and consequently not in essential oils (17)).

CONTACT ALLERGY

General

The SCCS (Scientific Committee on Consumer Safety), in a 2012 Opinion on Fragrance allergens in cosmetic products, has marked trimethylbenzenepropanol as 'established contact allergen in humans' (2,10). The sensitizing potency of trimethylbenzenepropanol was classified as 'weak' based on an EC3 value of 30% in the LLNA (local lymph node assay) in animal experiments (2,10). In other animal and human tests, trimethylbenzenepropanol showed no sensitizing potential (15).

Hence, is was hypothesized that impurities, specifically organochlorines, in Majantol® may be the actual sensitizers in the commercial products. However, testing with both 'normal' and purified trimethylbenzenepropanol resulted in comparable rates of positive patch tests and it was concluded that organochlorine impurities are very probably not the cause of allergic reactions to Majantol® (15).

Patch testing in groups of patients

Results of patch testing trimethylbenzenepropanol in consecutive patients suspected of contact dermatitis (routine testing) and those of testing in groups of *selected* patients (e.g. patients with suspected cosmetic intolerance, individuals with known of suspected fragrance allergy) are shown in table 3.159.2.

Patch testing in consecutive patients suspected of contact dermatitis: routine testing

In nine studies in which routine testing with trimethylbenzenepropanol was performed, frequencies of sensitization have ranged from 0.2% to 1.4%, but were 0.8% or lower in seven of the nine investigations (table 3.159.2). In 6 studies, no specific relevance data were provided. In two NACDG studies, 'definite + probable' relevance was 9% and 23%, respectively (5,6). In a Danish study, 4 out of 6 positive patch test reactions to trimethylbenzenepropanol were scored as 'probably relevant' (13).

In an IVDK study, the hypothesis that organochlorine compounds in commercial Majantol ® are the allergenic culprits could not be confirmed (15).

Patch testing in groups of selected patients

Results of studies patch testing trimethylbenzenepropanol in groups of selected patients (e.g. patients with suspected cosmetic intolerance, individuals with known of suspected fragrance allergy) are shown in table 3.159.2.

Frequencies of sensitization in 5 such studies ranged from 0.8% to 5.4% (1,3,7,11,19). The highest rates (3.2% and 5.4%) were found in two international studies in groups of patients with proven or suspected fragrance sensitivity (1,3), but relevance was not discussed in any study. These studies probably stimulated the interest in trimethylbenzenepropanol as a new 'important' fragrance allergen (12), which obviously proved not to be the case (table 3.159.2).

Table 3.159.2 Patch testing in groups of patients

Years and Country	Test conc. & vehicle	Number of patients tested | positive (%)		Selection of patients (S); Relevance (R); Comments (C)	Ref.
Routine testing					
2015-2016 UK	5% pet.	2084	4 (0.2%)	R: not specified for individual fragrances; 25% of patients who reacted to any fragrance or fragrance marker had a positive history of fragrance sensitivity	18
2013-2014 IVDK	5% pet., 'normal'	8005	45 (0.6%)	R: not stated; C: the 'normal' patch test material contained organochlorine impurities (11 ppm), the purified material did	15
	5% pet., purified	8005	40 (0.5%)	not; 32 patients reacted to both preparations, 13 only to the normal and 8 only to the purified test substance; hence, it was concluded that organochlorine impurities are very probably not the cause of allergic reactions to Majantol®	
2011-2012 NACDG	5% pet.	4231	53 (1.3%)	R: definite + probable relevance: 9%	5
2011-2012 UK	5% pet.	1951	15 (0.8%)	R: not stated	9
2009-2012, Six European countries [a]	5% pet.	3643	(0.7%)	R: not stated; C: range per country: 0.3-1.5%	8
2009-2010 NACDG	5% pet.	4303	(1.4%)	R: definite + probable relevance: 23%	6
2008-2009 Denmark	5% pet.	722	6 (0.8%)	R: 4 (67%) probably relevant	13
2005-2008 IVDK	5% pet.	2189	(0.4%)	R: not stated	11
2003-2005 IVDK	5% pet.	6573	36 (0.5%)	R: not stated; C: there were 40 doubtful or irritant reactions	12
Testing in groups of selected patients					
2011-2015 Spain	5% pet.	607	13 (2.1%)	S: patients previously reacting to FM I, FM II, Myroxylon pereirae resin or hydroxyisohexyl 3-cyclohexene carboxaldehyde in the baseline series and subsequently tested with a fragrance series; R: not stated	19
2006-2011 IVDK	5% pet.	516	7 (1.4%)	S: patients with suspected cosmetic intolerance; R: not stated	7
2005-2008 IVDK	5% pet.	4974	(0.8%)	S: not specified; R: not stated	11
<2002 Japan, Europe, USA		218	7 (3.2%)	S: patients with known fragrance sensitivity; R: not stated	3
<1996 Japan, Europe, USA	5% pet.	167	9 (5.4%)	S: patients known or suspected to be allergic to fragrances; R: not stated	1

[a] study of the ESSCA (European Surveillance System on Contact Allergy network)
FM: Fragrance mix; IVDK: Informationsverbund Dermatologischer Kliniken (Germany, Switzerland, Austria); NACDG: North American Contact Dermatitis Group (USA, Canada)

Case reports and case series

In 2016, 3 cases of 'clinically relevant allergy' to trimethylbenzenepropanol in adolescent children were presented. Quite curiously, the culprit products containing the fragrance were not mentioned (14).

Trimethylbenzenepropanol was stated to be the (or an) allergen in one patient in a group of 603 individuals suffering from cosmetic dermatitis, seen in the period 2010-2015 in Leuven, Belgium (4).

LITERATURE

1   Larsen W, Nakayama H, Fischer T, Elsner P, Burrows D, Jordan W, et al. Fragrance contact dermatitis: A worldwide multicenter investigation (Part I). Am J Cont Dermat 1996;7:77-83

2   SCCS (Scientific Committee on Consumer Safety). Opinion on Fragrance allergens in cosmetic products, 26-27 June 2012, SCCS/1459/11. Available at: https://ec.europa.eu/health/sites/health/files/scientific_committees/consumer_safety/docs/sccs_o_102.pdf

3   Larsen W, Nakayama H, Fischer T, Elsner P, Frosch P, Burrows D, et al. Fragrance contact dermatitis - a worldwide multicenter investigation (Part III). Contact Dermatitis 2002;46:141-144

4   Goossens A. Cosmetic contact allergens. Cosmetics 2016, 3, 5; doi:10.3390/cosmetics3010005

5   Warshaw EM, Maibach HI, Taylor JS, Sasseville D, DeKoven JG, Zirwas MJ, et al. North American Contact Dermatitis Group patch test results: 2011-2012. Dermatitis 2015;26:49-59

6   Warshaw EM, Belsito DV, Taylor JS, Sasseville D, DeKoven JG, Zirwas MJ, et al. North American Contact Dermatitis Group patch test results: 2009 to 2010. Dermatitis 2013;24:50-59

7   Dinkloh A, Worm M, Geier J, Schnuch A, Wollenberg A. Contact sensitization in patients with suspected cosmetic intolerance: results of the IVDK 2006-2011. J Eur Acad Dermatol Venereol 2015;29:1071-1081

8   Frosch PJ, Johansen JD, Schuttelaar M-LA, Silvestre JF, Sánchez-Pérez J, Weisshaar E, et al. (on behalf of the ESSCA network). Patch test results with fragrance markers of the baseline series – analysis of the European Surveillance System on Contact Allergies (ESSCA) network 2009–2012. Contact Dermatitis 2015;73:163-171

9   Mann J, McFadden JP, White JML, White IR, Banerjee P. Baseline series fragrance markers fail to predict contact allergy. Contact Dermatitis 2014;70:276-281

10 Uter W, Johansen JD, Börje A, Karlberg A-T, Lidén C, Rastogi S, Roberts D, White IR. Categorization of fragrance contact allergens for prioritization of preventive measures: clinical and experimental data and consideration of structure–activity relationships. Contact Dermatitis 2013;69:196-230

11 Uter W, Geier J, Frosch P, Schnuch A. Contact allergy to fragrances: current patch test results (2005–2008) from the Information Network of Departments of Dermatology. Contact Dermatitis 2010;63:254-261

12 Schnuch A, Geier J, Uter W, Frosch PJ. Majantol® – a new important fragrance allergen. Contact Dermatitis 2007;57:48-50

13 Heisterberg MV, Johansen JD. Contact allergy to trimethyl-benzenepropanol (Majantol). Contact Dermatitis 2009;61:360-361

14 Norris P, Hill H, Morton K, Jacob SE. Majantol is a relevant fragrance allergy in adolescent children. Dermatitis 2016;27:233-234

15 Schnuch A, Müller BP, Geier J, Grabbe J, Worm M, Simon D, et al. Differences in contents of organochlorine impurities do not influence responses to patch testing with Majantol®. Contact Dermatitis 2017;76:11-18

16 Herro E, Jacob SE. Majantol. Dermatitis 2011;22:112-113

17 De Groot AC, Schmidt E. Essential oils: contact allergy and chemical composition. Boca Raton, Fl., USA: CRC Press, Taylor and Francis Group, 2016 (ISBN 9781482246407)

18 Ung CY, White JML, White IR, Banerjee P, McFadden JP. Patch testing with the European baseline series fragrance markers: a 2016 update. Br J Dermatol 2018;178:776-780

19 Silvestre JF, Mercader P, González-Pérez R, Hervella-Garcés M, Sanz-Sánchez T, Córdoba S, et al. Sensitization to fragrances in Spain: A 5-year multicentre study (2011-2015). Contact Dermatitis. 2018 Nov 14. doi: 10.1111/cod.13152. [Epub ahead of print]

Chapter 3.160   5,5,6-TRIMETHYLBICYCLOHEPT-2-YLCYCLOHEXANOL

IDENTIFICATION

Description/definition : 5,5,6-Trimethylbicyclohept-2-ylcyclohexanol is the bicyclic alcohol that conforms to the structural formula shown below

Chemical class(es) : Bicyclic organic compounds; alcohols

INCI name USA : Not in the Personal Care Products Council Ingredient Database

Chemical/IUPAC name : 3-(2,2,3-Trimethyl-5-bicyclo[2.2.1]heptanyl)cyclohexan-1-ol

Other names : Isobornyl cyclohexanol; isocamphyl cyclohexanol (mixed isomers); sandal hexanol; 3-(5,5,6-trimethylbicyclo[2.2.1]heptan-2-yl)cyclohexanol

CAS registry number(s) : 3407-42-9; 4105-12-8

EC number(s) : 222-294-1; 223-879-4

Function(s) in cosmetics : EU: perfuming

Patch testing : 10% pet. (6); 2% pet. (7)

Molecular formula : $C_{16}H_{28}O$

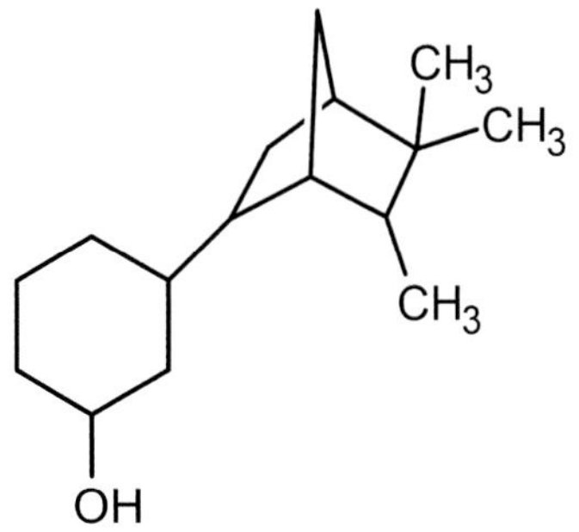

GENERAL

5,5,6-Trimethylbicyclohept-2-ylcyclohexanol is a colorless to pale yellow clear viscous liquid; its odor type is woody and its odor at 100% is described as 'sandalwood clean sweet woody' (www.thegoodscentscompany.com). It is a synthetic chemical, not found in nature (and consequently not in essential oils).

CONTACT ALLERGY

In Japan, between 1979 and 1990, 25 of 1949 (1.3%) patients (probably selected) tested with isobornyl cyclohexanol (synthetic sandalwood) had positive patch test reactions (1). Details are unknown. Other patch test results from Japan with synthetic sandalwood may have been reported in ref. 8.

Pigmented cosmetic dermatitis

In Japan, in the 1960s and 1970s, many female patients developed pigmentation of the face after having facial dermatitis (3). The skin manifestations of this so-called pigmented cosmetic dermatitis consisted of diffuse or patchy brown hyperpigmentation on the cheeks and/or forehead, sometimes the entire face was involved. In severe cases, the pigmentation was black, purple, or blue-black, and in mild cases, it was pale brown. Occasionally, erythematous macules or papules, suggesting a mild contact dermatitis, were observed and itching was also noted at varying times.

Pigmented cosmetic dermatitis was shown to be caused by contact allergy to components of cosmetic products, notably essential oils, other fragrance materials, antimicrobials, preservatives and coloring materials (2,3,4). 'Synthetic sandalwood' was one the of main contact sensitizers (6).

The number of patients with pigmented cosmetic dermatitis decreased strongly after 1978, when major cosmetic companies began to eliminate strong contact sensitizers from their products (2). Since 1980, pigmented cosmetic dermatitis became a rare disease in Japan (5).

LITERATURE

1   Utsumi M, Sugai T, Shoji A, Watanabe K, Asoh S, Hashimoto Y. Incidence of positive reactions to sandalwood oil and its related fragrance materials in patch tests and a case of contact allergy to natural and synthetic sandalwood oil in a museum worker. Skin Res 1992;34(suppl.14):209-213 (article in Japanese). Data cited in ref. 7

2   Nakayama H, Matsuo S, Hayakawa K, Takhashi K, Shigematsu T, Ota S. Pigmented cosmetic dermatitis. Int J Dermatol 1984;23:299-305

3   Nakayama H, Harada R, Toda M. Pigmented cosmetic dermatitis. Int J Dermatol 1976;15:673-675
4   Nakayama H, Hanaoka H, Ohshiro A. Allergen Controlled System. Tokyo: Kanehara Shuppan, 1974
5   Ebihara T, Nakayama H. Pigmented contact dermatitis. Clin Dermatol 1997;15:593-599
6   Nakayama H. Pigmented contact dermatitis and chemical depigmentation. In: Johansen JD, Frosch PJ, LePoittevin J-P, Eds. Contact Dermatitis, 5th Edition. Heidelberg: Springer, Chapter 19:377-393
7   De Groot AC, Frosch PJ. Adverse reactions to fragrances: a clinical review. Contact Dermatitis 1997;36:57-86
8   Sugai T. Historical data of the JSCD. Group study III - Fragrance materials. Environ Dermatol 1994;1:209-212 (article in Japanese). Data cited in ref. 7

Chapter 3.161 2,4,6-TRIMETHYL-4-PHENYL-1,3-DIOXANE

IDENTIFICATION

Description/definition   : 2,4,6-Trimethyl-4-phenyl-1,3-dioxane is the heterocyclic organic compound that conforms to the structural formula shown below

Chemical class(es)   : Heterocyclic organic compounds; aromatic compounds

INCI name USA   : Not in the Personal Care Products Council Ingredient Database

Chemical/IUPAC name   : 2,4,6-Trimethyl-4-phenyl-1,3-dioxane

Other name(s)   : Gardenia acetal; Floropal®

CAS registry number(s)   : 5182-36-5

EC number(s)   : 225-963-6

Function(s) in cosmetics : EU: perfuming

Patch testing   : 5% pet. (2)

Molecular formula   : $C_{13}H_{18}O_2$

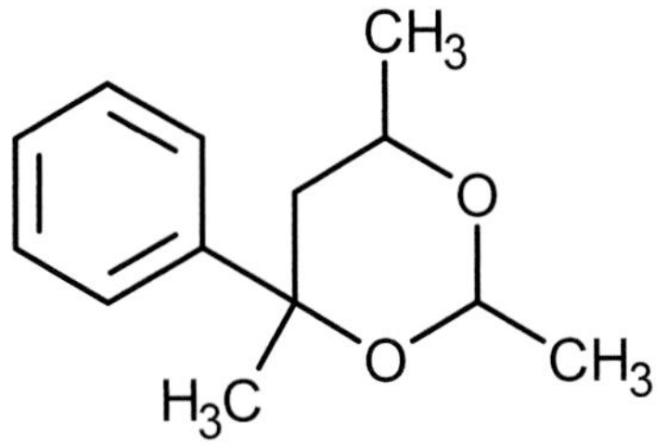

GENERAL

2,4,6-Trimethyl-4-phenyl-1,3-dioxane is a colorless to pale yellow clear liquid; its odor type is floral and its odor at 100% is described as 'fresh citrus gardenia green natural' (www.thegoodscentscompany.com). 2,4,6-Trimethyl-4-phenyl-1,3-dioxane is a synthetic chemical, not found in nature (and consequently not in essential oils (3)).

CONTACT ALLERGY

Patch testing in groups of patients

Patch testing in consecutive patients suspected of contact dermatitis: routine testing
Studies in which 2,4,6-trimethyl-4-phenyl-1,3-dioxane was patch tested in consecutive patients suspected of contact dermatitis (routine testing) with positive results have not been found.

Patch testing in groups of selected patients
Before 1996, in Japan, some European countries and the USA, 167 patients known or suspected to be allergic to fragrances were patch tested with 2,4,6-trimethyl-4-phenyl-1,3-dioxane 5% pet. and there were two (1.2%) positive reactions; their relevance was not mentioned (1).

Case reports and case series
Case reports of allergic contact dermatitis from 2,4,6-trimethyl-4-phenyl-1,3-dioxane have not been found.

LITERATURE

1   Larsen W, Nakayama H, Fischer T, Elsner P, Burrows D, Jordan W, et al. Fragrance contact dermatitis: A worldwide multicenter investigation (Part I). Am J Cont Dermat 1996;7:77-83
2   De Groot AC. Patch Testing, 4th Edition. Wapserveen, The Netherlands: acdegroot publishing, 2018 (ISBN 978-90-813233-4-5)
3   De Groot AC, Schmidt E. Essential oils: contact allergy and chemical composition. Boca Raton, Fl., USA: CRC Press, Taylor and Francis Group, 2016 (ISBN 9781482246407)

Chapter 3.162 VANILLIN

IDENTIFICATION

Description/definition   : Vanillin is the substituted aromatic aldehyde that conforms to the structural formula
                              shown below
Chemical class(es)   : Aldehydes; phenols
Chemical/IUPAC name   : 4-Hydroxy-3-methoxybenzaldehyde
Other names   : Vanillaldehyde; vanillic aldehyde
CAS registry number(s)   : 121-33-5
EC number(s)   : 204-465-2
RIFM monograph(s)   : Food Cosmet Toxicol 1977;15:633
Merck Index monograph   : 11390
Function(s) in cosmetics   : EU: masking. USA: flavoring agents; fragrance ingredients
Patch testing   : 10% Pet. (SmartPracticeEurope, Chemotechnique, SmartPracticeCanada)
Molecular formula   : $C_8H_8O_3$

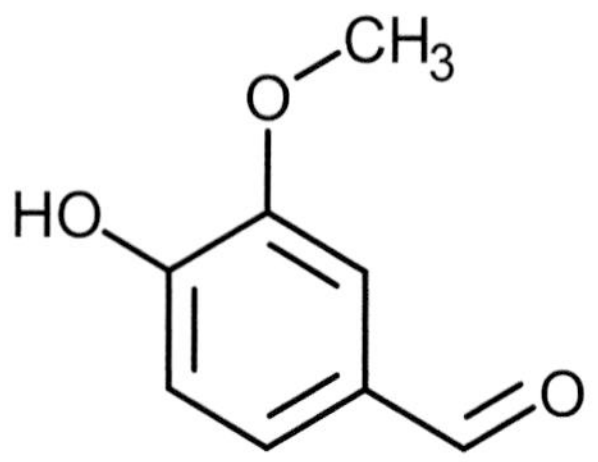

GENERAL

Vanillin is a white to off-white crystalline powder; its odor type is vanilla and its odor at 100% is described as 'sweet, vanilla, vanillin, creamy and phenolic' (www.thegoodscentscompany.com). Vanillin occurs widely in nature and has been identified in propolis and Myroxylon pereirae resin (balsam of Peru) (12,19,20,21). It is present in tobacco, tobacco smoke and tobacco substitute smoke. Vanillin is an important commercial chemical that is used for flavoring confectionaries, beverages, foods, and animal feeds. Small quantities are used in perfumery to round and fix sweet, balsamic fragrances. Vanillin is also used as a brightener in galvanotechnical processes and is an important intermediate in, for example, the production of pharmaceuticals such as *l*-3,4-dihydroxyphenylalanine (*l*-DOPA) and methyldopa. It is an ingredient in pet care products and bug sprays for in-home use (U.S. National Library of Medicine).

Presence in essential oils, Myroxylon pereirae resin (balsam of Peru) and propolis

Vanillin has been identified by chemical analysis in 12 of 91 essential oils, which have caused contact allergy / allergic contact dermatitis. In none of these oils, it belonged to the 'Top-10' of ingredients with the highest concentrations (23). Vanillin may also be present in Myroxylon pereirae resin (balsam of Peru) (0.2-1.3%) (12,20,21) and in propolis (19).

CONTACT ALLERGY

General

In a 2012 SCCS Opinion, the sensitizing potency of vanillin could not be classified, because no EC3 value was established in the LLNA (local lymph node assay) in animal experiments; higher concentrations should also have been tested (17,18).

Patch testing in groups of patients

Results of studies testing vanillin in consecutive patients suspected of contact dermatitis (routine testing) and those of testing in groups of *selected* patients (e.g. patients with suspected fragrance or cosmetic dermatitis, individuals with eyelid dermatitis or allergic contact cheilitis, patients allergic to Myroxylon pereirae (balsam of Peru)) are shown in table 3.162.1.

Patch testing in consecutive patients suspected of contact dermatitis: routine testing

In China, in the period 2010-2011, 296 consecutive patients were patch tested with vanillin 10% pet. and there was one (0.3%) positive reaction; its relevance was not mentioned (9).

Patch testing in groups of selected patients
In nine studies testing patients suspected of cosmetic or fragrance intolerance, patients with fragrance allergy, or individuals with eyelid dermatitis or contact cheilitis with vanillin (mostly 10% pet.), mostly low frequencies of sensitization, ranging from 0.1% to 5% have been observed (1,2,3,7,8,10,13,26,27). The high percentage of 5 consisted of 2 positive reactions in 41 patients with proven allergic contact cheilitis (26). The relevance of the positive reactions was mentioned in two studies, both 100% (1,26), but one of these investigations (1) had certain flaws (table 3.162.1).

In patients known to be allergic to Myroxylon pereirae resin (balsam of Peru) who were tested with vanillin, higher rates of sensitization ranging from 5.6% to 17% were observed (12,16,22). This is not unexpected, as vanillin is a constituent of balsam of Peru (Chapter 3.126 Myroxylon pereirae resin).

Table 3.162.1 Patch testing in groups of patients

Years and Country	Test conc. & vehicle	Number of patients tested | positive (%)		Selection of patients (S); Relevance (R); Comments (C)	Ref.
Routine testing					
2010-2011 China	10% pet.	296	1 (0.3%)	R: 67% for all fragrances tested together (excluding FM I)	9
Testing in groups of selected patients					
2011-2015 Spain	10% pet.	607	7 (1.1%)	S: patients previously reacting to FM I, FM II, Myroxylon pereirae resin or hydroxyisohexyl 3-cyclohexene carboxaldehyde in the baseline series and subsequently tested with a fragrance series; R: not stated	27
2006-2011 IVDK	10% pet.	664	2 (0.3%)	S: patients with suspected cosmetic intolerance; R: not stated	8
2001-2011 USA	10% pet.	41	2 (5%)	S: patients with allergic contact cheilitis; R: 100%	26
2006-2010 USA	10% pet.	100	2 (2%)	S: patients with eyelid dermatitis; R: not stated	3
2005-2008 IVDK	10% pet.	4377	(0.2%)	S: not specified; R: not stated	10
2000-2007 USA	10% pet.	871	7 (0.8%)	S: patients who were tested with a supplemental cosmetic screening series; R: 100%; C: weak study: a. high rate of macular erythema and weak reactions; b. relevance figures included 'questionable' and 'past' relevance	1
<2003 Israel		91	1 (1%)	S: patients with a positive or doubtful reaction to the fragrance mix and/or Myroxylon pereirae resin and/or to one or two commercial fine fragrances; R: not stated	7
1997-2000 Austria	10% pet.	747	1 (0.1%)	S: patients suspected of fragrance allergy; R: not stated	2
1994-1995 UK	2% pet.	40	1 (2.5%)	S: patients reacting to the FM I and tested with an extended fragrance series; R: not stated	13
Testing in patients allergic to Myroxylon pereirae resin (balsam of Peru)					
<1982 Poland	10% pet.	12	2 (17%)	S: patients allergic to Myroxylon pereirae resin and to propolis; C: vanillin may be an ingredient of both substances	12
<1976 USA, Canada, Europe		142	8 (5.6%)	S: patients allergic to balsam of Peru	22
1955-1960 Denmark	10% pet. or as is	164	21 (12.8%)	S: patients allergic to balsam of Peru	16

FM: Fragrance mix; IVDK: Informationsverbund Dermatologischer Kliniken (Germany, Switzerland, Austria)

Case reports and case series
A man had allergic contact dermatitis from vanillin and coumarin in a topical pharmaceutical preparation used on a traumatic leg ulcer (11). A worker involved in producing vanillin became sensitized to this material (25).

Cross-reactions, pseudo-cross-reactions and co-reactions
For general information on cross-/pseudo-cross-/co-reactivity of fragrance chemicals with other fragrances, fragrance markers (fragrance mix I, fragrance mix II, colophonium, Myroxylon pereirae resin [balsam of Peru]) and essential oils see Chapter 1.2 General information on cross-reactions, pseudo-cross-reactions and co-reactions. Co-reactivity with Myroxylon pereirae resin (MP) may be explained by the presence of vanillin (0.2-1.3%) in MP (pseudo-cross-reactions).

Reactions to vanillin in patients allergic to Myroxylon pereirae resin (balsam of Peru) in one study only occurred in those also reacting to natural vanilla. However, patients allergic to vanilla do not necessarily react to vanillin (16).

Patch test sensitization

In 3 patients out of 230 with contact allergy to Myroxylon pereirae resin (balsam of Peru), there was a positive patch test to vanillin (5% pet., 10% pet. or pure), that developed 6 days or later after application. Whether this was simply a 'delayed' reaction or indicative of patch test sensitization was not well investigated (16).

Presence in products and chemical analyses

In 2008, 66 different fragrance components (including 39 essential oils) were identified in 370 (10% of the total) topical pharmaceutical products marketed in Belgium; 8 of these (2.2%) contained vanillin (4).

In 2000, fifty-nine domestic and occupational products, purchased in retail outlets in Denmark, England, Germany and Italy were analyzed by GC-MS for the presence of fragrances. The product categories were liquid soap and soap bars (n=13), soft/hard surface cleaners (n=23), fabric conditioners/laundry detergents for hand wash (n=8), dish wash (n=10), furniture polish, car shampoo, stain remover (each n=1) and 2 products used in occupational environments. Vanillin and related aromatic aldehydes were present in 3 products (5%); quantification was not performed (5).

In 1997, 71 deodorants (22 vapo-spray, 22 aerosol spray and 27 roll-on products) were collected in Denmark, England, France, Germany and Sweden and analyzed by gas chromatography – mass spectrometry (GC-MS) for the presence of fragrances and other materials. Vanillin was present in 27 (38%) of the products (6).

OTHER SIDE EFFECTS

Immediate-type reactions

Two patients with positive immediate tests to Myroxylon pereirae resin (balsam of Peru) co-reacted to its ingredient vanillin 2% in water (15).

Miscellaneous side effects

Vanillin caused bronchospasm in a controlled double-blind challenge test in one asthmatic patient (24).

LITERATURE

1   Wetter DA, Yiannias JA, Prakash AV, Davis MDP, Farmer SA, el-Azhary RA. Results of patch testing to personal care product allergens in a standard series and a supplemental cosmetic series: an analysis of 945 patients from the Mayo Clinic Contact Dermatitis Group, 2000-2007. J Am Acad Dermatol 2010;63:789-798

2   Wöhrl S, Hemmer W, Focke M, Götz M, Jarisch R. The significance of fragrance mix, balsam of Peru, colophony and propolis as screening tools in the detection of fragrance allergy. Br J Dermatol 2001;145:268-273

3   Wenk KS, Ehrlich AE. Fragrance series testing in eyelid dermatitis. Dermatitis 2012;23:22-26

4   Nardelli A, D'Hooge E, Drieghe J, Dooms M, Goossens A. Allergic contact dermatitis from fragrance components in specific topical pharmaceutical products in Belgium. Contact Dermatitis 2009;60:303-313

5   Rastogi SC, Heydorn S, Johansen JD, Basketter DA. Fragrance chemicals in domestic and occupational products. Contact Dermatitis 2001;45:221-225

6   Rastogi SC, Lepoittevin J-P, Johansen JD, Frosch PJ, Menné T, Bruze M, et al. Fragrances and other materials in deodorants: search for potentially sensitizing molecules using combined GC-MS and structure activity relationship (SAR) analysis. Contact Dermatitis 1998;39:293-303

7   Trattner A, David M. Patch testing with fine fragrances: comparison with fragrance mix, balsam of Peru and a fragrance series. Contact Dermatitis 2003:49:287-289

8   Dinkloh A, Worm M, Geier J, Schnuch A, Wollenberg A. Contact sensitization in patients with suspected cosmetic intolerance: results of the IVDK 2006-2011. J Eur Acad Dermatol Venereol 2015;29:1071-1081

9   Liu J, Li L-F. Contact sensitization to fragrances other than fragrance mix I in China. Contact Dermatitis 2015;73:252-253

10 Uter W, Geier J, Frosch P, Schnuch A. Contact allergy to fragrances: current patch test results (2005–2008) from the Information Network of Departments of Dermatology. Contact Dermatitis 2010;63:254-261

11 Van Ketel WG. Allergy to cumarin and cumarin-derivatives. Contact Dermatitis Newsletter 1973;13:355

12 Rudzki E, Grzywa Z. Dermatitis from propolis. Contact Dermatitis 1983;9:40-45

13 Katsarma G, Gawkrodger DJ. Suspected fragrance allergy requires extended patch testing to individual fragrance allergens. Contact Dermatitis 1999;41:193-197

14 Ferguson JE, Beck MH. Contact sensitivity to vanilla in a lip salve. Contact Dermatitis 1995;33:352

15 Temesvári E, Soos G, Podányi B, Kovács I, Nemeth I. Contact urticaria provoked by balsam of Peru. Contact Dermatitis 1978;4:65-68

16 Hjorth N. Eczematous allergy to balsams. Acta Derm Venereol 1961;41(suppl.46):1-216

17 SCCS (Scientific Committee on Consumer Safety). Opinion on Fragrance allergens in cosmetic products, 26-27 June 2012, SCCS/1459/11. Available at: https://ec.europa.eu/health/sites/health/files/scientific_committees/consumer_safety/docs/sccs_o_102.pdf

18 Uter W, Johansen JD, Börje A, Karlberg A-T, Lidén C, Rastogi S, Roberts D, White IR. Categorization of fragrance contact allergens for prioritization of preventive measures: clinical and experimental data and consideration of structure–activity relationships. Contact Dermatitis 2013;69:196-230

19 De Groot AC, Popova MP, Bankova VS. An update on the constituents of poplar-type propolis. Wapserveen, The Netherlands: acdegroot publishing, 2014, 11 pages. ISBN/EAN: 978-90-813233-0-7. Available at: https://www.researchgate.net/publication/262851225_AN_UPDATE_ON_THE_CONSTITUENTS_OF_POPLAR-TYPE_PROPOLIS

20 Hausen BM. Contact allergy to Balsam of Peru. II. Patch test results in 102 patients with selected balsam of Peru constituents. Am J Cont Derm 2001;12:93-102

21 Hausen BM, Simatupang T, Bruhn G, Evers P, Koenig WA. Identification of new allergenic constituents and proof of evidence for coniferyl benzoate in Balsam of Peru. Am J Cont Derm 1995;6:199-208

22 Mitchell JC, Calnan CD, Clendenning WE, Cronin E, Hjorth N, Magnusson B, et al. Patch testing with some components of balsam of Peru. Contact Dermatitis 1976;2:57-58

23 De Groot AC, Schmidt E. Essential oils: contact allergy and chemical composition. Boca Raton, Fl., USA: CRC Press, Taylor and Francis Group, 2016 (ISBN 9781482246407)

24 Van Assendelft AH. Bronchospasm induced by vanillin and lactose. Eur J Respir Dis 1984;65:468-472

25 Wang XS, Xue YS, Jiang Y, Ni HL, Zhu H, Luo BG, Luo SQ. Occupational contact dermatitis in manufacture of vanillin. Chin Med J (Engl) 1987;100:250-254

26 O'Gorman SM, Torgerson RR. Contact allergy in cheilitis. Int J Dermatol 2016;55:e386-e391

27 Silvestre JF, Mercader P, González-Pérez R, Hervella-Garcés M, Sanz-Sánchez T, Córdoba S, et al. Sensitization to fragrances in Spain: A 5-year multicentre study (2011-2015). Contact Dermatitis. 2018 Nov 14. doi: 10.1111/cod.13152. [Epub ahead of print]

Chapter 3.163　VERDYL ACETATE *

* Not officially an INCI name but perfuming name

IDENTIFICATION

Description/definition	: Verdyl acetate is the tricyclic ester that conforms to the structural formula shown below
Chemical class(es)	: Tricyclic organic compounds; unsaturated compounds; esters
INCI name USA	: Not in the Personal Care Products Council Ingredient Database
Chemical/IUPAC name	: 3a,4,5,6,7,7a-Hexahydro-4,7-methanoinden-6-yl acetate
Synonym(s)	: Cyclacet ®; cycloverdyl acetate; greenyl acetate; tricyclo(5.2.1.02,6)dec-4-en-8-yl acetate; tricyclo decenyl acetate
CAS registry number(s)	: 5413-60-5; 2500-83-6; 54830-99-8
EC number(s)	: 226-501-6; 219-700-4; 259-367-2
RIFM monograph(s)	: Food Chem Toxicol 2008;46(12)(suppl.):S100-S101 (tricyclo[5.2.1.02,6]dec-4-en-8-yl acetate); Food Chem Toxicol 2008;46(12)(suppl.):S93-S96 (tricyclodecenyl acetate); Food Cosmet Toxicol 1976;14:889 (special issue III)
Function(s) in cosmetics	: EU: perfuming
Patch testing	: 5% pet. (1,2)
Molecular formula	: $C_{12}H_{16}O_2$

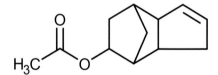

GENERAL

Verdyl acetate is a colorless to pale yellow clear liquid; its odor type is floral and its odor at 100% is described as 'floral green soapy cedar pine woody' (www.thegoodscentscompany.com). Verdyl acetate is a synthetic chemical, not found in nature (and consequently not in essential oils (3)).

CONTACT ALLERGY

Patch testing in groups of patients

Results of studies patch testing verdyl acetate in groups of consecutive patients (routine testing) are shown in table 3.163.1. In two studies, very low frequencies of sensitization (0.1% and 0.3%, in both investigations one patient) were observed (1,2). One reaction was not relevant (1), the relevance of the other was not specified (2).

Studies in which verdyl acetate was patch tested in in groups of *selected* patients with positive results have not been found.

Table 3.163.1 Patch testing in groups of patients: Routine testing

Years and Country	Test conc. & vehicle	Number of patients tested	positive (%)	Selection of patients (S); Relevance (R); Comments (C)	Ref.
1997-8 Six European countries	5% pet.	1855	1　(0.1%)	R: not stated / specified	2
<1995 France and UK	5% pet.	313	1　(0.3%)	R: not relevant	1

Case reports and case series

Case reports of allergic contact dermatitis from verdyl acetate have not been found.

LITERATURE

1　Frosch PJ, Pilz B, Andersen KE, Burrows D, Camarasa JG, Dooms-Goossens A, et al. Patch testing with fragrances: results of a multicenter study of the European Environmental and Contact Dermatitis Research Group with 48 frequently used constituents of perfumes. Contact Dermatitis 1995;33:333-342

2　Frosch PJ, Johansen JD, Menné T, Pirker C, Rastogi SC, Andersen KE, et al. Further important sensitizers in patients sensitive to fragrances. I. Reactivity to 14 frequently used chemicals. Contact Dermatitis 2002;47:78-85

3　De Groot AC, Schmidt E. Essential oils: contact allergy and chemical composition. Boca Raton, Fl., USA: CRC Press, Taylor and Francis Group, 2016 (ISBN 9781482246407)

Chapter 3.164 VETIVERYL ACETATE

IDENTIFICATION

Description/definition	: Vetiveryl acetate is the ester that conforms to the structural formula shown below
Chemical class(es)	: Bicyclic organic compounds; unsaturated compounds; esters
INCI name USA	: Not in the Personal Care Products Council Ingredient Database
Chemical/IUPAC name	: (4,8-Dimethyl-2-propan-2-ylidene-3,3a,4,5,6,8a-hexahydro-1*H*-azulen-6-yl) acetate
Other names	: Acetivenol ®; vetiverol acetate; vetiver acetate
CAS registry number(s)	: 117-98-6; 62563-80-8
EC number(s)	: 204-225-7; 263-597-9
RIFM monograph(s)	: Food Cosmet Toxicol 1974;12:1011 (special issue I) (binder, page 726)
SCCS opinion(s)	: SCCS/1541/14 (3)
Function(s) in cosmetics	: EU: perfuming
Patch testing	: No patch test data available; based on RIFM data, 20% 'vetiver acetate' is probably not irritant (1)
Molecular formula	: $C_{17}H_{26}O_2$

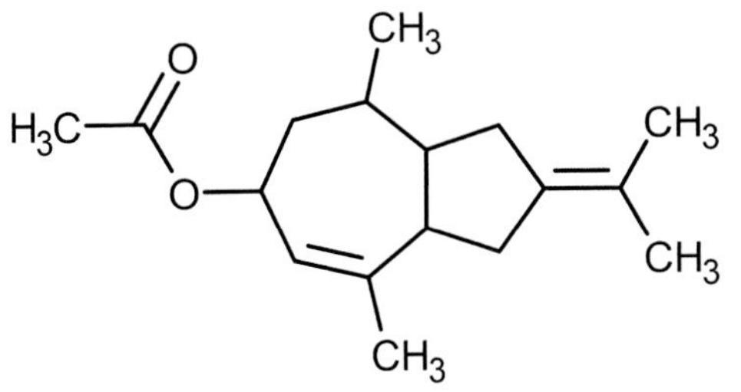

GENERAL

Vetiveryl acetate is a pale yellow clear viscous liquid to solid; its odor type is woody and its odor at 100% is described as 'woody powdery root vetiver sweet dry sandal' (www.thegoodscentscompany.com). Vetiveryl acetate tested in the murine local lymph node assay (LLNA) has been shown to be a moderate skin sensitizer (3).

Presence in essential oils

Vetiveryl acetate has been identified by chemical analysis in zero of 91 essential oils (including vetiver oil), which have caused contact allergy / allergic contact dermatitis (4).

CONTACT ALLERGY

Patch testing in groups of selected patients: Pigmented cosmetic dermatitis

While searching for causative ingredients of pigmented cosmetic dermatitis in Japan in the 1970s, both patients with ordinary (nonpigmented) cosmetic dermatitis and women with pigmented cosmetic dermatitis were tested with a large number of fragrance materials. In 1980 the accumulated data enabled the classification of fragrant materials into 4 groups: common sensitizers, rare sensitizers, virtually non-sensitizing fragrances and fragrances considered as non-sensitizers. Vetiveryl acetate (Acetivenol) was classified in the group of rare sensitizers, indicating that one or more cases of contact allergy / allergic contact dermatitis to it have been observed (2). More specific data are lacking, the results have largely or solely been published in Japanese journals only.

Case reports and case series

Case reports of allergic contact dermatitis from vetiveryl acetate have not been found.

LITERATURE

1   De Groot AC. Patch Testing, 4th Edition. Wapserveen, The Netherlands: acdegroot publishing, 2018
2   Nakayama H. Fragrance hypersensitivity and its control. In: Frosch PJ, Johansen JD, White IR, Eds. Fragrances - beneficial and adverse effects. Berlin Heidelberg New York: Springer-Verlag, 1998:83-91
3   SCCS (Scientific Committee on Consumer Safety). Opinion on the fragrance ingredient vetiveryl acetate, 26-27 June 2012, SCCS/1541/14. Available at:
    http://ec.europa.eu/health/scientific_committees/consumer_safety/docs/sccs_o_167.pdf
4   De Groot AC, Schmidt E. Essential oils: contact allergy and chemical composition. Boca Raton, Fl., USA: CRC Press, Taylor and Francis Group, 2016 (ISBN 9781482246407)

Chapter 3.165 VIOLA ODORATA LEAF EXTRACT

IDENTIFICATION

Description/definition	: Viola odorata leaf extract is an extract of the leaves of the sweet violet, *Viola odorata* L., Violaceae
Chemical class(es)	: Botanical products and botanical derivatives
Other names	: Violet leaves absolute
CAS registry number(s)	: 90147-36-7
EC number(s)	: 290-427-0
RIFM monograph(s)	: Food Cosmet Toxicol 1976;14:893 (special issue III) (violet leaves absolute)
Function(s) in cosmetics	: EU: masking. USA: fragrance ingredients
Patch testing	: 2% pet. (1)

GENERAL

Viola odorata leaf extract is a dark green amber viscous liquid to semi-solid; its odor type is green and its odor is described as 'green, melon, earthy, waxy, fresh, vegetative with floral nuances' (www.thegoodscentscompany.com).

CONTACT ALLERGY

Patch testing in groups of patients

Patch testing in consecutive patients suspected of contact dermatitis: routine testing
Studies in which Viola odorata leaf extract was patch tested in consecutive patients suspected of contact dermatitis (routine testing) with positive results have not been found.

Patch testing in groups of selected patients
Before 1996, in Japan, some European countries and the USA, 167 patients known or suspected to be allergic to fragrances were patch tested with Viola odorata leaf extract and there were two (1.2%) positive reactions; their relevance was not mentioned (1).

Case reports and case series
Case reports of allergic contact dermatitis from Viola odorata leaf extract have not been found.

LITERATURE

1   Larsen W, Nakayama H, Fischer T, Elsner P, Burrows D, Jordan W, et al. Fragrance contact dermatitis: A worldwide multicenter investigation (Part I). Am J Cont Dermat 1996;7:77-83

CHAPTER 4 MONOGRAPHS OF CHEMICALS NOT USED AS FRAGRANCES PER SE BUT PRESENT AS ALLERGENS IN BOTANICAL PRODUCTS USED AS FRAGRANCES

4.0 INTRODUCTION

In this chapter, monographs are presented of sixteen chemicals that are not used as fragrances *per se*, but that may be present as allergenic ingredients in botanical products that are themselves used as fragrance materials such as Evernia furfuracea (treemoss) extract, Evernia prunastri (oakmoss) extract, tea tree oil (Melaleuca alternifolia leaf oil), and Myroxylon pereirae resin (balsam of Peru) (derivatives). These are summarized in table 4.0.1.

Table 4.0.1 Allergenic non-fragrance ingredients in botanical products used as fragrances

Botanical product	Allergenic non-fragrance ingredients
Evernia furfuracea (treemoss) extract	Atranol; atranorin; chloroatranol; fumarprotocetraric acid; physodalic acid; physodic acid
Evernia prunastri (oakmoss) extract	Atranol; atranorin; chloroatranol; evernic acid; physodic acid (?); usnic acid
Tea tree oil (Melaleuca alternifolia leaf oil)	Aromadendrene; ascaridole; ledene; 1,2,4-trihydroxymenthane
Myroxylon pereirae resin (balsam of Peru)	Benzyl isoferulate; coniferyl alcohol; coniferyl benzoate; isoferulic acid

The data in the monographs are largely limited to those that have a direct or indirect relationship with the botanical products in which they may be present as haptens; they do not constitute full literature reviews. In the case of the lichen acids for example (evernic acid, fumarprotocetraric acid, physodalic acid, physodic acid, usnic acid), reports of sensitization from contact with the lichens in nature are not discussed.

Monographs of the botanical products themselves are presented elsewhere in this book: Chapter 3.66 (Evernia furfuracea [treemoss] extract), Chapter 3.67 (Evernia prunastri [oakmoss] extract), Chapter 6.71 (tea tree oil [Melaleuca alternifolia leaf oil]), and Chapter 3.126 (Myroxylon pereirae resin [balsam of Peru]). The literature on contact allergy to tea tree oil and its allergenic ingredients (1) and on the oil's chemical composition (2) has been fully reviewed in 2016 by the author (1,2).

LITERATURE

1   De Groot AC, Schmidt E. Tea tree oil: contact allergy and chemical composition. Contact Dermatitis 2016;75:129-143
2   De Groot AC, Schmidt E. Essential oils: contact allergy and chemical composition. Boca Raton, Fl., USA: CRC Press, Taylor and Francis Group, 2016 (ISBN 9781482246407)

Chapter 4.1   AROMADENDRENE

IDENTIFICATION

Description/definition   : Aromadendrene is the tricyclic organic compound that conforms to the structural
                              formula shown below
Chemical class(es)   : Tricyclic organic compounds; unsaturated compounds
INCI name USA   : Neither in Cosing nor in the Personal Care Products Council Ingredient Database
Chemical/IUPAC name   : 1,1,7-Trimethyl-4-methylene-2,3,4a,5,6,7,7a,7b-octahydro-1aH-cyclopropa[e]azulene
CAS registry number(s)   : 72747-25-2
EC number(s)   : 207-694-6
Patch testing   : 5% in diethyl phthalate (2); concentrations of 5% or higher in alcohol may be strongly
                              irritant (1)
Molecular formula   : $C_{15}H_{24}$

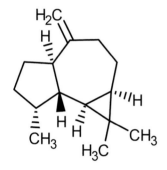

GENERAL

Aromadendrene per se is not used as a fragrance material, but is discussed here as it is a constituent of botanical products which may be applied in perfumery, notably Melaleuca alternifolia (tea tree) leaf oil.

Presence in essential oils

Aromadendrene has been identified by chemical analysis in 57 of 91 essential oils, which have caused contact allergy / allergic contact dermatitis. In one oil, aromadendrene belonged to the 'Top-10' of ingredients with the highest concentrations which may be expected in commercial essential oils of this type: Eucalyptus globulus oil (0.01-1.8%) (4).

CONTACT ALLERGY

General

Aromadendrene is a minor allergen in tea tree oil. Of 61 patients allergic to tea tree oil and tested with a number of its ingredients in various studies, 6 (10%) reacted to aromadendrene (3).

Patch testing in groups of patients

Patch testing in consecutive patients suspected of contact dermatitis: routine testing

Studies in which aromadendrene was patch tested in consecutive patients suspected of contact dermatitis (routine testing) with positive results have not been found.

Patch testing in groups of selected patients

Results of studies testing aromadendrene in groups of selected patients (individuals previously shown to have a positive patch test reaction to tea tree oil) are shown in table 4.1.1. In two studies, the frequencies of sensitization to aromadendrene were 5% (2) and 71% (1). The latter high concentration was in a small study in which seven patients were patch tested with 1% and 5% in alcohol, the latter of which was shown to induce irritant reactions. Of all patients tested with aromadendrene (other studies in which no positive reactions to aromadendrene were seen are not discussed here but are shown in ref. 3), some 10% reacted to aromadendrene, which indicates that it is a minor sensitizing component of tea tree oil (3, see also Chapter 6.71 tea tree oil).

Case reports

Case reports of allergic contact dermatitis from aromadendrene have not been found.

Table 4.1.1 Patch testing in groups of patients: Selected patient groups

Years and Country	Test conc. & vehicle	Number of patients tested	positive (%)	Selection of patients (S); Relevance (R); Comments (C)	Ref.
1999-2003 Germany	5% DEP	20	1 (5%)	S: patients with a positive patch test reaction to oxidized tea tree oil 5% DEP	2
1990-1992 Germany	1% and 5% alc.	7	5 (71%)	S: patients with a positive patch test reaction to tea tree oil 1% alc.	1

DEP: Diethyl phthalate

LITERATURE

1   Knight TE, Hausen BM. Melaleuca oil (tea tree oil) dermatitis. J Am Acad Dermatol 1994;30:423-427
2   Hausen BM. Evaluation of the main contact allergens in oxidized tea tree oil. Dermatitis 2004;15:213-214
3   De Groot AC, Schmidt E. Tea tree oil: contact allergy and chemical composition. Contact Dermatitis 2016;75:129-143
4   De Groot AC, Schmidt E. Essential oils: contact allergy and chemical composition. Boca Raton, Fl., USA: CRC Press, Taylor and Francis Group, 2016 (ISBN 9781482246407)

Chapter 4.2   ASCARIDOLE

IDENTIFICATION

Description/definition : Ascaridole is a monoterpene endoperoxide that conforms to the structural formula shown below

Chemical class(es) : Heterocyclic organic compounds; unsaturated compounds; peroxides

USA INCI name : Neither in Cosing nor in the Personal Care Products Council Ingredient Database

Chemical/IUPAC name : 1-Methyl-4-propan-2-yl-2,3-dioxabicyclo[2.2.2]oct-5-ene

Other names : 1,4-Peroxido-p-menthene-2

CAS registry number(s) : 512-85-6

EC number(s) : 208-147-4

Patch testing : 2% pet. (4,7); 5% in water or diethyl phthalate (1,3,5,6); 5% pet. causes irritant reactions (4,7,9)

Molecular formula : $C_{10}H_{16}O_2$

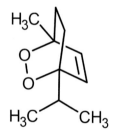

GENERAL

Ascaridole *per se* is not used as a fragrance material, but is discussed here as it is a constituent of botanical products which may be applied in perfumery, notably Melaleuca alternifolia (tea tree) leaf oil. Next to tea tree oil, the best known source of ascaridole is *Chenopodium ambrosioides* (24). The essential oil of *C. ambrosioides* contains 40-70% ascaridole, and was formerly used as an anthelminthic. Because of its toxicity, this oil is no longer used in humans (7). Another potential source of ascaridole, boldo leaf (*Peumus boldus* Molina) is used as a herbal remedy for various conditions (7). Boldo leaf essential oil is banned from use in cosmetics (prohibited by IFRA: www.ifraorg.org/en-us/standards-library), and its use as a herbal remedy is discouraged, in view of the potential risks associated with the toxicity of ascaridole (11).

Presence in essential oils

Ascaridole has been identified by chemical analysis in four of 91 essential oils, which have caused contact allergy / allergic contact dermatitis: bergamot oil, laurel leaf oil, sweet marjoram oil and tea tree oil (12).

CONTACT ALLERGY

Ascaridole is an important allergen in tea tree oil. Of 61 patients allergic to tea tree oil and tested with a number of its ingredients in various studies, 51 (84%) reacted to ascaridole (8).

Patch testing in groups of patients

Results of studies testing ascaridole in consecutive patients suspected of contact dermatitis (routine testing) and those of testing in groups of *selected* patients (patients allergic to tea tree oil, patients with known or suspected fragrance or cosmetic allergy) are shown in table 4.2.1.

Patch testing in consecutive patients suspected of contact dermatitis: routine testing

Routine testing with ascaridole has been done in one study, performed in The Netherlands in the period 2011-2013, in a group of 290 dermatitis patients (7) (table 4.2.1). Test concentrations used were 1%, 2% and 5% in petrolatum. Frequencies of sensitization were 1.4% for the 1% test material, 5.5% for 2% and even 7.2% for the 5% petrolatum test substance. The 5% concentration and to a lesser degree the 2% material caused many irritant and dubious reactions; therefore, it is very likely that a number of 'positive' reactions were in fact false-positive. This also shows from the relevance figures, which decreased from 100% with the 1% test material (albeit only one patient), through 33% for the middle concentration to 19% for the 5% test material. The authors advised a test concentration of 2% in petrolatum (7).

Patch testing in groups of selected patients

Results of studies testing ascaridole in groups of selected patients (patients allergic to tea tree oil, patients with known or suspected fragrance or cosmetic allergy) are shown in table 4.2.1. Five studies investigated ascaridole contact allergy in patients previously shown to be allergic to (oxidized) tea tree oil (1,3,5,6,7). In groups of 6 to 15 tea tree-allergic patients tested with a battery of its ingredients, 75 to 100% reacted to ascaridole, mostly tested 5% in various vehicles, with a mean of 84% (8), attesting to the fact that ascaridole is a very important sensitizing ingredient of tea tree oil (8). In two studies in which groups of patients suspected of cosmetic or fragrance allergy were tested with ascaridole, the rates of sensitization were – as expected – far lower: 1.5% (4) and 14.6% (4). However, the latter group was tested with ascaridole 5% pet., which concentration obviously caused many irritant reactions (4). Accordingly, only about one in 10 reactions were considered to be relevant (4).

Table 4.2.1 Patch testing in groups of patients

Years and Country	Test conc. & vehicle	Number of patients tested | positive (%)		Selection of patients (S); Relevance (R); Comments (C)	Ref.
Routine testing					
2011-13 Netherlands	1% pet.	290	1 (1.4%)	R: 100%	7
	2% pet.	290	16 (5.5%)	R: 33%	
	5% pet.	290	21 (7.2%)	R: 19%; C: the 5% concentration and to a lesser degree 2% causes many irritant and dubious reactions; it is very likely that a number of 'positive' reactions were in fact false-positive	
Testing in groups of selected patients					
2011-13 Netherlands	1%, 2% and 5% pet.	6	6 (100%)	S: patients allergic to tea tree oil; C: all reacted to ascaridole 1% and/or 2% and/or 5% in petrolatum; as test concentration 2% pet. was advised	7
2008-10 Netherlands	1% pet.	602	9 (1.5%)	S: patients suspected of cosmetic or fragrance allergy; R: 1/8 (12.5%)	4
2010-11 Netherlands	5% pet.	144	21 (14.6%)	S: patients suspected of cosmetic or fragrance allergy; R: 2/21 (9.5%); C: the test concentration was considered too high; 2% was suggested	4
1999-2003 Germany	5% DEP	20	15 (75%)	S: patients with a positive patch test reaction to oxidized tea tree oil 5% DEP	6
1999-2000 Germany, Austria	5% DEP	10	10 (100%)	S: patients with a positive patch test reaction to oxidized tea tree oil 5% DEP	1
1999 Germany	5% water	8	7 (88%)	S: patients with a positive patch test reaction to oxidized tea tree oil 20% in olive oil	3
<1999 Germany	5% vehicle?	16	12 (75%)	S: patients allergic to tea tree oil	5

DEP: Diethyl phthalate

Case reports

A man became sensitized after using tea tree oil in his shampoo and for blisters on his face. When patch tested, he reacted to tea tree oil; in a second session, het was tested with its ingredients and now had positive reactions to ascaridole (10%, vehicle unknown), terpinolene (10%, vehicle unknown) and alpha-terpinene (5%, vehicle unknown) (2,5).

Another patient had treated warts on his hands with tea tree oil and became sensitized within three weeks. When patch tested, he reacted to tea tree oil and its ingredients ascaridole (5%, vehicle unknown), terpinolene (10%, vehicle unknown) and alpha-terpinene (5%, vehicle unknown) (5). A woman, who treated her atopic dermatitis with tea tree oil, also became sensitized to the essential oil from contact allergy to the same ingredients (5).

Six more patients were presented by the same authors, who had used tea tree oil for various reasons and indications, who developed allergic contact dermatitis from it and reacted on ingredient patch testing to ascaridole and 1-5 other oil components (5).

A woman with periorbital dermatitis had positive patch tests to oxidized tea tree oil and its ingredient ascaridole, tested 1%, 2% and 5% pet. (the latter concentration caused an irritant reaction). Tea tree oil was present in a cream, a herbal remedy against eczema. When she stopped using it, the dermatitis disappeared (9).

A male patient suffered from periorbital dermatitis and persistent folliculitis barbae. Patch testing revealed contact allergy to tea tree oil (oxidized, 5% pet.) and its ingredient ascaridole, tested 1%, 2% and 5% pet. Tea tree oil turned out to be a component of the patient's shaving oil. He switched to another shaving product, and tacrolimus ointment was prescribed, which resolved his skin problems (9).

LITERATURE

1   Pirker C, Hausen BM, Uter W, Hillen U, Brasch J, Bayerl C, et al. Sensitization to tea tree oil in Germany and Austria. A multicenter Study of the German Contact Dermatitis group. J Dtsch Dermatol Ges 2003;1:629-634 (article in German)

2   Hausen BM. Kontaktallergie auf Teebaumöl und Ascaridol. Akt Dermatol 1998;24:60-62

3   Lippert U, Walter A, Hausen BM, Fuchs Th. Increasing incidence of contact dermatitis to tea tree oil. J Allergy Clin Immunol 2000;105;S43 (abstract 127)

4   Bakker C, Blömeke B, Coenraads PJ, Schuttelaar M-L. Ascaridole, a sensitizing component of tea tree oil, patch tested at 1% and 5% in two series of patients. Contact Dermatitis 2012;65:240-241

5   Hausen BM, Reichling J, Harkenthal M. Degradation products of monoterpenes are the sensitizing agents in tea tree oil. Am J Contact Dermat 1999;10:68-77

6   Hausen BM. Evaluation of the main contact allergens in oxidized tea tree oil. Dermatitis 2004;15:213-214

7   Christoffers WA, Blömeke B, Coenraads P-J, Schuttelaar M-LA. The optimal patch test concentration for ascaridole as a sensitizing component of tea tree oil. Contact Dermatitis 2014;71:129-137

8   De Groot AC, Schmidt E. Tea tree oil: contact allergy and chemical composition. Contact Dermatitis 2016;75:129-143

9   Christoffers WA, Blömeke B, Coenraads PJ, Schuttelaar M-LA. Co-sensitization to ascaridole and tea tree oil. Contact Dermatitis 2013;69:187-189

10 Dembitsky V, Shkrob I, Hanus LO. Ascaridole and related peroxides from the genus *Chenopodium*. Biomed Pap Med Fac Univ Palacky Olomouc, Czech Repub 2008;152:209-215

11 European Medicines Agency, Committee on Herbal Medicinal Products (HMPC). Final European Union herbal monograph on *Peumus boldus* Molina, folium. EMA/810459/2016, 31 January 2017

12 De Groot AC, Schmidt E. Essential oils: contact allergy and chemical composition. Boca Raton, Fl., USA: CRC Press, Taylor and Francis Group, 2016 (ISBN 9781482246407)

Chapter 4.3   ATRANOL *

* Not an INCI name

IDENTIFICATION

Description/definition   : Atranol is the hydroxylated benzaldehyde that conforms to the structural formula
                            shown below
Chemical class(es)   : Aromatic compounds; phenols; aldehydes
INCI name USA   : Not in the Personal Care Products Council Ingredient Database
Chemical/IUPAC name   : 2,6-Dihydroxy-4-methylbenzaldehyde
CAS registry number(s)   : 526-37-4
EC number(s)   : Not available
SCCS Opinion(s)   : SCCP/00847/04 (11)
EU cosmetic restrictions : Regulated in Annex II/1381 of the Regulation (EC) No. 1223/2009 (Prohibited)
Patch testing   : 0.0163% alc. (15)
Molecular formula   : $C_8H_8O_3$

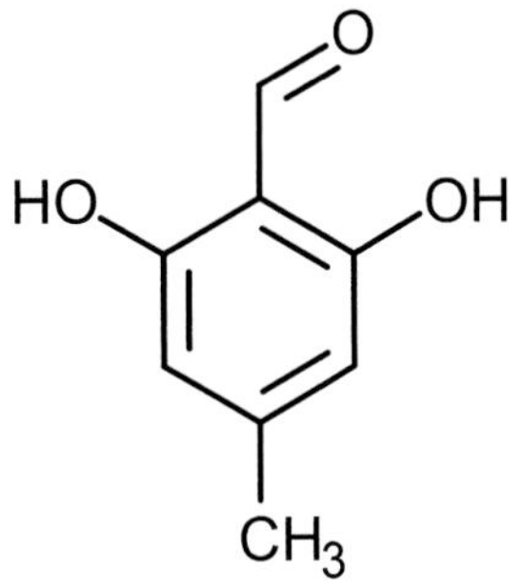

GENERAL

Atranol *per se* is not used as a fragrance material, but is discussed here as it is a constituent of certain botanical products which may be applied in perfumery, e.g. Evernia prunastri (oakmoss) extract and Evernia furfuracea (treemoss) extract (4,5). The chemical is not present in essential oils (6).

In animal experiments, atranol has been found to be a sensitizer (8) and a 'strong' sensitizer when analyzed with the local lymph node assay (LLNA), under the conditions of the test (11). In treemoss and oakmoss extract atranol and chloroatranol are the main sensitizers (9), albeit not the only ones (7).

Formerly, oakmoss absolutes used for fragrances contained high concentrations of atranol (2.1%-2.9%) and chloroatranol (0.9%-1.4%) (4,9,10). Industry has made great efforts to reduce their levels and the contents of atranol and chloroatranol in IFRA-compliant oakmoss absolutes (http://www.ifraorg.org/en-us/standards-library) offered on the market today are below 100 ppm (0.01%) each. These low-level absolutes are far less reactive in patch tests and ROATs (Repeated Open Application Tests) than the conventional untreated oakmoss samples with high (chloro) atranol content (7,12,13,14, discussed in Chapter 3.67 Evernia prunastri [oakmoss] extract).

Consumers using cosmetic products containing these extracts are exposed to atranol and chloroatranol at concentrations of ≤0.1 ppm (12). However, in one study, it has been found that 10% of oakmoss-sensitized patients react to patch tests with an estimated concentration of atranol as low as 0.017 ppm (15). Therefore, it is very likely that some highly sensitized patients will develop clinically manifest allergic contact dermatitis from fragranced cosmetics containing such (≤0.1 ppm) low concentrations of atranol. This study (15) therefore corroborated the 2004 recommendation of the EC Scientific Committee on Consumer Products (SCCP) that atranol and chloroatranol should not be present in cosmetic products at all (11).

As a consequence (15 years later), the presence of atranol in cosmetic products in the EU will be prohibited from August 2021 on; starting August 2019, cosmetic products containing atranol are not allowed to be placed on the Union market (16). This will probably result in oakmoss extracts and treemoss extracts not being used at all anymore in fragrances.

See also Chapter 3.67 Evernia prunastri (oakmoss) extract and Chapter 3.66 Evernia furfuracea (treemoss) extract.

Presence in products and chemical analyses

In Denmark, in 2006, 25 perfume products (13 eaux de parfum, 8 eaux de toilette, one perfume spray, one perfume, and 2 aftershave lotions) for both men and women were purchased from Danish retail outlets and investigated for the presence of atranol and chloroatranol. Atranol was present in 15 products (60%) in a concentration range of 0.6

ppb (detection level)-1055 ppb (parts per billion, ng/ml; 1 ppb = 0.0000001%). The highest concentration was found – as expected - in an aftershave (1).

In Denmark, in the period 2000-2003, 31 popular fragranced cosmetics (12 perfumes, 6 eaux de parfum, 11 eaux de toilette and 2 aftershave lotions) were analyzed for the content of atranol and chloroatranol by liquid chromato-graphy-tandem mass spectrometry (LC-MS-MS) with electrospray ionization (ESI) (2). Atranol was identified in 24 products (77%) in a concentration range of 0.012-190 µg/ml. The median concentrations of atranol were higher in perfumes (0.502 µg/ml) as compared to eaux de toilette (0.012 µg/ml). As expected, the highest concentrations of atranol were found in the 2 aftershave lotions (3).

The contents of atranol and chloroatranol in *untreated* oakmoss absolutes (atranol and chloroatranol not removed) have been reported to be in the ranges of 2.1-2.9% and 0.9-1.4%, respectively (4,9,10).

Serial dilution tests

To investigate and compare the elicitation potential of atranol and chloroatranol, in 2004, in Denmark, ten patients with dermatitis and known sensitization to chloroatranol and oakmoss absolute were tested simultaneously to a serial dilution series of chloroatranol and atranol in ethanol in equimolar concentrations. Concentrations ranged from 200 ppm to 0.00063 ppm for chloroatranol and from 163 ppm to 0.00052 ppm for atranol, which means that the doses varied from 0.0034 to 1072 mM. Dose–response curves were estimated and analyzed by logistic regression. Both substances elicited reactions at very low levels of exposure. The estimated concentration eliciting a reaction in half of the tested individuals ($ED_{50\%}$) was 1.1 ppm for atranol and 0.28 ppm for chloroatranol. The estimated $ED_{10\%}$ (elicitation dose in 10% of tested individuals) was 0.017 ppm for atranol and 0.0137 ppm for chloroatranol. The estimated difference in elicitation potency of chloroatranol relative to atranol was 217%. This is counterbalanced by exposure being greater to atranol than to chloroatranol in oakmoss extract. Thus, it was concluded that both substances contribute to the clinical problems seen in oakmoss absolute-sensitized individuals (15).

Tests with oakmoss extracts with varying concentrations of atranol and chloroatranol

The results of 4 studies performing serial dilution tests and repeated Open Application Tests (ROATs) with oakmoss extracts containing high and low concentrations of atranol and chloroatranol (7,12,13,14) are discussed in Chapter 3.67 Evernia prunastri (oakmoss) extract.

LITERATURE

1   Rastogi SC, Johansen JD, Bossi R. Selected important fragrance sensitizers in perfumes: current exposures. Contact Dermatitis 2007;56:201-204

2   Bossi R, Rastogi SC, Bernard G, Gimenez-Arnau E, Johansen JD, Lepoittevin JP, et al. A liquid chromatography-mass spectrometric method for the determination of oak moss allergens atranol and chloroatranol in perfumes. J Sep Sci 2003;27:537-540

3   Rastogi SC, Bossi R, Johansen JD, Menné T, Bernard T, Giménez-Arnau E, Lepoittevin J-P. Content of oak moss allergens atranol and chloroatranol in perfumes and similar products. Contact Dermatitis 2004;50:367-370

4   Joulain D, Tabacchi R. Lichen extracts as raw materials in perfumery. Part 1: oakmoss. Flavour Fragr J 2009;24:49-61

5   Joulain D, Tabacchi R. Lichen extracts as raw materials in perfumery. Part 2: treemoss. Flavour Fragr J 2009;24:105-116

6   De Groot AC, Schmidt E. Essential oils: contact allergy and chemical composition. Boca Raton, Fl., USA: CRC Press, Taylor and Francis Group, 2016 (ISBN 9781482246407)

7   Mowitz M, Zimerson E, Svedman C, Bruze M. Patch testing with serial dilutions and thin-layer chromatograms of oak moss absolutes containing high and low levels of atranol and chloroatranol. Contact Dermatitis 2013;69:342-349

8   Menné Bonefeld C, Nielsen MM, Giménéz-Arnau E, Lang M, Vennegaard T, et al. An immune response study of oakmoss absolute and its constituents atranol and chloroatranol. Contact Dermatitis 2014;70:282-290

9   Bernard G, Giménez-Arnau E, Rastogi SC, Heydorn S, Johansen JD, Menné T, et al. Contact allergy to oak moss: search for sensitizing molecules using combined bioassay-guided chemical fractionation, GC-MS, and structure-activity relationship analysis. Arch Dermatol Res 2003;295:229-235

10 Ehret C, Maupetit P, Petrzilka M, Klecak G. Preparation of an oakmoss absolute with reduced allergenic potential. Int J Cosmet Sci 1992;14:121-130

11 SCCP (Scientific Committee on Consumer Products). Opinion on Atrranol and Chloroatranol present in natural extracts (e.g. oak moss and tree moss extract), 7 December 2004, SCCP/00847/04. Available at: http://ec.europa.eu/health/ph_risk/committees/04_sccp/docs/sccp_o_006.pdf

12   Mowitz M, Svedman C, Zimerson E, Bruze M. Usage tests of oak moss absolutes containing high and low levels of atranol and chloroatranol. Acta Derm Venereol 2014;94:398-402

13   Andersen F, Andersen KH, Bernois A, Brault C, Bruze M, Eudes H, et al. Reduced content of chloroatranol and atranol in oak moss absolute significantly reduces the elicitation potential of this fragrance material. Contact Dermatitis 2015;72:75-83

14   Nardelli A, Giménez-Arnau E, Bernard G, Lepoittevin J-P, Goossens A. Is a low content in atranol/chloroatranol safe in oak moss-sensitized individuals? Contact Dermatitis 2009;60:91-95

15   Johansen JD, Bernard G, Giménez-Arnau E, Lepoittevin J-P, Bruze M, Andersen KE. Comparison of elicitation potential of chloroatranol and atranol – 2 allergens in oak moss absolute. Contact Dermatitis 2006;54:192-195

16   Directorate-General for Internal Market, Industry, Entrepreneurship and SMEs (European Commission). Commission Regulation (EU) 2017/1410 of 2 August 2017 amending Annexes II and III to Regulation (EC) No 1223/2009 of the European Parliament and of the Council on cosmetic products. Official J European Union 2017;L202:1-3

Chapter 4.4   ATRANORIN

IDENTIFICATION

Description/definition   : Atranorin is the lichen acid that conforms to the structural formula shown below
Chemical class(es)   : Aromatic compounds; alcohols; esters; ketones
INCI name USA   : Neither in Cosing nor in the Personal Care Products Council Ingredient Database
Chemical/IUPAC name   : (3-Hydroxy-4-methoxycarbonyl-2,5-dimethylphenyl) 3-formyl-2,4-dihydroxy-6-methylbenzoate
Other names   : Parmelin; parmelin acid; usmarin; usmarin acid; atranoric acid
CAS registry number(s)   : 479-20-9
EC number(s)   : 207-527-7
Merck Index monograph : 2130
Patch testing   : 0.1% pet. (SmartPracticeEurope, Chemotechnique, SmartPracticeCanada)
Molecular formula   : $C_{19}H_{18}O_8$

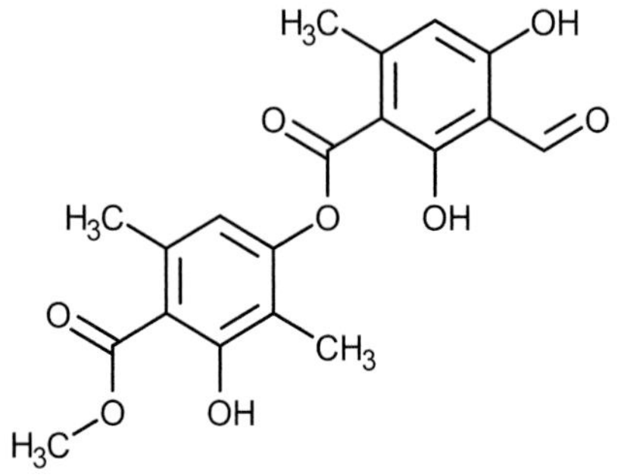

GENERAL

Atranorin *per se* is not used as a fragrance material, but is discussed here as it is a constituent of botanical products which may be applied in perfumery, e.g. Evernia prunastri (oakmoss) extract and Evernia furfuracea (treemoss) extract (6,7). Atranorin is not present in essential oils, which have caused contact allergy (16).

See also Chapter 3.67 Evernia prunastri (oakmoss) extract and Chapter 3.66 Evernia furfuracea (treemoss) extract.

CONTACT ALLERGY

General
Atranorin was shown to be a moderate sensitizer in animal experiments under the conditions of the test (11).

Patch testing in groups of patients

Patch testing in consecutive patients suspected of contact dermatitis: routine testing
In Sweden, before 1981, 951 consecutive dermatitis patients were patch tested with atranorin 0.1% pet. and 10 (1.1%) had a positive reaction. Relevance is discussed in the section 'Case reports and case series' below and co-reactivity in the section 'Cross-reactions, pseudo-cross-reactions and co-reactions', also below (8).

Also in Sweden, before 1979, 760 consecutive dermatitis patients were patch tested with atranorin 1% pet. and 8 (1.1%) had a positive reaction. Three of the patients had reacted to their own fragranced products (perfumes, deodorant, aftershave). In one case, a woman reacted to the perfumes with which her husband experimented at work and at home (5).

Patch testing in groups of selected patients
Before 1987, in Norway, 55 patients with sensitivity to different brands of perfumes, deodorants, aftershave lotions *et cetera* verified by repeated questioning and/or patch testing were tested with atranorin 0.1% (vehicle not mentioned) and there were 21 (38%) positive reactions. Their relevance was not mentioned. Thirty-five of the 55 subjects (64%) also reacted to oakmoss absolute, of which atranorin is an ingredient (17).

Case reports and case series

Before 1981, ten patients (6 women, 4 men) in Sweden were shown to be allergic to atranorin 0.1% pet. by routine testing. Eight of the 10 had a history of hand dermatitis. A nurse had occupational allergic hand dermatitis from an aftershave lotion which she applied on disabled patients in a hospital. Another woman on several occasions had observed itching on her face after dancing 'cheek to cheek', caused by allergy to aftershave used by her partner(s). Three of the four men allergic to atranorin had suffered from dermatitis of the face from aftershave lotions. Nine of the subjects had a history of perfume dermatitis at sites other than the hands. Relapses of dermatitis were explained by lichen exposure in three cases. One developed dermatitis between the fingers when handling logs grilling in a forest. Another suffered from dermatitis on his arms when handling old logs and on the thighs when sitting on a wet stone covered by lichens. A third subject reacted to atranorin-containing reindeer moss (*Cladonia alpestris*) on her hands and forearms, when she arranged Christmas decorations (8).

In Bologna, Italy, 12 cases of contact dermatitis to lichens were observed in the period 1990-1996. Six individuals reacted to atranorin. All 6 co-reacted to the Fragrance mix M I (FM I), 5 to oakmoss (which is present in the FM I and contains atranorin), and 3 to other fragrances. In 3 patients, the reactions were caused by oakmoss extract in aftershave preparations, in the other 3, the source of sensitization remained unknown (1).

A man had suffered from a mild itchy, erythematous eruption above the sternum for the last 18 months. His dermatitis increased and spread over the sides of the neck during the summer months. The patient had a long beard and had been using an eau de cologne every day for the past 18 months. The day before his consultation, he developed a spread with a drop-like configuration to the xiphoid area suggesting that the lotion applied was the cause. Patch testing and photopatch testing showed contact allergy to the eau de cologne, oakmoss extract, oakmoss (lichen, pure), tree moss (lichen, pure) and atranorin and photocontact allergy to evernic acid; whether the fragrance contained oak moss extract (a source of atranorin) was not mentioned (4,10).

A male patient, who had allergic contact dermatitis from oakmoss extract in aftershave lotions, experienced exacerbations of his hand dermatitis when handling firewood or trees in the forest, and he had allergic reactions to atranorin and evernic acid on patch testing (13).

A female student had a one-month-history of an itchy, erythematosquamous eruption mainly on the left side of her face, with associated eyelid swelling. She had a personal history of atopy, and associated recurrences of dermatitis with perfume use. When patch tested, she reacted to oakmoss extract 1% pet., atranorin 1% pet. and to an oakmoss-containing perfume that she wore only on 'special occasions'. Enquiries with the manufacturer of the perfume used by the patient revealed that it indeed contained atranorin. She was advised to stop using the allergenic perfume. Following this, she had no more severe outbreaks, but would show some less severe symptoms, particularly on the face, when being in a perfumed atmosphere (15).

Cross-reactions, pseudo-cross-reactions and co-reactions

Oakmoss extract

Of 8 patients allergic to oakmoss absolute, 6 (75%) co-reacted to atranorin (2). In 7 patients allergic to oakmoss, patch tests were also performed with lichen acids and there were 4 reactions to atranorin (3). Of 5 patients allergic to oakmoss extract, all co-reacted to atranorin; conversely, of 6 patients allergic to atranorin, 5 co-reacted to oakmoss extract (1).

Of 10 patients reacting to an acetone extract of oakmoss 7% in petrolatum, all co-reacted to atranorin (9). Of 20 patients allergic to oakmoss extract (identified by ingredient testing of the fragrance mix I), 10 co-reacted to atranorin (12). Of 15 patients allergic to oakmoss absolute, 4 co-reacted to atranorin (14). Of 7 patients reacting to atranorin 1% pet., all 7 co-reacted to the lichen *Evernia prunastri* itself and to an oakmoss perfume (5).

Other co-reactions

Of 8 patients reacting to atranorin 1% pet., all co-reacted to fumarprotocetraric acid and 5 (63%) to evernic acid, both tested 0.1% in acetone (5).

Of 10 patients reacting to atranorin 0.1% pet. seen in Sweden before 1981, all co-reacted to the fragrance mix I (containing 2% oakmoss extract), to oakmoss perfume and to fumarprotocetraric acid; 9/10 co-reacted to acetone oakmoss extract 7% pet., 7 to evernic acid, and 4 of 9 to *d*-usnic acid (8).

Of 8 patients allergic to *Frullania* (and oakmoss absolute), 6 (75%) co-reacted to atranorin (2).

Patch test sensitization

One of 951 patients tested with atranorin 0.1% pet. developed a late reaction at D11, possibly indicating patch test sensitization; however, the patient was not retested for verification (8).

Serial dilution testing

Eight consecutive patients reacting to patch testing with atranorin 1% pet. were subsequently tested with a dilution series with concentrations ranging from 0.1% down to 0.000001% in acetone. All reacted to 0.1%, 7/8 to 0.01%. Of the 5 who were tested with the complete dilution series, one reacted to 0.1% only, two reacted down to 0.0001% and the other 2 had atranorin 0.00001% in acetone as lower threshold for a positive patch test (5).

Two patients allergic to atranorin were patch tested with a dilution series of 1% down to 0.001% in petrolatum; they reacted down to 0.05% and 0.001%, respectively (11).

Two other individuals allergic to atranorin were also tested with a dilution series: one reacted to 0.032% in acetone as lower threshold and the other down to 0.0032% (14).

OTHER SIDE EFFECTS

Photosensitivity

Photopatch testing in groups of patients

Before 1987, in Norway, 5 patients with sensitivity to different brands of perfumes, deodorants, aftershave lotions *et cetera* verified by repeated questioning and/or patch testing were photopatch tested with atranorin 0.1% and 0.01% (vehicle not mentioned) and there were 2 (40%) positive reactions. Their relevance was not mentioned (17).

LITERATURE

1   Stinchi C, Gulrrini V, Guetti E, Tosti A. Contact dermatitis from lichens. Contact Dermatitis 1997;36:309-310
2   Gonçalo S. Contact sensitivity to lichens and Compositae in *Frullania* dermatitis. Contact Dermatitis 1987;16: 84-86
3   Thune P, Solberg Y, McFadden N, Stærfeet F, Sandberg M. Perfume allergy due to oak moss and other lichens. Contact Dermatitis 1982;8:396-400
4   Fernández de Corres L, Muñoz D, Leaniz-Barrutia I, Corrales JL. Photocontact dermatitis from oak moss. Contact Dermatitis 1983;9:528-529
5   Dahlquist I, Fregert S. Contact allergy to atranorin in lichens and perfumes. Contact Dermatitis 1980;6:111-119
6   Joulain D, Tabacchi R. Lichen extracts as raw materials in perfumery. Part 1: oakmoss. Flavour Fragr J 2009;24:49-61
7   Joulain D, Tabacchi R. Lichen extracts as raw materials in perfumery. Part 2: treemoss. Flavour Fragr J 2009;24:105-116
8   Dahlquist I, Fregert S. Atranorin and oak moss contact allergy. Contact Dermatitis 1981;7:168-169
9   Fregert S, Dahlquist I. Patch testing with oak moss extract. Contact Dermatitis 1983;9:227
10   Fernández de Corres L. Photosensitivity to oak moss. Contact Dermatitis 1986;15:118
11   Sandberg M, Thune P. The sensitizing capacity of atranorin. Contact Dermatitis 1984;11:168-173
12   Gonçalo S, Cabral F, Gonçalo M. Contact sensitivity to oak moss. Contact Dermatitis 1988;19:355-357
13   Aalto-Korte K, Lauerma A, Alanko K. Occupational allergic contact dermatitis from lichens in present-day Finland. Contact Dermatitis 2005;52:36-38
14   Mowitz M, Zimerson E, Svedman C, Bruze M. Patch testing with serial dilutions and thin-layer chromatograms of oak moss absolutes containing high and low levels of atranol and chloroatranol. Contact Dermatitis 2013;69:342-349
15   Lorenzi S, Guerra L, Vezzani C, Vincenzi C. Airborne contact dermatitis from atranorin. Contact Dermatitis 1995;32:315-316
16   De Groot AC, Schmidt E. Essential oils: contact allergy and chemical composition. Boca Raton, Fl., USA: CRC Press, Taylor and Francis Group, 2016 (ISBN 9781482246407)
17   Thune P, Sandberg M. Allergy to lichen and compositae compounds in perfumes. Investigations on the sensitizing, toxic and mutagenic potential. Acta Derm Venereol 1987;134(suppl.):87-89

Chapter 4.5   BENZYL ISOFERULATE

IDENTIFICATION

Description/definition   : Benzyl isoferulate is the benzyl ester of isoferulic acid that conforms to the structural
                             formula shown below
Chemical class(es)   : Aromatic compounds; unsaturated compounds; esters; phenols; ethers
INCI name USA   : Neither in Cosing nor in the Personal Care Products Council Ingredient Database
Chemical/IUPAC name   : Benzyl (*E* or *Z*)-3-(3-hydroxy-4-methoxyphenyl)prop-2-enoate
CAS registry number(s)   : no CAS number found
EC number(s)   : no EC number found
Patch testing   : 1% pet. (1)
Molecular formula   : $C_{17}H_{16}O_4$

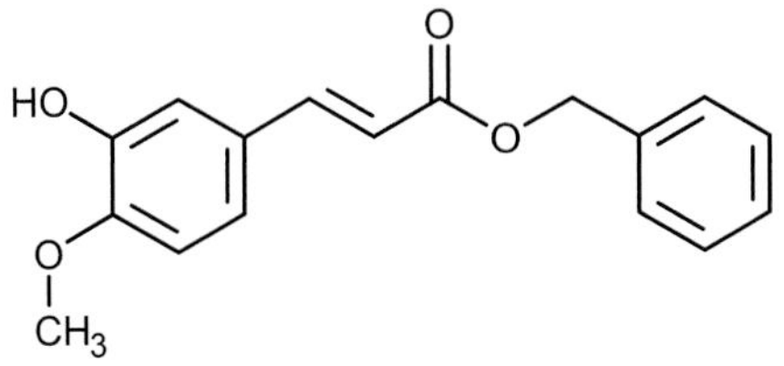

GENERAL

Benzyl isoferulate *per se* is not used as a fragrance material, but is discussed here as it is a constituent of botanical products which may be applied in perfumery, e.g. (derivatives of) Myroxylon pereirae resin (balsam of Peru) (1) and propolis (2,3).

Presence in essential oils, Myroxylon pereirae resin (balsam of Peru) and propolis

Benzyl isoferulate has been identified by chemical analysis in none of 91 essential oils, which have caused contact allergy / allergic contact dermatitis (5). Benzyl isoferulate may be present in Myroxylon pereirae resin (balsam of Peru) (0.2%, in fraction 'BP3' up to 18%) (1) and in propolis (2,3).

CONTACT ALLERGY

Patch testing in groups of patients

In Germany, in the period 1995-1998, 102 patients allergic to Myroxylon pereirae resin (balsam of Peru) were tested with a battery of its ingredients and there were 2 reactions (2%) to benzyl isoferulate 1% pet. (1). It can be concluded that this chemical is not an important sensitizer in Myroxylon pereirae resin.

Also in Germany, in the period 1988-1990, 4 patients allergic to propolis have been tested with a number of its ingredients and one (25%) had a positive patch test reaction to benzyl isoferulate 1% pet. (4). Benzyl isoferulate is not an important sensitizer in propolis; the main allergens are esters of caffeic acid (2)

Case reports and case series

Case reports of allergic contact dermatitis from benzyl isoferulate have not been found.

LITERATURE

1   Hausen BM. Contact allergy to Balsam of Peru. II. Patch test results in 102 patients with selected balsam of Peru constituents. Am J Cont Derm 2001;12:93-102
2   De Groot AC. Propolis: a review of properties, applications, chemical composition, contact allergy, and other adverse effects. Dermatitis 2013;24:263-282
3   De Groot AC, Popova MP, Bankova VS. An update on the constituents of poplar-type propolis. Wapserveen, The Netherlands: acdegroot publishing, 2014. ISBN/EAN: 978-90-813233-0-7 (pdf booklet). Available at: https://www.researchgate.net/publication/262851225_AN_UPDATE_ON_THE_CONSTITUENTS_OF_POPLAR-TYPE_PROPOLIS
4   Hausen BM, Evers P, Stüwe H-T, König WA, Wollenweber E. Propolis allergy (IV) Studies with further sensitizers from propolis and constituents common to propolis, poplar buds and balsam of Peru. Contact Dermatitis 1992;26:34-44
5   De Groot AC, Schmidt E. Essential oils: contact allergy and chemical composition. Boca Raton, Fl., USA: CRC Press, Taylor and Francis Group, 2016 (ISBN 9781482246407)

Chapter 4.6   CHLOROATRANOL *

* Not an INCI name

IDENTIFICATION

Description/definition	: Chloroatranol is the chlorinated hydroxylated benzaldehyde that conforms to the structural formula shown below
Chemical class(es)	: Aromatic compounds; phenols; aldehydes; organochlorine compounds
INCI name USA	: Not in the Personal Care Products Council Ingredient Database
Chemical/IUPAC name	: 3-Chloro-2,6-Dihydroxy-4-methylbenzaldehyde
CAS registry number(s)	: 57074-21-2
EC number(s)	: Not available
SCCS Opinion(s)	: SCCP/00847/04 (11)
EU cosmetic restrictions	: Regulated in Annex II/1382 of the Regulation (EC) No. 1223/2009 (Prohibited)
Patch testing	: 0.02% alc. (16)
Molecular formula	: $C_8H_7ClO_3$

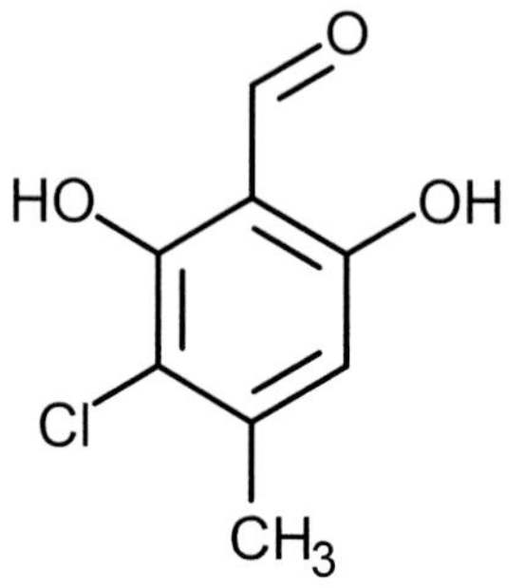

GENERAL

Chloroatranol *per se* is not used as a fragrance material, but is discussed here as it is a constituent of botanical products which may be applied in perfumery, e.g. Evernia prunastri (oakmoss) extract and Evernia furfuracea (treemoss) extract (4,5). Chloroatranol is not present in essential oils (6).

In animal experiments, chloroatranol has been found to be a sensitizer (8) and a 'strong' sensitizer when analyzed with the local lymph node assay (LLNA), under the conditions of the test (11). In treemoss and oakmoss extract chloroatranol and atranol are the main sensitizers (9), albeit not the only ones (7).

Formerly, oakmoss absolutes used for fragrances contained high concentrations of chloroatranol (0.9%-1.4%) and atranol (2.1%-2.9%) (4,9,10). Industry has made great efforts to reduce their levels and the contents of chloroatranol and atranol in IFRA-compliant oakmoss absolutes (http://www.ifraorg.org/en-us/standards-library) offered on the market today are below 100 ppm (0.01%) each. These are far less reactive in patch tests and ROATs (Repeated Open Application Tests) than the conventional untreated oakmoss samples with high chloroatranol and atranol content (7,12,13,14, discussed in Chapter 3.67 Evernia prunastri [oakmoss] extract).

Consumers using cosmetic products containing these extracts are exposed to atranol and chloroatranol at concentrations of ≤0.1 ppm (12). However, as it has been found that 10% of oakmoss-sensitized patients react to patch tests with an estimated concentration of chloroatranol as low as 0.0137 ppm (15) and 0.013 ppm (16), it is very likely that some highly sensitized patients will develop clinically manifest allergic contact dermatitis from fragranced cosmetics containing such (≤0.1 ppm) low concentrations. These studies (15,16) therefore corroborate the 2004 recommendation of the EC Scientific Committee on Consumer Products (SCCP) that atranol and chloroatranol should not be present in cosmetic products at all (11).

As a consequence (15 years later), the presence of chloroatranol in cosmetic products in the EU will be prohibited from August 2021 on; starting August 2019, cosmetic products containing chloroatranol are not allowed to be placed on the Union market (17). This will probably result in oakmoss extracts and treemoss extracts not being used at all anymore in fragrances.

See also Chapter 3.67 Evernia prunastri (oakmoss) extract and Chapter 3.66 Evernia furfuracea (treemoss) extract.

Presence in products and chemical analyses

The contents of chloroatranol and atranol in untreated oakmoss absolutes have been reported to be in the ranges of 0.9-1.4% and 2.1-2.9%, respectively (4,9,10).

In Denmark, in 2006, 25 perfume products (13 eaux de parfum, 8 eaux de toilette, one perfume spray, one perfume, and 2 aftershave lotions) for both men and women were purchased from Danish retail outlets and investigated for the presence of chloroatranol and atranol. Chloroatranol was present in 9 products (36%) in a concentration range of 0.6 ppb (detection level)-735 ppb (parts per billion, ng/ml; 1 ppb = 0.0000001%). The highest concentration was found – as expected – in an aftershave (1).

In Denmark, in the period 2000-2003, 31 popular fragranced cosmetics (12 perfumes, 6 eaux de parfum, 11 eaux de toilette and 2 aftershave lotions) were analyzed for the content of chloroatranol and atranol by liquid chromatography-tandem mass spectrometry (LC-MS-MS) with electrospray ionization (ESI) (2). Chloroatranol was identified in 27 products (87%) in a concentration range of 0.004-53 µg/ml. The median concentrations of chloroatranol were higher in perfumes (0.235 µg/ml) as compared to eaux de toilette (0.006 µg/ml). As expected, the highest concentrations of chloroatranol were found in the 2 aftershave lotions) (3).

Serial dilution tests

In Denmark and Sweden, in 2002-2003, in thirteen patients previously showing a positive patch test to oakmoss absolute and chloroatranol, serial dilution tests and use tests were performed with chloroatranol (16). The serial dilution patch test concentrations ranged from 200 to 0.0063 ppm of chloroatranol in ethanol. Simultaneously with patch testing, the subjects performed an open test simulating the use of perfumes on the volar aspect of the forearms with a solution of 5 ppm chloroatranol for 14 days, and, in case of no reaction, the applications were continued for another 14 days with a solution containing 25 ppm. All subjects had one or more reactions to the chloroatranol solution. Based on the dose-response curve, the dose of chloroatranol eliciting a reaction in 10% of the test group was determined to be 0.013 ppm and to be 0.15 ppm in 50% of the test group. In the use test, 12/13 (92%) gave a positive reaction to the 5 ppm solution and one to the 25 ppm solution. The use test was terminated (= when positive) at median day 4. It was concluded that, judged from the elicitation profile, chloroatranol is the most potent allergen present in consumer products (16).

To investigate and compare the elicitation potential of chloroatranol and atranol, in 2004, in Denmark, ten patients with dermatitis and known sensitization to chloroatranol and oakmoss absolute were tested simultaneously to a serial dilution series of chloroatranol and atranol in ethanol in equimolar concentrations. Concentrations ranged from 200 ppm to 0.00063 ppm for chloroatranol and from 163 ppm to 0.00052 ppm for atranol, which means that the doses varied from 0.0034 to 1072 mM. Dose–response curves were estimated and analysed by logistic regression. Both substances elicited reactions at very low levels of exposure. The estimated concentration eliciting a reaction in half of the tested individuals ($ED_{50\%}$) was 0.28 ppm for chloroatranol and 1.1 ppm for atranol. The estimated $ED_{10\%}$ (elicitation dose in 10% of tested individuals) was 0.0137 ppm for chloroatranol and 0.017 ppm for atranol. The estimated difference in elicitation potency of chloroatranol relative to atranol was 217%. This is counterbalanced by exposure being greater to atranol than to chloroatranol in oakmoss extract. Thus, it was concluded that both substances contribute to the clinical problems seen in oakmoss absolute-sensitized individuals (15).

Tests with oakmoss extracts with varying concentrations of chloroatranol and atranol

The results of 4 studies performing serial dilution tests and repeated Open Application Tests (ROATs) with oakmoss extracts containing high and low concentrations of chloroatranol and atranol (7,12,13,14) are discussed in Chapter 3.67 Evernia prunastri (oakmoss) extract.

LITERATURE

1   Rastogi SC, Johansen JD, Bossi R. Selected important fragrance sensitizers in perfumes: current exposures. Contact Dermatitis 2007;56:201-204

2   Bossi R, Rastogi SC, Bernard G, Giménez-Arnau E, Johansen JD, Lepoittevin JP, et al. A liquid chromatography-mass spectrometric method for the determination of oak moss allergens atranol and chloroatranol in perfumes. J Sep Sci 2003;27:537-540

3   Rastogi SC, Bossi R, Johansen JD, Menné T, Bernard T, Giménez-Arnau E, Lepoittevin J-P. Content of oak moss allergens atranol and chloroatranol in perfumes and similar products. Contact Dermatitis 2004;50:367-370

4   Joulain D, Tabacchi R. Lichen extracts as raw materials in perfumery. Part 1: oakmoss. Flavour Fragr J 2009;24:49-61

5   Joulain D, Tabacchi R. Lichen extracts as raw materials in perfumery. Part 2: treemoss. Flavour Fragr J 2009;24:105-116

6   De Groot AC, Schmidt E. Essential oils: contact allergy and chemical composition. Boca Raton, Fl., USA: CRC Press, Taylor and Francis Group, 2016 (ISBN 9781482246407)

7   Mowitz M, Zimerson E, Svedman C, Bruze M. Patch testing with serial dilutions and thin-layer chromatograms of oak moss absolutes containing high and low levels of atranol and chloroatranol. Contact Dermatitis 2013;69:342-349

8   Menné Bonefeld C, Nielsen MM, Gimenéz-Arnau E, Lang M, Vennegaard T, et al. An immune response study of oakmoss absolute and its constituents atranol and chloroatranol. Contact Dermatitis 2014;70:282-290

9   Bernard G, Giménez-Arnau E, Rastogi SC, Heydorn S, Johansen JD, Menné T, et al. Contact allergy to oak moss: search for sensitizing molecules using combined bioassay-guided chemical fractionation, GC-MS, and structure-activity relationship analysis. Arch Dermatol Res 2003;295:229-235

10   Ehret C, Maupetit P, Petrzilka M, Klecak G. Preparation of an oakmoss absolute with reduced allergenic potential. Int J Cosmet Sci 1992;14:121-130

11   SCCP (Scientific Committee on Consumer Products). Opinion on Atrranol and Chloroatranol present in natural extracts (e.g. oak moss and tree moss extract), 7 December 2004, SCCP/00847/04. Available at: http://ec.europa.eu/health/ph_risk/committees/04_sccp/docs/sccp_o_006.pdf

12   Mowitz M, Svedman C, Zimerson E, Bruze M. Usage tests of oak moss absolutes containing high and low levels of atranol and chloroatranol. Acta Derm Venereol 2014;94:398-402

13   Andersen F, Andersen KH, Bernois A, Brault C, Bruze M, Eudes H, et al. Reduced content of chloroatranol and atranol in oak moss absolute significantly reduces the elicitation potential of this fragrance material. Contact Dermatitis 2015;72:75-83

14   Nardelli A, Giménez-Arnau E, Bernard G, Lepoittevin J-P, Goossens A. Is a low content in atranol/chloroatranol safe in oak moss-sensitized individuals? Contact Dermatitis 2009;60:91-95

15   Johansen JD, Bernard G, Giménez-Arnau E, Lepoittevin J-P, Bruze M, Andersen KE. Comparison of elicitation potential of chloroatranol and atranol – 2 allergens in oak moss absolute. Contact Dermatitis 2006;54:192-195

16   Johansen JD, Andersen KE, Svedman C, Bruze M, Bernard G, Giménez-Arnau E, et al. Chloroatranol, an extremely potent allergen hidden in perfumes: a dose-response elicitation study. Contact Dermatitis 2003;49:180-184

17   Directorate-General for Internal Market, Industry, Entrepreneurship and SMEs (European Commission). Commission Regulation (EU) 2017/1410 of 2 August 2017 amending Annexes II and III to Regulation (EC) No 1223/2009 of the European Parliament and of the Council on cosmetic products. Official J European Union 2017;L202:1-3

Chapter 4.7 CONIFERYL ALCOHOL

IDENTIFICATION

Description/definition : Coniferyl alcohol is the dihydroxybenzene derivative that conforms to the structural formula shown below
Chemical class(es) : Aromatic compounds; ethers; alcohols
INCI name USA : Neither in Cosing nor in the Personal Care Products Council Ingredient Database
Chemical/IUPAC name : 4-(3-Hydroxyprop-1-enyl)-2-methoxyphenol
Other names : Coniferol; γ-hydroxyisoeugenol; 3-(4-hydroxy-3-methoxyphenyl)-2-propen-1-ol; 4-hydroxy-3-methoxycinnamyl alcohol
CAS registry number(s) : 458-35-5
EC number(s) : 207-277-9
Merck Index monograph : 3758
Patch testing : 1% pet. (1); 2% pet. (4)
Molecular formula : $C_{10}H_{12}O_3$

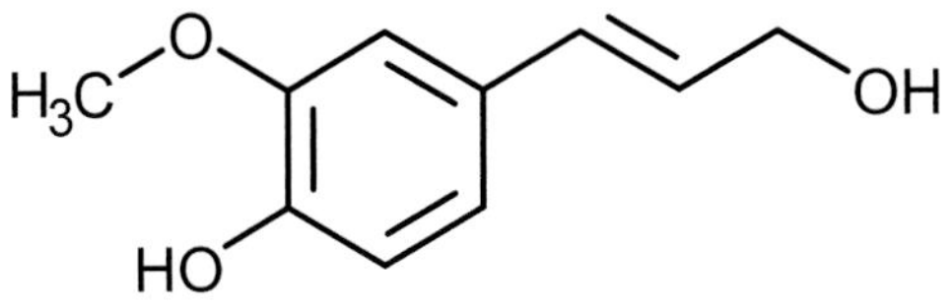

GENERAL

Coniferyl alcohol *per se* is not used as a fragrance material, but is discussed here as it is a constituent of botanical products which may be applied in perfumery, e.g. Myroxylon pereirae resin (balsam of Peru) and benzoin gum.

Presence in essential oils and Myroxylon pereirae resin (balsam of Peru)

Coniferyl alcohol has been identified by chemical analysis in none of 91 essential oils, which have caused contact allergy / allergic contact dermatitis (2). Coniferyl alcohol may be present in Myroxylon pereirae resin (balsam of Peru) (0.2%) (1). It can also be found in foods, e.g. tomatoes (3).

CONTACT ALLERGY

Patch testing in groups of patients

Studies in which coniferyl alcohol was patch tested in consecutive patients suspected of contact dermatitis (routine testing) with positive results have not been found.

In Germany, in the period 1995-1998, 102 patients allergic to Myroxylon pereirae resin (balsam of Peru) were patch tested with a battery of its ingredients including coniferyl alcohol 1% pet. and there were 13 (13%) positive reactions (1).

Case reports and case series

Case reports of allergic contact dermatitis from coniferyl alcohol have not been found.

Cross-reactions, pseudo-cross-reactions and co-reactions

Co-reactivity with Myroxylon pereirae resin (MP) may be explained by the presence of coniferyl alcohol (0.2%) in MP (pseudo-cross-reactions).

LITERATURE

1   Hausen BM. Contact allergy to Balsam of Peru. II. Patch test results in 102 patients with selected Balsam of Peru constituents. Am J Contact Derm 2001;12:93-102
2   De Groot AC, Schmidt E. Essential oils: contact allergy and chemical composition. Boca Raton, Fl., USA: CRC Press, Taylor and Francis Group, 2016 (ISBN 9781482246407)
3   Srivastava D, Cohen DE. Identification of the constituents of balsam of peru in tomatoes. Dermatitis 2009;20:99-105
4   De Groot AC. Patch Testing, 4th Edition. Wapserveen, The Netherlands: acdegroot publishing, 2018 (ISBN 978-90-813233-4-5)

Chapter 4.8   CONIFERYL BENZOATE

IDENTIFICATION

Description/definition   : Coniferyl benzoate is the coniferyl alcohol ester of benzoic acid
Chemical class(es)   : Aromatic compounds; esters; ethers; alcohols
INCI name USA   : Neither in Cosing nor in the Personal Care Products Council Ingredient Database
Chemical/IUPAC name   : 3-(4-Hydroxy-3-methoxyphenyl)prop-2-enyl benzoate
Other names   : Phenol, 4-(3-(benzoyloxy)-1-propenyl)-2-methoxy-
CAS registry number(s)   : 4159-29-9
EC number(s)   : Not available
Patch testing   : 1% pet. (2,3); 0.5% pet. (5); the material should be kept in a deep-freezer to avoid
                            degradation; high risk of patch test sensitization at 2% pet. (5)
Molecular formula   : $C_{17}H_{16}O_4$

GENERAL

Coniferyl benzoate *per se* is not used as a fragrance material, but is discussed here as it is a constituent of botanical products which may be applied in perfumery, e.g. Siam benzoin (Styrax tonkinensis resin) (65-75% [5]) and (derivatives of) Myroxylon pereirae resin (balsam of Peru) (1-8.5% [2]).

Coniferyl benzoate is labile, oxidizing with polymerization and browning on exposure to air, by treatment with solvents, and by saponification (5). As a result of instability it is destroyed in Myroxylon pereirae resin and in a commercial test syringe within a short time; it should be prepared freshly and kept in a refrigerator at -20 degrees Celsius (3). At 2% in petrolatum, there is a high risk of patch test sensitization (5).

Presence in essential oils and propolis

Coniferyl benzoate has been identified by chemical analysis in none of 91 essential oils, which have caused contact allergy / allergic contact dermatitis (6). Coniferyl benzoate may be present in balsam of Peru (3) and in propolis (1).

CONTACT ALLERGY

Coniferyl benzoate was reported to be a strong sensitizer based on animal experiments (3,5). It is an important (2), if not the main (5) sensitizer in Myroxylon pereirae resin.

Patch testing in groups of patients

Studies in which coniferyl benzoate was patch tested in consecutive patients suspected of contact dermatitis (routine testing) with positive results have not been found. Studies in which coniferyl benzoate was tested in groups of selected patients are shown in table 4.8.1.

In two studies, patients allergic to Myroxylon pereirae (MP) resin (2,5) and in one, individuals allergic to propolis (4) have been patch tested with coniferyl benzoate, which may be present in both substances. In the Myroxylon pereirae resin studies, 29 of 102 (28%) and 68 of 82 (81%) individuals allergic to MP reacted to coniferyl benzoate 0.5%, 1% or 2% pet. (2,5), suggesting it is an important allergenic ingredient in this material. Of 2 patients allergic to propolis, one reacted to coniferyl benzoate (4). The major sensitizers in propolis, however, are esters of caffeic acid (7).

Table 4.8.1 Patch testing in groups of patients: Selected patient groups

Years and Country	Test conc. & vehicle	Number of patients tested	positive (%)	Selection of patients (S); Relevance (R); Comments (C)	Ref.
1995-1998 Germany	1% pet.	102	29 (28%)	S: patients allergic to Myroxylon pereirae resin	2
1988-1990 Germany	1% pet.	2	1 (50%)	S: patients allergic to propolis	4
1955-1959 Denmark	2% or 0.5% pet.	82	68 (81%)	S: patients allergic to Myroxylon pereirae resin	5

Case reports and case series
Case reports of allergic contact dermatitis from coniferyl benzoate have not been found.

Cross-reactions, pseudo-cross-reactions and co-reactions
For general information on cross-/pseudo-cross-/co-reactivity of fragrance chemicals with other fragrances, fragrance markers (fragrance mix I, fragrance mix II, colophonium, Myroxylon pereirae resin [balsam of Peru]) and essential oils see Chapter 1.2 General information on cross-reactions, pseudo-cross-reactions and co-reactions.

Co-reactions are frequently observed to Myroxylon pereirae resin (in which it is an important or the most important sensitizer), to other chemicals in this material (coniferyl alcohol, eugenol, cinnamic acid, benzoic acid, benzyl alcohol, benzyl cinnamate) and to other balsams / resins: wood tar, styrax (INCI name: Liquidambar orientalis resin), balsam of Tolu (INCI name: Myroxylon balsamum resin) and Siam benzoin (INCI name: Styrax tonkinensis resin) (5).

Patch test sensitization
Of 82 patients allergic to Myroxylon pereirae resin and patch tested with coniferyl benzoate (approx. 2/3 with 2% pet., 1/3 with 0.5% pet.), 4 developed late reactions on the 7th, 8th, 10th and 24th day (5). Of 30 control patients tested with coniferyl benzoate 2% pet., 7 (23%) had positive delayed reactions after 14-27 days. Four of these were retested and now reacted after 2-4 days, proving patch test sensitization (5). Another two, who were negative in the first test, were positive at re-testing after 3-4 weeks (5).

LITERATURE

1   De Groot AC, Popova MP, Bankova VS. An update on the constituents of poplar-type propolis. Wapserveen, The Netherlands: acdegroot publishing, 2014, 11 pages. ISBN/EAN: 978-90-813233-0-7. Available at: https://www.researchgate.net/publication/262851225_AN_UPDATE_ON_THE_CONSTITUENTS_OF_POPLAR-TYPE_PROPOLIS

2   Hausen BM. Contact allergy to Balsam of Peru. II. Patch test results in 102 patients with selected Balsam of Peru constituents. Am J Contact Derm 2001;12:93-102

3   Hausen BM, Simatupang T, Bruhn G, Evers P, Koenig WA. Identification of new allergenic constituents and proof of evidence for coniferyl benzoate in Balsam of Peru. Am J Cont Dermat 1995;6:199-208

4   Hausen BM, Evers P, Stüwe H-T, König WA, Wollenweber E. Propolis allergy (IV) Studies with further sensitizers from propolis and constituents common to propolis, poplar buds and balsam of Peru. Contact Dermatitis 1992;26:34-44

5   Hjorth N. Eczematous allergy to balsams. Acta Derm Venereol 1961;41(suppl.46):1-216

6   De Groot AC, Schmidt E. Essential oils: contact allergy and chemical composition. Boca Raton, Fl., USA: CRC Press, Taylor and Francis Group, 2016 (ISBN 9781482246407)

7   De Groot AC. Propolis: a review of properties, applications, chemical composition, contact allergy, and other adverse effects. Dermatitis 2013;24:263-82

Chapter 4.9   EVERNIC ACID

IDENTIFICATION

Description/definition : Evernic acid is the lichen acid that conforms to the structural formula shown below
Chemical class(es) : Aromatic acids
INCI name USA : Neither in Cosing nor in the Personal Care Products Council Ingredient Database
Chemical/IUPAC name : 2-Hydroxy-4-(2-hydroxy-4-methoxy-6-methylbenzoyl)oxy-6-methylbenzoic acid
CAS registry number(s) : 537-09-7
EC number(s) : 208-658-2
Patch testing : 0.1% Pet. (Chemotechnique)
Molecular formula : $C_{17}H_{16}O_7$

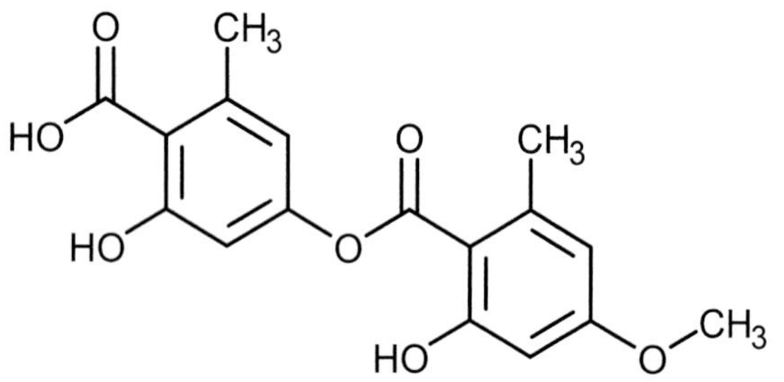

GENERAL

Evernic acid *per se* is not used as a fragrance material, but is discussed here as it is a constituent of botanical products which may be applied in perfumery, e.g. Evernia prunastri (oakmoss) extract (5). It is not present in Evernia furfuracea (treemoss) extract (6) nor in essential oils (7). See also Chapter 3.67 Evernia prunastri (oakmoss) extract.

CONTACT ALLERGY

Patch testing in groups of patients

Patch testing in consecutive patients suspected of contact dermatitis: routine testing
Studies in which evernic acid was patch tested in consecutive patients suspected of contact dermatitis (routine testing) with positive results have not been found.

Patch testing in groups of selected patients
Before 1987, in Norway, 55 patients with sensitivity to different brands of perfumes, deodorants, aftershave lotions *et cetera* verified by repeated questioning and/or patch testing were tested with evernic acid 0.1% (vehicle not mentioned) and there were 12 (22%) positive reactions. Their relevance was not mentioned. Thirty-five of the 55 subjects (64%) also reacted to oakmoss absolute, of which evernic acid is an ingredient (15).

Case report
A male patient, who had allergic contact dermatitis from oak moss in aftershave lotions, experienced exacerbations of his hand dermatitis when handling firewood or trees in the forest, and he had allergic reactions to evernic acid and atranorin on patch testing. Whether he actually had contact with evernic acid, e.g. from lichens on the firewood or trees, was not mentioned (13).

Cross-reactions, pseudo-cross-reactions and co-reactions

Oakmoss extracts
In 7 patients allergic to oakmoss, patch tests were also performed with lichen acids and there were 4 reactions to evernic acid (2). Of 7 patients reacting to an acetone extract of oakmoss 7% in petrolatum, 4 co-reacted to evernic acid (9). Of 20 patients allergic to oakmoss extract (identified by ingredient testing of the fragrance mix I), 6 co-reacted to evernic acid (12). Of 15 patients allergic to oakmoss absolute, 2 co-reacted to evernic acid 0.1% pet. (14).

Atranorin
Of 8 patients reacting to atranorin 1% pet., 5 (63%) co-reacted to evernic acid 0.1% in acetone (4). Of 10 patients allergic to atranorin 0.1% pet. seen in Sweden before 1981, 7 co-reacted to evernic acid (8).

Serial dilution testing
Three patients allergic to evernic acid were patch tested with a dilution series of 1% down to 0.001% in petrolatum; the lower thresholds for positive reactions were 0.01%, 0.005% and 0.001%, respectively (11).

OTHER SIDE EFFECTS

Photosensitivity

Photopatch testing in groups of patients
In Italy, between 1985 and 1993, 1050 patients suspected of photoallergic contact dermatitis were patch tested with evernic acid (test concentration and vehicle not stated) and there was one (0.1%) positive photopatch test; its relevance was not specified (78% for all photoallergens together) (1).

Case report
A man had suffered from a mild itchy, erythematous eruption above the sternum for the last 18 months. His dermatitis increased and spread over the sides of the neck during the summer months. The patient had a long beard and had been using an eau de cologne every day for the past 18 months. The day before his consultation, he developed a spread with a drop-like configuration to the xiphoid area suggesting that the lotion applied was the cause. Patch testing and photopatch testing showed photocontact allergy to the eau de cologne and evernic acid and photoaggravated contact allergy to oakmoss and atranorin (3). This patient was later retested, he now had plain contact allergy to oakmoss extract, oakmoss (lichen, pure), treemoss (lichen, pure) and atranorin, but photocontact allergy only to evernic acid (10). Whether the eau de cologne actually contained evernic acid (through its presence in oakmoss extract), is unknown.

LITERATURE

1 Pigatto PD, Legori A, Bigardi AS,Guarrera M, Tosti A, Santucci B, et al. Gruppo Italiano recerca dermatiti da contatto ed ambientali Italian multicenter study of allergic contact photodermatitis: epidemiological aspects. Am J Contact Dermatitis 1996;7:158-163
2 Thune P, Solberg Y, McFadden N, Stærfeet F, Sandberg M. Perfume allergy due to oak moss and other lichens. Contact Dermatitis 1982;8:396-400
3 Fernández de Corres L, Muñoz D, Leaniz-Barrutia I, Corrales JL. Photocontact dermatitis from oak moss. Contact Dermatitis 1983;9:528-529
4 Dahlquist I, Fregert S. Contact allergy to atranorin in lichens and perfumes. Contact Dermatitis 1980;6:111-119
5 Joulain D, Tabacchi R. Lichen extracts as raw materials in perfumery. Part 1: oakmoss. Flavour Fragr J 2009;24:49-61
6 Joulain D, Tabacchi R. Lichen extracts as raw materials in perfumery. Part 2: treemoss. Flavour Fragr J 2009;24:105-116
7 De Groot AC, Schmidt E. Essential oils: contact allergy and chemical composition. Boca Raton, Fl., USA: CRC Press, Taylor and Francis Group, 2016 (ISBN 9781482246407)
8 Dahlquist I, Fregert S. Atranorin and oak moss contact allergy. Contact Dermatitis 1981;7:168-169
9 Fregert S, Dahlquist I. Patch testing with oak moss extract. Contact Dermatitis 1983;9:227
10 Fernández de Corres L. Photosensitivity to oak moss. Contact Dermatitis 1986;15:118
11 Sandberg M, Thune P. The sensitizing capacity of atranorin. Contact Dermatitis 1984;11:168-173
12 Gonçalo S, Cabral F, Gonçalo M. Contact sensitivity to oak moss. Contact Dermatitis 1988;19:355-357
13 Aalto-Korte K, Lauerma A, Alanko K. Occupational allergic contact dermatitis from lichens in present-day Finland. Contact Dermatitis 2005;52:36-38
14 Mowitz M, Zimerson E, Svedman C, Bruze M. Patch testing with serial dilutions and thin-layer chromatograms of oak moss absolutes containing high and low levels of atranol and chloroatranol. Contact Dermatitis 2013;69:342-349
15 Thune P, Sandberg M. Allergy to lichen and compositae compounds in perfumes. Investigations on the sensitizing, toxic and mutagenic potential. Acta Derm Venereol 1987;134(suppl.):87-89

Chapter 4.10   FUMARPROTOCETRARIC ACID

IDENTIFICATION

Description/definition	: Fumarprotocetraric acid is the tricyclic organic acid that conforms to the structural formula shown below
Chemical class(es)	: Tricyclic organic compounds; carboxylic acids; esters
INCI name USA	: Neither in Cosing nor in the Personal Care Products Council Ingredient Database
Chemical/IUPAC name	: 4-[[(E)-3-Carboxyprop-2-enoyl]oxymethyl]-10-formyl-3,9-dihydroxy-1,7-dimethyl-6-oxobenzo[b][1,4]benzodioxepine-2-carboxylic acid
CAS registry number(s)	: 489-50-9
EC number(s)	: 207-698-8
Patch testing	: 0.1% acet. or 0.1%-1% pet. (1)
Molecular formula	: $C_{22}H_{16}O_{12}$

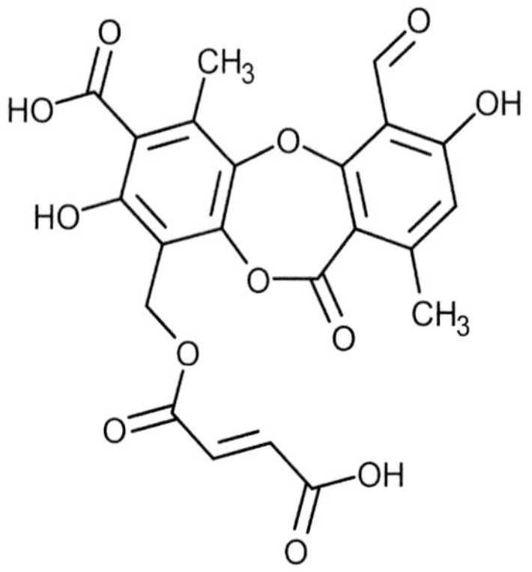

GENERAL

Fumarprotocetraric acid *per se* is not used as a fragrance material, but is discussed here as it is a constituent of botanical products which may be applied in perfumery. Fumarprotocetraric acid may be present in Evernia furfuracea (treemoss) extract but not in Evernia prunastri (oakmoss) extract (3,4). It is also not present in essential oils which have caused contact allergy / allergic contact dermatitis.

See also Chapter 3.66 Evernia furfuracea (treemoss) extract.

CONTACT ALLERGY

Patch testing in groups of patients and case reports

Studies in which fumarprotocetraric acid was patch tested in either consecutive patients suspected of contact dermatitis (routine testing) or in groups of selected patients with positive results have not been found, nor have case reports of allergic contact dermatitis from fumarprotocetraric acid.

Cross-reactions, pseudo-cross-reactions and co-reactions

Of 8 patients reacting to atranorin 1% pet., all co-reacted to fumarprotocetraric acid 0.1% in acetone (2). Of 10 patients reacting to atranorin 0.1% pet. seen in Sweden before 1981, all co-reacted to fumarprotocetraric acid (6).

Of 7 patients reacting to an acetone extract of oakmoss 7% in petrolatum, all co-reacted to fumarprotocetraric acid (7). Of 20 patients allergic to oakmoss extract (identified by ingredient testing of the fragrance mix I), 3 co-reacted to fumarprotocetraric acid (5).

LITERATURE

1   De Groot AC. Patch Testing, 4th Edition. Wapserveen, The Netherlands: acdegroot publishing, 2018 (ISBN 978-90-813233-4-5)
2   Dahlquist I, Fregert S. Contact allergy to atranorin in lichens and perfumes. Contact Dermatitis 1980;6:111-119
3   Joulain D, Tabacchi R. Lichen extracts as raw materials in perfumery. Part 1: oakmoss. Flavour Fragr J 2009;24:49-61
4   Joulain D, Tabacchi R. Lichen extracts as raw materials in perfumery. Part 2: treemoss. Flavour Fragr J 2009;24:105-116
5   Gonçalo S, Cabral F, Gonçalo M. Contact sensitivity to oak moss. Contact Dermatitis 1988;19:355-357
6   Dahlquist I, Fregert S. Atranorin and oak moss contact allergy. Contact Dermatitis 1981;7:168-169
7   Fregert S, Dahlquist I. Patch testing with oak moss extract. Contact Dermatitis 1983;9:227

Chapter 4.11   ISOFERULIC ACID

IDENTIFICATION

Description/definition : Isoferulic acid is the dihydroxybenzene derivative that conforms to the structural formula shown below
Chemical class(es) : Aromatic organic compounds; unsaturated compounds; carboxylic acids; phenols; ethers
INCI name USA : Neither in Cosing nor in the Personal Care Products Council Ingredient Database
Chemical/IUPAC name : (*E*)-3-(3-Hydroxy-4-methoxyphenyl)prop-2-enoic acid
Other names : 3-Hydroxy-4-methoxycinnamic acid; hesperetic acid
CAS registry number(s) : 537-73-5; 25522-33-2
EC number(s) : 208-676-0; 247-071-6
Patch testing : 5% pet. (1)
Molecular formula : $C_{10}H_{10}O_4$

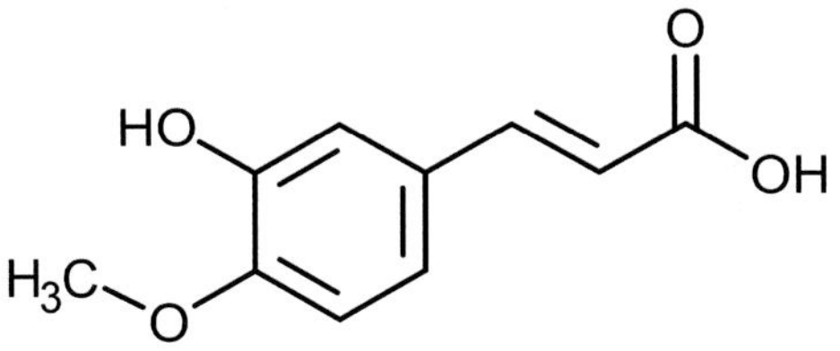

GENERAL

Isoferulic acid *per se* is not used as a fragrance material, but is discussed here as it is a constituent of botanical products which may be applied in perfumery, e.g. (derivatives of) Myroxylon pereirae resin (balsam of Peru, in traces) (1). It may also be present in propolis (2,4), but it has not been found in essential oils which have caused contact allergy / allergic contact dermatitis (3).

CONTACT ALLERGY

Patch testing in consecutive patients suspected of contact dermatitis: routine testing

Studies in which isoferulic acid was patch tested in consecutive patients suspected of contact dermatitis (routine testing) with positive results have not been found.

Testing in groups of selected patients

In Germany, in the period 1995-1998, 102 patients allergic to Myroxylon pereirae resin (balsam of Peru) were patch tested with a battery of its ingredients and there was one (1%) positive reaction to isoferulic acid 5% pet., showing that this compound is not an important allergen in balsam of Peru (1).

Case reports

Case reports of allergic contact dermatitis from isoferulic acid have not been found.

LITERATURE

1   Hausen BM. Contact allergy to Balsam of Peru. II. Patch test results in 102 patients with selected balsam of Peru constituents. Am J Cont Derm 2001;12:93-102
2   De Groot AC, Popova MP, Bankova VS. An update on the constituents of poplar-type propolis. Wapserveen, The Netherlands: acdegroot publishing, 2014, 11 pages. ISBN/EAN: 978-90-813233-0-7. Available at: https://www.researchgate.net/publication/262851225_AN_UPDATE_ON_THE_CONSTITUENTS_OF_POPLAR-TYPE_PROPOLIS
3   De Groot AC, Schmidt E. Essential oils: contact allergy and chemical composition. Boca Raton, Fl., USA: CRC Press, Taylor and Francis Group, 2016 (ISBN 9781482246407)
4   Xuan H, Wang Y, Li A, Fu C, Wang Y, Peng W. Bioactive components of Chinese propolis water extract on antitumor activity and quality control. Evid Based Complement Alternat Med 2016;9641965, Article ID 9641965, 9 pages

Chapter 4.12   LEDENE

IDENTIFICATION

Description/definition   : Ledene is the tricyclic organic compound that conforms to the structural formula shown
                             below
Chemical class(es)   : Tricyclic organic compounds; unsaturated organic compounds
INCI name USA   : Neither in Cosing nor in the Personal Care Products Council Ingredient Database
Chemical/IUPAC name   : 1,1,4,7-Tetramethyl-1a,2,3,5,6,7,7a,7b-octahydrocyclopropa[e]azulene
Other names   : 3,3,7,11-Tetramethyltricyclo[6.3.0.02.4]undec-7-ene; viridiflorene; viridiflorine;
                             viridoflorene
CAS registry number(s)   : 21747-46-6
EC number(s)   : 244-565-3
Patch testing   : 5% diethyl phthalate (1,3); suggested: 5% pet.
Molecular formula   : $C_{15}H_{24}$

GENERAL

Ledene is a colorless clear liquid. Ledene *per se* is not used as a fragrance material, but is discussed here as it is a
constituent of botanical products which may be applied in perfumery, e.g. Melaleuca alternifolia (tea tree) leaf oil.

Presence in essential oils

Ledene has been identified by chemical analysis in 31 of 91 essential oils, which have caused contact allergy / allergic
contact dermatitis. In none of these oils, it belonged to the 'Top-10' of ingredients with the highest concentrations
(5).

CONTACT ALLERGY

General

Ledene is a minor allergen in tea tree oil. Of 54 patients allergic to tea tree oil and tested with a number of its
ingredients in various studies, 3 (6%) reacted to ledene (4).

Patch testing in consecutive patients suspected of contact dermatitis: routine testing

Studies in which ledene was patch tested in consecutive patients suspected of contact dermatitis (routine testing)
with positive results have not been found.

Patch testing in groups of selected patients

Results of studies patch testing ledene in groups of selected patients are shown in table 4.12.1. In three studies,
small groups of individuals allergic to (oxidized) tea tree oil were tested with a battery of its ingredients and 5-10%
had positive reactions to ledene 5% in diethyl phthalate, attesting to the fact that ledene is a minor allergen in the oil
(4).

Table 4.12.1 Patch testing in groups of patients: Selected patient groups

Years and Country	Test conc. & vehicle	Number of patients tested	positive (%)	Selection of patients (S); Relevance (R); Comments (C)	Ref.
1999-2003 Germany,	5% DEP	20	1 (5%)	S: patients with a positive patch test reaction to oxidized tea tree oil 5% DEP	3
1999-2000 Germany, Austria	5% DEP	10	1 (10%)	S: patients with a positive patch test reaction to oxidized tea tree oil 5% DEP	1
<1999 Germany	5% vehicle?	16	1 (7%)	S: patients allergic to tea tree oil	2

DEP: Diethyl phthalate

Case report

A woman became strongly sensitized to tea tree oil after treating insect bites, herpes simplex, and other lesions of the skin with tea tree oil. When patch tested with the essential oil and 15 of its ingredients, she had a (weak) positive reaction to ledene (viridiflorene) (5%, vehicle unknown) and to six other components, of which 4 were very strong. Hence, a false-positive reaction to ledene cannot be excluded (2).

LITERATURE

1   Pirker C, Hausen BM, Uter W, Hillen U, Brasch J, Bayeret C, et al. Sensitization to tea tree oil in Germany and Austria. A multicenter Study of the German Contact Dermatitis group. J Dtsch Dermatol Ges 2003;1:629-634 (article in German)
2   Hausen BM, Reichling J, Harkenthal M. Degradation products of monoterpenes are the sensitizing agents in tea tree oil. Am J Contact Dermat 1999;10:68-77
3   Hausen BM. Evaluation of the main contact allergens in oxidized tea tree oil. Dermatitis 2004;15:213-214
4   De Groot AC, Schmidt E. Tea tree oil: contact allergy and chemical composition. Contact Dermatitis 2016;75:129-143
5   De Groot AC, Schmidt E. Essential oils: contact allergy and chemical composition. Boca Raton, Fl., USA: CRC Press, Taylor and Francis Group, 2016 (ISBN 9781482246407)

Chapter 4.13   PHYSODALIC ACID

IDENTIFICATION

Description/definition	: Physodalic acid is the heterocyclic aromatic compound that conforms to the structural formula shown below
Chemical class(es)	: Aromatic compounds; heterocyclic compounds; esters; carboxylic acids; alcohols
INCI name USA	: Neither in Cosing nor in the Personal Care Products Council Ingredient Database
Chemical/IUPAC name	: 4-(Acetyloxymethyl)-10-formyl-3,9-dihydroxy-1,7-dimethyl-6-oxobenzo[b][1,4]benzo-dioxepine-2-carboxylic acid
CAS registry number(s)	: 90689-60-4
EC number(s)	: Not available
Patch testing	: 1% pet. (1)
Molecular formula	: $C_{20}H_{16}O_{10}$

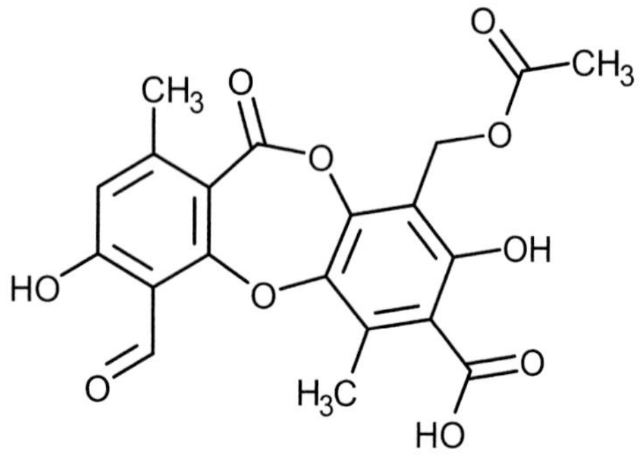

GENERAL

Physodalic acid *per se* is not used as a fragrance material, but is discussed here as it is a constituent of botanical products which may be applied in perfumery including Evernia furfuracea (treemoss) extract. It is apparently not present in Evernia prunastri (oakmoss) extract (2,3) and physodalic acid has not been identified in essential oils that have caused contact allergy (4).

Older literature on contact allergy to physodalic acid from its presence in lichens is not discussed here. See also Chapter... Evernia furfuracea (treemoss) extract.

CONTACT ALLERGY

Case reports and case series
In the period 1980-1982, in a clinic in Norway, 7 of 2000 routinely tested patients revealed contact allergy to oak moss in perfumes. In three, the reactions to the perfumes were positive, in the others, they were not tested. Patch tests were also performed with lichen acids and there were 3 reactions to physodic/physodalic acid, 4 to evernic acid, 5 reactions to usnic acid, 4 to atranorin, and one to diffractaic acid, all tested 1% pet. The authors suggested that cosmetics containing lichen extracts are a much more important source of contact allergy than lichens encountered in nature, but whether the reactions to physodic/physodalic acid were relevant was not mentioned (1).

Cross-reactions, pseudo-cross-reactions and co-reactions
In 7 patients allergic to oakmoss extract, patch tests were also performed with lichen acids and there were 3 reactions to physodic/physodalic acid 1% pet. (1). Physodalic acid is not present in oakmoss extracts (2), but physodic acid has been identified in oakmoss extracts (Chapter 4.14 Physodic acid).

LITERATURE

1   Thune P, Solberg Y, McFadden N, Stærfeet F, Sandberg M. Perfume allergy due to oak moss and other lichens. Contact Dermatitis 1982;8:396-400
2   Joulain D, Tabacchi R. Lichen extracts as raw materials in perfumery. Part 1: oakmoss. Flavour Fragr J 2009;24:49-61
3   Joulain D, Tabacchi R. Lichen extracts as raw materials in perfumery. Part 2: treemoss. Flavour Fragr J 2009;24:105-116
4   De Groot AC, Schmidt E. Essential oils: contact allergy and chemical composition. Boca Raton, Fl., USA: CRC Press, Taylor and Francis Group, 2016 (ISBN 9781482246407)

Chapter 4.14   PHYSODIC ACID

IDENTIFICATION

Description/definition : Physodic acid is the heterocyclic aromatic compound that conforms to the structural formula shown below

Chemical class(es) : Aromatic compounds; heterocyclic compounds; carboxylic acids; alcohols; esters; ketones

INCI name USA : Neither in Cosing nor in the Personal Care Products Council Ingredient Database

Chemical/IUPAC name : 3,9-Dihydroxy-6-oxo-7-(2-oxoheptyl)-1-pentylbenzo[b][1,4]benzodioxepine-2-carboxylic acid

Other names : Physodalin

CAS registry number(s) : 84-24-2

EC number(s) : Not available

Patch testing : 1% pet. (1)

Molecular formula : $C_{26}H_{30}O_8$

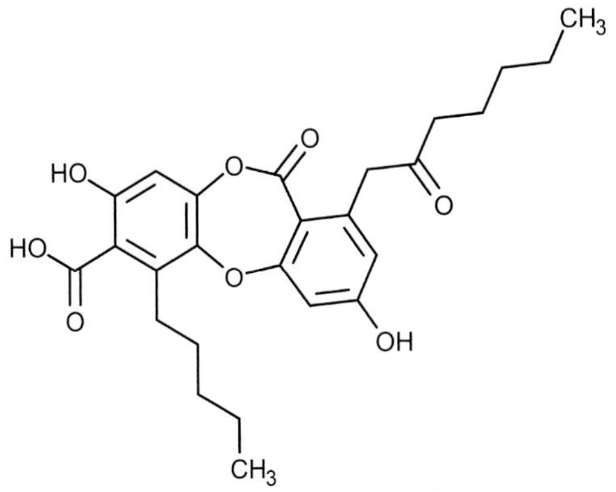

GENERAL

Physodic acid *per se* is not used as a fragrance material, but is discussed here as it is a constituent of botanical products which may be applied in perfumery. Physodic acid may be present in Evernia furfuracea (treemoss) extract (2). According to some authors, it is not an ingredient of Evernia prunastri (oakmoss) extract (2,3), but others have identified it in acetone extracts of oakmoss (6). Physodic acid is not present in essential oils that have caused contact allergy (4).

See also Chapter 3.66 Evernia furfuracea (treemoss) extract.

CONTACT ALLERGY

Patch testing in groups of patients

Studies in which physodic acid was patch tested in either consecutive patients suspected of contact dermatitis (routine testing) or in groups of selected patients with positive results have not been found.

Case reports and case series

In the period 1980-1982, in a clinic in Norway, 7 of 2000 routinely tested patients revealed contact allergy to oak moss in perfumes. In three, the patch test reactions to the perfumes were positive, in the others, they were not tested. Patch tests were also performed with lichen acids and there were 3 reactions to physodic/physodalic acid, 4 to evernic acid, 5 reactions to usnic acid, 4 to atranorin, and one to diffractaic acid, all tested 1% pet. The authors suggested that cosmetics containing lichen extracts are a much more important source of contact allergy than lichens encountered in nature, but whether the reactions to physodic/physodalic acid were relevant was not mentioned (1).

Cross-reactions, pseudo-cross-reactions and co-reactions

In 7 patients allergic to oakmoss extract, patch tests were also performed with lichen acids and there were 3 reactions to physodic/physodalic acid 1% pet. (1). Physodalic acid is not present in oakmoss extracts (2), but physodic acid has been identified in it (6).

Serial dilution testing

One patient allergic to physodic acid was patch tested with a dilution series of 1% down to 0.001% in petrolatum; the lower threshold for a positive patch test was 0.005% (5).

LITERATURE

1   Thune P, Solberg Y, McFadden N, Stærfeet F, Sandberg M. Perfume allergy due to oak moss and other lichens. Contact Dermatitis 1982;8:396-400

2   Joulain D, Tabacchi R. Lichen extracts as raw materials in perfumery. Part 1: oakmoss. Flavour Fragr J 2009;24:49-61

3   Joulain D, Tabacchi R. Lichen extracts as raw materials in perfumery. Part 2: treemoss. Flavour Fragr J 2009;24:105-116

4   De Groot AC, Schmidt E. Essential oils: contact allergy and chemical composition. Boca Raton, Fl., USA: CRC Press, Taylor and Francis Group, 2016 (ISBN 9781482246407)

5   Sandberg M, Thune P. The sensitizing capacity of atranorin. Contact Dermatitis 1984;11:168-173

6   Kosanić M, Manojlović N, Janković S, Stanojković T, Ranković B. *Evernia prunastri* and *Pseudoevernia furfuraceae* lichens and their major metabolites as antioxidant, antimicrobial and anticancer agents. Food Chem Toxicol 2013;53:112-118

Chapter 4.15 1,2,4-TRIHYDROXYMENTHANE

IDENTIFICATION

Description/definition : 1,2,4-Trihydroxymenthane is the cyclic alcohol that conforms to the structural formula shown below
Chemical class(es) : Cyclic organic compounds; alcohols
INCI name USA : Neither in Cosing nor in the Personal Care Products Council Ingredient Database
Chemical/IUPAC name : 1-Methyl-4-propan-2-ylcyclohexane-1,2,4-triol
Other name(s) : 4-Isopropyl-1-methylcyclohexane-1,2,4-triol
CAS registry number(s) : 61073-90-3
EC number(s) : Not available
Patch testing : 5% pet.
Molecular formula : $C_{10}H_{20}O_3$

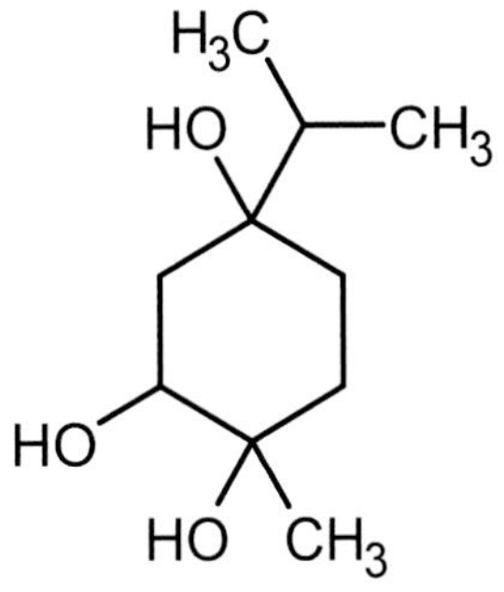

GENERAL

1,2,4-Trihydroxymenthane *per se* is not used as a fragrance material, but is discussed here as it is a constituent of botanical products which may be applied in perfumery, notably Melaleuca alternifolia (tea tree) leaf oil. 1,2,4-Trihydroxymenthane is the oxidation product of 4-terpineol (3) and an important allergenic ingredient of photo-oxidized or air-oxidized tea tree oil (Chapter 6.71 Tea tree oil).

Presence in essential oils

1,2,4-Trihydroxymenthane has been identified by chemical analysis in one of 91 essential oils, which have caused contact allergy / allergic contact dermatitis: tea tree oil (7).

CONTACT ALLERGY

General

1,2,4-Trihydroxymenthane is an important allergen in tea tree oil. Of 69 patients allergic to tea tree oil and tested with a number of its ingredients in various studies, 43 (62%) reacted to 1,2,4-trihydroxymenthane (6).

Patch testing in groups of patients

Patch testing in consecutive patients suspected of contact dermatitis: routine testing
Studies in which 1,2,4-trihydroxymenthane was patch tested in consecutive patients suspected of contact dermatitis (routine testing) with positive results have not been found.

Patch testing in groups of selected patients
Results of studies patch testing 1,2,4-trihydroxymenthane in groups of selected patients (in all studies: patients previously shown to be allergic to (oxidized) tea tree oil) are shown in table 4.15.1. In the period 1990-2003, five small series of 8-20 patients allergic to (oxidized) tea tree oil have been tested with a battery of its ingredients, including 1,2,4-trihydroxymenthane 5% in various vehicles (1,2,3,4,5). Frequencies of sensitization have ranged from 25 to 90%, with a mean percentage of 62% (6), attesting to the fact that 1,2,4-trihydroxymenthane is an important allergenic ingredient of tea tree oil (6).

Case reports and case series

A woman washed her mouth with a tincture of tea tree oil in warm water to treat her tooth pain, and she treated other skin lesions with the undiluted oil. Another female patient treated a sunburn with tea tree oil. A third one used tea tree oil for pain of the neck and eczematous lesions of the heels. A man used only herbal extracts for hygiene and cosmetic purposes, including several bottles of tea tree oil. All four patients became sensitized to tea tree oil and had positive patch tests to the oil, its ingredient 1,2,4-trihydroxymenthane (5%, vehicle unknown) and 1-6 other oil components (4).

Table 4.15.1 Patch testing in groups of patients: Selected patient groups

Years and Country	Test conc. & vehicle	Number of patients tested	positive (%)	Selection of patients (S); Relevance (R); Comments (C)	Ref.
1999-2003 Germany	5% pet.	20	13 (65%)	S: patients with a positive patch test reaction to oxidized tea tree oil 5% DEP	5
2000 Germany		15	11 (73%)	S: patients with a positive patch test reaction to oxidized tea tree oil	3
1999-2000 Germany, Austria	5% DEP	10	9 (90%)	S: patients with a positive patch test reaction to oxidized tea tree oil 5% DEP	1
1999 Germany	5% pet.	8	2 (25%)	S: patients with a positive patch test reaction to oxidized tea tree oil 20% in olive oil	2
<1999 Germany	5% vehicle?	16	8 (50%)	S: patients allergic to tea tree oil	4

DEP: Diethyl phthalate

LITERATURE

1   Pirker C, Hausen BM, Uter W, Hillen U, Brasch J, Bayeret C, et al. Sensitization to tea tree oil in Germany and Austria. A multicenter Study of the German Contact Dermatitis group. J Dtsch Dermatol Ges 2003;1:629-634 (article in German)
2   Lippert U, Walter A, Hausen BM, Fuchs Th. Increasing incidence of contact dermatitis to tea tree oil. J Allergy Clin Immunol 2000;105;S43 (abstract 127)
3   Harkenthal M, Hausen BM, Reichling J. 1,2,4-Trihydroxy menthane, a contact allergen from oxidized Australian tea tree oil. Pharmazie 2000;55:153-154 (article in German)
4   Hausen BM, Reichling J, Harkenthal M. Degradation products of monoterpenes are the sensitizing agents in tea tree oil. Am J Contact Dermat 1999;10:68-77
5   Hausen BM. Evaluation of the main contact allergens in oxidized tea tree oil. Dermatitis 2004;15:213-214
6   De Groot AC, Schmidt E. Tea tree oil: contact allergy and chemical composition. Contact Dermatitis 2016;75:129-143
7   De Groot AC, Schmidt E. Essential oils: contact allergy and chemical composition. Boca Raton, Fl., USA: CRC Press, Taylor and Francis Group, 2016 (ISBN 9781482246407)

Chapter 4.16   USNIC ACID

IDENTIFICATION

Description/definition   : Usnic acid is the organic compound that conforms to the formula shown below
Chemical class(es)   : Heterocyclic compounds; phenols
Chemical/IUPAC name   : 2,6-Diacetyl-7,9-dihydroxy-8,9b-dimethyldibenzofuran-1,3-dione
CAS registry number(s)   : 125-46-2
EC number(s)   : 204-740-7
Merck Index monograph : 11348
Function(s) in cosmetics : EU: antimicrobial. USA: cosmetic biocides
Patch testing   : 0.1% pet. (Chemotechnique, SmartPracticeEurope, SmartPracticeCanada)
Molecular formula   : $C_{18}H_{16}O_7$

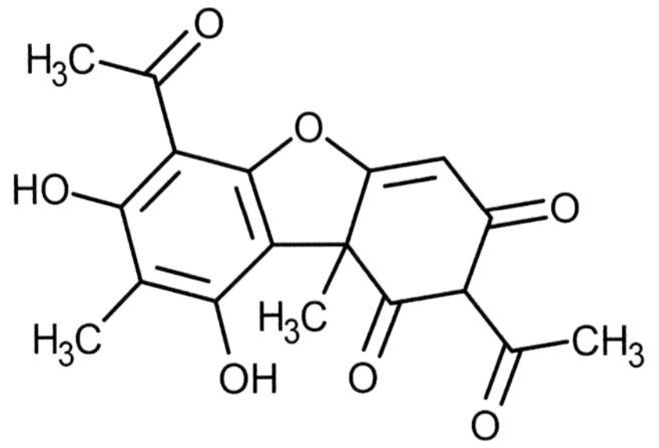

GENERAL

Usnic acid, a lichen acid, is a yellow crystalline solid (www.thegoodscentscompany.com). It is a monobasic acid (dibenzofuran) that accumulates in lichens. In nature, usnic acid occurs in *D-* and *L-*stereoisomers. Usnic acids have antimicrobial properties against bacteria, viruses, fungi, and protozoa (3). These properties have led to their use in personal care products including deodorants, creams, toothpaste, mouthwash, and sunscreens, especially in Europe (13). They also are used in clothing dyes and funeral wreaths. The dye used in litmus paper is derived from lichens (14).

Usnic acid *per se* is not used as a fragrance material, but is discussed here as it is a constituent of botanical products which may be applied in perfumery. It may be present in many lichens (22), including *Evernia prunastri* (oakmoss) but not in *Pseudoevernia furfuracea* (treemoss) (5,6). It is not present in essential oils (7).

Discussion of contact allergy / allergic contact dermatitis to usnic acid, which is probably the main allergen in lichens, is focused on its role in fragrances, relation with oakmoss extract and its use in pharmaceutical products. Literature of contact allergy to usnic acid from contact with lichens in nature, which is often occupational (e.g. 18,20; older literature reviewed in ref. 22) is not discussed here.

The biological properties and toxicity of usnic acid have been reviewed in 2015 (17). See also Chapter 3.67 Evernia prunastri (oakmoss) extract.

CONTACT ALLERGY

General

In human and animal studies, usnic acid has been shown to be a weak sensitizer (22). Contact allergy to usnic acid is caused more frequently by *D-*usnic acid ([+]-) than by its *L-*enantiomer ([-]-)- (19,22), although the latter appears to have stronger sensitizing capacities (22).

Patch testing in groups of patients

Patch testing in consecutive patients suspected of contact dermatitis: routine testing

Studies in which usnic acid was patch tested in consecutive patients suspected of contact dermatitis (routine testing) with positive results have not been found.

Patch testing in groups of selected patients

Before 1987, in Norway, 55 patients with sensitivity to different brands of perfumes, deodorants, aftershave lotions *et cetera* verified by repeated questioning and/or testing, were patch tested with usnic acid 0.1% (vehicle not mentioned) and there were 9 (16%) positive reactions. The relevance of these reactions was not mentioned. Thirty-five of the 55 patients (64%) also reacted to oakmoss absolute, of which usnic acid is an ingredient. The authors concluded that 'the present study has shown that plant extract particularly from lichens are important allergenic constituents in cosmetics' (15).

Case reports and case series

Eight patients developed allergic contact dermatitis of the axillae from usnic acid present in deodorant sprays (1).

Four patients had allergic contact dermatitis from a natural deodorant. Three had axillary dermatitis, the 4th patient developed allergic contact dermatitis of the earlobe after night-time contact with the natural deodorant present on her husband's axilla. All 4 patients reacted to lichen acid mix and D-usnic acid; 3 patients had positive reactions to the natural deodorant that they (or their spouse) were using; the remaining patient was not tested to the cosmetic product. The natural deodorant contained 'lichen extract' as one of its ingredients, but it could not be ascertained that – although likely – the deodorants contained usnic acid or one of the other ingredients of the lichen acid mix, atranorin and evernic acid (14).

A woman developed dermatitis in the genital area, accompanied by fever, from contact allergy to usnic acid in vaginal ovules (2).

Another female patient suffered from a recurrent facial eruption. She had positive patch tests the fragrance mix I and the lichen acid mix; photopatch tests were negative. Testing to the individual ingredients of these mixes demonstrated positive reactions to oakmoss absolute and usnic acid (part of the lichen acid mix and present in oakmoss absolute). The patient now admitted to regular use of fragrances, which matched her history of dermatitis. The constituents of her fragrances were not determined, but avoidance led to clinical resolution. Later, the patient had an acute vesicular flare affecting the face and hands following an afternoon in the garden. She had not used any fragrances but, on this occasion, was aware of exposure to lichens growing on several shrubs (16).

Cross-reactions, pseudo-cross-reactions and co-reactions

Usnic acid is a constituent of oakmoss extract, and co-reactivity can be expected. In 7 patients allergic to oakmoss extract, patch tests were also performed with lichen acids and there were 5 reactions to usnic acid (4). Of 20 patients allergic to oakmoss extract (identified by ingredient testing of the fragrance mix I), 8 co-reacted to usnic acid (11). Of 15 patients allergic to oakmoss absolute, one co-reacted to usnic acid 0.1% pet. (12). Of 10 patients reacting to an acetone extract of oakmoss 7% in petrolatum, 2 co-reacted to D-usnic acid (9).

Of 9 patients reacting to atranorin 0.1% pet. seen in Sweden before 1981, 4 co-reacted to D-usnic acid (8).

Serial dilution testing

Two patients allergic to usnic acid were patch tested with a dilution series of 1% down to 0.001% in petrolatum; they both reacted to all concentrations (10).

OTHER SIDE EFFECTS

Photosensitivity

Photopatch testing in groups of patients

Before 1987, in Norway, 5 patients with sensitivity to different brands of perfumes, deodorants, aftershave lotions et cetera verified by repeated questioning, and/or testing were photopatch tested with usnic acid 0.1% and 0.01% (vehicle not mentioned) and there were 2 (40%) positive reactions. The relevance of these reactions was not mentioned (15).

Case reports

Case reports of photoallergic contact dermatitis from usnic acid have not been found.

LITERATURE

1   Heine A, Tarnick M. Allergisches Kontaktekzem durch Usninsäure in Deodorant Sprays. Derm Monatsschr 1987;173:221-225 (article in German)
2   Rafanelli S, Bacchillga R, Stanganelli I, Rafanelli A. Contact dermatitis from usnic acid in vaginal ovules. Contact Dermatitis 1995;33:271
3   Cocchietto M, Skert N, Nimis PL, Sava G. A review on usnic acid, an interesting natural compound. Naturwissenschaften 2002;89:137-146
4   Thune P, Solberg Y, McFadden N, Stærfeet F, Sandberg M. Perfume allergy due to oak moss and other lichens. Contact Dermatitis 1982;8:396-400
5   Joulain D, Tabacchi R. Lichen extracts as raw materials in perfumery. Part 1: oakmoss. Flavour Fragr J 2009;24:49-61

6   Joulain D, Tabacchi R. Lichen extracts as raw materials in perfumery. Part 2: treemoss. Flavour Fragr J 2009;24:105-116

7   De Groot AC, Schmidt E. Essential oils: contact allergy and chemical composition. Boca Raton, Fl., USA: CRC Press, Taylor and Francis Group, 2016 (ISBN 9781482246407)

8   Dahlquist I, Fregert S. Atranorin and oak moss contact allergy. Contact Dermatitis 1981;7:168-169

9   Fregert S, Dahlquist I. Patch testing with oak moss extract. Contact Dermatitis 1983;9:227

10   Sandberg M, Thune P. The sensitizing capacity of atranorin. Contact Dermatitis 1984;11:168-173

11   Gonçalo S, Cabral F, Gonçalo M. Contact sensitivity to oak moss. Contact Dermatitis 1988;19:355-357

12   Mowitz M, Zimerson E, Svedman C, Bruze M. Patch testing with serial dilutions and thin-layer chromatograms of oak moss absolutes containing high and low levels of atranol and chloroatranol. Contact Dermatitis 2013;69:342-349

13   Ingolfsdottir K. Usnic acid. Phytochemistry 2002;61:729-736

14   Sheu M, Simpson EL, Law SV, Storrs FJ. Allergic contact dermatitis from a natural deodorant: a report of 4 cases associated with lichen acid mix allergy. J Am Acad Dermatol 2006;55:332-337

15   Thune P, Sandberg M. Allergy to lichen and compositae compounds in perfumes. Investigations on the sensitizing, toxic and mutagenic potential. Acta Derm Venereol 1987;134(suppl.):87-89

16   Rademaker M. Allergy to lichen acids in a fragrance. Australas J Dermatol 2000;41:50-51

17   Araújo AA, de Melo MG, Rabelo TK, Nunes PS, Santos SL, Serafini MR, et al. Review of the biological properties and toxicity of usnic acid. Nat Prod Res 2015;29:2167-2180

18   Mitchell JC. Allergic contact dermatitis from usnic acid produced by lichenized fungi. Arch Dermatol 1965;92:142-146

19   Mitchell JC. Stereoisomeric specificity of usnic acid in delayed hypersensitivity. J Invest Dermatol 1966;47:167-168

20   Pacheco D, Travassos AR, Antunes J, Soares de Almeida L, Filipe P, Correia T. Occupational airborne contact dermatitis caused by usnic acid in a domestic worker. Allergol Immunopathol (Madr) 2014;42:80-82

21   Aalto-Korte K, Lauerma A, Alanko K. Occupational allergic contact dermatitis from lichens in present-day Finland. Contact Dermatitis 2005;52:36-38

22   Hausen BM, Emde L, Marks V. An investigation of the allergenic constituents of Cladonia stellaris (Opiz) Pous & Vezda ('silver moss', 'reindeer moss' or 'reindeer lichen'). Contact Dermatitis 1993;28:70-76

Monographs in Contact Allergy, Volume 2
Fragrances and Essential oils

SECTION 3

ESSENTIAL OILS

Chapter 5   ESSENTIAL OILS: GENERAL ASPECTS

5.1 INTRODUCTION

Essential oils are complex substances, which are usually obtained by steam-distillation of plant material. Citrus oils, originating from the peels of *Citrus* species such as grapefruit, lemon, mandarin, orange, or tangerine, are produced by a process called cold-pressing. Essential oils are produced in many parts and countries of the world and are very important trade commodities. It is estimated that essential oils can be obtained from around 30,000 plant species, but, currently, the number of oils produced is limited to approximately 150, of which 70-80 are high-volume products. Essential oils have many applications in foods, beverages, perfumes, and cosmetics. They are also widely employed as pharmacological agents in various forms of medicine, e.g. traditional medicine, folk medicine, Ayurveda and more recently aromatherapy. In the latter form, the oils are usually applied to the skin, but can also be given orally, by inhalation, by distribution through the air or by other means (8,9).

In everyday life man has frequent contact with essential oils or products containing their source materials, e.g., toothpaste, deodorant, perfumes, other cosmetics, oranges, foods flavored with essential oils, spices and plants. Under normal conditions of established use, most oils appear to have a good safety profile. However, toxicity may sometimes occur. The majority of adverse events are mild, but serious toxic reactions have been observed, including abortions or abnormalities in pregnancy, neurotoxicity manifesting as seizures or retardation of infant development, bronchial hyperreactivity and hepatotoxicity. Accidental ingestion by young children has occasionally proved fatal (12). Allergic reactions to essential oils have long been known to occur and are the subject of the Monographs of Essential oils presented in this part of the book.

This introductory chapter provides a brief discussion of what essential oils are, their applications, the chemistry of essential oils and a broad introduction to and survey of various aspects of contact allergy to and allergic contact dermatitis from essential oils. The data in this chapter – with the exception of recent 2015-2018 updated and new data – largely originate from the author's previous articles in the journal *Dermatitis* (2,3,4,5; reproduced and adapted with kind permission of Dr. Ponciano Cruz, Editor-in-Chief of *Dermatitis*) and from a book, written by the author together with Erich Schmidt: De Groot AC, Schmidt E. Essential oils: contact allergy and chemical composition, Boca Raton, Fl., USA: CRC Press, Taylor and Francis Group, 2016 (ISBN 9781482246407) (1). This book provides an extensive discussion of the subjects briefly reviewed in this chapter, other relevant issues (e.g., history of essential oils, production, quality, adulteration *et cetera*) and a full literature review of the chemicals that have been identified in essential oils up to 2015.

The focus in this Essential oils part of the book is on contact allergy / allergic contact dermatitis, which is reviewed up to September 2018. Other side effects, including immediate contact reactions, photosensitivity and systemic reactions from percutaneous absorption, are discussed only when encountered while searching for literature on contact allergy to essential oils, but not reviewed *in extenso*.

5.2 WHAT ARE ESSENTIAL OILS?

An essential oil is defined by the International Organization for Standardization (ISO) as a 'product obtained from a natural raw material of plant origin, by steam-distillation (which includes hydrodistillation), by mechanical processes from the pericarp (peel) of citrus fruits, or by dry distillation, after separation of the aqueous phase - if any - by physical processes' (7). Essential oils may undergo physical treatments, if they do not result in any significant change in its composition, such as filtration, decantation or centrifugation. Citrus oils (bergamot, grapefruit, lemon, mandarin, tangerine, sweet orange, bitter orange) are so-called cold-pressed essential oils; they are obtained by mechanical processes from the peels of the fruit of a citrus. Essential oils should come from one clearly defined plant source and species; breeding, cultivation and harvest must be optimized, production has to be done according to GMP (Good Manufacturing Practices) (10) and they have to fulfill the requirements as laid down in relevant ISO standards.

Sometimes, essential oils undergo one or more physical processes to alter their chemical composition; these are called 'post-treatment essential oils'. One such treatment is fractional distillation, resulting in 'rectified' oils. The objective of post-treatments can be to eliminate certain individual chemicals (e.g., phototoxic furocoumarins [psoralens] from bergamot oil, methyl eugenol from rose oils), lower the concentration of certain fractions, such as the terpenes or sesquiterpenes, to concentrate one or more chemicals or change the color of the essential oil (1,3).

Products obtained from plants which are *not* essential oils

In older literature, but still today, both in the lay press and in scientific literature, the term essential oil is often incorrectly used for a variety of products obtained from plant material by methods other than distillation or cold-pressing, e.g., by solvent extraction, supercritical fluid extraction or simultaneous distillation and extraction. Reports of essential oils that were 'extracted' are by definition wrong. Examples of other products obtained from plant material, which are *not* essential oils, include the following (1,3):

Absolutes are products obtained from concretes, resinoids, supercritical fluid extracts or pomades by extraction with ethanol (alcohol). These products contain all the fragrance compounds, but also some fatty materials. Absolutes are widely used in the fine fragrance industries, notably jasmine and violet leaf absolutes.

Aromatic waters (synonym: hydrolates) are aqueous distillates which remain after steam-distillation of plant material and removal (separation) of the essential oil (e.g., 'rose water').

Concretes are products obtained from fresh plant material by extraction with one or more solvents (usually hexane or supercritical fluids such as CO_2), which are subsequently partly or totally removed. These products are obtained from flowers and other plant material, for which conventional steam-distillation is considered unsuitable, since it induces thermal degradation of many fragrant compounds contained in the plant. Examples include jasmine, narcissus and violet leaves. Concretes are the main source material for the production of absolutes.

Extracts are products obtained from plant biomass by treating them with one or more solvents.

Pomades are fragrant products obtained by a very old method using fat. In cold enfleurage (enfleurage à froid) flowers are pressed into a layer of animal fat for diffusion of the odoriferous compounds of the flower in the fat. Flowers can also be immersed in warm melted fat (enfleurage à chaud). Nowadays, pomades are hardly produced anymore because of very high cost.

Resinoids are products obtained by extracting dry plant material, usually gum resins like myrrh or olibanum, with one or more solvents.

Vegetable oils are oils that consist mainly of fatty acids and their glycerol esters (acylglycerols, glycerides). They are usually obtained by pressing certain plant parts, usually fruits or seeds (including nuts) and sometimes by solvent extraction. Contrary to essential oils they are fixed, non-volatile oils. Many are edible and used for cooking, e.g., coconut, olive, sesame and sunflower oil. Other examples are nut oils such as almond, cashew, hazelnut and walnut oil. Some vegetable oils are used in cosmetics (mainly as emollients and skin-conditioners), for medicinal purposes, as fuel and in a variety of other (industrial) applications, e.g., oil painting and wood finishing.

5.3 WHAT ARE ESSENTIAL OILS USED FOR?
Essential oils have a wide field of applications; examples are shown in table 5.1 (1,3). The largest buyer of essential oils is the flavor industry, making flavors which are widely used by the food, fragrance and cosmetics industries. In the food industry, essential oils and chemicals derived from them are added to a vast array of products including non-alcoholic (fruit juice preparations, flavored waters, many other soft drinks) and alcoholic beverages, and foods (e.g., milk drinks, yoghurt, candies, chocolate, quick meals, baking mixtures, meats, sausages, teas, and even spices and herbs) for flavoring purposes. Essential oils may also be added to foods (e.g., to meat) for (longer) preservation and are widely employed by the tobacco industry (1,3). Another major application of essential oils is in perfumes (perfume, eau de parfum, eau de toilette, eau de cologne), cosmetics, household products such as detergents, softeners, cleaning products and other consumer commodities including room scents, candles, incense and bouquets (a bouquet is a potpourri existing of dried flowers, barks and leaves, perfumed by adding perfume mixtures supplied separately).

Table 5.1 Examples of essential oils applications (1,3)

Flavor industry: flavors for the food industry
Food industry: soft drinks, foods, alcoholic beverages, spices, herbs, tea, food preservation
Fragrance industry: perfumes, fragrances for other products
Cosmetics industry
Household products: detergents, softeners, room scents, candles, incense
Tobacco industry: cigarettes
Medicinal use: folk medicine, traditional medicine, phytotherapy, balneotherapy, aromatherapy
Pharmaceutical industry: masking agent
Animal food

Essential oils are often incorporated to give the desired scent to cosmetics products and fragrances. In general, fragrances contain between 5 and 10% of essential oils. Most commonly used are orange, bergamot, lemon, lavender, patchouli, and cedarwood oils. Spice oils are employed in small concentrations and others in traces. Expensive oils are only used in fine fragrances (1,3). However, essential oils are also employed as 'masking fragrance', to mask the smell of certain cosmetic ingredients such as fatty acids, lipid balancing bases, aqueous plant extracts, fatty oils and surfactants. All cosmetics can be presumed to contain fragrances, unless they are specifically labeled as 'fragrance-free', 'contains no perfume', 'non-scented' or have similar indications. However, even then, they may sometimes contain (masking) fragrance materials (11).

Essential oils are also widely employed to promote health and combat diseases, e.g., in forms of traditional and folk medicine, phytotherapy (the use of extracts of natural origin as medicines or health-promoting agents) and aromatherapy. Aromatherapy, which appears to be gaining in popularity, has been defined by aromatherapy and essential oils book authors as 'The therapeutic application of essential oils and aromatic plant extracts in a holistic context, to maintain or improve physical, emotional and mental well-being' (8), 'the use of essential oils, applied topically, orally, by inhalation or by other means, to promote health, hygiene and psychological wellbeing' (12) or - more shortly - 'the therapeutic use of essential oils' (9).

Essential oils are also used in animal feeding (13). It may be employed as appetizer and for preservation purposes, as certain essential oils, that contain high concentrations of carvacrol such as origanum and thyme oil, have been shown to have antimicrobial effects (6). Herbs and essential oils may, according to some authors, even be able to partly substitute antibiotic growth promoters (14).

5.4 CHEMISTRY OF ESSENTIAL OILS

5.4.1 General

Essential oils are multi-component mixtures; in individual oil samples, over a hundred chemicals may be identified or even more, when sophisticated analytical equipment and the proper detection methods are used (1,4). The largest group of chemicals found in essential oils consists of terpenes. Terpenes are hydrocarbon chemicals produced from five-carbon isoprene units (C_5H_8). From these units, numerous molecules can be constructed in biosynthesis, both linear-chained chemicals and molecules with one or more ring structures. There are several classes of terpenes based on their number of isoprene units; in essential oils, the most important ones are the monoterpenes and the sesquiterpenes. Monoterpenes possess 10 carbon atoms and are built from two isoprene units ($C_{10}H_{16}$) which can form various carbon skeletons. There are three forms of monoterpenes: linear (acyclic), monocyclic and bicyclic.

Sesquiterpenes possess 15 carbon atoms; they are built form three isoprene units ($C_{15}H_{24}$) and may occur in acyclic, monocyclic, bicyclic and tricyclic forms. These are the terpenes with higher boiling temperatures. Mono- and sesquiterpenes are the main components in essential oils, sesquiterpenes comprising about 25% of the terpene fraction. Volatility and the typical odor of essential oils are created through both groups. Chemical modification of terpenes and sesquiterpenes, e.g., by rearranging carbon skeletons or by oxidation, produces compounds generally termed terpenoids. The oxidation products are the most important, creating subgroups like alcohols, aldehydes, phenols, ethers and ketones. Infrequently, during biosynthesis, functional groups like sulfur or nitrogen are bond to or integrated in the carbon skeleton (1,4).

The most important chemical classes and some examples of compounds belonging to the various groups found in essential oils are show in table 5.2 (1,4).

Table 5.2 Chemical classes of compounds present in essential oils with examples (1,4)

Chemical class	Examples of chemicals from this class
Terpenes	
Acyclic terpenes	Myrcene, (*E*)-ocimene, (*Z*)-ocimene
Monocyclic monoterpenes	*p*-Cymene, α-fenchene, limonene, β-phellandrene, α-terpinene, γ-terpinene, terpinolene
Bicyclic monoterpenes	Camphene, δ3-carene, α-pinene, β-pinene, sabinene, α-thujene
Tricyclic monoterpenes	Tricyclene
Acyclic sesquiterpenes	α-Farnesene, (*E,E*)-α-farnesene, (*E*)-β-farnesene,
Monocyclic sesquiterpenes	α-Bisabolene, β-bisabolene, curcumene, β-elemene, α-humulene, α-zingiberene
Bicyclic sesquiterpenes	α-Cadinene, γ-cadinene, δ-cadinene, β-caryophyllene, β-selinene, valencene
Tricyclic sesquiterpenes	Aromadendrene, β-bourbonene, α-cedrene, β-cedrene, α-gurjunene, β-gurjunene, α-patchoulene, β-patchoulene, α-santalene, viridiflorene
Alcohols	
Monocyclic monoterpene alcohols	(*Z*)-Carveol, menthol, pulegol, terpineol
Bicyclic monoterpene alcohols	Borneol, myrtenol, pinocarveol, verbenol (*cis*- and *trans*-)
Monocyclic sesquiterpene alcohols	α-Bisabolol, β-bisabolol, γ-bisabolol, elemol, lanceol
Tricyclic sesquiterpene alcohols	Patchoulol, α-santalol, β-santalol, viridiflorol
Acyclic monoterpene alcohols	Citronellol, geraniol, lavandulol, linalool, nerol
Bicyclic sesquiterpene alcohols	α-Cadinol, δ-cadinol, τ-cadinol, chrysanthemol, α-eudesmol, β-eudesmol, γ-eudesmol, 10-epi-γ-eudesmol, α-muurolol, τ-muurolol
Aromatic alcohols	Benzyl alcohol, cinnamyl alcohol, 2-phenethyl alcohol

Table 5.2 Chemical classes of compounds present in essential oils with examples (1,4) (continued)

Chemical class	Examples of chemicals from this class
Aldehydes	
Bicyclic monoterpene aldehydes	Myrtenal
Bicyclic sesquiterpene aldehydes	Isovalencenal, zizanal
Aromatic aldehydes	Benzaldehyde, cinnamal ((*E*)-, (*Z*)-), cuminaldehyde, vanillin
Acyclic monoterpene aldehydes	Citronellal, geranial, neral
Ketones	
Monocyclic monoterpene ketones	Carvone, menthone, piperitone, pulegone
Bicyclic terpene ketones	Camphor (α-camphor, *d*-camphor, *dl*-camphor), fenchone
Bicyclic sesquiterpene ketones	(*E,E*)-Germacrone, khushimone, nootkatone, valeranone, α-vetivone, β-vetivone
Others	
Acids	Geranic acid, isovaleric acid, zizanoic (khusenic) acid
Acyclic monoterpene esters	Citronellyl acetate, geranyl acetate, linalyl acetate, neryl acetate, terpinyl acetate
Aromatic esters	(*Z*)-Methylcinnamate, methyl salicylate
Monocyclic monoterpene phenols	Carvacrol, eugenol, thymol
Oxides	Bisabolol oxide A, bisabolol oxide B, 1,8-cineole (eucalyptol), linalool oxide (*cis-*, *trans-*, furanoid, pyranoid), menthofuran
Phenolic ethers	(*E*)-Anethole, (*Z*)-anethole, methyl chavicol (estragole), safrole

The composition of essential oils can vary considerably from country to country, from producer to producer, and even from year to year for the same producer and crop. Factors that may influence the oils' chemical composition include plant parameters (e.g., species, cultivated or wild plants, chemotype), environmental parameters (e.g., origin of plant, climate, soil conditions, fertilization), harvest and post-harvest / pre-distillation parameters (e.g., season of harvest, pretreatment of biomass, storage conditions of source plant material), production parameters (e.g., mode of production, distillation parameters, commercial oil or laboratory-produced), and other parameters (e.g., storage condition and storage time of essential oils, age of essential oil, aging by exposure to oxygen and ultraviolet light, analytical parameters) (1,3).

5.4.2 Chemicals identified in essential oils
In a literature review of contact allergy to and chemical composition of essential oils, approximately 4,350 chemicals were found to have been identified in 93 essential oils and jasmine absolutes that have caused contact allergy (1,4). Many chemicals are present in a large number of oils. Ninety of them have been identified in at least 40 of the 93 (43%) essential oils. In fact, 23 (25%) are present in >80% of all oils, and 6 (7%) may be components of >90% of all oils, with scores of 97% for limonene and 98% for β-caryophyllene (table 5.3) (1,4). This means that many essential oils have many ingredients in common. Of the 23 that are present in >80% of the oils, 14 (61%) have been reported to cause contact allergy (from any source). The presence of these chemicals in a large number of oils may be one explanation for the fact that allergic patients often react to more than one or even a large number of essential oils. This is usually termed cross-reactivity, but, in the case of positive patch test reactions caused by contact allergy to common ingredients, we prefer the term pseudo-cross-reactivity (1,4).

Conversely, many of the 4,350 chemicals have been identified in only one (55%) or a few oils. Sometimes, these are part of specific essential oils, which have a characteristic composition much unlike most other oils. Examples include calamus oil, chamomile oil (both German and Roman), costus root oil, guaiacwood oil, lovage oil, myrrh oil, sandalwood oil, valerian oil, vetiver oil and zdravetz oil. However, many of the chemicals found in *one oil only* (including a large number of components of spike lavender oils and lavender oils) were also identified in *one study only*, probably indicating that a number of these have been incorrectly identified, especially in older studies when analytical equipment was less sophisticated and reliable than at the present time (1,4).

5.4.3 Number of chemicals in essential oils
The (approximate) number of chemicals identified by chemical analysis in essential oils (types of oil that have caused contact allergy) varies considerably (1,4). On the low end of the spectrum are guaiacwood oil (25 chemicals identified), clove stem oil (n=35), cedarwood oil Texas (n=45), elemi oil (n=45), cedarwood oil Virginia (n=55), cedar-

Table 5.3 Chemicals which are present in at least 50% of 93 reviewed essential oils and absolutes (1,4)

Chemical	% Oils [a]	CA [b]	Chemical	% Oils [a]	CA [b]
β-Caryophyllene	98%	+	β-Selinene	70%	
Limonene	97%	+	Linalyl acetate	67%	+
α-Pinene	94%	+	α-Muurolene	67%	
α-Terpineol	94%	+	(E)-Nerolidol	67%	+
δ-Cadinene	91%		Spathulenol	66%	
α-Humulene	91%		γ-Muurolene	65%	
p-Cymene	89%	+	Nerol	65%	+
Linalool	88%	+	Bornyl acetate	63%	
Myrcene	87%	+	τ-Cadinol	63%	
Sabinene	87%	+	α-Cubebene	63%	
Camphene	86%		(E)-β-Farnesene	63%	
trans-Caryophyllene oxide	86%	+	β-Phellandrene	63%	
Terpinen-4-ol	86%	+	Aromadendrene	62%	+
1,8-Cineole (eucalyptol)	85%	+	Eugenol	59%	+
γ-Terpinene	85%		trans-α-Bergamotene	57%	
γ-Cadinene	84%		Bicyclogermacrene	57%	
β-Pinene	83%	+	α-Cadinol	56%	
α-Terpinene	83%	+	Citronellol	56%	+
Terpinolene	83%	+	β-Cubebene	56%	
Germacrene D	82%		trans-Sabinene hydrate	56%	
α-Copaene	81%		α-Selinene	55%	
(E)-β-Ocimene	81%		Carvacrol	54%	+
α-Thujene	81%		α-Terpinyl acetate	54%	+
β-Elemene	77%		Carvone	53%	+
δ3-Carene	76%	+	p-Cymen-8-ol	53%	
(Z)-β-Ocimene	76%		Neryl acetate	53%	
dl-Camphor	73%	+	p-Cymenene	52%	
Geranyl acetate	73%	+	Methyl eugenol	52%	+
α-Phellandrene	73%	+	Geranial	51%	+
Borneol	72%		α-Gurjunene	51%	
β-Bisabolene	70%		cis-Sabinene hydrate	51%	
Geraniol	70%	+			

[a] Percentage of 93 essential oils and absolutes in which the chemical may be present
[b] Contact allergy to this chemical has been reported (from any source, not necessarily from essential oils)

wood oil Himalaya (n=60), rosewood oil (n=60) and neem oil (n=65). For most of these, this can be explained by the small number of published analytical reports (n=2-5). In the majority of essential oils, the number of identified components ranges from 100-250. Thirteen oils had 250-300 chemical identifications, ten ranged from 300 to 400 and five oils scored 400-500 identified chemicals (table 5.4) (1,4). At the high end of the spectrum finally, in geranium oil some 500 chemicals have been identified and 505 in rosemary essential oils.

Table 5.4 Number of chemicals identified in essential oils and percentage found in one study only (1,4) [a]

Essential oil	Nr. Chem. [b]	% Single [c]	Essential oil	Nr. Chem. [b]	% Single [c]
Rosemary oil	505	53%	Orange oil sweet	335	NK
Geranium oil	500	60%	Peppermint oil	335	59%
Lavender oil	450	64%	Valerian oil	330	50%
Vetiver oil	445	55%	Thyme oil	325	50%
Rose oil	440	56%	Carrot seed oil	315	60%
Basil oil sweet	435	53%	Melissa oil	310	49%
Laurel leaf oil	425	54%	Sage oil Dalmatian	310	47%
Spike lavender oil	395	63%	Black pepper oil	305	58%
Black cumin oil	340	62%			

[a] Only oils with >300 identified components are listed here; [b] Number of chemicals found in the essential oil by chemical analyses
[c] Percentage of chemicals which were identified in one analytical study only; NK Not Known; the percentage of chemicals found in one study only cannot be calculated, as a result of the data collection method

Of these components in oils containing over 300 ingredients, 47-64% have been identified in one study only (table 5.4) (1,4). Such high percentages of 'unique, one-time-only' chemicals were also found in most other essential oils (generally 40-60%). These chemicals may well be genuine, for example in laboratory-prepared oils from plant material collected in the wild or in one or more oil samples analyzed in-depth with highly sophisticated analytical equipment, for example nitrogen-containing compounds in particular fractions of the oil. However, it may be assumed that, in many cases, these unique chemicals are in fact artefacts caused by botanical misinterpretation (wrong biomass), incorrectly prepared oils, misidentification of small peaks in chromatograms or by other causes. Some data have been generated over 30 years ago when analytical results were far less reliable than they are now. But even today, many reports are of rather poor quality and incorrect interpretation of analytical results appears to be by no means rare.

5.4.4 The major chemicals in specific essential oils

In most essential oils, there are two to five components which together constitute over 50-60% of the oil. The 'Top-10' ingredients of each essential oil, as shown by analyses of commercial essential oil samples, are shown in the individual essential oil chapters.

In some oils, however, there is one dominant ingredient that always constitutes >50% (wt./wt.) of the product. In 6,350 samples of 91 commercial essential oils and two jasmine absolutes, investigated by GC-MS between 1998 and 2014, thirteen such dominant components were found in 26 oils (table 5.5) (1,4). Limonene is highly dominant in all *Citrus* essential oils with maximum concentrations of >95% in grapefruit, orange (both bitter and sweet) and tangerine oils. Aniseed oils may contain up to 99% (*E*)-anethole and clove oils up to 90% eugenol (1,4).

Table 5.5 Chemicals which are dominant ingredients (>50%) in essential oils (1,4)

Dominant chem.[a]	Conc. range [b]	Essential oil	Dominant Chem.[a]	Conc. Range[b]	Essential oil
(*E*)-Anethole	91-99%	Aniseed oil	Limonene (cont.)	54-73%	Lemon oil
	84-90%	Star anise oil		64-76%	Mandarin oil
Carvone	61-82%	Spearmint oil		92-96%	Orange oil bitter
1,8-Cineole	62-89%	Eucalyptus globulus oil		95-96%	Orange oil sweet
(*E*)-Cinnamal	75-83%	Cassia oil		82-98%	Tangerine oil
	43-72%	Cinnamon bark oil	Linalool	55-81%	Coriander fruit oil
Citronellal	69-84%	Eucalyptus citriodora oil		73-88%	Rosewood oil
			β-Phellandrene	52-76%	Angelica fruit oil
Eugenol	72-82%	Cinnamon leaf oil	α-Pinene	>80%	Angelica root oil (Indian)
	82-92%	Clove bud oil			
	76-89%	Clove leaf oil		57-74%	Turpentine oil Chinese
	87-90%	Clove stem oil		68-82%	Turpentine oil Iberian
Geraniol	74-87%	Palmarosa oil	β-Pinene	51-81%	Galbanum resin oil
Limonene	81-96%	Grapefruit oil	α-Thujone	50-66%	Thuja oil

[a] Dominant chemical; [b] Concentration range; cont. continued

5.5 CONTACT ALLERGY TO AND ALLERGIC CONTACT DERMATITIS FROM ESSENTIAL OILS

Dermatologists interested in contact allergy have been confronted in increasing frequency with allergic reactions to essential oils in the recent past. This development may be explained by increasing use of essential oils on the skin and the availability of commercial patch test preparations, which stimulates more liberal patch testing of essential oils in selected patients or in routine testing. In the USA, for example, four essential oils (tea tree oil, lavender oil, peppermint oil, ylang-ylang oil) and one absolute (jasmine absolute) are currently present in the screening series of the North American Contact Dermatitis Group (NACDG) (15). This inevitably results in more cases of contact allergy to essential oils being detected. Additionally, there is increased awareness of possible allergic reactions to essential oils, resulting from for example the large number of publications on tea tree oil allergy.

Seventy-eight essential oils have caused contact allergy (as demonstrated by positive patch test reactions) or allergic contact dermatitis (table 5.6) (1,2). All these oils and jasmine absolute, which is included because there are many reports of contact allergy to this material, are discussed in separate chapters. For some oils, only one or two reports on contact allergy are available. For others, however, there is a considerable amount of literature on contact allergy and allergic contact dermatitis, e.g., in the cases of tea tree oil, ylang-ylang oil, lavender oil, peppermint oil, jasmine absolute, geranium oil, rose oil, turpentine oil and sandalwood oil. Due to the selection criterion (contact allergy reported), the group of 78 oils is very heterogeneous. Some are high volume essential oils, such as orange oil and lemon oil, others are produced and commercialized in very small quantities, e.g., zdravetz oil. Costus root oil may apparently still be used in aromatherapy (9), but has been prohibited by IFRA (International Fragrance Association) for use in fragrances and cosmetics since decades because of its sensitizing properties. Others are prohibited or restricted by governmental regulations and laws, as in the case of rosewood oil, guaiacwood oil and East Indian sandalwood oil, which are produced from endangered species of trees (1,2).

Table 5.6 List of essential oils and jasmine absolutes with botanical sources, plant part(s) used and ISO numbers [b]

Common name		Botanical source(s)	Part(s) of plant used	ISO [a]
Angelica oil	- fruit	*Angelica archangelica* L.	Fruit	
	- root	*Angelica archangelica* L.	Rhizome and root	
Aniseed oil		*Pimpinella anisum* L.	Fruit	3475
Basil oil sweet		*Ocimum basilicum* L.	Flowering aerial top	11043
Bay oil		*Pimenta racemosa* (Mill.) J.W. Moore	Leaf	3045
Bergamot oil		*Citrus bergamia* (Risso et Poit.)	Pericarp (peel)	3520
Bitter almond oil		*Prunus dulcis* (Mill.) D. A. Webb. (*Prunus amygdalus* var. *amara*)	Fruit kernel	
Black cumin oil		*Nigella sativa* L.	Seed	
Black pepper oil		*Piper nigrum* L.	Fruit	3061
Cajeput oil		*Melaleuca cajuputi* Powell	Leaf, terminal branchlet	
Calamus oil		*Acorus calamus* L.	Rhizome	
Cananga oil		*Cananga odorata* (Lam.) Hook f. et Thomson, forma *macrophylla*	Flower	3523
Cardamom oil		*Elettaria cardamomum* (L.) Maton	Fruit	4733
Carrot seed oil		*Daucus carota* L.	Fruit	
Cassia oil	- bark	*Cinnamomum cassia* (Nees & T. Nees) J.Presl	Bark	3216
	- leaf	*Cinnamomum cassia* (Nees & T. Nees) J.Presl	Leaf	
Cedarwood oil	- Atlas	*Cedrus atlantica* (Endl.) G. Manetti ex Carrière	Wood	
	- China	*Cupressus funebris* (Endl.)	Wood	9843
	- Himalaya	*Cedrus deodara* (Roxb. ex D.Don) G.Don	Wood	
	- Texas	*Juniperus ashei* J. Buchholz	Wood	4725
	- Virginia	*Juniperus virginiana* L.	Wood	4724
Chamomile oil	- German	*Chamomilla recutita* (L.) Rauschert	Flowering tops	19332
	- Roman	*Chamaemelum nobile* (L.)	Flowering tops	
Cinnamon oil	- bark	*Cinnamomum zeylanicum* Blume	Twig and bark of stem	
	- leaf	*Cinnamomum zeylanicum* Blume	Leaf	3524
Citronella oil	- Java	*Cymbopogon winterianus* Jowitt.	Aerial part (leaves)	3848
	- Sri Lanka	*Cymbopogon nardus* (L.) Rendle	Aerial part (leaves)	3849
Clary sage oil		*Salvia sclarea* L.	Flowering top, leaf	
Clove oil	- bud	*Syzygium aromaticum* (L.) Merr. & L.M. Perry	Bud	3142
	- leaf	*Syzygium aromaticum* (L.) Merr. & L.M. Perry	Leaf	3141
	- stem	*Syzygium aromaticum* (L.) Merr. & L.M. Perry	Stem	3143
Coriander fruit oil		*Coriandrum sativum* L.	Fruit	3516
Costus root oil		*Saussurea costus* (Falc.) Lipsch.	Root	
Cypress oil		*Cupressus sempervirens* L.	Twig with leaves	20809
Dwarf pine oil		*Pinus mugo* Turra	Leaf, terminal branchlets	21093
Elemi oil		*Canarium luzonicum* (Blume) A. Gray	Wood exudate	10624
Eucalyptus oil	- globulus	*Eucalyptus globulus* Labill.	Leaf, terminal branch	770
	- citriodora	*Corymbia citriodora* (Hook.) K.D. Hill & L.A.S. Johnson	Leaf, terminal branch	3044
Galbanum resin oil		*Ferula gummosa* Boiss.	Root exudate	40716
Geranium oil		*Pelargonium* x spp.	Herbaceous part	4731
Ginger oil		*Zingiber officinale* Roscoe.	Rhizome	16928
Grapefruit oil		*Citrus paradisi* Macfad.	Pericarp (peel)	3053
Guaiacwood oil		*Bulnesia sarmientoi* Lorentz ex Griseb.	Wood	
Hinoki oil		*Chamaecyparis obtusa* (Siebold & Zucc.) Endl.	Wood	
Hyssop oil		*Hyssopus officinalis* L. ssp. *officinalis*	Flowering top and leaf	9841
Jasmine abs.	- grandiflorum	*Jasminum grandiflorum* L.	Flower	
	- sambac	*Jasminum sambac* (L.) Aiton.	Flower	
Juniper berry oil		*Juniperus communis* L.	Fruit, terminal branchlets	8897
Laurel leaf oil		*Laurus nobilis* L.	Leaf	
Lavandin oil	- lavandin oil	*Lavandula angustifolia* Mill. x *Lavandula latifolia* Medik.	Flowering top	
	- Abrial	*Lavandula angustifolia* Mill. x *Lavandula latifolia* Medik. 'Abrial'	Flowering top	3054
	- Grosso	*Lavandula angustifolia* Mill. x *Lavandula latifolia* Medik. 'Grosso'	Flowering top	8902
Lavender oil		*Lavandula angustifolia* Mill.	Flowering top	3515
Lemon oil		*Citrus limon* (L.) Burm. f.	Pericarp (peel)	855
Lemongrass oil	- East Indian	*Cymbopogon flexuosus* (Nees ex Steudel) J.F. Watson	Aerial part (leaves)	4718
	- West Indian	*Cymbopogon citratus* (DC) Stapf.	Whole aerial part (leaves)	3217
Litsea cubeba oil		*Litsea cubeba* (Lour) Pers.	Fruit	3214
Lovage oil		*Levisticum officinale* W.D.J. Koch	Root	11019
Mandarin oil		*Citrus reticulata* Blanco	Pericarp (peel)	3528

Table 5.6 List of essential oils and jasmine absolutes with botanical sources, plant part(s) used and ISO numbers [b] (continued)

Common name		Botanical source(s)	Part(s) of plant used	ISO [a]
Marjoram oil sweet		*Origanum majorana* L.	Flowering top	
Melissa oil (lemon balm oil)		*Melissa officinalis* L.	Aerial parts	
Myrrh oil		*Commiphora myrrha* (Nees) Engl. and related *Commiphora* species	Wood exudate	
Neem oil		*Azadirachta indica* A. Juss.	Seed	
Neroli oil		*Citrus aurantium* L.	Flower	3517
Niaouli oil		*Melaleuca quinquenervia* (Cav.) S.T. Blake	Leaves, terminal branchlets	
Nutmeg oil		*Myristica fragrans* Houtt.	Seed	3215
Olibanum (frankincense) oil		*Boswellia sacra* Flueck.	Wood exudate	
Orange oil	- bitter	*Citrus aurantium* L.	Pericarp (peel)	9844
	- sweet	*Citrus sinensis* (L.) Osbeck	Pericarp (peel)	3140
Oregano oil		*Origanum vulgare* L. subsp. *hirtum* (Link) letsw.	Leaves with flowers	13171
Palmarosa oil		*Cymbopogon martini* (Roxb.) Will. Watson	Aerial part (leaves)	4727
Patchouli oil		*Pogostemon cablin* (Blanco) Benth.	Leaf	3757
Peppermint oil		*Mentha* x *piperita* L.	Aerial parts, leaf	856
Petitgrain bigarade oil		*Citrus aurantium* L.	Leaf, twig, little green fruit	8901
Pine needle oil (Scots pine oil)		*Pinus sylvestris* L.	Needle, twig	
Ravensara oil		*Ravensara aromatica* Sonn.	Twig with leaves	
Rosemary oil		*Rosmarinus officinalis* L.	Flowering top, leaf	1342
Rose oil		*Rosa* x *damascena* Mill.	Flower	9842
Rosewood oil		*Aniba rosaeodora* Ducke, *Aniba parviflora* (Meisn.) Mez.	Wood	3761
Sage oil	- Dalmatian	*Salvia officinalis* L.	Flowering top	9909
	- Spanish	*Salvia lavandulifolia* Vahl	Flowering top	3526
Sandalwood oil	- East India	*Santalum album* L.	Wood	3518
	- Australia	*Santalum spicatum* (R. Br.) A.DC.	Wood	22769
	- New Caledonia	*Santalum austrocaledonicum* Vieill.	Wood	
Silver fir oil		*Abies alba* Mill.	Needles	
Spearmint oil		*Mentha spicata* L.	Flowering aerial part, leaf	3033
Spike lavender oil		*Lavandula latifolia* Medik.	Flowering top	4719
Spruce oil (black)		Unknown: can be obtained from various species	Leaves (needles) with twigs	
Star anise oil		*Illicium verum* Hook. f.	Fruit	11016
Tangerine oil		*Citrus tangerina* Hort. ex Tan.	Peel	
Tea tree oil		*Melaleuca alternifolia* (Maiden et Betche) Cheel; *Melaleuca linariifolia* Smith; *Melaleuca dissitiflora* F. Muell.	Leaf, terminal branchlet	4730
Thuja oil		*Thuja occidentalis* L.	Twig with leaves	
Thyme oil	- thyme oil	*Thymus vulgaris* L.	Flowering top	
	- Spanish	*Thymus zygis* L.	Flowering top	14715
Turmeric oil		*Curcuma longa* L.	Rhizomes	
Turpentine oil	- Iberian	*Pinus pinaster* Aiton	Oleoresin	11020
	- Chinese	*Pinus massoniana* Lamb.	Oleoresin	21389
Valerian oil		*Valeriana officinalis* L.	Rhizome, root	
Vetiver oil		*Chrysopogon zizanioides* (L.) Roberty	Root	4716
Ylang-ylang oil		*Cananga odorata* (Lam.) Hook f. et Thomson, forma *genuina*	Flower	3063
Zdravetz oil		*Geranium macrorrhizum* L.	Aerial part	

[a] Number of ISO standard; International Organization for Standardization, Geneva, Switzerland, www.iso.org
[b] Adapted from refs. 1 and 2

Of the79 oils (from here on jasmine absolute is termed 'oil' for convenience sake), 45 have been tested in groups of consecutive patients suspected of contact dermatitis. Testing in groups of *selected* patients has been performed with 53 essential oils, usually in patients suspected of fragrance allergy, of cosmetic dermatitis, or patients who previously had a positive reaction to the fragrance mix I or to one of the other indicators of fragrance allergy such as Myroxylon pereirae resin (balsam of Peru). Case reports and case seriess of allergic contact dermatitis were found for 68 oils.

Contact allergy to fourteen oils was mentioned in one publication only; more extensive literature is available for oils of cananga, clove, eucalyptus, geranium, jasmine, lavender, lemon, lemongrass, peppermint, rose, sandalwood, spearmint, turpentine, tea tree and ylang-ylang. Most case report publications (with one or more patients described) were found for tea tree oil (n=35), followed by oils of lavender (n=26), peppermint (n=21), geranium (n=15), turpentine (n=12, not fully reviewed), spearmint (n=11), ylang-ylang (n=10), eucalyptus (n=10), lemongrass (n=9), lemon (n=9) and cananga, clove, eucalyptus, jasmine absolute and rose oils (8 publications each).

5.5.1 Frequency of contact allergy to essentials oils

For the frequency of contact allergy to essential oils, prevalence rates of positive patch test reactions, tested in consecutive patients suspected of contact dermatitis, can be used as an indication. Of the 45 essential oils that have been tested in consecutive patients (number of studies per oil ranging from one to 19), ten have had maximum rates of positive patch test reactions between 1% and 1.5% and in another ten, rates of over 2% have been observed. These are, in order of descending maximum values, laurel oil 6.9% (old data, cited in ref. 19), turpentine oil 4.2%, orange oil 3.2%, lavender oil (oxidized) 2.8%, tea tree oil 2.7%, citronella oil 2.5%, ylang-ylang oil 2.6%, sandalwood oil 2.4%, clove oil 2.1% and costus root oil 2.1% (historical allergen).

Thus, it appears that contact allergy to essential oils as a group is not very frequent. Nevertheless, in the general German adult population, 2.5% of 1141 test subjects reacted to oil of turpentine, 4.3% of the women and 0.7% of the men (20). Currently, the highest observed prevalences of positive patch test reactions – depending of the country and which oils are patch tested – are observed with tea tree oil, ylang-ylang oil and sandalwood oil. The latter observation is surprizing, because the price of sandalwood oil is so high that it is virtually only used in fine fragrances.

5.5.2 Clinical relevance of positive patch test reactions to essential oils

Determining the clinical relevance of positive patch test reactions to essential oils appears to be difficult. In many studies presenting results of patch testing with essential oils, no relevance data were provided. The NACDG provides relevance data for the essential oils which are included in the NACDG screening series (22). Percentages for 'definite' + 'probable' relevance in various NACDG studies were as follows: lavender oil 30-69%, tea tree oil 20-56%, peppermint oil 22-39%, jasmine absolute 14-37% and ylang-ylang oil 0-27%. Rates for 'definite' relevance were usually <10-15% and sometimes zero.

This indicates that, in the majority of cases of positive patch test reactions, no source of contact with the oil can be found. Indeed, the oils or their ingredients can be present in a large array of applications and are often 'hidden' in products where no details on composition are available, e.g., in perfumes or in household products. Reliable data on the relevance of positive patch test reactions to essential oils as reported in literature are therefore largely lacking or inadequate. Insufficient knowledge of the chemical composition of essential oils and difficulties in ascertaining whether oils or their ingredients are present in materials with which the patients have contact, may partly be responsible. In addition, a previously acquired contact allergy to a fragrance chemical *per se* may result in a positive patch test to an essential oil containing it. Thus, previous sensitization to geraniol from any source may result in non-relevant positive patch test reactions to rose oil and geranium oil, both of which contain high concentrations of geraniol (23). Previously acquired contact allergy to limonene has resulted in non-relevant positive patch tests to tea tree oil (24).

5.5.3 Products responsible for allergic contact dermatitis from essential oils

The categories of products most frequently responsible for allergic contact dermatitis from essential oils are shown in table 5.7 (1,5).

Table 5.7 Categories of products most frequently responsible for allergic contact dermatitis from essential oils [a]

Product category	Causative essential oils reported / products
Pure essential oils	Black cumin, citronella, hinoki, laurel, lavender, lovage, neem, patchouli, peppermint, tea tree
Massage products	Mostly occupational allergic contact dermatitis to a large number of essential oils
Cosmetic products	Angelica root, black cumin, citronella, eucalyptus, geranium, jasmine absolute, laurel, lavender, lemon, neroli, niaouli, orange, peppermint, rose, tea tree, ylang-ylang
Toothpastes and other oral preparations	Aniseed, cassia, cinnamon, cloves, laurel, peppermint, spearmint
Pharmaceutical products	Cinnamon, dwarf pine, eucalyptus, geranium, laurel, lavender, neroli, pine needle, Roman chamomile, rose, sandalwood, tea tree, thyme, peppermint
Other products	Immersion oil, mud bath, aromatherapy lamps, wax polish

[a] Adapted from refs. 1 and 5

Pure oils are usually applied to the skin for alleged therapeutic actions. This is certainly the case with tea tree oil; overt 100 patients with allergic contact dermatitis from tea tree oil have been described in case reports, mostly by the application of neat oil. A separate category of patients who become sensitized to pure oils or diluted oils in high concentrations is that of people who have frequent contact with such products at work, e.g. aromatherapists and masseurs. Many such cases of occupational contact dermatitis to essential oils have been described. Essential oils are also widely used in cosmetic products and the development of allergic cosmetic dermatitis from them has been reported in 23 publications. However, related to their widespread use, the role of cosmetics in essential oil contact allergy is modest.

Although toothpastes are diluted under normal use circumstances and the contact time with the oral mucosa, lips, and perioral skin is short, essential oils in these products have been reported to cause contact allergic reactions repeatedly (26). Essential oils in topical pharmaceutical preparations are mostly used as masking fragrance, not as active ingredient. Sensitization is facilitated by application of these products on damaged skin (27).

5.5.4 Clinical picture of allergic contact dermatitis from essential oils

There are no descriptions of the clinical picture of allergic contact dermatitis from essential oils in larger groups of patients. As the products in which the oils may be present vary considerably, as do the sites of application and the goals of applying the oils to the skin, the presentation of patients with allergic contact dermatitis from essential oils may take various forms.

Undiluted oils may be applied for therapeutic purposes, notably tea tree oil and eucalyptus oil. Dermatitis will appear at the site of application and may stay limited to the primary site, but spreading of dermatitis is not infrequent and even generalisation occurs occasionally (1). The same applies to topical pharmaceutical products. In a group of 127 patients with iatrogenic allergic contact dermatitis from essential oils and other fragrances in topical pharmaceutical drugs, women were more frequently affected than men, and legs, hands, and face were the most commonly affected body sites (27).

Essential oils are frequently added to toothpastes, especially spearmint, peppermint and cinnamon oils. Contact allergy may lead to symptoms of the oral mucosa, the lips and the perioral skin including perioral eczema, cheilitis, burning/sore mouth, stomatitis, swelling of the tongue, lips and gingival mucosa and ulceration of the mouth (26). There are some indications that oral lichen planus may be worsened by contact allergy to essential oils (28). Rare cases of pigmented contact dermatitis, airborne allergic contact dermatitis, systemic contact dermatitis (29) and erythema multiforme-like reactions (25) from contact allergy to essential oils have been reported.

Dermatitis from occupational exposure

There have been many case reports of patients who developed occupational allergic contact dermatitis from oils used for massaging clients, including aromatherapists (16,30), masseurs (31), beauticians and physiotherapists (31). The patients are usually women and present with dermatitis of the hands and sometimes of the forearms. In a number of them, dermatitis spreads to other parts of the body and may become generalized (30). The use of products such as massage oils, creams or lotions containing essential oils has been shown to be a significant independent risk factor for hand dermatitis in this population (32). Occupational allergic contact dermatitis from essential oils has also been observed in workers in the fragrance and cosmetic industries (33), in the food industries and in several other occupations including hairdressers.

5.5.5 The allergens in essential oils

In patients with established allergic contact dermatitis from essential oils, virtually never attempts have been made to identify the allergenic component(s). With the exception of tea tree oil and turpentine oil, large-scale patch testing with components of essential oils in allergic patients in order to determine the major sensitizers, has not been performed. Few investigators have performed analyses of oils that caused allergic contact dermatitis (16). Thus, tea tree oil (17,18) and turpentine oil (34) excepted, the allergens in essential oils are largely unknown.

Tea tree oil, stored in open bottles or in a bottle opened for several times, suffers an aging process resulting in photo-oxidation leading to degradation products (peroxides, epoxides and endoperoxides), which are strong sensitizers. The most important sensitizers in tea tree oil appear to be terpinolene, ascaridole, α-terpinene (and its oxidation products), 1,2,4-trihydroxymenthane, α-phellandrene, *d*-limonene and myrcene (17,18,40). In turpentine oil, the allergens are δ3-carene hydroperoxides (in oils from Scandinavia [probably hardly used anymore] and Indonesia), α-pinene, oxidized limonene, β-pinene, α-terpineol, and rarely α-phellandrene (34).

For some other oils, their major allergens can tentatively be identified on the basis of their general composition and co-reactions to important ingredients in patch testing as documented in literature. For example, 50% of 94 patients allergic to clove oil co-reacted to eugenol, which is the major ingredient (>82%) of this essential oil (35). Eugenol is also an important component of bay oil (40-55%). Of seven patients reacting to bay oil and tested with eugenol, five (71%) co-reacted to eugenol (36). In the case of lemongrass oil, of 67 patients reacting to this oil, 34 (51%) also reacted to citral (35). Citral consists of geranial + neral, both of which are the dominant ingredients of lemongrass oils (1). Similar combinations include geraniol and geranium oil (23), geraniol and rose oil (23), cinnamal and cinnamon oil, cinnamal and cassia oil, menthol and peppermint oil, and carvone and spearmint oil.

In citrus peel oils (bergamot, grapefruit, lemon, orange, mandarin, tangerine), limonene is by far the most important constituent (70-98%), but has thus far not been identified as main allergen. The reason may be that patients allergic to citrus peel oils have not yet been tested with oxidized limonene, which is the allergenic form of limonene (see Chapter 3.95 Limonene) (37). Probably for the same reason, linalool has as yet not been found as major allergenic ingredient of lavender and ylang-ylang oils, in which high concentrations of linalool and linalyl acetate are present (see Chapter 3.96 Linalool and Chapter 3.97 Linalyl acetate).

Table 5.8 Essential oils which have caused contact allergy / allergic contact dermatitis and probable allergens identified (1,5)

Name of essential oil	Probable allergen(s) identified [a]
Angelica oil	α-Pinene
Aniseed oil	Anethole
Basil oil sweet	Linalool
Bay oil	Eugenol
Bergamot oil	Limonene, linalool, β-pinene
Black pepper oil	Caryophyllene, α-pinene
Cajeput oil	Caryophyllene, α-pinene
Cassia oil	Cinnamal
Cinnamon oil	Cinnamal, eugenol
Citronella oil	Citronellal, citronellol, geraniol, geranyl acetate, limonene
Clary sage oil	Geraniol, linalool
Clove oil	Eugenol
Coriander fruit oil	Linalool, α-pinene
Cypress oil	α-Pinene
Eucalyptus oil	α-Pinene
Galbanum resin oil	α-Pinene
Geranium oil	Caryophyllene, citral (neral + geranial), citronellol, geraniol, linalool
Jasmine absolute	Eugenol, linalool
Juniper berry oil	α-Pinene
Lavender oil	Caryophyllene, linalool, linalyl acetate
Lemongrass oil	Citral (geranial + neral), geraniol
Lemon oil	Limonene, β-pinene
Marjoram oil sweet	Caryophyllene, linalool, α-pinene
Melissa oil	Caryophyllene, geraniol
Neroli oil	Geraniol
Niaouli oil	α-Pinene
Olibanum oil	Caryophyllene, α-pinene
Orange oil sweet	Limonene
Peppermint oil	Caryophyllene, limonene, menthofuran, menthol, menthyl acetate, α-pinene, piperitone, pulegone
Petitgrain bigarade oil	Geraniol, linalool
Pine needle oil	α-Pinene
Ravensara oil	Linalool, α-pinene
Rosemary oil	Linalool, α-pinene
Rose oil	Citronellol, geraniol, linalool
Rosewood oil	Linalool
Sandalwood oil	Santalol
Spearmint oil	Carvone
Star anise oil	Anethole, methyl chavicol, limonene
Tea tree oil	Aromadendrene, ascaridole, d-carvone, l-carvone, 1,8-cineole, p-cymene, limonene, myrcene, α-phellandrene, α-terpinene, terpinen-4-ol, terpinolene, 1,2,4-trihydroxymenthane, sabinene, viridiflorene
Thyme oil	Linalool, α-pinene
Turpentine oil	δ3-Carene, dipentene (dl-limonene), α-phellandrene, α-pinene, β-pinene, α-terpineol
Ylang-ylang oil	Caryophyllene, linalool

[a] Patch test reactivity to one or more chemicals which have been demonstrated in the essential oil used by the patient by chemical analysis, or known to be present in such oils in high concentrations (e.g., geraniol in geranium and rose oils, citronellal and citronellol in citronella oils, cinnamal in cassia and cinnamon oils), or which have been demonstrated in commercial samples of the essential oil in question in concentrations >3% (1)

Determination of the allergenic ingredients of essential oils by analyzing oils that caused allergic contact dermatitis has been performed in a few studies only (e.g., 16). Possible or probable allergens identified in patients reacting to essential oils are shown in table 5.8.

5.5.6 Patch testing with essential oils and their ingredients

Essential oils should be patch tested in any patient suspected of contact allergy to these oils on the basis of the patient's history and the clinical picture. Suspicion is high in cases of hand dermatitis in aromatherapists, masseurs *et cetera*, in patients working in the fragrance industry, the food industry and in individuals who have applied essential oils to their skin, e.g., for therapeutic purposes (notably tea tree oil and eucalyptus oil). In addition, in any patient with symptoms of the oral mucosa, lips (cheilitis) and the perioral skin, contact allergy to essential oils in toothpastes or other oral preparations should be considered. However, the range of products in which essential oils can be present is broad and localisation and aspect of essential oil-induced allergic contact dermatitis are often not specific.

Several essential oils are available as commercial patch test substances (table 5.9). Four essential oils and jasmine absolute are currently present in the screening series of the North American Contact Dermatitis Group and tested in all consecutive patients suspected of contact dermatitis (15). Many other investigators test a series of essential oils and other fragrance materials when fragrance contact allergy is suspected. Another indication for further testing is when a patient has previously shown positive patch test reactions to one or more of the fragrance indicator allergens, such as the fragrance mix(es) and Myroxylon pereirae resin, to an essential oil, to other fragrance materials, or to the patient's personal fragrances or fragranced cosmetics.

For screening purposes, these series of commercial allergens are very useful. However, when patients have a history of contact with one or more oils, it is preferable (if not imperative) to test these products themselves, because of the strong variability that may occur in the composition of essential oils. In addition, in aged oils that have been exposed to light, oxygen and temperature changes, new allergenic chemicals may have formed (which is well known in for example tea tree oil and lavender oil), which are not or in lower concentrations present in adequately stored (cool, dark, unexposed to air) commercial test substances.

For most essential oils, testing at 2-5% in petrolatum (or both, unless many oils are tested, risk of great number of reactions with false-positives due to the excited skin syndrome) will likely be adequate. Lower concentrations may be appropriate for costus root oil (0.1%, very unlikely to encounter, historical allergen), black cumin oil (0.5%), star anise oil (0.5%, it may be preferable to test the main ingredient anethole 5%), and cassia and cinnamon (bark) oils (1%, because of the very high concentrations of cinnamal). When obtaining positive patch tests to one or more essential oils, a search for the allergenic ingredients should preferably be initiated. Likely candidates are discussed in table 5.8, right column. A list of all chemicals which can be present in essential oils and which have caused contact allergy (either from their presence in essential oils or from other sources, n=>100) is provided in ref. 1.

Co-reactivity to other test substances in patients reacting to essential oils
In most publications, patients reacting positively to an essential oil co-reacted – if tested – to other essential oils, the fragrance mix I, the fragrance mix II, Myroxylon pereirae resin (balsam of Peru), one or more individual fragrance chemicals, or a combination of these.

Essential oils
Many patients in case reports react to a great number of essential oils, which is certainly true for aromatherapists and other professionals using oils and essential oil-containing products for massaging their clients. Of two aromatherapists, for example, one reacted to 32 and the other to 21 essential oils (16). Another aromatherapist was patch test positive to 17 of 20 oils used at her work (38). In a group of 19 patients allergic to fragrances and tested with a series of essential oils, 6 reacted to one oil only, three to 2 oils, three to 3, three to 4, two to 5, one reacted to 7 oils and one even had positive patch test reactions to nine oils (36).

Fragrance mixes
Co-reactivity to the fragrance mix I (FM I) (and to a lesser degree to the fragrance mix II [FM II]) in patients with contact allergy to or allergic contact dermatitis from essential oils is very frequent, both in case reports and in investigations in groups of patients. Of 637 patients reacting to at least one essential oil seen by the IVDK (Germany, Austria, Switzerland), 55% co-reacted to FM I, 35% to FM II and 63% to one of these two (35). Of 15 patients reacting to ylang-ylang oil in The Netherlands, 15 (83%) co-reacted to FM I (39). Co-reactivity to FM for individual essential oils as observed in a European multicenter study was as follows: ylang-ylang oil 36/42 (86%), lemongrass oil 18/25 (72%), jasmine absolute 11/20 (55%) and patchouli oil 9/13 (69%) (21).

Fragrance chemicals
Patients allergic to perfumes often react to many fragrance materials, which is also the case in individuals reacting to essential oils. These may both be chemicals which are important ingredients of the oils themselves (especially to be

found when they are routinely tested) such as cinnamal in cassia and cinnamon oil, eugenol in clove and bay oil, and geraniol in geranium and rose oil, but also to other fragrance materials which are either not present in the allergenic oil or only at (very) low concentrations.

There are (at least) three possible explanations for these co-reactivities. In many such cases, co-reactivity probably results from pseudo-cross-reactivity, meaning that the test substances share common components responsible for the positive patch test reactions. In a number of cases, real cross-reactivity may play a role. Thirdly, as many patients (e.g. in the case of occupational contact allergy) are exposed to a large number of essential oils and possibly individual fragrances, concomitant or successive sensitization to various products and chemicals can be anticipated.

Table 5.9 Essential oils which are commercially available for patch testing [d]

Essential oil	Chemo	SPEurope	SP Canada
Bergamot oil			2%
Cananga oil	2%		
Cedarwood oil		10% (*J. virginiana*)	10% ('Cedar oil')
Cinnamon oil			0.5%
Clove oil			2%
Eucalyptus oil		2% (*E. globulus*)	2% (unspecified)
Geranium oil	2%		
Jasmine absolute	2% (*J. grandiflorum*)	5% (*J. officinale*)	2% [a]
Laurel leaf oil		2%	2% [b]
Lavender oil	2% (absolute)		2%
Lemongrass oil		2% [c]	2%
Lemon oil		2%	2%
Neroli oil			2% and 5%
Orange oil		2% (sweet)	2% (sweet)
Patchouli oil		10%	10%
Peppermint oil	2%	2%	2%
Petitgrain bigarade oil		5%	
Rosemary oil			0.5%
Rose oil	2% (absolute)		0.5%
Sandalwood oil	2% (*S. album*)	10% (*S. album*)	10% (unspecified)
Tea tree oil	5% (ox.)		5% (ox.)
Turpentine oil	0.4% (ox.)	10%	10%
Ylang-ylang oil	2%	10%	2%

[a] Termed 'Jasminum officinale oil (*Jasminum grandiflorum*)': this is incorrect as it is an abstract (not an essential oil) and *Jasminum grandiflorum* is not a synonym for *Jasminum officinale*. The CAS number given refers to *J. grandiflorum*; [b] Incorrectly termed 'Bay leaf oil'; [c] Prepared from *Cymbopogon schoenanthus*; [d] All test substances in petrolatum
Chemo: Chemotechnique Diagnostics, www.chemotechnique.se; SPCanada: SmartPractice Canada, www.smartpracticecanada.com; SPEurope: SmartPractice Europe, www.smartpracticeeurope.com

LITERATURE

1   De Groot AC, Schmidt E. Essential oils: contact allergy and chemical composition. Boca Raton, Fl., USA: CRC Press, Taylor and Francis Group, 2016 (ISBN 9781482246407)
2   De Groot AC, Schmidt E. Essential Oils, Part I: Introduction. Dermatitis 2016;27:39-42
3   De Groot AC, Schmidt E. Essential Oils, Part II: General aspects. Dermatitis 2016;27:43-49
4   De Groot AC, Schmidt E. Essential Oils, Part III: Chemical composition. Dermatitis 2016;27:161-169
5   De Groot AC, Schmidt E. Essential oils, Part IV: Contact allergy. Dermatitis 2016;27:170-175
6   Franz C, Baser KHC, Windisch W. Essential oils and aromatic plants in animal feeding – a European perspective. A review. Flavour Fragr J 2010;25:327-340
7   ISO 9235:2013 Aromatic natural raw materials – Vocabulary. International Organization for Standardization, Geneva, Switzerland. www.iso.org
8   Rhind JP. Essential oils. A handbook for aromatherapy practice, 2nd Edition. London: Singing Dragon, 2012
9   Lawless J. The encyclopedia of essential oils, 2nd Edition. London: Harper Thorsons, 2014
10 ISO 22716:2007 Cosmetics -- Good Manufacturing Practices (GMP) -- Guidelines on Good Manufacturing Practices. International Organization for Standardization, Geneva, Switzerland, www.iso.org
11 Nardelli A, Thijs L, Janssen K, Goossens A. Rosa centifolia in a 'non-scented' moisturizing body lotion as a cause of allergic contact dermatitis. Contact Dermatitis 2009;61:306-309
12 Tisserand R, Young R. Essential oil safety, 2nd Edition. Edinburgh, UK: Churchill Livingstone Elsevier, 2014

13 Becker PM, Galetti S. Food and feed components for gut health-promoting adhesion of *E. coli* and *Salmonella enterica*. J Sci Food Agric 2008;88:2026-2035

14 Ehrlinger M. Phytogene Zusatzstoffe in der Tierernährung. Inaugural-Dissertation, Tierärztliche Fakultät der Ludwig-Maximilians-Universität, München, Germany, 2007:235-247

15 Cheng J, Zug KA. Fragrance allergic contact dermatitis. Dermatitis 2014;25:232-245

16 Dharmagunawardena B, Takwale A, Sanders KJ, Cannan S, Roger A, Ilchyshyn A. Gas chromatography: an investigative tool in multiple allergies to essential oils. Contact Dermatitis 2002;47:288-292

17 Hausen BM, Reichling J, Harkenthal M. Degradation products of monoterpenes are the sensitizing agents in tea tree oil. Am J Cont Derm 1999;10:68-77

18 Pirker C, Hausen BM, Uter W, Hillen U, Brasch J, Bayerl C, et al. Sensitization to tea tree oil in Germany and Austria. A multicenter study of the German Contact Dermatitis Group. J Dtsch Dermatol Ges 2003;1:629-634

19 Foussereau J, Benezra C, Ourisson G. Contact dermatitis from laurel. I. Clinical aspects. Transactions of the St John's Hospital Dermatological Society 1967;53:141-146

20 Schäfer T, Böhler E, Ruhdorfer S, Weigl L, Wessner D, Filipiak B, et al. Epidemiology of contact allergy in adults. Allergy 2001;56:1192-1196

21 Frosch PJ, Johansen JD, Menné T, Pirker C, Rastogi SC, Andersen KE, et al. Further important sensitizers in patients sensitive to fragrances. II. Reactivity to essential oils. Contact Dermatitis 2002;47:279-287

22 Warshaw EM, Maibach HI, Taylor JS, Sasseville D, DeKoven JG, Zirwas MJ, et al. North American Contact Dermatitis Group patch test results: 2011-2012. Dermatitis 2015;26:49-59

23 Juarez A, Goiriz R, Sanchez-Perez J, Garcia-Diez A. Disseminated allergic contact dermatitis after exposure to a topical medication containing geraniol. Dermatitis 2008;19:163

24 Pesonen M, Suomela S, Kuuliala O, Henriks-Eckerman M-L, Aalto-Korte K. Occupational contact dermatitis caused by D-limonene. Contact Dermatitis 2014;71:273-279

25 Athanasiadis GI, Pfab F, Klein A, Braun-Falco M, Ring J, Ollert M. Erythema multiforme due to contact with laurel oil. Contact Dermatitis 2007;57:116-118

26 De Groot AC. Contact allergy to (ingredients of) toothpastes. Dermatitis 2017;28:95-114

27 Nardelli A, D'Hooge E, Drieghe J, Dooms M, Goossens A. Allergic contact dermatitis from fragrance components in specific topical pharmaceutical products in Belgium. Contact Dermatitis 2009;60:303-313

28 Gunatheesan S, Tam MM, Tate B, Tversky J, Nixon R. Retrospective study of oral lichen planus and allergy to spearmint oil. Australas J Dermatol 2012;53:224-228

29 De Groot AC, Weijland JW. Systemic contact dermatitis from tea tree oil. Contact Dermatitis 1992;27:279-280

30 Boonchai W, Lamtharachai P, Sunthonpalin P. Occupational allergic contact dermatitis from essential oils in aromatherapists. Contact Dermatitis 2007;56:181-182

31 Trattner A, David M, Lazarov A. Occupational contact dermatitis due to essential oils. Contact Dermatitis 2008;58:282-284

32 Crawford GH, Katz KA, Ellis E, James WD. Use of aromatherapy products and increased risk of hand dermatitis in massage therapists. Arch Dermatol 2004;140:991-996

33 Schubert HJ. Skin diseases in workers at a perfume factory. Contact Dermatitis 2006;55:81-83

34 Cachao P, Menezes Brandao F, Carmo M, Frazao S, Silva M. Allergy to oil of turpentine in Portugal. Contact Dermatitis 1986;14:205-208

35 Uter W, Schmidt E, Geier J, Lessmann H, Schnuch A, Frosch P. Contact allergy to essential oils: current patch test results (2000–2008) from the Information Network of Departments of Dermatology (IVDK). Contact Dermatitis 2010;63:277-283

36 Meynadier JM, Meynadier J, Peyron JL, Peyron L. Formes cliniques des manifestations cutanées d'allergie aux parfums. Ann Dermatol Venereol 1986;113:31-39

37 Karlberg A-T, Börje A, Johansen JD, Lidén C, Rastogi S, Roberts D, et al. Activation of non-sensitizing or low-sensitizing fragrance substances into potent sensitizers – prehaptens and prohaptens. Contact Dermatitis 2013;69:323-334

38 Selvaag E, Holm J, Thune P. Allergic contact dermatitis in an aromatherapist with multiple sensitizations to essential oils. Contact Dermatitis 1995;33:354-355

39 De Groot AC, Coenraads PJ, Bruynzeel DP, Jagtman BA, van Ginkel CJW, Noz K, van der Valk PGM, et al. Routine patch testing with fragrance chemicals in The Netherlands. Contact Dermatitis 2000;42:184-185

40 De Groot AC, Schmidt E. Tea tree oil: contact allergy and chemical composition. Contact Dermatitis 2016;75:129-143

Chapter 6   Monographs of essential oils that have caused contact allergy / allergic contact dermatitis

6.0 INTRODUCTION

In this chapter, Monographs of 97 essential oils that have caused contact allergy / allergic contact dermatitis are presented. They have a standardized format, which is explained and detailed in Chapter 1.2. The essential oils discussed here are shown in table 6.0.1. A short summary of these data and other general aspects of essential oils allergy (frequency of contact allergy to essentials oils; clinical relevance of positive patch test reactions to essential oils; products responsible for allergic contact dermatitis from essential oils; clinical picture of allergic contact dermatitis from essential oils; the allergens in essential oils; patch testing with essential oils and their ingredients) can be found in Chapter 5. Monographs on fragrances and exctracts are shown in Chapter 3 and Monographs of chemicals not used as fragrances themselves but present as allergenic ingredients of botanical fragrance materials are in Chapter 4.

Table 6.0.1 Essential oils presented in Monographs in Chapter 6

Angelica oil	Litsea cubeba oil
Aniseed oil	Lovage oil
Basil oil	Mandarin oil
Bay oil	Marjoram oil (sweet)
Bergamot oil	Melissa oil (lemon balm oil)
Bitter almond oil	Myrrh oil
Black cumin oil	Neem oil
Black pepper oil	Neroli oil
Cajeput oil	Niaouli oil
Calamus oil	Nutmeg oil
Cananga oil	Olibanum oil (frankincense oil)
Cardamom oil	Orange oil
Carrot seed oil	Oregano oil
Cassia oil	Palmarosa oil
Cedarwood oil	Patchouli oil
Chamomile oil	Peppermint oil
Cinnamon oil	Petitgrain bigarade oil
Citronella oil	Pine needle oil
Clary sage oil	Ravensara oil
Clove oil	Rose oil
Coriander fruit oil	Rosemary oil
Costus root oil	Rosewood oil
Cypress oil	Sage oil
Dwarf pine oil	Sandalwood oil
Elemi oil	Silver fir oil
Eucalyptus oil	Spearmint oil
Galbanum resin oil	Spike lavender oil
Geranium oil	Spruce oil
Ginger oil	Star anise oil
Grapefruit oil	Tangerine oil
Guaiacwood oil	Tea tree oil
Hinoki oil	Thuja oil
Hyssop oil	Thyme oil
Jasmine absolute	Turmeric oil
Juniper berry oil	Turpentine oil
Laurel leaf oil	Valerian oil
Lavandin oil	Vetiver oil
Lavender oil	Ylang-ylang oil
Lemon oil	Zdravetz oil
Lemongrass oil	

Chapter 6.1   ANGELICA OIL

There are two forms of Angelica essential oils, fruit and root oil. The fruits and seeds are often considered as synonymous, but the seeds are contained within the fruits. The seed oil mentioned in INCI is probably synonymous with the fruit oil.

6.1.1   ANGELICA FRUIT OIL

IDENTIFICATION

Description/definition   : Angelica fruit oil is the essential oil obtained from the fruit of the angelica (wild
                             parsnip), *Angelica archangelica* L.
INCI name(S) EU & USA   : Angelica archangelica seed oil
CAS registry number(s)   : 8015-64-3; 84775-41-7
EC number(s)   : 283-871-1
RIFM monograph(s)   : Food Cosmet Toxicol 1974;12:821 (special issue I) (binder, page 96)
SCCS opinion(s)   : SCCNFP/0389/00, final (4)
Merck Index monograph   : 1908 (Angelica)
Function(s) in cosmetics   : EU: skin conditioning. USA: fragrance ingredients
Patch testing   : 2% pet.

GENERAL

Angelica archangelica L. is an aromatic, perennial herb that grows up to 2 meter tall. The plant is native to the temperate regions of Asia (Caucasus, Siberia), northern, middle and east Europe, and the Himalayas, and has become widely naturalized in northern temperate regions. The plant is cultivated in Italy, Germany, Finland, Hungary, and several other countries including Korea, India and North America (GRIN Taxonomy for Plants; www.kew.org). Commercial angelica root and fruit oils are mostly obtained from cultivated *Angelica archangelica* L. ssp. *angelica* var. *sativa* (10). Essential oils of the fruits (often incorrectly referred to as 'seeds', as the seeds are contained within the fruits) and roots of *Angelica archangelica* are used for healing purposes, as spice and as fragrance component in perfumery (7) and cosmetics. Angelica root oils are also part of aromatherapy practices (9). The biological activities and medicinal uses of *Angelica archangelica* L. have been reviewed in references 6 and 8.

CHEMICAL COMPOSITION

Angelica fruit oil is a clear, mobile, pale yellow to amber liquid which has a fresh, pungent, terpenic odor. In angelica fruit oils from various origins, over 120 chemicals have been identified. About 57 per cent of these were found in a single reviewed publication only. The ten chemicals that had the highest maximum concentrations in 11 commercial angelica fruit essential oil samples are shown in table 6.1.1.1 (Erich Schmidt, analytical data presented in ref. 5).

A full literature review of the qualitative and quantitative composition of commercial and non-commercial angelica fruit oils of various origins has been published in 2016 (5).

Table 6.1.1.1 Ten ingredients with the highest concentrations in commercial angelica fruit oils (5)

Name	Concentration range	Name	Concentration range
β-Phellandrene	52.1 - 76.0%	(*E*)-β-Ocimene	0.5 - 1.8%
α-Pinene	2.3 - 13.3%	Bicyclogermacrene	0.4 - 1.5%
Myrcene	0.6 - 5.0%	Camphene	0.1 - 1.2%
α-Phellandrene	0.7 - 3.7%	Cryptone	0.01 - 1.2%
Limonene	2.3 - 2.9%	α-Humulene	0.5 - 1.1%

6.1.2   ANGELICA ROOT OIL

IDENTIFICATION

Description/definition   : Angelica root oil is the essential oil obtained from the roots and rhizomes of the
                             angelica (wild parsnip), *Angelica archangelica* L.
INCI name(s) EU and USA : Angelica archangelica root oil
CAS registry number(s)   : 8015-64-3; 84775-41-7
EC number(s)   : 283-871-1

RIFM monograph(s)	: Food Cosmet Toxicol 1975;13:713 (special issue II) (binder, page 94)
IFRA standard	: Restricted (www.ifraorg.org/en-us/standards-library) (table 6.1.2.1)
SCCS opinion(s)	: SCCNFP/0392/00, final (13); SCCNFP/0389/00, final (4)
Merck Index monograph	: 1908 (Angelica)
Function(s) in cosmetics	: EU: masking; perfuming; tonic. USA: fragrance ingredients
Patch testing	: 2% pet.

Table 6.1.2.1 IFRA restrictions for Angelica root oil

Leave-on products:	0.8%
Rinse-off products:	no restriction
Non-skin contact products:	no restriction

The limit only applies to applications on skin exposed to sunshine, excluding rinse-off products. If combinations of phototoxic fragrance ingredients are used, the use levels have to be reduced accordingly. The sum of the concentrations of all phototoxic ingredients, expressed in percentage of their recommended maximum level in the consumer product shall not exceed 100

GENERAL

General aspects of *Angelica* and Angelica root oil are discussed in the section 'General' of Angelica fruit oil above.

CHEMICAL COMPOSITION

Angelica root oil is, when freshly distilled, a colorless, mobile liquid; with storage, its color changes from yellowish to brownish. The odor is aromatic, spicy with a peppery touch and a typical earthy-rooty character. In angelica root oils from various origins, over 165 chemicals have been identified. About 40 per cent of these were found in a single reviewed publication only. The ten chemicals that had the highest maximum concentrations in 31 commercial angelica root essential oil samples are shown in table 6.1.2.2 (Erich Schmidt, analytical data presented in ref. 5). The composition of *Indian* angelica oils is quite different from oils produced elsewhere (other chemotype) (5).

A full literature review of the qualitative and quantitative composition of commercial and non-commercial angelica root oils of various origins has been published in 2016 (5).

Table 6.1.2.2 Ten ingredients with the highest concentrations in commercial angelica root oils (5)

Name	Concentration range	Name	Concentration range
α-Pinene	11.4 - 27.0%	Sabinene	0.6 - 11.3%
α-Phellandrene	4.5 - 22.0%	*p*-Cymene	1.3 - 8.4%
β-Phellandrene	9.4 - 18.7%	(*E*)-Ocimene	0 - 5.9%
δ3-Carene	6.4 - 17.5%	Myrcene	1.4 - 5.4%
Limonene	6.4 – 15.0%	(*Z*)-β-Ocimene	0.7 - 4.6%

CONTACT ALLERGY / ALLERGIC CONTACT DERMATITIS

Angelica oil (unspecified)

General

Contact allergy to / allergic contact dermatitis from angelica oil (plant part unspecified) has been reported in two publications only.

Testing in groups of patients

Two hundred dermatitis patients from Poland were tested with angelica oil 2% in petrolatum and two (1%) reacted; relevance data were not provided (2). In a group of 51 patients allergic to Myroxylon pereirae resin (balsam of Peru) and/or turpentine and/or wood tar and/or colophony and tested with angelica oil 2% in petrolatum, three (5.9%) had a positive patch test; relevance data were not provided (2).

Case reports and case series

A female aromatherapist developed occupational contact dermatitis of the hands from contact allergy to angelica oil; she also reacted to ylang-ylang oil and geraniol, which were also used at her work (1).

<u>Angelica fruit oil</u>

General
Contact allergy to / possible allergic contact dermatitis from angelica fruit oil has been reported in one publication only. A false-positive patch test reaction due to the excited skin syndrome cannot be excluded. In the same case report, α-pinene may have been an allergen in angelica fruit oil.

Case reports and case series
A case of non-occupational contact dermatitis in an aromatherapist with allergies to multiple essential oils used at work, including angelica seed oil, has been reported. The patient also reacted to geraniol, linalool, linalyl acetate, α-pinene, the fragrance mix and various other fragrance materials. α-Pinene, linalool, and geraniol were demonstrated by GC-MS in angelica seed oil (3). α-Pinene may be an important constituent in angelica fruit oils and has been found in concentrations of up to 13.3% in commercial angelica fruit oils (5).

<u>Angelica root oil</u>

General
Contact allergy to / allergic contact dermatitis from angelica root oil has been reported in two publications only.

Testing in groups of patients
A group of 86 patients from Poland previously reacting to the fragrance mix was tested with angelica root oil and two (2.3%) had a positive patch test reaction; relevance data were not provided (11).

Case reports and case series
A patient developed allergic contact dermatitis from the perfume in an eye cream; she was patch tested with all 94 components of the perfume and reacted to angelica root oil (test concentration unknown) and eleven of the other chemicals in the perfume (12).

Photosensitivity
Photosensitivity from Angelica root oil has been cited in ref. 14

LITERATURE

1   Keane FM, Smith HR, White IR, Rycroft RJG. Occupational allergic contact dermatitis in two aromatherapists. Contact Dermatitis 2000;43:49-51
2   Rudzki E, Grzywa Z, Bruo WS. Sensitivity to 35 essential oils. Contact Dermatitis 1976;2:196-200
3   Dharmagunawardena B, Takwale A, Sanders KJ, Cannan S, Roger A, Ilchyshyn A. Gas chromatography: an investigative tool in multiple allergies to essential oils. Contact Dermatitis 2002;47:288-292
4   Opinion of the Scientific Committee on Cosmetic Products and Non-Food Products Intended for Consumers concerning 'The 1st update of the inventory of ingredients employed in cosmetic products. Section II: Perfume and aromatic raw materials', 24 October 2000, SCCNFP/0389/00, final. Available at: http://ec.europa.eu/health/ph_risk/committees/sccp/documents/out131_en.pdf
5   De Groot AC, Schmidt E. Essential oils: contact allergy and chemical composition. Boca Raton, Fl., USA: CRC Press, Taylor and Francis Group, 2016 (ISBN 9781482246407)
6   Bhat ZA, Kumar D, Shah MY. *Angelica archangelica* Linn. is an angel on earth for the treatment of diseases: a review. Int J Nutr Pharm Neurol Dis 2011;1:35-49
7   Lopes D, Strobl H, Kolodziejczyk P. 14-Methylpentadecano-15-lactone (Muscolide): A new macrocyclic lactone from the oil of *Angelica archangelica* L. Chem Biodivers 2004;1:1880-1887
8   Sarker SD, Nahar L. Natural medicine: the genus *Angelica*. Curr Med Chem 2004;11:1479-500
9   Nivinskienė O, Butkienė R, Mockutė D. The chemical composition of the essential oil of *Angelica archangelica* L. roots growing wild in Lithuania. J Essent Oil Res 2005;17:373-377
10   Lawrence BM. Progress in essential oils. Angelica root and seed oils. Perfum Flavor 1999;24:47-49
11   Rudzki E, Grzywa Z. Allergy to perfume mixture. Contact Dermatitis 1986;15:115-116
12   Larsen WG. Cosmetic dermatitis due to a perfume. Contact Dermatitis 1975;1:142-145
13   Opinion of the Scientific Committee on Cosmetic Products and Non-Food Products Intended for Consumers concerning 'An initial list of perfumery materials which must not form part of cosmetic products except subject to the Restrictions and Conditions laid down, 25 September 2001, SCCNFP/0392/00, final. Available at: http://ec.europa.eu/health/archive/ph_risk/committees/sccp/documents/out150_en.pdf
14   De Groot AC. Patch Testing, 4th Edition. Wapserveen, The Netherlands: acdegroot publishing, 2018 (ISBN 978-90-813233-4-5)

Chapter 6.2   ANISEED OIL

IDENTIFICATION

Description/definition	: Aniseed oil (essential oil of aniseed) is the essential oil obtained from the fruit of the anise, *Pimpinella anisum* L.
INCI name(s) EU	: Pimpinella anisum fruit oil
INCI name(s) USA	: Pimpinella anisum (anise) fruit oil
CAS registry number(s)	: 8007-70-3; 84775-42-8
EC number(s)	: 283-872-7
RIFM monograph(s)	: Food Cosmet Toxicol 1973;11:865 (binder, page 97)
ISO standard	: ISO 3475 Essential oil of aniseed, 2002; Geneva, Switzerland, www.iso.org
Merck Index monograph	: 1927 (Anise)
Function(s) in cosmetics	: EU: flavouring; masking; perfuming. USA: flavoring agents; fragrance ingredients
Patch testing	: 1% pet.; test also anethole (see Chapter 3.11 Anethole)

GENERAL

Pimpinella anisum L. is a herbaceous annual plant growing to one meter tall or higher. It probably originates from the eastern Mediterranean region and south-west Asia and is now widely cultivated in the Mediterranean rim, Russia, South Africa, and Brazil (1,2, GRIN Taxonomy for Plants). Western cuisines have long used anise to flavor some dishes, drinks, and candies and aniseed is also used as a breath freshener. The essential oil obtained from the fruits (commercially called seeds [aniseeds]) is used in perfumery, toothpastes, medicinally, as a food flavoring, as an insecticide against head-lice and mites and is also utilized in aromatherapy (6), though some warn for its toxicity (7).

The pharmacological activities of *Pimpinella anisum* have been reviewed (3,4). The European Medicines Agency in 2013 concluded that 'Medicinal use of aniseed and anise oil is not supported by clinical evidence' (5).

Aniseed oil should not be confused with star anise oil, obtained from *Illicium verum* (Chapter 6.69 Star anise oil).

CHEMICAL COMPOSITION

Aniseed oil is a clear, more or less mobile liquid or solid crystalline mass, which has a spicy and sweet odor from the high amounts of anethole. In aniseed oils from various origins, over 120 chemicals have been identified. Nearly half of these were found in a single reviewed publication only (14). Aniseed oil is always dominated by (*E*)-anethole. The ten chemicals that had the highest maximum concentrations in 81 commercial aniseed essential oil samples are shown in table 6.2.1 (Erich Schmidt, analytical data presented in ref. 14).

A full literature review of the qualitative and quantitative composition of commercial and non-commercial aniseed oils of various origins and with data from the ISO standard has been published in 2016 (14).

Table 6.2.1 Ten ingredients with the highest concentrations in commercial aniseed oils (14)

Name	Concentration range	Name	Concentration range
(*E*)-Anethole	91.0 - 98.6%	*trans*-Pseudoisoeugenyl 2-methylbutyrate	0.4 - 1.3%
Limonene	0.01 - 3.5%		
Methyl chavicol	0.01 - 3.2%	*p*-Anisic acid	0 - 0.9%
γ-Himachalene	1.4 - 2.9%	α-Zingiberene	0.2 - 0.5%
p-Anisaldehyde	0.1 - 1.4%	(*Z*)-Anethole	0.03 - 0.3%
p-Methoxyphenylacetone	0 - 1.4%		

CONTACT ALLERGY / ALLERGIC CONTACT DERMATITIS

General
Contact allergy to / allergic contact dermatitis from aniseed oil has been reported in a few studies, including some patients with occupational allergic contact dermatitis. In one case report, anethole may have been the allergen in aniseed oil.

Testing in groups of patients
In a group of 21 patients with dermatitis caused by perfumes and tested with a series of essential oils, one (5%) reacted to 'anise oil' 2%; relevance data were not provided (13).

Case reports and case series

One patient had psoriasis-like dermatitis from contact allergy to aniseed oil (8). Two patients working in the food industry developed occupational allergic contact dermatitis from aniseed oil (tested 5% olive oil) and its main ingredient anethole (19). A case of dermatitis and stomatitis was caused by contact allergy to aniseed oil in denture cream (12).

A porcelain painter had occupational allergic contact dermatitis from oil of anise, oil of turpentine and lavender oil, that were mixed with pigments for painting (11). One positive patch test to aniseed oil (relevance unknown) was observed in a patient working in a cosmetic factory, who had occupational dermatitis from a fragrance mixture he was handling daily (9).

Patch test sensitization

Patch test sensitization from aniseed oil has been cited in ref. 15.

LITERATURE

1   Saibi S, Belhadj M, El-Hadi B. Essential oil composition of *Pimpinella anisum* from Algeria. Anal Chem Lett 2012;2:401-404

2   Orav A, Raal A, Arak E. Essential oil composition of *Pimpinella anisum* L. fruits from various European countries. Nat Prod Res 2008;22:227-232

3   Shojaii A, Abdollahi Fard M. Review of pharmacological properties and chemical constituents of *Pimpinella anisum*. International Scholarly Research Network. ISRN Pharmaceutics, Volume 2012, Article ID 510795, 8 pages. doi:10.5402/2012/510795

4   Silano V, Delbò M. Assessment Report on *Pimpinella Anisum* L. European Medicines Agency, Evaluation of Medicines for Human Use. Doc. Ref: EMEA/HMPC/137421/2006.

5   European Medicines Agency, Committee on Herbal Medicinal Products (HMPC). Assessment report on *Pimpinella anisum* L., fructus and *Pimpinella anisum* L., aetheroleum. EMEA/HMPC/321181/2012, November 2013

6   Rhind JP. Essential oils. A handbook for aromatherapy practice, 2nd Edition. London: Singing Dragon, 2012

7   Davis P. Aromatherapy. An A-Z, 3rd Edition. London: Vermilion, 2005

8   Assalve D, Caraffini S, Lisi P. Psoriasis-like allergic contact dermatitis from aniseed oil. Annali Italiani di Dermatologia Clinica e Sperimentale 1987;41:411-414

9   Rudzki E, Rebandel P, Grzywa Z. Occupational dermatitis from cosmetic creams. Contact Dermatitis 1993;29:210

10 Garcia-Bravo B, Pérez Bernal A, Garcia-Hernandez MJ, Camacho F. Occupational contact dermatitis from anethole in food handlers. Contact Dermatitis 1997;37:38

11 Vente C, Fuchs T. Contact dermatitis due to oil of turpentine in a porcelain painter. Contact Dermatitis 1997;37:187

12 Loveman AB. Stomatitis venenata. Report of a case of sensitivity of the mucous membranes and the skin to oil of anise. Arch Derm Syph 1938;37:70-81

13 Meynadier JM, Meynadier J, Peyron JL, Peyron L. Formes cliniques des manifestations cutanées d'allergie aux parfums. Ann Dermatol Venereol 1986;113:31-39

14 De Groot AC, Schmidt E. Essential oils: contact allergy and chemical composition. Boca Raton, Fl., USA: CRC Press, Taylor and Francis Group, 2016 (ISBN 9781482246407)

15 De Groot AC. Patch Testing, 4th Edition. Wapserveen, The Netherlands: acdegroot publishing, 2018 (ISBN 978-90-813233-4-5)

Chapter 6.3   BASIL OIL

IDENTIFICATION

Description/definition	: Sweet basil oil (essential oil of basil) is the essential oil obtained from the flowering aerial tops of the (sweet) basil, *Ocimum basilicum* L.
INCI name(s) EU	: Ocimum basilicum herb oil (perfuming name, not an INCI name proper); Ocimum basilicum flower/leaf extract
INCI name(s) USA	: Ocimum basilicum (basil) flower/leaf extract
CAS registry number(s)	: 84775-71-3; 8015-73-4
EC number(s)	: 283-900-8
RIFM monograph(s)	: Food Cosmet Toxicol 1973;11:867 (binder, page 110) (estragole [= methyl chavicol] chemotype)
ISO standard	: ISO 11043 Essential oil of basil, methyl chavicol type, 1998; Geneva, Switzerland, www.iso.org
Merck Index monograph	: 8137
Function(s) in cosmetics	: EU: perfuming; masking; tonic. USA: fragrance ingredients; skin-conditioning agents – miscellaneous
Patch testing	: 5% pet.

GENERAL

Ocimum basilicum L. is an aromatic, erect, almost glabrous annual herb, which grows to between 0.3 and 0.5 meters. The plant is native to India, Iran and tropical Asia, and now grows wild in tropical and sub-tropical regions. Basil is cultivated for commercial use in many countries around the world, including France, Hungary, Greece, Italy, Egypt, Morocco, Indonesia and several states in the USA (3). *Ocimum basilicum* L. is the major essential oil crop around the world.

The essential oil, which may be obtained from the leaves, the aerial parts or the flowering tops, is used to flavor various food products, liquors and non-alcoholic beverages. In addition, *Ocimum basilicum* essential oils, notably those from the flowering tops, are widely used in the pharmaceutical, cosmetic, aromatherapy and perfumery industries (3).

CHEMICAL COMPOSITION

Basil oil is a pale yellow to ambery yellow clear mobile liquid, which has a spicy, slightly anisic to spicy woody or to spicy cinnamic odor. In basil oils from various origins, over 435 chemicals have been identified. About half of these were found in a single reviewed publication only. There are several types of basil oil in international commerce, each derived principally from different cultivars or chemotypes of sweet basil. The chemotype heavily influences the chemical composition of the essential oil (3).

The ten chemicals that had the highest maximum concentrations in 47 commercial sweet basil essential oil samples are shown in table 6.3.1 (Erich Schmidt, analytical data presented in ref. 3).

A full literature review of the qualitative and quantitative composition of commercial and non-commercial basil oils of various origins, their chemotypes and with data from the ISO standard, has been published in 2016 (3).

Table 6.3.1 Ten ingredients with the highest concentrations in commercial sweet basil oils (3)

Name	Concentration range	Name	Concentration range
Methyl chavicol	0.2 - 87.0%	Eugenol	0.03 - 15.3%
Linalool	0.6 - 55.8%	1,8-Cineole	0.03 - 13.7%
Methyl eugenol	0 - 24.7%	τ-Cadinol	0 - 7.1%
(Z)-Methyl cinnamate	0 - 23.6%	β-Elemene	0 - 5.5%
trans-α-Bergamotene	0.01 - 19.8%	α-Guaiene	0 - 4.3%

CONTACT ALLERGY / ALLERGIC CONTACT DERMATITIS

General

Contact allergy to / allergic contact dermatitis from basil oil has been reported in two publications only, both from occupational exposure in aromatherapists. In neither can a false-positive reaction due to the excited skin syndrome be excluded. In one case report, linalool may have been an allergen in basil oil (2).

Case reports and case series

An aromatherapist had chronic hand dermatitis and was patch test positive to 17 of 20 oils used at her work (tested 1% and 5% in petrolatum), including basil oil (1).

Two other aromatherapists had contact dermatitis (occupational in one) with allergies to multiple essential oils used at their work, including basil oil. Both patients also reacted to geraniol, α-pinene, the fragrance mix and various other fragrance materials. In addition, one proved to be allergic to linalool and linalyl acetate, the other to caryophyllene; α-pinene, linalool, geraniol and caryophyllene were demonstrated by GC-MS in basil oil (2). Linalool may be an important component of basil oil and has been found in concentrations of up to 55.8% in commercial basil oils (3). In neither of these case reports can a false-positive reaction due to the excited skin syndrome be excluded.

LITERATURE

1   Selvaag E, Holm J, Thune P. Allergic contact dermatitis in an aromatherapist with multiple sensitizations to essential oils. Contact Dermatitis 1995;33:354-355
2   Dharmagunawardena B, Takwale A, Sanders KJ, Cannan S, Roger A, Ilchyshyn A. Gas chromatography: an investigative tool in multiple allergies to essential oils. Contact Dermatitis 2002;47:288-292
3   De Groot AC, Schmidt E. Essential oils: contact allergy and chemical composition. Boca Raton, Fl., USA: CRC Press, Taylor and Francis Group, 2016 (ISBN 9781482246407)

Chapter 6.4   BAY OIL

IDENTIFICATION

Description/definition	: Bay oil (essential oil of bay) is the essential oil obtained from the leaves of the bay rum tree (West Indian bay), *Pimenta racemosa* (Mill.) J.W. Moore
INCI name(s) EU	: Pimenta acris leaf oil
INCI name(s) USA	: Pimenta acris (bay) leaf oil
Other names	: Bay leaf oil
CAS registry number(s)	: 8006-78-8; 85085-61-6; 91721-75-4
EC number(s)	: 294-376-5; 285-385-5
RIFM monograph(s)	: Food Cosmet Toxicol 1973;11:869 (binder, page 112)
ISO standard	: ISO 3045 Essential oil of bay, 2004; Geneva, Switzerland, www.iso.org
Function(s) in cosmetics	: EU: masking. USA: fragrance ingredients
Patch testing	: 2% pet.

GENERAL

Pimenta racemosa (Mill.) J.W. Moore, commonly known as bay, bayrum tree or West Indian bay, is a shrub or small slender tree 7.5-15 meter tall with very aromatic leaves. It is native to the Caribbean (West Indies) and northern South America, and is cultivated widely in tropical countries including Indonesia, West Indies, Venezuela, Mexico, Puerto Rico, Guyana, Jamaica, Tanzania (Zanzibar and Pemba) and Cameroon.

Essential oils may be obtained from the leaves and the fruits. They are used in perfumes, aftershaves, lotions enhancing hair growth and strength or acting against hair loss, for commercial food flavoring, in Caribbean folk medicine and aromatherapy practices (2).

Bay oil should not be confused with *sweet* bay oil, which is obtained from the leaves of *Laurus nobilis* L. (see Laurel leaf oil, Chapter 6.36).

CHEMICAL COMPOSITION

Bay oil is a clear mobile liquid of brownish to dark brown color, which has a spicy odor, reminding of cloves. There appear to be (at least) three chemotypes of bay oil, of which the eugenol-chavicol chemotype is the commercial type. The ten chemicals that had the highest maximum concentrations in 33 commercial bay essential oil samples are shown in table 6.4.1 (Erich Schmidt, analytical data presented in ref. 2).

A full literature review of the qualitative and quantitative composition of commercial and non-commercial bay oils of various origins, their chemotypes and with data from the ISO standard, has been published in 2016 (2).

Table 6.4.1 Ten ingredients with the highest concentrations in commercial bay oils (2)

Name	Concentration range	Name	Concentration range
Eugenol	41.4 - 54.0%	Terpinolene	0.1 - 2.1%
Myrcene	20.5 - 32.0%	β-Caryophyllene	0.4 - 1.9%
Chavicol	6.6 - 10.8%	β-Pinene	0.05 - 1.8%
Limonene	2.4 - 3.2%	Dimyrcene	0.2 - 1.5%
Linalool	0.5 - 2.7%	(*E*)-Ocimene	0.7 - 1.3%

CONTACT ALLERGY / ALLERGIC CONTACT DERMATITIS

Testing in groups of patients

In a group of 21 patients with dermatitis caused by perfumes and tested with a series of essential oils, nine (43%) reacted to oil of bay 1.5% in petrolatum; relevance data were not provided (1). Bay oil consists for 41-54% of eugenol, and as eugenol is an important cause of fragrance sensitivity, the high percentage of positive reactions to bay oil (43%) in this fragrance-sensitive population may largely be ascribed to contact allergy to eugenol. Indeed, of the 7 patients reacting to bay oil and tested with eugenol, five (71%) co-reacted to eugenol (1).

LITERATURE

1   Meynadier JM, Meynadier J, Peyron JL, Peyron L. Formes cliniques des manifestations cutanées d'allergie aux parfums. Ann Dermatol Venereol 1986;113:31-39.
2   De Groot AC, Schmidt E. Essential oils: contact allergy and chemical composition. Boca Raton, Fl., USA: CRC Press, Taylor and Francis Group, 2016 (ISBN 9781482246407)

Chapter 6.5   BERGAMOT OIL

IDENTIFICATION

Description/definition	: Bergamot oil (essential oil of bergamot) is the essential oil obtained by expression from the pericarp (peel) of the bergamot orange, *Citrus bergamia* (Risso et Poit.)
INCI name(s) EU	: Citrus aurantium bergamia fruit oil; Citrus aurantium bergamia peel oil
INCI name(s) USA	: Citrus aurantium bergamia (bergamot) fruit oil; Citrus aurantium bergamia (bergamot) peel oil
Other names	: Bergamot oil bergaptene free; bergamot oil rectified; bergamot orange oil
CAS registry number(s)	: 8007-75-8; 68648-33-9; 89957-91-5; 85049-52-1
EC number(s)	: 289-612-9
RIFM monograph(s)	: Food Cosmet Toxicol 1973;11:1031 (binder, page 143) (bergamot oil expressed); Food Cosmet Toxicol 1973;11:1035 (binder, page 146) (bergamot oil, furocoumarin free)
SCCS opinion(s)	: SCCNFP/0392/00, final (19); SCCNFP/0389/00, final (20); SCCS/1459/11 (21)
IFRA standard	: Restricted (www.ifraorg.org/en-us/standards-library) (table 6.5.1)
ISO standard	: ISO 3520 Essential oil of bergamot, Italian type,1998; Geneva, Switzerland, www.iso.org
Merck Index monograph	: 8135
Function(s) in cosmetics	: EU: masking; perfuming. USA: fragrance ingredients
Patch testing	: 2% pet. (SPCanada)

Table 6.5.1 IFRA restrictions for bergamot oil

Leave-on products:	0.4%
Rinse-off products:	no restriction
Non-skin contact products:	no restriction

The limit only applies to applications on skin exposed to sunshine, excluding rinse-off products. If combinations of phototoxic fragrance ingredients are used, the use levels have to be reduced accordingly. The sum of the concentrations of all phototoxic ingredients, expressed in percentage of their recommended maximum level in the consumer product shall not exceed 100

GENERAL

Bergamot is the common name of the fruit and plant of *Citrus bergamia* Risso et Poiteau, a small tree that blossoms during the winter, producing a fragrant pale yellow, spherical fruit 7.5-10 cm in diameter. Its origin is uncertain, but probably lies in the Mediterranean region. *Citrus bergamia* is commercially grown mainly in the southern Italian region of Calabria, where more than 90% of the world production is realized. Among the *Citrus* peel oils, because of its unique fragrance and freshness, bergamot essential oil is the most valuable and is therefore mainly employed in the perfumery (e.g. in the original Eau de Cologne) and cosmetic industries. The oil also serves for the flavoring of foods, tobacco, liqueur, tea e.g., Earl Grey tea) and soft drinks. Because of its antiseptic and antibacterial properties, bergamot oil is part of the pharmacopoeia of several countries and is used in the pharmaceutical industry and in sanitary preparations. It is also applied in folk medicine and is very popular in aromatherapy (23).

Bergamot oils are phototoxic, causing skin reactions (burns) and secondary hyperpigmentation when the skin to which products (notably fragrances) containing bergamot oils are applied, are exposed to sunlight (1). These reactions are caused by furocoumarins (psoralens) present in the non-volatile fraction of the oils, notably bergapten (5-methoxypsoralen). Therefore, also to adhere to cosmetic legislation, current oils are 'furocoumarin-free', 'bergapten-free' or 'bergamot FCF' (furocoumarin-free) (5), maintaining the composition of the volatile fraction and a bouquet very similar to cold-pressed oils (2). For aromatherapy oils, however, there are currently no official limits to 5-MOP concentrations and the use of such oils still results in occasional cases of phototoxic dermatitis from exposure to sunlight or artificial ultraviolet radiation (5).

The biological properties and cosmetic and medical uses have been reviewed in 2012 (1), clinical applications in 2017 (26).

CHEMICAL COMPOSITION

Bergamot oil is a greenish to yellow, clear mobile liquid which has a fresh, citrusy, soft green and fruity odor with floral accent. In bergamot oils from various origins, over 250 chemicals have been identified. About half of these were found in a single reviewed publication only (23). The ten chemicals that had the highest maximum concentrations in 103 commercial bergamot essential oil samples are shown in table 6.5.2 (Erich Schmidt, analytical data presented in ref. 23).

Ranges for the chemicals in cold-pressed oils, bergapten-free bergamot oils and distilled bergamot oils are provided in ref. 4. A full literature review of the qualitative and quantitative composition of commercial and non-commercial bergamot oils of various origin and with data from the ISO standard has been published in 2016 (23).

Table 6.5.2 Ten ingredients with the highest concentrations in commercial bergamot oils (23)

Name	Concentration range	Name	Concentration range
Limonene	31.4 - 45.1%	Myrcene	0.7 - 1.8%
Linalyl acetate	20.3 - 35.6%	α-Pinene	0.6 - 1.7%
Linalool	4.7 - 16.7%	Sabinene	0.03 - 1.3%
β-Pinene	4.8 - 9.3%	α-*trans*-Bergamotene	0.02 - 1.2%
γ-Terpinene	5.1 - 8.5%	Camphene	0.02 - 1.1%

CONTACT ALLERGY / ALLERGIC CONTACT DERMATITIS

General

The SCCS (Scientific Committee on Consumer Safety), in a 2012 Opinion on Fragrance allergens in cosmetic products, has marked bergamot oil as 'established contact allergen in humans' (21,22).

Contact allergy to / allergic contact dermatitis from bergamot oil has been reported repeatedly. In groups of consecutive patients suspected of contact dermatitis, prevalence rates of up to 1.5% positive patch test reactions have been observed, but reliable data on relevance are lacking. Most cases of allergic contact dermatitis to bergamot oil have been the result of occupational exposure in masseuses / aromatherapists and the fragrance industry. Linalool and β-pinene may have been allergens in bergamot oils in two case reports (7,15). Co-reactivity to limonene, the main component of bergamot oil, has been observed once (6). Phototoxicity due to the psoralens in bergamot oils used to be frequent, but has become rare nowadays.

Testing in groups of patients

The results of patch tests with bergamot oil in routine testing (consecutive patients suspected of contact dermatitis) and in groups of selected patients are shown in table 6.5.3. In routine testing, rates of positive reactions ranged from 0.2% to 1.5%, whereas between 1.5% and 2.0% of patients in selected groups had positive patch tests.

Table 6.5.3 Patch testing in groups of patients

Years and Country	Test conc. & vehicle	Number of patients tested | positive (%)		Selection of patients (S); Relevance (R); Comments (C)	Ref.
Routine testing					
2000-2007 USA	2% pet.	500	6 (1.2%)	R: 100%; C: see Comments below; tested was 'bergamot – natural'	10
2000-2007 USA	2% pet.	500	4 (0.8%)	R: 100%; C: weak study: a. high rate of macular erythema and weak reactions, b. relevance figures include 'questionable' and 'past' relevance; tested was 'bergamot – synthetic'	10
1983-1984 Italy	2% pet.	1200	2 (0.2%)	R: not stated	16
<1976 Poland	2% pet.	200	3 (1.5%)	R: not stated	9
<1973 Poland	10% pet.	200	3 (1.5%)	R: not stated	25
1967-1970	10% pet.	590	3 (0.5%)	R: unknown	17
Testing in groups of selected patients					
<1994 Japan	?	?	? (1.5%)	S: unknown; R: unknown	14
<1976 Poland	2% pet.	51	1 (2.0%)	S: patients allergic to Myroxylon pereirae (balsam of Peru) and/or turpentine and/or wood tar and/or colophony; R: not stated	9

pet.: petrolatum

Case reports and case series

Two aromatherapists had contact dermatitis (occupational in one) with allergies to multiple essential oils used at their work, including bergamot oil. Both patients also reacted to geraniol, α-pinene, the fragrance mix and various other fragrance materials. In addition, one proved to be allergic to linalool and linalyl acetate, the other to caryophyllene; α-pinene, linalool, geraniol and caryophyllene were demonstrated by GC-MS in bergamot oil (7). Linalool may be an important component of bergamot oil and has been found in concentrations of up to 16.7% in commercial bergamot oils (23).

One masseuse had occupational contact dermatitis from contact allergy to bergamot oil; she also reacted to other essential oils and fragrance materials (8). Bergamot oil sensitized one worker in the fragrance industry; she also reacted to α-pinene and β-pinene. Commercial bergamot oils were investigated for the presence of these chemicals and they were identified in maximum concentrations of 1.7% (α-pinene) and 9.3% (β-pinene) (15).

In a group of 70 patients with proven allergic cosmetic dermatitis, bergamot oil was the allergen in one (18). One positive patch test to bergamot oil and its main ingredient limonene was found in a confectioner with occupational contact dermatitis from cardamom (which also contains limonene) (6).

Photosensitivity

Formerly, the most frequent side effect of bergamot oil present in cosmetics was phototoxicity due to its content of furocoumarines, notably 5-methoxypsoralen (bergapten). Its presence in fragrances caused 'Berloque' pigmentation, sometimes preceded by erythema, classically assuming a drop-like or pendant-like configuration over the sides of the neck in adult females from perfumes dripping down. However, pigmentation of the face from perfumes or aftershaves or at other body parts where perfumes were applied have also been observed. Concentrations of 12 ppm of 5-methoxypsoralen could induce phototoxicity with hyperpigmentation (24). Already in the 1970s, the incidence of such reactions decreased from lowering the concentration of bergamot oil in perfumes and using bergapten-free oil. Yet, at the end of the 1970s, 8 cases of phototoxic hyperpigmentation from 5-methoxypsoralen in perfumes were seen in one clinic in Lebanon (24).

Currently, psoralens are (largely) removed from the crude oil before being used in fragrances and other cosmetics, including bronzing and sun-protecting products (which should not contain bergapten in quantities >1 ppm in the European Union). There are no regulations, however, for its content in essential oils used in aromatherapy. Indeed, several cases of phototoxicity from such use have been reported (12,13). One patient developed phototoxicity from bath oil, which was shown to contain 5-methoxypsoralen (12). Two patients developed bullous phototoxic dermatitis from aromatherapy with bergamot oil, of which one from its use in a sauna. One of the preparations used proved to contain 2400 ppm (0.24%) bergapten (13).

Two cases of photo*allergy* from bergamot oil were reported from Italy (11).

LITERATURE

1   Forlot P, Pevet P. Bergamot (*Citrus bergamia* Risso et Poiteau) essential oil: Biological properties, cosmetic and medical use. A review. J Essent Oil Res 2012;24:195-201
2   Dugo G, Bonaccorsi I, Sciarrone D, Schipilliti L, Russo M, Cotroneo A, et al. Characterization of cold-pressed and processed bergamot oils by using GC-FID, GC-MS, GC-C-IRMS, enantio-GC, MDGC, HPLC and HPLC-MS-IT-TOF. J Essent Oil Res 2012;24:93-117
3   Russo M, Torre G, Carnovale C, Bonaccorsi I, Mondello L, Dugo P. A new HPLC method developed for the analysis of oxygen heterocyclic compounds in Citrus essential oils. J Essent Oil Res 2012;24:119-129
4   Schipilliti L, Dugo G, Santi L, Dugo P, Mondello L. Authentication of bergamot essential oil by gas chromatography-combustion-isotope ratio mass spectrometer (GC-C-IRMS). J Essent Oil Res 2011;23:60-71
5   Kaddu S, Kerl H, Wolf P. Accidental bullous phototoxic reactions to bergamot aromatherapy oil. J Am Acad Dermatol 2001;45:458-461
6   Mobacken H, Fregert S. Allergic contact dermatitis from cardamom. Contact Dermatitis 1975;1:175-176
7   Dharmagunawardena B, Takwale A, Sanders KJ, Cannan S, Roger A, Ilchyshyn A. Gas chromatography: an investigative tool in multiple allergies to essential oils. Contact Dermatitis 2002;47:288-292
8   Trattner A, David M, Lazarov A. Occupational contact dermatitis due to essential oils. Contact Dermatitis 2008;58:282-284
9   Rudzki E, Grzywa Z, Bruo WS. Sensitivity to 35 essential oils. Contact Dermatitis 1976;2:196-200
10 Wetter DA, Yiannias JA, Prakash AV, Davis MD, Farmer SA, el-Azhary RA, et al. Results of patch testing to personal care product allergens in a standard series and a supplemental cosmetic series: an analysis of 945 patients from the Mayo Clinic Contact Dermatitis Group, 2000-2007. J Am Acad Dermatol 2010;63:789-798
11 Pigatto PD, Legori A, Bigardi AS, Guarrera M, Tosti A, Santucci B, et al. Gruppo Italiano recerca dermatiti da contatto ed ambientali Italian multicenter study of allergic contact photodermatitis: epidemiological aspects. Am J Contact Dermatitis 1996;7:158-163
12 Clark SM, Wilkinson SM. Phototoxic contact dermatitis from 5-methoxypsoralen in aromatherapy oil. Contact Dermatitis 1998;38:289-290
13 Kaddu S, Kerl H, Wolf P. Accidental bullous phototoxic reactions to bergamot aromatherapy oil. J Am Acad Dermatol 2001;45:458-461
14 Sugai T. Group study IV – farnesol and lily aldehyde. Environ Dermatol 1994;1:213-214
15 Zacher KD, Ippen H. Kontaktekzem durch Bergamottöl. Derm Beruf Umwelt 1984;32:95-97
16 Santucci B, Cristaudo A, Cannistraci C, Picardo M. Contact dermatitis to fragrances. Contact Dermatitis 1987;16:93-95
17 Meneghini CL, Rantuccio F, Lomuto M. Additives, vehicles and active drugs of topical medicaments as causes of delayed-type allergic dermatitis. Dermatologica 1971;143:137-147

18 Schorr WF. Cosmetic allergy: Diagnosis, incidence, and management. Cutis 1974;14:844-850

19 Opinion of the Scientific Committee on Cosmetic Products and Non-Food Products Intended for Consumers concerning 'An initial list of perfumery materials which must not form part of cosmetic products except subject to the Restrictions and Conditions laid down, 25 September 2001, SCCNFP/0392/00, final. Available at: http://ec.europa.eu/health/archive/ph_risk/committees/sccp/documents/out150_en.pdf

20 Opinion of the Scientific Committee on Cosmetic Products and Non-Food Products Intended for Consumers concerning 'The 1st update of the inventory of ingredients employed in cosmetic products. Section II: Perfume and aromatic raw materials', 24 October 2000, SCCNFP/0389/00, final. Available at: http://ec.europa.eu/health/ph_risk/committees/sccp/documents/out131_en.pdf

21 SCCS (Scientific Committee on Consumer Safety). Opinion on Fragrance allergens in cosmetic products, 26-27 June 2012, SCCS/1459/11. Available at: https://ec.europa.eu/health/sites/health/files/scientific_committees/consumer_safety/docs/sccs_o_102.pdf

22 Uter W, Johansen JD, Börje A, Karlberg A-T, Lidén C, Rastogi S, Roberts D, White IR. Categorization of fragrance contact allergens for prioritization of preventive measures: clinical and experimental data and consideration of structure–activity relationships. Contact Dermatitis 2013;69:196-230

23 De Groot AC, Schmidt E. Essential oils: contact allergy and chemical composition. Boca Raton, Fl., USA: CRC Press, Taylor and Francis Group, 2016 (ISBN 9781482246407)

24 Zaynoun ST, Aftimos BA, Tenekjian KK, Kurban AK. Berloque dermatitis – A continuing cosmetic problem. Contact Dermatitis 1981;7:111-116

25 Rudzki E, Kielak D. Sensitivity to some compounds related to Balsam of Peru. Contact Dermatitis Newsletter 1972;nr.13:335-336

26 Mannucci C, Navarra M, Calapai F, Squeri R, Gangemi S, Calapai G. Clinical pharmacology of *Citrus bergamia*: A systematic review. Phytother Res 2017;31:27-39

Chapter 6.6   BITTER ALMOND OIL

IDENTIFICATION

Description/definition   : Bitter almond oil is the volatile oil obtained from the kernels of the bitter almond, *Prunus amygdalus* var. *amara*, Rosaceae
INCI name USA   : Prunus amygdalus amara kernel oil
CAS registry number(s)   : 8013-76-1; 8015-75-6; 90320-35-7
EC number(s)   : 291-060-9
RIFM monograph(s)   : Food Cosmet Toxicol 1979;17:705,707 (special issue V)
Merck Index monograph   : 8139
Function(s) in cosmetics : EU: masking; perfuming. USA: flavoring agents, fragrance ingredients
Patch testing   : 5% pet.

GENERAL

The correct botanical name *for Prunus amygdalus amara* and *Prunus amygdalus* var. *amara* is *Prunus dulcis* (Mill.) D. A. Webb. (U.S. National Plant Germplasm System; www.theplantlist.org).

The almond is a deciduous tree, growing 4-10 meter in height, with a trunk of up to 30 cm in diameter. Almond grows best in Mediterranean climates with warm, dry summers and mild, wet winters. The almond is native to the Mediterranean climate region of the Middle East, from Syria and Turkey eastward to Pakistan and India. It was spread by humans in ancient times along the shores of the Mediterranean into northern Africa and southern Europe, and more recently transported to other parts of the world, notably California.

The almond's velvety, fleshy fruit measures 3.5-6 cm. In botanical terms, it is not a nut but a drupe (Wikipedia). The seed contained in the drupe kernel contains a very fragrant essential oil. The fruit kernels of other trees of the *Prunus* genus also contain bitter almonds such as the apricot tree (*Prunus armeniaca*), peach tree (*Prunus persica*), plum tree (*Prunus domestica*) and cherry tree (*Prunus cerasus*). Once stripped of their hard shells, the kernels are pressed once, releasing a vegetable oil. The solid residue of this expression, called the 'defatted meal', is then hydro-distilled to produce bitter almond essential oil.

Bitter almonds naturally contain traces of hydrogen cyanide (HCN, prussic acid), recognized as a lethal compound worldwide. The reported lethal dose of HCN is 1 mg/kg body weight. Therefore, the oils are rectified to remove the toxic hydrogen cyanide (www.thegoodscentscompany.com) and may be used for food flavoring, e.g. in marzipan. Bitter almond oil is no longer used for internal medication and is not used in the fragrance and cosmetics industry or in aromatherapy. The oil is increasingly being replaced by synthetic benzaldehyde in food flavorings.

CHEMICAL COMPOSITION

Bitter almond oil is a pale yellow to yellow clear liquid; its odor type is fruity is and its odor at 100% is described as 'bitter almond cherry' (www.thegoodscentscompany.com). The chemical composition of the essential oil from bitter almond has hardly ever been investigated; the main components are benzaldehyde (60-90%) and benzoic acid (3).

CONTACT ALLERGY

Case reports and case series

In the 1930s, two cases of allergic contact dermatitis from toilet soap perfumed with bitter almond essential oil have been reported. Both patients had positive patch tests to the oil and to benzaldehyde, its main ingredient (1). Because of the very high price of bitter almond oil (far too high for soap), it is likely that technical grade benzaldehyde had been used (Erich Schmidt, personal communication, September 2018).

Of 12 patients allergic to Myroxylon pereirae resin (balsam of Peru) and tested with oil of bitter almonds (10% in olive oil) and benzaldehyde 5% pet. (present in both bitter almond oil and in balsam of Peru), 6 reacted to both substances and one to the essential oil only (2).

LITERATURE

1   Hansen (1936) and Bonnevie (1939), cited in ref 2 (page 96)
2   Hjorth N. Eczematous allergy to balsams. Acta Derm Venereol 1961;41(suppl.46):1-216
3   Geng H, Yu X, Lu A, Cao H, Zhou B, Zhou L, Zhao Z. Extraction, chemical composition, and antifungal activity of essential oil of bitter almond. Int J Mol Sci 2016 Aug 29;17(9). pii: E1421. doi: 10.3390/ijms17091421

Chapter 6.7   BLACK CUMIN OIL

DEFINITION

Description/definition : Black cumin oil is the essential oil obtained from the seeds of the black caraway (black cumin), *Nigella sativa* L.
INCI name(s) EU and USA : Nigella sativa seed extract
CAS registry number(s) : 90064-32-7
EC number(s)   : 290-094-1
Function(s) in cosmetics : EU: perfuming; skin conditioning. USA: skin-conditioning agents - miscellaneous
Patch testing   : 0.5% -1% pet. (12); may sometimes result in false negative reactions (15)

GENERAL

Nigella sativa L. (black caraway, black cumin) is an annual flowering plant, which grows to 20-30 cm tall. The plant is native to Turkey and Iraq and is sometimes naturalized from the Mediterranean region to central Asia. It is widely cultivated in different parts of the world, mainly in countries bordering the Mediterranean Sea (2); Egypt is one of the main producers of *N. sativa* seeds.

The essential black cumin oil is used as condiment, carminative, analgesic and food preservative and has been recommended as a remedy for various medical conditions (12). The possible health effects of *Nigella sativa* (products) have been reviewed (1,3,4), pharmacological properties summarized (5) and clinical trials of *Nigella sativa* products and its important constituent thymoquinone assessed (14).

Black cumin essential oil should not be confused with Nigella sativa *seed* oil (INCI name EU and USA), which is the *fixed* (vegetable) oil expressed from the seeds of *Nigella sativa* L. (CAS 90064-32-7, EC 290-094-1).

CHEMICAL COMPOSITION

Black cumin oil is a yellow to brown, clear mobile liquid, which has a spicy, herbaceous and phenolic odor. In black cumin oils from various origins, over 340 chemicals have been identified. About 62 per cent of these were found in a single reviewed publication only. The ten chemicals that had the highest maximum concentrations in 13 commercial black cumin essential oil samples are shown in table 6.7.1 (Erich Schmidt, analytical data presented in ref. 12).

A full literature review of the qualitative and quantitative composition of commercial and non-commercial black cumin oils of various origins has been published in 2016 (12).

Table 6.7.1 Ten ingredients with the highest concentrations in commercial black cumin oils (12)

Name	Concentration range	Name	Concentration range
p-Cymene	19.9 - 57.5%	β-Pinene	0.7 - 4.4%
Thymoquinone	0.6 - 24.5%	α-Pinene	0.7 - 4.1%
α-Thujene	8.9 - 17.0%	Limonene	0.08 - 3.7%
trans-p-Menth-2-en-1-ol	0 - 6.1%	Longifolene	0.4 - 0.6%
Carvacrol	trace - 5.8%	γ-Terpinene	0.1 - 2.4%

CONTACT ALLERGY / ALLERGIC CONTACT DERMATITIS

General

Eleven cases of allergic contact dermatitis from black cumin oil have been reported. The dermatitis tends to be extensive and may lead to serious erythema multiforme-like eruptions with fever, progressing to Stevens-Johnson syndrome / toxic epidermal necrolysis (TEN) from oral ingestion, combined oral and topical application and even topical application alone (6,7,13,15). Patch test reactions are usually strongly positive.

Case reports and case series

Case series

In one reference center for toxic bullous dermatoses in France, in the period 2009-2017, three female patients were seen who had developed severe acute contact dermatitis due to topically applied black cumin oil (13). They showed polymorphic lesions that mimicked erythema multiforme, bullous fixed drug eruption, Stevens-Johnson syndrome, or toxic epidermal necrolysis (TEN). All 3 patients had severe impairment with more than 15% of the body surface area involved, with Nikolsky sign and fever, and had a hospital length of stay of more than 10 days. Histologic examination of a skin biopsy was performed in all cases and revealed epidermal apoptosis characterized by confluent nests of apoptotic keratinocytes, with subepidermal detachment or epidermal regenerative changes, and a slight to moderate perivascular infiltrate of lymphocytes in the superficial dermis. Results from direct immunofluorescence were negative. All later had strongly positive patch tests to their own black cumin oils, diluted 1% in petrolatum. The severity of the cases suggests, according to the authors, a systemic effect of black cumin oil, inducing an extension of the lesions away from the area of application, even after topical use alone (13).

In the same period, 4 other patients were also hospitalized with acute allergic contact dermatitis from black cumin oil, but in these individuals, no patch tests were performed (13).

Case reports

One patient developed allergic contact dermatitis from the application of undiluted black cumin oil on the neck for a sore throat; positive patch test reactions were obtained with the pure oil and with 1% and 0.5% black cumin oil (8). A woman developed allergic contact dermatitis from a skin care product containing black cumin oil; upon patch testing she reacted to the cosmetic and to black cumin. There was a negative reaction, however, to black cumin oil itself, but this can easily be explained by the fact that a *cold-pressed* oil, not the essential oil, was used for testing (9).

Another female patient developed generalized dermatitis from contact allergy to black cumin oil applied to the face (10). One individual had pigmented dermatitis of the face and a second had generalized dermatitis from contact allergy to *Nigella sativa* black seed oil, which was confirmed by an open test (11). One case of a bullous erythema multiforme / toxic epidermal necrolysis –like eruption was reported in a patient who had ingested *Nigella sativa* oil and had applied it to the skin; there was a strongly positive patch test reaction to the oil (6).

One individual had allergic contact dermatitis expressing as generalized erythema multiforme with both ingestion and topical application of the oil; a patch test and ROAT with the pure oil were strongly positive (7). In the same article, an unpublished case of Stevens-Johnson syndrome from black cumin oil (contact allergy?) was mentioned as a personal communication (7).

In one female patient, oral use of black cumin oil resulted in the progression of an atypical Stevens–Johnson syndrome / toxic epidermal necrolysis overlap into bullous pemphigoid. Patch tests were later positive to the undiluted oil, but negative to 1% and 10% aqueous dilutions (15).

LITERATURE

1 Butt MS. *Nigella sativa*: Reduces the risk of various maladies. Crit Rev Food Sci Nutrit 2010;50:654-665
2 Bourgou S, Pichette A, Marzouk B, Legault J. Bioactivities of black cumin essential oil and its main terpenes from Tunisia. South Afr J Bot 2010;76:210-216
3 Ahmad A, Husain A, Mujeeb M, Khan SA, Najmi AK, Siddique NA, et al. A review on therapeutic potential of *Nigella sativa*: A miracle herb. Asian Pac J Trop Biomed 2013;3:337-352
4 Hassanien MF, Assiri AM, Alzohairy AM, Oraby HF. Health-promoting value and food applications of black cumin essential oil: an overview. J Food Sci Technol 2015;52:6136-6142
5 Dajani EZ, Shahwan TG, Dajani NE. Overview of the preclinical pharmacological properties of *Nigella sativa* (black seeds): a complementary drug with historical and clinical significance. J Physiol Pharmacol 2016;67:801-817
6 Gelot P, Bara-Passot C, Gimenez-Arnau E, Beneton N, Maillard H, Celerier P. Bullous drug eruption with *Nigella sativa* oil. Ann Dermatol Venereol 2012;139:287-291
7 Nosbaum A, Ben Said B, Halpern S-J, Nicolas J-F, Bérard F. Systemic allergic contact dermatitis to black cumin essential oil expressing as generalized erythema multiforme. Eur J Dermatol 2011;21:447-448
8 Steinmann A, Schätzle M, Agathos M, Breit R. Allergic contact dermatitis from black cumin (*Nigella sativa*) oil after topical use. Contact Dermatitis 1997;36:268-269
9 Zedlitz S, Kaufmann R, Boehncke W. Allergic contact dermatitis from black cumin (*Nigella sativa*) oil-containing ointment. Contact Dermatitis 2002;46:188
10 Lleonart R, Andrés B, Molinero J, Corominas M. Systemic allergic contact dermatitis due to black cumin oil. Contact Dermatitis 2014;70(Suppl. 1):45
11 Gad El-Rab MO, Al-Sheikh OA. Is the European standard series suitable for patch testing in Riyadh, Saudi Arabia? Contact Dermatitis 1995;33:310-314
12 De Groot AC, Schmidt E. Essential oils: contact allergy and chemical composition. Boca Raton, Fl., USA: CRC Press, Taylor and Francis Group, 2016 (ISBN 9781482246407)
13 Gaudin O, Toukal F, Hua C, Ortonne N, Assier H, Jannic A, et al. Association between severe acute contact dermatitis due to Nigella sativa oil and epidermal apoptosis. JAMA Dermatol 2018;154:1062-1065
14 Tavakkoli A, Mahdian V, Razavi BM, Hosseinzadeh H. Review on clinical trials of black seed (Nigella sativa) and its active constituent, thymoquinone. J Pharmacopuncture 2017;20:179-193
15 Bonhomme A, Poreaux C, Jouen F, Schmutz JL, Gillet P, Barbaud A. Bullous drug eruption to *Nigella sativa* oil: consideration of the use of a herbal medicine—clinical report and review of the literature. J Eur Acad Dermatol Venereol 2017;31:e217-e219

Chapter 6.8   BLACK PEPPER OIL

IDENTIFICATION

Description/definition   : Black pepper oil (essential oil of black pepper) is the essential oil obtained from the fruit of the (black) pepper, *Piper nigrum* L.
INCI name(s) EU   : Piper nigrum fruit oil
INCI name(s) USA   : Piper nigrum (pepper) fruit oil
CAS registry number(s)   : 8006-82-4; 84929-41-9
EC number(s)   : 284-524-7
RIFM monograph(s)   : Food Cosmet Toxicol 1978;16:651 (special issue IV)
ISO standard   : ISO 3061 Essential oil of black pepper, 2008; Geneva, Switzerland, www.iso.org
Merck Index monograph   : 2584 (Black pepper)
Function(s) in cosmetics : EU: masking; perfuming. USA: fragrance ingredients
Patch testing   : 2% pet.; based on RIFM data, 4% pet. is probably not irritant (2)

GENERAL

Black pepper (*Piper nigrum* L.) is a perennial woody evergreen plant that can grow to a height of 50-60 cm. The tropical forest of the Malabar region of southern India is considered to be the center of its origin; it is now widely cultivated in the tropics. The most important exporters of black pepper are India, Indonesia, Brazil, Malaysia, Sri Lanka and Vietnam. 'Black pepper' is obtained by sun-drying green berries harvested before full maturity is reached, whereas fully ripe dried fruits devoid of pericarp form the commercial 'white pepper'. Pepper is the most widely used spice throughout the world, appreciated for both its aroma and its pungency. The 'king of spices' is not only used for culinary, but also for medicinal and other purposes (10).

The essential oil of black pepper is obtained by hydrodistillation of the (powdered) black pepper fruits. Pepper essential oil has important applications in the food and pharmacological industries, perfumery, cosmetics, and home remedies (3,4,5). Externally, the oil is used as a rubefacient and anti-rheumatic, and as gargling agent for sore throat (7). It is also employed in aromatherapy practice (8). The biological activities (6,7) and health claims (1) of black pepper have been reviewed.

Black pepper essential oil should not be confused with Piper nigrum (pepper) seed oil (also CAS 84929-41-9, EC 284-524-7), which is a fatty, expressed (vegetable, fixed) oil from black pepper seeds.

CHEMICAL COMPOSITION

Black pepper oil is a colorless or light yellow to blue, mobile liquid which has a terpenic, aromatic, somewhat spicy and herbaceous odor. In black pepper oils from various origins, over 305 chemicals have been identified. About 58 percent of these were found in a single publication reviewed only. The ten chemicals that had the highest maximum concentrations in 46 commercial black pepper essential oil samples are shown in table 6.8.1 (Erich Schmidt, analytical data presented in ref. 10).

A full literature review of the qualitative and quantitative composition of commercial and non-commercial black pepper oils of various origins, their chemotypes and with data from the ISO standard, has been published in 2016 (10).

Table 6.8.1 Ten ingredients with the highest concentrations in commercial black pepper oils (10)

Name	Concentration range	Name	Concentration range
β-Caryophyllene	0.9 - 32.4%	α-Phellandrene	0.8 - 17.4%
α-Pinene	5.1 - 29.5%	Sabinene	0.1 - 15.4%
Limonene	10.2 - 24.7%	Camphene	0.1 - 8.0%
β-Pinene	6.7 - 20.3%	Myrcene	1.5 - 6.3%
δ3-Carene	4.3 - 17.6%	*p*-Cymene	0.2 - 6.0%

CONTACT ALLERGY / ALLERGIC CONTACT DERMATITIS

General

Contact allergy to and possible allergic contact dermatitis from black pepper oil have been reported in one publication only. A false-positive patch test reaction due to the excited skin syndrome cannot be excluded. In the same case report, α-pinene and caryophyllene may have been allergens in black pepper oil (9).

Case reports and case series

Two aromatherapists had contact dermatitis (occupational in one) with allergies to multiple essential oils used at their work, including black pepper oil. Both patients also reacted to geraniol, α-pinene, the fragrance mix and various other fragrance materials. In addition, one proved to be allergic to linalool and linalyl acetate, the other to caryophyllene; α-pinene and caryophyllene were demonstrated by GC-MS in black pepper oil (9). Both chemicals are the main components of black pepper oils with concentrations found in commercial oils in maximum concentrations of 32% for caryophyllene and 29% for α-pinene (see the section 'Chemical composition' above).

REFERENCES

1   Butt MS, Pasha I, Tauseef Sultan M, Randhawa MA, Saeed F, Ahmed W. Black pepper and health claims: a comprehensive treatise. Crit Rev Food Sci Nutrit 2013;53:875-886

2   De Groot AC. Patch Testing, 4th Edition. Wapserveen, The Netherlands: acdegroot publishing, 2018 (ISBN 978-90-813233-4-5)

3   Singh G, Marimuthu P, Catalan C, deLampasona MP. Chemical, antioxidant and antifungal activities of volatile oil of black pepper and its acetone extract. J Sci Food Agric 2004;84:1878-1884

4   Bagheri H, Bin Abdul Manap MY, Solati Z. Antioxidant activity of *Piper nigrum* L. essential oil extracted by supercritical CO2 extraction and hydrodistillation. Talanta 2014;121:220-228

5   Abd El Mageed MA, Mansour AF, El Massry KF, Ramadan MM, Shaheen MS. The effect of microwaves on essential oils of white and black pepper (*Piper nigrum* L.) and their antioxidant activities. J Essent Oil Bear Plants 2011;14:214-223

6   Ahmad N, Fazal H, Haider Abbasi B, Farooq S, Ali M, Ali Khan M. Biological role of *Piper nigrum* L. (Black pepper): A review. Asian Pac J Trop Biomed 2012;2(Suppl.):S1945-S1953

7   Meghwal M, Goswami TK. *Piper nigrum* and piperine: An update. Phytother Res 2013;27:1121-1130

8   Lawless J. The encyclopedia of essential oils, 2nd Edition. London: Harper Thorsons, 2014

9   Dharmagunawardena B, Takwale A, Sanders KJ, Cannan S, Roger A, Ilchyshyn A. Gas chromatography: an investigative tool in multiple allergies to essential oils. Contact Dermatitis 2002;47:288-292

10 De Groot AC, Schmidt E. Essential oils: contact allergy and chemical composition. Boca Raton, Fl., USA: CRC Press, Taylor and Francis Group, 2016 (ISBN 9781482246407)

Chapter 6.9   CAJEPUT OIL

IDENTIFICATION

Description/definition	: Cajeput oil [b] is the essential oil obtained from the leaves and the terminal branchlets (twigs) of the cajaput tree, *Melaleuca cajuputi* Powell (synonyms: *Melaleuca minor* Smith., *Melaleuca leucodendra* auct. nonn.)
INCI name(s) EU	: Melaleuca leucadendron cajaput oil [a,b]; Melaleuca leucadendron cajuputi leaf oil [a] (perfuming name, not an INCI name proper)
INCI name(s) USA	: Melaleuca leucadendron cajaput oil [a,b]
Other names	: Cajuput oil [b]; cajaput oil [b]
CAS registry number(s)	: 8008-98-8; 85480-37-1
EC number(s)	: 287-316-4
RIFM monograph(s)	: Food Cosmet Toxicol 1976;14:701 (special Issue III)
Function(s) in cosmetics	: EU: masking; perfuming. USA: fragrance ingredients
Patch testing	: 2% pet.; based on RIFM data, 4% pet. is probably not irritant (11)

[a] The source of cajeput oil is *Melaleuca cajuputi* Powell, not *Melaleuca leucadendra* (sometimes termed *Melaleuca leucadendron*) (2). This earlier nomenclature confusion stems from the fact that the trees of both *Melaleuca* species are known in Indonesia and Malaysia under a same name, gelam (2,5). However, the composition of the oil of *Melaleuca leucadendra* differs considerably from that of cajeput oil (6,7).

[b] The terms cajaput, cajuput and cajeput are synonymously used for both the tree and the oil

GENERAL

Melaleuca cajuputi Powell (swamp tea tree, paperbark tea tree) is an evergreen shrub or tree which may measure up to 25 meters in height. The tree is native to tropical Asia and northern Australia and is cultivated in Indonesia (especially Sulawezi, the former Celebes), Vietnam and Malaysia (GRIN taxonomy for plants). The name 'cajeput' is derived from its Indonesian name, '*kayu putih*' or 'white wood'.

The essential oil made from the leaves and twigs of the tree is extremely pungent and has the odor of a mixture of turpentine and camphor. It is frequently employed externally as a counterirritant and as an ingredient in some liniments for sore muscles such as Tiger Balm and the Indonesian traditional medicine Minyak Telon. Cajeput oil has been used in Vietnam, Indonesia, China and elsewhere for the treatment of various ailments and is also employed by aromatherapists. Other applications include its use as a treatment against skin mites, as insect repellent and the oil may have anti-termite activity and has shown some promise in dengue vector control (1,3,4,6,10, Wikipedia).

CHEMICAL COMPOSITION

Cajeput oil is a colorless to yellowish easily mobile clear liquid which has a fresh, camphoraceus, minty and eucalyptus-like odor. In cajeput oils from various origins, over 130 chemicals have been identified. About half of these were found in a single reviewed publication only. The ten chemicals that had the highest maximum concentrations in 51 commercial cajeput essential oil samples are shown in table 6.9.1 (Erich Schmidt, analytical data presented in ref. 10).

A full literature review of the qualitative and quantitative composition of commercial and non-commercial cajeput oils of various origins, their chemotypes and with data from the ISO standard, has been published in 2016 (10).

Table 6.9.1 Ten ingredients with the highest concentrations in commercial cajeput oils (10)

Name	Concentration range	Name	Concentration range
1,8-Cineole	46.0 - 70.2%	γ-Terpinene	0.7 - 5.4%
α-Terpineol	2.5 - 11.6%	Terpinolene	0.4 - 5.3%
Limonene	1.8 - 10.2%	β-Caryophyllene	0.08 - 5.2%
p-Cymene	0.1 - 9.5%	Sabinene	0.01 - 4.5%
α-Pinene	0.6 - 7.6%	β-Pinene	0.7 - 4.4%

CONTACT ALLERGY / ALLERGIC CONTACT DERMATITIS

General

Allergic contact dermatitis from cajeput oil has been observed in two publications only. In both reports, false-positive patch test reactions due to the excited skin syndrome cannot be excluded. In one case report, α-pinene and caryophyllene may have been allergens in cajeput oil (9).

Case reports and case series

An aromatherapist had chronic hand dermatitis and was patch test positive to 17 of 20 oils used at her work (tested 1% and 5% in petrolatum), including cajeput oil; cajeput was given as synonym for tea tree oil, which is incorrect (8).

Two other aromatherapists had contact dermatitis (occupational in one) with allergies to multiple essential oils used at their work including cajeput oil. Both patients also reacted to geraniol, α-pinene, the fragrance mix and various other fragrance materials. In addition, one proved to be allergic to linalool and linalyl acetate, the other to caryophyllene; α-pinene and caryophyllene were demonstrated by GC-MS in cajeput oil (9). Both chemicals have been found in commercial cajeput oils in maximum concentrations of 5.2% (caryophyllene) and 7.6% (α-pinene) (see the section 'Chemical composition' above).

LITERATURE

1   Barbosa LCA, Silva CJ, Teixeira RR, Alves Meira MAS, Pinheiro AL. Chemistry and biological activities of essential oils from *Melaleuca* L. species. Agriculturae Conspectus Scientificus 2013;78:11-23
    Available at: http://www.agr.unizg.hr/smotra/pdf_78/acs78_02.pdf
2   Lawrence BM. Progress in essential oils. Perfum Flav 2012;37 (april):56-57
3   Abu Bakar A, Sulaiman S, Omar B, Mat Ali R. Evaluation of *Melaleuca cajuputi* (Family: Myrtaceae) essential oil in aerosol spray cans against dengue vectors in low cost housing flats. J Arthropod-Borne Dis 2012;6:28-35
4   Cuong ND, Xuyen TT, Motl O, Stransky K, Presslova J, Jedlikova Z, et al. Antibacterial properties of Vietnamese cajuput oil. J Essent Oil Res 1994;6:63-67
5   Roszaini K, Nor Azah MA, Mailina J, Zaini S, Faridz ZM. Toxicity and antitermite activity of the essential oils from *Cinnamomum camphora*, *Cymbopogon nardus*, *Melaleuca cajuputi* and *Dipterocarpus* sp. against *Coptotermes curvignathus*. Wood Sci Technol 2013;47:1273-1284
6   Sakasegawa M, Hori K, Yatagai M. Composition and antitermite activities of essential oils from *Melaleuca* species. J Wood Sci 2003;49:181-187
7   Brophy JJ, Lassak EV. *Melaleuca leucadendra* L. leaf oil: Two phenylpropanoid chemotypes. Flavour Fragr J 1988;3:43-46
8   Selvaag E, Holm J, Thune P. Allergic contact dermatitis in an aromatherapist with multiple sensitizations to essential oils. Contact Dermatitis 1995;33:354-355
9   Dharmagunawardena B, Takwale A, Sanders KJ, Cannan S, Roger A, Ilchyshyn A. Gas chromatography: an investigative tool in multiple allergies to essential oils. Contact Dermatitis 2002;47:288-292
10 De Groot AC, Schmidt E. Essential oils: contact allergy and chemical composition. Boca Raton, Fl., USA: CRC Press, Taylor and Francis Group, 2016 (ISBN 9781482246407)
11 De Groot AC. Patch Testing, 4th Edition. Wapserveen, The Netherlands: acdegroot publishing, 2018 (ISBN 978-90-813233-4-5)

Chapter 6.10   CALAMUS OIL

IDENTIFICATION

Description/definition : Calamus oil is the essential oil obtained from the rhizomes of the calamus (flagroot,
myrtle flag, sweet flag), *Acorus calamus* L.

INCI name(s) EU : Acorus calamus root oil (perfuming name, not an INCI name proper)

INCI name(s) USA : Not in the Personal Care Products Council Ingredient Database

Other names : Sweet flag oil

CAS registry number(s) : 8015-79-0; 84775-39-3

EC number(s) : 283-869-0

RIFM monograph(s) : Food Cosmet Toxicol 1977;15:623

IFRA standard : Restricted: the total level of *cis-* (beta) and *trans-* (alpha) asarone resulting from natural
presence in essential oils (e.g. calamus oil) should not exceed 0.01% in the finished
product (www.ifraorg.org/en-us/standards-library)

SCCS opinion(s) : SCCNFP/0389/00, final (16); SCCS/1459/11 (17)

Merck Index monograph : 2910 (Calamus)

Function(s) in cosmetics : EU: perfuming

Patch testing : 2% pet.; based on RIFM data, 4% pet. is probably not irritant (20)

GENERAL

Acorus calamus L. or 'sweet flag' is a reed-like semiaquatic perennial plant, which is native to India. It is found growing wild in abundance there, ascending to 2200 meters in the Himalayas. It also grows in the temperate zones of Europe, East Asia and North America. Calamus inhabits perpetually wet areas such as the banks of streams and rivers and around ponds, lakes, and swamps. The stout aromatic roots of *A. calamus* spread horizontally (rhizomes) and can grow to almost 0.5-1.25 m in length (1,2,3). It is cultivated in South Africa (GRIN Taxonomy for Plants).

In India, *A. calamus* and its essential oil serve mainly as an insecticide and insect repellent (4). The rhizomes and their oils are in addition used in Ayurvedic, Unani and folk medicines (3,5).

The essential oil from the rhizomes may sometimes be found in beer and aromatic cordial and liqueur preparations (3,5) and the rhizomes of the European *A. calamus* and calamus essential oil are used in the flavoring industry. Because of the toxicity of its ingredient β-asarone, calamus products for human use should contain no or negligible amounts of β-asarone (6). In several countries including the USA, *A. calamus* and its oil have been prohibited as a food additive, and in the EU it is not used anymore in perfumery. Also, in recent years many herbal shops have stopped recommending or dispensing it (2). It is also considered too toxic for aromatherapy (13). However, calamus products are available for recreational (hallucinogenic) use on the internet and acute intoxications from abuse of such substances, mainly characterized by prolonged vomiting, have been reported and are not rare (10). Several review articles on pharmacological activities, medicinal applications and biological properties have been published (6,7,9,11,12).

CHEMICAL COMPOSITION

Calamus oil is a yellowish to yellowish brown, clear liquid which has an aromatic, herbaceous, spicy and creamy odor. In calamus oils from various origins, over 275 chemicals have been identified. Nearly half of these were found in a single reviewed publication only. The ten chemicals that had the highest maximum concentrations in 14 commercial calamus essential oil samples are shown in table 6.10.1 (Erich Schmidt, analytical data presented in ref. 19).

Acorus calamus includes four cytotypes distinguished by chromosome number: diploid (2x =24), triploid (3x =36), tetraploid (4x = 48) and hexaploid (6x = 72). The distinction is important, as the ploidy determines the amount of the toxic chemical β-asarone in the rhizomes and the rhizome oil (1,2,3,5,7,8).

A full literature review of the qualitative and quantitative composition of commercial and non-commercial calamus oils of various origins and their chemotypes has been published in 2016 (19).

Table 6.10.1 Ten ingredients with the highest concentrations in commercial calamus oils (19)

Name	Concentration range	Name	Concentration range
α-Asarone	1.8 - 79.6%	Camphene	trace - 7.3%
β-Asarone	1.6 - 13.9%	Isoshyobunone	0.2 - 7.2%
(*Z*)-Methyl isoeugenol	0.3 - 13.7%	Methyl eugenol	0.03 - 6.5%
α-Pinene	0.02 - 12.4%	Camphor	0.02 - 5.9%
α-Calacorene	1.7 - 8.5%	*trans*-Calamene	2.5 - 5.4%

CONTACT ALLERGY / ALLERGIC CONTACT DERMATITIS

General
The SCCS (Scientific Committee on Consumer Safety), in a 2012 Opinion on Fragrance allergens in cosmetic products, has categorized calamus root oil as 'possible fragrance contact allergen' (17,18). Contact allergy to calamus oil has been reported in two publications, but no cases of allergic contact dermatitis from the oil have been identified.

Testing in groups of patients
A group of 86 patients from Poland previously reacting to the fragrance mix was tested with calamus oil and seven (8.1%) had a positive patch test reaction to calamus oil 2% in petrolatum; relevance data were not provided (14). In a group of 21 patients with dermatitis caused by perfumes and tested with a series of essential oils, one (5%) reacted to calamus oil; relevance data were not provided (15).

LITERATURE

1   Özcan M, Akgül A, Chalchat JC. Volatile constituents of the essential oil of *Acorus calamus* L. grown in Konya Province (Turkey). J Ess Oil Res 2002;14:366-368
2   Venskutonis PR, Dagilyte A. Composition of essential oil of sweet flag (*Acorus calamus* L.) leaves at different growing phases. J Essent Oil Res 2003;15:313-318
3   Raina VK, Srivastava SK, Syamasunder KV. Essential oil composition of *Acorus calamus* L. from the lower region of the Himalayas. Flavour Fragr J 2003;18:18-20
4   Marongiu B, Piras A, Porcedda S, Scorciapino A. Chemical composition of the essential oil and supercritical CO_2 extract of *Commiphora myrrha* (Nees) Engl. and of *Acorus calamus* L. J Agric Food Chem 2005;53:7939-7943
5   Ahlawat A, Katoch M, Ram G, Ahuja A. Genetic diversity in *Acorus calamus* L. as revealed by RAPD markers and its relationship with β-asarone content and ploidy level. Scientiae Horticulturae 2010;124:294-297
6   Singh C, Jamwal U, Sing P. *Acorus calamus* (sweet flag): an overview of oil composition, biological activity and usage. J Medic Arom Plant Sci 2001;23:687-708
7   Sharma V, Singh I, Chaudhary P. *Acorus calamus* (The Healing Plant): a review on its medicinal potential, micropropagation and conservation. Nat Prod Res 2014;28:1454-1466
8   Dušek K, Galambosi B, Hethelyi EB, Korany K, Karlová K. Morphological and chemical variations of sweet flag (*Acorus calamus* L.) in the Czech and Finnish gene bank collection. Hort Sci (Prague) 2007;34:17-25
9   Rajput SB, Tonge MB, Karuppayil SM. An overview on traditional uses and pharmacological profile of *Acorus calamus* Linn. (sweet flag) and other *Acorus* species. Phytomed 2014;21:268-276
10   Björnstad K, Helander A, Hultén P, Beck O. Bioanalytical investigation of asarone in connection with *Acorus calamus* oil intoxications. J Anal Toxicol 2009;33:604-609
11   Mukherjee PK, Kumar V, Mal M, Houghton PJ. *Acorus calamus*: Scientific validation of Ayurvedic tradition from natural resources. Pharm Biol 2007;45:651-666
12   Devis A, Bawankar R, Babu S. Current status on biological activities of *Acorus calamus* - a review. Int J Pharm Pharm Sci 2014;6(10):66-71
13   Davis P. Aromatherapy. An A-Z, 3rd Edition. London: Vermilion, 2005
14   Rudzki E, Grzywa Z. Allergy to perfume mixture. Contact Dermatitis 1986;15:115-116
15   Meynadier JM, Meynadier J, Peyron JL, Peyron L. Formes cliniques des manifestations cutanées d'allergie aux parfums. Ann Dermatol Venereol 1986;113:31-39
16   Opinion of the Scientific Committee on Cosmetic Products and Non-Food Products Intended for Consumers concerning 'The 1st update of the inventory of ingredients employed in cosmetic products. Section II: Perfume and aromatic raw materials', 24 October 2000, SCCNFP/0389/00, final. Available at: http://ec.europa.eu/health/ph_risk/committees/sccp/documents/out131_en.pdf
17   SCCS (Scientific Committee on Consumer Safety). Opinion on Fragrance allergens in cosmetic products, 26-27 June 2012, SCCS/1459/11. Available at: https://ec.europa.eu/health/sites/health/files/scientific_committees/consumer_safety/docs/sccs_o_102.pdf
18   Uter W, Johansen JD, Börje A, Karlberg A-T, Lidén C, Rastogi S, Roberts D, White IR. Categorization of fragrance contact allergens for prioritization of preventive measures: clinical and experimental data and consideration of structure–activity relationships. Contact Dermatitis 2013;69:196-230
19   De Groot AC, Schmidt E. Essential oils: contact allergy and chemical composition. Boca Raton, Fl., USA: CRC Press, Taylor and Francis Group, 2016 (ISBN 9781482246407)
20   De Groot AC. Patch Testing, 4th Edition. Wapserveen, The Netherlands: acdegroot publishing, 2018 (ISBN 978-90-813233-4-5)

Chapter 6.11 CANANGA OIL

IDENTIFICATION

Description/definition	: Cananga oil (essential oil of cananga) is the essential oil obtained from the flowers of the perfume tree (Macassar oil tree), *Cananga odorata* (Lam.) Hook f. et Thomson, forma *macrophylla*
INCI name(s) EU	: Cananga odorata macrophylla flower extract (perfuming name, not an INCI name proper)
INCI name(s) USA	: Not in the Personal Care Products Council Ingredient Database
CAS registry number(s)	: 93686-30-7; 68606-83-7
EC number(s)	: 297-681-1
RIFM monograph(s)	: Food Cosmet Toxicol 1973;11:1049 (binder, page 178)
SCCS opinion(s)	: SCCS/1459/11 (32)
ISO standard	: ISO 3523 Essential oil of cananga, 2002; Geneva, Switzerland, www.iso.org
Function(s) in cosmetics	: EU: perfuming
Patch testing	: 2-5% pet. (36)

GENERAL

Cananga oil should not be confused with ylang-ylang oil, obtained from *Cananga odorata* (Lam.) Hook f. et Thomson, forma *genuina.* These oils were originally thought to be identical and are still often used – incorrectly – as synonyms. See also Chapter 6.78 Ylang-ylang oil.

For a general introduction to the *Cananga odorata* tree see Chapter 6.78 Ylang-ylang oil. Ylang-Ylang oil is of higher quality than and is mostly preferred by the fragrance industry over cananga oil. In general, however, their applications are similar. Cananga oil is produced commercially mainly in Indonesia and to a much lesser extent in Vietnam (4). It is used as fragrance in perfumes and cosmetics, as flavor in foods and beverages, in pharmaceuticals and in aromatherapy (1,2,3,5,6).

CHEMICAL COMPOSITION

Cananga oil is a clear mobile liquid with a faint yellow to darker yellow color, which has a floral and woody, slightly aromatic odor. In cananga oils from various origins, over 100 chemicals have been identified. About 22 per cent of these were found in a single reviewed publication only. The ten chemicals that had the highest maximum concentrations in 25 commercial cananga essential oil samples are shown in table 6.11.1 (Erich Schmidt, analytical data presented in ref. 34).

A full literature review of the qualitative and quantitative composition of commercial and non-commercial cananga oils of various origins and with data from the ISO standard, has been published in 2016 (34).

Table 6.11.1 Ten ingredients with the highest concentrations in commercial cananga oils (34)

Name	Concentration range	Name	Concentration range
β-Caryophyllene	32.9 - 38.0%	Benzyl benzoate	2.6 - 5.6%
Germacrene D	4.5 - 9.5%	Linalool	1.2 - 2.8%
α-Humulene	8.3 - 9.4%	γ-Muurolene	0.6 - 2.2%
(*E,E*)-α-Farnesene	2.3 - 7.1%	*p*-Cresyl methyl ether	1.2 - 2.1%
δ-Cadinene	4.5 - 6.1%	α-Cadinol	0.2 - 2.1%

CONTACT ALLERGY / ALLERGIC CONTACT DERMATITIS

General

The SCCS (Scientific Committee on Consumer Safety), in a 2012 Opinion on Fragrance allergens in cosmetic products, has marked cananga oil as 'established contact allergen in humans' (32,33).

Contact allergy to / allergic contact dermatitis from cananga oil has been reported in over 25 publications. In groups of consecutive patients suspected of contact dermatitis, prevalence rates of up to 1.2% positive patch test reactions have been observed, but reliable data on relevance are lacking. Case reports of allergic contact dermatitis to cananga oil are all from occupational exposure in massage therapists / aromatherapists. Co-reactions to the related ylang-ylang oil (also prepared from the *Cananga odorata* tree, but from the forma *genuina*) are frequent. Cananga oil used to be a frequent cause of pigmented cosmetic dermatitis in Japan.

Testing in groups of patients

The results of patch tests with cananga oil in routine testing (consecutive patients suspected of contact dermatitis) and in groups of selected patients are shown in table 6.11.2. In routine testing, rates of positive reactions ranged from 0.5% to 1.2%, whereas between 0.2% and 33% of patients in selected groups had positive patch tests. The very high positivity rate of 33% was found in a small group of 21 patients previously shown to have allergic contact dermatitis from fragrances (7).

Table 6.11.2 Patch testing in groups of patients

Years and Country	Test conc. & vehicle	Number of patients tested | positive (%)		Selection of patients (S); Relevance (R); Comments (C)	Ref.
Routine testing					
2000-2007 USA	2% pet.	486	5 (1.0%)	R: 100%; C: weak study: a. high rate of macular erythema and weak reactions, b. relevance figures include 'questionable' and 'past' relevance	8
2002-2003 Korea	2% pet.	422	5 (1.2%)	R: not stated	20
<1976 Poland	2% pet.	200	1 (0.5%)	R: not stated	27
Testing in groups of selected patients					
2011-2015 Spain	2% pet.	607	12 (2.0%)	S: patients previously reacting to FM I, FM II, Myroxylon pereirae resin or hydroxyisohexyl 3-cyclohexene carboxaldehyde in the baseline series and subsequently tested with a fragrance series; R: not stated	37
2008-2014 UK	2% pet.	471	1 (0.2%)	S: patients tested with a fragrance series; R: not stated	35
2001-2010 Australia	2% pet.	823	39 (4.7%)	S: not specified; R: 31%	29
2004-2008 Spain	2% pet.	86	3 (3.5%)	S: patients previously reacting to the fragrance mix I or Myroxylon pereirae (n=54) or suspected of fragrance contact allergy (n=32); R: not stated	15
<2004 Israel	2% pet.	91	1 (1.1%)	S: patients who had shown a doubtful or positive reaction to the fragrance mix I and/or Myroxylon pereirae resin and/or one or two commercial fine fragrances; R: not stated	21
1989-1999 Portugal	2% pet.	67	7 (10.4%)	S: patients who had a positive patch test to the fragrance mix; R: not stated	22
1990-1998 Japan	5% pet.	1483	16 (1.1%)	S: patients suspected of cosmetic contact dermatitis, virtually all were women; range of annual frequency of sensitization: 0-1.9%; R: not stated	16
1996-1997 UK	2% pet.	10	2 (20%)	S: patients suspected of cosmetic dermatitis and reacting to the fragrance mix; R: not stated	10
<1986 Poland	2% pet.	86	10 (11.6%)	S: patients previously reacting to the fragrance mix; R: not stated	13
<1986 France	2.5% pet.	21	7 (33%)	S: patients with dermatitis caused by perfumes; R: not stated	7
<1983 Poland	2% pet.	16	3 (19%)	S: patients known to be allergic to propolis and Myroxylon pereirae; R: not stated	30
1971-1980 Japan	5% pet.	477	4 (0.8%)	S: patients with dermatoses other than pigmented cosmetic dermatitis and volunteers; R: not stated	11
<1976 Poland	2% pet.	51	1 (2.0%)	S: patients allergic to Myroxylon pereirae resin (balsam of Peru) and/or turpentine and/or wood tar and/or colophony	27
<1974 Japan	?	183	26 (14.2%)	S: patients suspected of cosmetic dermatitis; R: unknown; in many, there was co-reactivity with benzyl salicylate, which may be present in commercial cananga oils in concentration of up to 0.5%	23

pet.: petrolatum

Case reports and case series

An aromatherapist / massage therapist developed occupational contact dermatitis from contact allergy to multiple essential oils; she reacted to both cananga oil and ylang-ylang oil in the fragrance series, which reactions were considered to be relevant (18). A similar case was seen in another aromatherapist (28). Two massage therapists / aromatherapists with occupational contact dermatitis from (multiple) essential oils had positive patch tests to cananga oil; it was uncertain whether this oil had been used by these patients (17).

In a number of publications, positive patch tests to cananga oil have been reported with unknown, uncertain or unstated relevance. These include (literature screened up to 2014 [34]) the following. Of seven patients allergic to the fragrance farnesol, 4 (57%) co-reacted to cananga oil (and various other fragrances) (31). One positive patch test reaction to cananga oil was seen in a patient primarily sensitized to compound tincture of benzoin (19). Among 819 patients suspected of contact dermatitis, two had positive patch tests to cananga oil (9). A naturopathic therapist with occupational contact dermatitis to multiple essential oils also reacted to cananga oil in the fragrance series (26).

Positive patch tests to cananga oil were observed in two aromatherapists with occupational allergic contact dermatitis from multiple essential oils, who did not use cananga oils at work (25). One positive patch test reaction to cananga oil was seen in a patient with allergic contact dermatitis from lovage oil and jasmine absolute (14). Two patients had positive patch tests to cananga oil; they both also reacted to ylang-ylang oil (24).

Pigmented cosmetic dermatitis

In Japan, in the 1960s and 1970s, many female patients developed pigmentation of the face after having facial dermatitis (12). This so-called pigmented cosmetic dermatitis was shown to be caused by contact allergy to components of cosmetic products, notably essential oils, other fragrance materials, antimicrobials, preservatives and coloring materials (11,12). In a group of 620 Japanese patients with this condition investigated between 1970 and 1980, 7-11 % had positive patch test reactions to cananga oil 15% in petrolatum in various time periods (11). The number of patients with pigmented cosmetic dermatitis decreased strongly after 1978, when major cosmetic companies began to eliminate strong contact sensitizers from their products (11).

Co-reactivity to ylang-ylang oil

Of eight patients with dermatitis from fragrances and reacting to ylang-ylang oil, seven (88%) also reacted to cananga oil (7). Of seven patients with dermatitis from fragrances and reacting to cananga oil, all also reacted to ylang-ylang oil (7). In various other reports (e.g., 9,17,18,24,28) patients had positive patch tests to both ylang-ylang oil and cananga oil, which may indicate cross-sensitivity or can be explained by pseudo-cross-sensitivity due to the presence of the same allergenic component(s).

LITERATURE

1 Kristiawan M, Sobolik V, Allaf K. Isolation of Indonesian cananga oil by instantaneous controlled pressure drop. J Essent Oil Res 2008;20:135-146

2 Kristiawan M, Sobolik V, Al-Haddad M, Allaf K. Effect of pressure-drop rate on the isolation of cananga oil using instantaneous controlled pressure-drop process. Chemical Engineering and Processing 2008;47:66-75

3 Megawati, Saputra SWD. A combination of water-steam distillation and solvent extraction of *Cananga odorata* essential oil. IOSR J Engin 2012;2:5-12

4 Lawrence BM. Progress in essential oils. Perfum Flavor 2004;29(6):80-90

5 Kristiawan M, Sobolik V, Allaf K. Isolation of Indonesian cananga oil using multi-cycle pressure drop process. J Chromatogr A 2008;1192:306-318

6 Kristiawan M, Sobolik V, Allaf K. Yield and composition of Indonesian cananga oil obtained by steam distillation and organic solvent extraction. Int J Food Engin 2012;8(3):article 28 (19 pages). DOI: 10.1515/1556-3758.1412

7 Meynadier JM, Meynadier J, Peyron JL, Peyron L. Formes cliniques des manifestations cutanées d'allergie aux parfums. Ann Dermatol Venereol 1986;113:31-39

8 Wetter DA, Yiannias JA, Prakash AV, Davis MD, Farmer SA, el-Azhary RA, et al. Results of patch testing to personal care product allergens in a standard series and a supplemental cosmetic series: an analysis of 945 patients from the Mayo Clinic Contact Dermatitis Group, 2000-2007. J Am Acad Dermatol 2010;63:789-798

9 Kohl L, Blondeel A, Song M. Allergic contact dermatitis from cosmetics: retrospective analysis of 819 patch-tested patients. Dermatology 2002;204:334-337

10 Thomson KF, Wilkinson SM. Allergic contact dermatitis to plant extracts in patients with cosmetic dermatitis. Br J Dermatol 2000;142:84-88

11 Nakayama H, Matsuo S, Hayakawa K, Takhashi K, Shigematsu T, Ota S. Pigmented cosmetic dermatitis. Int J Dermatol 1984;23:299-305

12 Nakayama H, Harada R, Toda M. Pigmented cosmetic dermatitis. Int J Dermatol 1976;15:673-675

13 Rudzki E, Grzywa Z. Allergy to perfume mixture. Contact Dermatitis 1986;15:115-116

14 Lapeere H, Boone B, Verhaeghe E, Ongenae K, Lambert J. Contact dermatitis caused by lovage (*Levisticum officinalis*) essential oil. Contact Dermatitis 2013;69:181-182

15 Cuesta L, Silvestre JF, Toledo F, Lucas A, Pérez-Crespo M, Ballester I. Fragrance contact allergy: a 4-year retrospective study. Contact Dermatitis 2010; 63:77-84

16 Sugiura M, Hayakawa R, Kato Y, Sigiura K, Hashimoto R. Results of patch testing with lavender oil in Japan. Contact Dermatitis 2000;43:157-160

17 Bleasel N, Tate B, Rademaker M. Allergic contact dermatitis following exposure to essential oils. Australas J Dermatol 2002;43:211-213

18 Boonchai W, Lamtharachai P, Sunthonpalin P. Occupational allergic contact dermatitis from essential oils in aromatherapists. Contact Dermatitis 2007;56:181-182

19 Sasseville D, Saber M, Lessard L. Allergic contact dermatitis from tincture of benzoin with multiple concomitant reactions. Contact Dermatitis 2009;61:358-360

20 An S, Lee AY, Lee CH, Kim D-W, Hahm JH, Kim K-J, et al. Fragrance contact dermatitis in Korea: a joint study. Contact Dermatitis 2005;53:320-323

21 Trattner A, David M. Patch testing with fine fragrances: comparison with fragrance mix, balsam of Peru and a fragrance series. Contact Dermatitis 2004;49:287-289

22 Manuel Brites M, Goncalo M, Figueiredo A. Contact allergy to fragrance mix - a 10-year study. Contact Dermatitis 2000;43:181-182

23 Nakayama H, Hanaoka H, Ohshiro A. Allergen Controlled System (ACS). Tokyo, Japan: Kanehara Shuppan, 1974:42. Data cited in ref. 12

24 Srivastava PK, Bajaj AK. Ylang-ylang oil not an uncommon sensitizer in India. Indian J Dermatol 2014;59:200-201

25 Dharmagunawardena B, Takwale A, Sanders KJ, Cannan S, Roger A, Ilchyshyn A. Gas chromatography: an investigative tool in multiple allergies to essential oils. Contact Dermatitis 2002;47:288-292

26 Trattner A, David M, Lazarov A. Occupational contact dermatitis due to essential oils. Contact Dermatitis 2008;58:282-284

27 Rudzki E, Grzywa Z, Bruo WS. Sensitivity to 35 essential oils. Contact Dermatitis 1976;2:196-200

28 Cockayne SE, Gawkrodger DJ. Occupational contact dermatitis in an aromatherapist. Contact Dermatitis 1997;37:306-307

29 Toholka R, Wang Y-S, Tate B, Tam M, Cahill J, Palmer A, Nixon R. The first Australian Baseline Series: Recommendations for patch testing in suspected contact dermatitis. Australas J Dermatol 2015;56:107-115

30 Rudzki E, Grzywa Z. Dermatitis from propolis. Contact Dermatitis 1983;9:40-45

31 Goossens A, Merckx L. Allergic contact dermatitis from farnesol in a deodorant. Contact Dermatitis 1997;37:179-180

32 SCCS (Scientific Committee on Consumer Safety). Opinion on Fragrance allergens in cosmetic products, 26-27 June 2012, SCCS/1459/11. Available at: https://ec.europa.eu/health/sites/health/files/scientific_committees/consumer_safety/docs/sccs_o_102.pdf

33 Uter W, Johansen JD, Börje A, Karlberg A-T, Lidén C, Rastogi S, Roberts D, White IR. Categorization of fragrance contact allergens for prioritization of preventive measures: clinical and experimental data and consideration of structure–activity relationships. Contact Dermatitis 2013;69:196-230

34 De Groot AC, Schmidt E. Essential oils: contact allergy and chemical composition. Boca Raton, Fl., USA: CRC Press, Taylor and Francis Group, 2016 (ISBN 9781482246407)

35 Sabroe RA, Holden CR, Gawkrodger DJ. Contact allergy to essential oils cannot always be predicted from allergy to fragrance markers in the baseline series. Contact Dermatitis 2016;74:236-241

36 De Groot AC. Patch Testing, 4th Edition. Wapserveen, The Netherlands: acdegroot publishing, 2018 (ISBN 978-90-813233-4-5)

37 Silvestre JF, Mercader P, González-Pérez R, Hervella-Garcés M, Sanz-Sánchez T, Córdoba S, et al. Sensitization to fragrances in Spain: A 5-year multicentre study (2011-2015). Contact Dermatitis. 2018 Nov 14. doi: 10.1111/cod.13152. [Epub ahead of print]

Chapter 6.12   CARDAMOM OIL

IDENTIFICATION

Description/definition	: Cardamom oil (essential oil of cardamom, cardamom seed oil) is the essential oil obtained from the fruits of the cardamom, *Elettaria cardamomum*, Zingiberaceae
INCI name(s) EU & USA	: Elettaria cardamomum seed oil
CAS registry number(s)	: 8000-66-6
EC number(s)	: 288-922-1
RIFM monograph(s)	: Food Cosmet Toxicol 1974;12:837 (special issue I) (binder, page 180)
ISO standard	: ISO 4733 Essential oil of cardamom, 2004; Geneva, Switzerland, www.iso.org
Merck Index monograph	: 3103 (Cardamom)
Function(s) in cosmetics	: EU: masking; perfuming; tonic. USA: fragrance ingredients; skin-conditioning agents – miscellaneous
Patch testing	: 2% pet.; based on RIFM data, 4% pet. is probably not irritant (3)

GENERAL

Cardamom (*Elettaria cardamomum* L. (Maton)) is a tall, perennial herbaceous plant belonging to the Zingiberaceae family. Its dried fruit is one of the most highly priced spices in the world. It takes 3-4 years before the plant starts bearing the yellow-grey capsules containing many small black seeds (2).

Cardamom essential oil, extracted from the fruits by distillation, is utilized in perfumery and in tobacco products as well as for flavoring liqueur and food. According to some researchers, cardamom oil has pharmacological properties It also has applications in aromatherapy (2).

CHEMICAL COMPOSITION

Cardamom oil is a colorless to pale, mobile liquid which has a strong aromatic, spicy and eucalyptus-like, discreet woody odor. The ten major constituents found in 101 commercial cardamom essential oils are shown in table 6.12.1 (Erich Schmidt, analytical data presented in ref. 2)

Table 6.12.1 Ten ingredients with the highest concentrations in commercial cardamom oils (2)

Name	Concentration range	Name	Concentration range
Terpinyl acetate	31.3 - 46.1%	Limonene	1.4 - 6.0%
1,8-Cineole	20.9 - 38.2%	Sabinene	1.8 - 5.5%
Linalool	0.2 - 8.7%	α-Terpinolene	0.09 - 5.4%
Linalyl acetate	0.4 - 8.5%	α-Pinene	1.0 - 4.0%
α-Terpineol	1.7 - 6.7%	Myrcene	0.04 - 3.2%

CONTACT ALLERGY / ALLERGIC CONTACT DERMATITIS

General
Contact allergy to cardamom oil has been reported in one case report only. Dipentene (*dl*-limonene) may have been an allergen in that case (1).

Case reports and case series
A male confectioner developed occupational contact dermatitis which was ascribed to working with cardamom powder. He reacted to cardamom powder, cardamom oil 2% in petrolatum, δ-carene (δ2, δ3?), dipentene (*dl*-limonene), bergamot oil and turpentine peroxides (1). Limonene is the main component of bergamot oil, can be present in cardamom oil in concentrations up to 6% (table 6.12.1) and has been found in commercial turpentine oils in concentrations up to 13.6% (2). The reaction to δ-carene may also explain the co-reactivity to turpentine peroxides (see Chapter 6.75 Turpentine oil).

LITERATURE

1   Mobacken H, Fregert S. Allergic contact dermatitis from cardamom. Contact Dermatitis 1975;1:175-176
2   De Groot AC, Schmidt E. Essential oils: contact allergy and chemical composition. Boca Raton, Fl., USA: CRC Press, Taylor and Francis Group, 2016 (ISBN 9781482246407)
3   De Groot AC. Patch Testing, 4th Edition. Wapserveen, The Netherlands: acdegroot publishing, 2018 (ISBN 978-90-813233-4-5)

Chapter 6.13   CARROT SEED OIL

IDENTIFICATION

Description/definition	: Carrot seed oil is the essential oil obtained from the fruits of the carrot, *Daucus carota* L.
INCI name(s) EU	: Daucus carota fruit oil (perfuming name, not an INCI name proper)
INCI name(s) USA	: Not in the Personal Care Council Ingredient Database
CAS registry number(s)	: 84929-61-3
EC number(s)	: 284-545-1
RIFM monograph(s)	: Food Cosmet Toxicol 1976;14:705 (special issue III)
Function(s) in cosmetics	: EU: perfuming
Patch testing	: 4% pet. (3)

GENERAL

Daucus carota L. is a biennial flowering herb, which grows to a height of 20-60 cm. It is native to Europe, northern Africa, western Asia, and tropical Asia (Pakistan) and is widely naturalized elsewhere. Carrot seed oil is obtained from the fruits of various subspecies of *Daucus carota* L., but not from the seeds *per se*. The terms seeds and fruits are often used as synonyms, but the seeds are contained within the fruits (ripe umbels). Carrot seed oil is widely used as an aromatic and fragrance component in the formulation of alcoholic liquors, food products, perfumes, cosmetics and soaps. It has also been used in folk medicine and aromatherapy (2).

It should be noted that the Cosing and Personal Care Council Ingredient Database entry Daucus carota sativa seed oil (CAS registry numbers 8015-88-1 and 84929-61-3; EC number 284-545-1) is not an essential (volatile) oil but a fixed (vegetable) oil.

CHEMICAL COMPOSITION

Carrot seed oil is a clear mobile, colorless to yellowish liquid which has a terpeny, slightly fatty herbaceous and aromatic odor. In carrot seed oils from various origins, over 315 chemicals have been identified. About 60 per cent of these were found in a single reviewed publication only. The ten chemicals that had the highest maximum concentrations in 41 commercial carrot seed essential oil samples are shown in table 6.13.1 (Erich Schmidt, analytical data presented in ref. 2).

A full literature review of the qualitative and quantitative composition of commercial and non-commercial carrot seed oils of various origins and their chemotypes has been published in 2016 (2).

Table 6.13.1 Ten ingredients with the highest concentrations in commercial carrot seed oils (2)

Name	Concentration range	Name	Concentration range
Carotol	10.2 - 36.8%	β-Bisabolene	1.6 - 7.8%
Geranyl acetate	0.9 - 13.9%	*p*-Cymene	0.4 - 6.0%
β-Caryophyllene	1.9 - 12.6%	β-Pinene	0.4 - 4.4%
α-Pinene	1.9 - 12.5%	Caryophyllene oxide	0.1 - 3.1%
Sabinene	0.2 - 12.2%	β-Selinene	0.4 - 3.0%

CONTACT ALLERGY / ALLERGIC CONTACT DERMATITIS

General
Only one case of allergic contact dermatitis from carrot seed oil has been reported (1).

Case reports and case series
A female 'complementary therapist' developed occupational contact dermatitis from a multitude of essential oils used at work, including carrot seed oil (1).

LITERATURE

1   Newsham J, Rai S, Williams JDL. Two cases of allergic contact dermatitis to neroli oil. Br J Dermatol 2011;165(suppl.1):76

2   De Groot AC, Schmidt E. Essential oils: contact allergy and chemical composition. Boca Raton, Fl., USA: CRC Press, Taylor and Francis Group, 2016 (ISBN 9781482246407)

3   De Groot AC. Patch Testing, 4th Edition. Wapserveen, The Netherlands: acdegroot publishing, 2018 (ISBN 978-90-813233-4-5)

Chapter 6.14   CASSIA OIL

INTRODUCTION

Cassia oil (essential oil of cassia) is the essential oil obtained from the leaves, twigs and terminal branchlets of the Chinese cinnamon, *Cinnamomum cassia* (Nees & T. Nees) J.Presl (synonyms: *Cinnamomum aromaticum* Nees; *Cinnamomum cassia* Nees ex Blume, *Cinnamomum cassia* auct). Enquiries with commercial parties – those providing cassia oils to the fragrance industries - generally confirm that the plant parts used for producing cassia oils are the leaves, twigs and terminal branchlets. In spite of this, two separate oils with difference source material are presented here, cassia *bark* oil and cassia *leaf* oil for the following reasons:
1. many authors of studies analyzing cassia oils specifically mention bark as the source of the cassia oils, and in a number of studies only the leaves were investigated. However: 'leaves, twigs and terminal branchlets' is never mentioned as the plant parts from which the cassia oils were obtained
2. on-line commercial parties offer both cassia bark oils and cassia leaf oils.

In non-botanical literature, cassia oil is often termed 'cinnamon oil'. However, cassia oil should not be confused with cinnamon bark oil and cinnamon leaf oil Sri Lanka type, which are obtained from the 'true cinnamon', *Cinnamomum zeylanicum* Blume (see Chapter 6.16). The chemical profile of the oils and also their uses (including medicinal) have many similarities, though.

6.14.1 CASSIA BARK OIL

IDENTIFICATION

Description/definition	: Cassia bark oil (essential oil of cassia bark) is the essential oil obtained from the bark of the Chinese cinnamon, *Cinnamomum cassia* (Nees & T. Nees) J.Presl (synonyms: *Cinnamomum aromaticum* Nees; *Cinnamomum cassia* Nees ex Blume, *Cinnamomum cassia* auct)
INCI name(s) EU & USA	: Cinnamomum cassia oil
Other names	: Chinese cinnamon oil
CAS registry number(s)	: 84961-46-6; 8007-80-5
EC number(s)	: 284-635-0
RIFM monograph(s)	: Food Cosmet Toxicol 1975;13:109 (binder, page 194)
SCCS opinion(s)	: SCCNFP/0392/00, final (14); SCCNFP/0389/00, final (15)
ISO standard	: ISO 3216 Essential oil of cassia, 1997; Geneva, Switzerland, www.iso.org
Merck Index monograph	: 3570 (Cinnamon)
Function(s) in cosmetics	: EU: masking; perfuming. USA: fragrance ingredients
Patch testing	: 1% pet. (18); test also cinnamal (see Chapter 3.34 Cinnamal)

GENERAL

Cinnamomum cassia (Nees & T. Nees*)* J. Presl, also called Chinese cinnamon, is a medium-sized (10-15 meter tall) evergreen tree, with greyish bark and hard elongated leaves that are 10-15 cm long, belonging to the Lauraceae. It is native to China and is widely distributed in China, Vietnam, Sri Lanka, Madagascar, Seychelles and India. The tree is cultivated in China, Laos, Thailand, Vietnam, Indonesia and Malaysia. It is one of the most important economic plant resources in tropical and subtropical areas (18).

Essential oils are important products from *C. cassia*, and they may be obtained from barks, twigs, leaves, calyces and seeds, the most important one apparently being cassia bark oil (3). The bark essential oil is used as a food and drink flavoring agent, in the cosmetics industry and for medicinal purposes. *C. cassia* leaves also contain large amounts of oils (cassia leaf oil), and are used similarly to cassia bark oil in flavoring, medicine and especially cola-type drinks. Cassia oils are not used in aromatherapy because of risk of dermal sensitization to cinnamal (4,5).

Possible health effects of 'cinnamon' have been reviewed (1). A comprehensive review of all aspects of *Cinnamomum cassia* is provided in ref. 2. It should be realized that 'cinnamon' (or what is called 'cinnamon') may have been obtained either from *Cinnamomum cassia* (Nees & T. Nees*)* J. Presl or from *Cinnamomum zeylanicum* Blume (true cinnamon).

CHEMICAL COMPOSITION

Cassia oil is a mobile liquid with yellowish to reddish brown color, which has a spicy sweet odor, reminding of cinnamon bark. In cassia oils from various origins, over 245 chemicals have been identified. About 60 per cent of these were found in a single reviewed publication only. The ten chemicals that had the highest maximum concentrations in 38 commercial cassia essential oil samples, probably prepared from leaves, twigs and terminal branchlets, are shown in table 6.14.1.1 (Erich Schmidt, analytical data presented in ref. 18).

A full literature review of the qualitative and quantitative composition of commercial and non-commercial cassia oils of various origins with data from the ISO standard has been published in 2016 (18).

Table 6.14.1.1 Ten ingredients with the highest concentrations in commercial cassia oils (18)

Name	Concentration range	Name	Concentration range
(E)-Cinnamal(dehyde)	75.4 - 83.1%	Limonene	0.03 - 1.1%
(E)-o-Methoxycinnamal-dehyde	6.8 - 11.1%	Camphene	0.05 - 0.8%
		(E)-Cinnamic acid	0.2 - 0.7%
(E)-Cinnamyl acetate	1.1 - 4.7%	2-Methoxybenzaldehyde	0.2 - 0.7%
Coumarin	0.6 - 2.6%	2-Phenethyl alcohol	0.2 - 0.7%
Benzaldehyde	0.9 - 2.3%		

6.14.2 CASSIA LEAF OIL

IDENTIFICATION

Description/definition   : Cassia leaf oil is the essential oil obtained from the leaves and twigs of the Chinese cinnamon, *Cinnamomum cassia* (Nees & T. Nees) J.Presl (synonyms: *Cinnamomum aromaticum* Nees, *Cinnamomum cassia* Nees ex Blume, *Cinnamomum cassia* auct)
INCI name(s) EU & USA   : Cinnamomum cassia leaf oil
Other names   : Cassia oil; cinnamon oil chinense
CAS registry number(s)   : 8007-80-5; 84961-46-6
EC number(s)   : 284-635-0
RIFM monograph(s)   : Food Cosmet Toxicol 1975;13:109 (binder, page 194)
SCCS opinion(s)   : SCCNFP/0392/00, final (14); SCCNFP/0389/00, final (15); SCCS/1459/11 (16)
Merck Index monograph   : 3570 (Cinnamon)
Function(s) in cosmetics   : EU: denaturant; masking; perfuming. USA: denaturants; flavoring agents; fragrance ingredients
Patch testing   : 1% pet. (18); test also cinnamal (see Chapter 3.34 Cinnamal)

GENERAL

See the section 'General' of Cinnamon bark oil above.

CHEMICAL COMPOSITION

Cassia leaf oil is a yellow to brown liquid with the characteristic odor and taste of cassia cinnamon. On aging or exposure to air it darkens and thickens. In cassia leaf oils from various origins (only few analytical studies found), over 115 chemicals have been identified. About 69 per cent of these were found in a single reviewed publication only. The major compounds found in cassia leaf oils from different sources include (highest concentrations in any study given) (E)-cinnamaldehyde (cinnamal) (78.4%), 2-methoxycinnamaldehyde (25.4%) and cinnamyl acetate (12.5%). Ingredients of cassia leaf oils that were present in high concentrations (>6%) in one or two studies were 3-methoxy-1,2-propanediol (29.3%) and coumarin (6.4% and 15.3%) (18).

A full literature review of the qualitative and quantitative composition of commercial and non-commercial cassia leaf oils of various origins has been published in 2016 (18).

CONTACT ALLERGY / ALLERGIC CONTACT DERMATITIS

Cassia oil (unspecified)

General

Contact allergy to / allergic contact dermatitis from cassia oil has been reported in a few publications. In groups of consecutive patients suspected of contact dermatitis, prevalence rates of up to 1% positive patch test reactions have been observed, but the relevance is unknown. Most case reports were patients with oral symptoms, cheilitis and/or perioral dermatitis from contact allergy to cassia oil in toothpastes. Although unproven, the most important sensitizer is likely to be (E)-cinnamaldehyde (cinnamal) , the major component in both the cassia bark oil (75-85%) and cassia leaf oil (60-70%). In literature, no good distinction is made between cassia oil and cinnamon oil (from *Cinnamomum zeylanicum*), and sometimes they are used as synonyms.

Testing in groups of patients

Routine testing
Two hundred dermatitis patients from Poland were patch tested with cassia oil 2% in petrolatum and two (1%) reacted (6). Of 750 consecutive dermatitis patients tested with 2% cassia oil, 5 (0.7%) had a positive patch test (11). In neither report were relevance data provided.

Testing in groups of selected patients
Fifty-one patients allergic to Myroxylon pereirae resin (balsam of Peru) and/or turpentine and/or wood tar and/or colophony were tested with cassia oil 2% in petrolatum and ten (19.6%) had a positive patch test; relevance data were not provided (6). A group of 86 patients from Poland previously reacting to the fragrance mix was tested with cassia oil and 24 (27.9%) had a positive patch test reaction; relevance data were not provided (7). In this group of 86, there were 16 reactions to cinnamic aldehyde (cinnamal), which is by far the most important constituent of cassia oil (7). In 16 patients known to be allergic to propolis and Myroxylon pereirae resin, three (19%) had positive patch tests to cassia oil 2% in petrolatum; the relevance was not mentioned (13).

Case reports and case series
One patient was described with stomatitis from contact allergy to cassia oil and cinnamon oil in toothpaste, who was negative, however, to their main component cinnamal (8). One female individual had burning mouth and soreness and swelling of the tongue from contact allergy to her toothpaste; the patient also reacted to cassia oil and its main ingredient cinnamal, but it was not stated whether these compounds were present in the toothpaste (8). Another patient had mucosal inflammation and purpuric perioral macules associated with the use of a prophylactic dental tablet and was found to be contact allergic to its components oil of cassia and oil of cloves (9). One case of cheilitis from allergy to cinnamon (cassia) oil in toothpaste has been reported (10). Another patient developed contact stomatitis and dermatitis from contact allergy to cinnamal and cinnamon (cassia) oil in toothpaste (12).

Cassia bark oil
No reports on contact allergy to cassia bark oil, specifically mentioned to be obtained from the bark of *Cinnamomum cassia*, have been found.

Cassia leaf oil
The SCCS (Scientific Committee on Consumer Safety), in a 2012 Opinion on Fragrance allergens in cosmetic products, has marked cassia leaf oil as 'established contact allergen in humans' (16,17).

No reports of contact allergy to cassia leaf oil, specifically mentioned to be obtained from the leaves of *Cinnamomum cassia*, have been found.

OTHER SIDE EFFECTS

Immediate contact reactions
Immediate contact reactions (contact urticaria) from cassia oil have been cited in ref. 19.

Photosensitivity
Photosensitivity from cassia oil has been cited in ref. 19.

LITERATURE
1   Gruenwald J, Freder J, Armbruester N. Cinnamon and health. Crit Rev Food Sc Nutrit 2010;50:822-834
2   Cinnamon and Cassia. PN Ravindran, K Nirmal Babu and M Shylaja, eds. Boca Raton – London – New York – Washington: CRC Press, 2004
3   Deng X, Liao Q, Xu X, Yao M, Zhou Y, Lin M, Zhang P, Xie Z. Analysis of essential oils from cassia bark and cassia twig samples by GC-MS combined with multivariate data analysis. Food Anal Methods 2014;7:1840-1847
4   Rhind JP. Essential oils. A handbook for aromatherapy practice, 2nd Edition. London: Singing Dragon, 2012
5   Lawless J. The encyclopedia of essential oils, 2nd Edition. London: Harper Thorsons, 2014
6   Rudzki E, Grzywa Z, Bruo WS. Sensitivity to 35 essential oils. Contact Dermatitis 1976;2:196-200
7   Rudzki E, Grzywa Z. Allergy to perfume mixture. Contact Dermatitis 1986;15:115-116
8   Magnusson B, Wilkinson DS. Cinnamic aldehyde in toothpaste. 1. Clinical aspects and patch tests. Contact Dermatitis 1975;1:70-76
9   Silvers SH. Stomatitis and dermatitis venenata with purpura, resulting from oil of cloves and oil of cassia. Dental Items of Interest 1939;61:649-651. Data cited in ref. 8

10   Laubach JL, Malkenson FD, Ringrose EJ. Cheilitis caused by cinnamon (cassia) oil in toothpaste. JAMA 1953;152:404-405. Data cited in ref. 8

11   Rudzki E, Grzywa Z. The value of a mixture of cassia and citronella oils for detection of hypersensitivity to essential oils. Dermatosen 1985;33:59-62

12   Drake TE, Maibach HI. Allergic contact dermatitis and stomatitis caused by a cinnamic aldehyde-flavored toothpaste. Arch Dermatol 1976;112:202-203

13   Rudzki E, Grzywa Z. Dermatitis from propolis. Contact Dermatitis 1983;9:40-45

14   Opinion of the Scientific Committee on Cosmetic Products and Non-Food Products Intended for Consumers concerning 'An initial list of perfumery materials which must not form part of cosmetic products except subject to the Restrictions and Conditions laid down, 25 September 2001, SCCNFP/0392/00, final. Available at: http://ec.europa.eu/health/archive/ph_risk/committees/sccp/documents/out150_en.pdf

15   Opinion of the Scientific Committee on Cosmetic Products and Non-Food Products Intended for Consumers concerning 'The 1st update of the inventory of ingredients employed in cosmetic products. Section II: Perfume and aromatic raw materials', 24 October 2000, SCCNFP/0389/00, final. Available at: http://ec.europa.eu/health/ph_risk/committees/sccp/documents/out131_en.pdf

16   SCCS (Scientific Committee on Consumer Safety). Opinion on Fragrance allergens in cosmetic products, 26-27 June 2012, SCCS/1459/11. Available at: https://ec.europa.eu/health/sites/health/files/scientific_committees/consumer_safety/docs/sccs_o_102.pdf

17   Uter W, Johansen JD, Börje A, Karlberg A-T, Lidén C, Rastogi S, Roberts D, White IR. Categorization of fragrance contact allergens for prioritization of preventive measures: clinical and experimental data and consideration of structure–activity relationships. Contact Dermatitis 2013;69:196-230

18   De Groot AC, Schmidt E. Essential oils: contact allergy and chemical composition. Boca Raton, Fl., USA: CRC Press, Taylor and Francis Group, 2016 (ISBN 9781482246407)

19   De Groot AC. Patch Testing, 4th Edition. Wapserveen, The Netherlands: acdegroot publishing, 2018 (ISBN 978-90-813233-4-5)

Chapter 6.15 CEDARWOOD OIL

There are five major cedarwood essential oils: cedarwood oil Atlas, cedarwood oil China, cedarwood oil Himalaya, cedarwood oil Texas, and cedarwood oil Virginia. These are obtained from different botanical species, and as a consequence, their chemical compositions differ both qualitatively and quantitatively. Unfortunately, in non-botanical literature, usually the term 'cedarwood oil' is used, lacking information on the botanical origin.

6.15.1 CEDARWOOD OIL ATLAS

IDENTIFICATION

Description/definition : Cedarwood oil Atlas is the essential oil obtained from the wood of the Atlantic cedar (Atlas cedar), *Cedrus atlantica* (Endl.) G. Manetti ex Carrière
INCI name(s) EU : Cedrus atlantica wood oil (perfuming name, not an INCI name proper)
INCI name(s) USA : Not in the Personal Care Products Council Ingredient Database
CAS registry number(s) : 92201-55-3
EC number(s) : 295-985-9
SCCS opinion(s) : SCCNFP/0392/00, final (9); SCCNFP/0389/00, final (10); SCCS/1459/11 (11)
RIFM monograph(s) : Food Cosmet Toxicol 1976;14:709 (special issue III)
Function(s) in cosmetics : EU: perfuming
EU cosmetic restrictions : Regulated in Annex III/122 of the Regulation (EC) No. 344/2013
Patch testing : 5% pet. (6,8)

GENERAL

Cedrus atlantica is an evergreen coniferous tree which can grow up to 40 meter high and 2 meter in diameter. It is native to the Atlas Mountains in Morocco and Algeria. Atlas cedar is the principal species in Moroccan forests used for production of timber. It is also cultivated in southern France for this purpose. The machining waste, sawdust (estimated to be 8-30%) is the ground material for the production of Atlas cedarwood essential oil, which is used in the perfumery and flavor industry and for its medicinal properties, especially for their content of himachalenes. It is also used in aromatherapy (14).

CHEMICAL COMPOSITION

Cedarwood oil Atlas is a pale to dark yellow, clear mobile liquid which has a balsamic, soft woody odor reminding of sandalwood. In cedarwood oils Atlas from various origins, over 135 chemicals have been identified. About half of these were found in a single reviewed publication only. The ten chemicals that had the highest maximum concentrations in 24 commercial cedarwood Atlas essential oil samples are shown in table 6.15.1.1 (Erich Schmidt, analytical data presented in ref. 13).

A full literature review of the qualitative and quantitative composition of commercial and non-commercial cedarwood Atlas oils of various origins and their chemotypes has been published in 2016 (13).

Table 6.15.1.1 Ten ingredients with the highest concentrations in commercial cedarwood Atlas oils (13)

Name	Concentration range	Name	Concentration range
β-Himachalene	40.0 - 52.0%	γ-Dehydro-ar-himachalene	0.2 – 3.0%
α-*cis*-Himachalene	15.5 - 19.3%	(*E*)-α-Atlantone	0.03 - 2.7%
γ-Himachalene	9.5 - 12.0%	Deodarone	1.1 - 2.3%
α-Terpineol	0 - 6.0%	α-Cedrene	0.5 - 2.3%
Himachalol	0.4 - 3.1%	δ-Cadinene	0.7 - 2.2%

6.15.2 CEDARWOOD OIL CHINA

IDENTIFICATION

Description/definition : Cedarwood oil China (essential oil of cedarwood, Chinese type) is the essential oil obtained from the wood of the Chinese weeping cypress (mourning cypress), *Cupressus funebris* (Endl.)
INCI name(s) EU : Cupressus funebris wood oil
INCI name(s) USA : Not in the Personal Care Products Council Ingredients Database

IDENTIFICATION   (continued)

Other names   : Chinese cedarwood oil
CAS registry number(s)   : 85085-29-6
EC number(s)   : 285-360-9
ISO standard   : ISO 9843 Essential oil of cedarwood, Chinese type, 2002; Geneva, Switzerland,
                                www.iso.org
Function(s) in cosmetics : EU: perfuming
Patch testing   : 5% pet. (6,8)

GENERAL

Cupressus funebris Endl. (synonyms: *Chamaecyparis funebris* (Endl.) Franco; Chinese weeping cypress) is an evergreen coniferous tree up to 35 meter tall and with a trunk up to 2 meter in diameter, which is native to China and Vietnam and is cultivated widely in south China. The general source of Chinese cedarwood oil is from stumps after logging. Chinese cedarwood oil and wood are used to prepare incense in China. In medicine, specially thickened varieties of cedarwood oils are used as immersion oil and for clarification in microscopy, because they have the same refraction index as glass (13). It is not used in aromatherapy (14).

CHEMICAL COMPOSITION

Cedarwood oil China is an almost colorless to light yellow, clear mobile liquid which has a smoky, crude woody odor. In cedarwood oils China from various origins over 135 chemicals have been identified. About 58 per cent of these were found in a single reviewed publication only. The ten chemicals that had the highest maximum concentrations in 21 commercial cedarwood China essential oil samples are shown in table 6.15.2.1 (Erich Schmidt, analytical data published in ref. 13).

A full literature review of the qualitative and quantitative composition of commercial and non-commercial Chinese cedarwood oils of various origins and with data from the ISO standard has been published in 2016 (13).

Table 6.15.2.1 Ten ingredients with the highest concentrations in commercial cedarwood China oils (13)

Name	Concentration range	Name	Concentration range
Thujopsene	16.5 - 40.9%	Cuparene	1.9 - 2.8%
α-Cedrene	10.3 - 38.4%	Methylcarvacrol	0.1 - 2.1%
Cedrol	9.5 - 14.5%	β-Himachalene	1.2 - 2.1%
β-Cedrene	3.4 - 8.2%	γ-Acoradiene	0.8 - 1.9%
β-Funebrene	1.8 - 3.4%	β-Chamigrene	0.6 - 1.8%

6.15.3 CEDARWOOD OIL HIMALAYA

IDENTIFICATION

Description/definition   : Himalayan cedarwood oil (essential oil of cedarwood Himalaya) is the essential oil
                                 obtained from the wood of the Himalayan cedar (deodar, deodar cedar) *Cedrus deodara*
                                 (Roxb. ex D.Don) G.Don.
INCI name(s) EU & USA   : Cedrus deodara wood oil
CAS registry number(s)   : 91771-47-0
EC number(s)   : 294-939-5
SCCS opinion(s)   : SCCS/1459/11 (11)
Function(s) in cosmetics : EU: masking. USA: fragrance ingredients
Patch testing   : 2% pet.

GENERAL

Cedrus deodara (Himalayan cedar, deodar, deodar cedar) is a graceful, ornamental evergreen tree which can grow up to 60 meters and develop a diameter of three meters. It is native to the temperate (Afghanistan, China) and tropical (India, Nepal, Pakistan) regions of Asia and grows extensively on the slopes of the western Himalayas at altitudes of 1200-3000 meter. The tree is cultivated in China as ornamental plant and for its timber. The essential oil of the Himalayan cedar finds use in Ayurvedic medicine, as an anthelmintic and in aromatherapy, but not in perfumes or other cosmetics. The oil sold to aromatherapists is usually rectified (13).

The traditional and folklore medicinal uses, phytochemistry and biological activities of *Cedrus deodara* have been reviewed (16).

CHEMICAL COMPOSITION

Cedarwood oil Himalaya is a yellowish to brownish slightly viscous clear liquid, which has a pleasant, typical, mild and woody cedar connotation odor. In Himalayan cedarwood oils from various origins, over 65 chemicals have been identified. About 60 per cent of these were found in a single reviewed publication only, but it should be realized that very few analytical studies have been performed on this essential oil. The ten chemicals that had the highest maximum concentrations in 8 commercial Himalayan cedarwood essential oil samples are shown in table 6.15.3.1 (Erich Schmidt, analytical data presented in ref. 13).

A full literature review of the qualitative and quantitative composition of commercial and non-commercial cedarwood Himalaya oils of various origins has been published in 2016 (13).

Table 6.15.3.1 Ten ingredients with the highest concentrations in commercial cedarwood Himalaya oils (13)

Name	Concentration range	Name	Concentration range
β-Himachalene	32.8 - 46.7%	(Z)-γ-Atlantone	0.6 - 2.7%
α-Himachalene	16.6 - 20.3%	(Z)-α-Atlantone	0.8 - 2.6%
γ-Himachalene	9.8 - 11.6%	(E)-γ-Atlantone	0.5 - 2.1%
(E)-α-Atlantone	4.4 - 9.7%	Deodarone	0.7 - 2.2%
Himachalol	0.5 - 8.5%	δ-Cadinene	0.3 - 1.9%

6.15.4 CEDARWOOD OIL TEXAS

IDENTIFICATION

Description/definition	: Cedarwood oil Texas (essential oil of cedarwood oil, Texas type) is the essential oil obtained from the wood of the Mexican juniper (Mexican cedar, mountain cedar), *Juniperus ashei* J. Buchholz (synonym: *Juniperus mexicana* auct.)
INCI name(s) EU	: Juniperus mexicana oil; Juniperus mexicana wood oil (perfuming name, not an INCI name proper)
INCI name(s) USA	: Juniperus mexicana oil
CAS registry number(s)	: 68990-83-0; 91722-61-1
EC number(s)	: 294-461-7
RIFM monograph(s)	: Food Cosmet Toxicol 1976;14:711 (special issue III)
ISO standard	: ISO 4725 Essential oil of cedarwood, Texas type, 2004; Geneva, Switzerland, www.iso.org
Function(s) in cosmetics	: EU: masking; perfuming. USA: fragrance ingredients
Patch testing	: 2% pet.; based on RIFM data, 6% pet. is probably not irritant (19)

GENERAL

Juniperus ashei J. Buchholz is a dioecious (biparental reproductive) large evergreen shrub or small tree, 6-15 meters tall, and up to 50 cm in diameter. The tree is native to the USA and northern Mexico. Its wood is steam-distilled to produce Texas cedarwood oil, which is used in a range of fragrance applications such as soap perfumes, candles, cosmetics, household sprays, and floor polishes. It is also used in aromatherapy, as an insecticide and in medicine as immersion oil and for clarification in microscopy. Another very important application is as feedstock for the manufacture of chemical derivatives, such as cedrol, cedryl methyl ether, acetyl cedrene, and cedryl acetate (13).

CHEMICAL COMPOSITION

Cedarwood oil Texas is a brown to reddish viscous liquid, which has a woody, dry and soft odor with slightly smoky top note. In cedarwood oils Texas from various origins (we could find only a few publications), over 45 chemicals have been identified. About 43 per cent of these were found in a single reviewed publication only. The ten chemicals that had the highest maximum concentrations in 119 commercial cedarwood Texas essential oil samples are shown in table 6.15.4.1 (Erich Schmidt, analytical data presented in ref. 13).

A full literature review of the qualitative and quantitative composition of commercial and non-commercial cedarwood Texas oils of various origins and with data from the ISO standard, has been published in 2016 (13).

Table 6.15.4.1 Ten ingredients with the highest concentrations in commercial cedarwood Texas oils (13)

Name	Concentration range	Name	Concentration range
Thujopsene	31.6 - 49.2%	Cuparene	1.3 - 2.9%
Cedrol	14.3 - 33.7%	β-Caryophyllene	0.08 - 1.9%
α-Cedrene	1.8 - 21.3%	β-Himachalene	0.5 - 1.9%
β-Cedrene	1.5 - 5.2%	α-Acorenol	0.7 - 1.8%
Widdrol	0.4 - 3.2%	α-Acoradiene	0.5 - 1.4%

6.15.5 CEDARWOOD OIL VIRGINIA

IDENTIFICATION

Description/definition	: Cedarwood oil Virginia (essential oil of cedarwood, Virginian type; Virginian cedarwood oil; red cedarwood oil) is the essential oil obtained from the wood of the (eastern) red cedar (coastal cedar), *Juniperus virginiana* L.
INCI name(s) EU	: Juniperus virginiana wood oil (perfuming name, not an INCI name proper)
INCI name(s) USA	: Juniperus virginiana oil
Other names	: Red cedarwood oil
CAS registry number(s)	: 8000-27-9; 85085-41-2
EC number(s)	: 285-370-3
RIFM monograph(s)	: Food Cosmet Toxicol 1974;12:845 (special issue I) (binder, page 201)
SCCS opinion(s)	: SCCS/1459/11 (11)
ISO standard	: ISO 4724 Essential oil of cedarwood, Virginian type, 2004; Geneva, Switzerland, www.iso.org
Function(s) in cosmetics	: EU: perfuming. USA: fragrance ingredients
Patch testing	: 10% pet. (SPEurope, SPCanada)

GENERAL

Juniperus virginiana L., commonly called eastern red cedar, is a single-stemmed coniferous evergreen tree which can grow to 30 meters tall. The tree is native to the USA and Canada, naturalized elsewhere and is also cultivated. Virginia cedarwood oils, which are obtained by steam-distillation of sawdust, waste shavings, old stumps, and chipped logs of eastern red cedar, are used in polishes to restore the smell of cedar to furniture and as fragrance in cosmetic formulations, including shampoos for humans and animals, aftershave lotions, soap bars, and perfumes. They are also found in insect repellents, massage oils, cleaning products, room deodorants, disinfectants, liniments, incense oils, in medicine as immersion oil and for clarification in microscopy, and in numerous other industrial products and may be used for medicinal purposes and in aromatherapy (13,14,17).

CHEMICAL COMPOSITION

Cedarwood oil Virginia is a slightly viscous liquid, sometimes containing crystals from cedrol, colorless to pale yellow, which has a mild woody, warm and dry odor. In cedarwood oils Virginia from various origins, over 55 chemicals have been identified. About 54 per cent of these were found in a single reviewed publication only. The ten chemicals that had the highest maximum concentrations in 36 commercial cedarwood Virginia essential oil samples are shown in table 6.15.5.1 (Erich Schmidt, analytical data presented in ref. 13).

A review of various aspects of Virginian cedarwood oils is provided in ref. 17. A full literature review of the qualitative and quantitative composition of commercial and non-commercial cedarwood oils Virginia of various origins and with data from the ISO standard has been published in 2016 (13).

Table 6.15.5.1 Ten ingredients with the highest concentrations in commercial cedarwood Virginia oils (13)

Name	Concentration range	Name	Concentration range
Thujopsene	22.2 - 33.2%	β-Funebrene	1.6 - 4.8%
α-Cedrene	12.8 - 27.2%	Widdrol	1.0 - 4.0%
Cedrol	15.8 - 25.9%	α-Acoradiene	0.5 - 2.3%
β-Cedrene	3.6 - 7.7%	β-Caryophyllene	0.5 - 1.9%
Cuparene	1.1 - 6.3%	β-Chamigrene	1.1 - 1.8%

CONTACT ALLERGY / ALLERGIC CONTACT DERMATITIS

The SCCS (Scientific Committee on Consumer Safety), in a 2012 Opinion on Fragrance allergens in cosmetic products, has marked cedarwood oil Atlas and Juniperus virginiana extract (cedarwood Virginia extract) as 'established contact allergen in humans' and Cedrus deodara wood oil as 'possible fragrance contact allergen' (11,12).

Cedarwood oil, unspecified or partly specified

General

Contact allergy to / allergic contact dermatitis from cedarwood oil has been reported in several publications. In groups of consecutive patients suspected of contact dermatitis, prevalence rates of up to 1.5% positive patch test reactions have been observed, but relevance data are lacking. In most publications, the botanical origin of the cedarwood oil was not mentioned. In two publications (6,8, both parts of the same study) the test substance was prepared from 50% Moroccan cedarwood oil (presumably cedarwood oil, Atlas, *ex Cedrus atlantica*) and 50% Chinese cedarwood oil (presumably *ex Cupressus funebris*). One large study from Germany, Austria and Switzerland used Virginian cedarwood oil (*ex Juniperus virginiana*) for patch testing. Reports of contact allergy to cedarwood specified to be obtained from *Juniperus ashei* J. Buchholz (cedarwood oil, Texas) have not been found.

Testing in groups of patients

The results of patch tests with cedarwood oil in routine testing (consecutive patients suspected of contact dermatitis) and in groups of selected patients are shown in table 6.15.5.2. In routine testing, rates of positive reactions ranged from 0.6% to 1.5%, whereas between 0.2% and 5.9% of patients in selected groups had positive patch tests.

Table 6.15.5.2 Patch testing in groups of patients

Years and Country	Test conc. & vehicle	Number of patients tested | positive (%)		Selection of patients (S); Relevance (R); Comments (C)	Ref.
Routine testing					
1999-2000 Denmark	10% pet.	318	3 (0.9%)	R: not specified; C: this study was part of the international study mentioned below (23); C: the test substance was prepared from 50% Moroccan and 50% Chinese cedar-wood oil	8
1998-2000 six European countries	10% pet.	1606	10 (0.6%)	R: not specified for individual oils/chemicals; C: the test substance was prepared from 50% Moroccan and 50% Chinese cedarwood oil	6
<1976 Poland	2% pet.	200	3 (1.5%)	R: not stated	3
Testing in groups of selected patients					
2008-2014 UK	10% pet.	471	1 (0.2%)	S: patients tested with a fragrance series; R: not stated; the test material was from *Juniperus virginiana*	18
2000-2008 IVDK	10% pet.	6223	52 (0.8%)	S: patients with dermatitis suspected of causal exposure to fragrances; R: not stated; C: the cedarwood oil was prepared from *Juniperus virginiana* (cedarwood oil Virginia)	5
1997-2000 Austria	2% pet.	747	5 (0.7%)	S: patients suspected of fragrance allergy; R: not stated	1
<1976 Poland	2% pet.	51	3 (5.9%)	S: patients allergic to Myroxylon pereirae resin and/or turpentine and/or wood tar and/or colophony; R: not stated	3

IVDK Information Network of Departments of Dermatology, Germany, Switzerland, Austria (www.ivdk.org). pet.: petrolatum

Case reports and case series

An aromatherapist had occupational contact dermatitis with allergies to multiple essential oils used at work, including cedarwood oil. The patient also reacted to geraniol, α-pinene, caryophyllene, the fragrance mix and various other fragrance materials; caryophyllene was demonstrated by GC-MS in cedarwood oil (2), but in none of the cedarwood oils is caryophyllene an important component. One case of allergic contact dermatitis was caused by cedarwood oil present as a contaminant in immersion oil for dermatoscopy (4).

One patient developed allergic contact dermatitis from cedarwood oil used as the vehicle for applying a black henna temporary tattoo (7).

Cedarwood oil Atlas

Possible contact allergy to cedarwood oil Atlas has been reported in two publications, where patients were tested with a mixture of cedarwood oil Morocco (presumably a synonym of Atlas) and Chinese cedarwood oil. Their data are presented in table 6.15.1.1.

Cedarwood oil China
Possible contact allergy to cedarwood oil China has been reported in two publications, where patients were tested with a mixture of Chinese cedarwood oil and cedarwood oil Morocco (presumably a synonym of Atlas). Their data are presented in table 6.15.2.1.

Cedarwood oil Himalaya

Testing in groups of patients
Two hundred dermatitis patients from Poland were tested with 'cedarwood oil' 2% in petrolatum and three (1.5%) reacted (3). Although not explicitly stated, from the information given in this study and from a later study by the same authors (15) it is very likely that the cedarwood oil tested was Himalayan cedarwood oil. A group of 86 patients reacting to the fragrance mix was tested with Himalayan cedarwood oil 2% in petrolatum and 3 (3.5%) reacted (15). In neither of these studies were relevance data provided.

Cedarwood oil Texas
No reports on contact allergy to cedarwood oil Texas specifically mentioned to be obtained from the wood of *Juniperus ashei* J. Buchholz have been found.

Cedarwood oil Virginia
Contact allergy to cedarwood oil Virginia, has been reported in two publications (5,18); its data are presented in table 6.15.5.1.

OTHER SIDE EFFECTS

Photosensitivity
Photosensitivity from cedarwood oil Atlas, Texas and Virginia has been cited in ref. 19.

LITERATURE
1   Wöhrl S, Hemmer W, Focke M, Götz M, Jarisch R. The significance of fragrance mix, balsam of Peru, colophonium and propolis as screening tools in the detection of fragrance allergy. Br J Dermatol 2001;145:268-273
2   Dharmagunawardena B, Takwale A, Sanders KJ, Cannan S, Roger A, Ilchyshyn A. Gas chromatography: an investigative tool in multiple allergies to essential oils. Contact Dermatitis 2002;47:288-292
3   Rudzki E, Grzywa Z, Bruo WS. Sensitivity to 35 essential oils. Contact Dermatitis 1976;2:196-200
4   Franz H, Frank R, Rytter M, Haustein UF. Allergic contact dermatitis due to cedarwood oil after dermatoscopy. Contact Dermatitis 1998;38:182-183
5   Uter W, Schmidt E, Geier J, Lessmann H, Schnuch A, Frosch P. Contact allergy to essential oils: current patch test results (2000–2008) from the Information Network of Departments of Dermatology (IVDK). Contact Dermatitis 2010;63:277-283
6   Frosch PJ, Johansen JD, Menné T, Pirker C, Rastogi SC, Andersen KE, et al. Further important sensitizers in patients sensitive to fragrances. II. Reactivity to essential oils. Contact Dermatitis 2002;47:279-287
7   Temesvári E, Podányi B, Pónyai G, Németh I. Fragrance sensitization caused by temporary henna tattoo. Contact Dermatitis 2002;47:240
8   Paulsen E, Andersen KE. Colophonium and Compositae mix as markers of fragrance allergy: Cross-reactivity between fragrance terpenes, colophonium and Compositae plant extracts. Contact Dermatitis 2005;53:285-291
9   Opinion of the Scientific Committee on Cosmetic Products and Non-Food Products Intended for Consumers concerning 'An initial list of perfumery materials which must not form part of cosmetic products except subject to the Restrictions and Conditions laid down, 25 September 2001, SCCNFP/0392/00, final. Available at: http://ec.europa.eu/health/archive/ph_risk/committees/sccp/documents/out150_en.pdf
10 Opinion of the Scientific Committee on Cosmetic Products and Non-Food Products Intended for Consumers concerning 'The 1st update of the inventory of ingredients employed in cosmetic products. Section II: Perfume and aromatic raw materials', 24 October 2000, SCCNFP/0389/00 Final. Available at: http://ec.europa.eu/health/ph_risk/committees/sccp/documents/out131_en.pdf
11 SCCS (Scientific Committee on Consumer Safety). Opinion on Fragrance allergens in cosmetic products, 26-27 June 2012, SCCS/1459/11. Available at: https://ec.europa.eu/health/sites/health/files/scientific_committees/consumer_safety/docs/sccs_o_102.pdf
12 Uter W, Johansen JD, Börje A, Karlberg A-T, Lidén C, Rastogi S, Roberts D, White IR. Categorization of fragrance contact allergens for prioritization of preventive measures: clinical and experimental data and consideration of structure–activity relationships. Contact Dermatitis 2013;69:196-230

13 De Groot AC, Schmidt E. Essential oils: contact allergy and chemical composition. Boca Raton, Fl., USA: CRC Press, Taylor and Francis Group, 2016 (ISBN 9781482246407)

14 Lawless J. The encyclopedia of essential oils, 2nd Edition. London: Harper Thorsons, 2014

15 Rudzki E, Grzywa Z. Allergy to perfume mixture. Contact Dermatitis 1986;15:115-116

16 Chaudhary AK, Ahmad S, Mazumder A. *Cedrus deodara* (Roxb.) Loud.: A review on its ethnobotany, phytochemical and pharmacological profile. Pharmacogn J 2011;3:12-17

17 Semen E, Hiziroglu S. Production, yield and derivatives of volatile oils from eastern red cedar (Juniperus Virginiana L.). Am J Environ Sci 2005;1:133-138

18 Sabroe RA, Holden CR, Gawkrodger DJ. Contact allergy to essential oils cannot always be predicted from allergy to fragrance markers in the baseline series. Contact Dermatitis 2016;74:236-241

19 De Groot AC. Patch Testing, 4th Edition. Wapserveen, The Netherlands: acdegroot publishing, 2018 (ISBN 978-90-813233-4-5)

Chapter 6.16   CHAMOMILE OIL

Chamomile oil (may also be spelled camomile sometimes) may refer either to German chamomile oil obtained from *Chamomilla recutita* L. Rauschert or to chamomile oil Roman (synonym: English) obtained from *Chamaemelum nobile* (L.) All., better known as *Anthemis nobilis* L. In non-botanical literature, the nature of the oil and the botanical source are often not specified.

6.16.1 CHAMOMILE OIL GERMAN

IDENTIFICATION

Description/definition	: German chamomile oil (essential oil of German chamomile, essential oil of blue chamomile) is the essential oil obtained from the flowering tops of the (blue, common, Hungarian, German) chamomile, *Chamomilla recutita* (L.) Rauschert (synonyms: *Matricaria chamomilla* auct., *Matricaria recutita*)
INCI name(s) EU	: Chamomilla recutita flower oil; Matricaria recutita flower oil (perfuming name, not an INCI name proper)
INCI name(s) USA	: Chamomilla recutita (matricaria) flower oil
Other names	: Chamomile oil, Hungarian; matricaria oil; camomile oil German, Hungarian
CAS registry number(s)	: 8002-66-2; 8053-34-7; 84082-60-0
EC number(s)	: 282-006-5
RIFM monograph(s)	: Food Cosmet Toxicol 1974;12:851 (special issue I) (binder, page 209)
ISO standard	: ISO 19332 Essential oil of German / blue chamomile, 2007; Geneva, Switzerland, www.iso.org
Merck Index monograph	: 3310 (Chamomile)
Function(s) in cosmetics	: EU: masking; perfuming; skin conditioning. USA: fragrance ingredients; skin-conditioning agents - miscellaneous
Patch testing	: 2% pet.; based on RIFM data, 4% pet. is probably not irritant (19)

GENERAL

Chamomilla recutita (L.) Rauschert (syn. *Matricaria chamomilla* L., *Matricaria recutita* L.), popularly known as German chamomile, is a perennial plant belonging to the Asteraceae family. Native to Europe and adjoining Asian countries, the plant is cultivated all over the world for the flowers and the flower oil, particularly in European countries such as Hungary, France, Germany, Czech Republic, Slowakia and the former Yugoslavia, and in Egypt and Argentina. German chamomile is an important medicinal and aromatic plant of both traditional and modern systems of medicine and chamomile flowers are still an official drug in the pharmacopoeia of some 20 countries (11).

The essential oil of *Chamomilla recutita*, which is obtained by steam-distillation of the flowering tops, has a blue color, hence the common term 'blue oil'. The color is caused by the compound chamazulene, which is actually an artefact component formed during the steam-distillation of the oil from matricin (proazulene). The oil has wide application in medicine, cosmetics, aromatherapy and foodstuffs and in the flavoring of alcoholic and non-alcoholic beverages. The possible health effects of 'chamomile' and chamomile tea have been reviewed (1,2,3,20).

CHEMICAL COMPOSITION

German chamomile oil is a greenish blue to dark blue clear and slightly viscous liquid which has a herbaceous, fresh and slightly fruity odor. In German chamomile oils from various origins, over 280 chemicals have been identified. About 56 per cent of these were found in a single reviewed publication only. The ten chemicals that had the highest maximum concentrations in 85 commercial German chamomile essential oil samples are shown in table 6.16.1.1 (Erich Schmidt, analytical data presented in ref. 11).

Table 6.16.1.1 Ten ingredients with the highest concentrations in commercial German chamomile oils (11)

Name	Concentration range	Name	Concentration range
α-Bisabolol oxide A	1.0 - 46.0%	Bisabolol oxide B	3.1 - 12.1%
α-Bisabolol	1.5 - 38.3%	*cis*-Spiroether	2.5 - 10.5%
(*E*)-β-Farnesene	18.4 - 35.4%	α-Bisabolone oxide A	0.1 - 8.5%
Chamazulene	0.6 - 21.6%	(*E,E*)-α-Farnesene	0.1 - 5.8%
trans-Spiroether	0.2 - 16.8%	Spathulenol	0.5 - 5.8%

A full literature review of the qualitative and quantitative composition of commercial and non-commercial German chamomile oils of various origins, their chemotypes and with data from the ISO standard, has been published in 2016 (11).

6.16.2 CHAMOMILE OIL ROMAN

IDENTIFICATION

Description/definition : Chamomile oil Roman (English) is the essential oil obtained from the flowering tops of the (common, corn, garden, English, Roman) chamomile, *Chamaemelum nobile* (L.) All. (synonyms: *Anthemis nobilis* L., *Ortmenis nobilis* (L.) J. Gay ex Coss. et Germ.)
INCI name(s) EU & USA : Anthemis nobilis flower oil
Other names : Roman chamomile oil; English chamomile oil; camomile oil Roman
CAS registry number(s) : 8015-92-7; 84649-86-5
EC number(s) : 283-467-5
CIR review(s) : Int J Toxicol 2017;36(suppl.1):S57-S66 (access: www.cir-safety.org/ingredients)
RIFM monograph(s) : Food Cosmet Toxicol 1974;12:853 (special issue I) (binder, page 210)
Merck Index monograph : 3310 (Chamomile)
Function(s) in cosmetics : EU: masking; perfuming; skin conditioning. USA: fragrance ingredients; skin-conditioning agents - miscellaneous
Patch testing : 2% pet.; based on RIFM data, 4% pet. is probably not irritant (19)

GENERAL

Chamaemelum nobile (L.) All. is a low perennial herb with daisy-like white flowers, native to the Portuguese Azores, northern Africa (Algeria, Morocco), and Europe (Ireland, United Kingdom, France, Portugal, Spain). It is naturalized in Australia, New Zealand, other parts of Europe and the USA and also widely cultivated. One variety with full flowers and containing a large amount of essential oil is preferred for cultivation: *C. nobile* var. *flora plena* (synonym: var. *ligulosa*) (11). Traditionally, chamomile has been widely used for medicinal purposes. The possible health effects of chamomile (not properly differentiated between the German and Roman varieties) have been reviewed (1). However, the European Medicines Agency in 2011 concluded that 'The provided clinical and non-clinical data do not fulfil the requirements of a well-established medicinal use with recognised efficacy and an acceptable level of safety of Roman chamomile products' (12).

Essential oils of chamomile are used extensively in the cosmetics and perfume industries. It is also popular in aromatherapy, practitioners of which believe it to be a calming agent to end stress and aid in sleep (11).

CHEMICAL COMPOSITION

Roman chamomile oil is a clear mobile liquid which may be colorless or have a yellowish color with a tinge of blue and which has a fruity, etheric and herbal green odor. In Roman chamomile oils from various origins, over 165 chemicals have been identified. About 58% of these were found in a single reviewed publication only. The ten chemicals that had the highest maximum concentrations in 22 commercial Roman chamomile essential oil samples are shown in table 6.16.2.1 (Erich Schmidt, analytical data presented in ref. 11).

A full literature review of the qualitative and quantitative composition of commercial and non-commercial Roman chamomile oils of various origins has been published in 2016 (11). Older literature from before 1992 has been reviewed in refs. 13 and 14.

Table 6.16.2.1 Ten ingredients with the highest concentrations in commercial Roman chamomile oils (11)

Name	Concentration range	Name	Concentration range
Isobutyl angelate	11.2 - 34.4%	Methallyl angelate	6.8 - 8.0%
Isoamyl angelate	2.2 - 22.3%	Isobutyl isobutyrate	1.5 - 7.1%
3-Methylpentyl angelate	0.4 - 12.8%	Pinocarvone	2.3 - 5.6%
α-Pinene	2.2 - 11.5%	*trans*-Pinocarveol	1.7 - 5.2%
2-Methylbutyl angelate	2.0 - 9.7%	2-Methylbutyl isobutyrate	0.5 - 4.7%

CONTACT ALLERGY / ALLERGIC CONTACT DERMATITIS

Chamomile oil (unspecified)

General

Contact allergy to / allergic contact dermatitis from chamomile oil (botanical source not specified) has been reported in a few publications only. In groups of consecutive patients suspected of contact dermatitis (and in one study [10] also other forms of dermatitis), prevalence rates of up to 0.5% positive patch test reactions have been observed, but relevance data are lacking. Both cases of (possible) allergic contact dermatitis were from occupational exposure in aromatherapists (4,5). In one of these case reports, α-pinene may have been an allergen in chamomile oil (5).

Testing in groups of patients

Routine testing

Two hundred dermatitis patients from Poland were patch tested with 'camomile oil' 2% in petrolatum and one (0.5%) reacted (6). Between 1967 and 1970, 290 patients with various forms of dermatitis were tested in south Italy and 1 (0.3%) had a positive patch test (10). In neither of these studies was the relevance mentioned.

Testing in groups of selected patients

Fifty-one patients allergic to Myroxylon pereirae resin (balsam of Peru) and/or turpentine and/or wood tar and/or colophony were tested with 'camomile oil' 2% in petrolatum and one (2.0%) had a positive patch test; relevance data were not provided (6). One relevant positive patch test reaction to chamomile oil 1% in petrolatum was found among 122 patients (0.8%), who reported adverse cutaneous reactions to products (notably cosmetics) containing botanical ingredients in a questionnaire and who were subsequently tested with a 'botanical series' (7).

Case reports and case series

An aromatherapist had chronic hand dermatitis and was patch test positive to 17 of 20 oils used at her work (tested 1% and 5% in petrolatum), including chamomile oil (4). Another aromatherapist had non-occupational contact dermatitis with allergies to multiple essential oils used at work, including chamomile oil. The patient also reacted to geraniol, linalool, linalyl acetate, α-pinene, the fragrance mix and various other fragrance materials; α-pinene was demonstrated by GC-MS in the chamomile oil (5). In commercial *Roman* chamomile oil, α-pinene has been found in a maximum concentration of 11.5% (11).

<u>Chamomile oil German</u>

General

Contact allergy to German chamomile oil has been reported in a few publications, but relevance data were lacking and no cases of allergic contact dermatitis have been identified.

Testing in groups of patients

A group of 51 patients from Poland allergic to Myroxylon pereirae resin (balsam of Peru) and/or turpentine and/or wood tar and/or colophony was tested with German chamomile oil 2% in petrolatum and one (2.0%) had a positive patch test; relevance data were not provided (6). Another group of 86 patients from Poland previously reacting to the fragrance mix was tested with chamomile oil and three (3.4%) had a positive patch test reaction; relevance data were not provided (8).

Nine patients from Denmark who had previously tested positive to a short ether extract of German chamomile were tested with blue chamomile oil 1% and 4% in petrolatum and one (11%) had a positive reaction; the relevance of this was not mentioned (9).

<u>Chamomile oil, Roman</u>

General

Contact allergy to / allergic contact dermatitis from Roman chamomile oil has been reported in a few studies only.

Testing in groups of patients

In a group of 271 patient with dermatitis, who used products containing *Anthemis nobilis* and were tested with *Anthemis nobilis* 1% in petrolatum, there were eight positive patch test reactions (3.0%); these were 'at least possibly relevant'; not certain it was essential oil (17).

Case reports and case series

In one clinic in Belgium, in the period 1990-2016, six cases of dermatitis caused by contact allergy to Roman chamomile oil from its presence as active principle in 'topical botanical medicines' have been observed (18).

One patient developed generalized dermatitis from *Anthemis nobilis* oil in a homeopathic preparation; she also applied chamomile compresses and drank chamomile tea (15). Two cases of allergic contact dermatitis were caused by Roman chamomile oil in the topical pharmaceutical preparation Kamillosan® (16).

LITERATURE

1   Srivastava JK, Shankar E, Gupta S. Chamomile: a herbal medicine of the past with bright future. Mol Med Report 2010;3:895-901

2   Singh O, Khanam Z, Misra N, Srivastava MK. Chamomile (*Matricaria chamomilla* L.): an overview. Pharmacogn Rev 2011;5:82-95

3   McKay DL, Blumberg JB. A review of the bioactivity and potential health benefits of chamomile tea (*Matricaria recutita* L.). Phytother Res 2006;20:519-530

4   Selvaag E, Holm J, Thune P. Allergic contact dermatitis in an aromatherapist with multiple sensitizations to essential oils. Contact Dermatitis 1995;33:354-355

5   Dharmagunawardena B, Takwale A, Sanders KJ, Cannan S, Roger A, Ilchyshyn A. Gas chromatography: an investigative tool in multiple allergies to essential oils. Contact Dermatitis 2002;47:288-292

6   Rudzki E, Grzywa Z, Bruo WS. Sensitivity to 35 essential oils. Contact Dermatitis 1976;2:196-200

7   Corazza M, Borghi A, Gallo R, Schena D, Pigatto P, Lauriola MM, et al. Topical botanically derived products: use, skin reactions, and usefulness of patch tests. A multicentre Italian study. Contact Dermatitis 2014;70:90-97

8   Rudzki E, Grzywa Z. Allergy to perfume mixture. Contact Dermatitis 1986;15:115-116

9   Paulsen E, Christensen LP, Andersen KE. Cosmetics and herbal remedies with Compositae plant extracts – are they tolerated by Compositae-allergic patients? Contact Dermatitis 2008;58:15-23

10   Meneghini CL, Rantuccio F, Lomuto M. Additives, vehicles and active drugs of topical medicaments as causes of delayed-type allergic dermatitis. Dermatologica 1971;143:137-147

11   De Groot AC, Schmidt E. Essential oils: contact allergy and chemical composition. Boca Raton, Fl., USA: CRC Press, Taylor and Francis Group, 2016 (ISBN 9781482246407)

12   European Medicines Agency. Assessment report on Chamaemelum nobile (L.) All., flos. EMA/HMPC/560906/2010, Committee on Herbal Medicinal Products (HMPC), 27 January 2011

13   Lawrence BM. Progress in essential oils. Perfum Flavor 1992;17(5):131-146

14   Lawrence BM. Progress in essential oils. Perfum Flavor 1990;15(4):63-71

15   Giordano-Labadie F, Schwarze HP, Bazex J. Allergic contact dermatitis from chamomile used in phytotherapy. Contact Dermatitis 2000;42:247

16   McGeorge BCL, Steele MC. Allergic contact dermatitis of the nipple from Roman chamomile ointment. Contact Dermatitis 1991;24:139-140

17   Guin JD. Use of consumer product ingredients for patch testing. Dermatitis 2005;16:71-77

18   Gilissen L, Huygens S, Goossens A. Allergic contact dermatitis caused by topical herbal remedies: importance of patch testing with the patients' own products. Contact Dermatitis 2018;78:177-184

19   De Groot AC. Patch Testing, 4th Edition. Wapserveen, The Netherlands: acdegroot publishing, 2018 (ISBN 978-90-813233-4-5)

20   Miraj S, Alesaeidi S. A systematic review study of therapeutic effects of *Matricaria recutita* chamomile (chamomile). Electron Physician 2016;8:3024-3031

Chapter 6.17   CINNAMON OIL

There are two types of cinnamon oils derived from *Cinnamomum zeylanicum* Blume, cinnamon bark oil Sri Lanka and cinnamon leaf oil Sri Lanka. Cinnamon oils should not be confused with cassia oils, which are obtained from the Chinese cinnamon, *Cinnamomum cassia* (Nees & T. Nees) J. Presl (see Chapter 6.14).

It should be realized that 'cinnamon' may be obtained either from the true cinnamon *Cinnamomum zeylanicum* Blume, from the cassia (Chinese cinnamon) *Cinnamomum cassia* (Nees & T. Nees) J. Presl. or from other *Cinnamomum* species.

6.17.1 CINNAMON BARK OIL SRI LANKA

IDENTIFICATION
Description/definition   : Cinnamon bark oil, Sri Lanka type (essential oil of cinnamon bark, Sri Lanka type), is the
                             essential oil obtained from the twigs and bark of stem of the cinnamon, *Cinnamomum
                             zeylanicum* Blume (synonym: *Cinnamomum verum* J. Presl)
INCI name(s) EU & USA   : Cinnamomum zeylanicum bark oil
Other names   : Cinnamon oil Ceylon
CAS registry number(s)   : 8015-91-6; 84649-98-9
EC number(s)   : 283-479-0
RIFM monograph(s)   : Food Cosmet Toxicol 1975;13:111 (binder, page 216)
SCCS opinion(s)   : SCCNFP/0389/00, final (24); SCCS/1459/11 (25)
Merck Index monograph   : 3570 (Cinnamon)
Function(s) in cosmetics   : EU: masking; perfuming; tonic. USA: fragrance ingredients
Patch testing   : 1% pet. (27); 0.5% pet. (SPCanada); test also cinnamal (see Chapter 3.34 Cinnamal)

GENERAL
Cinnamomum zeylanicum Blume is an evergreen small tree, up to 10 meter tall with a black-brown bark, and an inner bark with cinnamon flavor. The tree is native to Sri Lanka. It is naturalized on islands in the western Indian Ocean, the Pacific and the Caribbean (West Indies). The cinnamon is cultivated in Africa (Madagascar, Seychelles), Asia (China, Taiwan, India, Sri Lanka, Vietnam, Indonesia, Malaysia), Mexico, the Caribbean (Jamaica, Martinique), French Guiana and Brazil (27).

The essential oil, extracted from the bark by distillation (cinnamon bark oil), serves as flavor for bakery and confectionary products, meat, liqueur, chewing-gum, ice-cream, beverages, soup and pharmaceutical products. Cinnamon bark oil is not used in aromatherapy because the risk of skin sensitization from the high content of cinnamal (5,6).

A comprehensive review of all aspects of *Cinnamomum zeylanicum* is provided in ref. 1. Other useful reviews include refs. 2,3 and 4.

CHEMICAL COMPOSITION
Cinnamon bark oil is an amber to brown, clear mobile liquid which has a strong sweet spicy, characteristic odor. In cinnamon bark oils from various origins, over 160 chemicals have been identified. About 46 per cent of these were found in a single reviewed publication only. The ten chemicals that had the highest maximum concentrations in 43 commercial cinnamon bark Sri Lanka essential oil samples are shown in table 6.17.1.1 (Erich Schmidt, analytical data presented in ref. 27).

A full literature review of the qualitative and quantitative composition of commercial and non-commercial cinnamon bark oils Sri Lanka of various origins and chemotypes has been published in 2016 (27).

Table 6.17.1.1 Ten ingredients with the highest concentrations in commercial cinnamon bark oils (27)

Name	Concentration range	Name	Concentration range
(*E*)-Cinnamal(dehyde)	43.0 - 72.7%	β-Phellandrene	1.1 - 4.6%
Eugenol	0.2 - 16.4%	(*Z*)-β-Ocimene	0.01 - 3.6%
(*E*)-Cinnamyl acetate	0.9 - 7.8%	α-Phellandrene	0.5 - 3.2%
β-Caryophyllene	2.7 - 7.5%	*p*-Cymene	2.2 - 2.8%
Linalool	2.1 - 7.2%	α-Terpinene	0.3 - 2.6%

6.17.2 CINNAMON LEAF OIL SRI LANKA

IDENTIFICATION

Description/definition   : Cinnamon leaf oil, Sri Lanka type (essential oil of cinnamon leaf, Sri Lanka type), is the essential oil obtained from the leaves of the cinnamon, *Cinnamomum zeylanicum* Blume (synonym: *Cinnamomum verum* J. Presl.)
INCI name(s) EU & USA   : Cinnamomum zeylanicum leaf oil
Other names   : Ceylon cinnamon leaf oil
CAS registry number(s)   : 8015-91-6; 84649-98-9
EC number(s)   : 283-479-0
RIFM monograph(s)   : Food Cosmet Toxicol 1975;13:749 (special issue II) (binder, page 218)
SCCS opinion(s)   : SCCNFP/0389/00, final (24)
ISO standard   : Essential oil of cinnamon leaf, Sri Lanka type, 2003; Geneva, Switzerland, www.iso.org
Merck Index monograph   : 3570 (Cinnamon)
Function(s) in cosmetics : EU: masking; perfuming. USA: fragrance ingredients
Patch testing   : 2% pet.; test also eugenol (see Chapter 3.65 Eugenol)

GENERAL

General aspects are discussed in the section 'General' of cinnamon bark oil above. Bark oils may be adulterated with leaf oils (27).

CHEMICAL COMPOSITION

Cinnamon leaf oil is a light to dark amber clear and mobile liquid, which has a strong spicy odor, reminding of fresh crushed cloves with tender cinnamic notes. In cinnamon leaf oils from various origins, over 160 chemicals have been identified. About 52 per cent of these were found in a single reviewed publication only. The ten chemicals that had the highest maximum concentrations in 30 commercial cinnamon leaf essential oil samples (concentration ranges provided) are shown in table 6.17.2.1 (Erich Schmidt, analytical data presented in ref. 27).

A full literature review of the qualitative and quantitative composition of commercial and non-commercial cinnamon leaf oils Sri Lanka of various origins, chemotypes and with data from the ISO standard, has been published in 2016 (27).

Table 6.17.2.1 Ten ingredients with the highest concentrations in commercial cinnamon leaf oils (27)

Name	Concentration range	Name	Concentration range
Eugenol	72.2 - 81.6%	Linalool	1.8 - 2.8%
β-Caryophyllene	1.3 - 4.6%	(*E*)-Cinnamyl acetate	1.0 - 2.0%
Eugenyl acetate	1.2 - 4.1%	α-Phellandrene	0.5 - 1.5%
Benzyl benzoate	0.6 - 3.6%	α-Pinene	0.4 - 1.4%
(*E*)-Cinnamal(dehyde)	0.8 - 2.8%	Safrole	0.8 - 1.3%

CONTACT ALLERGY / ALLERGIC CONTACT DERMATITIS

The SCCS (Scientific Committee on Consumer Safety), in a 2012 Opinion on Fragrance allergens in cosmetic products, has marked cinnamon bark oil Sri Lanka as 'established contact allergen in humans' (25,26).

Cinnamon oil, unspecified

General

Contact allergy to / allergic contact dermatitis from cinnamon has been reported in over 15 publications. Routine testing in unselected dermatitis patients has not been performed. Many case reports of allergy to cinnamon oil relate to its presence in toothpastes, and there were also some patients with occupational allergic contact dermatitis. We assume (but cannot be certain), that most reports of contact allergy to 'cinnamon oil' concern cinnamon *bark* oil, dominated by (*E*)-cinnamaldehyde (cinnamal) (versus the *leaf* oil, which has eugenol as major component). Indeed, several authors have found concomitant reactions to cinnamon oil and cinnamal (14,15,20). However, there must be other allergenic ingredients in cinnamon oil (e.g. eugenol [22], which can be present in concentrations of up to 16% in commercial cinnamon bark oils [see the section 'Chemical composition' above]), as cinnamal is sometimes tested negative (16,21).

In literature, no good distinction is made between cinnamon oil and cassia oil, sometimes they are used as synonyms.

Testing in groups of patients

In a group of 21 patients with dermatitis caused by perfumes and tested with a series of essential oils, nine (43%) reacted to oil of cinnamon, Ceylon (=Sri Lanka). In four cinnamon oil-allergic patients who were also tested with eugenol, three (75%) had a concomitant positive patch test reaction; cinnamal was not tested. Because of the high percentage of positive reactions to eugenol and it is unknown whether cinnamal would be positive, it is possible that the oil used for testing was cinnamon *leaf* oil (22).

Of 15 patients allergic to balsam of Peru and tested with cinnamon oil 5% pet., all reacted to the oil. Three out of 6 had positive tests to cinnamon oil 1% pet. and 3/3 reacted to a 2.5% in alcohol test material (29). The concentrations of 5% and 2.5% in alcohol may be irritant.

Case reports and case series

A physiotherapist developed occupational contact dermatitis from a massage cream and its ingredients cinnamon oil and clove oil; the patient was also allergic to eugenol, which may well have been the causative allergen, as it is the major ingredient of clove oil and can be present in commercial cinnamon bark oils in a concentration of up to 16% (see the section 'Chemical composition' above) (23). One patient had cheilitis from contact allergy to the vapor of cinnamon oil to which she was occupationally exposed while making bubble gum (17). Another individual developed dermatitis and stomatitis attributed to cinnamon oil and clove oil (7).

A woman developed erythematous vulvitis, thick leucorrhoea and patches of dermatitis on the buttocks after the use of a galenic vaginal suppository containing 3% cinnamon oil; there were positive patch test reactions to the fragrance-mix, the suppository, its ingredient cinnamon oil (3% and 1% positive, 0.5% negative) and cinnamyl alcohol (not an important component of cinnamon oil). The reaction to cinnamal, its major ingredient was, however, negative (21).

A baker with hand dermatitis had a positive patch test to cinnamon oil 5% in petrolatum, judged to be relevant (13). One case of generalized allergic contact dermatitis from cinnamon oil added to a mud bath in a spa has been reported; the patient reacted to cinnamon 'essence', eugenol, cinnamyl alcohol and cinnamic aldehyde (cinnamal) (14). An individual with cheilitis from contact allergy to cinnamon oil developed a recurrence of dermatitis after eating cinnamon (10).

In older literature, occupational allergic contact dermatitis from oil of cinnamon has been described in bakers, candy makers and cooks, but also in housewives. Oil of cinnamon has further been reported as the cause of eczema in lipsticks. After an allergic dermatitis from cinnamon, ingestion of cinnamon oil may provoke a relapse (data cited in ref. 29).

In a number of publications, positive patch tests to cinnamon oil have been reported with unknown, uncertain or unstated relevance. These include (literature screened up to 2014 [27]) the following. A positive patch test to cinnamon oil was seen in a patient working in a cosmetic factory who had occupational dermatitis from 2-bromo-2-nitropropane-1,3-diol (8). Two patients with contact dermatitis reacted to both cinnamon oil and its main ingredient, cinnamal (15). Another individual showed a positive patch test reaction to cinnamon oil, possibly from its presence in a topical pharmaceutical preparation (12).

Toothpastes

One patient had stomatitis from contact allergy to cinnamon oil and cassia oil in toothpaste, who was negative, however, to their main component cinnamal (16). One case of cheilitis from allergy to cinnamon (cassia) oil in toothpaste was reported (11). Three patients became sensitized to cinnamon oil in their toothpaste; one had perioral dermatitis, the second unilateral angular cheilitis, while case 3 had marked ulceration of the mucous membranes without external involvement of the lips (18,19). One individual had allergic contact stomatitis and dermatitis from cinnamal and cinnamon (cassia) oil in toothpaste (20). Another one developed dermatitis of some fingers from cinnamon oil in toothpaste, which ran along the tooth-brush on his hand; there was no cheilitis or stomatitis (9).

Cinnamon bark oil Sri Lanka

No reports on contact allergy to cinnamon bark oil, specifically mentioned to be obtained from the *bark* of *Cinnamomum zeylanicum*, have been found.

Cinnamon leaf oil Sri Lanka

General

Contact allergy to cinnamon leaf oil has been rarely reported and there are no cases of proven allergic contact dermatitis/stomatitis.

Testing in groups of patients

Routine testing
The members of the International Contact Dermatitis Research Group before 1975 tested 1382 dermatitis patients with cinnamon leaf oil 1% in petrolatum and saw 15 (1.1%) positive reactions. Three (20%) were also positive to eugenol, the major component of cinnamon leaf oil; relevance is unknown (data cited in ref. 16).

Testing in groups of selected patients
In a group of 21 patients with dermatitis caused by perfumes and tested with a series of essential oils, nine (43%) reacted to oil of cinnamon, Ceylon (=Sri Lanka) (not specified whether it was bark or of leaf oil). In four cinnamon oil-allergic patients who were also tested with eugenol, three (75%) had a concomitant positive patch test reaction. Cinnamal was not tested. Because of the high percentage of positive reactions to eugenol and as it was unknown whether there were positive reactions to cinnamal, it is possible that the oil used for testing was cinnamon *leaf* oil (22).

Case reports and case series
One positive patch test reaction to cinnamon leaf oil was observed in a patient with an allergic reaction to toothpaste; however, the presence of the oil in the toothpaste was not ascertained (16).

OTHER SIDE EFFECTS

Irritant contact dermatitis
Cinnamal is well-known to be able to cause irritant dermatitis, e.g., when patch tested at 2% or higher. As cinnamon bark oil may contain up to 70% cinnamal, irritant reactions from this oil may be expected. Indeed, a woman developed an 8% total body surface area superficial, partial thickness chemical burn to her bilateral posterior thighs and buttocks after spilling cinnamon oil onto her seat cushion and sitting on it for 2 hours (31). A similar case is that of a boy who sustained a second-degree burn after a vial of cinnamon oil broke in his pocket and the area was unwashed for 2 days (32).

Immediate-type reactions
Two patients had immediate positive patch tests to cinnamon oil and to Myroxylon pereirae resin (balsam of Peru). They both had urticarial reactions from contact with perfumes and both of them experienced gastrointestinal symptoms when eating cinnamon-flavored products or having drinks flavored with cinnamon such as coca-cola and vermouth (28).

Photosensitivity
Photosensitivity from cinnamon bark oil has been cited in ref. 30.

LITERATURE
1   Cinnamon and Cassia. PN Ravindran, K Nirmal Babu and M Shylaja, eds. Boca Raton – London – New York – Washington: CRC Press, 2004
2   Jayaprakasha GK, Mohan Rao LJ. Chemistry, biogenesis, and biological activities of *Cinnamomum zeylanicum*. Crit Rev Food Sc Nutrit 2011;51:547-562
3   Barceloux DG. Cinnamon (Cinnamomum species). DM-Dis Mon 2009;55:327-335
4   Manosi D, Suvra M, Budhimanta N, Jayram H. Ethnobotany, phytochemical and pharmacological aspects of *Cinnamomum zeylanicum* Blume. Int Res J Pharm 2013;4:58-63
5   Rhind JP. Essential oils. A handbook for aromatherapy practice, 2nd Edition. London: Singing Dragon, 2012
6   Lawless J. The encyclopedia of essential oils, 2nd Edition. London: Harper Thorsons, 2014
7   Silvers SH. Stomatitis and dermatitis venenata with purpura, resulting from oil of cloves and oil of cassia. Dental Items of Interest 1939;61:649-651. Data cited in ref. 23
8   Rudzki E, Rebandel P, Grzywa Z. Occupational dermatitis from cosmetic creams. Contact Dermatitis 1993;29:210
9   Cummer CL. Dermatitis due to oil of cinnamon. Arch Dermatol Syphilol 1940;42:674-675
10 Leifer W. Contact dermatitis due to cinnamon. Recurrence of dermatitis following oral administration of cinnamon oil. Arch Dermatol Syphylol 1951;64:52-55. Data cited in ref. 16
11 Laubach JL, Malkinson FD, Ringrose EJ. Cheilitis caused by cinnamon (cassia) oil in toothpaste. JAMA 1953;152:404-405. Data cited in ref. 16
12 Nardelli A, D'Hooge E, Drieghe J, Dooms M, Goossens A. Allergic contact dermatitis from fragrance components in specific topical pharmaceutical products in Belgium. Contact Dermatitis 2009;60:303-313

13　Nethercott JR, Holness DL. Occupational dermatitis in food handlers and bakers. J Am Acad Dermatol 1989;21:485-490

14　Garcia-Abujeta JL, de Larramendi CH, Pomares Berna J, Munoz Palomino E. Mud bath dermatitis due to cinnamon oil. Contact Dermatitis 2005;52:234

15　Kirton V, Wilkinson DS. Sensitivity to cinnamic aldehyde in a toothpaste. 2. Further studies. Contact Dermatitis 1975;1:77-80

16　Magnusson B, Wilkinson DS. Cinnamic aldehyde in toothpaste. 1. Clinical aspects and patch tests. Contact Dermatitis 1975;1:70-76

17　Miller J. Cheilitis from sensitivity to oil of cinnamon present in bubble gum. JAMA 1941;116:131-132. Data cited in ref. 16

18　Millard LG. Acute contact sensitivity to a new toothpaste. J Dentistry 1973;1:168-170

19　Millard LG. Contact sensitivity to toothpaste. Brit Med J 1973;1:676

20　Drake TE, Maibach HI. Allergic contact dermatitis and stomatitis caused by a cinnamic aldehyde-flavored toothpaste. Arch Dermatol 1976;112:202-203

21　Lauriola MM, De Bitonto A, Sena P. Allergic contact dermatitis due to cinnamon oil in galenic vaginal suppositories. Acta Derm Venereol 2010;90:187-188

22　Meynadier JM, Meynadier J, Peyron JL, Peyron L. Formes cliniques des manifestations cutanées d'allergie aux parfums. Ann Dermatol Venereol 1986;113:31-39

23　Sánchez-Pérez J, García-Díez A. Occupational allergic contact dermatitis from eugenol, oil of cinnamon and oil of cloves in a physiotherapist. Contact Dermatitis 1999;41:346-347

24　Opinion of the Scientific Committee on Cosmetic Products and Non-Food Products Intended for Consumers concerning 'The 1st update of the inventory of ingredients employed in cosmetic products. Section II: Perfume and aromatic raw materials', 24 October 2000, SCCNFP/0389/00, final. Available at: http://ec.europa.eu/health/ph_risk/committees/sccp/documents/out131_en.pdf

25　SCCS (Scientific Committee on Consumer Safety). Opinion on Fragrance allergens in cosmetic products, 26-27 June 2012, SCCS/1459/11. Available at: https://ec.europa.eu/health/sites/health/files/scientific_committees/consumer_safety/docs/sccs_o_102.pdf

26　Uter W, Johansen JD, Börje A, Karlberg A-T, Lidén C, Rastogi S, Roberts D, White IR. Categorization of fragrance contact allergens for prioritization of preventive measures: clinical and experimental data and consideration of structure–activity relationships. Contact Dermatitis 2013;69:196-230

27　De Groot AC, Schmidt E. Essential oils: contact allergy and chemical composition. Boca Raton, Fl., USA: CRC Press, Taylor and Francis Group, 2016 (ISBN 9781482246407)

28　Temesvári E, Soos G, Podányi B, Kovács I, Nemeth I. Contact urticaria provoked by balsam of Peru. Contact Dermatitis 1978;4:65-68

29　Hjorth N. Eczematous allergy to balsams. Acta Derm Venereol (Stockh.) 1961;41(suppl.46):1-216

30　De Groot AC. Patch Testing, 4th Edition. Wapserveen, The Netherlands: acdegroot publishing, 2018 (ISBN 978-90-813233-4-5)

31　Connolly M, Axtell A, Hickey S, Whalen A, McNamara L, Albright D, et al. Chemical burn from cinnamon oil. Eplasty 2017;17:ic11

32　Sparks T. Cinnamon oil burn. West J Med 1985;142:835 (data cited in ref. 31)

Chapter 6.18 CITRONELLA OIL

There are two major citronella oils: citronella oil, Java type, obtained from *Cymbopogon winterianus* Jowitt and citronella oil, Sri Lanka type, which is obtained from *Cymbopogon nardus* (L.).

6.18.1 CITRONELLA OIL JAVA

IDENTIFICATION

Description/definition	: Citronella oil Java is the essential oil obtained from the aerial parts (leaves) of the Java (Burma) citronella, *Cymbopogon winterianus* Jowitt.
INCI name(s) EU	: Cymbopogon winterianus herb oil (perfuming name, not an INCI name proper)
INCI name(s) USA	: Not in the Personal Care Products Council Ingredient Database
CAS registry number(s)	: 8000-29-1; 91771-61-8
EC number(s)	: 294-954-7
RIFM monograph(s)	: Food Cosmet Toxicol 1973;11:1067 (binder, page 231)
SCCS opinion(s)	: SCCS/1459/11 (10)
ISO standard	: ISO 3848 Essential oil of citronella, Java type, 2016 and 2001; Geneva, Switzerland, www.iso.org
Function(s) in cosmetics	: EU: perfuming
Patch testing	: 2% pet.; based on RIFM data, 8% pet. is probably not irritant (13)

GENERAL

Cymbopogon winterianus Jowitt (Java citronella, also known as Java lemongrass) is an aromatic perennial herb (grass) with fibrous roots, which seems to have arisen as a distinct form of the Sri Lanka citronella, *Cymbopogon nardus*. It is erecting over two meter tall with smooth and shiny leaves that are up to one meter long; the plant has a fresh, green, lemony odor. The Java citronella is cultivated in Africa (Ghana), Asia (China, India, Vietnam, Indonesia, Malaysia), South-America (Guatemala, Honduras, Brazil), and elsewhere (12).

'Citronella oil' is the essential oil obtained by steam-distillation from the leaves of different species of *Cymbopogon*, of which *Cymbopogon winterianus* Jowitt and *Cymbopogon nardus* L. (Rendle) (produces citronella oil, Sri Lanka type) are the most important. The oil is used on a large scale as a source of perfumery chemicals such as citronellal, citronellol and geraniol. These aroma chemicals, isolated from the essential oil, are further employed for producing high value semi-synthetic aroma chemicals including hydroxycitronellal, synthetic menthol and esters of geraniol and citronellol such as geranyl acetate and citronellyl acetate (1,12). The chemicals find extensive use in soap, candles and incense, perfumery, and in the cosmetic, flavoring and pharmaceutical industries. Citronella oil is also a renowned plant-based insect repellent and has many traditional and Chinese medicinal uses and is very popular in aromatherapy (1,12).

CHEMICAL COMPOSITION

Citronella oil Java is a pale yellow to yellowish, clear mobile liquid which has a fresh floral and sweet rosy lemon-like odor. In citronella oils Java from various origins, over 165 chemicals have been identified. About 53 per cent of these were found in a single reviewed publication only. The ten chemicals that had the highest maximum concentrations in 138 commercial citronella oil Java essential oil samples are shown in table 6.18.1.1 (Erich Schmidt, analytical data presented in ref. 12).

A full literature review of the qualitative and quantitative composition of commercial and non-commercial citronella Java oils of various origins and with data from the ISO standard, has been published in 2016 (12).

Table 6.18.1.1 Ten ingredients with the highest concentrations in commercial citronella Java oils (12)

Name	Concentration range	Name	Concentration range
Citronellal	31.5 - 49.6%	Limonene	2.5 - 5.9%
Geraniol	17.3 - 25.2%	Citronellyl acetate	1.6 - 4.5%
Citronellol	8.7 - 13.5%	β-Elemene	0.7 - 3.2%
Geranyl acetate	1.9 - 8.7%	Germacrene D	0.4 - 2.9%
α-Elemol	1.3 - 7.0%	δ-Cadinene	1.4 - 2.8%

6.18.2 CITRONELLA OIL SRI LANKA

IDENTIFICATION

Description/definition	: Citronella oil, Sri Lanka type, is the essential oil obtained from the aerial parts (leaves) of the Ceylon citronella (citronella grass), *Cymbopogon nardus* (L.) Rendle
INCI name(s) EU	: Cymbopogon nardus oil
INCI name(s) USA	: Cymbopogon nardus (citronella) oil
CAS registry number(s)	: 8000-29-1; 89998-15-2
EC number(s)	: 289-753-6
SCCS opinion(s)	: SCCS/1459/11 (10)
ISO standard	: ISO 3849 Essential oil of citronella, Sri Lanka type, 2002; Geneva, Switzerland, www.iso.org
Function(s) in cosmetics	: EU: masking; tonic. USA: fragrance ingredients
Patch testing	: 2% pet.; based on RIFM data, 8% pet. is probably not irritant (13)

GENERAL

Cymbopogon nardus (L.) Rendle (syn. *Andropogon nardus* L.), commonly known as citronella grass or Ceylon (Sri Lanka) citronella, is a perennial from the Poaceae (Gramineae) grass family, which has stems of 75-300 cm and aromatic leaves 20-60 cm long. It is native to tropical Africa, India and Sri Lanka and is cultivated in China, Sri Lanka, Myanmar and Indonesia (12). For the uses of citronella oils see the section 'General' of citronella Java oil above. The biological properties of citronella oil *ex C. nardus* have been reviewed in 2018 (14).

CHEMICAL COMPOSITION

Citronella oil Sri Lanka is a pale yellowish to pale brownish, clear mobile liquid which has a floral, rosy warm and slightly woody odor. In citronella oils Sri Lanka from various origins, over 145 chemicals have been identified. About half of these were found in a single reviewed publication only. The ten chemicals that had the highest maximum concentrations in 29 commercial citronella oil Sri Lanka essential oil samples are shown in table 6.18.2.1 (Erich Schmidt, analytical data presented in ref. 12).

A full literature review of the qualitative and quantitative composition of commercial and non-commercial citronella Sri Lanka oils of various origins and with data from the ISO standard has been published in 2016 (12).

Table 6.18.2.1 Ten ingredients with the highest concentrations in commercial citronella Sri Lanka oils (12)

Name	Concentration range	Name	Concentration range
Geraniol	18.0 - 48.7%	Limonene	3.0 - 10.4%
Citronellal	1.0 - 12.0%	(Z)-Methylisoeugenol	0.4 - 9.9%
Geranial	0.5 - 11.3%	Citronellol	1.7 - 9.6%
Camphene	7.0 - 10.9%	Borneol	5.0 - 7.6%
(E)-Methylisoeugenol	6.7 - 10.7%	Methyl eugenol	0.4 - 7.2%

CONTACT ALLERGY / ALLERGIC CONTACT DERMATITIS

Citronella oil (unspecified)

General

Contact allergy to / allergic contact dermatitis from citronella oil has been reported infrequently. In one group of consecutive patients suspected of contact dermatitis, the prevalence rate of positive patch test reactions was 2.5%, but relevance data are lacking. In all but one publication, the botanical source of the oil (Java, Sri Lanka = Ceylon) was not mentioned. In case reports, geraniol, citronellal, citronellol, geranyl acetate and limonene may have been allergens in citronella oils (2,8).

Testing in groups of patients

Routine testing

Two hundred dermatitis patients from Poland were patch tested with citronella oil 2% in petrolatum and five (2.5%) reacted; relevance data were not provided (3).

Testing in groups of selected patients

In a group of 51 patients allergic to Myroxylon pereirae resin (balsam of Peru) and/or turpentine and/or wood tar and/or colophony and tested with citronella oil 2% in petrolatum, two (3.9%) had a positive patch test; relevance data were not provided (3). A group of 86 patients from Poland previously reacting to the fragrance mix was tested with citronella oil and one (1.1%) had a positive patch test reaction; relevance data were not provided (4).

Case reports and case series

An aromatherapist had occupational contact dermatitis with allergies to multiple essential oils used at work, including citronella oil. The patient also reacted to geraniol, α-pinene, caryophyllene, the fragrance mix and various other fragrance materials; geraniol and caryophyllene were demonstrated by GC-MS in the citronella oil (2). Geraniol may be present in commercial citronella oils in concentrations up to 49% (Sri Lanka) and 25% (Java) (12).

A woman changed the urinary bag from her child daily and thereby used an ostomy deodorant; she developed dermatitis on the hands and the face. On patch testing she reacted to the deodorant and subsequently to one ingredient, which consisted mainly of citronella oil and citronellal (but according to the manufacturer also pine oil derivatives) (6). One patient allergic to a topical pharmaceutical product intended to treat osteomuscular pain reacted to the active ingredients and to 'citronella', one of the product's base ingredients (7).

Two patients had used oil of citronella for protection against mosquitos and developed dermatitis. They reacted to oil of citronella (pure and 50% in mineral oil, concentrations are slightly irritant), citronellal, citronellol, hydroxycitronellal, citral and geranyl acetate (8). Citronellal and citronellol are both important components of citronella oils and geranyl acetate may be present in concentrations up to 11% in commercial citronella oil Sri Lanka (12).

One positive patch test to citronella oil was seen in a patient working in a cosmetic factory who had occupational dermatitis from 2-bromo-2-nitropropane-1,3-diol; its relevance was not stated (5). Additional information on allergy to citronella oil may be found in ref. 9 (article not read).

Citronella oil Java

General

The SCCS (Scientific Committee on Consumer Safety), in a 2012 Opinion on Fragrance allergens in cosmetic products, has categorized Cymbopogon winterianus herb oil as 'possible fragrance contact allergen' (10,11).

There is only one documented case of contact allergy to citronella oil Java (8).

Case reports and case series

A patient occupationally sensitized to lemon oil and limonene also had positive patch test reactions to oil of citronella Java, oil of citronella Ceylon (= Sri Lanka) (both probably undiluted, may be irritant), turpentine and its component β-pinene (8). Limonene is the dominant component of lemon oil and may be present in citronella oils in concentrations up to 6% (Java) and 10.4% (Sri Lanka) (12).

Citronella oil Sri Lanka

General

The SCCS (Scientific Committee on Consumer Safety), in a 2012 Opinion on Fragrance allergens in cosmetic products, has categorized Cymbopogon nardus herb oil as 'possible fragrance contact allergen' (10,11).

There is only one documented case of contact allergy to citronella oil, Sri Lanka (8).

Case reports and case series

A patient occupationally sensitized to lemon oil and limonene, also had positive patch test reactions to oil of citronella Ceylon (= Sri Lanka), oil of citronella Java, (both probably undiluted, may be irritant), turpentine and its component β-pinene (8). Limonene is the dominant component of lemon oil and may be present in citronella oils in concentrations up to 6% (Java) and 10.4% (Sri Lanka) (12).

LITERATURE

1   Katiyar R, Gupta S, Yadav KR. *Cymbopogon winterianus*: An important species for essential Java citronella oil and medicinal value. National Conference on Forest Biodiversity: Earth's Living Treasure, 22 May, 2011. Available at: http://www.upsbdb.org/pdf/Souvenir2011/16.pdf
2   Dharmagunawardena B, Takwale A, Sanders KJ, Cannan S, Roger A, Ilchyshyn A. Gas chromatography: an investigative tool in multiple allergies to essential oils. Contact Dermatitis 2002;47:288-292
3   Rudzki E, Grzywa Z, Bruo WS. Sensitivity to 35 essential oils. Contact Dermatitis 1976;2:196-200

4   Rudzki E, Grzywa Z. Allergy to perfume mixture. Contact Dermatitis 1986;15:115-116

5   Rudzki E, Rebandel P, Grzywa Z. Occupational dermatitis from cosmetic creams. Contact Dermatitis 1993;29:210

6   Davies MG, Hodgson GA, Evans E. Contact dermatitis from an ostomy deodorant. Contact Dermatitis 1978;4:11-13

7   Bilbao I, Aguirre A, Zabala R, Gonzalez R, Raton J, Diaz Perez JL. Allergic contact dermatitis from butoxyethyl nicotinic acid and Centella asiatica extract. Contact Dermatitis 1995;33:435-436

8   Keil H. Contact dermatitis due to oil of citronellal. J Invest Dermatol 1947;8:327-334

9   Rudzki E, Grzywa Z. The value of a mixture of cassia and citronella oils for detection of hypersensitivity to essential oils. Dermatosen 1985;33:59-62

10   SCCS (Scientific Committee on Consumer Safety). Opinion on Fragrance allergens in cosmetic products, 26-27 June 2012, SCCS/1459/11. Available at: https://ec.europa.eu/health/sites/health/files/scientific_committees/consumer_safety/docs/sccs_o_102.pdf

11   Uter W, Johansen JD, Börje A, Karlberg A-T, Lidén C, Rastogi S, Roberts D, White IR. Categorization of fragrance contact allergens for prioritization of preventive measures: clinical and experimental data and consideration of structure–activity relationships. Contact Dermatitis 2013;69:196-230

12   De Groot AC, Schmidt E. Essential oils: contact allergy and chemical composition. Boca Raton, Fl., USA: CRC Press, Taylor and Francis Group, 2016 (ISBN 9781482246407)

13   De Groot AC. Patch Testing, 4th Edition. Wapserveen, The Netherlands: acdegroot publishing, 2018 (ISBN 978-90-813233-4-5)

14   Sharma R, Rao R, Kumar S, Mahant S, Khatkar S. Therapeutic potential of citronella essential oil: a review. Curr Drug Discov Technol 2018 Jul 17. doi: 10.2174/1570163815666180718095041. [Epub ahead of print]

Chapter 6.19 CLARY SAGE OIL

IDENTIFICATION

Description/definition	: Clary sage oil is the essential oil obtained from the flowering tops of the clary (clary sage), *Salvia sclarea* L. (synonym: *Salvia sclarea* var. *turkestaniana* Mottet)
INCI name(s) EU	: Salvia sclarea oil; Salvia sclarea flower oil (perfuming name, not an INCI name proper)
INCI name(s) USA	: Salvia sclarea (clary) oil
Other name(s)	: Clary oil
CAS registry number(s)	: 8016-63-5; 84775-83-7
EC number(s)	: 283-911-8
RIFM monograph(s)	: Food Cosmet Toxicol 1974;12:865 (special issue I); Food Cosmet Toxicol 1982;20: 823 (special issue)
Function(s) in cosmetics	: EU: masking; perfuming; tonic. USA: fragrance ingredients
Patch testing	: 2% pet.; based on RIFM data, 8% pet. is probably not irritant (9)

GENERAL

Salvia sclarea L., commonly known as clary sage or clary, is a biennial or short-lived herbaceous perennial, which reaches 0.9 to 1.2 meter in height and is one of the most valuable aromatic plants of the temperate region. It is native to southern Europe, central Asia and to Africa up to the Atlantic Ocean and is cultivated all over the world, commonly in the former USSR, Bulgaria, France, Morocco, USA, England, central Europe and West China. The essential oil of the clary sage serves as flavoring agent in food, liqueurs, non-alcoholic beverages and tobacco, and is used in perfumery, in the cosmetic industries and for pharmaceutical and medicinal purposes (8).

CHEMICAL COMPOSITION

Clary sage oil is a mobile, clear and colorless to light yellowish or light brown liquid which has a fresh herbaceous, soft floral to woody ambery changing odor. In clary sage oils from various origins, over 295 chemicals have been identified. About 60 per cent of these were found in a single reviewed publication only. The ten chemicals that had the highest maximum concentrations in 34 commercial clary sage essential oil samples are shown in table 6.19.1 (Erich Schmidt, analytical data presented in ref. 8).

Quality clary sage oil is preferably made solely from the flowering tops of *Salvia sclarea* L. but many commercially available oils are produced from the flowering tops *and* the leaves (aerial parts, above-ground plant). The composition of clary sage *leaf* oils considerably differs from that of the oils obtained from the flowering tops. The usual main components of leaf oils are germacrene D (with concentrations up to 69%) and β-caryophyllene (8).

A full literature review of the qualitative and quantitative composition of commercial and non-commercial clary sage oils of various origins has been published in 2016 (8).

Table 6.19.1 Ten ingredients with the highest concentrations in commercial clary sage oils (8)

Name	Concentration range	Name	Concentration range
Linalyl acetate	31.2 - 64.2%	(*Z*)-β-Ocimene	0.2 - 4.8%
Linalool	18.6 - 31.0%	Bicyclogermacrene	0.2 - 4.8%
α-Copaene	0.2 - 7.8%	Geranyl acetate	0.5 - 4.0%
Germacrene D	0.4 - 5.4%	β-Caryophyllene	0.6 - 4.0%
α-Terpineol	0.6 - 5.1%	Geraniol	0.2 - 3.6%

CONTACT ALLERGY / ALLERGIC CONTACT DERMATITIS

General

Contact allergy to / allergic contact dermatitis from clary sage oil has been reported in a few publications only. In a group of consecutive patients suspected of contact dermatitis, the prevalence rate of positive patch test reactions was 0.5%, but relevance data were lacking. All four case reports concerned occupational allergic contact dermatitis in aroma- / massage- / complementary therapists and perfume factory workers. In one case report, linalool and geraniol may have been allergens in clary sage oil (1).

Testing in groups of patients

Routine testing
Two hundred dermatitis patients from Poland were tested with clary sage oil 2% in petrolatum and one (0.5%) reacted; relevance data were not provided (2).

Testing in groups of selected patients
In a group of 51 patients allergic to Myroxylon pereirae resin (balsam of Peru) and/or turpentine and/or wood tar and/or colophony and tested with clary sage oil 2% in petrolatum, four (4.9%) had a positive patch test; relevance data were not provided (2). A group of 86 patients from Poland previously reacting to the fragrance mix was tested with clary sage oil and four (4.6%) had a positive patch test reaction; relevance data were not provided (5).

Three patients in a group of 16 (19%) known to be allergic to propolis and Myroxylon pereirae resin had positive patch test reactions to clary sage oil; relevance data were not provided (6).

Case reports and case series
Two aromatherapists had contact dermatitis (one occupational) with allergies to multiple essential oils used at their work, including clary sage oil. Both patients also reacted to geraniol, α-pinene, the fragrance mix and various other fragrance materials. In addition, one proved to be allergic to linalool and linalyl acetate, the other to caryophyllene; α-pinene, linalool, geraniol and caryophyllene were demonstrated by GC-MS in clary sage oils (1). Linalool and to a lesser degree geraniol may be important components of clary sage oil, with maximum concentrations of 31.0% and 3.6% resp. found in clary sage essential oils (see the section 'Chemical composition' above).

Occupational contact dermatitis developed in a massage therapist with allergies to various essential oils, including clary sage oil (3). A 'complementary therapist' developed occupational contact dermatitis from a multitude of essential oils used at work, including clary sage oil (4). Clary sage oil caused dermatitis in an unknown number of perfumery workers (7, article not read).

LITERATURE
1   Dharmagunawardena B, Takwale A, Sanders KJ, Cannan S, Roger A, Ilchyshyn A. Gas chromatography: an investigative tool in multiple allergies to essential oils. Contact Dermatitis 2002;47:288-292
2   Rudzki E, Grzywa Z, Bruo WS. Sensitivity to 35 essential oils. Contact Dermatitis 1976;2:196-200
3   Cockayne SE, Gawkrodger DJ. Occupational contact dermatitis in an aromatherapist. Contact Dermatitis 1997;37:306-307
4   Newsham J, Rai S, Williams JDL. Two cases of allergic contact dermatitis to neroli oil. Br J Dermatol 2011;165(suppl.1):76
5   Rudzki E, Grzywa Z. Allergy to perfume mixture. Contact Dermatitis 1986;15:115-116
6   Rudzki E, Grzywa Z. Dermatitis from propolis. Contact Dermatitis 1983;9:40-45
7   Gutman SG, Somov BA. Allergic reactions caused by components of perfumery preparations. Vestnik Dermatologii i Venerologii 1968;42:62 (in Russian)
8   De Groot AC, Schmidt E. Essential oils: contact allergy and chemical composition. Boca Raton, Fl., USA: CRC Press, Taylor and Francis Group, 2016 (ISBN 9781482246407)
9   De Groot AC. Patch Testing, 4th Edition. Wapserveen, The Netherlands: acdegroot publishing, 2018 (ISBN 978-90-813233-4-5)

Chapter 6.20   CLOVE OIL

There are three types of clove essential oils: those made from the buds (clove bud oil), leaves (clove leaf oil) and from the stems (clove stem oil) of *Syzygium aromaticum* L. Eugenol is the main ingredient in all three clove oils. Although there is a wide variation in concentrations, generally increasing percentages of eugenol are observed from bud (ISO norm: 75.0-87.0%) to leaf (ISO norm: 80.0-92.0%) and to stem (ISO norm: 83.0-92.0%) oils (2,5).

6.20.1 CLOVE BUD OIL

IDENTIFICATION

Description/definition	: Clove bud oil (essential oil of clove buds) is the essential oil obtained from the buds of the clove (clove tree) *Syzygium aromaticum* (L.) Merr. & L.M. Perry
INCI name(s) EU	: Eugenia caryophyllus bud oil
INCI name(s) USA	: Eugenia caryophyllus (clove) bud oil
CAS registry number(s)	: 8000-34-8; 84961-50-2
EC number(s)	: 284-638-7
RIFM monograph(s)	: Food Cosmet Toxicol 1975;13:761 (special issue II) (binder, page 247)
SCCS opinion(s)	: SCCS/1459/11 (33)
ISO standard	: ISO 3142 Essential oil of clove buds, 1997; Geneva, Switzerland, www.iso.org
Merck Index monograph	: 3672 (Clove)
Function(s) in cosmetics	: EU: masking; perfuming. USA: fragrance ingredients
Patch testing	: 2% pet. (SPCanada, 'clove oil'); test also eugenol (see Chapter 3.65 Eugenol)

GENERAL

The clove tree *Syzygium aromaticum* (L.) Merril and Perry (synonyms: *Eugenia caryophyllus* (Spreng.) Bullock and S.G. Harrison; *Caryophyllus aromaticus* L.; *Eugenia aromatica* (L.) Baill.; *Eugenia caryophyllata* Thunb.), is a perennial tropical plant which grows to a height ranging from 10 to 20 meter. The clove tree is native to the Maluku Islands in Indonesia, also known as the Moluccas or the Spice Islands. Two major products are available and marketed from clove tree: the cloves, which are the unopened dried fully-grown buds, and the essential oil extracted either from bud, leaf or stem. Today the most important producers of cloves are Tanzania (Zanzibar and Pemba islands), Madagascar, Indonesia, Sri Lanka and Brazil (35).

Clove oil is used traditionally in dental care as an antiseptic and analgesic, where the undiluted oil may be rubbed on the gums to treat toothache. It is active against oral bacteria associated with dental caries and periodontal disease and effective against a large number of other bacteria. Most of these biological activities are ascribed to its main ingredient eugenol, which is also used as a starting material for the production of vanillin (1). An overview of potential health benefits of clove is provided in ref. 4.

Clove essential oils are also used as flavoring agents and antimicrobial materials in food and alcoholic and soft drinks and in cosmetic products. In addition, clove oil finds extensive use in dental formulations, toothpaste, breath freshener, mouth washes, soaps, and insect repellents. Clove *bud* oils are used in aromatherapy (35).

CHEMICAL COMPOSITION

Clove bud oil is a yellowish to brown, clear, mobile, sometimes slightly viscous liquid which has an intense spicy and aromatic odor, reminding of fresh crushed cloves. In clove bud oils from various origins, over 200 chemicals have been identified. About 67 per cent of these were found in a single reviewed publication only. The ten chemicals that had the highest maximum concentrations in 31 commercial clove bud essential oil samples are shown in table 6.20.1.1 (Erich Schmidt, analytical data presented in ref. 35).

A full literature review of the qualitative and quantitative composition of commercial and non-commercial clove bud oils of various origins and with data from the ISO standard, has been published in 2016 (35).

Table 6.20.1.1 Ten ingredients with the highest concentrations in commercial clove bud oils (35)

Name	Concentration range	Name	Concentration range
Eugenol	82.0 - 90.4%	Caryophyllene alcohol	0.01 - 0.3%
β-Caryophyllene	2.6 - 12.0%	Methyl salicylate	0.02 - 0.3%
Eugenyl acetate	0.3 - 6.4%	Chavicol	0.04 - 0.2%
α-Humulene	0.5 - 2.1%	Methyl eugenol	0.04 - 0.2%
Caryophyllene oxide	0.06 - 0.4%	Furfural	0.01 - 0.1%

6.20.2 CLOVE LEAF OIL

IDENTIFICATION

Description/definition	: Clove leaf oil (essential oil of clove leaves) is the essential oil obtained from the leaves of the clove (clove tree), *Syzygium aromaticum* (L.) Merr. & L.M. Perry
INCI name(s) EU	: Eugenia caryophyllus leaf oil
INCI name(s) USA	: Eugenia caryophyllus (clove) leaf oil
CAS registry number(s)	: 8000-34-8; 84961-50-2
EC number(s)	: 284-638-7
RIFM monograph(s)	: Food Cosmet Toxicol 1978;16:695 (special issue IV)
ISO standard	: ISO Essential oil of clove leaf, 1997; Geneva, Switzerland, www.iso.org
Merck Index monograph	: 3672 (Clove)
Function(s) in cosmetics	: EU: masking; perfuming; skin conditioning; tonic. USA: fragrance ingredients; skin-conditioning agents - miscellaneous
Patch testing	: 2% pet. (SPCanada, 'clove oil'); test also eugenol (see Chapter 3.65 Eugenol)

CHEMICAL COMPOSITION

Clove leaf oil is a yellow to slightly brown mobile to slight viscous liquid which has a spicy, aromatic and sweet odor. In clove leaf oils from various origins, over 110 chemicals have been identified. About 65 per cent of these were found in a single reviewed publication only. The ten chemicals that had the highest maximum concentrations in 201 commercial clove leaf essential oil samples are shown in table 6.20.2.1 (Erich Schmidt, analytical data presented in ref. 35).

A full literature review of the qualitative and quantitative composition of commercial and non-commercial clove leaf oils of various origins and with data from the ISO standard has been published in 2016 (35).

Table 6.20.2.1 Ten ingredients with the highest concentrations in commercial clove leaf oils (35)

Name	Concentration range	Name	Concentration range
Eugenol	75.7 - 89.1%	Benzyl benzoate	0.03 - 0.6%
β-Caryophyllene	2.6 - 19.5%	Caryophyllene oxide	0.2 - 0.6%
Eugenyl acetate	0.08 - 5.9%	α-Copaene	0.01 - 0.6%
α-Humulene	0.5 - 3.0%	δ-Cadinene	0.1 - 0.6%
(*E,E*)-Farnesyl acetate	0.01 - 0.7%	Caryophyllene alcohol	0.02 - 0.4%

6.20.3 CLOVE STEM OIL

IDENTIFICATION

Description/definition	: Clove stem oil (essential oil of clove stem) is the essential oil obtained from the stem of the clove (clove tree), *Syzygium aromaticum* (L.) Merr. & L.M. Perry
INCI name(s) EU	: Eugenia caryophyllus stem oil
INCI name(s) USA	: Eugenia caryophyllus (clove) stem oil
CAS registry number(s)	: 8000-34-8; 84961-50-2
EC number(s)	: 284-638-7
RIFM monograph(s)	: Food Cosmet Toxicol 1975;13:765 (special issue II) (binder, page 250)
ISO standard	: ISO 3143 Essential oil of clove stem, 1997; Geneva, Switzerland, www.iso.org
Merck Index monograph	: 3672 (Clove)
Function(s) in cosmetics	: EU: perfuming; skin conditioning. USA: flavoring agents; fragrance ingredients
Patch testing	: 2% pet. (SPCanada, 'clove oil'); test also eugenol (see Chapter 3.65 Eugenol)

CHEMICAL COMPOSITION

Clove stem oil is a yellowish to light brown, clear mobile, sometimes slightly viscous liquid which has a spicy, aromatic odor, reminding of fresh crushed cloves. In clove stem oils from various origins over 35 chemicals have been identified. About 73 per cent of these were found in a single reviewed publication only; this high percentage may partly be explained by the low number of analytical studies performed. The ten chemicals that had the highest maximum concentrations in 29 commercial clove stem essential oil samples are shown in table 6.20.3.1 (Erich Schmidt, analytical data presented in ref. 35).

A full literature review of the qualitative and quantitative composition of commercial and non-commercial clove stem oils of various origins and with data from the ISO standard has been published in 2016 (35).

Table 6.20.3.1 Ten ingredients with the highest concentrations in commercial clove stem oils (35)

Name	Concentration range	Name	Concentration range
Eugenol	86.5 - 90.1%	Methyl salicylate	0.03 - 0.3%
β-Caryophyllene	2.4 - 9.5%	Furfural	0.01 - 0.2%
Eugenyl acetate	0.2 - 5.9%	Methyl eugenol	0.04 - 0.1%
α-Humulene	0.5 - 1.4%	Caryophyllene alcohol	0.03 - 0.1%
Caryophyllene oxide	0.2 - 0.6%	(E,E)-α-Farnesene	0.01 - 0.1%

CONTACT ALLERGY / ALLERGIC CONTACT DERMATITIS

The SCCS (Scientific Committee on Consumer Safety), in a 2012 Opinion on Fragrance allergens in cosmetic products, has marked clove bud oil (termed Eugenia caryophyllus flower oil) as 'established contact allergen in humans' (33,34).

Clove oil (unspecified)

General

Contact allergy to / allergic contact dermatitis from clove oil has been reported in over 25 publications. In groups of consecutive patients suspected of contact dermatitis, prevalence rates of up to 2.1% positive patch test reactions have been observed, but adequate relevance data are lacking. Case reports have included patients with cosmetic allergy, stomatitis and two cases of occupational contact dermatitis in a physiotherapist and a masseuse. In several studies, there were concomitant reactions to eugenol, the main component of clove oil.

Table 6.20.3.2 Patch testing in groups of patients

Years and Country	Test conc. & vehicle	Number of patients tested | positive (%)		Selection of patients (S); Relevance (R); Comments (C)	Ref.
Routine testing					
2000-2007 USA	2% pet.	326	7 (2.1%)	R: 100%; C: weak study: a. high rate of macular erythema and weak reactions, b. relevance figures include 'questionable' and 'past' relevance	9
<1976 Poland	2% pet.	200	1 (0.5%)	R: not stated	14
<1973 Poland	5% pet.	200	4 (2.0%)	R: not stated	3
1967-1970 Italy	1% pet.	380	1 (0.3%)	R: not stated; C: patients who had forms of dermatitis other than contact dermatitis were also tested	31
Testing in groups of selected patients					
2008-2014 UK	2% pet.	471	4 (0.8%)	S: patients tested with a fragrance series; R: not stated	7
2000-2008 IVDK	2% pet.	6,893	105 (1.5%)	S: patients with dermatitis suspected of causal exposure to fragrances; R: not stated; C: 50% of the patients allergic to clove oil who were also tested with eugenol, co-reacted to this major (>82%) component of the oil; the oil tested was a clove BUD oil	21
<2002 Japan, USA and 5 European countries	10% pet.	218	42 (19.3%)	S: patients previously shown to be allergic to fragrances; R: not stated; C: tested was clove BUD oil	22
1997-2000 Austria	2% pet.	747	12 (1.6%)	S: patients suspected of fragrance allergy; R: not stated	10
1989-1999 Portugal	2% pet.	67	9 (13.4%)	S: patients who had a positive patch test to the fragrance mix; R: not stated	23
1994-1995 UK	2% pet.	40	2 (5%)	S: patients previously reacting to the fragrance mix; R: not stated	24
<1986 Poland	2% pet.	86	12 (14.0%)	S: patients previously reacting to the fragrance mix; R: not stated; in the group of 86, 25% reacted to eugenol, which constitutes >80% of the oil	16
<1983 Poland	2% pet.	16	13 (81%)	S: patients known to be allergic to propolis and Myroxylon pereirae; R: not stated; C: 6 patients also reacted to eugenol, which is the main ingredient of clove oil and is present in Myroxylon pereirae and may also be present in propolis	29
<1976 Poland	2% pet.	51	1 (2.0%)	S: patients allergic to Myroxylon pereirae resin (balsam of Peru) and/or turpentine and/or wood tar and/or colophony; R: not stated	14

IVDK Information Network of Departments of Dermatology, Germany, Switzerland, Austria (www.ivdk.org); pet.: petrolatum

Testing in groups of patients

The results of patch tests with clove oil in routine testing (consecutive patients suspected of contact dermatitis) and in groups of selected patients are shown in table 6.20.3.2. In routine testing, rates of positive reactions ranged from 0.5% to 2.1%, whereas between 0.8% and 81% of patients in selected groups had positive patch tests. The very high positivity rate of 81% was seen in a small group of 16 patients previously reacting to Myroxylon pereirae resin and propolis (29).

Case reports and case series

Clove oil was responsible for 1 out of 399 cases of cosmetic allergy where the causal allergen was identified in a study of the NACDG, USA, 1977-1983 (8). In a group of 70 patients with proven allergic cosmetic dermatitis, clove oil was the allergen in one (32). A physiotherapist had occupational contact dermatitis from a massage cream and its ingredients cinnamon oil and clove oil; the patient was also allergic to eugenol, the main component of clove oil (11). One patient had dermatitis and stomatitis which was attributed to clove oil and cinnamon oil (12).

A masseuse/reflexologist developed occupational contact dermatitis from clove oil and two other essential oils (13). In a group of 63 patients with facial dermatitis, one had a relevant positive patch test reaction to clove oil (25). One patient with mucosal inflammation and purpuric perioral macules associated with the use of a prophylactic dental tablet from contact allergy to its components oil of cloves and oil of cassia, was reported (27). Another individual suffering from oral lichenoid mucositis had relevant positive patch test reactions to clove oil, lemon oil and metals (30).

In a number of publications, positive patch tests to clove oil have been reported with unknown, uncertain or unstated relevance. These include (literature screened up to 2014 [35]) the following. One patient with burning mouth syndrome reacting to clove oil, eugenol, isoeugenol, Myroxylon pereirae resin and the fragrance mix (19). One positive patch test to clove oil in 20 perfume factory workers without dermatitis (15). Two positive patch test reactions in patients allergic to ascaridole, an allergen in tea tree oil (negative to tea tree oil itself) (20).

Additional information in older literature on contact allergy to clove oil can be found in refs. 17,18 and 28 (articles not read).

Clove bud oil

In only two articles, it was specified that the clove oil used for testing was obtained from clove buds (clove bud oil) (21,22). Their data are presented in in table 6.20.3.2.

Clove leaf oil

The SCCS (Scientific Committee on Consumer Safety), in a 2012 Opinion on Fragrance allergens in cosmetic products, has marked clove leaf oil as 'established contact allergen in humans' (33,34).

Articles on contact allergy to clove oil, specified as being clove *leaf* oil, have not been found.

Clove stem oil

Articles on contact allergy to clove oil specified as being clove *stem* oil have not been found.

OTHER SIDE EFFECTS

Miscellaneous side effects

Spillage of clove oil under the right eye caused minor, transient irritation followed by permanent local anesthesia and anhidrosis in one patient. The side effect was ascribed to a direct neurotoxic effect of its main ingredient, eugenol (which is used as an anodyne in cases of toothache) (6).

LITERATURE

1   Chaieb K, Hajlaoui H, Zmantar T, Kahla-Nakbi AB, Rouabhia M, Mahdouani K, et al. The chemical composition and biological activity of clove essential oil, *Eugenia caryophyllata* (*Syzigium aromaticum* L. Myrtaceae): A short review. Phytother Res 2007;21:501-506

2   Razafimamonjison G, Jahiel M, Duclos T, Ramanoelina P, Fawbush F, Danthu P. Bud, leaf and stem essential oil composition of clove (*Syzygium aromaticum* L.) from Indonesia, Madagascar and Zanzibar. Int J Basic Appl Sci 2014;3(3):224-233

3   Rudzki E, Kielak D. Sensitivity to some compounds related to Balsam of Peru. Contact Dermatitis Newsletter 1972;nr.13:335-336

4   Singletary K. Clove: Overview of potential health benefits. Nutrition Today 2014;49(4):207-224

5   Lawrence BM. Progress in essential oils. Perfum Flavor 2013;38(November):46-52

6   Isaacs G. Permanent local anaesthesia and anhidrosis after clove oil spillage. Lancet 1983;321(8329):882

7   Sabroe RA, Holden CR, Gawkrodger DJ. Contact allergy to essential oils cannot always be predicted from allergy to fragrance markers in the baseline series. Contact Dermatitis 2016;74:236-241

8   Adams RM, Maibach HI. A five-year study of cosmetic reactions. J Am Acad Dermatol 1985;13:1062-1069

9   Wetter DA, Yiannias JA, Prakash AV, Davis MD, Farmer SA, el-Azhary RA, et al. Results of patch testing to personal care product allergens in a standard series and a supplemental cosmetic series: an analysis of 945 patients from the Mayo Clinic Contact Dermatitis Group, 2000-2007. J Am Acad Dermatol 2010;63:789-798

10   Wöhrl S, Hemmer W, Focke M, Götz M, Jarisch R. The significance of fragrance mix, balsam of Peru, colophonium and propolis as screening tools in the detection of fragrance allergy. Br J Dermatol 2001;145:268-273

11   Sánchez-Pérez J, García-Díez A. Occupational allergic contact dermatitis from eugenol, oil of cinnamon and oil of cloves in a physiotherapist. Contact Dermatitis 1999;41:346-347

12   Silvers SH. Stomatitis and dermatitis venenata with purpura, resulting from oil of cloves and oil of cassia. Dental Items of Interest 1939;61:649-651. Data cited in ref. 26

13   Trattner A, David M, Lazarov A. Occupational contact dermatitis due to essential oils. Contact Dermatitis 2008;58:282-284

14   Rudzki E, Grzywa Z, Bruo WS. Sensitivity to 35 essential oils. Contact Dermatitis 1976;2:196-200

15   Schubert HJ. Skin diseases in workers at a perfume factory. Contact Dermatitis 2006;55:81-83

16   Rudzki E, Grzywa Z. Allergy to perfume mixture. Contact Dermatitis 1986;15:115-116

17   Sternberg L. Contact Dermatitis. Cases caused by oil of cloves and by oil of camomile tea (*Anthemis Cotula*). J Allergy 1937;8:185-186

18   Gaul LE. Dermatitis of the hands from oil of cloves. Skin (Los Angeles) 1963;2:314

19   Steele JC, Bruce AJ, Davis MDP, Torgerson RR, Drage LA, Rogers RS III. Clinically relevant patch test results in patients with burning mouth syndrome. Dermatitis 2012;23:61-70

20   Christoffers WA, Blömeke B, Coenraads P-J, Schuttelaar M-LA. The optimal patch test concentration for ascaridole as a sensitizing component of tea tree oil. Contact Dermatitis 2014;71:129-137

21   Uter W, Schmidt E, Geier J, Lessmann H, Schnuch A, Frosch P. Contact allergy to essential oils: current patch test results (2000–2008) from the Information Network of Departments of Dermatology (IVDK). Contact Dermatitis 2010;63:277-283

22   Larsen W, Nakayama H, Fischer T, Elsner P, Frosch P, Burrows D, et al. Fragrance contact dermatitis – a worldwide multicenter investigation (Part III). Contact Dermatitis 2002;46:141-144

23   Manuel Brites M, Goncalo M, Figueiredo A. Contact allergy to fragrance mix - a 10-year study. Contact Dermatitis 2000;43:181-182

24   Katsarma G, Gawkrodger DJ. Suspected fragrance allergy requires extended patch testing to individual fragrance allergens. Contact Dermatitis 1999;41:193-197

25   Sha M, Lewis FM, Gawkrodger DJ. Facial dermatitis and eyelid dermatitis: a comparison of patch test results and final diagnoses. Contact Dermatitis 1996;34:140-141

26   Magnusson B, Wilkinson DS. Cinnamic aldehyde in toothpaste. 1. Clinical aspects and patch tests. Contact Dermatitis 1975;1:70-76

27   Silvers SH. Stomatitis and dermatitis venenata with purpura, resulting from oil of cloves and oil of cassia. Dental Items of Interest 1939;61:649-651. Data cited in ref. 26

28   Calnan CD. Oil of cloves, laurel, lavender, peppermint. Contact Dermatitis Newsletter 1970;7:148

29   Rudzki E, Grzywa Z. Dermatitis from propolis. Contact Dermatitis 1983;9:40-45

30   Yiannias JA, el-Azhary RA, Hand JH, Pakzad SY, Rogers RS III. Relevant contact sensitivities in patients with the diagnosis of oral lichen planus. J Am Acad Dermatol 2000;42:177-182

31   Meneghini CL, Rantuccio F, Lomuto M. Additives, vehicles and active drugs of topical medicaments as causes of delayed-type allergic dermatitis. Dermatologica 1971;143:137-147

32   Schorr WF. Cosmetic allergy: Diagnosis, incidence, and management. Cutis 1974;14:844-850

33   SCCS (Scientific Committee on Consumer Safety). Opinion on Fragrance allergens in cosmetic products, 26-27 June 2012, SCCS/1459/11. Available at: https://ec.europa.eu/health/sites/health/files/scientific_committees/consumer_safety/docs/sccs_o_102.pdf

34   Uter W, Johansen JD, Börje A, Karlberg A-T, Lidén C, Rastogi S, Roberts D, White IR. Categorization of fragrance contact allergens for prioritization of preventive measures: clinical and experimental data and consideration of structure–activity relationships. Contact Dermatitis 2013;69:196-230

35   De Groot AC, Schmidt E. Essential oils: contact allergy and chemical composition. Boca Raton, Fl., USA: CRC Press, Taylor and Francis Group, 2016 (ISBN 9781482246407)

Chapter 6.21   CORIANDER FRUIT OIL

IDENTIFICATION

Description/definition	: Coriander fruit oil (essential oil of coriander fruits) is the essential oil obtained from the fruit of the coriander, *Coriandrum sativum* L.
INCI name(s) EU	: Coriandrum sativum fruit oil
INCI name(s) USA	: Coriandrum sativum (coriander) fruit oil
CAS registry number(s)	: 8008-52-4; 84775-50-8
EC number(s)	: 283-880-0
RIFM monograph(s)	: Food Cosmet Toxicol 1973;11:1077 (binder, page 257)
ISO standard	: ISO 3516 Essential oil of coriander fruits, 1997; Geneva, Switzerland, www.iso.org
Merck Index monograph	: 3787 (Coriander)
Function(s) in cosmetics	: EU: masking; perfuming. USA: flavoring agents; fragrance ingredients; skin-conditioning agents - miscellaneous
Patch testing	: 2% pet.; based on RIFM data, 6% pet. is probably not irritant (10); test also linalool (see Chapter 3.96 Linalool)

GENERAL

Coriander (synonyms: Chinese parsley, cilantro) is a glabrous, aromatic, herbaceous annual plant with a height of 30 - 90 cm. It is native to Mediterranean Europe and Western Asia and naturalized worldwide. It is now extensively cultivated as an important vegetable (leaves), spice and medicinal plant (fruits). The main exporters of coriander fruits are Russia, Egypt, India, Bulgaria, Morocco, Canada, China, Romania, Poland, the USA and Italy (9).

Coriander fruit essential oil, obtained by steam-distillation of the ripe fruits containing seeds, is included among the 20 major essential oils in the world market. The oil is extensively used as a flavoring agent in all types of food products, including alcoholic beverages, candy, pickles and meat sauce, in tobacco, in seasonings and in perfumes. Many medicinal properties have been attributed to coriander essential oil and the oil is used in aromatherapy (9). Reviews of coriander, its products, their properties and their uses are provided in refs. 1-4.

The fruit of the coriander is often (also) termed seed, but they are not synonymous: the seeds are contained within the ripe fruits. Thus, the fruit essential oil should not be confused with Coriandrum sativum *seed* oil (INCI name, CAS 84775-50-8, EC 283-880-0), which is the *fixed* (vegetable) oil of the coriander seed and is used as an emollient.

CHEMICAL COMPOSITION

Coriander fruit oil is a colorless to pale yellow, clear mobile liquid which has a floral, fresh and herbaceous odor, reminding of linalool. In coriander fruit oils from various origins, over 200 chemicals have been identified. About 48 per cent of these were found in a single reviewed publication only. The ten chemicals that had the highest maximum concentrations in 38 commercial coriander essential oil samples are shown in table 6.21.1 (Erich Schmidt, analytical data presented in ref. 9).

A full literature review of the qualitative and quantitative composition of commercial and non-commercial coriander fruit oils of various origins with data from the ISO standard, has been published in 2016 (9).

Table 6.21.1 Ten ingredients with the highest concentrations in commercial coriander fruit oils (9)

Name	Concentration range	Name	Concentration range
Linalool	55.0 - 81.2%	γ-Terpinene	0.4 - 6.6%
α-Pinene	0.9 - 8.7%	Geranyl acetate	1.4 - 5.0%
Camphor	2.2 - 8.0%	Camphene	0.2 - 4.8%
p-Cymene	0.2 - 7.8%	Limonene	1.0 - 3.6%
Geraniol	0.2 - 7.0%	Hexadecanoic acid	0 - 2.8%

CONTACT ALLERGY / ALLERGIC CONTACT DERMATITIS

General

Contact allergy to / allergic contact dermatitis from coriander fruit oil has been reported in a few studies only. In a group of consecutive patients suspected of contact dermatitis, the prevalence rate of positive patch test reactions was 1.0%, but relevance data were lacking (5). In one case report of occupational allergic contact dermatitis in an aromatherapist, the patient co-reacted to linalool and α-pinene, the two major ingredients of coriander oil (6).

Testing in groups of patients

Routine testing
Two hundred dermatitis patients from Poland were tested with coriander oil 2% in petrolatum and two (1%) reacted; relevance data were not provided (5).

Testing in groups of selected patients
In a group of 51 patients allergic to Myroxylon pereirae resin (balsam of Peru) and/or turpentine and/or wood tar and/or colophony and tested with coriander oil 2% in petrolatum, there were four (7.8%) positive patch test reactions (5). A group of 86 patients from Poland previously reacting to the fragrance mix was tested with coriander oil and three (3.4%) had a positive patch test reaction (7). In a group of 16 patients known to be allergic to propolis and Myroxylon pereirae resin there were four (25%) reactions to coriander oil (8). In none of these three studies were relevance data provided.

Case reports and case series
An aromatherapist had occupational contact dermatitis with allergies to multiple essential oils used at work, including coriander seed oil (indicating fruit oil). The patient also reacted to geraniol, α-pinene, caryophyllene, linalool, the fragrance mix and various other fragrance materials; linalool and α-pinene were demonstrated by GC-MS in the coriander seed oil and is are in fact the major ingredients of commercial coriander oils (see table 6.21.1) (6).

LITERATURE

1　Sharma MM, Sharma RK. Coriander. In: Peter KV, Ed. Handbook of herbs and spices, 2nd Ed., Vol. 1. Oxford-Cambridge-Philadelhpia-New Delhi: Woodhead Publishing Ltd, 2012: Chapter 12, 216-249
2　Shavandi MA, Haddadian Z, Shah Ismail MH. *Eryngium foetidum* L., *Coriandrum sativum* and *Persicaria odorata* L.: a review. J Asian Sci Res 2012;2:410-426
3　Mahendra P, Bisht S. *Coriandrum sativum*: A daily use spice with great medicinal effect. Pharmacogn J 2011;3:84-88
4　Msaada K, Hosni K, Ben Taarit M, Ouchikh O, Marzouk B. Variations in essential oil composition during maturation of coriander (*Coriandrum sativum* L.) fruits. J Food Biochem 2009;33:603-612
5　Rudzki E, Grzywa Z, Bruo WS. Sensitivity to 35 essential oils. Contact Dermatitis 1976;2:196-200
6　Dharmagunawardena B, Takwale A, Sanders KJ, Cannan S, Roger A, Ilchyshyn A. Gas chromatography: an investigative tool in multiple allergies to essential oils. Contact Dermatitis 2002;47:288-292
7　Rudzki E, Grzywa Z. Allergy to perfume mixture. Contact Dermatitis 1986;15:115-116
8　Rudzki E, Grzywa Z. Dermatitis from propolis. Contact Dermatitis 1983;9:40-45
9　De Groot AC, Schmidt E. Essential oils: contact allergy and chemical composition. Boca Raton, Fl., USA: CRC Press, Taylor and Francis Group, 2016 (ISBN 9781482246407)
10　De Groot AC. Patch Testing, 4th Edition. Wapserveen, The Netherlands: acdegroot publishing, 2018 (ISBN 978-90-813233-4-5)

Chapter 6.22   COSTUS ROOT OIL

IDENTIFICATION

Description/definition   : Costus root oil is the essential oil obtained from the roots of the costus, *Saussurea costus* (Falc.) Lipsch. (synonyms: *Aplotaxis lappa* Decne.; *Aucklandia costus* Falck.; *Saussurea lappa* (Decne.) C.B. Clarke)

INCI name(s) EU   : Costus root oil (perfuming name, not an INCI name proper)
INCI name(s) USA   : Not in the Personal Care Products Council Ingredient Database
CAS registry number(s)   : 8023-88-9; 90106-55-1
EC number(s)   : 290-278-1
RIFM monograph(s)   : Food Cosmet Toxicol 1974;12:867 (special issue I) (binder, page 260)
IFRA standard   : Prohibited (www.ifraorg.org/en-us/standards-library)
SCCS opinion(s)   : SCCNFP/0771/03 (4)
EU cosmetic restrictions   : Regulated in Annex II/1133 of the Regulation (EC) No. 1223/2009, regulated by 2005/42/EC (prohibited)
Patch testing   : 0.1% pet. (2)

GENERAL

Saussurea costus (Falc.) Lipsch. is a perennial herb with a stout simple stem 1-2 meters high. The costus is endemic In India (where it is called kuth in Hindi) in the sub-alpine regions of Jammu and Kashmir, Himachal Pradesh and Uttaranchal, in altitudes of 2500-4000 meter. The major producers of cultivated *Saussurea costus* are India, China and Vietnam. The costus is a well-known medicinal plant used in the indigenous systems of medicine in India, Korea, Tibet, China, and Japan (2).

Costus root essential oil may apparently be used as a flavoring component in foods and beverages. In cosmetics, costus root oil used to serve as a fixative and fragrance. Already 40 years ago it was demonstrated that the oil (through its ingredients costunolide and dehydrocostus lactone) is a very powerful sensitizer. Dermal application may also cause (severe) skin irritation (2). Because of these dangers, IFRA (International Fragrance Association) banned the use of costus root oil in cosmetics and fragrances in 1974 (5). In the EU, the use of costus root essential oil as a fragrance ingredient is prohibited. Quite curiously, according to some, the oil can be used in aromatherapy (6); others, however, consider its use (quite rightfully) contra-indicated (7).

CHEMICAL COMPOSITION

Costus root oil is a yellow to brown, viscous liquid which has a woody, erogenic animal, balsamic and slightly sweet odor. In costus root oils from various origins, over 135 chemicals have been identified. About 59 per cent of these were found in a single reviewed publication only. The ten chemicals that had the highest maximum concentrations in 6 commercial costus root essential oil samples are shown in table 6.22.1 (Erich Schmidt, analytical data presented in ref. 2).

A full literature review of the qualitative and quantitative composition of commercial and non-commercial costus root oils of various origins has been published in 2016 (2).

Table 6.22.1 Ten ingredients with the highest concentrations in commercial costus root oils (2)

Name	Concentration range	Name	Concentration range
n-Heptadeca-1,8,11,14-tetraene	26.1 - 35.4%	γ-Costol	1.5 - 7.6%
		β-Elemene	0.1 - 4.8%
Dehydrocostunolide	1.8 - 20.5%	β-Costol	3.5 - 4.7%
Dihydrodehydrocostus lactone	2.5 - 7.9%	*trans*-Caryophyllene oxide	0.5 - 4.3%
		β-Selinene	1.8 - 4.2%
β-Elemenol	2.6 - 7.7%	β-Caryophyllene	1.1 - 3.7%

CONTACT ALLERGY / ALLERGIC CONTACT DERMATITIS

General

Contact allergy to / allergic contact dermatitis from costus root oil has been reported in a few older studies only. Costus oil pure causes irritation and patch test sensitization, 1% in petrolatum was considered suitable for patch testing (12,13).

Testing in groups of patients

The members of the North American Contact Dermatitis Group (NACDG) saw 6 positive patch test reactions to 'essence costus notre distillate' in a group of 282 (2.1%) patch tested dermatitis patients. Despite the high rate of sensitization, patch testing with it was abandoned (3). In a group of 96 patients suffering from photosensitivity dermatitis with actinic reticuloid syndrome, 17 (18%) had positive patch tests to costus root oil 1% in petrolatum. The relevance of these vast numbers of reactions was not mentioned (1).

Case reports and case series

Costus root oil in cosmetics was reported to be the cause of contact dermatitis of the face in some Japanese women (10,11). 'Costus oil' was responsible for 1 out of 399 cases of cosmetic allergy where the causal allergen was identified in a study of the NACDG, USA, 1977-1983 (8).

In a number of publications, positive patch tests to costus root oil have been reported with unknown, uncertain or unstated relevance. These include (literature screened up to 2014 [2]) the following. One positive patch test reaction to 'costus oil' was observed in a group of 460 patients with positive patch tests related to cosmetics; relevance data were not provided (9). Five patients reacted to costus root oil 1% in petrolatum, but had never had contact with the oil. However, they were all allergic to *Chrysanthemum* x *morifolium* (Compositae) or to the liverwort *Frullania* (Jubuilaceae). These plants are known to yield sesquiterpene lactones, and the five patients also showed positive patch test reactions to alantolactone and to some related lactones, which may indicate cross-sensitization to costus root oil (12). Of 3 patients allergic to laurel oil (leaf extract) and laurel essential oil, all co-reacted to costus oil and costunolide (ref. lost during writing).

OTHER SIDE EFFECTS

Photosensitivity

Two patients with photosensitivity dermatitis with actinic reticuloid syndrome had a positive photopatch test to costus root oil 1% in petrolatum. The relevance of these reactions was not mentioned (1).

LITERATURE

1 Addo HA, Ferguson J, Johnson BF, Frain-Bell W. The relationship between exposure to fragrance materials and persistent light reaction in photosensitivity dermatitis with actinic reticuloid syndrome. Br J Dermatol 1982;107:261-274

2 De Groot AC, Schmidt E. Essential oils: contact allergy and chemical composition. Boca Raton, Fl., USA: CRC Press, Taylor and Francis Group, 2016 (ISBN 9781482246407)

3 Mitchell JC, Adams RM, Glendenning WE, Fisher A, Kanof N, Larsen W, et al. Results of standard patch tests with substances abandoned. Contact Dermatitis 1982;8:336-337

4 SCCFNP (Scientific Committee on Cosmetic Products and Non-Food Products Intended for Consumers). Opinion concerning An update of the initial list of perfumery materials which must not form part of fragrance compounds used in cosmetic products, 9 December 2003, SCCNFP/0771/03.
   Available at: http://ec.europa.eu/health/ph_risk/committees/sccp/documents/out251_en.pdf

5 RIFM. Fragrance raw materials monographs. Costus root, essential oil, absolute and concrete. Food Cosmet Toxicol 1974;12:867-868

6 Lawless J. The encyclopedia of essential oils, 2nd Edition. London: Harper Thorsons, 2014

7 Davis P. Aromatherapy. An A-Z, 3rd Edition. London: Vermilion, 2005

8 Adams RM, Maibach HI. A five-year study of cosmetic reactions. J Am Acad Dermatol 1985;13:1062-1069

9 Romaguera C, Camarasa JMG, Alomar A, Grimalt F. Patch tests with allergens related to cosmetics. Contact Dermatitis 1983;9:167-168

10 Nakayama H. Fragrance hypersensitivity and its control. In: Frosch PJ, Dooms-Goossens A, Lachapelle J-M, Rycroft RJG, Scheper RJ, Eds. Current Topics in contact dermatitis. Heidelberg: Springer Verlag, 1989:83-91

11 Nakayama H. Cosmetic dermatitis in Japan. Read before the First Annual Clinical Chemical Correlation Seminar, Pacific Dermatological Association, Vancouver, British Columbia, Canada, 1973. Data cited in ref. 3

12 Mitchell JC. Contact sensitivity to costusroot oil, an ingredient of some perfumes. Arch Dermatol 1974;109:572

13 Mitchell JC, Epstein WL. Contact hypersensitivity to a perfume material, Costus absolute. Arch Dermatol 1974;110:871-873

Chapter 6.23   CYPRESS OIL

IDENTIFICATION

Description/definition	: Cypress oil is the essential oil obtained from the twigs with leaves of the Italian (Mediterranean) cypress, *Cupressus sempervirens* L.
INCI name(s) EU & USA	: Cupressus sempervirens oil; Cupressus sempervirens leaf oil
CAS registry number(s)	: 8013-86-3; 84696-07-1
EC number(s)	: 283-626-9
RIFM monograph(s)	: Food Cosmet Toxicol 1978;16:699 (special Issue IV)
ISO standard	: ISO 20809 Essential oil of cypress, 2017; Geneva, Switzerland, www.iso.org
SCCS opinion(s)	: SCCNFP/0389/00, final (6); SCCNFP/0392/00, final (5)
Function(s) in cosmetics	: EU: masking; perfuming; skin conditioning. USA: fragrance ingredients; skin-conditioning agents - miscellaneous
EU cosmetic restrictions	: Regulated in Annex III/123 of the Regulation (EC) No. 344/2013
Patch testing	: 5% pet. (8)

GENERAL

The Italian (common) cypress (*Cupressus sempervirens* L.) is native to northern Africa (Libya), Asia (Cyprus, Iran, Israel, Jordan, Lebanon, Syria, Turkey), Italy and Greece; it is also cultivated. This tree is mainly used as an ornamental tree due to its conical crown shape, but it can also be used for timber, as a privacy screen, and protection against wind as well. Moreover, cypress has proved to be very suitable as a pioneer species for reforestation as it can tolerate poor, barren, and superficial soils. Cypress products are used in traditional medicine.

Commercial cypress essential oils, which are obtained from the young twigs with leaves of the cypress, are mainly used in perfumes, but can be used as flavors as well; another application is in aromatherapy (1,7).

CHEMICAL COMPOSITION

Cypress oil is a very pale to yellowish orange, clear, easily mobile liquid which has a terpeny, fresh   and   coniferous, slightly herbal odor. In cypress oils from various origins, over 205 chemicals have been identified. About 57 per cent of these were found in a single reviewed publication only. The ten chemicals that had the highest maximum concentrations in 33 commercial cypress essential oil samples are shown in table 6.23.1 (Erich Schmidt, analytical data presented in ref. 7).

A full literature review of the qualitative and quantitative composition of commercial and non-commercial cypress oils of various origins and chemotypes has been published in 2016 (7).

Table 6.23.1 Ten ingredients with the highest concentrations in commercial cypress oils (7)

Name	Concentration range	Name	Concentration range
α-Pinene	43.2 - 68.0%	Terpinyl acetate	1.2 - 3.2%
δ3-Carene	7.2 - 25.9%	Myrcene	1.0 - 2.9%
Limonene	0.1 - 10.8%	Sabinene	0.5 - 2.2%
Cedrol	0.4 - 4.2%	β-Caryophyllene	0.2 - 2.1%
Terpinolene	0.8 - 3.5%	Germacrene D	0.02 - 2%

CONTACT ALLERGY / ALLERGIC CONTACT DERMATITIS

General

Reports on routine testing with cypress oil have not been found. Allergic contact dermatitis to cypress oil has been reported in three studies only, describing occupational allergic contact dermatitis from cypress oils in two aromatherapists and a naturopathic therapist. One of these patients was also allergic to α-pinene, which is the dominant component of cypress oils and may have been the allergen in that case (3).

Case reports and case series

A naturopathic therapist had occupational contact dermatitis from cypress oil; she also reacted to other essential oils and fragrance materials (4). An aromatherapist had chronic hand dermatitis and was patch test positive to 17 of 20 oils used at her work (tested 1% and 5% in petrolatum), including cypress oil (2).

Another aromatherapist had non-occupational contact dermatitis with allergies to multiple essential oils used at work, including cypress oil. The patient also reacted to geraniol, linalool, linalyl acetate, α-pinene, the fragrance mix and various other fragrance materials; α-pinene, linalool, terpineol and caryophyllene were demonstrated by GC-MS in the cypress oil (3). α-Pinene is indeed the dominant ingredient in commercial cypress essential oils with concentrations ranging from 43% to 68% (table 6.23.1). It should be appreciated that, in the latter two patients, false-positive reactions due to an excited skin syndrome cannot be excluded.

LITERATURE

1   Rhind JP. Essential oils. A handbook for aromatherapy practice, 2nd Edition. London: Singing Dragon, 2012
2   Selvaag E, Holm J, Thune P. Allergic contact dermatitis in an aromatherapist with multiple sensitizations to essential oils. Contact Dermatitis 1995;33:354-355
3   Dharmagunawardena B, Takwale A, Sanders KJ, Cannan S, Roger A, Ilchyshyn A. Gas chromatography: an investigative tool in multiple allergies to essential oils. Contact Dermatitis 2002;47:288-292
4   Trattner A, David M, Lazarov A. Occupational contact dermatitis due to essential oils. Contact Dermatitis 2008;58:282-284
5   Opinion of the Scientific Committee on Cosmetic Products and Non-Food Products Intended for Consumers concerning 'An initial list of perfumery materials which must not form part of cosmetic products except subject to the Restrictions and Conditions laid down, 25 September 2001, SCCNFP/0392/00, final. Available at: http://ec.europa.eu/health/archive/ph_risk/committees/sccp/documents/out150_en.pdf
6   Opinion of the Scientific Committee on Cosmetic Products and Non-Food Products Intended for Consumers concerning 'The 1st update of the inventory of ingredients employed in cosmetic products. Section II: Perfume and aromatic raw materials', 24 October 2000, SCCNFP/0389/00, final. Available at: http://ec.europa.eu/health/ph_risk/committees/sccp/documents/out131_en.pdf
7   De Groot AC, Schmidt E. Essential oils: contact allergy and chemical composition. Boca Raton, Fl., USA: CRC Press, Taylor and Francis Group, 2016 (ISBN 9781482246407)
8   De Groot AC. Patch Testing, 4th Edition. Wapserveen, The Netherlands: acdegroot publishing, 2018 (ISBN 978-90-813233-4-5)

Chapter 6.24 DWARF PINE OIL

IDENTIFICATION

Description/definition : Dwarf pine oil (essential oil of dwarf pine) is the essential oil obtained from needles with twigs (leaves and terminal branchlets) of the (dwarf) mountain pine, *Pinus mugo* Turra

INCI name(s) EU & USA : Pinus pumilio branch/leaf oil; Pinus mugo leaf oil
CAS registry number(s) : 90082-73-8; 8000-26-8; 90082-72-7
EC number(s) : 290-164-1; 290-163-6
RIFM monograph(s) : Food Cosmet Toxicol 1976;14:843 (special issue III)
IFRA standard : Essential oils and isolates derived from the Pinacea family, including *Pinus* and *Abies* genera, should only be used when the level of peroxides is kept to the lowest practicable level, for instance by adding antioxidants at the time of production; such products should have a peroxide value of less than 10 millimoles peroxide per liter, determined according to the FMA method (www.ifraorg.org/en-us/standards-library)
SCCS opinion(s) : SCCNFP/0392/00, final (9); SCCNFP/0389/00, final (10); SCCS/1459/11 (11)
ISO standard : ISO 21093 Essential oil of dwarf pine, 2002; Geneva, Switzerland, www.iso.org
Merck Index monograph : 8153
Function(s) in cosmetics : EU: masking; perfuming. USA: fragrance ingredients
EU cosmetic restrictions : Regulated in Annex III/109 of the Regulation (EC) No. 344/2013
Patch testing : 2% pet.; 12% pet. induces irritant reactions (14)

GENERAL

The dwarf mountain pine (synonyms: mountain pine, mugo pine) *Pinus mugo* Turra (synonyms: *Pinus montana* Mill., *Pinus montana* var. *pumilio* (Haenke) Willk., *Pinus mugo* var. *pumilio*, *Pinus pumilio* Haenke, and *Pinus mugo* Turra var. *pumilio* (Haenke) Zenari) is an evergreen shrub (rarely a tree) 1-5 meter tall, with one or more curved trunks and long branches. It is found in the Pyrenees, Alps, Erzgebirge, Carpathians, northern Apennines and the Balkan Peninsula mountains, mostly at altitudes between 1,000 and 2,200 meter.

Dwarf pine oil (synonym: mountain pine oil) is obtained from the needles and twigs of the dwarf mountain pine. It has been used to treat acute and chronic respiratory diseases by steam or cold inhalation. It is also added to bath oils and may be used as air freshener (13). Dwarf pine oil is considered a dermal irritant and sensitizer (from its high δ3-carene content, air-oxidized chemicals which are important allergens in some turpentine oils) and is therefore not used in aromatherapy (1,2).

CHEMICAL COMPOSITION

Dwarf pine oil is a clear and transparent, mobile liquid which has a discreet green, slightly fatty odor with terpenic background (turpentine-like smell). In dwarf pine oils from various origins, over 170 chemicals have been identified. About 57 per cent of these were found in a single reviewed publication only. The ten chemicals that had the highest maximum concentrations in 283 commercial dwarf pine essential oil samples are shown in table 6.24.1 (Erich Schmidt, analytical data presented in ref. 13).

A full literature review of the qualitative and quantitative composition of commercial and non-commercial dwarf pine oils of various origins and with data from the ISO standard has been published in 2016 (13).

Table 6.24.1 Ten ingredients with the highest concentrations in commercial dwarf pine oils (13)

Name	Concentration range	Name	Concentration range
α-Pinene	0.3 - 38.8%	β-Phellandrene	0.8 - 20.6%
δ3-Carene	0.6 - 34.4%	Terpinolene	0.4 - 8.3%
Myrcene	1.6 - 30.2%	β-Caryophyllene	0.5 - 5.7%
β-Pinene	0.01 - 29.0%	*p*-Cymene	0.2 - 4.3%
Limonene	0.6 - 24.2%	α-Terpinene	0.07 - 4.2%

CONTACT ALLERGY / ALLERGIC CONTACT DERMATITIS

General

The SCCS (Scientific Committee on Consumer Safety), in a 2012 Opinion on Fragrance allergens in cosmetic products, has marked Pinus mugo extract as 'established contact allergen in humans' (11,12).

Contact allergy to / allergic contact dermatitis from dwarf pine oil has been reported in a few publications only. In groups of consecutive patients suspected of contact dermatitis, prevalence rates of up to 0.7% positive patch test reactions have been observed, but relevance data are lacking.

Testing in groups of patients

Between 1998 and 2000, dwarf pine oil 2% in petrolatum was tested in 1606 consecutive patient suspected of contact dermatitis in six European countries and there were 12 (0.7%) positive patch test reactions (6). In the same period and as part of this international study, 318 patients were tested in Denmark and two (0.6%) reacted (8). The relevance was not specified in either study.

In a group of 21 patients with dermatitis caused by perfumes and tested with a series of essential oils, four (19%) reacted to dwarf pine oil; relevance data were not provided (7).

Case reports and case series

Allergic contact dermatitis (probably one case) to a pharmaceutical cream containing the NSAID etofenamate was caused by its base ingredient dwarf pine oil (5).

In two publications, positive patch tests to dwarf pine oil have been reported with unknown, uncertain or unstated relevance. These include (literature screened up to 2014 [13]) the following. One positive patch test to dwarf pine oil was observed in a patient with contact allergy to Melaleuca alternifolia (tea tree) oil (3). One positive patch test reaction to dwarf pine oil occurred among 20 workers in a perfume factory without dermatitis patch tested with the oil (4).

LITERATURE

1 Lawless J. The encyclopedia of essential oils, 2nd Edition. London: Harper Thorsons, 2014
2 Davis P. Aromatherapy. An A-Z, 3rd Edition. London: Vermilion, 2005
3 Hausen BM, Reichling J, Harkenthal M. Degradation products of monoterpenes are the sensitizing agents in tea tree oil. Am J Contact Dermat 1999;10: 68-77
4 Schubert HJ. Skin diseases in workers at a perfume factory. Contact Dermatitis 2006;55:81-83
5 Knöll R, Ulrich R, Spallek W. Allergic contact eczema to etofenamate and dwarf pine oil. Sportverletz Sportschaden 1990;4(2):96-98 (article in German)
6 Frosch PJ, Johansen JD, Menné T, Pirker C, Rastogi SC, Andersen KE, et al. Further important sensitizers in patients sensitive to fragrances. II. Reactivity to essential oils. Contact Dermatitis 2002;47:279-287
7 Meynadier JM, Meynadier J, Peyron JL, Peyron L. Formes cliniques des manifestations cutanées d'allergie aux parfums. Ann Dermatol Venereol 1986;113:31-39
8 Paulsen E, Andersen KE. Colophonium and Compositae mix as markers of fragrance allergy: Cross-reactivity between fragrance terpenes, colophonium and Compositae plant extracts. Contact Dermatitis 2005;53:285-291
9 Opinion of the Scientific Committee on Cosmetic Products and Non-Food Products Intended for Consumers concerning 'An initial list of perfumery materials which must not form part of cosmetic products except subject to the Restrictions and Conditions laid down, 25 September 2001, SCCNFP/0392/00, final. Available at: http://ec.europa.eu/health/archive/ph_risk/committees/sccp/documents/out150_en.pdf
10 Opinion of the Scientific Committee on Cosmetic Products and Non-Food Products Intended for Consumers concerning 'The 1st update of the inventory of ingredients employed in cosmetic products. Section II: Perfume and aromatic raw materials', 24 October 2000, SCCNFP/0389/00, final. Available at: http://ec.europa.eu/health/ph_risk/committees/sccp/documents/out131_en.pdf
11 SCCS (Scientific Committee on Consumer Safety). Opinion on Fragrance allergens in cosmetic products, 26-27 June 2012, SCCS/1459/11. Available at: https://ec.europa.eu/health/sites/health/files/scientific_committees/consumer_safety/docs/sccs_o_102.pdf
12 Uter W, Johansen JD, Börje A, Karlberg A-T, Lidén C, Rastogi S, Roberts D, White IR. Categorization of fragrance contact allergens for prioritization of preventive measures: clinical and experimental data and consideration of structure–activity relationships. Contact Dermatitis 2013;69:196-230
13 De Groot AC, Schmidt E. Essential oils: contact allergy and chemical composition. Boca Raton, Fl., USA: CRC Press, Taylor and Francis Group, 2016 (ISBN 9781482246407)
14 De Groot AC. Patch Testing, 4th Edition. Wapserveen, The Netherlands: acdegroot publishing, 2018 (ISBN 978-90-813233-4-5)

Chapter 6.25   ELEMI OIL

IDENTIFICATION

Description/definition   : Elemi oil (essential oil of elemi) is the essential oil obtained from the wood exudate of the Manila elemi tree (elemi canary tree), *Canarium luzonicum* (Blume) A. Gray (synonym: *Canarium luzonicum* Miq.)
INCI name(s) EU   : Canarium luzonicum gum oil (perfuming name, not an INCI name proper)
INCI name(s) USA   : Not in the Personal Care Products Council Ingredient Database
Other name(s)   : Elemi resin oil
CAS registry number(s)   : 8031-63-8
EC number(s)   : None found
RIFM monograph(s)   : Food Cosmet Toxicol 1976;14:755 (special issue III)
ISO standard   : ISO 10624 Essential oil of elemi, 1998; Geneva, Switzerland, www.iso.org
Function(s) in cosmetics : EU: perfuming
Patch testing   : 2% pet.; based on RIFM data, 4% pet. is probably not irritant (8)

GENERAL

Canarium luzonicum (Blume) A. Gray (also indicated as *Canarium luzonicum* Miq., *Canarium luzonicum* (Miq.) A. Gray; synonym: *Pimela luzonica* Blume), commonly known as Manila elemi, is an evergreen tree native to the Philippines. An oleoresin is harvested from it, elemi resin, a yellow substance of honey-like consistency. It should be stressed that the name elemi is a term applied to a variety of resinous products obtained from different countries and having different botanical origins (1). The species concerned all belong to the family Burseraceae. However, the greater part of the world's supply is coming from the Philippine Islands (Manila elemi) and is obtained from the trunk of *Canarium luzonicum*.

Steam-distillation of the elemi resin yields the essential oil of elemi. A variety of foodstuffs are flavored with elemi oil and in Europe it is used in spices and seasonings. In the US, elemi oil is also used in fragrances (3). Additionally, it has applications in aromatherapy (5).

CHEMICAL COMPOSITION

Elemi oil is a colorless to pale yellow clear mobile liquid which has a terpenic, woody, somewhat spicy and balsamic odor. In elemi oils from various origins, over 45 chemicals have been identified (very few analytical publications available[1,2,4]). About 30 per cent of these were found in a single reviewed publication only. The ten chemicals that had the highest maximum concentrations in 39 commercial elemi essential oil samples are shown in table 6.25.1 (Erich Schmidt, analytical data presented in ref. 7).

A full literature review of the qualitative and quantitative composition of commercial and non-commercial elemi oils of various origins and with data from the ISO standard has been published in 2016 (7).

Table 6.25.1 Ten ingredients with the highest concentrations in commercial elemi oils (7)

Name	Concentration range	Name	Concentration range
Limonene	33.0 - 58.4%	Sabinene	2.5 - 6.6%
α-Phellandrene	10.3 - 23.9%	β-Phellandrene	1.7 - 3.9%
Elemol	6.1 - 22.1%	Terpinolene	0.7 - 3.1%
Elemicin	0.5 - 8.7%	α-Terpineol	0.4 - 3.1%
p-Cymene	0.9 - 7.1%	α-Eudesmol	0.3 - 1.6%

CONTACT ALLERGY / ALLERGIC CONTACT DERMATITIS

General

Contact allergy to and possible allergic contact dermatitis from elemi oil have been reported in one publication only (6). A false-positive patch test reaction due to the excited skin syndrome cannot be excluded.

Case reports and case series

An aromatherapist had occupational contact dermatitis with allergies to multiple essential oils used at work, including elemi oil. The patient also reacted to geraniol, α-pinene, caryophyllene, the fragrance mix and various other fragrance materials. α-Pinene and caryophyllene were demonstrated by GC-MS in the elemi oil (6), but are not important components of commercial elemi oils (table 6.25.1).

LITERATURE

1   Villanueva MA, Torres RC, Can Başer KH, Oztek T, Kurkcuoglu M. The composition of Manila elemi oil. Flavour Fragr J 1993;8:35-37

2   Moyler DA, Clery RA. The aromatic resins: their chemistry and uses. In: KAD Swift, ed. Flavors and Fragrances. Cambridge, UK: Royal Society of Chemistry, 1997:46-115. Data cited in ref. 4

3   Mogana R, Wiart C. *Canarium* L. A phytochemical and pharmacological review. J Pharm Res 2011;4:2482-2489.

4   Lawrence BM. Essential oils 2001-2004. Carol Stream, USA: Allured Publishing Corporation, 2006:215-6

5   Lawless J. The encyclopedia of essential oils, 2nd Edition. London: Harper Thorsons, 2014

6   Dharmagunawardena B, Takwale A, Sanders KJ, Cannan S, Roger A, Ilchyshyn A. Gas chromatography: an investigative tool in multiple allergies to essential oils. Contact Dermatitis 2002;47:288-292

7   De Groot AC, Schmidt E. Essential oils: contact allergy and chemical composition. Boca Raton, Fl., USA: CRC Press, Taylor and Francis Group, 2016 (ISBN 9781482246407)

8   De Groot AC. Patch Testing, 4th Edition. Wapserveen, The Netherlands: acdegroot publishing, 2018 (ISBN 978-90-813233-4-5)

Chapter 6.26   EUCALYPTUS OIL

There are two major eucalyptus oils: Eucalyptus globulus oil, obtained from *Eucalyptus globulus* Labill. and Eucalyptus citriodora oil. However, Eucalyptus citriodora oil is a misnomer (31). This oil is obtained from the citron-scent gum (lemon-scent gum) *Corymbia citriodora* (Hook) K.D. Hill & L.A.S. Johnson, which was formerly (and is still often today) incorrectly termed *Eucalyptus citriodora* Hook (31). This oil has a composition that is completely different (main components 69-84% citronellal and up to 12% neoisopulegol + isoisopulegol in the commercial chemotype oil) from that of oils obtained from *Eucalyptus* species (main component 62-89% 1,8-cineole [eucalyptol]) (31). Nevertheless, as both oils are termed 'eucalyptus oil', they are discussed here in this chapter 'Eucalyptus oil'.

In non-botanical literature, the botanical source of 'eucalyptus oil' is hardly ever specified. In the case of contact allergic reactions, we consider it likely to be Eucalyptus globulus oil with high eucalyptol (1,8-cineole) content in most cases, which certainly holds true for patients sensitized to eucalyptus oils in topical pharmaceutical preparations. Short reviews of contact allergy to eucalyptus oils have been published in 2015 (31,32).

6.26.1 EUCALYPTUS GLOBULUS OIL

IDENTIFICATION

Description/definition	: Eucalyptus globulus oil (essential oil of Eucalyptus globulus) is the essential oil obtained from the leaves and terminal branches of the (southern, Victorian) blue gum, *Eucalyptus globulus* Labill.
INCI name(s) EU &USA	: Eucalyptus globulus leaf/twig oil; Eucalyptus globulus leaf oil
CAS registry number(s)	: 8000-48-4; 84625-32-1; 92502-70-0
EC number(s)	: 283-406-2
CIR review(s)	: Final report 06/05/2018 (access: www.cir-safety.org/ingredients)
RIFM monograph(s)	: Food Cosmet Toxicol 1975;13:107 (binder, page 374)
SCCS opinion(s)	: SCCS/1459/11 (23)
ISO standard	: ISO 770 Essential oil of eucalyptus globulus, 2002; Geneva, Switzerland, www.iso.org
Merck Index monograph	: 5209 (Eucalyptus)
Function(s) in cosmetics	: EU: masking; perfuming; skin conditioning. USA: fragrance ingredients; skin-conditioning agents - miscellaneous
Patch testing	: 2% pet. (SPEurope, SPCanada)

GENERAL

Eucalyptus globulus (Tasmanian blue gum) is a tall, evergreen tree native to Tasmania and Victoria (Australia). It has been widely planted in temperate South America, China and sub-Saharan Africa. Vast plantations have been established in southern Australia, Spain, Chile and elsewhere, notably for paper pulp and timber production.

From the leaves (with twigs) of *Eucalyptus globulus* an essential oil is produced which has a high 1,8-cineole (eucalyptol) content. Eucalyptus globulus oils are widely used in pharmaceutical, confectionery and cosmetic industries. The oil is medicinally used as a decongestant for treating catarrh, bronchitis, sore throat and influenza, but may also be employed in the treatment of other diseases. Other applications include in liniments for bruises, sprains and muscular pains. Eucalyptus oils are also used as a general disinfectant, cleaner and deodorizer about the house and is utilized in aromatherapy (25).

Table 6.26.1.1 Ten ingredients with the highest concentrations in commercial Eucalyptus globulus oils (25)

Name	Concentration range	Name	Concentration range
1,8-Cineole (eucalyptol)	61.6 - 88.7%	Terpinolene	0.02 - 3.6%
Limonene	4.5 - 12.9%	*p*-Cymene	1.1 - 3.1%
α-Pinene	0.3 - 8.2%	α-Terpineol	0.02 - 1.9%
β-Pinene	0.3 - 5.8%	Aromadendrene	0.01 - 1.8%
γ-Terpinene	0.2 - 4.9%	*trans*-Pinocarveol	0.01 - 1.7%

CHEMICAL COMPOSITION

Eucalyptus globulus oil is a mobile, colorless to pale yellow colored liquid which has a fresh, aromatic, and minty odor. In Eucalyptus globulus oils from various origins, over 250 chemicals have been identified. About 58 per cent of these were found in a single reviewed publication only. The ten chemicals that had the highest maximum concentrations in 185 commercial Eucalyptus globulus essential oil samples are shown in table 6.26.1.1 (Erich Schmidt, analytical data presented in ref. 25).

A full literature review of the qualitative and quantitative composition of commercial and non-commercial Eucalyptus globulus oils of various origins and with data from the ISO standard has been published in 2016 (25). Literature data on the chemical composition of eucalyptus globulus oils from before 1990 can be found in refs. 1-3.

6.26.2 EUCALYPTUS CITRIODORA OIL

IDENTIFICATION

Description/definition	: Eucalyptus citriodora oil (essential oil of eucalyptus citriodora) is the essential oil obtained from the leaves and terminal branches of the citron-scent gum (lemon-scent gum), *Corymbia citriodora* (Hook) K.D. Hill & L.A.S. Johnson (synonym: *Eucalyptus citriodora* Hook.)
INCI name(s) EU & USA	: Eucalyptus citriodora oil
CAS registry number(s)	: 85203-56-1; 129828-24-6
EC number(s)	: 286-249-8
RIFM monograph(s)	: Food Chem Toxicol 1988;26:323 (special issue VII)
ISO standard	: ISO 3044 Essential oil of eucalyptus citriodora, 1997; Geneva, Switzerland, www.iso.org
Merck Index monograph	: 5209 (Eucalyptus)
Function(s) in cosmetics	: EU: masking; tonic. USA: fragrance ingredients
Patch testing	: 2% pet.; based on RIFM data, 4% pet. is probably not irritant (5); test also citronellal (see Chapter 3.41 Citronellal)

GENERAL

Corymbia citriodora (Hook.) K.D. Hill & L.A.S. Johnson, also known as broad leaved peppermint tree, citron-scent gum, lemon-scent gum or spotted gum, is a tall tree, growing to 40-60 meters in height. This tree is native to Australia and is cultivated mainly in Brazil, south China, India, Sri Lanka, Zaire, Kenya, South Africa, Fiji and in other (sub)tropical countries. It is a graceful tree having strong lemon-scented leaves, used mainly as timber plant (25).

The leaves and terminal branches serve for the production of the essential Eucalyptus citriodora oil, which has wide applications in perfumery, pharmaceutical, chemical and other industries. It is used in perfumes, soaps, hair oils and other cosmetics, disinfectants and room fresheners. The chemical industries use the oil as source material to produce citronellol, hydroxycitronellol and menthol. A rectified form of this oil is used in insect repellents. The oil also has pharmacological applications in anti-inflammatory and antipyretic remedies and against the symptoms of respiratory infections, such as colds, flu and sinus congestion. In addition, it is administered internally for a wide range of complaints. Eucalyptus citriodora oil also has applications in aromatherapy (25).

CHEMICAL COMPOSITION

Eucalyptus citriodora oil is a mobile, colorless to yellow or yellowish green liquid which has a fresh, slightly citrusy odor reminding of citronellal. In eucalyptus citriodora oils from various origins, over 220 chemicals have been identified. About 60 per cent of these were found in a single reviewed publication only. The ten chemicals that had the highest maximum concentrations in 57 commercial Eucalyptus citriodora essential oil samples are shown in table 6.26.2.1 (Erich Schmidt, analytical data presented in ref. 25).

A full literature review of the qualitative and quantitative composition of commercial and non-commercial Eucalyptus citriodora oils of various origins, their chemotypes and with data from the ISO standard, has been published in 2016 (25).

Table 6.26.2.1 Ten ingredients with the highest concentrations in commercial Eucalyptus citriodora oils (25)

Name	Concentration range	Name	Concentration range
Citronellal	68.6 - 84.4%	α-Pinene	0.2 - 3.5%
Neoisopulegol	3.7 - 9.4%	β-Caryophyllene	0.5 - 2.6%
Citronellol	3.9 - 8.0%	1,8-Cineole	0.1 - 2.0%
Citronellyl acetate	0.3 - 3.7%	β-Pinene	0.4 - 1.3%
Isoisopulegol	0.9 - 3.7%	β-Phellandrene	0.07 - 0.8%

CONTACT ALLERGY / ALLERGIC CONTACT DERMATITIS

Eucalyptus oil (unspecified)

General

Contact allergy to / allergic contact dermatitis from eucalyptus oil has been reported in over 20 publications. In all but two (6,32; *Eucalyptus globulus* oil) the botanical origin of the eucalyptus oil was not specified, but is likely to be Eucalyptus globulus oil with high eucalyptol (1,8-cineole) content. In groups of consecutive patients suspected of contact dermatitis, prevalence rates of up to 10.5% positive patch test reactions have been observed, but reliable relevance data are lacking.

Most cases of allergic contact dermatitis were in patients sensitized to eucalyptus oil in topical pharmaceutical products; in others, cosmetics were the culprit. There were also two aromatherapists with occupational allergic contact dermatitis, in one of whom α-pinene may have been an allergen in eucalyptus oil (11).

Testing in groups of patients

The results of patch tests with eucalyptus oil in routine testing (consecutive patients suspected of contact dermatitis) and in groups of selected patients are shown in table 6.26.2.2. In routine testing, rates of positive reactions ranged from 0.6% to 10.5%. The extremely high percentage of 10.5% was observed in an early Polish study and included undoubtedly many irritant reactions (34). In groups of selected patients, between 0.2% and 5.9% had positive patch tests.

Table 6.26.2.2 Patch testing in groups of patients

Years and Country	Test conc. & vehicle	Number of patients tested | positive (%)		Selection of patients (S); Relevance (R); Comments (C)	Ref.
Routine testing					
2000-2007 USA	2% pet.	679	4 (0.6%)	R: 100%; C: weak study: a. high rate of macular erythema and weak reactions, b. relevance figures include 'questionable' and 'past' relevance	7
<1976 Poland	2% pet.	200	3 (1.5%)	R: not stated	12
<1973 Poland	10% pet.	200	21 (10.5%)	R: not stated; C: undoubtedly many irritant reactions	34
Testing in groups of selected patients					
1993-2013 Australia	5% pet.	596	2 (0.3%)	S: not stated; R: not found; C: the test substances was prepared from *E. globulus*	32
2000-2008 IVDK	2% pet.	6680	16 (0.2%)	S: patients with dermatitis suspected of causal exposure to fragrances; R: not stated	18
<2005 USA	2% pet.	96	3 (3.1%)	S: patients using consumer products containing eucalyptus oil; R: 'at least possibly relevant'	16
<2002 Japan, USA and 5 European countries	10% pet.	218	4 (1.8%)	S: patients previously shown to be allergic to fragrances; R: not stated	19
1997-2000 Austria	2% pet.	747	4 (0.5%)	S: patients suspected of fragrance allergy; R: not stated	8
1994-1995 UK	2% pet.	40	1 (2.5%)	S: patients previously reacting to the fragrance mix; R: not stated; C: there was also one positive reaction in a patient negative to the fragrance mix	21
<1986 Poland	2% pet.	86	1 (1.2%)	S: patients previously reacting to the fragrance mix; R: not stated	14
<1976 Poland	2% pet.	51	3 (5.9%)	S: patients allergic to Myroxylon pereirae resin (balsam of Peru) and/or turpentine and/or wood tar and/or colophony; R: not stated	12

IVDK Information Network of Departments of Dermatology, Germany, Switzerland, Austria (www.ivdk.org); pet.: petrolatum

Case reports and case series

An aromatherapist had chronic hand dermatitis and was patch test positive to 17 of 20 oils used at her work (tested 1% and 5% in petrolatum), including eucalyptus oil (13). Another aromatherapist had non-occupational contact dermatitis with allergies to multiple essential oils used at work, including eucalyptus oil. The patient also reacted to geraniol, linalool, linalyl acetate, α-pinene, the fragrance mix and various other fragrance materials; α-pinene was demonstrated by GC-MS in the eucalyptus oil (11). α-Pinene may be an important component of *E. globulus* oil (maximum concentration of 8.2% found in commercial oils) and to a lesser degree of *E. citriodora* oil (maximum concentration found 3.5%) (25).

Two patients had positive patch test reactions to eucalyptus oil, which was present in cosmetics that had given a positive patch test or had been positive in a usage test, seen in a 9-year period in one clinic in Belgium (17). In a group of 70 patients with proven allergic cosmetic dermatitis, eucalyptus oil was the allergen in one (22). One patient had allergic contact dermatitis from eucalyptus oil in Vicks Vaporub (15). Another one developed with allergic contact dermatitis from eucalyptus oil present in an anti-inflammatory cream (20). Two cases of contact sensitization to eucalyptus oil in topical pharmaceutical products have been reported (9). A positive patch test to eucalyptus oil was observed in a patient with of airborne allergic contact dermatitis from aromatherapy caused by other essential oils (10).

An inhalant ointment, consisting entirely of eucalyptus oil and spruce oil, that helps to relieve nasal congestion due to upper respiratory tract infections was applied to the collar of the pajamas of a female child and caused dermatitis in the neck and on the upper chest. Patch tests were positive to eucalyptus oil (probably tested 2% pet.) and spruce oil 5% pet. Three controls were negative (28).

In one clinic in Belgium, in the period 1990-2016, five cases of dermatitis caused by contact allergy to eucalyptus oil (ex E. globulus) from its presence as active principle in 'topical botanical medicines' have been observed (33).

Out of 6 patients having airborne contact dermatitis, 2 showed a positive patch test to eucalyptus oil; out of 26 patients having contact dermatitis due to other agents such as cosmetics, topical drugs and wearing apparel, one was positive to eucalyptus oil (4). Details are lacking (article not read).

Eucalyptus globulus oil

The SCCS (Scientific Committee on Consumer Safety), in a 2012 Opinion on Fragrance allergens in cosmetic products, has marked Eucalyptus species leaf oils as 'established contact allergen in humans' (23,24).

Occupational allergic contact dermatitis from eucalyptus oil (ex E. globulus) was observed in one patient with hand dermatitis working in the food industry (6). The results of patch testing with E. globulus oil in Australia is shown in table 6.26.2.2 (32).

Eucalyptus citriodora oil

No reports on contact allergy to eucalyptus oil, specifically mentioned to be obtained from Eucalyptus citriodora, have been found.

OTHER SIDE EFFECTS

Systemic side effects

A 12-month-old healthy girl may have developed systemic toxicity with convulsion, irregular breathing, cyanosis and seizures from five prolonged baths containing an unknown quantity of essential oils of eucalyptus, pine, and thyme over a 4-day period for a benign and afebrile upper respiratory tract infection (30).

In France, two children aged 2 years and 3 months, who received a cosmetic baby balm on the skin of their thorax containing eucalyptus, rosemary and lavender essential oils, developed convulsions. As there was no other explanation for this and the 'neurologic toxicity of terpene derivatives is well known' (referring to studies on camphor toxicity), the cosmetic was suspected to be the culprit product. Although no specific terpene ingredient was blamed, the authors discussed the possible role of camphor, menthol and eucalyptol (1,8-cineole). On the basis of these 2 hardly convincing cases, the product was withdrawn from the market (26).

Eucalyptus oil is well documented as being very toxic if ingested and was leading cause of hospital admissions for childhood poisoning in Victoria, Australia in the 1990s (29). A possible case of systemic eucalyptus oil toxicity from topical application has been reported, also from Australia. A 6-year-old girl was treated topically with a home remedy for urticaria consisting of apple cider vinegar (200 ml), olive oil (200 ml), methylated spirits (200 ml), 95% ethanol and Eucalyptus globulus leaf oil (50 ml, containing 80% to 85% eucalyptol). The concoction (approximately 400 ml) had been applied to her limbs and trunk under plastic wrap and the dressing changed every 2 to 4 hours for 2 days. When she was not improving, the amount of Eucalyptus globulus leaf oil was doubled. Within 10 to 15 minutes of applying the bandages, the patient was noted by her father to appear 'intoxicated', with slurred speech and an unsteady gait. Over the next 30 minutes the patient became drowsy, eventually lost consciousness and was unarousable. After a night in the hospital, her symptoms resolved, with no long-term effects. The side effect was ascribed to eucalyptus oil, although the authors admitted that her symptoms may have been, in part, contributed to by an elevated blood ethanol level of 0.05 g/dL (27).

LITERATURE

1   Lawrence BM. Progress in essential oils. Eucalyptus oil (cineole type). Perfum Flav 1990;15(6):58-61
2   Boelens MH. Essential oils and aroma chemicals from Eucalyptus globulus L. Perfum Flav 1985;9(6):1-14
3   Lawrence BM. Progress in essential oils. Eucalyptus oil (cineole-rich). Perfum Flav 1986;11(6):39-40
4   Pasricha JS, Puri A. Contact dermatitis due to eucalyptus oil. Indian J Dermatol Venereol Leprol 1986;52:201-202

5 De Groot AC. Patch Testing, 4th Edition. Wapserveen, The Netherlands: acdegroot publishing, 2018 (ISBN 978-90-813233-4-5)

6 Peltonen L, Wickstrom G, Vaahtoranta M. Occupational dermatoses in the food industry. Dermatosen 1985;33:166-169

7 Wetter DA, Yiannias JA, Prakash AV, Davis MD, Farmer SA, el-Azhary RA, et al. Results of patch testing to personal care product allergens in a standard series and a supplemental cosmetic series: an analysis of 945 patients from the Mayo Clinic Contact Dermatitis Group, 2000-2007. J Am Acad Dermatol 2010;63:789-798

8 Wöhrl S, Hemmer W, Focke M, Götz M, Jarisch R. The significance of fragrance mix, balsam of Peru, colophonium and propolis as screening tools in the detection of fragrance allergy. Br J Dermatol 2001;145:268-273

9 Devleeschouwer V, Roelandts R, Garmyn M, Goossens A. Allergic and photoallergic contact dermatitis from ketoprofen: results of (photo) patch testing and follow-up of 42 patients. Contact Dermatitis 2008;58:159-166

10 Schaller M, Korting HC. Allergic airborne contact dermatitis from essential oils used in aromatherapy. Clin Exp Dermatol 1995;20:143-145

11 Dharmagunawardena B, Takwale A, Sanders KJ, Cannan S, Roger A, Ilchyshyn A. Gas chromatography: an investigative tool in multiple allergies to essential oils. Contact Dermatitis 2002;47:288-292

12 Rudzki E, Grzywa Z, Bruo WS. Sensitivity to 35 essential oils. Contact Dermatitis 1976;2:196-200

13 Selvaag E, Holm J, Thune P. Allergic contact dermatitis in an aromatherapist with multiple sensitizations to essential oils. Contact Dermatitis 1995;33:354-355

14 Rudzki E, Grzywa Z. Allergy to perfume mixture. Contact Dermatitis 1986;15:115-116

15 Noiles K, Pratt M. Contact dermatitis to Vicks VapoRub. Dermatitis 2010;21:167-169

16 Guin JD. Use of consumer product ingredients for patch testing. Dermatitis 2005;16:71-77

17 Nardelli A, Drieghe J, Claes L, Boey L, Goossens A. Fragrance allergens in 'specific' cosmetic products. Contact Dermatitis 2011;64:212-219

18 Uter W, Schmidt E, Geier J, Lessmann H, Schnuch A, Frosch P. Contact allergy to essential oils: current patch test results (2000–2008) from the Information Network of Departments of Dermatology (IVDK). Contact Dermatitis 2010;63:277-283

19 Larsen W, Nakayama H, Fischer T, Elsner P, Frosch P, Burrows D, et al. Fragrance contact dermatitis – a worldwide multicenter investigation (Part III). Contact Dermatitis 2002;46:141-144

20 Vilaplana J, Romaguera C. Allergic contact dermatitis due to eucalyptol in an anti-inflammatory cream. Contact Dermatitis 2000;43:118

21 Katsarma G, Gawkrodger DJ. Suspected fragrance allergy requires extended patch testing to individual fragrance allergens. Contact Dermatitis 1999;41:193-197

22 Schorr WF. Cosmetic allergy: Diagnosis, incidence, and management. Cutis 1974;14:844-850

23 SCCS (Scientific Committee on Consumer Safety). Opinion on Fragrance allergens in cosmetic products, 26-27 June 2012, SCCS/1459/11. Available at: https://ec.europa.eu/health/sites/health/files/scientific_committees/consumer_safety/docs/sccs_o_102.pdf

24 Uter W, Johansen JD, Börje A, Karlberg A-T, Lidén C, Rastogi S, Roberts D, White IR. Categorization of fragrance contact allergens for prioritization of preventive measures: clinical and experimental data and consideration of structure–activity relationships. Contact Dermatitis 2013;69:196-230

25 De Groot AC, Schmidt E. Essential oils: contact allergy and chemical composition. Boca Raton, Fl., USA: CRC Press, Taylor and Francis Group, 2016 (ISBN 9781482246407)

26 Laribière A, Miremont-Salamé G, Bertrand S, François C, Haramburu F. Terpènes dans les cosmétiques: 2 cas d'épilepsie. Thérapie 2005;60: 607-609

27 Darben T, Cominos B, Lee C. Topical eucalyptus oil poisoning. Australas J Dermatol 1998;39:265-267

28 Kartal D, Kartal L, Çinar S, Borlu M. Allergic contact dermatitis caused by both eucalyptus oil and spruce oil. Int J Med Pharm Case Rep 2016;7:1-3

29 Day LM, Ozanne-Smiith J, Parsons BJ, Doblin M, Tibballs J. Eucalyptus oil poisoning among young children: mechanisms of access and the potential for prevention. Aust NZ J Public Health 1997;21:297-301

30 Burkhard PR, Burkhardt K, Haenggeli CA, Landis T. Plant-induced seizures: Reappearance of an old problem. J Neurol 1999;246:667-670

31 De Groot AC, Schmidt E. Eucalyptus oil and tea tree oil. Contact Dermatitis 2015;73:381-386

32 Higgins C, Palmer A, Nixon R. Eucalyptus oil: contact allergy and safety. Contact Dermatitis 2015;72:344-346

33 Gilissen L, Huygens S, Goossens A. Allergic contact dermatitis caused by topical herbal remedies: importance of patch testing with the patients' own products. Contact Dermatitis 2018;78:177-184

34 Rudzki E, Kielak D. Sensitivity to some compounds related to Balsam of Peru. Contact Dermatitis Newsletter 1972;nr.13:335-336

Chapter 6.27   GALBANUM RESIN OIL

IDENTIFICATION

Description/definition : Galbanum resin oil is the essential oil obtained from the resin of the galbanum, *Ferula gummosa* Boiss. (synonym: *Ferula galbaniflua* Boiss. & Buhse)
INCI name(s) EU : Ferula galbaniflua resin oil
INCI name(s) USA : Ferula galbaniflua (galbanum) resin oil
CAS registry number(s) : 8023-91-4; 93165-40-3
EC number(s) : 296-925-4
RIFM monograph(s) : Food Cosmet Toxicol 1978;16:765 (special issue IV)
ISO standard : ISO 14716 Essential oil of galbanum, 1998; Geneva, Switzerland, www.iso.org
Function(s) in cosmetics : EU: antimicrobial; perfuming; tonic. USA: fragrance ingredients; skin-conditioning agents - miscellaneous
Patch testing : 2% pet.; based on RIFM data, 4% pet. is probably not irritant (8)

GENERAL

Ferula gummosa Boiss. is a perennial, herbaceous, very resinous plant of the Apiaceae family, indigenous to Iran and possibly Turkmenistan, generally growing up to one meter tall and wide. It can be found in the wild mainly in Iran, Turkey, Afghanistan and neighboring countries, and can become three meter tall when growing naturally (1,3). The major producer of *Ferula gummosa* is Iran. The resin of this plant, called 'galbanum', has a strong scent and is used in the preparation of various types of incense. It is collected either by exposing the upper part of the root and cutting it into strips or by making incisions in the trunk (GRIN Taxonomy for Plants). The galbanum from *F. gummosa* is said to have many bioactive properties including antimicrobial, anti-inflammatory, anticonvulsant, carminative, expectorant, anti-catarrh, anti-rheumatic, anti-nociceptive, anti-hysteric, laxative, aphrodisiac, antiseptic, and analgesic, and is therefore widely used for numerous afflictions in folk medicine (1). In addition, galbanum is also used in the manufacture of glues, textiles and cosmetics, and due to its transparency and high-power bond, it is employed to glue gems to jewelry (1,2). The resin can also be utilized in food flavoring, where it contributes to the savory notes of curries and sauces (3).

The essential oil of galbanum (galbanum essential oil), obtained from the resin by steam- distillation, is widely used in aromatherapy (4,5) and in perfumery.

CHEMICAL COMPOSITION

Galbanum resin oil is a colorless to light yellow, clear, easily mobile liquid which has a terpenic green, aromatic and woody note with sometimes sulfurous odor. In galbanum resin oils from various origins, over 225 chemicals have been identified. About 75 per cent of these were found in a single reviewed publication only. Most of these 'single' chemicals were identified in one of two studies (1,2), in which the sesquiterpene composition and the monoterpene composition of a lab-hydrodistilled oil from galbanum, harvested from 50 *F. gummosa* plants in north Iran, were investigated; the chemical composition of this oil was entirely different from all other studies.

The ten chemicals that had the highest maximum concentrations in 21 commercial galbanum resin essential oil samples are shown in table 6.27.1 (Erich Schmidt, analytical data presented in ref. 7).

A full literature review of the qualitative and quantitative composition of commercial and non-commercial galbanum resin oils of various origins and with data from the ISO standard has been published in 2016 (7).

Table 6.27.1 Ten ingredients with the highest concentrations in commercial galbanum resin oils (7)

Name	Concentration range	Name	Concentration range
β-Pinene	51.0 - 81.2%	Bulnesol	0.4 - 3.4%
α-Pinene	2.3 - 10.1%	*trans*-Pinocarveol	0.1 - 3.3%
δ3-Carene	1.6 - 9.5%	Limonene	0.4 - 3.2%
Myrcene	0.1 - 6.6%	β-Phellandrene	0.3 - 2.8%
α-Phellandrene	0.2 - 3.6%	Myrtenol	0.06 - 2.2%

CONTACT ALLERGY / ALLERGIC CONTACT DERMATITIS

General

Contact allergy to and possible allergic contact dermatitis from galbanum resin oil has been reported in one publication only. A false-positive patch test reaction due to the excited skin syndrome cannot be excluded, but α-pinene may have been an allergen in galbanum resin oil in this case (6).

Case reports and case series

An aromatherapist had non-occupational allergic contact dermatitis with allergies to multiple essential oils used at work, including 'galbanum oil'. The patient also reacted to geraniol, linalool, linalyl acetate, α-pinene, the fragrance mix and various other fragrance materials; α-pinene and linalool were demonstrated by GC-MS in the galbanum oil (15). α-Pinene is an important component of galbanum resin oil and has been found in a maximum concentration of 10.1% in commercial galbanum resin oils (table 6.27.1).

LITERATURE

1   Jalali HT, Petronilho S, Villaverde JJ, Coimbra MA, Domingues MRM, Ebrahimian ZJ et al. Assessment of the sesquiterpenic profile of *Ferula gummosa* oleo-gum-resin (galbanum) from Iran. Contributes to its valuation as a potential source of sesquiterpenic compounds. Ind Crops Prod 2013;44:185-191

2   Jalali HT, Petronilho S, Villaverde JJ, Coimbra MA, Domingues MRM, Ebrahimian ZJ, et al. Deeper insight into the monoterpenic composition of *Ferula gummosa* oleo-gum-resin from Iran. Ind Crops Prod 2012;36:500-507

3   Miyazawa N, Nakanishi A, Tomita N, Ohkubo Y, Maeda T, Fujita A. Novel key aroma components of galbanum oil. J Agric Food Chem 2009;57:1433-1439

4   Rhind JP. Essential oils. A handbook for aromatherapy practice, 2nd Edition. London: Singing Dragon, 2012

5   Lawless J. The encyclopedia of essential oils, 2nd Edition. London: Harper Thorsons, 2014

6   Dharmagunawardena B, Takwale A, Sanders KJ, Cannan S, Roger A, Ilchyshyn A. Gas chromatography: an investigative tool in multiple allergies to essential oils. Contact Dermatitis 2002;47:288-292

7   De Groot AC, Schmidt E. Essential oils: contact allergy and chemical composition. Boca Raton, Fl., USA: CRC Press, Taylor and Francis Group, 2016 (ISBN 9781482246407)

8   De Groot AC. Patch Testing, 4th Edition. Wapserveen, The Netherlands: acdegroot publishing, 2018 (ISBN 978-90-813233-4-5)

Chapter 6.28   GERANIUM OIL

IDENTIFICATION

Description/definition	: Geranium oil (essential oil of geranium) is the essential oil obtained from the herbaceous part of *Pelargonium* x spp.
INCI name(s) EU & USA	: Pelargonium graveolens oil
CAS registry number(s)	: 8000-46-2; 90082-51-2
EC number(s)	: 290-140-0
RIFM monograph(s)	: Food Cosmet Toxicol 1974;12:883 (special issue I) (binder, page 396); Food Cosmet Toxicol 1975;13:451; Food Cosmet Toxicol 1976;14:781 (special issue III) (the latter two Geranium oil African)
SCCS opinion(s)	: SCCS/1459/11 (33)
ISO standard	: ISO 4731 Essential oil of geranium, 2012; Geneva, Switzerland, www.iso.org
Merck Index monograph	: 5708 (Geranium)
Function(s) in cosmetics	: EU: masking; perfuming. USA: fragrance ingredients
Patch testing	: 2% pet. (Chemo)

GENERAL

Pelargonium graveolens L' Hér. is an erect, multi-branched shrub, which can reach a height of up to 1.3 meter and a spread of one meter. The hairy stems are herbaceous when young, becoming woody with age. The deeply incised leaves are velvety and soft to the touch and scent strongly like roses. This species and other *Pelargonium* species are native to south tropical Africa (Mozambique, Zimbabwe) and South Africa. Plants cultivated under this name differ from wild plants and may be of hybrid origin. In fact, for the production of geranium oils not one plant species is employed, but several *Pelargonium* species and especially their hybrids are used, which are often called rose geraniums or rose-scented geraniums. These scented *Pelargonium* hybrid cultivars (e.g., 'Bourbon' or 'Rosé') are widely cultivated in Madagascar, China, Algeria, Tunisia, Morocco, South Africa and India and various other countries (35).

Essential oil of geranium is obtained by steam- or hydrodistillation of the leaves plus stems of *Pelargonium* cultivars (sometimes during flowering, as the minty fragrance turns to a smell resembling roses), or (according to ISO criteria) from the herbaceous part (leaf, stem, stalk, petiole, flower). It is one of the most valuable natural materials for the perfumery and cosmetic industries. It is also used in flavoring tobacco products and pharmaceutical preparations. The essential oil is sparingly used in food and drinks, not only as flavor but also as a food preservative. Geranium oil is popular in Chinese medicine and aromatherapy, and it is even said that the French medicinal community treats diabetes and a variety of other ailments with this oil (35).

CHEMICAL COMPOSITION

Geranium oil is an amber to greenish yellow, clear mobile liquid which has an odor with floral rosy notes and green and minty accents. In geranium oils from various origins, over 500 chemicals have been identified. About 60 per cent of these were found in a single reviewed publication only. The ten chemicals that had the highest maximum concentrations in 97 commercial geranium essential oil samples are shown in table 6.28.1 (Erich Schmidt, analytical data presented in ref. 35).

A full literature review of the qualitative and quantitative composition of commercial and non-commercial geranium oils of various origins, their chemotypes and with data from the ISO standard has been published in 2016 (35).

Table 6.28.1 Ten ingredients with the highest concentrations in commercial geranium oils (35)

Name	Concentration range	Name	Concentration range
Citronellol	20.1 - 49.4%	Isomenthone	0.1 - 8.9%
Geraniol	5.6 - 31.8%	Guaia-6,9-diene	0 - 8.4%
Citronellyl formate	2.7 - 15.0%	Geranyl formate	0.5 - 7.2%
Linalool	1.4 - 11.1%	Geranyl propionate	0.4 - 5.9%
Geranial	0.1 - 10.3%	10-epi-γ-Eudesmol	0 - 5.6%

CONTACT ALLERGY / ALLERGIC CONTACT DERMATITIS

General

The SCCS (Scientific Committee on Consumer Safety), in a 2012 Opinion on Fragrance allergens in cosmetic products, has marked Pelargonium graveolens extract as 'established' and Pelargonium roseum extract as 'possible' contact allergen in humans (33,34).

Contact allergy to / allergic contact dermatitis from geranium oil has been reported in over 30 publications. In a group of consecutive patients suspected of contact dermatitis, a prevalence rate of 1.2% positive patch test reactions has been observed, but reliable relevance data are lacking (3). There have been many case reports of allergic contact dermatitis from geranium oil, mostly in cosmetics and some in pharmaceutical preparations. In addition, there at least five descriptions of occupational allergic contact dermatitis from geranium oil in aromatherapists, a masseuse and a physiotherapist. Often, there was co-reactivity with geraniol, which is an important component of geranium oil, and with rose oils, which also contain high concentrations of geraniol. Other co-reacting chemicals which may be present in concentrations >3% in commercial geranium oils (table 6.28.1) include citronellol (the dominant ingredient), citral (neral + geranial), linalool and caryophyllene.

Table 6.28.2 Patch testing in groups of patients

Years and Country	Test conc. & vehicle	Number of patients tested | positive (%)		Selection of patients (S); Relevance (R); Comments (C)	Ref.
Routine testing					
2000-2007 USA	2% pet.	486	6 (1.2%)	R: 100%; C: weak study: a. high rate of macular erythema and weak reactions, b. relevance figures include 'questionable' and 'past' relevance	3
Testing in groups of selected patients					
2011-2015 Spain	2% pet.	607	37 (6.1%)	S: patients previously reacting to FM I, FM II, Myroxylon pereirae resin or hydroxyisohexyl 3-cyclohexene carboxaldehyde in the baseline series and subsequently tested with a fragrance series; R: not stated	37
2006-2010 USA	2% pet.	100	1 (1.0%)	S: patients with eyelid dermatitis; R: not stated	16
2004-2008 Spain	2% pet.	86	8 (9.3%)	S: patients previously reacting to the fragrance mix I or Myroxylon pereirae (n=54) or suspected of fragrance contact allergy (n=32); R: not stated; C: almost all patients also reacted to geraniol, one of its major components	18
<2004 Israel	2% pet.	91	1 (1.1%)	S: patients who had shown a doubtful or positive reaction to the fragrance mix I and/or Myroxylon pereirae resin and/or one or two commercial fine fragrances; R: not stated	21
2000 USA, Japan and 4 European countries	10% pet.	178	15 (8.4%)	S: patients previously shown to be allergic to fragrances; R: not stated	22
1989-1999 Portugal	2% pet.	67	5 (7.5%)	S: patients who had a positive patch test to the fragrance mix; R: not stated	24
1990-1998 Japan	20% pet.	1483	31 (2.1%)	S: patients suspected of cosmetic contact dermatitis, virtually all were women; range of annual frequency of sensitization: 0-4.0%; R: not stated	5
1996-1997 UK	2% pet.	10	3 (30%)	S: patients strongly suspected of fragrance allergy; all also reacted to the fragrance mix; R: not stated	4
<1986 Poland	2% pet.	86	2 (2.3%)	S: patients previously reacting to the fragrance mix; R: not stated	14
<1986 France	2% pet.	21	3 (14%)	S: patients with dermatitis caused by perfumes; R; not stated; C: the patients reacted to Egyptian geranium oil; two (67%) co-reacted to geraniol; there was also one patient who reacted to Bourbon geranium oil	32
1971-1980 Japan	20% pet.	477	4 (0.8%)	S: patients with dermatoses other than pigmented cosmetic dermatitis and volunteers; R: not stated	12
<1976 Poland	2% pet.	51	2 (3.9%)	S: patients allergic to Myroxylon pereirae resin (balsam of Peru) and/or turpentine and/or wood tar and/or colophony	10
<1974 Japan	?	183	3 (1.6%)	S: patients suspected of cosmetic dermatitis; R: unknown; C: in (probably) all there was co-reactivity with geraniol, which may be present in commercial geranium oils in concentrations of up to 32% (table 6.28.1)	26

pet.: petrolatum

Testing in groups of patients

The results of patch tests with geranium oil in routine testing (consecutive patients suspected of contact dermatitis) and in groups of selected patients are shown in table 6.28.2. In routine testing, the rate of positive reactions was 1.2% (one study only [3]). In groups of selected patients, between 0.8% and 30% had positive patch tests. The very high positivity rate of 30% was found in a very small group of 10 patients strongly suspected of fragrance allergy and reacting to the fragrance mix (4).

Case reports and case series

Occupational exposure

Two aromatherapists had contact dermatitis (one occupational) with allergies to multiple essential oils used at their work, including geranium oil. Both patients also reacted to geraniol, α-pinene, the fragrance mix and various other fragrance materials. In addition, one proved to be allergic to linalool and linalyl acetate, the other to caryophyllene; α-pinene, linalool, geraniol and caryophyllene were demonstrated by GC-MS in geranium oil (8). Linalool and geraniol may be important components of geranium oil (maximum linalool concentration in commercial geranium essential oils found: 11.1%, maximum geraniol concentration: 31.8%) and caryophyllene to a lesser degree (max. 3.2%, table 6.28.1).

Another aromatherapist had chronic hand dermatitis and was patch test positive to 17 of 20 oils used at her work (tested 1% and 5% in petrolatum), including geranium oil (7). Yet another aromatherapist developed occupational contact dermatitis from contact allergy to multiple essential oils; she reacted to geranium oil, Bourbon in the fragrance series, which reaction was considered to be relevant (11). A masseuse had occupational contact dermatitis from (other) essential oils; she also reacted to geranium oil Bourbon and other fragrance materials (9).

A female beautician had occupational allergic hand dermatitis from products containing citral and essential oils; she reacted to geranium oil, citral, citronellol, geraniol, and limonene (17); citronellol and geraniol are the main components of geranium oil (table 6.28.1).

Cosmetics

A man had allergic contact dermatitis from geranium oil, Bourbon, in an aftershave; the patient also had *photo*contact allergy to sandalwood (*Santalum album*) oil (2). A patient with hand dermatitis reacted to geranium oil Bourbon, rose oil, geraniol and several other fragrances and essential oils; she used a 'fragrance-free' hand soap containing rose oil (15).

Another individual developed allergic contact dermatitis from 'Rose Absolute' perfume and a body lotion containing *Rosa centifolia*; she reacted to her own products, geranium oil Bourbon, *Rosa centifolia*, rose oil Bulgarian, several indicators of fragrance allergy, lavender oil and various individual fragrance chemicals including linalool, which may be present in commercial geranium oils up to a concentration of 11.1% (table 6.28.1), citral (combination of neral [maximum 4.7%] and geranial [maximum concentration 10.3%, table 6.28.1]) and limonene, which may be present in lower concentrations in geranium oil (19).

Three patients developed allergic cosmetic dermatitis from geranium oil in hair dye, face cream and nail polish, one reaction each (23). An individual with allergic contact cheilitis from geranium oil in a lip balm has been described; although the title of the article suggests otherwise, geraniol itself was either negative or not tested (25). Another patient developed disseminated allergic contact dermatitis from geraniol and lavender essence in a cream; the patient also reacted to geranium oil Bourbon and Bulgarian rose oil (28).

Pharmaceutical preparations and other exposures

Twelve cases of contact allergy to geranium oil present in topical pharmaceutical preparations were reported from Belgium (1). One of three patients allergic to a topical preparation to promote wound healing and prevent scar formation (active ingredient: *Centella asiatica* extract) reacted to geranium oil present in the ointment (30).

In one clinic in Belgium, in the period 1990-2016, nine cases of dermatitis caused by contact allergy to geranium oil from their presence as active principle in 'topical botanical medicines' have been observed (36, possibly overlap with ref. 1).

Other

In a number of publications, positive patch tests to geranium oil have been reported with unknown, uncertain or unstated relevance. These include (literature screened up to 2014 [35]) the following. A patient had allergic contact cheilitis from lime in gin and tonic; she reacted to lime, geranium oil Bulgarian, rose oil, and their important component geraniol (20). Three positive patch tests were seen to geranium oil Bourbon in massage therapists / aromatherapists with occupational contact dermatitis from (multiple) essential oils; it was uncertain whether these oils had been used at work by the patients (6). One patient with erythema on the face reacted upon patch testing to geranium oil and other essential oils (29). Of seven patients allergic to the fragrance farnesol, 3 (43%) co-reacted to geranium oil (and various other fragrances) (31).

Pigmented cosmetic dermatitis
In Japan, in the 1960s and 1970s, many female patients developed pigmentation following dermatitis of the face (13). This so-called pigmented cosmetic dermatitis was shown to be caused by contact allergy to components of cosmetic products, notably essential oils, other fragrance materials, antimicrobials, preservatives and coloring materials (12,13). In a group of 620 Japanese patients with this condition investigated between 1970 and 1980, 2% had positive patch test reactions to geranium oil 20% in petrolatum (12). The number of patients with pigmented cosmetic dermatitis decreased strongly after 1978, when major cosmetic companies began to eliminate strong contact sensitizers from their products (12).

LITERATURE

1   Nardelli A, D'Hooge E, Drieghe J, Dooms M, Goossens A. Allergic contact dermatitis from fragrance components in specific topical pharmaceutical products in Belgium. Contact Dermatitis 2009;60:303-313
2   Starke JC. Photoallergy to sandalwood oil. Arch Dermatol 1967;96:62-63
3   Wetter DA, Yiannias JA, Prakash AV, Davis MD, Farmer SA, el-Azhary RA, et al. Results of patch testing to personal care product allergens in a standard series and a supplemental cosmetic series: an analysis of 945 patients from the Mayo Clinic Contact Dermatitis Group, 2000-2007. J Am Acad Dermatol 2010;63:789-798
4   Thomson KF, Wilkinson SM. Allergic contact dermatitis to plant extracts in patients with cosmetic dermatitis. Br J Dermatol 2000;142:84-88
5   Sugiura M, Hayakawa R, Kato Y, Sigiura K, Hashimoto R. Results of patch testing with lavender oil in Japan. Contact Dermatitis 2000;43:157-160
6   Bleasel N, Tate B, Rademaker M. Allergic contact dermatitis following exposure to essential oils. Australas J Dermatol 2002;43:211-213
7   Selvaag E, Holm J, Thune P. Allergic contact dermatitis in an aromatherapist with multiple sensitizations to essential oils. Contact Dermatitis 1995;33:354-355
8   Dharmagunawardena B, Takwale A, Sanders KJ, Cannan S, Roger A, Ilchyshyn A. Gas chromatography: an investigative tool in multiple allergies to essential oils. Contact Dermatitis 2002;47:288-292
9   Trattner A, David M, Lazarov A. Occupational contact dermatitis due to essential oils. Contact Dermatitis 2008;58:282-284
10 Rudzki E, Grzywa Z, Bruo WS. Sensitivity to 35 essential oils. Contact Dermatitis 1976;2:196-200
11 Boonchai W, Lamtharachai P, Sunthonpalin P. Occupational allergic contact dermatitis from essential oils in aromatherapists. Contact Dermatitis 2007;56:181-182
12 Nakayama H, Matsuo S, Hayakawa K, Takhashi K, Shigematsu T, Ota S. Pigmented cosmetic dermatitis. Int J Dermatol 1984;23:299-305
13 Nakayama H, Harada R, Toda M. Pigmented cosmetic dermatitis. Int J Dermatol 1976;15:673-675
14 Rudzki E, Grzywa Z. Allergy to perfume mixture. Contact Dermatitis 1986;15:115-116
15 Scheinman PL. Is it really fragrance free? Am J Cont Derm 1997;8:239-242
16 Wenk KS, Ehrlich AE. Fragrance series testing in eyelid dermatitis. Dermatitis 2012;23:22-26
17 De Mozzi P, Johnston GA. An outbreak of allergic contact dermatitis caused by citral in beauticians working in a health spa. Contact Dermatitis 2014;70:377-379
18 Cuesta L, Silvestre JF, Toledo F, Lucas A, Pérez-Crespo M, Ballester I. Fragrance contact allergy: a 4-year retrospective study. Contact Dermatitis 2010; 63:77-84
19 Nardelli A, Thijs L, Janssen K, Goossens A. *Rosa centifolia* in a 'non-scented' moisturizing body lotion as a cause of allergic contact dermatitis. Contact Dermatitis 2009;61:306-309
20 Thomson MA, Preston PW, Prais L, Foulds IS. Lime dermatitis from gin and tonic with a twist of lime. Contact Dermatitis 2007;56:114-115
21 Trattner A, David M. Patch testing with fine fragrances: comparison with fragrance mix, balsam of Peru and a fragrance series. Contact Dermatitis 2004;49:287-289
22 Larsen W, Nakayama H, Fischer T, Elsner P, Frosch P, Burrows D, et al. Fragrance contact dermatitis: a worldwide multicenter investigation (Part II). Contact Dermatitis 2001;44:344-346
23 Penchalaiah K, Handa S, Lakshmi SB, Sharma VK, Kumar B. Sensitizers commonly causing allergic contact dermatitis from cosmetics. Contact Dermatitis 2000;43:311-313
24 Manuel Brites M, Goncalo M, Figueiredo A. Contact allergy to fragrance mix - a 10-year study. Contact Dermatitis 2000;43:181-182
25 Chang Y-C, Maibach HI. Pseudo flautist's lip: allergic contact cheilitis from geraniol. Contact Dermatitis 1997;37:39

26   Nakayama H, Hanaoka H, Ohshiro A. Allergen Controlled System (ACS). Tokyo, Japan: Kanehara Shuppan, 1974:42. Data cited in ref. 27

27   Mitchell JC. Contact hypersensitivity to some perfume materials. Contact Dermatitis 1975;1:196-199

28   Juarez A, Goiriz R, Sanchez-Perez J, Garcia-Diez A. Disseminated allergic contact dermatitis after exposure to a topical medication containing geraniol. Dermatitis 2008;19:163

29   Srivastava PK, Bajaj AK. Ylang-ylang oil not an uncommon sensitizer in India. Indian J Dermatol 2014;59:200-201

30   Eun HC, Lee AY. Contact dermatitis due to Madecassol. Contact Dermatitis 1985;13:310-313

31   Goossens A, Merckx L. Allergic contact dermatitis from farnesol in a deodorant. Contact Dermatitis 1997;37:179-180

32   Meynadier JM, Meynadier J, Peyron JL, Peyron L. Formes cliniques des manifestations cutanées d'allergie aux parfums. Ann Dermatol Venereol 1986;113:31-39

33   SCCS (Scientific Committee on Consumer Safety). Opinion on Fragrance allergens in cosmetic products, 26-27 June 2012, SCCS/1459/11. Available at: https://ec.europa.eu/health/sites/health/files/scientific_committees/consumer_safety/docs/sccs_o_102.pdf

34   Uter W, Johansen JD, Börje A, Karlberg A-T, Lidén C, Rastogi S, Roberts D, White IR. Categorization of fragrance contact allergens for prioritization of preventive measures: clinical and experimental data and consideration of structure–activity relationships. Contact Dermatitis 2013;69:196-230

35   De Groot AC, Schmidt E. Essential oils: contact allergy and chemical composition. Boca Raton, Fl., USA: CRC Press, Taylor and Francis Group, 2016 (ISBN 9781482246407)

36   Gilissen L, Huygens S, Goossens A. Allergic contact dermatitis caused by topical herbal remedies: importance of patch testing with the patients' own products. Contact Dermatitis 2018;78:177-184

37   Silvestre JF, Mercader P, González-Pérez R, Hervella-Garcés M, Sanz-Sánchez T, Córdoba S, et al. Sensitization to fragrances in Spain: A 5-year multicentre study (2011-2015). Contact Dermatitis. 2018 Nov 14. doi: 10.1111/cod.13152. [Epub ahead of print]

Chapter 6.29   GINGER OIL

IDENTIFICATION

Description/definition	: Ginger oil (essential oil of ginger) is the essential oil obtained from the rhizomes of the ginger, *Zingiber officinale* Roscoe.
INCI name(s) EU	: Zingiber officinale root oil
INCI name(s) USA	: Zingiber officinale (ginger) root oil
CAS registry number(s)	: 8007-08-7; 84696-15-1
EC number(s)	: 283-634-2
RIFM monograph(s)	: Food Cosmet Toxicol 1974;12:901 (special issue I) (binder, page 411) (ginger oil Nigeria)
ISO standard	: ISO 16928 Essential oil of ginger, 2014; Geneva, Switzerland, www.iso.org
Merck Index monograph	: 5728 (Ginger)
Function(s) in cosmetics	: EU: masking; perfuming; skin conditioning; tonic. USA: flavoring agents; fragrance ingredients; skin-conditioning agents - miscellaneous
Patch testing	: 4% pet. (15)

GENERAL

Zingiber officinale is a tropical herbaceous plant, possibly native to India. It is widely grown as a commercial crop in south and south-east Asia, tropical Africa (especially Sierra Leone and Nigeria), Latin America, the Caribbean (especially Jamaica) and Australia (1,8). *Zingiber officinale* is best known as the source of the pungent, aromatic spice called ginger, produced from the knotted and branched rhizome (underground stem, commonly called the 'root'), which is used to add flavor in cooking (4). Ginger has also many applications in traditional medicine (e.g., in China, where ginger products are also recorded in the official Pharmacopoeia [5]), Ayurveda formulations and Arabic herbal traditions (3).

Ginger essential oil is used to flavor ginger beer and ginger ale, and is commonly used as an ingredient in perfumery, cosmetics and pharmaceuticals, including in topical applications as an analgesic. In addition, the oil is employed by aromatherapists (11,12).

Ginger and *Zingiber officinale* have been extensively reviewed in refs. 10 (chemical constituents, traditional medical uses, pharmacological activities), 6 (technology, chemistry, and biological activities), 2 and 9 (prevention of [chemotherapy-induced] nausea and vomiting), and 7 (botany and horticulture).

CHEMICAL COMPOSITION

Ginger oil is a pale yellow to amber, clear mobile liquid which has a spicy, fresh citrusy and peppery odor. In ginger oils from various origins, over 295 chemicals have been identified. About half these were found in a single reviewed publication only. The ten chemicals that had the highest maximum concentrations in 41 commercial ginger essential oil samples are shown in table 6.29.1 (Erich Schmidt, analytical data published in ref. 14).

A full literature review of the qualitative and quantitative composition of commercial and non-commercial ginger oils of various origins and with data from the ISO standard has been published in 2016 (14).

Table 6.29.1 Ten ingredients with the highest concentrations in commercial ginger oils (14)

Name	Concentration range	Name	Concentration range
α-Zingiberene	17.0 - 32.4%	β-Sesquiphellandrene	4.5 - 9.1%
Geranial	0.06 - 12.6%	1,8-Cineole	0.4 - 8.9%
Camphene	0.3 - 12.1%	α-Copaene	0.2 - 6.4%
Neral	0.3 - 10.2%	β-Bisabolene	5.1 - 6.3%
2-Heptanone	0.01 - 9.7%	Curcumene	2.5 - 5.8%

CONTACT ALLERGY / ALLERGIC CONTACT DERMATITIS

General

Contact allergy to and possible allergic contact dermatitis from ginger oil has been reported in one publication only (13). A false-positive patch test reaction due to the excited skin syndrome cannot be excluded.

Case reports and case series

An aromatherapist had non-occupational contact dermatitis with allergies to multiple essential oils used at work, including ginger oil. The patient also reacted to geraniol, linalool, linalyl acetate, α-pinene, the fragrance mix and various other fragrance materials. Linalool and geraniol were demonstrated by GC-MS in the ginger oil (13), but neither of these is an important component of commercial ginger oils (table 6.29.1).

OTHER SIDE EFFECTS

Photosensitivity
Photosensitivity from ginger oil has been cited in ref. 15.

LITERATURE

1   Kiran CR, Kumar Chakka A, Padmakumari Amma KP, Nirmala Menon A, Sree Kumar MM, Venugopalan VV. Essential oil composition of fresh ginger cultivars from North-East India. J Essent Oil Res 2013;25:380-387

2   Palatty P, Haniadka R, Valder B, Arora R, Baliga MS. Ginger in the prevention of nausea and vomiting: A review. Crit Rev Food Sci Nutrit 2013;53:659-669

3   El-Ghorab AH, Nauman M, Anjum FM, Hussain S, Nadeem M. A comparative study on chemical composition and antioxidant activity of ginger (*Zingiber officinale*) and cumin (*Cuminum cyminum*). J Agric Food Chem 2010;58: 8231-8237

4   Kiran CR, Chakka AK, Padmakumari Amma KP, Nirmala Menon A, Sree Kumar MM, Venugopalan VV. Influence of cultivar and maturity at harvest on the essential oil composition, oleoresin and [6]-gingerol contents in fresh ginger from Northeast India. J Agric Food Chem 2013;61:4145-4154

5   Huang B, Wang G, Chu Z, Qin L. Effect of oven drying, microwave drying, and silica gel drying methods on the volatile components of ginger (*Zingiber officinale* Roscoe) by HS-SPME-GC-MS. Drying Technol 2012;30:248-255

6   Kubra IR, Mohan Rao LJ. An Impression on current developments in the technology, chemistry, and biological activities of ginger (*Zingiber officinale* Roscoe). Crit Rev Food Sci Nutrit 2012;52:651-688

7   Parthasarathy VA, Srinivasan V, Nair RR, Zachariah TJ, Kumar A, Prasath D. Ginger: botany and horticulture. In: J Janick, Ed. Horticultural Reviews, Volume 39, First Edition. Wiley-Blackwell, 2012:273-388

8   Kubra IR, Rao LJM. Effect of microwave drying on the phytochemical composition of volatiles of ginger. Int J Food Sci Technol 2012;47: 53-60

9   Marx WM, Teleni L, McCarthy AL, Vitetta L, McKavanagh D, Thomson D, Isenring E. Ginger (*Zingiber officinale*) and chemotherapy-induced nausea and vomiting: a systematic literature review. Nutrit Rev 2013;71:245-254

10 Ross IA. *Zingiber officinale* Roscoe. In: Medicinal plants of the world, vol. 3: Chemical constituents, traditional and modern medicinal uses. Totowa, NJ, USA: Humana Press Inc, 2005:507-560

11 Rhind JP. Essential oils. A handbook for aromatherapy practice, 2nd Edition. London: Singing Dragon, 2012

12 Lawless J. The encyclopedia of essential oils, 2nd Edition. London: Harper Thorsons, 2014

13 Dharmagunawardena B, Takwale A, Sanders KJ, Cannan S, Roger A, Ilchyshyn A. Gas chromatography: an investigative tool in multiple allergies to essential oils. Contact Dermatitis 2002;47:288-292

14 De Groot AC, Schmidt E. Essential oils: contact allergy and chemical composition. Boca Raton, Fl., USA: CRC Press, Taylor and Francis Group, 2016 (ISBN 9781482246407)

15 De Groot AC. Patch Testing, 4th Edition. Wapserveen, The Netherlands: acdegroot publishing, 2018 (ISBN 978-90-813233-4-5)

Chapter 6.30   GRAPEFRUIT OIL

IDENTIFICATION

Description/definition	: Grapefruit oil (essential oil of grapefruit) is the essential oil obtained from the pericarp (peel) of the grapefruit, *Citrus paradisi* Macfad.
INCI name(s) EU	: Citrus paradisi peel oil
INCI name(s) USA	: Citrus paradisi (grapefruit) peel oil
CAS registry number(s)	: 8016-20-4; 90045-43-5
EC number(s)	: 289-904-6
RIFM monograph(s)	: Food Cosmet Toxicol 1974;12:723 (binder, page 412)
IFRA standard	: Restricted (www.ifraorg.org/en-us/standards-library) (table 6.30.1)
SCCS opinion(s)	: Various (10); SCCNFP/0392/00, final (11); SCCNFP/0389/00, final (12)
ISO standard	: ISO 3053 Essential oil of grapefruit, 2004; Geneva, Switzerland, www.iso.org
Function(s) in cosmetics	: EU: masking; perfuming. USA: fragrance ingredients
EU cosmetic restrictions	: Regulated in Annex II/358 of the Regulation (EC) No. 1223/2009, regulated by 95/34/EC
Patch testing	: 2% pet.; test also limonene (see Chapter 3.95 Limonene)

Table 6.30.1 IFRA restrictions for grapefruit oil expressed

Leave-on products:	4%
Rinse-off products:	no restriction
Non-skin contact products:	no restriction

The limit only applies to applications on skin exposed to sunshine, excluding rinse-off products. If combinations of phototoxic fragrance ingredients are used, the use levels have to be reduced accordingly. The sum of the concentrations of all phototoxic ingredients, expressed in % of their recommended maximum level in the consumer product shall not exceed 100.
Note: See remark on phototoxic ingredients in the Introduction to the IFRA Standards (Appendix 8 to the IFRA Code of Practice) and the Standard on Citrus oil and other furocoumarins-containing essential oils. For qualities of the expressed oil in which less volatile components have been concentrated by partial or total removal of the terpene fraction, this limit should be reduced in proportion to the degree of concentration.

GENERAL

Citrus paradisi Macfad. is regarded as the result of a spontaneous crossing of *Citrus maxima* (Burm.) Merrill (pumelo, syn. *Citrus grandis* Osbeck) and *Citrus sinensis* (L.) Osbeck (sweet orange). The hybrid probably originated on the West Indies (Barbados, Jamaica), where it was reported growing around 1750 (4). It is a tree, 5-9 m tall, with spreading branches, and sometimes spines which are usually blunt; it produces fruits 10-15 centimeter in diameter. Commercial grapefruit varieties were mainly developed in Florida, and several types are currently cultivated in many tropical and subtropical regions of warm and humid climates. The main producing countries are the USA (Florida, to a lesser extent the west coast), Israel, Mexico, Cuba, Argentina, Morocco, Brazil, the Philippines, the Caribbean Islands, and South Africa (13).

From the byproduct of the grapefruits, the peels (rinds), essential oils of grapefruit are obtained by cold pressing (3). The peel oil has a strong and desirable aroma, useful in industrial flavoring of foods (chewing gum, sweets, baked goods, ice cream *et cetera*), beverages, perfumes, and cosmetics (2,4). It is also employed in the pharmaceutical industry and in aromatherapy (7,8).

The pharmacological potentials of *Citrus paradisi* have been discussed in ref. 6. The history, global distribution, and nutritional importance of *Citrus* fruits have been reviewed in ref. 5.

CHEMICAL COMPOSITION

Grapefruit oil is a yellow to pinkish orange mobile clear liquid, which has a fresh juicy and bitter-sweet citrus peel-like odor. Depending of the quantity of waxes in the oil, it may sometimes have a tight foggy appearance. In grapefruit oils from various origins, over 210 chemicals have been identified. The ten chemicals that had the highest maximum concentrations in 122 commercial grapefruit essential oil samples are shown in table 6.30.2 (Erich Schmidt, analytical data presented in ref. 13).

A full literature review of the qualitative and quantitative composition of commercial and non-commercial grapefruit oils of various origins and with data from the ISO standard has been published in 2016 (13). Older reviews can be found in refs. 1 and 2.

Table 6.30.2 Ten ingredients with the highest concentrations in commercial grapefruit oils (13)

Name	Concentration range	Name	Concentration range
Limonene	81.1 - 95.5%	(E)-β-Ocimene	trace - 0.6%
Myrcene	1.3 - 3.5%	n-Octanal	0.1 - 0.5%
β-Caryophyllene	0.1 - 1.2%	Decanal	0.2 - 0.4%
α-Pinene	0.2 - 1.0%	Germacrene D	0.02 - 0.4%
Sabinene	0.2 - 0.8%	Neral	0.01 - 0.4%

CONTACT ALLERGY / ALLERGIC CONTACT DERMATITIS

General
Contact allergy to and possible allergic contact dermatitis from grapefruit oil has been reported in one publication only (9). A false-positive patch test reaction due to the excited skin syndrome cannot be excluded.

Case reports and case series
Two aromatherapists had contact dermatitis (one occupational) with allergies to multiple essential oils used at their work, including grapefruit oil. Both patients also reacted to geraniol, α-pinene, the fragrance mix and various other fragrance materials. In addition, one proved to be allergic to linalool and linalyl acetate, the other to caryophyllene. α-Pinene and caryophyllene were demonstrated by GC-MS in grapefruit oil (9), but neither of these is an important component of grapefruit oil (table 6.30.2). Limonene, the dominant chemical in essential oils of *Citrus paradisi*, was not tested.

LITERATURE

1   Dugo G, Cotroneo A, Bonaccorsi I, Trozzi A. Composition of the volatile fraction of citrus peel oils. In: G Dugo and L Mondello, eds. Citrus oils: composition, advanced analytical techniques, contaminants, and biological activity. Boca Raton, USA: CRC Press, Taylor & Francis Group, 2011:20-29

2   Kirbaşlar I, Boz I, Kirbaşlar G. Composition of Turkish lemon and grapefruit peel oils. J Essent Oil Res 2006;18:525-543

3   Pino JA, Acevedo A, Rabelo J, González C, Escandon J. Chemical composition of distilled grapefruit oil. J Essent Oil Res 1999;11:75-76

4   Njoroge SM, Koaze H, Karanja PN, Sawamura M. Volatile constituents of redblush grapefruit (*Citrus paradisi*) and pummelo (*Citrus grandis*) peel essential oils from Kenya. J Agric Food Chem 2005;53:9790-9794

5   Liu YQ, Heying E, Tanumihardjo SA. History, global distribution, and nutritional importance of *Citrus* fruits. Compreh Rev Food Sci Food Saf 2012;11:530-545

6   Gupta V, Kohli K, Ghaiye P, Bansal P, Lather A. Pharmacological potentials of *Citrus paradisi* - an overview Int J Photother res 2011;1:8-17

7   Rhind JP. Essential oils. A handbook for aromatherapy practice, 2nd Edition. London: Singing Dragon, 2012

8   Lawless J. The encyclopedia of essential oils, 2nd Edition. London: Harper Thorsons, 2014

9   Dharmagunawardena B, Takwale A, Sanders KJ, Cannan S, Roger A, Ilchyshyn A. Gas chromatography: an investigative tool in multiple allergies to essential oils. Contact Dermatitis 2002;47:288-292

10 Various SCCS Opinions, available at: http://ec.europa.eu/growth/tools-databases/cosing/index.cfm?fuseaction =search.details_v2&id=28697

11 Opinion of the Scientific Committee on Cosmetic Products and Non-Food Products Intended for Consumers concerning 'An initial list of perfumery materials which must not form part of cosmetic products except subject to the Restrictions and Conditions laid down, 25 September 2001, SCCNFP/0392/00, final. Available at: http://ec.europa.eu/health/archive/ph_risk/committees/sccp/documents/out150_en.pdf

12 Opinion of the Scientific Committee on Cosmetic Products and Non-Food Products Intended for Consumers concerning 'The 1st update of the inventory of ingredients employed in cosmetic products. Section II: Perfume and aromatic raw materials', 24 October 2000, SCCNFP/0389/00, final. Available at: http://ec.europa.eu/health/ph_risk/committees/sccp/documents/out131_en.pdf

13 De Groot AC, Schmidt E. Essential oils: contact allergy and chemical composition. Boca Raton, Fl., USA: CRC Press, Taylor and Francis Group, 2016 (ISBN 9781482246407)

Chapter 6.31   GUAIACWOOD OIL

IDENTIFICATION

Description/definition : Guaiacwood oil is the essential oil obtained from the wood of the guaiacwood (true guaiac; in Spanish: palo santo), *Bulnesia sarmientoi* Lorentz ex Griseb.
INCI name(s) EU & USA : Bulnesia sarmientoi wood oil
CAS registry number(s) : 8016-23-7
EC number(s) : Not available
RIFM monograph(s) : Food Cosmet Toxicol 1974;12:905 (special issue I) (binder, page 415)
Function(s) in cosmetics : EU: masking; skin conditioning. USA: fragrance ingredients; skin-conditioning agents – miscellaneous
Patch testing : 2% pet.; based on RIFM data, 8% pet. is probably not irritant (11)

GENERAL

Bulnesia sarmientoi Lorentz ex Griseb. (often misspelled as *Bulnesia sarmienti*) (synonyms: guaiac wood, Paraguay lignum vitae) is a deciduous tree that grows 6-20 meters tall. It inhabits the Gran Chaco region of Argentina, Bolivia, Paraguay and - marginally - Brazil (2,3). The species, called Palo Santo (holy tree) by the local population throughout the Gran Chaco region, is highly valued as a medicinal plant for the many healing powers attributed to infusions brewed from its bark, crust or leaves.

The essential guaiacwood oil (also known as 'lignum vitae oil', 'guaiac oil', 'guayacol', 'guajol', or 'guayaco'), which is obtained by steam-distillation of a mixture of the heartwood and sawdust from the tree, is used in fragrances. The oil has a soft rose-like odor, and has thus been used as an adulterant for rose oil (3,4). In addition, it has been used to perfume luxury soaps by masking the unpleasant smell of synthetic components and as an excipient in the manufacturing of cosmetics (4). The oil of Palo Santo is also highly valued in aromatherapy (4). Paraguay currently supplies most of the international demand of guaiacwood oil (4,5).

Guaiacwood oil should not be confused with Guaiacum officinale wood oil (CAS 84650-13-5; EC 283-494-2), the essential oil obtained from *Guaiacum officinale* L. This too is a member of the family Zygophyllaceae and is *also* known as guaiacwood.

CHEMICAL COMPOSITION

Guaiacwood oil is a yellow greenish to ambery semisolid mass which has a woody, balsamic, mild rosy and medicinal odor. In guaiacwood oils from various origins, over 110 chemicals have been identified (1,3,6,10,12,13).The ten chemicals that had the highest maximum concentrations in 22 commercial guaiacwood essential oil samples are shown in table 6.31.1 (Erich Schmidt, analytical data presented in ref. 10).

A full literature review of the qualitative and quantitative composition of commercial and non-commercial guaiacwood oils of various origins has been published in 2016 (10).

Table 6.31.1 Ten ingredients with the highest concentrations in commercial guaiacwood oil (10)

Name	Concentration range	Name	Concentration range
Bulnesol	30.5 - 49.8%	β-Eudesmol	0.2 - 3.6%
Guaiol	25.6 - 38.7%	10-epi-γ-Eudesmol	1.2 - 3.5%
α-Eudesmol	2.3 - 4.7%	Guaioxide	0.3 - 1.9%
α-Bulnesene	0.8 - 4.5%	Elemol	0.5 - 1.7%
γ-Eudesmol	1.6 - 3.8%	Guaiol isomer	0 - 1.0%

CONTACT ALLERGY / ALLERGIC CONTACT DERMATITIS

General

Contact allergy to guaiacwood oil has been reported in two publications, but no cases of allergic contact dermatitis from the oil have been identified.

Testing in groups of patients

Two positive patch test reactions to guaiacwood oil 2% petrolatum were observed in 51 patients (3.9%) allergic to Myroxylon pereirae resin (balsam of Peru) and/or turpentine and/or wood tar and/or colophony (8). A group of 86 patients from Poland previously reacting to the fragrance mix was tested with guaiacwood oil and one (1.1%) had a positive patch test reaction (9). In neither of these studies were relevance data provided.

LITERATURE

1 Marongiu B, Piras A, Porcedda S, Tuveri E. Isolation of *Guaiacum bulnesia* volatile oil by supercritical carbon dioxide extraction. J Essent Oil Bear Plants 2007;10:221-228

2 Kamruzzaman SM, Endale M, Oh WJ, Park S-C, Kim K-S, Hong JH, et al. Inhibitory effects of *Bulnesia sarmienti* aqueous extract on agonist-induced platelet activation and thrombus formation involves mitogen-activated protein kinases. J Ethnopharmacol 2010;130:614-620

3 Rodilla JM, Silva LA, Martinez N, Lorenzo D, Davyt D, Castillo L, et al. Advances in the identification and agrochemical importance of sesquiterpenoids from *Bulnesia sarmientoi* essential oil. Ind Crops Prod 2011;33:497-503

4 Waller T, Barros M, Draque J, Micucci P. Conservation of the Palo Santo tree, *Bulnesia sarmientoi* Lorentz ex Griseb, in the South America Chaco Region. Medicinal Plant Conservation 2012;15:4-8. Available at: http://www.academia.edu/2120881/Conservation_of_the_Palo_Santo_tree_Bulnesia_sarmientoi_Lorentz_ex_G riseb_in_the_South_American_Chaco_Region

5 Janzen HKJ. Guaiac wood oil, Paraguay and CITES. Paper presented at the IFEAT International Conference in Marrakech, 26-30 Sept. 2010 'North African and Mediterranean essential oils and aromas: 2010 tales and realities of our industry – a new decade of challenges and opportunities'. Pages 317-324 in the Conference Proceedings. Available at: http://www.ifeat.org/wp-content/uploads/2012/10/Janzen+-+Guaiac+wood.pdf

6 Prudent D, Perineau F, Bravo R, Delmas M. Preparation et characterisation d'extraits volatils de bois de guaiac (*Bulnesia sarmientoi* Lor.). Rivist Ital EPPOS 1991;5:35-43. Data cited in ref. 7

7 Lawrence BM. Progress in essential oils. Perfum Flavor 1992;17(6):51

8 Rudzki E, Grzywa Z, Bruo WS. Sensitivity to 35 essential oils. Contact Dermatitis 1976;2:196-200

9 Rudzki E, Grzywa Z. Allergy to perfume mixture. Contact Dermatitis 1986;15:115-116

10 De Groot AC, Schmidt E. Essential oils: contact allergy and chemical composition. Boca Raton, Fl., USA: CRC Press, Taylor and Francis Group, 2016 (ISBN 9781482246407)

11 De Groot AC. Patch Testing, 4th Edition. Wapserveen, The Netherlands: acdegroot publishing, 2018 (ISBN 978-90-813233-4-5)

12 Tissandié L, Viciana S, Brevard H, Meierhenrich UJ, Filippi JJ. Towards a complete characterisation of guaiacwood oil. Phytochemistry 2018;149:64-81

13 Tissandié L, Gaysinski M, Brévard H, Meierhenrich UJ, Filippi JJ. Revisiting the chemistry of guaiacwood oil: identification and formation pathways of 5,11- and 10,11-epoxyguaianes. J Nat Prod 2017;80:526-537

Chapter 6.32　　HINOKI OIL

IDENTIFICATION

Description/definition　　　: Hinoki oil is the essential oil obtained from the wood of the hinoki tree, *Chamaecyparis obtusa*, Cupressaceae
INCI name USA and EU　　: Chamaecyparis obtusa wood oil
CAS registry number(s)　　: 91745-97-0
EC number(s)　　　　　　: 294-769-1
Function(s) in cosmetics　: EU: masking; tonic. USA: fragrance ingredients
Patch testing　　　　　　: 5% pet. (1)

GENERAL

Chamaecyparis obtusa, also called Hinoki (meaning 'white cedar') is a slow-growing, evergreen cypress tree that grows in Japan, Korea and Taiwan. It can be as tall as 35 meters with a trunk up to 1 meter in diameter. The tree is a major plantation species for timber production. Hinoki wood, which is highly resistant to decay, is held in high esteem in Japan. Over centuries, wood from the Hinoki tree has been used for building palaces, temples, religious shrines, bathtubs, table tennis blades, and the masu, an indigenous square wooden box used to measure rice. Hinoki wood is used as a traditional Japanese stick incense for its light, earthy aroma (Wikipedia).

The essential oil of hinoki, which is mostly made of the wood (but can also be obtained from the bark, the leaves and the roots), is hardly used in the perfume industry, because it is too expensive. In aromatherapy it is used for its perceived relaxing effects on the body and to help relieve tension and stress. Medicinally, it is used in a variety of diseases (http://ultranl.com/hinoki-oil/). The essential oil of *C. obtusa* shows relatively strong antibacterial activity against Gram-positive bacteria, and good antifungal activity. These properties have led patients to use hinoki oil for acne and fungal disease (1).

According to INCI definitions, hinoki oil is 'expressed' from the bark (INCI EU) or the aerial parts (INCI USA) of *Chamaecyparis obtusa*. This is incorrect, as essential oils – with the exception of *Citrus* species – are not expressed but are but obtained by steam-distillation or hydrodistillation.

CHEMICAL COMPOSITION

Hinoki wood oil is a pale yellow to yellow clear liquid; its odor type is woody and its odor at 100% is described as 'dry woody camphor sweet spicy'. Hinoki *leaf* oil is a yellow clear liquid; its odor type is camphoreous and its odor at 100% is described as 'strong camphor fresh pine green'. Hinoki *root* oil is a pale yellow clear liquid; its odor type is woody and its odor at 100% is described as 'dry woody camphor sweet spicy' (www.thegoodscentscompany.com).

The ingredients of hinoki wood essential oil that were found to be present in two commercial oils in concentrations higher than 1% are shown in table 6.32.1 (Erich Schmidt, personal communication, September 2018)

Table 6.32.1 Ingredients with concentrations higher than 1% found in two commercial hinoki wood oil samples

Name	Concentration range	Name	Concentration range
δ-Cadinene	12.4 - 19.5%	Myrtenol	0 - 3.3%
α-Pinene	0.5 - 14.0%	τ-Cadinol	0 - 2.8%
α-Muurolene	0 - 12.2%	*trans*-Pinocarveol + Iso-	0 - 2.3%
τ-Cadinol+ τ-Muurolol	0 - 10.1%	pulegol	
α-Cadinol	4.4 - 9.1%	Terpinolene	0.7 - 1.6%
Limonene	2.6 - 9.1%	β-Cadinene	0 - 1.5%
Myrtanol	0.1 - 6.6%	β-Elemene	0.6 - 1.4%
γ-Cadinene	5.8 - 6.4%	γ-Costol	0 - 1.3%
α-Terpineol	2.0 - 4.4%	α-Calacorene	0 - 1.2%
α-Cadinene	0 - 3.9%	10-epi-γ-Eudesmol	0.2 - 1.2%
δ-Cadinol+ τ-Muurolol	0 - 3.6%	Borneol	0 - 1.1%
γ-Muurolene	0 - 3.3%	Cadina-1,4-diene	0 - 1.1%

CONTACT ALLERGY

General
There is only one report of allergic contact dermatitis from hinoki oil (1).

Case reports and case series
A female patient presented with a 2-week history of pruritic, eczematous dermatitis affecting the periungual area of her first and second toes. Twenty-one days previously, she had begun using over-the-counter hinoki essential oil on a nightly basis, in an attempt to treat a fungal infection of the feet and toenails. After several days of applying the oil, she developed a pruritic, erythematous peri-ungual eruption. With treatment and stopping the use of the oil, the eruption resolved within a few days. Patch testing with the baseline series and the patient's own products (5% of the essential oil preparations in pet.) revealed a positive reaction to colophonium (+) and an extreme positive reaction (+++) to the essential oil of hinoki 5% pet.; 8 controls were negative (1).

LITERATURE
1   Kim M, Hwang SW, Cho BK, Park HJ. Allergic contact dermatitis caused by essential oil of Hinoki (*Chamaecyparis obtusa*) on the periungual area. Contact Dermatitis 2015;73:250-251

Chapter 6.33   HYSSOP OIL

IDENTIFICATION

Description/definition	: Hyssop oil (essential oil of hyssop) is the essential oil obtained from the leaves and flowering tops (the aerial parts) of the hyssop, *Hyssopus officinalis* L. ssp. *officinalis*
INCI name(s) EU & USA	: Hyssopus officinalis leaf oil
CAS registry number(s)	: 8006-83-5; 84603-66-7
EC number(s)	: 283-266-2
RIFM monograph(s)	: Food Cosmet Toxicol 1978;16:783 (special issue IV)
ISO standard	: ISO 9841 Essential oil of hyssop (*Hyssopus officinalis* L. ssp. *officinalis*), 2013; Geneva, Switzerland, www.iso.org
Merck Index monograph	: 8159
Function(s) in cosmetics	: EU: skin conditioning. USA: fragrance ingredients; skin-conditioning agents – miscellaneous
Patch testing	: 2% pet.; based on RIFM data, 4% pet. is probably not irritant (3)

GENERAL

Hyssopus officinalis L. is an aromatic perennial subshrub belonging to the Lamiaceae family. Hyssop is native to Northern Africa (Algeria, Morocco), temperate regions of Asia (Iran, Turkey, Caucasus) and middle, southern and eastern Europe. It is an important medicinal and culinary plant extensively cultivated in Russia, various European countries, the United States and China. The leaves and flowering tops produce a pleasantly smelling essential oil used for flavoring and food preservation, in liqueurs, cosmetic products, in perfumery, in the pharmaceutical field in several antiseptic preparations and for phytotherapeutic uses in folk medicine and aromatherapy (2).

CHEMICAL COMPOSITION

Hyssop oil is a pale yellow to brownish yellow clear mobile liquid, which has an herbaceous, fresh minty and camphoraceous odor. In hyssop oils from various origins, over 285 chemicals have been identified. About 52 per cent of these were found in a single reviewed publication only. The ten chemicals that had the highest maximum concentrations in 26 commercial hyssop essential oil samples are shown in table 6.33.1 (Erich Schmidt, analytical data presented in ref. 2).

A full literature review of the qualitative and quantitative composition of commercial and non-commercial hyssop oils of various origins, their chemotypes and with data from the ISO standard, has been published in 2016 (2).

Table 6.33.1 Ten ingredients with the highest concentrations in commercial hyssop oils (2)

Name	Concentration range	Name	Concentration range
Isopinocamphone	0.5 - 47.3%	Germacrene D	0.1 - 3.6%
trans-Pinocarvone	5.9 - 37.9%	Limonene	1.0 - 3.5%
Pinocarveol	0.1 - 19.2%	Caryophyllene oxide	0.2 - 3.4%
β-Pinene	8.2 - 17.2%	β-Caryophyllene	0.8 - 3%
β-Phellandrene	0.9 - 6.0%	γ-Cadinene	trace - 2.9%

CONTACT ALLERGY / ALLERGIC CONTACT DERMATITIS

General

Contact allergy to and possible allergic contact dermatitis from hyssop oil has been reported in one publication only. A false-positive patch test reaction due to the excited skin syndrome cannot be excluded (1).

Case reports and case series

An aromatherapist had non-occupational contact dermatitis with allergies to multiple essential oils used at work, including hyssop oil. The patient also reacted to geraniol, linalool, linalyl acetate, α-pinene, the fragrance mix and various other fragrance materials. α-Pinene and geraniol were demonstrated by GC-MS in hyssop oil (1), but neither of these are important components of commercial hyssop oils (table 6.33.1).

LITERATURE

1   Dharmagunawardena B, Takwale A, Sanders KJ, Cannan S, Roger A, Ilchyshyn A. Gas chromatography: an
     investigative tool in multiple allergies to essential oils. Contact Dermatitis 2002;47:288-292
2   De Groot AC, Schmidt E. Essential oils: contact allergy and chemical composition. Boca Raton, Fl., USA: CRC Press,
     Taylor and Francis Group, 2016 (ISBN 9781482246407)
3   De Groot AC. Patch Testing, 4th Edition. Wapserveen, The Netherlands: acdegroot publishing, 2018 (ISBN 978-90-
     813233-4-5)

Chapter 6.34   JASMINE ABSOLUTE

GENERAL

The volatile chemicals in jasmine flowers are much appreciated in the perfumery industries. Conventional steam-distillation is generally considered unsuitable to process such materials, since it induces thermal degradation of many compounds contained in the flowers. Therefore, solvents, usually hexane or supercritical fluids such as CO_2, are used to extract the fragrant chemicals. After the solvent has evaporated, a viscose product remains called a 'concrete'; these concretes may sometimes be used 'as is' in soaps (45,46). Concretes contain not only fragrance compounds, but also fatty acids, their methyl esters and paraffins (up to 50% by weight), originating from the cuticular waxes covering the surface of the jasmine flowers (45,46). As these fatty materials do not contribute to the fragrance but do cause solubility problems, they have to be removed, which is done by solubilisation of the concrete in a large excess of ethyl alcohol. The solution is then cooled and filtered to eliminate the precipitated waxes. After removing the ethyl alcohol and thereafter concentration of the solution by vacuum distillation, a product remains which is called an 'absolute'. This product contains all the fragrance compounds, but still also some fatty acid methyl esters and paraffins (45). These absolutes are the jasmine products used in the fragrance industries.

Jasmine absolutes can be obtained from the flowers of several species of the genus *Jasminum*, but are mainly derived from *Jasminum grandiflorum* L. (Spanish jasmine) and *Jasminum sambac* (L.) Aiton (Arabia, China, sambac jasmine) (46,47); hence, only these two (and not *J. officinale*) are discussed here. *J. grandiflorum* flowers are mainly grown for production of jasmine absolute in India, Egypt and Morocco. *J. sambac* flowers are harvested in India mostly for ornamental purposes, garlands and religious offerings. Only some 5% of the annual flower harvest in India is used to produce absolute (60), but the sambac absolute appears to be gaining in popularity in the fragrance industries (48)

6.34.1 JASMINUM GRANDIFLORUM ABSOLUTE

IDENTIFICATION

Description/definition	: Jasminum grandiflorum absolute is the absolute obtained from the flowers of the Spanish jasmine, *Jasminum grandiflorum* L.
INCI name(s) EU	: Jasminum grandiflorum flower extract
INCI name(s) USA	: Jasminum grandiflorum (jasmine) flower extract
CAS registry number(s)	: 84776-64-7
EC number(s)	: 283-993-5
RIFM monograph(s)	: Food Cosmet Toxicol 1976;14:331(binder, page 477)
SCCS opinion(s)	: SCCS/1459/11 (43)
IFRA standard	: Restricted (www.ifraorg.org/en-us/standards-library) (table 6.34.1.1)
Function(s) in cosmetics	: EU: masking; perfuming. USA: fragrance ingredients
Patch testing	: 2% pet. (Chemo, SPEurope, SPCanada)

Table 6.34.1.1 IFRA restrictions for Jasminum grandiflorum absolute

Category ª	Limits ᵇ	Category ª	Limits ᵇ	Category ª	Limits ᵇ
1	0.04%	5	0.40%	9	5.00%
2	0.05%	6	1.10%	10	2.50%
3	0.22%	7	0.10%	11	not restricted
4	0.70%	8	1.50%		

ª For explanation of categories see pages 6-8
ᵇ Limits in the finished products

GENERAL

Jasminum grandiflorum L. (Spanish jasmine, royal jasmine, Catalonian jasmine) is a scrambling deciduous shrub growing to 2-4 meter tall, with flowers that have an intensely floral, warm, rich and highly diffusive odor. It is native to Africa (Djibouti, Eritrea, Ethiopia, Somalia, Sudan, Kenya, Uganda, Rwanda) and Asia (Oman, Saudi Arabia, Yemen, India, Pakistan). It is occasionally naturalized in the tropics and is cultivated in Africa (Algeria, Egypt, Morocco), India, Italy and France (48). By method of solvent extraction, the jasmine flowers are converted into jasmine concrete and by separating the waxes with alcohol, filtration and removal of the ethanol, jasmine absolute is obtained, for which there is a great demand in the perfume industry. Jasmine absolute is also employed in aromatherapy (1,2).

CHEMICAL COMPOSITION

Jasmine absolute from *Jasminum grandiflorum* L. is a mobile to viscous light orange to reddish-brown colored liquid, which has an intensive blooming, flowery and long lasting odor. In Jasminum grandiflorum absolutes from various origins, over 220 chemicals have been identified. About 68 per cent of these were found in a single reviewed publication only. The ten chemicals that had the highest maximum concentrations in 41 commercial Jasminum grandiflorum absolute samples are shown in table 6.34.1.2 (Erich Schmidt, analytical data presented in ref. 48).

A full literature review of the qualitative and quantitative composition of commercial and non-commercial Jasminum grandiflorum absolutes of various origins has been published in 2016 (48). Older literature findings have been summarized in references 50 (up to 1992) and 49 (up to 1980).

Table 6.34.1.2 Ten ingredients with the highest concentrations in commercial Jasminum grandiflorum absolutes (48)

Name	Concentration range	Name	Concentration range
Benzyl acetate	9.5 - 32.9%	Phytyl acetate	1.4 - 11.0%
Benzyl benzoate	7.5 - 25.6%	Geranyllinalool	1.1 - 10.2%
(*E*)-Phytol	4.1 - 16.9%	Linalool	3.0 - 9.3%
(*Z*)-Phytol	0.2 - 13.3%	Squalene 2,3-oxide	5.9 - 9.2%
Isophytol	0.4 - 11.3%	Methyl benzoate	0.06 - 8.1%

6.34.2 JASMINUM SAMBAC ABSOLUTE

IDENTIFICATION

Description/definition	: Jasminum sambac absolute is the absolute obtained from the flowers of the Arabian / China jasmine, *Jasminum sambac* (L.) Aiton
INCI name(s) EU	: Jasminum sambac flower extract
INCI name(s) USA	: Jasminum sambac (jasmine) flower extract
CAS registry number(s)	: 91770-14-8
EC number(s)	: 294-797-4
RIFM monograph(s)	: Food Cosmet Toxicol 1976;14:331 (binder, page 477)
IFRA standard	: Restricted (www.ifraorg.org/en-us/standards-library) (table 6.34.2.1)
Function(s) in cosmetics	: EU: masking; perfuming. USA: fragrance ingredients
Patch testing	: 2% pet. (Chemo, SPEurope, SPCanada) (*Jasminum grandiflorum*)

Table 6.34.2.1 IFRA restrictions for Jasminum sambac absolute

Category [a]	Limits [b]	Category [a]	Limits [b]	Category [a]	Limits [b]
1	0.25%	5	2.10%	9	5.00%
2	0.32%	6	6.40%	10	2.50%
3	1.33%	7	0.70%	11	not restricted
4	4.00%	8	2.00%		

[a] For explanation of categories see pages 6-8
[b] Limits in the finished products

GENERAL

Jasminum sambac (L.) Aiton (Arabian jasmine, China jasmine, sambac jasmine) is an evergreen vine or shrub reaching up to 0.5-3 meter tall with white, strongly scented flowers that bloom all through the year. It is native to India and widely cultivated, e.g., in India and China. The flowers open only at night and are picked in the morning when the tiny petals are tightly closed. Harvested buds are taken to auction markets and then stored in a cool place until dark. Between 6.00 pm and 8.00 p.m., when the temperature drops, the petals begin to open, releasing the fullness of the fragrance at midnight. Jasmine sambac absolutes are highly appreciated in the fragrances industries and are also used in aromatherapy (48).

CHEMICAL COMPOSITION

Jasminum sambac (L.) Aiton absolute is a mobile to viscous light orange to reddish brown colored liquid which has an intensive flowery and slightly animalist and long-lasting odor. In Chinese jasmine absolutes from various origins, over 270 chemicals have been identified. About 61 per cent of these were found in a single reviewed publication only. The ten chemicals that had the highest maximum concentrations in 11 commercial Jasminum sambac absolute samples are shown in table 6.34.2.2 (Erich Schmidt, analytical data presented in ref. 48).

A full literature review of the qualitative and quantitative composition of commercial and non-commercial Jasminum sambac absolute of various origins has been published in 2016 (48).

Table 6.34.2.2 Ten ingredients with the highest concentrations in commercial Jasminum sambac absolutes (48)

Name	Concentration range	Name	Concentration range
Linalool	11.5 - 34.2%	[1(10)E,5E]-Germacradien-	0.9 - 7.6%
Benzyl acetate	10.5 - 21.0%	4α-ol	
(E,E)-α-Farnesene	10.6 - 17.1%	Methyl anthranilate	0.5 - 7.6%
(Z)-3-Hexenyl benzoate	3.9 - 14.9%	Benzyl alcohol	1.2 - 6.3%
1H-Indole	0.9 - 12.2%	Tricosene	0.2 - 5.4%
Methyl linolenate	0.4 - 8.6%		

CONTACT ALLERGY / ALLERGIC CONTACT DERMATITIS

Jasminum grandiflorum absolute and Jasmine absolute (unspecified)
The SCCS (Scientific Committee on Consumer Safety), in a 2012 Opinion on Fragrance allergens in cosmetic products, has marked Jasminum grandiflorum extract and Jasminum officinale extract as 'established contact allergen in humans' (43,44).

A short review of contact allergy to jasmine absolute has been provided in 2016 (54).

General
Contact allergy to / allergic contact dermatitis from jasmine absolute has been reported in at least 46 publications. Jasmine absolute has been included in the screening series of the North American Contact Dermatitis Group (NACDG) since 2001 (but not anymore in the period 2015-2017 [58]) and in the German baseline series in 2010 (52). In most publications, the botanical origin of the jasmine absolute was not mentioned. In the most recent NACDG publications the test substance is called Jasminum officinale (J. grandiflorum) oil, which cannot be correct, as it is not an oil but an absolute and Jasminum grandiflorum is not a synonym of Jasminum officinale. In a German publication it is called Jasminum grandiflorum / officinale extract (52).

In groups of consecutive patients suspected of contact dermatitis, prevalence rates of up to 1.9% positive patch test reactions have been observed. Rarely, reactions are considered to be of definite relevance. In the NACDG studies, 'definite + probable relevance' was reported in only 9% (2001-2002) to 37% (2011-2012) of positive patients. In two case reports, linalool and eugenol may have been allergens in jasmine absolute.

Testing in groups of patients
The results of patch tests with jasmine absolute in routine testing (consecutive patients suspected of contact dermatitis) are shown in table 6.34.2.3; those in groups of selected patients are shown in table 6.34.2.4. In routine testing, rates of positive reactions ranged from 0.3% to 1.9%, whereas between 1.0% and 35% of patients in selected groups had positive patch tests. The very high positivity rate of 35% was found in a small group of 20 patients previously shown to be allergic to fragrances (35).

Table 6.34.2.3 Patch testing in groups of patients: Routine testing

Years and Country	Test conc. & vehicle	Number of patients tested | positive (%)		Selection of patients (S); Relevance (R); Comments (C)	Ref.
2013-14 USA, Canada	2% pet.	4859	25 (0.5%)	R: definite + probable relevance: 24%	55
2010-2014 IVDK	5% pet.	48,956	703 (1.4%)	R: not stated	53
2009-14 USA, Canada	2% pet.	13,398	89 (0.7%)	R: of 23 patients reacting, but negative to FM I, FM II and balsam of Peru, 30% had definite + probable relevance	53
2011-12 USA, Canada	2% pet.	4230	19 (0.4%)	R: definite + probable relevance: 37%; C: origin: Jasminum officinale (J. grandiflorum) 'oil'; Jasminum officinale and Jasminum grandiflorum are not synonyms	25
2010-2012, Germany, Austria, Switzerland	5% pet.	9601	(1.9%)	R: not stated; C: range per country: 1.4-2.6%; the test substances was J. grandiflorum/officinale extract	52
2009-10 USA, Canada	2% pet.	4302	43 (1.0%)	R: definite + probable relevance 18%; C: origin: Jasminum officinale (J. grandiflorum) 'oil'; see comments above (25)	16
2000-2008 IVDK	5% pet.	3668	56 (1.5%)	R: not stated	23
2000-2007 USA	2% pet.	869	12 (1.4%)	R: 92%; C: weak study: a. high rate of macular erythema and weak reactions, b. relevance figures include 'questionable' and 'past' relevance	13

Table 6.34.2.3 Patch testing in groups of patients: Routine testing (continued)

Years and Country	Test conc. & vehicle	Number of patients tested	positive (%)		Selection of patients (S); Relevance (R); Comments (C)	Ref.
2005-6 USA, Canada	2% pet.	4447	49	(1.1%)	R: definite + probable relevance 25%	9
<2006 USA, Canada	2% pet.	1603	7	(0.4%)	R: definite + probable relevance: 14%	19
2003-4 USA, Canada	2% pet.	5143	44	(0.9%)	R: not stated	10
2002-2003 Korea	2% pet.	422	5	(1.2%)	R: not stated; C: tested was 'Jasmine officinale oil'	41
2001-2 USA, Canada	2% pet.	4900	34	(0.7%)	R: definite + probable relevance 9.4%	11
1999-2000 Denmark	5% pet.	318	1	(0.3%)	R: not specified; C: this study was part of the international study mentioned below (ref. 27)	40
1998-2000 six European countries	5% pet.	1606	20	(1.2%)	R: not specified for individual oils/chemicals	27
1983-1984 Italy	2% pet.	1200	13	(1.1%)	R: not stated	31

Table 6.34.2.4 Testing groups of patients: Selected patient groups

Years and Country	Test conc. & vehicle	Number of patients tested	positive (%)		Selection of patients (S); Relevance (R); Comments (C)	Ref.
2011-2015 Spain	2% pet.	607	15	(2.4%)	S: patients previously reacting to FM I, FM II, Myroxylon pereirae resin or hydroxyisohexyl 3-cyclohexene carboxaldehyde in the baseline series and subsequently tested with a fragrance series; R: not stated	57
2003-2014 IVDK	5% pet.	5202		(3.6%)	S: patients with stasis dermatitis / chronic leg ulcers; R: not stated; C: percentage of reactions significantly higher than in a control group of routine testing	51
2007-2011 IVDK	5% pet.	100	6	(6%)	S: physical therapists; R: not stated	56
2006-2010 USA	2% pet.	100	2	(2.0%)	S: patients with eyelid dermatitis; R: not stated	18
2000-2008 IVDK	5% pet.	982	11	(1.1%)	S: patients with dermatitis suspected of causal exposure to fragrances; R: not stated	23
2004-2008 Spain	2% pet.	86	3	(3.5%)	S: patients previously reacting to the fragrance mix I or Myroxylon pereirae (n=54) or suspected of fragrance contact allergy (n=32); R: not stated	22
<2005 USA	2% or 10% pet.	51	1	(2.0%)	S: patients using consumer products containing jasmine absolute; R: 'at least possibly relevant'	20
<2004 Israel	2% pet.	91	2	(2.2%)	S: patients who had shown a doubtful or positive reaction to the fragrance mix I and/or Myroxylon pereirae resin and/or one or two commercial fine fragrances; R: not stated	26
2000 USA, Japan and 4 European countries	10% pet.	178	30	(16.9%)	S: patients previously shown to be allergic to fragrances; R: not stated	28
1990-1998 Japan	20% pet.	1483	15	(1.0%)	S: patients suspected of cosmetic contact dermatitis, virtually all were women; C: range of annual frequency of sensitization: 0-4.0%; R: not stated	5
1996-1997 UK	2% pet.	10	2	(20%)	S: patients suspected of cosmetic dermatitis and reacting to the fragrance mix; R: not stated	3
<1994 Japan	?	?	?	(7.3%)	S: unknown; R: unknown	30
1971-1980 Japan	10% pet.	477	10	(2.1%)	S: patients with dermatoses other than pigmented cosmetic dermatitis and volunteers; R: not stated	14
<1977 USA	10% pet.	185	20	(10.8%)	S: not specified; R: not stated	32
1975 USA	10% pet.	20	7	(35%)	S: patients with fragrance contact allergy; R: not stated	35
<1974 Japan	?	183	44	(24.0%)	S: patients suspected of cosmetic dermatitis; R: unknown; C: tested was 'jasmine oil'; in many, there was co-reactivity with benzyl salicylate, which may be present in commercial jasmine absolutes in low concentrations	33

IVDK Information Network of Departments of Dermatology, Germany, Switzerland, Austria (www.ivdk.org); pet.: petrolatum

Case reports and case series

In Belgium, in the years before 1986, of 5202 consecutive patients with dermatitis patch tested, 156 were diagnosed with pure cosmetic allergy. 'Oil of jasmine' was the 'dermatitic ingredient' in 4 of the 156 (2.6%) patients (frequency in the entire group: 0.4%). It should be realized, however, that only a very limited number of patients was tested with a fragrance series (39).

An aromatherapist developed occupational contact dermatitis from contact allergy to multiple essential oils; she reacted to jasmine absolute, Egyptian, in the fragrance series, which reaction was considered to be relevant (8). One case of airborne contact dermatitis from 'jasmine oil' and two essential oils from aromatherapy lamps, whereby the water vapour produced distributes the essential oils as an aerosol in the air, was reported; the patient also reacted to linalool (4); linalool is an important constituent of all three materials (48).

One individual developed allergic contact dermatitis from undiluted lovage oil and a mixture of essential oils containing jasmine absolute; she reacted to her own products, jasmine absolute, lovage oil, cananga oil, eugenol and isoeugenol (21); commercial jasmine absolutes (*grandiflorum*, not *sambac*) may contain up to 6.8% eugenol but no or very low concentrations of isoeugenol (48). One patient was shown to have allergic cosmetic dermatitis from '*Jasminum officinale*' in a face cream (29). Jasmine absolute was responsible for 3 out of 399 cases of cosmetic (photo)allergy where the causal allergen was identified in a study of the NACDG, USA, 1977-1983 (37).

In a number of publications, positive patch tests to jasmine absolutes have been reported with unknown, uncertain or unstated relevance. These include (literature screened up to 2014 [48]) the following. Of seven patients allergic to the fragrance farnesol, 5 (71%) co-reacted to jasmine absolute (and various other fragrances) (36). In a group of 91 patients with cosmetic allergy, there was one patch test reaction to 'jasmin oil'; the relevance was not ascertained, but felt by the authors to be 'indicative' (38). One positive patch test reaction to jasmine absolute was seen in 53 women with chronic anogenital dermatoses (24). Two positive patch test reactions to 'jasmine oil' were observed in 7 patients with allergic contact dermatitis from compound tincture of benzoin (17).

One positive patch test reaction was found to jasmine absolute in a patient with occupational hand dermatitis from working in a perfume factory, and one reaction in 20 workers of the same factory without dermatitis (12). A positive patch test to jasmine absolute Egyptian was observed in an aromatherapist allergic to multiple essential oils, who did not use jasmine absolute at work (6). A naturopathic therapist had occupational contact dermatitis from various essential oils; she also reacted to jasmine absolute in the fragrance series, but probably did not use it in her work (7). One positive patch test to 'jasmine oil', possibly from its presence in a topical pharmaceutical preparation, has been observed (42).

Pigmented cosmetic dermatitis
In Japan, in the 1960s and 1970s, many female patients developed pigmentation following dermatitis of the face (15). This so-called pigmented cosmetic dermatitis was shown to be caused by contact allergy to components of cosmetic products, notably essential oils, other fragrance materials, antimicrobials, preservatives and coloring materials (14,15). In a group of 620 Japanese patients with this condition investigated between 1970 and 1980, 8-11% had positive patch test reactions to jasmine absolute 10% in petrolatum (14). The number of patients with pigmented cosmetic dermatitis decreased strongly after 1978, when major cosmetic companies began to eliminate strong contact sensitizers from their products (14).

Jasminum sambac absolute
No publications on contact allergy to or allergic contact dermatitis from jasmine absolute specified to have been obtained from the Arabian / China jasmine, *Jasminum sambac* (L.) Aiton have been found.

LITERATURE
1   Rhind JP. Essential oils. A handbook for aromatherapy practice, 2nd Edition. London: Singing Dragon, 2012
2   Lawless J. The encyclopedia of essential oils, 2nd Edition. London: Harper Thorsons, 2014
3   Thomson KF, Wilkinson SM. Allergic contact dermatitis to plant extracts in patients with cosmetic dermatitis. Br J Dermatol 2000;142:84-88
4   Schaller M, Korting HC. Allergic airborne contact dermatitis from essential oils used in aromatherapy. Clin Exp Dermatol 1995;20:143-145
5   Sugiura M, Hayakawa R, Kato Y, Sugiura K, Hashimoto R. Results of patch testing with lavender oil in Japan. Contact Dermatitis 2000;43:157-160
6   Dharmagunawardena B, Takwale A, Sanders KJ, Cannan S, Roger A, Ilchyshyn A. Gas chromatography: an investigative tool in multiple allergies to essential oils. Contact Dermatitis 2002;47:288-292
7   Trattner A, David M, Lazarov A. Occupational contact dermatitis due to essential oils. Contact Dermatitis 2008;58:282-284
8   Boonchai W, Lamtharachai P, Sunthonpalin P. Occupational allergic contact dermatitis from essential oils in aromatherapists. Contact Dermatitis 2007;56:181-182
9   Zug KA, Warshaw EM, Fowler JF Jr, Maibach HI, Belsito DL, Pratt MD, et al. Patch-test results of the North American Contact Dermatitis Group 2005-2006. Dermatitis 2009;20:149-160
10   Warshaw EM, Belsito DV, DeLeo VA, Fowler JF Jr, Maibach HI, Marks JG, et al. North American Contact Dermatitis Group patch-test results, 2003-2004 study period. Dermatitis 2008;19:129-136
11   Pratt MD, Belsito DV, DeLeo VA, Fowler JF Jr, Fransway AF, Maibach HI, et al. North American Contact Dermatitis Group patch-test results, 2001–2002 study period. Dermatitis 2004;15:176-183
12   Schubert HJ. Skin diseases in workers at a perfume factory. Contact Dermatitis 2006;55:81-83

13 Wetter DA, Yiannias JA, Prakash AV, Davis MD, Farmer SA, el-Azhary RA, et al. Results of patch testing to personal care product allergens in a standard series and a supplemental cosmetic series: an analysis of 945 patients from the Mayo Clinic Contact Dermatitis Group, 2000-2007. J Am Acad Dermatol 2010;63:789-798

14 Nakayama H, Matsuo S, Hayakawa K, Takhashi K, Shigematsu T, Ota S. Pigmented cosmetic dermatitis. Int J Dermatol 1984;23:299-305

15 Nakayama H, Harada R, Toda M. Pigmented cosmetic dermatitis. Int J Dermatol 1976;15:673-675

16 Warshaw EM, Belsito DV, Taylor JS, Sasseville D, DeKoven JG, Zirwas MJ, et al. North American Contact Dermatitis Group patch test results: 2009 to 2010. Dermatitis 2013;24:50-59

17 Fettig J, Taylor J, Sood A. Post-surgical allergic contact dermatitis to compound tincture of benzoin and association with reactions to fragrances and essential oils. Dermatitis 2014;25:211-212

18 Wenk KS, Ehrlich AE. Fragrance series testing in eyelid dermatitis. Dermatitis 2012;23:22-26

19 Belsito DV, Fowler JF Jr, Sasseville D, Marks JG Jr, De Leo VA, Storrs FJ. Delayed-type hypersensitivity to fragrance materials in a select North American population. Dermatitis 2006;17:23-28

20 Guin JD. Use of consumer product ingredients for patch testing. Dermatitis 2005;16:71-77

21 Lapeere H, Boone B, Verhaeghe E, Ongenae K, Lambert J. Contact dermatitis caused by lovage (Levisticum officinalis) essential oil. Contact Dermatitis 2013;69:181-182

22 Cuesta L, Silvestre JF, Toledo F, Lucas A, Pérez-Crespo M, Ballester I. Fragrance contact allergy: a 4-year retrospective study. Contact Dermatitis 2010;63:77-84

23 Uter W, Schmidt E, Geier J, Lessmann H, Schnuch A, Frosch P. Contact allergy to essential oils: current patch test results (2000–2008) from the Information Network of Departments of Dermatology (IVDK). Contact Dermatitis 2010;63:277-283

24 Vermaat H, Smienk F, Rustemeyer Th, Bruynzeel DP, Kirtschig G. Anogenital allergic contact dermatitis, the role of spices and flavour allergy. Contact Dermatitis 2008;59:233-237

25 Warshaw EM, Maibach HI, Taylor JS, Sasseville D, DeKoven JG, Zirwas MJ, et al. North American Contact Dermatitis Group patch test results: 2011-2012. Dermatitis 2015;26:49-59

26 Trattner A, David M. Patch testing with fine fragrances: comparison with fragrance mix, balsam of Peru and a fragrance series. Contact Dermatitis 2004;49:287-289

27 Frosch PJ, Johansen JD, Menné T, Pirker C, Rastogi SC, Andersen KE, et al. Further important sensitizers in patients sensitive to fragrances. II. Reactivity to essential oils. Contact Dermatitis 2002;47:279-287

28 Larsen W, Nakayama H, Fischer T, Elsner P, Frosch P, Burrows D, et al. Fragrance contact dermatitis: a worldwide multicenter investigation (Part II). Contact Dermatitis 2001;44:344-346

29 Penchalaiah K, Handa S, Lakshmi SB, Sharma VK, Kumar B. Sensitizers commonly causing allergic contact dermatitis from cosmetics. Contact Dermatitis 2000;43:311-313

30 Sugai T. Group study IV – farnesol and lily aldehyde. Environ Dermatol 1994;1:213-214

31 Santucci B, Cristaudo A, Cannistraci C, Picardo M. Contact dermatitis to fragrances. Contact Dermatitis 1987;16:93-95

32 Rudner EJ. North American Group results. Contact Dermatitis 1977;3:208-209

33 Nakayama H, Hanaoka H, Ohshiro A. Allergen Controlled System (ACS). Tokyo, Japan: Kanehara Shuppan, 1974:42 Data cited in ref. 34

34 Mitchell JC. Contact hypersensitivity to some perfume materials. Contact Dermatitis 1975;1:196-199

35 Larsen WG. Perfume dermatitis. A study of 20 patients. Arch Dermatol 1977;113:623-626

36 Goossens A, Merckx L. Allergic contact dermatitis from farnesol in a deodorant. Contact Dermatitis 1997;37:179-180

37 Adams RM, Maibach HI. A five-year study of cosmetic reactions. J Am Acad Dermatol 1985;13:1062-1069

38 Ngangu Z, Samsoen M, Foussereau J. Einige Aspekte zur Kosmetika-allergie in Strassburg. Dermatosen 1983;31:126-129

39 Broeckx W, Blondeel A, Dooms-Goossens A, Achten G. Cosmetic intolerance. Contact Dermatitis 1987;16:189-194

40 Paulsen E, Andersen KE. Colophonium and Compositae mix as markers of fragrance allergy: Cross-reactivity between fragrance terpenes, colophonium and Compositae plant extracts. Contact Dermatitis 2005;53:285-291

41 An S, Lee AY, Lee CH, Kim D-W, Hahm JH, Kim K-J, et al. Fragrance contact dermatitis in Korea: a joint study. Contact Dermatitis 2005;53:320-323

42 Nardelli A, D'Hooge E, Drieghe J, Dooms M, Goossens A. Allergic contact dermatitis from fragrance components in specific topical pharmaceutical products in Belgium. Contact Dermatitis 2009;60:303-313

43 SCCS (Scientific Committee on Consumer Safety). Opinion on Fragrance allergens in cosmetic products, 26-27 June 2012, SCCS/1459/11. Available at:
    https://ec.europa.eu/health/sites/health/files/scientific_committees/consumer_safety/docs/sccs_o_102.pdf

44 Uter W, Johansen JD, Börje A, Karlberg A-T, Lidén C, Rastogi S, Roberts D, White IR. Categorization of fragrance contact allergens for prioritization of preventive measures: clinical and experimental data and consideration of structure–activity relationships. Contact Dermatitis 2013;69:196-230

45 Reverchon E, Della Porta G, Gorgoglione D. Supercritical CO2 fractionation of jasmine concrete. J Supercr Fluids 1995;8:60-65

46 Hellivan P-J. Jasmine. Reinventing the 'king of perfumes'. Perfum Flavor 2009;34(October):42-52

47 Braun NA, Sim S. *Jasminum sambac* flower absolutes from India and China – geographic variations. Nat Prod Commun 2012;7:645-650

48 De Groot AC, Schmidt E. Essential oils: contact allergy and chemical composition. Boca Raton, Fl., USA: CRC Press, Taylor and Francis Group, 2016 (ISBN 9781482246407)

49 Verzele M, Maes G, Vuye A, Godefroot M, van Alboom M, Vervisch J, et al. Chromatographic investigation of jasmin absolutes. J Chromatogr A 1981;205:367-386

50 Verghese J, Sunny TP. Seasonal studies on the concrete and absolute of Indian *Jasminum grandiflorum* L. flowers Flavour Fragr J 1992;7:323-327

51 Erfurt-Berge C, Geier J, Mahler V. The current spectrum of contact sensitization in patients with chronic leg ulcers or stasis dermatitis - new data from the Information Network of Departments of Dermatology (IVDK). Contact Dermatitis 2017;77:151-158

52 Frosch PJ, Johansen JD, Schuttelaar M-LA, Silvestre JF, Sánchez-Pérez J, Weisshaar E, et al. (on behalf of the ESSCA network). Patch test results with fragrance markers of the baseline series – analysis of the European Surveillance System on Contact Allergies (ESSCA) network 2009–2012. Contact Dermatitis 2015;73:163-171

53 Warshaw EM, Zug KA, Belsito DV, Fowler JF Jr, DeKoven JG, Sasseville D, et al. Positive patch-test reactions to essential oils in consecutive patients: Results from North America and Central Europe. Dermatitis 2017;28:246-252

54 De Groot AC, Schmidt E. Essential oils, Part VI: Sandalwood oil, ylang-ylang oil, and jasmine absolute. Dermatitis 2017;28:14-21

55 DeKoven JG, Warshaw EM, Belsito DV, Sasseville D, Maibach HI, Taylor JS, et al. North American Contact Dermatitis Group Patch Test Results: 2013-2014. Dermatitis 2017;28:33-46

56 Girbig M, Hegewald J, Seidler A, Bauer A, Uter W, Schmitt J. Type IV sensitizations in physical therapists: patch test results of the Information Network of Departments of Dermatology (IVDK) 2007-2011. J Dtsch Dermatol Ges 2013;11:1185-1192

57 Silvestre JF, Mercader P, González-Pérez R, Hervella-Garcés M, Sanz-Sánchez T, Córdoba S, et al. Sensitization to fragrances in Spain: A 5-year multicentre study (2011-2015). Contact Dermatitis. 2018 Nov 14. doi: 10.1111/cod.13152. [Epub ahead of print]

58 DeKoven JG, Warshaw EM, Zug KA, Maibach HI, Belsito DV, Sasseville D, et al. North American Contact Dermatitis Group patch test results: 2015-2016. Dermatitis 2018;29:297-309

Chapter 6.35 JUNIPER BERRY OIL

IDENTIFICATION

Description/definition	: Juniper berry oil (essential oil of juniper berry) is the essential oil obtained from the fruit and the terminal branchlets of the (common) juniper, *Juniperus communis* L.
INCI name(s) EU & USA	: Juniperus communis fruit oil
CAS registry number(s)	: 8002-68-4; 84603-69-0; 73049-62-4
EC number(s)	: 283-268-3
RIFM monograph(s)	: Food Cosmet Toxicol 1976;14:333 (binder, page 479)
SCCS opinion(s)	: SCCNFP/0389/00, final (7)
ISO standard	: ISO 8897 Essential oil of juniper berry, 2010; Geneva, Switzerland, www.iso.org
Merck Index monograph	: 6588 (Juniper)
Function(s) in cosmetics	: EU: masking; perfuming. USA: cosmetic astringents; fragrance ingredients
Patch testing	: 2% pet.; based on RIFM data, 8% pet. is probably not irritant (9)

GENERAL

The common juniper (*Juniperus communis* L.) is an aromatic and evergreen coniferous shrub or tree. It is widely distributed in Europe, North Africa, North America and north Asia southwards to the Himalayas. It produces blue-black 'berries', which are not true berries in the botanical sense, but are the female seed cones which have a berry-like appearance. The junipers are grown commercially in several countries, including the United States, Canada, northern Italy, and Croatia. Juniper berries are widely used in the food industry as flavorings (in tea, beer, brandy and marinades for meat, poultry and fish) and in the production of juniper-flavored spirits, such as gin (8).

The berries (*Juniperi fructus*) and needles (leaves) of juniper contain an essential oil that has a characteristic aromatic flavor and bitter taste. Juniper berry essential oil is used in the pharmaceutical and food industries (also in gin and liqueurs) and perfumery, as well as in cosmetics; the oils are also applied in aromatherapy practices (1,2). Juniper oil is stated to possess a wide range of pharmacological activities and is the subject of Pharmacopoeia monographs in various countries (8).

CHEMICAL COMPOSITION

Juniper berry oil is a colorless, sometimes greenish clear mobile liquid, which has a fresh and herbaceous, typical 'gin'- note odor with fruity-woody note. In juniper berry oils from various origins, over 295 chemicals have been identified. About 45 per cent of these were found in a single reviewed publication only. The ten chemicals that had the highest maximum concentrations in 395 commercial juniper berry essential oil samples are shown in table 6.35.1 (Erich Schmidt, analytical data presented in ref. 8).

A full literature review of the qualitative and quantitative composition of commercial and non-commercial juniper berry oils of various origins, their chemotypes and with data from the ISO standard, has been published in 2016 (8).

Table 6.35.1 Ten ingredients with the highest concentrations in commercial juniper berry oils (8)

Name	Concentration range	Name	Concentration range
α-Pinene	18.1 - 66.6%	β-Caryophyllene	2.0 - 5.9%
Myrcene	11.6 - 21.6%	Terpinen-4-ol	1.9 - 5.4%
Sabinene	1.0 - 17.7%	γ-Terpinene	0.4 - 4.5%
β-Pinene	1.8 - 7.8%	δ-Cadinene	0.3 - 2.7%
Limonene	2.5 - 7.6%	Germacrene D	0.07 - 2.6%

CONTACT ALLERGY / ALLERGIC CONTACT DERMATITIS

General

Contact allergy to / allergic contact dermatitis from juniper berry oil has been reported in four publications only. In a group of consecutive patients suspected of contact dermatitis (only one study), the prevalence rate of positive patch test reactions to juniper berry oil was 0.5%; relevance data were not provided. In a case report, α-pinene may have been an allergen in juniper berry oil (3).

Testing in groups of patients
Two hundred dermatitis patients from Poland were tested with 'juniper oil' 2% in petrolatum and one (0.5%) reacted. The same authors also patch tested 51 patients allergic to Myroxylon pereirae resin (balsam of Peru) and/or turpentine and/or wood tar and/or colophony and two (3.9%) had a positive patch test; relevance data were not provided (4). A group of 86 patients from Poland previously reacting to the fragrance mix was tested with juniper berries oil and six (7.0%) had a positive patch test reaction; relevance data were not provided (5).

Case reports and case series
Two aromatherapists had contact dermatitis (occupational in one) with allergies to multiple essential oils used at their work, including juniper oil. Both patients also reacted to geraniol, α-pinene, the fragrance mix and various other fragrance materials. In addition, one proved to be allergic to linalool and linalyl acetate, the other to caryophyllene. α-Pinene was demonstrated by GC-MS in the juniper oils (3) and is the dominant ingredient of the oil (table 6.35.1).
        Additional information on allergy to juniper berry oil can be found in ref. 6 (article not read).

LITERATURE

1   Rhind JP. Essential oils. A handbook for aromatherapy practice, 2nd Edition. London: Singing Dragon, 2012
2   Lawless J. The encyclopedia of essential oils, 2nd Edition. London: Harper Thorsons, 2014
3   Dharmagunawardena B, Takwale A, Sanders KJ, Cannan S, Roger A, Ilchyshyn A. Gas chromatography: an investigative tool in multiple allergies to essential oils. Contact Dermatitis 2002;47:288-292
4   Rudzki E, Grzywa Z, Bruo WS. Sensitivity to 35 essential oils. Contact Dermatitis 1976;2:196-200
5   Rudzki E, Grzywa Z. Allergy to perfume mixture. Contact Dermatitis 1986;15:115-116
6   Rothe A, Heine A, Rebohle E. Oil from juniper berries as an occupational allergen for the skin and respiratory tract. Berufsdermatosen 1973;21:11-16 (in German)
7   Opinion of the Scientific Committee on Cosmetic Products and Non-Food Products Intended for Consumers concerning 'The 1st update of the inventory of ingredients employed in cosmetic products. Section II: Perfume and aromatic raw materials', 24 October 2000, SCCNFP/0389/00, final. Available at: http://ec.europa.eu/health/ph_risk/committees/sccp/documents/out131_en.pdf
8   De Groot AC, Schmidt E. Essential oils: contact allergy and chemical composition. Boca Raton, Fl., USA: CRC Press, Taylor and Francis Group, 2016 (ISBN 9781482246407)
9   De Groot AC. Patch Testing, 4th Edition. Wapserveen, The Netherlands: acdegroot publishing, 2018 (ISBN 978-90-813233-4-5)

Chapter 6.36   LAUREL LEAF OIL

IDENTIFICATION

Description/definition : Laurel leaf oil is the essential oil obtained from the leaves of the laurel (bay, bay laurel), *Laurus nobilis* L.
INCI name(s) EU & USA : Laurus nobilis leaf oil
Other names : Bay oil, sweet; sweet bay oil
CAS registry number(s) : 8002-41-3; 84603-73-6; 8007-48-5
EC number(s) : 283-272-5
RIFM monograph(s) : Food Cosmet Toxicol 1976;14:337 (binder, page 481)
SCCS opinion(s) : SCCS/1459/11 (26)
Merck Index monograph : 6707 (Laurel)
Function(s) in cosmetics : EU: masking; perfuming. USA: fragrance ingredients; skin bleaching agents
Patch testing : 2% pet. (SPEurope, SPCanada; incorrectly termed 'bay leaf oil' by SPCanada)

GENERAL

Laurus nobilis L. is an evergreen shrub up to 8 meter in height and commonly named bay laurel. This tree belongs to the Lauraceae family and is native to the southern Mediterranean region and widely cultivated in Europe and the USA as an ornamental plant. In North African countries (Tunisia, Algeria, Morocco), bay laurel is a common species. It is grown commercially for its aromatic leaves in Turkey, Algeria, Morocco, Portugal, Spain, Italy, France and Mexico (28). The (fresh and dried) leaves are commonly used as a spicy, aromatic flavouring for soups, fish, meats, stews, puddings, vinegars, and beverages and also has food preserving properties from its antibacterial effects. Benzene compounds such as eugenol, methyl eugenol and elemicin are responsible for the spicy aroma of bay leaves (1). The leaves are also widely used in folk medicine to treat a variety of diseases.

The essential laurel leaf oil is said to cure rheumatic pain and dermatitis and is used by the cosmetic industry in creams, perfumes and soaps (1). It is also used in aromatherapy practices (2,3).

Laurel leaf oil is also termed bay oil, sweet (sweet bay oil), not to be confused with 'bay oil', which is obtained from *Pimenta racemosa* (Mill.) J.W. Moore (see Chapter 6.4 Bay oil).

CHEMICAL COMPOSITION

Laurel leaf oil is a slightly yellowish to greenish, clear mobile liquid, which has a fresh, aromatic odor with connotations of eucalyptus and clove leaves. In laurel leaf oils from various origins, over 425 chemicals have been identified. About 54 per cent of these were found in a single reviewed publication only. The ten chemicals that had the highest maximum concentrations in 23 commercial laurel leaf essential oil samples are shown in table 6.36.1 (Erich Schmidt, analytical data presented in ref. 28).

A full literature review of the qualitative and quantitative composition of commercial and non-commercial laurel leaf oils of various origins and their chemotypes has been published in 2016 (28).

Table 6.36.1 Ten ingredients with the highest concentrations in commercial laurel leaf oils (28)

Name	Concentration range	Name	Concentration range
1,8-Cineole	38.4 - 52.0%	β-Pinene	3.2 - 5.0%
Terpinyl acetate	6.3 - 12.0%	Limonene	1.0 - 4.0%
Sabinene	7.3 - 11.8%	Terpinen-4-ol	1.7 - 3.4%
Linalool	1.1 - 7.8%	Methyl eugenol	1.0 - 3.0%
α-Pinene	4.4 - 7.5%	*p*-Cymene	0.04 - 2.7%

CONTACT ALLERGY / ALLERGIC CONTACT DERMATITIS

General

The SCCS (Scientific Committee on Consumer Safety), in a 2012 Opinion on Fragrance allergens in cosmetic products, has marked Laurus nobilis extract as 'established contact allergen in humans' (26,27).

Contact allergy to / allergic contact dermatitis from laurel oil has been reported in over 25 publications. Laurel oil used to be a frequent contact allergen in the middle of the 20th century. At that time, the oil was used to improve the luster of felt hats, which frequently caused hatband dermatitis in the wearer (22,29). Laurel-based ointments were also a frequent cause of allergic contact dermatitis in those years, especially in France, Germany and Switzerland (24,29). Between 1953 and 1962, several thousands of dermatitis patients have been tested with 'laurel oil' in Germany and positive reactions were seen in 3.1-6.9% of patients (22,30,31,32). However, it should be appreciated that that most cases of early reports of contact allergy to laurel oil (<1960) were due to vegetable (not essential) oil from laurel *berries* (10,18,24). However, in some publications, distinction was made between laurel oil and laurel essential oil; both were made from the leaves, the 'oils' being extracts and the 'essential oils' being steam-distillates (29).

Laurel *berry* oils from *L. nobilis* are prohibited in cosmetics in the EU.

Testing in groups of patients

The results of patch tests with 'laurel oil' and laurel leaf oil in routine testing (consecutive patients suspected of contact dermatitis) and in groups of selected patients are shown in table 6.36.2. In routine testing, rates of positive reactions ranged from 2.0% to 6.9% (data from half a century ago, probably mostly laurel berries oil), whereas in more recent studies between 0.4% and 50.5% (but the latter was also *vegetable* laurel *berries* oil) patients in selected groups had positive patch tests.

Table 6.36.2 Patch testing in groups of patients

Years and Country	Test conc. & vehicle	Number of patients tested | positive (%)		Selection of patients (S); Relevance (R); Comments (C)	Ref.
Routine testing					
<1973 Poland	2% pet.	200	4 (2.0%)	R: not stated; C: tested was 'laurel oil'	37
1953-1962 Germany	?	>1,000	see right column	Between 1953 and 1962, several thousands of dermatitis patients have been tested with 'laurel oil' in Germany; positive reactions were seen in 3.1-6.9% of patients (data cited in ref. 22); most likely *vegetable* oil from laurel *berries*	22
Testing in groups of selected patients					
2008-2014 UK	2% pet.	471	2 (0.4%)	S: patients tested with a fragrance series; R: not stated	33
2001-2010 Australia	2% pet.	681	31 (4.6%)	S: not specified; R: 32%	23
2000-2008 IVDK	2% pet.	6297	63 (1.0%)	S: patients with dermatitis suspected of causal exposure to fragrances; R: not stated	13
1997-2000 Austria	2% pet.	747	4 (0.6%)	S: patients suspected of fragrance allergy; R: not stated	5
1994-1995 UK	2% pet.	40	2 (5%)	S: patients previously reacting to the fragrance mix; R: not stated	14
1985-1990 Germany	2% pet.	99	50 (50.5%)	S: patients with a positive reaction to the Compositae mix; R: not stated; the reactions to laurel oil were considered as indicators for Compositae allergy; C: laurel oil contains sesquiterpene lactones such as in Compositae, ergo cross-reactivity or pseudo-cross-reactivity can be expected (10); the test substances was not an essential oil, but *vegetable* laurel *berries* oil	18
1967-1972 France	20% pet.	276	49 (17.8%)	S: patients with plant contact allergy; R: not stated	29

IVDK Information Network of Departments of Dermatology, Germany, Switzerland, Austria (www.ivdk.org); pet.: petrolatum

Case reports and case series

In one clinic in Belgium, in the period 1990-2016, five cases of dermatitis caused by contact allergy to laurel leaf oil from its presence as active principle in 'topical botanical medicines' have been observed (35).

A patient developed erythema multiforme from contact allergy to laurel oil used for knee arthropathy; the patch test had a target-like appearance and had the histopathology of erythema multiforme (6). Generalized allergic contact dermatitis was caused by contact allergy to a mixture of laurel oil and olive oil used for massage in one patient (8). Another patient had allergic contact dermatitis from the topical use of laurel oil for rheumatic complaints (11). One individual suffered from dermatitis as a result of contact allergy to laurel oil in a face mask (84).

Two cases of allergic contact dermatitis from laurel oil in a topical pharmaceutical preparation have also been observed (4). A female patient developed extensive dermatitis of the face which proved to have been caused by contact allergy to laurel leaf oil in a cosmetic oil (34). Contact allergy to laurel oil in toothpaste was described in the 1950s (16, data cited in ref. 15).

In a number of publications, positive patch tests to laurel (leaf) oil have been reported with unknown, uncertain or unstated relevance. These include (literature screened up to 2014 [28]) the following. One positive patch test to laurel oil in an aromatherapists with occupational contact dermatitis from (multiple) essential oils; it was uncertain whether this oil had been used by the patient (7). One positive patch test reaction to laurel leaf oil in a patient known to be allergic to oak moss (25). A positive patch test reaction to laurel oil was observed in a patient who had airborne allergic contact dermatitis from tea tree oil and lavender oil (12). One positive patch test to laurel oil in a patient suffering from airborne allergic contact dermatitis from aromatherapy with other essential oils (9).

Additional literature on contact allergy to laurel (leaf) oil may be found in refs. 17,19,20 and 21 (articles not read).

Cross-reactions, pseudo-cross-reactions and co-reactions

Frullania and frullanolide; this probably related to leaf extracts, not essential oils (29). Of 3 patients allergic to laurel oil (leaf extract) and laurel essential oil, all co-reacted to costus oil and costunolide (29).

Patch test sensitization

Patch test sensitization from has been cited in ref. 36.

REFERENCES

1   Sellami IH, Aidi Wannes W, Bettaieb I, Berrima S, Chahed T, Marzouk B, et al. Qualitative and quantitative changes in the essential oil of *Laurus nobilis* L. leaves as affected by different drying methods. Food Chem 2011;126:691-697

2   Rhind JP. Essential oils. A handbook for aromatherapy practice, 2nd Edition. London: Singing Dragon, 2012

3   Lawless J. The encyclopedia of essential oils, 2nd Edition. London: Harper Thorsons, 2014

4   Nardelli A, D'Hooge E, Drieghe J, Dooms M, Goossens A. Allergic contact dermatitis from fragrance components in specific topical pharmaceutical products in Belgium. Contact Dermatitis 2009;60:303-313

5   Wöhrl S, Hemmer W, Focke M, Götz M, Jarisch R. The significance of fragrance mix, balsam of Peru, colophonium and propolis as screening tools in the detection of fragrance allergy. Br J Dermatol 2001;145:268-273

6   Athanasiadis GI, Pfab F, Klein A, Braun-Falco M, Ring J, Ollert M. Erythema multiforme due to contact with laurel oil. Contact Dermatitis 2007;57:116-118

7   Bleasel N, Tate B, Rademaker M. Allergic contact dermatitis following exposure to essential oils. Australas J Dermatol 2002;43:211-213

8   Adişen E, Önder M. Allergic contact dermatitis from *Laurus nobilis* oil induced by massage. Contact Dermatitis 2007;56:360-361

9   Schaller M, Korting HC. Allergic airborne contact dermatitis from essential oils used in aromatherapy. Clin Exp Dermatol 1995;20:143-145

10 Hausen BM. Lorbeer-Allergie Ursache, Wirkung und Folgen der äusserlichen Anwendung eines sogenannten Naturheilmittels. Dtsch Med Wschr 1985;110: 634-638

11 Özden MG, Öztaş P, Öztaş MO, Önder M. Allergic contact dermatitis from *Laurus nobilis* (laurel) oil. Contact Dermatitis 2001;45:178

12 De Groot AC. Airborne allergic contact dermatitis from tea tree oil. Contact Dermatitis 1996;35:304-305

13 Uter W, Schmidt E, Geier J, Lessmann H, Schnuch A, Frosch P. Contact allergy to essential oils: current patch test results (2000–2008) from the Information Network of Departments of Dermatology (IVDK). Contact Dermatitis 2010;63:277-283

14 Katsarma G, Gawkrodger DJ. Suspected fragrance allergy requires extended patch testing to individual fragrance allergens. Contact Dermatitis 1999;41:193-197

15 Sainio E-L, Kanerva L. Contact allergens in toothpastes and a review of their hypersensitivity. Contact Dermatitis 1995;33:100-105

16 Spier HW, Sixt I. Lorbeer als Träger eines wenig beachteten kontaktekzemotogenen Allergens. Derm Wochenschr 1953;128:805-810

17 Calnan CD. Oil of cloves, laurel, lavender, peppermint. Contact Dermatitis Newsletter 1970;7:148

18 Hausen BM. A 6-year experience with Compositae mix. Am J Cont Derm 1996;7:94-99

19 Larrègue M, Rat JP, Gallet P, Bressieux JM, Pousset JL. Contact dermatitis caused by dandelion, laurel oil and frullania by cross-allergy. Ann Dermatol Venereol 1978;105:547-548

20 Foussereau J. L'allergie de contact à l'huile de laurier (note préliminaire). Bull Soc Fr Dermatol Syphiligr 1963;70:698-701

21 Bandmann HJ, Dohn W. Laurel oil as a frequent cause of allergic contact eczema. Munch Med Wochenschr 1960;102:680-682 (in German)

22 Foussereau J, Benezra C, Ourisson G. Contact dermatitis from laurel. I. Clinical aspects. Transactions of the St John's Hospital Dermatological Society 1967;53:141-146. Data cited in ref. 24

23 Toholka R, Wang Y-S, Tate B, Tam M, Cahill J, Palmer A, Nixon R. The first Australian Baseline Series: Recommendations for patch testing in suspected contact dermatitis. Australas J Dermatol 2015;56:107-115

24 Tisserand R, Young R. Essential oil safety, 2nd Ed. Edinburgh: Churchill Livingstone, 2014:322

25 Benezra C, Schlewer G, Stampf JL. Lactones allergisantes naturelles et synthetiques. Rev Fr Allergol 1978;18:31-33. Data cited in ref. 24

26 SCCS (Scientific Committee on Consumer Safety). Opinion on Fragrance allergens in cosmetic products, 26-27 June 2012, SCCS/1459/11. Available at:
    https://ec.europa.eu/health/sites/health/files/scientific_committees/consumer_safety/docs/sccs_o_102.pdf

27 Uter W, Johansen JD, Börje A, Karlberg A-T, Lidén C, Rastogi S, Roberts D, White IR. Categorization of fragrance contact allergens for prioritization of preventive measures: clinical and experimental data and consideration of structure–activity relationships. Contact Dermatitis 2013;69:196-230

28 De Groot AC, Schmidt E. Essential oils: contact allergy and chemical composition. Boca Raton, Fl., USA: CRC Press, Taylor and Francis Group, 2016 (ISBN 9781482246407)

29 Foussereau J, Meller JC, Benezra C. Contact allergy to Frullania and Laurus nobilis: cross-sensitization and chemical structure of the allergens. Contact Dermatitis 1975;1:223-230

30 Paschoud JM. Kritische Bemerkungen zur Zusammensetzung der sogenannten Standard Reiben für epikutane Testproben. Dermatologica 1962;124:196-204 (article in German). Data cited in ref. 29

31 Schultheiss E. Gummi und Ekzem. Aulendorf: Cantor, 1959 (in German). Data cited in ref. 29

32 Bandmann HJ, Dohn W. Das Lorbeeröl als nicht seltene Ursache allergischer Kontakt Ekzeme. Münchener Med Wschr 1960;102:680-682 (article in German). Data cited in ref. 29

33 Sabroe RA, Holden CR, Gawkrodger DJ. Contact allergy to essential oils cannot always be predicted from allergy to fragrance markers in the baseline series. Contact Dermatitis 2016;74:236-241

34 Brás S, Mendes-Bastos P, Amaro C, Cardoso J. Allergic contact dermatitis caused by laurel leaf oil. Contact Dermatitis 2015;72:417-419

35 Gilissen L, Huygens S, Goossens A. Allergic contact dermatitis caused by topical herbal remedies: importance of patch testing with the patients' own products. Contact Dermatitis 2018;78:177-184

36 De Groot AC. Patch Testing, 4th Edition. Wapserveen, The Netherlands: acdegroot publishing, 2018 (ISBN 978-90-813233-4-5)

37 Rudzki E, Kielak D. Sensitivity to some compounds related to Balsam of Peru. Contact Dermatitis Newsletter 1972;nr.13:335-336

Chapter 6.37   LAVANDIN OIL

GENERAL

The lavandins (*Lavandula x intermedia* Emeric ex Loisel; *Lavandula hybrida*) are a class of sterile hybrids of the true (syn. English) lavender, *Lavandula angustifolia* P. Mill. and the spike lavender, *Lavandula latifolia* Medikus. They are perennial herbs, which may reach a height of 60 cm. The lavandin is native to the Mediterranean area and is widely cultivated for production of essential oils and as decorative plant in Spain, France, Bulgaria, Italy, the Balkan Peninsula, Morocco, South Africa, India, Argentina, Australia and Tasmania (2,3,5,6). The main lavandin cultivars are 'Grosso', 'Abrial' and 'Super' (2,3). In 2002, 'Grosso' accounted for 84% of lavandin production world-wide, 'Abrial' for 8%, 'Super' for 5% and others for 3% (6).

Lavandin essential oils are produced commercially by steam-distillation from the flowering tops of selected cultivars. They are used as fragrances in perfumes, soaps, detergents, cosmetics and air fresheners, and are also employed by the pharmaceutical industries (1,2,4,5,6). In food manufacturing, lavandin essential oil may be used in flavoring beverages, ice cream, baked goods and chewing gum (4,5,6). The oil is believed to have many pharmaceutical qualities, which render lavandin essential oils highly appreciated in phytotherapy and aromatherapy (4,5).

Lavandins are cultivated in far (5:1) larger quantities than lavenders (5), because they produce more oil (6), are easier to harvest and are hardier. However, they are considered of lesser quality, as they contain more camphor and less linalyl acetate and linalool than lavender oils. Nevertheless, lavandin oil is among the top ten most important essential oils by volume (6). A review of various aspects of lavenders (lavender, lavandin, spike lavender), written from the industry's perspective, can be found (on-line) in a dissertation from the International Centre for Aroma Trades Studies, Plymouth, UK (7).

6.37.1   LAVANDIN ABRIAL OIL

IDENTIFICATION

Description/definition	: Lavandin abrial oil (essential oil of lavandin Abrial, French type) is the essential oil obtained from the flowering tops of the lavandin (bastard lavender), *Lavandula angustifolia* Mill. x *Lavandula latifolia* Medik. 'Abrial'
INCI name(s) EU	: Lavandula hybrida abrial herb oil (perfuming name, not an INCI name proper)
INCI name(s) USA	: Not in the Personal Care Products Council Ingredient Database
CAS registry number(s)	: 8022-15-9; 93455-96-0
EC number(s)	: 297-384-7
RIFM monograph(s)	: Food Cosm Toxicol 1976;14:447 (binder, page 484)
SCCS opinion(s)	: SCCS/1459/11 (11)
ISO standard	: ISO 3054 Essential oil of Lavandin Abrial, French type, 2017; Geneva, Switzerland, www.iso.org
Merck Index monograph	: 6715 (Lavender)
Function(s) in cosmetics	: EU: perfuming
Patch testing	: 2% pet.; based on RIFM data, 5% pet. is probably not irritant (14)

CHEMICAL COMPOSITION

Lavandin abrial oil is a slightly yellow, clear mobile liquid which has a herbal, blooming and camphoraceous odor. In lavandin abrial oils from various origins, over 88 chemicals have been identified. About 45 per cent of these were found in a single reviewed publication only. The ten chemicals that had the highest maximum concentrations in 110 commercial lavandin abrial essential oil samples are shown in table 6.37.1.1 (Erich Schmidt, analytical data presented in ref. 13).

A full literature review of the qualitative and quantitative composition of commercial and non-commercial lavandin abrial oils of various origins and with data from the ISO standard has been published in 2016 (13).

Table 6.37.1.1 Ten ingredients with the highest concentrations in commercial lavandin abrial oils (13)

Name	Concentration range	Name	Concentration range
Linalool	35.1 - 56.2%	(Z)-β-Ocimene	1.0 - 3.7%
Linalyl acetate	14.9 - 26.1%	β-Caryophyllene	1.4 - 3.7%
1,8-Cineole	5.4 - 9.9%	(E)-β-Ocimene	1.4 - 3.3%
Camphor	7.6 - 9.9%	β -Pinene	0.5 - 1.9%
Borneol	2.3 - 4.2%	(E)-β-Farnesene	0.09 - 1.2%

6.37.2   LAVANDIN GROSSO OIL

IDENTIFICATION

Description/definition	: Lavandin grosso oil (essential oil of lavandin grosso, French type) is the essential oil obtained from the flowering tops of the lavandin (bastard lavender), *Lavandula angustifolia* Mill. x *Lavandula latifolia* Medik. 'Grosso'
INCI name(s) EU	: Lavandula hybrida grosso herb oil (perfuming name, not an INCI name proper)
INCI name(s) USA	: Not in the Personal Care Products Council Ingredient database
CAS registry number(s)	: 8022-15-9; 93455-97-1
EC number(s)	: 297-385-2
RIFM monograph(s)	: Food Cosm Toxicol 1976;14:447 (binder, page 484)
SCCS opinion(s)	: SCCS/1459/11 (11)
ISO standard	: ISO 8902 Essential oil of Lavandin grosso, French type, 2009; Geneva, Switzerland, www.iso.org
Merck Index monograph	: 6715 (Lavender)
Function(s) in cosmetics	: EU: perfuming
Patch testing	: 2% pet.; based on RIFM data, 5% pet. is probably not irritant (14)

GENERAL

General information on the lavandin and lavandin oil can be found in the section 'general' of Lavandin abrial oil above.

CHEMICAL COMPOSITION

Lavandin grosso oil is a light yellow, clear mobile liquid which has a fresh, herbal and floral, camphoraceous odor. In lavandin grosso oils from various origins, over 100 chemicals have been identified. About 44 per cent of these were found in a single reviewed publication only. The ten chemicals that had the highest maximum concentrations in 148 commercial lavandin grosso essential oil samples are shown in table 6.37.2.1 (Erich Schmidt, analytical data presented in ref. 13).

A full literature review of the qualitative and quantitative composition of commercial and non-commercial lavandin grosso oils of various origins and with data from the ISO standard has been published in 2016 (13).

Table 6.37.2.1 Ten ingredients with the highest concentrations in commercial lavandin grosso oils (13)

Name	Concentration range	Name	Concentration range
Linalool	26.0 - 38.6%	Borneol	1.3 - 3.7%
Linalyl acetate	23.9 - 36.0%	Lavandulyl acetate	1.5 - 3.2%
1,8-Cineole	3.0 - 9.5%	β-Caryophyllene	1.0 - 2.5%
Camphor	5.9 - 9.0%	(E)-β-Farnesene	0.6 - 1.7%
Terpinen-4-ol	2.0 - 5.5%	α-Terpineol	0.3 - 1.7%

6.37.3 LAVANDIN OIL (OTHER CULTIVARS AND CULTIVAR NOT SPECIFIED)

IDENTIFICATION

Description/definition : Lavandin oil is the essential oil obtained from the flowering tops of the lavandin, *Lavandula angustifolia* Mill. x *Lavandula latifolia* Medik.
INCI name(s) EU : Lavandula hybrida oil; Lavandula hybrida herb oil; Lavandula intermedia oil
INCI name(s) EU & USA : Lavandula hybrida oil; Lavandula intermedia oil
CAS registry number(s) : 8022-15-9; 91722-69-9; 92623-76-2
EC number(s) : 294-470-6; 296-408-3
RIFM monograph(s) : Food Cosm Toxicol 1976;14:447 (binder, page 484)
SCCS opinion(s) : SCCS/1459/11 (11)
Merck Index monograph : 6715 (Lavender)
Function(s) in cosmetics : EU: emollient; perfuming; masking. USA: fragrance ingredients
Patch testing : 2% pet.; based on RIFM data, 5% pet. is probably not irritant (14)

GENERAL

General information on the lavandin and lavandin oil can be found in the section 'general' of Lavandin abrial oil above.

CHEMICAL COMPOSITION

Lavandin oil is a colorless to slightly yellow, clear mobile liquid which has a floral, fresh lavender-like or herbal fresh camphoraceous odor, depending on the type of lavandin used to prepare the oil. In lavandin oils from various origins, over 180 chemicals have been identified. About 61 per cent of these were found in a single reviewed publication only. The ten chemicals that had the highest maximum concentrations in 26 commercial lavandin essential oil samples are shown in table 6.37.3.1 (Erich Schmidt, analytical data presented in ref. 13).

A full literature review of the qualitative and quantitative composition of commercial and non-commercial lavandin oils (cultivar unspecified) of various origins has been published in 2016 (13).

Table 6.37.3.1 Ten ingredients with the highest concentrations in commercial lavandin oils (13)

Name	Concentration range	Name	Concentration range
Linalool	35.1 - 56.2%	(Z)-β-Ocimene	1.0 - 3.7%
Linalyl acetate	14.9 - 26.1%	β-Caryophyllene	1.4 - 3.7%
1,8-Cineole	5.4 - 9.9%	(E)-β-Ocimene	1.4 - 3.3%
Camphor	7.6 - 9.9%	β-Pinene	0.5 - 1.9%
Borneol	2.3 - 4.2%	(E)-β-Farnesene	0.09 - 1.2%

CONTACT ALLERGY / ALLERGIC CONTACT DERMATITIS

Lavandin oil (unspecified)

General

The SCCS (Scientific Committee on Consumer Safety), in a 2012 Opinion on Fragrance allergens in cosmetic products, has marked Lavandula hybrida extract as 'established contact allergen in humans' (11,12).

Contact allergy to lavandin oil has been reported in two publications and there is one case report of possible allergic contact dermatitis (8). In the latter publication, however, a false-positive patch test to lavandin oil due to the excited skin syndrome cannot be excluded.

Testing in groups of patients

Two hundred dermatitis patients from Poland were tested with lavandin oil 2% in petrolatum and one (0.5%) reacted. The same authors also patch tested 51 patients allergic to Myroxylon pereirae resin (balsam of Peru) and/or turpentine and/or wood tar and/or colophony and one (2.0%) had a positive patch test; relevance data were not provided (9). A group of 86 patients from Poland previously reacting to the fragrance mix was tested with lavandin oil and four (4.6%) had a positive patch test reaction; relevance data were not provided (10).

Case reports and case series

An aromatherapist had non-occupational contact dermatitis with allergies to multiple essential oils used at work, including lavandin oil. The patient also reacted to geraniol, linalool, linalyl acetate, α-pinene, the fragrance mix and various other fragrance materials. α-Pinene was demonstrated by GC-MS in the lavandin oil, but curiously enough not linalool (8); α-pinene is not an important component of lavandin oils.

Lavandin abrial oil

No reports on contact allergy to or allergic contact dermatitis from lavandin oil, specified to have been obtained from *Lavandula angustifolia* Mill. x *Lavandula latifolia* Medik. 'Abrial' were found.

Lavandin grosso oil

No reports on contact allergy to or allergic contact dermatitis from lavandin oil, specified to have been obtained from *Lavandula angustifolia* Mill. x *Lavandula latifolia* Medik. 'Grosso' were found.

LITERATURE

1   Lammerink J, Wallace AR, Porter NG. Effects of harvest time and postharvest drying on oil from lavandin (*Lavandula × intermedia*). NZ J Crop Hortic Sc 1989;17:315-326
2   Baydar H, Kineci S. Scent composition of essential oil, concrete, absolute and hydrosol from lavandin (*Lavandula x intermedia* Emeric ex Loisel.). J Essent Oil Bear Plants 2009;12:131-136
3   Bombarda I, Dupuy N, Van Da JP, Gaydou EM. Comparative chemometric analyses of geographic origins and compositions of lavandin var. Grosso essential oils by mid infrared spectroscopy and gas chromatograpy. Anal Chim Acta 2008;613:31-39
4   Périno-Issartier S, Ginies C, Cravotto G, Chemat F. A comparison of essential oils obtained from lavandin via different extraction processes: Ultrasound, microwave, turbohydrodistillation, steam and hydrodistillation. J Chromatogr A 2013;1305:41- 47
5   Directorate Plant Production, Republic of South Africa. Lavender Production. Pretoria, South Africa: Directorate Agricultural Information Services, Department of Agriculture, Forestry and Fisheries, 2009. Available at: http://www.nda.agric.za/docs/brochures/essoilslavender.pdf
6   Bosilcov A. Lavender: A key perfumery material. Dissertation for the Postgraduate Diploma in Aroma Trades Studies of the International Federation of Essential Oils and Aroma Trades. University of Plymouth, 2010. Available at: http://www.ifeat.org/wp-content/uploads/2012/10/Bosilcov+-+Lavender.pdf
7   Bosilcov A. Lavender: A key perfumery material. Dissertation. International Centre for Aroma Trades Studies, Plymouth University, Plymouth, UK, 2010
8   Dharmagunawardena B, Takwale A, Sanders KJ, Cannan S, Roger A, Ilchyshyn A. Gas chromatography: an investigative tool in multiple allergies to essential oils. Contact Dermatitis 2002;47:288-292
9   Rudzki E, Grzywa Z, Bruo WS. Sensitivity to 35 essential oils. Contact Dermatitis 1976;2:196-200
10   Rudzki E, Grzywa Z. Allergy to perfume mixture. Contact Dermatitis 1986;15:115-116
11   SCCS (Scientific Committee on Consumer Safety). Opinion on Fragrance allergens in cosmetic products, 26-27 June 2012, SCCS/1459/11. Available at: https://ec.europa.eu/health/sites/health/files/scientific_committees/consumer_safety/docs/sccs_o_102.pdf
12   Uter W, Johansen JD, Börje A, Karlberg A-T, Lidén C, Rastogi S, Roberts D, White IR. Categorization of fragrance contact allergens for prioritization of preventive measures: clinical and experimental data and consideration of structure–activity relationships. Contact Dermatitis 2013;69:196-230
13   De Groot AC, Schmidt E. Essential oils: contact allergy and chemical composition. Boca Raton, Fl., USA: CRC Press, Taylor and Francis Group, 2016 (ISBN 9781482246407)
14   De Groot AC. Patch Testing, 4th Edition. Wapserveen, The Netherlands: acdegroot publishing, 2018 (ISBN 978-90-813233-4-5)

Chapter 6.38 LAVENDER OIL

IDENTIFICATION

Description/definition : Lavender oil (essential oil of lavender) is the essential oil obtained from the flowering tops of the (common, English, garden, true) lavender, *Lavandula angustifolia* Mill. (synonym: *Lavandula officinalis* Chaix)

INCI name(s) EU : Lavandula angustifolia oil; Lavandula officinalis flower oil (perfuming name, not an INCI name proper)

INCI name(s) USA : Lavandula angustifolia (lavender) oil

CAS registry number(s) : 8000-28-0; 90063-37-9; 84776-65-8

EC number(s) : 289-995-2; 283-994-0

RIFM monograph(s) : Food Cosmet Toxicol 1976;14:451 (binder, page 486)

SCCS opinion(s) : SCCS/1459/11 (45)

ISO standard : ISO 3515 Essential oil of lavender, 2001; Geneva, Switzerland, www.iso.org

Merck Index monograph : 6715

Function(s) in cosmetics : EU: masking; tonic; perfuming. USA: fragrance ingredients; skin-conditioning agents – miscellaneous

Patch testing : 2% pet. (Chemo [absolute], SPCanada); false-negative reactions occur with 2% (50,62); it may be preferable to test with oxidized lavender oil 6% pet. (66)

GENERAL

The lavender *Lavandula angustifolia* Mill. (synonyms: *Lavandula officinalis* Chaix, *Lavandula vera*), also known as medicinal lavender, true lavender, English lavender or common lavender, is an evergreen dwarf shrub, which can grow up to 75 centimeter. The plant is native to the Mediterranean region (France, Spain, Andorra, Italy), but is cultivated in many other countries as an ornamental and aromatic plant, including in Europe (especially France and Bulgaria, but also England, Moldova, Ukraine and former Yugoslavia), Africa, Australia and China (48).

The essential oil of lavender, which is obtained from the flowering tops by steam-distillation, is a very common fragrance ingredient. In food manufacturing, it is employed in flavoring beverages, ice-cream, candy, baked goods, and chewing gums. In traditional herbal medicine, it has many applications. In dermatology, lavender oil has been used for wounds, eczema, and psoriasis and even to promote hair growth in alopecia areata. Recent studies have investigated the effectiveness of lavender oils (sometimes in combination with other essential oils) in many health conditions. One of the major applications of lavender oil is in aromatherapy, especially for relief of anxiety, but also as a cure-all for mind, body and spirit, albeit with very little supportive evidence (48), although some would disagree to this statement (64,65).

Claimed biological properties of lavender and lavender oil have been reviewed in refs. 2 and 3. A useful review of various aspects of lavender (oil) is provided in ref. 25. Another review of various aspects of lavenders (lavender, lavandin, spike lavender), written from the industry's perspective, can be found (on-line) in a dissertation from the International Centre for Aroma Trades Studies, Plymouth, UK (1).

CHEMICAL COMPOSITION

Lavender oil is a pale yellowish liquid which has a fresh and floral to aromatic and woody odor. In lavender oils from various origins, over 450 chemicals have been identified. Nearly 110 of these were found in studies from before 1993 only. Of the more recent chemicals identified in lavender essential oils, about 52 per cent were found in a single reviewed publication only. The ten chemicals that had the highest maximum concentrations in 374 commercial lavender essential oil samples are shown in table 6.38.1 (Erich Schmidt, analytical data presented in ref. 48).

A full literature review of the qualitative and quantitative composition of commercial and non-commercial lavender oils of various origins, their chemotypes and with data from the ISO standard, has been published in 2016 (48).

Table 6.38.1 Ten ingredients with the highest concentrations in commercial lavender oils (48)

Name	Concentration range	Name	Concentration range
Linalool	26.0 - 44.8%	β-Caryophyllene	1.8 - 5.9%
Linalyl acetate	26.1 - 43.3%	(*E*)-β-Ocimene	0.7 - 4.7%
(*Z*)-β-Ocimene	0.3 - 7.5%	(*E*)-β-Farnesene	0.4 - 4.5%
Lavandulyl acetate	0.4 - 6.3%	Borneol	0.3 - 2.7%
Terpinen-4-ol	0.07 - 5.9%	1,8-Cineole	0.01 - 2.4%

CONTACT ALLERGY / ALLERGIC CONTACT DERMATITIS

General

The SCCS (Scientific Committee on Consumer Safety), in a 2012 Opinion on Fragrance allergens in cosmetic products, has marked Lavandula officinalis extract (synonym for angustifolia) as 'established contact allergen in humans' (45,46).

Fresh lavender oil is probably little allergenic. In this essential oil, the main ingredients are linalyl acetate (26-43%) and linalool (26-45%); caryophyllene (1.8-6%) is also an important constituent (48). It has been shown that lavender oil lacks protection against autoxidation and that 3 these terpenes are oxidized in air-exposed lavender oil to create hydroperoxides, which are strongly allergenic (30,49). Co-reactions between linalool and linalyl acetate may be explained by concurrent or successive sensitization, but also by the fact that linalyl acetate can be metabolically hydrolyzed in the skin to linalool (its corresponding alcohol) (49). See the chapters on linalool, linalyl acetate and caryophyllene.

Contact allergy to / allergic contact dermatitis from lavender oil has been reported in over 50 publications. In groups of consecutive patients suspected of contact dermatitis, prevalence rates of up to 2.8% positive patch test reactions have been observed, but definite relevance appears to be uncommon. The oil (2% in petrolatum) has been included in the screening series of the North American Contact Dermatitis Group (NACDG) since 2009. There have been many case reports of allergic contact dermatitis from lavender oil. Most cases were the result of their presence in topical pharmaceutical products. There are at least eleven cases of occupational allergic contact dermatitis from lavender oil, mostly in aromatherapists and other professionals who massage clients with the oil at their work. Cosmetics are an infrequent source of lavender contact allergy.

In several cases, there was a co-reaction to linalool, presumably the main allergen in lavender oil. Co-reactivity to linalyl acetate (oxidized) was sought for in one study and found in 34% of patients reacting to oxidized lavender oil (66). Caryophyllene may also have been an allergen. In the past, lavender oil was a frequent cause of pigmented cosmetic dermatitis in Japanese women.

A short review of contact allergy to lavender oil has been provided in 2016 (60).

Testing in groups of patients

The results of patch tests with lavender oil in routine testing (consecutive patients suspected of contact dermatitis) are shown in table 6.38.2 and those in groups of selected patients are shown in table 6.38.3. In routine testing, rates of positive reactions ranged from 0.2% to 2.8% (the highest rate was found when patients were tested with oxidized lavender oil 6% pet.) (66), whereas between 0.2% and 30% of patients in selected groups had positive patch tests. The very high positivity rate of 30% was found in a very small group of 10 patients strongly suspected of fragrance allergy and reacting to the fragrance mix (24).

Table 6.38.2 Patch testing in groups of patients: Routine testing

Years and Country	Test conc. & vehicle	Number of patients tested	positive (%)	Selection of patients (S); Relevance (R); Comments (C)	Ref.
2015-2017 NACDG	2% pet.	5594	28 (0.5%)	R: definite + probable relevance: 29%	71
2013-14 USA, Canada	2% pet.	4859	17 (0.3%)	R: definite + probable relevance: 42%	61
2009-14 USA, Canada	2% pet.	13,398	43 (0.3%)	R: of 11 patients reacting, but negative to FM I, FM II and balsam of Peru, 36% had definite + probable relevance	59
2011-12 USA, Canada	2% pet.	4229	16 (0.4%)	R: definite + probable relevance: 69%	32
2010-2011 China	2% pet.	296	2 (0.7%)	R: 82% for all fragrances tested together; C: the test substance was lavender absolute	54
2009-10 USA, Canada	2% pet.	4302	9 (0.2%)	R: definite + probable relevance: 30%	22
2008-2010 Sweden	6% pet., oxidized	1693	47 (2.8%)	R: not stated; C: 41% co-reacted to oxidized linalool 6%, 34% to oxidized linalyl acetate 6% and 20% to both	66
2002-2003 Korea	2% pet.	422	5 (1.2%)	R: not stated	33
<1973 Poland	2% pet.	200	4 (2.0%)	R: not stated	63

Case reports and case series

Occupational contact dermatitis

Two aromatherapists had contact dermatitis (one occupational) with allergies to multiple essential oils used at their work, including lavender oil. Both patients also reacted to geraniol, α-pinene, the fragrance mix and various other fragrance materials. In addition, one proved to be allergic to linalool and linalyl acetate, the other to caryophyllene; α-pinene, linalool, geraniol, and caryophyllene were demonstrated by GC-MS in the lavender oils (13). Linalool and linalyl acetate are the major ingredients of lavender oil and caryophyllene may be present in commercial lavender oils in concentrations up to 6%, but α-pinene and geraniol are not important components (48).

Table 6.38.3 Patch testing in groups of patients: Selected patient groups

Years and Country	Test conc. & vehicle	Number of patients tested | positive (%)		Selection of patients (S); Relevance (R); Comments (C)	Ref.
2014-2016 USA	2% pet.	45	1 (2%)	S: patients tested with a screening fragrance series; R: not stated; C: the test material was lavender absolute	72
2011-2015 Spain	2% pet.	607	22 (3.6%)	S: patients previously reacting to FM I, FM II, Myroxylon pereirae resin or hydroxyisohexyl 3-cyclohexene carboxaldehyde in the baseline series and subsequently tested with a fragrance series; R: not stated	70
2008-2014 UK	2% pet.	471	1 (0.2%)	S: patients tested with a fragrance series; R: not stated; C: the test material was an absolute	51
<2002 Japan, USA and 5 European countries	10% pet.	218	6 (2.8%)	S: patients previously shown to be allergic to fragrances; R: not stated	36
1990-1998 Japan	20% pet.	1443	53 (3.7%)	S: patients suspected of cosmetic contact dermatitis; virtu-all were women; R: 13/25 (52%) in 1997 and 1998; C: annual rates ranged from 0-13.9%; sudden increase in 1997 and 1998 from the placing of dried lavender flowers in pillows, drawers, cabinets or rooms and aromatherapy with lavender oil	6
1996-1997 UK	2% pet.	10	3 (30%)	S: patients strongly suspected of fragrance allergy; all also reacted to the fragrance mix; R: not stated	24
<1986 Poland	2% pet.	86	3 (3.5%)	S: patients previously reacting to the fragrance mix; R: not stated	23
<1974 Japan	?	183	6 (3.3%)	S: patients suspected of cosmetic dermatitis; R: unknown; in many, there was co-reactivity with geraniol, which is not an important component of commercial lavender oils	37

pet.: petrolatum

Another aromatherapist had occupational contact dermatitis from multiple essential oils, including lavender oil; the patient also reacted to lavender absolute (15). Yet another aromatherapist developed contact dermatitis from allergy to various essential oils, including lavender oil, used at work (16). Three cases of occupational allergic contact dermatitis in a masseuse, a physiotherapist and a reflexologist were caused by contact allergy to lavender oil and other essential oils (14).

An aromatherapist developed occupational contact dermatitis and proved to be allergic to lavender oil; she also reacted to neroli oil (4). A female 'complementary therapist' developed occupational contact dermatitis from a multitude of essential oils used at work, including lavender oil (17). A hairdresser who had occupational contact dermatitis of the hands developed contact allergy to lavender oil which was present in a shampoo used at work (9).

Another hairdresser developed occupational contact allergy to lavender oil from its presence in an eau de cologne (19). One case of occupational allergic contact dermatitis was observed in a porcelain painter due to lavender oil, oil of turpentine and oil of aniseed, which were mixed with pigments for painting (44).

Cosmetics

In a group of 70 patients with proven allergic cosmetic dermatitis, lavender oil was the allergen in two (42). Five positive patch test reactions to lavender oil, which was present in cosmetics that had given a positive patch test or had been positive in a usage test, were seen in a 9-year period in one clinic in Belgium (28). One patient had allergic contact dermatitis from 'Rose Absolute' perfume and a body lotion containing *Rosa centifolia*; she reacted to her own products, lavender oil, *Rosa centifolia*, several indicators of fragrance allergy, geranium oil Bourbon and various individual fragrance chemicals including linalool (29), which is a major component of commercial lavender oils, and limonene, which may be present in lower concentrations in commercial lavender oils (48).

Pharmaceutical products

In one clinic in Belgium, in the period 1990-2016, twenty cases of dermatitis caused by contact allergy to lavender oil from its presence as active principle in 'topical botanical medicines' have been observed (58). Twenty-four cases of contact sensitization to lavender oil present in topical pharmaceutical preparations were observed in Belgium (35). Two positive patch test reactions were seen to lavender oil which was present in a topical NSAID preparation used by patients suspected to be allergic to the NSAID; possible overlap with data from ref. 35 (34).

Allergy to lavender oil was the cause of allergic contact dermatitis from Phenergan cream in one patient (8). Another case of contact allergy to lavender oil in an antihistamine pharmaceutical cream was reported from France (18). Two patients developed allergic contact dermatitis from 'lavender essence' in topical pharmaceutical preparations (55,56). Another individual was allergic to a NSAID cream with lavender fragrance, and reacted to the cream and to lavender absolute (57)

Other products

One patient developed airborne contact dermatitis from contact allergy to lavender oil and two other products (jasmine absolute, rosewood oil) from aromatherapy lamps, whereby the water vapour produced distributes the essential oils as an aerosol in the air; the patient also reacted to linalool, which is an important constituent of all three oils (11). Two patients presented with dermatitis on their cheeks which proved to be caused by lavender drops applied on the pillow for their presumed hypnotic effects; a positive patch test to lavender oil was observed (12). One woman had eczema of the groins, vulva, and perianal area caused by tea tree oil and lavender gel containing lavender oil; the lavender gel reacted upon patch testing, as did lavender absolute 10% and 50% in petrolatum (26).

A man had extensive allergic airborne contact dermatitis from lemongrass, peppermint and possibly lavender oil from diffusing these essential oils at home and contact dermatitis from a lotion containing (unspecified) essential oils. As there were 22 positive patch test reactions, false-positives cannot be ruled out and are very likely (50). A woman had dermatitis on her face from contact allergy to neat lavender oil. The patch test to the product undiluted was positive, but there was no reaction to lavender oil 2% pet. (50)

A female patient presented with an 8-month history of facial dermatitis beginning on the malar cheeks and spreading to involve her forehead and chin. The patient applied essential oils, including lavender, macadamia nut (which is not an essential oil but vegetable oil), and sweet orange oil, to the affected areas. Patch tests gave positive reactions to the lavender oil used, tested undiluted, but not to sweet orange oil and macadamia nut oil. She was also tested with lavender oil 2%, which remained negative. The patient had several other reactions to plant products, but their relevance was not commented on (62).

A young boy treated his psoriasis with lavender oil which resulted in the clinical picture of allergic contact dermatitis, temporarily replacing psoriasis. Patch tests were positive to fragrance mixes I and II and to 'ylang ylang', which curiously were considered to be relevant. Apparently the patch test to lavender oil was negative, yet the authors suspected an immunologic reaction to a hapten in lavender oil (67).

Miscellaneous

Of 4 patients allergic to oxidized linalool, 4 (100%) co-reacted to oxidized lavender oil 4% pet. and 3 to oxidized linalyl acetate 4% pet. (30). The co-reactions to linalyl acetate was not unexpected, as linalyl acetate can be metabolically hydrolyzed in the skin to linalool (the corresponding alcohol) (49).

In a number of publications, positive patch tests to lavender oil have been reported with unknown, uncertain or unstated relevance. These include (literature screened up to 2014 [48]) the following. One positive patch test reaction to lavender oil 2% in petrolatum was found in a group of 31 patients allergic to oil of turpentine (5). Six positive patch test reactions to lavender oil were collected from various European patch test centers (7). A patient with airborne contact dermatitis from tea tree oil also reacted to lavender oil in patch testing (10). One beautician with occupational allergic hand dermatitis from products containing citral and certain essential oils also reacted to lavender oil and geranium oil; citral (neral + geranial) is not an important component of lavender oil (27).

One patient with erythema on the face reacted to lavender oil and other essential oils; their relevance was uncertain (39). Of seven patients allergic to the fragrance farnesol, 4 (57%) co-reacted to lavender oil (and various other fragrances) (40). In a group of 21 patients with dermatitis caused by perfumes and tested with a series of essential oils, five (24%) reacted to lavender absolute (41). In a group of 91 patients with cosmetic allergy, there was one patch test reaction to lavender oil; the relevance was not ascertained, but felt by the authors to be 'indicative' (43).

Pigmented cosmetic dermatitis

In Japan, in the 1960s and 1970s, many female patients developed pigmentation following dermatitis of the face (21). This so-called pigmented cosmetic dermatitis was shown to be caused by contact allergy to components of cosmetic products, notably essential oils, other fragrance materials, antimicrobials, preservatives and coloring materials (20,21). In a group of 620 Japanese patients with this condition investigated between 1970 and 1980, 4-7% had positive patch test reactions to lavender oil 20% in purified lanolin (20). The number of patients with pigmented cosmetic dermatitis decreased strongly after 1978, when major cosmetic companies began to eliminate strong contact sensitizers from their products (20).

OTHER SIDE EFFECTS

Photosensitivity

Photocontact allergy to lavender oil has been observed rarely (31).

Systemic side effects

In France, two children aged 2 years and 3 months who received a cosmetic baby balm on the skin of their thorax containing eucalyptus, rosemary and lavender essential oils, developed convulsions. As there was no other explanation for this and the 'neurologic toxicity of terpene derivatives is well known' (referring to studies on camphor toxicity), the cosmetic was suspected to be the culprit product. Although no specific terpene ingredient was blamed, the authors discussed the possible role of camphor, menthol and eucalyptol (1,8-cineole). On the basis of these 2 hardly convincing cases, the product was withdrawn from the market (47).

Repeated topical exposure to products containing lavender and tea tree oil was suggested to be the cause of prepubertal gynecomastia in three prepubertal boys. The explanation was that these oils may have estrogenic and antiandrogenic activity (52). The article received many critical reactions, but in a review article on side effects of essential oils in aromatherapy, the causality was classified as 'likely' (53). In another report, three more boys had prepubertal gynecomastia which was ascribed to 'lavender'. Two used a cologne called agua de violetas (violet water). Based on GC-MS, 'the appearance and the smell of the cologne', however, it was 'determined' that the cologne had lavender as an ingredient (68). In this article, too, the causal relationship between lavender (oil) and prepubertal gynecomastia is hardly convincing.

A 14-month old girl was found to have breast tissue of 2.5 cm bilaterally (premature thelarche). No cause was found. Over the next 12 months, the breast tissue enlarged to 3 cm bilaterally. Her parents then viewed a documentary discussing the link between lavender oil and breast development and revealed to medical staff that the child was exposed to a substantial amount of lavender oil body products. Her daily exposure included lavender wipes (20 wipes/day), lavender shampoo (5 mL alternate days), lavender body wash (5 mL daily), lavender moisturizing cream (10 mL daily) and lavender skin soothing lotion (10 mL daily). Specific lavender oil concentrations were unknown. The breast tissue, which was ascribed to endocrine disrupting estrogenic effects of lavender, receded 'immediately' following cessation of these products (69).

LITERATURE

1   Bosilcov A. Lavender: A key perfumery material. Dissertation. International Centre for Aroma Trades Studies, Plymouth University, Plymouth, UK, 2010

2   Prusinowska R, Śmigielski KB. Composition, biological properties and therapeutic effects of lavender (Lavandula angustifolia L.). A review. Herba Polonica 2014;60(2):56-66

3   Cavanagh HMA, Wilkinson JM. Biological activities of lavender essential oil. Phytother Res 2002;16:301-308

4   Keane FM, Smith HR, White IR, Rycroft RJG. Occupational allergic contact dermatitis in two aromatherapists. Contact Dermatitis 2000;43:49-51

5   Rudzki E, Grzywa Z, Bruo WS. Sensitivity to 35 essential oils. Contact Dermatitis 1976;2:196-200

6   Sugiura M, Hayakawa R, Kato Y, Sugiura K, Hashimoto R. Results of patch testing with lavender oil in Japan. Contact Dermatitis 2000;43:157-160

7   Calnan CD. Oil of cloves, laurel, lavender, peppermint. Contact Dermatitis Newsletter 1970;7:148

8   Zina G, Bonu G. Phenergan cream (role of base constituents). Contact Dermatitis Newsletter 1969;6:117

9   Brandao FM. Occupational allergy to lavender oil. Contact Dermatitis 1986;15:249-250

10 De Groot AC. Airborne allergic contact dermatitis from tea tree oil. Contact Dermatitis 1996;35:304-305

11 Schaller M, Korting HC. Allergic airborne contact dermatitis from essential oils used in aromatherapy. Clin Exp Dermatol 1995;20:143-145

12 Coulson IH, Ali Khan AS. Facial 'pillow' dermatitis due to lavender oil allergy. Contact Dermatitis 1999;41:111

13 Dharmagunawardena B, Takwale A, Sanders KJ, Cannan S, Roger A, Ilchyshyn A. Gas chromatography: an investigative tool in multiple allergies to essential oils. Contact Dermatitis 2002;47:288-292

14 Trattner A, David M, Lazarov A. Occupational contact dermatitis due to essential oils. Contact Dermatitis 2008;58:282-284

15 Bleasel N, Tate B, Rademaker M. Allergic contact dermatitis following exposure to essential oils. Australas J Dermatol 2002;43:211-213

16 Boonchai W, Lamtharachai P, Sunthonpalin P. Occupational allergic contact dermatitis from essential oils in aromatherapists. Contact Dermatitis 2007;56:181-182

17 Newsham J, Rai S, Williams JDL. Two cases of allergic contact dermatitis to neroli oil. Br J Dermatol 2011;165(suppl.1):76

18 Le Coulant P, Texier L, Malleville J, Doussy NN. Sensibilization à une crème antihistaminique. Bull Soc Franç Derm Syph 1964;71:234-237

19 Ménard E. Les dermatoses professionelles. Concours Médicale 1961;83:4308-4311

20 Nakayama H, Matsuo S, Hayakawa K, Takhashi K, Shigematsu T, Ota S. Pigmented cosmetic dermatitis. Int J Dermatol 1984;23:299-305

21 Nakayama H, Harada R, Toda M. Pigmented cosmetic dermatitis. Int J Dermatol 1976;15:673-675

22   Warshaw EM, Belsito DV, Taylor JS, Sasseville D, DeKoven JG, Zirwas MJ, et al. North American Contact Dermatitis Group patch test results: 2009 to 2010. Dermatitis 2013;24:50-59

23   Rudzki E, Grzywa Z. Allergy to perfume mixture. Contact Dermatitis 1986;15:115-116

24   Thomson KF, Wilkinson SM. Allergic contact dermatitis to plant extracts in patients with cosmetic dermatitis. Br J Dermatol 2000;142:84-88

25   Wu PA, James WD. Lavender. Dermatitis 2011;22:344-347

26   Varma S, Blackford S, Statham BN, Blackwell A. Combined contact allergy to tea tree oil and lavender oil complicating chronic vulvovaginitis. Contact Dermatitis 2000;42:309-310

27   De Mozzi P, Johnston GA. An outbreak of allergic contact dermatitis caused by citral in beauticians working in a health spa. Contact Dermatitis 2014;70:377-379

28   Nardelli A, Drieghe J, Claes L, Boey L, Goossens A. Fragrance allergens in 'specific' cosmetic products. Contact Dermatitis 2011;64:212-219

29   Nardelli A, Thijs L, Janssen K, Goossens A. Rosa centifolia in a 'non-scented' moisturizing body lotion as a cause of allergic contact dermatitis. Contact Dermatitis 2009;61:306-309

30   Hagvall L, Sköld M, Brared-Christensson J, Börje A, Karlberg A-T. Lavender oil lacks natural protection against autoxidation, forming strong contact allergens on air exposure. Contact Dermatitis 2008;59:143-150

31   Goiriz R, Delgado-Jiménez Y, Sánchez-Pérez J, García-Diez A. Photoallergic contact dermatitis from lavender oil in topical ketoprofen. Contact Dermatitis 2007;57:381-382

32   Warshaw EM, Maibach HI, Taylor JS, Sasseville D, DeKoven JG, Zirwas MJ, et al. North American Contact Dermatitis Group patch test results: 2011-2012. Dermatitis 2015;26:49-59

33   An S, Lee AY, Lee CH, Kim D-W, Hahm JH, Kim K-J, et al. Fragrance contact dermatitis in Korea: a joint study. Contact Dermatitis 2005;53:320-323

34   Matthieu L, Meuleman L, van Hecke E, Blondeel A, Dezfoulian B, Constandt L, Goossens A. Contact and photocontact allergy to ketoprofen. The Belgian experience. Contact Dermatitis 2004;50:238-241

35   Nardelli A, D'Hooge E, Drieghe J, Dooms M, Goossens A. Allergic contact dermatitis from fragrance components in specific topical pharmaceutical products in Belgium. Contact Dermatitis 2009;60:303-313

36   Larsen W, Nakayama H, Fischer T, Elsner P, Frosch P, Burrows D, et al. Fragrance contact dermatitis – a worldwide multicenter investigation (Part III). Contact Dermatitis 2002;46:141-144

37   Nakayama H, Hanaoka H, Ohshiro A. Allergen Controlled System (ACS). Tokyo, Japan: Kanehara Shuppan, 1974:42. Data cited in ref. 38

38   Mitchell JC. Contact hypersensitivity to some perfume materials. Contact Dermatitis 1975;1:196-199

39   Srivastava PK, Bajaj AK. Ylang-ylang oil not an uncommon sensitizer in India. Indian J Dermatol 2014;59:200-201

40   Goossens A, Merckx L. Allergic contact dermatitis from farnesol in a deodorant. Contact Dermatitis 1997;37:179-180

41   Meynadier JM, Meynadier J, Peyron JL, Peyron L. Formes cliniques des manifestations cutanées d'allergie aux parfums. Ann Dermatol Venereol 1986;113:31-39

42   Schorr WF. Cosmetic allergy: Diagnosis, incidence, and management. Cutis 1974;14:844-850

43   Ngangu Z, Samsoen M, Foussereau J. Einige Aspekte zur Kosmetika-allergie in Strassburg. Dermatosen 1983;31:126-129

44   Vente C, Fuchs T. Contact dermatitis due to oil of turpentine in a porcelain painter. Contact Dermatitis 1997;37:187

45   SCCS (Scientific Committee on Consumer Safety). Opinion on Fragrance allergens in cosmetic products, 26-27 June 2012, SCCS/1459/11. Available at: https://ec.europa.eu/health/sites/health/files/scientific_committees/consumer_safety/docs/sccs_o_102.pdf

46   Uter W, Johansen JD, Börje A, Karlberg A-T, Lidén C, Rastogi S, Roberts D, White IR. Categorization of fragrance contact allergens for prioritization of preventive measures: clinical and experimental data and consideration of structure–activity relationships. Contact Dermatitis 2013;69:196-230

47   Laribière A, Miremont-Salamé G, Bertrand S, François C, Haramburu F. Terpènes dans les cosmétiques: 2 cas d'épilepsie. Thérapie 2005;60: 607-609

48   De Groot AC, Schmidt E. Essential oils: contact allergy and chemical composition. Boca Raton, Fl., USA: CRC Press, Taylor and Francis Group, 2016 (ISBN 9781482246407)

49   Sköld M, Hagvall L, Karlberg AT. Autoxidation of linalyl acetate, the main component of lavender oil, creates potent contact allergens. Contact Dermatitis 2008;58:9-14

50   Grey KR, Hagen SL, Warshaw EM. Essential oils: emerging "medicaments". Dermatitis 2016;27:227-228

51   Sabroe RA, Holden CR, Gawkrodger DJ. Contact allergy to essential oils cannot always be predicted from allergy to fragrance markers in the baseline series. Contact Dermatitis 2016;74:236-241

52   Henley DV, Lipson N, Korach KS, Bloch CA. Brief report - Prepubertal gynecomastia linked to lavender and tea tree oils. N Engl J Med 2007;356:479-485

53 Posadzki P, Alotaibi A, Ernst E. Adverse effects of aromatherapy: a systematic review of case reports and case series. Int J Risk Saf Med 2012;24:147-161

54 Liu J, Li L-F. Contact sensitization to fragrances other than fragrance mix I in China. Contact Dermatitis 2015;73:252-253

55 Izu R, Aguirre A, Gil N, Díaz-Pérez JL. Allergic contact dermatitis from a cream containing Centella asiatica extract. Contact Dermatitis 1992;26:192-193

56 Aguirre A, Gardeazábal J, Izu R, Ratón JA, Díaz-Pérez JL. Allergic contact dermatitis due to plant extracts in a multisensitized patient. Contact Dermatitis 1993;28:186-187

57 Rademaker M. Allergic contact dermatitis from lavender fragrance in Difflam gel. Contact Dermatitis 1994;31:58-59

58 Gilissen L, Huygens S, Goossens A. Allergic contact dermatitis caused by topical herbal remedies: importance of patch testing with the patients' own products. Contact Dermatitis 2018;78:177-184

59 Warshaw EM, Zug KA, Belsito DV, Fowler JF Jr, DeKoven JG, Sasseville D, et al. Positive patch-test reactions to essential oils in consecutive patients: Results from North America and Central Europe. Dermatitis 2017;28:246-252

60 De Groot AC, Schmidt E. Essential Oils, Part V: Peppermint oil, lavender oil, and lemongrass oil. Dermatitis 2016; 27:325-332

61 DeKoven JG, Warshaw EM, Belsito DV, Sasseville D, Maibach HI, Taylor JS, et al. North American Contact Dermatitis Group Patch Test Results: 2013-2014. Dermatitis 2017;28:33-46

62 Grey KR, Hagen SL, Warshaw EM. Essential oils: Emerging "medicaments". Dermatitis 2016;27:227-228

63 Rudzki E, Kielak D. Sensitivity to some compounds related to Balsam of Peru. Contact Dermatitis Newsletter 1972;nr.13:335-336

64 Malcolm BJ, Tallian K. Essential oil of lavender in anxiety disorders: Ready for prime time? Ment Health Clin 2018;7:147-155

65 Ozkaraman A, Dügüm Ö, Özen Yılmaz H, Usta Yesilbalkan Ö. Aromatherapy: The effect of lavender on anxiety and sleep quality in patients treated with chemotherapy. Clin J Oncol Nurs 2018;22:203-210

66 Hagvall L, Christensson JB. Patch testing with main sensitizers does not detect all cases of contact allergy to oxidized lavender oil. Acta Derm Venereol 2016;96:679-683

67 Brown ME, Browning JC. A Case of psoriasis replaced by allergic contact dermatitis in a 12-year-old boy. Pediatr Dermatol 2016;33:e125-126

68 Diaz A, Luque L, Badar Z, Kornic S, Danon M. Prepubertal gynecomastia and chronic lavender exposure: report of three cases. J Pediatr Endocrinol Metab 2016;29:103-107

69 Linklater A, Hewitt JK. Premature thelarche in the setting of high lavender oil exposure. J Paediatr Child Health 2015;51:235

70 Silvestre JF, Mercader P, González-Pérez R, Hervella-Garcés M, Sanz-Sánchez T, Córdoba S, et al. Sensitization to fragrances in Spain: A 5-year multicentre study (2011-2015). Contact Dermatitis. 2018 Nov 14. doi: 10.1111/cod.13152. [Epub ahead of print]

71 DeKoven JG, Warshaw EM, Zug KA, Maibach HI, Belsito DV, Sasseville D, et al. North American Contact Dermatitis Group patch test results: 2015-2016. Dermatitis 2018;29:297-309

72 Nath NS, Liu B, Green C, Atwater AR. Contact allergy to hydroperoxides of linalool and d-limonene in a US population. Dermatitis 2017;28:313-316

Chapter 6.39   LEMON OIL

IDENTIFICATION

Description/definition	: Lemon oil (essential oil of lemon) is the essential oil obtained from the pericarp (peel) of the lemon, *Citrus limon* (L.) Burm. f.
INCI name(s) EU	: Citrus limon peel oil
INCI name(s) USA	: Citrus limon (lemon) peel oil
CAS registry number(s)	: 84929-31-7; 8008-56-8
EC number(s)	: 284-515-8
CIR review(s)	: Final report, 09/09/2014 (access: www.cir-safety.org/ingredients)
RIFM monograph(s)	: Food Cosmet Toxicol 1974;12:725 (binder, 491); Food Cosmet Toxicol 1974;12;727 (binder, page 493) (lemon oil, distilled)
IFRA standard	: Restricted (www.ifraorg.org/en-us/standards-library) (table 6.39.1)
SCCS opinion(s)	: Various (26); SCCNFP/0392/00, final (27); SCCNFP/0389/00, final (28); SCCS/1459/11 (29)
ISO standard	: ISO 855 Essential oil of lemon, obtained by expression, 2003; Geneva, Switzerland, www.iso.org
Merck Index monograph	: 8160
Function(s) in cosmetics	: EU: masking; perfuming; skin conditioning. USA: fragrance ingredients; skin-conditioning agents - miscellaneous
EU cosmetic restrictions	: Regulated in Annex II/358R1 of the Regulation (EC) No. 1223/2009, regulated by 95/34/EC
Patch testing	: 2% pet. (SPEurope [flower, leaf, stem extract], SPCanada); test also limonene (see Chapter 3.95 Limonene)

Table 6.39.1 IFRA restrictions for lemon oil cold pressed

Leave-on products:	2%
Rinse-off products:	no restriction
Non-skin contact products:	no restriction

The limit only applies to applications on skin exposed to sunshine, excluding rinse-off products. If combinations of phototoxic fragrance ingredients are used, the use levels have to be reduced accordingly. The sum of the concentrations of all phototoxic ingredients, expressed in % of their recommended maximum level in the consumer product shall not exceed 100

GENERAL

Citrus limon (L.) Burm. f. is a small evergreen tree that produces ellipsoidal yellow fruit, the lemon. The origin of the lemon tree is unknown, likely south China and Myanmar. It is cultivated in many subtropical countries. The main producing countries are China, Mexico, and India, followed by Argentina, Brazil, the USA, Turkey, Spain, Iran and Italy, notably the south (Calabria, Sicily). Most of the production of lemons is destined for extracting the juice from the fruits. Lemon juice has many applications in food and beverages, serves cosmetic, pharmaceutical and several technical purposes, is exploited as a source of vitamin C, pectin, and enzymes and may be used for cleaning (due to its acidity; the juice may contain up to 6% citric acid) (31).

After extraction of the juice many 'waste'-products, including peel, membranes and seeds, remain. From the peel of the fruits the essential oil of lemon is obtained by cold-pressing, which is widely used in the food and beverage industries as flavoring agent, e.g. in baked goods, confectionery, desserts, ice creams, and soft and alcoholic drinks. In the pharmaceutical industries it is used as flavoring agent to mask unpleasant tastes of drugs. In perfumery, it forms the base of many fragrance compositions and is employed in other cosmetic products as well.

The essential oil of lemon is also useful as a wood cleaner and polish, where its solvent properties are employed to dissolve old wax, fingerprints, and grime. In addition, lemon oil may serve as a nontoxic insecticide treatment, had some medical applications and is also employed in aromatherapy practices (4,5,31).

The history, global distribution, and nutritional importance of lemon and other *Citrus* fruits have been reviewed in ref. 1.

CHEMICAL COMPOSITION

Lemon oil is a pale yellow to dark green, clear mobile liquid, sometimes cloudy at lower temperature, which has a fresh citrusy green peel note odor. In lemon oils from various origins, over 245 chemicals have been identified. The ten chemicals that had the highest maximum concentrations in 178 commercial lemon essential oil samples are shown in table 6.39.2 (Erich Schmidt, analytical data presented in ref. 31).

A full literature review of the qualitative and quantitative composition of commercial and non-commercial lemon oils of various origins and with data from the ISO standard, has been published in 2016 (31). Older reviews can be found in refs. 2 and 3.

Table 6.39.2 Ten ingredients with the highest concentrations in commercial lemon oils (31)

Name	Concentration range	Name	Concentration range
Limonene	53.5 - 73.0%	Myrcene	1.2 - 2.2%
β-Pinene	7.4 - 17.8%	p-Cymene	0.1 - 2.2%
γ-Terpinene	3.1 - 12.4%	Geranial	0.6 - 2.1%
Sabinene	1.1 - 2.9%	Neral	0.3 - 1.4%
α-Pinene	1.5 - 2.4%	Geranyl acetate	0.1 - 1.3%

CONTACT ALLERGY / ALLERGIC CONTACT DERMATITIS

General

The SCCS (Scientific Committee on Consumer Safety), in a 2012 Opinion on Fragrance allergens in cosmetic products, has marked lemon oil as 'established contact allergen in humans' (29,30).

Contact allergy to / allergic contact dermatitis from lemon oil has been reported in 20 publications. In groups of consecutive patients suspected of contact dermatitis, prevalence rates of up to 0.9% positive patch test reactions have been observed, but adequate relevance data are lacking. There have been several case reports of allergic contact dermatitis from lemon oil, mostly from occupational exposure. In one such report, limonene and β-pinene may have been allergens in lemon oil.

Testing in groups of patients

The results of patch tests with lemon oil in routine testing (consecutive patients suspected of contact dermatitis) and in groups of selected patients are shown in table 6.39.3. In routine testing, rates of positive reactions ranged from 0.5% to 0.9%, whereas between 0.3% and 10% of patients in selected groups had positive patch tests.

Table 6.39.3 Patch testing in groups of patients

Years and Country	Test conc. & vehicle	Number of patients tested	positive (%)	Selection of patients (S); Relevance (R); Comments (C)	Ref.
Routine testing					
2000-2007 USA	2% pet.	345	3 (0.9%)	R: 100%; C: weak study: a. high rate of macular erythema and weak reactions, b. relevance figures include 'questionable' and 'past' relevance	6
<1976 Poland	2% pet.	200	1 (0.5%)	R: not stated	12
Testing in groups of selected patients					
2000-2008 IVDK	2% pet.	6467	17 (0.3%)	S: patients with dermatitis suspected of causal exposure to fragrances; R: not stated; C: no frequent co-reactivity to limonene, the main component of citrus oils	17
1997-2000 Austria	2% pet.	747	2 (0.3%)	S: patients suspected of fragrance allergy; R: not stated	8
1989-1999 Portugal	2% pet.	67	3 (4.5%)	S: patients who had a positive patch test to the fragrance mix; R: not stated	18
1996-1997 UK	2% pet.	10	1 (10%)	S: patients suspected of cosmetic dermatitis and reacting to the fragrance mix; R: not stated	7
1986 France	1% pet.	21	2 (10%)	S: patients with dermatitis caused by perfumes; R: not stated	22
<1986 Poland	2% pet.	86	2 (2.3%)	S: patients previously reacting to the fragrance mix; R: not stated	13
<1976 Poland	2% pet.	51	1 (2.0%)	S: patients allergic to Myroxylon pereirae resin (balsam of Peru) and/or turpentine and/or wood tar and/or colophony	12

IVDK Information Network of Departments of Dermatology, Germany, Switzerland, Austria (www.ivdk.org); pet.: petrolatum

Case reports and case series

Occupational contact dermatitis

An aromatherapist had chronic hand dermatitis and was patch test positive to 17 of 20 oils used at her work (tested 1% and 5% in petrolatum), including lemon oil (9). Two other aromatherapists had contact dermatitis (one occupational) with allergies to multiple essential oils used at their work, including lemon oil. Both patients also reacted to geraniol, α-pinene, the fragrance mix and various other fragrance materials. In addition, one proved to be allergic to linalool and linalyl acetate, the other to caryophyllene. α-Pinene and caryophyllene were demonstrated by GC-MS in one of the lemon oils, but limonene was not tested (10). α-Pinene may be present in commercial lemon oils in concentrations up to 2.5% (31).

One physiotherapist developed occupational contact dermatitis, which proved to be caused by contact allergy to lemon oil and other essential oils (11). Two cases of occupational allergic contact dermatitis to 'lemon oil terpenes' (tested 1% in olive oil) in bottle fillers in a perfume factory have been reported (15). A positive patch test to lemon oil considered to be relevant was observed in a case of occupational hand dermatitis in a cook / barman / fruit grower, who also reacted to lemongrass oil, neroli oil and geraniol. The patient was patch tested with 'essences' (no concentration mentioned), but from the text it seems that this would indicate essential oils. Geraniol is not an important constituent of lemon oil (16).

One case of occupational contact dermatitis of the fingers of both hands was considered to be caused by allergy to geraniol present in lemon oil and lemon peel, with which she came in contact while working in a company for baking ingredients (20); however, geraniol is not an important component of lemon oils (31). A porter became sensitized to oil of lemon, which he used occupationally; patch tests were positive to oil of lemon, limonene, oil of citronella Java, oil of citronella Ceylon (= Sri Lanka), turpentine and its component β-pinene (21). Limonene is the major ingredient in lemon oil and β-pinene can also be present in these oils in high concentrations (maximum concentration found in commercial lemon oils: 17.8%, table 6.39.2).

Non-occupational allergic contact dermatitis
One patient had developed pigmented contact dermatitis from contact allergy to lemon oil, geraniol and hydroxycitronellal present in a face compact powder (19). Another patient suffering from oral lichenoid mucositis had relevant positive patch test reactions to lemon oil, clove oil and metals (23).

Miscellaneous
In a number of publications, positive patch tests to lemon oil have been reported with unknown, uncertain or unstated relevance. These include (literature screened up to 2014 [31]) the following. One positive patch test reaction to lemon oil in a patient with airborne allergic contact dermatitis from tea tree oil and lavender oil (14). Two positive patch test reactions among 20 workers in a perfume factory without dermatitis (15). One patient had allergic contact dermatitis from a 'natural' deodorant containing lichen acids; reactions were seen to the deodorant, lichen acid mix, usnic acid and some essential oils including lemon oil (24). One positive patch test to lemon oil, possibly from its presence in a topical pharmaceutical preparation (25).

OTHER SIDE EFFECTS

Photosensitivity
Photosensitivity from lemon oil has been cited in ref. 32.

LITERATURE
1   Liu YQ, Heying E, Tanumihardjo SA. History, global distribution, and nutritional importance of Citrus fruits. Compreh Rev Food Sci Food Saf 2012;11:530-545
2   Kirbaşlar I, Boz I, Kirbaşlar G. Composition of Turkish lemon and grapefruit peel oils. J Essent Oil Res 2006;18:525-543
3   Baratta MT, Dorman HJD, Deans SG, Figueiredo AC, Barroso JG, Ruberto G. Antimicrobial and antioxidant properties of some commercial essential oils. Flavour Fragr J 1998;13:235-244
4   Rhind JP. Essential oils. A handbook for aromatherapy practice, 2nd Edition. London: Singing Dragon, 2012
5   Lawless J. The encyclopedia of essential oils, 2nd Edition. London: Harper Thorsons, 2014
6   Wetter DA, Yiannias JA, Prakash AV, Davis MD, Farmer SA, el-Azhary RA, et al. Results of patch testing to personal care product allergens in a standard series and a supplemental cosmetic series: an analysis of 945 patients from the Mayo Clinic Contact Dermatitis Group, 2000-2007. J Am Acad Dermatol 2010;63:789-798
7   Thomson KF, Wilkinson SM. Allergic contact dermatitis to plant extracts in patients with cosmetic dermatitis. Br J Dermatol 2000;142:84-88
8   Wöhrl S, Hemmer W, Focke M, Götz M, Jarisch R. The significance of fragrance mix, balsam of Peru, colophonium and propolis as screening tools in the detection of fragrance allergy. Br J Dermatol 2001;145:268-273
9   Selvaag E, Holm J, Thune P. Allergic contact dermatitis in an aromatherapist with multiple sensitizations to essential oils. Contact Dermatitis 1995;33:354-355
10 Dharmagunawardena B, Takwale A, Sanders KJ, Cannan S, Roger A, Ilchyshyn A. Gas chromatography: an investigative tool in multiple allergies to essential oils. Contact Dermatitis 2002;47:288-292

11 Trattner A, David M, Lazarov A. Occupational contact dermatitis due to essential oils. Contact Dermatitis 2008;58:282-284

12 Rudzki E, Grzywa Z, Bruo WS. Sensitivity to 35 essential oils. Contact Dermatitis 1976;2:196-200

13 Rudzki E, Grzywa Z. Allergy to perfume mixture. Contact Dermatitis 1986;15:115-116

14 De Groot AC. Airborne allergic contact dermatitis from tea tree oil. Contact Dermatitis 1996;35:304-305

15 Schubert HJ. Skin diseases in workers at a perfume factory. Contact Dermatitis 2006;55:81-83

16 Audicana M, Bernaola G. Occupational contact dermatitis from citrus fruits: Lemon essential oils. Contact Dermatitis 1994;31:183-185

17 Uter W, Schmidt E, Geier J, Lessmann H, Schnuch A, Frosch P. Contact allergy to essential oils: current patch test results (2000–2008) from the Information Network of Departments of Dermatology (IVDK). Contact Dermatitis 2010;63:277-283

18 Manuel Brites M, Goncalo M, Figueiredo A. Contact allergy to fragrance mix - a 10-year study. Contact Dermatitis 2000;43:181-182

19 Serrano G, Pujol C, Cuadra J, Gallo S, Aliaga A. Riehl's melanosis: Pigmented contact dermatitis caused by fragrances. J Am Acad Dermatol 1989;21:1057-1060

20 Hausen BM, Kulenkamp D. Geraniol-Kontaktallergie. Z Hautkr 1990;65:492-494

21 Keil H. Contact dermatitis due to oil of citronellal. J Invest Dermatol 1947;8:327-334

22 Meynadier JM, Meynadier J, Peyron JL, Peyron L. Formes cliniques des manifestations cutanées d'allergie aux parfums. Ann Dermatol Venereol 1986;113:31-39

23 Yiannias JA, el-Azhary RA, Hand JH, Pakzad SY, Rogers RS III. Relevant contact sensitivities in patients with the diagnosis of oral lichen planus. J Am Acad Dermatol 2000;42:177-182

24 Sheu M, Simpson EL, Law SV, Storrs FJ. Allergic contact dermatitis from a natural deodorant: A report of 4 cases associated with lichen acid mix allergy. J Am Acad Dermatol 2006;55:332-337

25 Nardelli A, D'Hooge E, Drieghe J, Dooms M, Goossens A. Allergic contact dermatitis from fragrance components in specific topical pharmaceutical products in Belgium. Contact Dermatitis 2009;60:303-313

26 Various SCCS Opinions, available at: http://ec.europa.eu/growth/tools-databases/cosing/index.cfm?fuseaction=search.details_v2&id=28697

27 Opinion of the Scientific Committee on Cosmetic Products and Non-Food Products Intended for Consumers concerning 'An initial list of perfumery materials which must not form part of cosmetic products except subject to the Restrictions and Conditions laid down, 25 September 2001, SCCNFP/0392/00, final. Available at: http://ec.europa.eu/health/archive/ph_risk/committees/sccp/documents/out150_en.pdf

28 Opinion of the Scientific Committee on Cosmetic Products and Non-Food Products Intended for Consumers concerning 'The 1st update of the inventory of ingredients employed in cosmetic products. Section II: Perfume and aromatic raw materials', 24 October 2000, SCCNFP/0389/00, final. Available at: http://ec.europa.eu/health/ph_risk/committees/sccp/documents/out131_en.pdf

29 SCCS (Scientific Committee on Consumer Safety). Opinion on Fragrance allergens in cosmetic products, 26-27 June 2012, SCCS/1459/11. Available at: https://ec.europa.eu/health/sites/health/files/scientific_committees/consumer_safety/docs/sccs_o_102.pdf

30 Uter W, Johansen JD, Börje A, Karlberg A-T, Lidén C, Rastogi S, Roberts D, White IR. Categorization of fragrance contact allergens for prioritization of preventive measures: clinical and experimental data and consideration of structure–activity relationships. Contact Dermatitis 2013;69:196-230

31 De Groot AC, Schmidt E. Essential oils: contact allergy and chemical composition. Boca Raton, Fl., USA: CRC Press, Taylor and Francis Group, 2016 (ISBN 9781482246407)

32 De Groot AC. Patch Testing, 4th Edition. Wapserveen, The Netherlands: acdegroot publishing, 2018 (ISBN 978-90-813233-4-5)

Chapter 6.40   LEMONGRASS OIL

There are two main lemongrass oils, derived from two species of the *Cymbopogon* family, lemongrass oil derived from *Cymbopogon flexuosus* (East Indian type) and West Indian type lemongrass oil, obtained from *Cymbopogon citratus*.

6.40.1 LEMONGRASS OIL EAST INDIAN

IDENTIFICATION

Description/definition	: Lemongrass oil (essential oil of lemongrass) East Indian is the essential oil obtained from the aerial part (leaves) of the (East Indian, Malabar) lemongrass, *Cymbopogon flexuosus* (Nees ex Steudel) J.F. Watson
INCI name(s) EU & USA	: Cymbopogon flexuosus oil
CAS registry number(s)	: 8007-02-1; 8055-93-4
EC number(s)	: 295-161-9
RIFM monograph(s)	: Food Cosmet Toxicol 1976;14:455 and 457 (binder, pages 489 and 490)
SCCS opinion(s)	: SCCS/1459/11 (23)
ISO standard	: ISO 4718 Oil of lemongrass, 2004; Geneva, Switzerland, www.iso.org
Function(s) in cosmetics	: EU: masking. USA: fragrance ingredients
Patch testing	: 2% pet. (SPEurope, SPCanada; formerly from C. flexuosus, currently from *C. Schoenanthus*)

GENERAL

Cymbopogon flexuosus (Nees ex Steudel) J.F. Watson is a perennial grass with stems that may measure 200-300 cm and aromatic leaves that may be 50-100 cm long. This so-called East Indian lemongrass is native to China, India, Nepal, Myanmar, Malaysia and Thailand and is cultivated in India, south-east Asia, Equatorial Africa, in the Caribbean and in Guatemala for the production of (East Indian) lemongrass oil (synonyms: Cochin lemongrass oil, Malabar oil).

The volatile essential oil obtained from lemongrass leaves by steam-distillation has a variety of uses in the perfumery, cosmetics and pharmaceutical industries and also for flavoring curries, wines, beverages and herbal teas. It may also be added to waxes, polishes, detergents and insecticides (25). However, lemongrass oil is mainly used for the isolation of citral. Citral is the major active component found in lemongrass oil and the quality of the oil is measured by the citral content. Citral is a mixture of geranial (citral A = (*E*)-citral = α-citral) and neral (citral B = (*Z*)-citral = β-citral), of which large quantities are being utilized for production of a number of chemicals such as α- and β-ionones, vitamins A and E and β-carotene. The oil is perceived to have efficacy to treat a wide variety of health conditions and is also used in aromatherapy (25).

CHEMICAL COMPOSITION

Lemongrass oil is a clear, mobile liquid with tender yellow to light yellowish brown color, which has a fresh citrusy, slightly green metallic odor, reminding of citral. In lemongrass oils from various origins, over 175 chemicals have been identified. About 52 per cent of these were found in a single reviewed publication only. The ten chemicals that had the highest maximum concentrations in 54 commercial lemongrass East Indian essential oil samples are shown in table 6.40.1.1 (Erich Schmidt, analytical data presented in ref. 25).

A full literature review of the qualitative and quantitative composition of commercial and non-commercial lemongrass East Indian oils of various origins, their chemotypes and with data from the ISO standard, has been published in 2016 (25).

Table 6.40.1.1 Ten ingredients with the highest concentrations in commercial citronella oils East Indian (25)

Name	Concentration range	Name	Concentration range
Geranial	35.8 - 46.3%	Myrcene	0.07 - 5.0%
Neral	27.5 - 35.5%	Camphene	0.08 - 2.6%
Geraniol	1.5 - 6.6%	(*E*)-Isocitral	0.5 - 2.3%
Geranyl acetate	1.0 - 6.0%	α-Terpinene	0.02 - 2.3%
Limonene	0.1 - 5.7%	6-Methyl-5-hepten-2-one	0.4 - 2.1%

6.40.2 LEMONGRASS OIL WEST INDIAN

IDENTIFICATION

Description/definition	: Lemongrass oil, West Indian type (essential oil of lemongrass) is the essential oil obtained from the whole aerial part (leaves) of the West Indian lemongrass, *Cymbopogon citratus* (DC) Stapf.
INCI name(s) EU & USA	: Cymbopogon citratus leaf oil
CAS registry number(s)	: 8007-02-1; 89998-14-1
EC number(s)	: 289-752-0
SCCS opinion(s)	: SCCS/1459/11 (23)
ISO standard	: ISO 3217 Essential oil of lemongrass, 2000; Geneva, Switzerland, www.iso.org
Function(s) in cosmetics	: EU: masking; perfuming. USA: antioxidants; fragrance ingredients; skin-conditioning agents - miscellaneous
Patch testing	: 2% pet.; based on RIFM data, 5% pet. is probably not irritant (29)

GENERAL

Cymbopogon citratus (DC) Stapf. is a tall, aromatic, perennial grass with culms (stems) up to two meter tall and linear leaves, up to one meter long and two centimeter wide. Lemongrass is native to India and Indonesia, and introduced and cultivated in most of the tropics, including Africa (Algeria, Egypt, Morocco), South America (including the Carribean islands and Central America) and Indo-China (25). A general introduction to lemongrass and lemongrass oils is provided in the section 'General' of lemongrass oil East Indian above.

CHEMICAL COMPOSITION

West Indian lemongrass oil is a clear mobile liquid with a soft yellow to yellowish orange color which has a strong lemon note, reminding of citral odor. In lemongrass oils, West Indian type, from various origins, over 245 chemicals have been identified. About 57 per cent of these were found in a single reviewed publication only. The ten chemicals that had the highest maximum concentrations in 32 commercial lemongrass West Indian essential oil samples are shown in table 6.40.2.1 (Erich Schmidt, analytical data provided in ref. 25).

A full literature review of the qualitative and quantitative composition of commercial and non-commercial lemongrass West Indian oils of various origins, their chemotypes and with data from the ISO standard, has been published in 2016 (25).

Table 6.40.2.1 Ten ingredients with the highest concentrations in commercial lemongrass West Indian oils (25)

Name	Concentration range	Name	Concentration range
Geranial	41.8 - 46.3%	β-Caryophyllene	0.4 - 3.0%
Neral	30.3 - 33.3%	Citronellal	0.2 - 1.9%
Geraniol	3.0 - 7.9%	Elemol	0.02 - 1.8%
Limonene	0.4 - 5.0%	(*E*)-Isocitral	1.4 - 1.7%
Geranyl acetate	1.0 - 4.3%	Linalool	0.6 - 1.4%

CONTACT ALLERGY / ALLERGIC CONTACT DERMATITIS

Lemongrass oil (unspecified)

General

Contact allergy to / allergic contact dermatitis from lemongrass oil has been reported in at least 25 publications. With three exceptions (15,19,27: test substances recorded as East Indian lemongrass oil) all studies have related to 'lemongrass oil', without specifying the botanical origin. In groups of consecutive patients suspected of contact dermatitis, prevalence rates of up to 1.6% positive patch test reactions have been observed, but adequate relevance data are lacking. There have been several case reports of allergic contact dermatitis from lemongrass oil, mostly from occupational exposure. In one case of a cosmetic reaction, citral (the combination of neral and geranial, both the dominant ingredients in lemongrass oils) was the allergenic component; in another report, geraniol may have been an allergen. Undiluted lemongrass oil is a strong irritant and may sensitize (21).

A short review of contact allergy to lemongrass oil has been provided in 2016 (28).

Testing in groups of patients

The results of patch tests with lemongrass oil in routine testing (consecutive patients suspected of contact dermatitis) and in groups of selected patients are shown in table 6.40.2.2. In routine testing, rates of positive reactions ranged from 0.6% to 1.6%, whereas between 0.8% and 20% of patients in selected groups had positive patch tests. The high positivity rate of 20% was seen in a very small group of 10 patients with fragrance contact allergy (2).

Table 6.40.2.2 Patch testing in groups of patients

Years and Country	Test conc. & vehicle	Number of patients tested	positive (%)	Selection of patients (S); Relevance (R); Comments (C)	Ref.
Routine testing					
2000-2008 IVDK	2% pet.	2435	14 (0.6%)	R: not stated	12
2000-2007 USA	2% pet.	868	11 (1.3%)	R: 100%; C: weak study: a. high rate of macular erythema and weak reactions, b. relevance figures include 'questionable' and 'past' relevance	1
1999-2000 Denmark	2% pet.	318	4 (1.3%)	R: not specified; C: this study was part of the international study mentioned below (ref. 15); the test preparation was East Indian lemongrass oil	19
1998-2000 six European countries	2% pet.	1606	25 (1.6%)	R: not specified for individual oils/chemicals; C: the test preparation was East Indian lemongrass oil	15
Testing in groups of selected patients					
2011-2015 Spain	2% pet.	406	11 (2.7%)	S: patients previously reacting to FM I, FM II, Myroxylon pereirae resin or hydroxyisohexyl 3-cyclohexene carboxaldehyde in the baseline series and subsequently tested with a fragrance series; R: not stated	31
2008-2014 UK	2% pet.	471	7 (1.5%)	S: patients tested with a fragrance series; R: not stated; the test material was from *C. flexuosus*	27
2007-2011 IVDK	2% pet.	45	6 (13.3%)	S: physical therapists; R: not stated	30
2001-2010 Australia	2% pet.	837	45 (5.4%)	S: not specified; R: 56%	18
2000-2008 IVDK	2% pet.	8445	190 (2.2%)	S: patients with dermatitis suspected of causal exposure to fragrances; R: not stated; C: 51% of the patients allergic to lemongrass oil who were also tested with citral, co-reacted to this important component of the oil	12
1997-2000 Austria	2% pet.	747	6 (0.8%)	S: patients suspected of fragrance allergy; R: not stated	3
1996-1997 UK	2% pet.	10	2 (20%)	S: patients suspected of cosmetic dermatitis and reacting to the fragrance mix; R: not stated	2
1994-1995 UK	2% pet.	40	3 (7.5%)	S: patients previously reacting to the fragrance mix; R: not stated; C: there was also one positive reaction in a patient negative to the fragrance mix	16

IVDK Information Network of Departments of Dermatology, Germany, Switzerland, Austria (www.ivdk.org); pet.: petrolatum

Case reports and case series

Occupational allergic contact dermatitis

Two aromatherapists had occupational contact dermatitis from multiple essential oils and reacted to lemongrass oil; one had used the oil, in the other patient this was uncertain (4). Another aromatherapist had occupational contact dermatitis from various essential oils, including lemongrass oil (5). Yet another aromatherapist had chronic hand dermatitis and was patch test positive to 17 of 20 oils used at her work (tested 1% and 5% in petrolatum); she also reacted to lemongrass oil, which was probably the primary sensitizer (6).

A massage therapist had occupational contact dermatitis from allergies to many essential oils; she reacted to lemongrass oil in the fragrance series, which reaction was considered to be relevant (7). A female 'complementary therapist' developed occupational contact dermatitis from a multitude of essential oils used at work, including lemongrass oil (9).

Eight of 30 men working on a boat developed dermatitis which was ascribed to lemongrass oil which had been spilled; four were patch tested with pine wood contaminated with the lemongrass oil (as there were no samples of the oil itself) and all reacted, with negative reactions to pinewood without the oil (20).

Non-occupational allergic contact dermatitis

One positive patch test reaction to lemongrass oil was seen in a patient who had allergic contact cheilitis from citral in a lip balm (14); citral is the combination of neral and geranial, which are the main components of lemongrass oil, both the West and the East Indian varieties (table 6.40.1.1. and 6.40.2.1). Two cases of contact allergy to lemongrass oil present in topical pharmaceutical preparations have been reported (22).

A male individual presented with a 1-month history of dermatitis that began on his dorsal hands with subsequent widespread involvement of his arms, trunk, legs, feet, and face. The patient treated his rash with a lotion made by his wife, which included essential oils (not specified). Furthermore, the patient diffused patchouli, lavender, lemongrass, and peppermint oils at home. When patch tested, he had 22 positive patch test reactions, including to the homemade lotion, including to lemongrass and peppermint oil but not to lavender oil; patchouli oil was not tested. It was not mentioned whether the reactions to other essential oils and fragrances were relevant. Obviously, some of the many weak (+) reactions may have been false-positive from the excited skin syndrome (26).

Miscellaneous

In a number of publications, positive patch tests to lemongrass oil have been reported with unknown, uncertain or not stated relevance. These include (literature screened up to 2014 [25]) the following. Irritant contact dermatitis of the hands was observed in a male masseur who worked with essential oils regularly; he had positive patch test reactions to lemongrass oil and orange oil, but it was not mentioned whether he had used these oils (8). One positive patch test to lemongrass oil was seen in a case of occupational hand dermatitis in a cook / barman / fruit grower caused by lemon oil, who also reacted to neroli oil and geraniol; the patient was patch tested with 'essences' (no concentration mentioned), but from the text it seems that this would indicate essential oils (10). Geraniol may be present in commercial lemongrass oils in concentrations up to 6% (25).

A positive patch test reaction to lemongrass oil was observed in a patient allergic to ascaridole, an allergen in tea tree oil (negative to tea tree oil itself) (11). One positive patch test reaction to lemongrass oil in 53 women with chronic anogenital dermatitis (13). One positive patch test reaction to lemongrass oil in a group of 475 patients with contact allergy to ingredients of cosmetics seen from January- April 1996 in 5 European dermatology centers; data on perfumes, toilet waters, aftershave lotions and deodorants were, however, excluded (17).

Lemongrass oil East Indian

The SCCS (Scientific Committee on Consumer Safety), in a 2012 Opinion on Fragrance allergens in cosmetic products, has marked Lemongrass oil East Indian (termed Cymbopogon schoenanthus oil) as 'established contact allergen in humans' (23,24).

Three studies have used East Indian lemongrass oil for patch testing (15,19,27). Their results are presented in table 6.40.2.2.

Lemongrass oil West Indian

The SCCS (Scientific Committee on Consumer Safety), in a 2012 Opinion on Fragrance allergens in cosmetic products, has marked Lemongrass oil West Indian as 'established contact allergen in humans' (23,24).

No reports on contact allergy to or allergic contact dermatitis from lemongrass oil, specified to have been obtained from *Cymbopogon citratus* (DC) Stapf. (West Indian lemongrass oil) have been found.

LITERATURE

1   Wetter DA, Yiannias JA, Prakash AV, Davis MD, Farmer SA, el-Azhary RA, et al. Results of patch testing to personal care product allergens in a standard series and a supplemental cosmetic series: an analysis of 945 patients from the Mayo Clinic Contact Dermatitis Group, 2000-2007. J Am Acad Dermatol 2010;63:789-798

2   Thomson KF, Wilkinson SM. Allergic contact dermatitis to plant extracts in patients with cosmetic dermatitis. Br J Dermatol 2000;142:84-88

3   Wöhrl S, Hemmer W, Focke M, Götz M, Jarisch R. The significance of fragrance mix, balsam of Peru, colophonium and propolis as screening tools in the detection of fragrance allergy. Br J Dermatol 2001;145:268-273

4   Bleasel N, Tate B, Rademaker M. Allergic contact dermatitis following exposure to essential oils. Australas J Dermatol 2002;43:211-213

5   Boonchai W, Lamtharachai P, Sunthonpalin P. Occupational allergic contact dermatitis from essential oils in aromatherapists. Contact Dermatitis 2007;56:181-182

6   Selvaag E, Holm J, Thune P. Allergic contact dermatitis in an aromatherapist with multiple sensitizations to essential oils. Contact Dermatitis 1995;33:354-355

7   Cockayne SE, Gawkrodger DJ. Occupational contact dermatitis in an aromatherapist. Contact Dermatitis 1997;:37:306-307

8   Jung P, Sesztak-Greinecker G, Wantke F, Götz M, Jarisch R, Hemmer W. Mechanical irritation triggering allergic contact dermatitis from essential oils in a masseur. Contact Dermatitis 2006;54:297-299

9   Newsham J, Rai S, Williams JDL. Two cases of allergic contact dermatitis to neroli oil. Br J Dermatol 2011;165(suppl.1):76

10 Audicana M, Bernaola G. Occupational contact dermatitis from citrus fruits: Lemon essential oils. Contact Dermatitis 1994;31:183-185

11 Christoffers WA, Blömeke B, Coenraads P-J, Schuttelaar M-LA. The optimal patch test concentration for ascaridole as a sensitizing component of tea tree oil. Contact Dermatitis 2014;71:129-137

12 Uter W, Schmidt E, Geier J, Lessmann H, Schnuch A, Frosch P. Contact allergy to essential oils: current patch test results (2000–2008) from the Information Network of Departments of Dermatology (IVDK). Contact Dermatitis 2010;63:277-283

13 Vermaat H, Smienk F, Rustemeyer Th, Bruynzeel DP, Kirtschig G. Anogenital allergic contact dermatitis, the role of spices and flavour allergy. Contact Dermatitis 2008;59:233-237

14 Hindle E, Ashworth J, Beck MH. Chelitis from contact allergy to citral in lip salve. Contact Dermatitis 2007;57:125-126

15 Frosch PJ, Johansen JD, Menné T, Pirker C, Rastogi SC, Andersen KE, et al. Further important sensitizers in patients sensitive to fragrances. II. Reactivity to essential oils. Contact Dermatitis 2002;47:279-287

16 Katsarma G, Gawkrodger DJ. Suspected fragrance allergy requires extended patch testing to individual fragrance allergens. Contact Dermatitis 1999;41:193-197

17 Goossens A, Beck MH, Haneke E, McFadden JP, Nolting S, Durupt G, Ries G. Adverse cutaneous reactions to cosmetic allergens. Contact Dermatitis 1999;40:112-113

18 Toholka R, Wang Y-S, Tate B, Tam M, Cahill J, Palmer A, Nixon R. The first Australian Baseline Series: Recommendations for patch testing in suspected contact dermatitis. Australas J Dermatol 2015;56:107-115

19 Paulsen E, Andersen KE. Colophonium and Compositae mix as markers of fragrance allergy: Cross-reactivity between fragrance terpenes, colophonium and Compositae plant extracts. Contact Dermatitis 2005;53:285-291

20 Mendelsohn HV. Dermatitis from lemon grass oil (*Cymbopogon citratus* or *Andropogon citratus*). Arch Dermatol 1944;50:34-35

21 Mendelsohn HV. Lemon grass oil. Arch Dermatol 1946;53:94-98

22 Nardelli A, D'Hooge E, Drieghe J, Dooms M, Goossens A. Allergic contact dermatitis from fragrance components in specific topical pharmaceutical products in Belgium. Contact Dermatitis 2009;60:303-313

23 SCCS (Scientific Committee on Consumer Safety). Opinion on Fragrance allergens in cosmetic products, 26-27 June 2012, SCCS/1459/11. Available at: https://ec.europa.eu/health/sites/health/files/scientific_committees/consumer_safety/docs/sccs_o_102.pdf

24 Uter W, Johansen JD, Börje A, Karlberg A-T, Lidén C, Rastogi S, Roberts D, White IR. Categorization of fragrance contact allergens for prioritization of preventive measures: clinical and experimental data and consideration of structure–activity relationships. Contact Dermatitis 2013;69:196-230

25 De Groot AC, Schmidt E. Essential oils: contact allergy and chemical composition. Boca Raton, Fl., USA: CRC Press, Taylor and Francis Group, 2016 (ISBN 9781482246407)

26 Grey KR, Hagen SL, Warshaw EM. Essential oils: emerging "medicaments". Dermatitis 2016;27:227-228

27 Sabroe RA, Holden CR, Gawkrodger DJ. Contact allergy to essential oils cannot always be predicted from allergy to fragrance markers in the baseline series. Contact Dermatitis 2016;74:236-241

28 De Groot AC, Schmidt E. Essential Oils, Part V: Peppermint oil, lavender oil, and lemongrass oil. Dermatitis 2016; 27:325-332

29 De Groot AC. Patch Testing, 4th Edition. Wapserveen, The Netherlands: acdegroot publishing, 2018 (ISBN 978-90-813233-4-5)

30 Girbig M, Hegewald J, Seidler A, Bauer A, Uter W, Schmitt J. Type IV sensitizations in physical therapists: patch test results of the Information Network of Departments of Dermatology (IVDK) 2007-2011. J Dtsch Dermatol Ges 2013;11:1185-1192

31 Silvestre JF, Mercader P, González-Pérez R, Hervella-Garcés M, Sanz-Sánchez T, Córdoba S, et al. Sensitization to fragrances in Spain: A 5-year multicentre study (2011-2015). Contact Dermatitis. 2018 Nov 14. doi: 10.1111/cod.13152. [Epub ahead of print]

Chapter 6.41 LITSEA CUBEBA OIL

IDENTIFICATION

Description/definition	: Litsea cubeba oil (essential oil of litsea cubeba) is the essential oil obtained from the fruit of the litsea (mountain pepper), *Litsea cubeba* (Lour) Pers.
INCI name(s) EU &USA	: Litsea cubeba fruit oil
CAS registry number(s)	: 68855-99-2; 90063-59-5
EC number(s)	: 290-018-7
RIFM monograph(s)	: Food Cosmet Toxicol 1982;20:731 (special issue VI)
SCCS opinion(s)	: SCCS/1459/11 (12)
ISO standard	: ISO 3214 Essential oil of litsea cubeba, 2000; Geneva, Switzerland, www.iso.org
Function(s) in cosmetics	: EU: masking; perfuming; tonic. USA: fragrance ingredients
Patch testing	: 2% pet.; based on RIFM data, 8% pet. is probably not irritant (15)

GENERAL

Litsea cubeba (Lour) Pers. is an evergreen, rarely deciduous, shrub or small tree 5-12 meter high. The plant is native to Asia (China, Japan, Taiwan, Bangladesh, Bhutan, India, Nepal, Cambodia, Laos, Myanmar, Thailand, Vietnam, Indonesia, Malaysia) and is cultivated in China, Indo-China, Japan, Indonesia and Taiwan. It is sometimes referred to as the May Chang tree or Chinese pepper, and has been used in traditional Chinese medicine for many diseases for thousands of years.

Litsea cubeba essential oil, also known as May Chang oil, is obtained from the small peppery-like fruits of the *Litsea cubeba* tree. It is widely used as a fragrance, especially in bar soaps, perfumes, household sprays and fresheners because of its intense lemon-like, fresh, sweet odor, which results from its high concentrations of citral (neral + geranial). Another major use of the oil is as a raw material source for the isolation of citral. This is used in its own right for flavor and fragrance purposes or converted by the chemical industry into a number of important derivatives including geranyl nitrile and the ionones, such as β-ionone, pseudo-ionone and methylionone (which are popular for their violet-like fragrance), and vitamins A, E and K (1,2,5,6,7).

Litsea cubeba oil is also a popular food-flavoring agent and preservative, particularly for sugar, cakes, drinks and spices (1). Other applications include their use as flavor enhancer in cigarettes, as a botanical antimicrobial and insecticidal agent (1,3,4,6) and in aromatherapy (8,9).

CHEMICAL COMPOSITION

Litsea cubeba oil is a clear and mobile liquid with pale to darker yellowish color, which has a fresh citrusy, slightly green odor. In litsea cubeba oils from various origins, over 170 chemicals have been identified. About 61 per cent of these were found in a single reviewed publication only. The ten chemicals that had the highest maximum concentrations in 101 commercial litsea cubeba essential oil samples are shown in table 6.41.1 (Erich Schmidt, analytical data presented in ref. 14).

A full literature review of the qualitative and quantitative composition of commercial and non-commercial litsea cubeba oils of various origins, their chemotypes and with data from the ISO standard, has been published in 2016 (14).

Table 6.41.1 Ten ingredients with the highest concentrations in commercial litsea cubeba oils (14)

Name	Concentration range	Name	Concentration range
Geranial	35.0 - 42.3%	Citronellal	0.4 - 3.8%
Neral	28.7 - 34.5%	α-Pinene	0.6 - 3.7%
Limonene	6.4 - 15.6%	(Z)-Isocitral	0.6 - 3.0%
Sabinene	0.2 - 5.1%	Linalool	1.0 - 2.4%
Methylheptenone	0.8 - 5.0%	(E)-Isocitral	0.9 - 2.0%

CONTACT ALLERGY / ALLERGIC CONTACT DERMATITIS

General

The SCCS (Scientific Committee on Consumer Safety), in a 2012 Opinion on Fragrance allergens in cosmetic products, has categorized Litsea cubeba extract as 'possible fragrance contact allergen' (12,13).

Contact allergy to litsea cubeba oil has been reported in two publications, but no cases of allergic contact dermatitis from the oil have been identified.

Testing in groups of patients

Two hundred dermatitis patients from Poland were tested with litsea cubeba oil 2% in petrolatum and three (1.5%) reacted. The same authors also patch tested 51 patients allergic to Myroxylon pereirae resin (balsam of Peru) and/or turpentine and/or wood tar and/or colophony and two (3.9%) had a positive patch test; relevance data were not provided (10). A group of 86 patients from Poland previously reacting to the fragrance mix was tested with litsea cubeba oil and seven (8.1%) had a positive patch test reaction; relevance data were not provided (11).

LITERATURE

1   Chen Y, Wang Y, Han X, Si L, Wu Q, Lin L. Biology and chemistry of *Litsea cubeba*, a promising industrial tree in China. J Essent Oil Res 2013;25:103-111

2   Wang Y, Jiang Z-T, Li R. Antioxidant activity, free radical scavenging potential and chemical composition of *Litsea cubeba* essential oil. J Essent Oil Bear Plants 2012;15:134-143

3   Si L, Chen Y, Han X, Zhan Z, Tian S, Cui Q, et al. Chemical composition of essential oils of *Litsea cubeba* harvested from its distribution areas in China. Molecules 2012;17:7057-7066

4   Yang Y, Jiang J, Qimei L, Yan X, Zhao J, Yuan H, Qin Z, Wang M. The fungicidal terpenoids and essential oil from *Litsea cubeba* in Tibet. Molecules 2010;15:7075-7082

5   Food and Agriculture Organization of the United Nations. Flavours and fragrances of plant origin. Chapter 7, Litsea cubeba oil. Rome: FAO, 1995. http://www.fao.org/docrep/018/v5350e/v5350e.pdf

6   Lawrence BM. Progress in essential oils. Perfum Flavor 2006;31(Jan/Feb):54-? (last page unknown)

7   Hu L, Du M, Zhang J, Wang Y. Chemistry of the main component of essential oil of *Litsea cubeba* and its derivatives. Open Journal of Forestry 2014;4:457-466

8   Rhind JP. Essential oils. A handbook for aromatherapy practice, 2nd Edition. London: Singing Dragon, 2012

9   Lawless J. The encyclopedia of essential oils, 2nd Edition. London: Harper Thorsons, 2014

10   Rudzki E, Grzywa Z, Bruo WS. Sensitivity to 35 essential oils. Contact Dermatitis 1976;2:196-200

11   Rudzki E, Grzywa Z. Allergy to perfume mixture. Contact Dermatitis 1986;15:115-116

12   SCCS (Scientific Committee on Consumer Safety). Opinion on Fragrance allergens in cosmetic products, 26-27 June 2012, SCCS/1459/11. Available at: https://ec.europa.eu/health/sites/health/files/scientific_committees/consumer_safety/docs/sccs_o_102.pdf

13   Uter W, Johansen JD, Börje A, Karlberg A-T, Lidén C, Rastogi S, Roberts D, White IR. Categorization of fragrance contact allergens for prioritization of preventive measures: clinical and experimental data and consideration of structure–activity relationships. Contact Dermatitis 2013;69:196-230

14   De Groot AC, Schmidt E. Essential oils: contact allergy and chemical composition. Boca Raton, Fl., USA: CRC Press, Taylor and Francis Group, 2016 (ISBN 9781482246407)

15   De Groot AC. Patch Testing, 4th Edition. Wapserveen, The Netherlands: acdegroot publishing, 2018 (ISBN 978-90-813233-4-5)

Chapter 6.42 LOVAGE OIL

IDENTIFICATION

Description/definition
: Lovage oil (essential oil of roots of lovage) is the essential oil obtained from the roots of the lovage, *Levisticum officinale* W.D.J. Koch

INCI name(s) EU & USA
: Levisticum officinale oil

CAS registry number(s)
: 8016-31-7; 84837-06-9

EC number(s)
: 284-292-7

RIFM monograph(s)
: Food Cosmet Toxicol 1978;16:813 (special issue IV)

Function(s) in cosmetics
: EU: masking; tonic. USA: fragrance ingredients

ISO standard
: ISO 11019 Essential oil of roots of lovage,1998: Geneva, Switzerland, www.iso.org; no chromatographic profile available

Patch testing
: 5% alc. (1)

GENERAL

Levisticum officinale Koch is an erect, tall perennial herbaceous plant, growing to 1.5 m or higher. It is native to Afghanistan and Iran. Lovage has escaped from cultivation and is sometimes naturalized in much of Europe, except the extreme north and south, and in eastern North America. The plant, all parts of which are strongly aromatic and have a characteristic celery-like flavor and smell, is cultivated in Europe and China as a spice and medicinal plant, mainly for its leaves and roots.

The essential oil from the roots, leaves and seeds of *L. officinale* are used in the food (condiments), beverage (liqueurs), perfumery, cosmetic (soaps and creams) and tobacco industries. The root oil is stated to have antispasmodic and anti-asthmatic properties and is also used in aromatherapy (3).

CHEMICAL COMPOSITION5

Lovage oil is a yellow to dark brown, clear mobile liquid which has an aromatic, herbaceous-spicy odor with celery aspects. In lovage oils from various origins, over 95 chemicals have been identified. About 52 per cent of these were found in a single reviewed publication only. The ten chemicals that had the highest maximum concentrations in 17 commercial lovage essential oil samples are shown in table 6.42.1 (Erich Schmidt, analytical data presented in ref. 3).

A full literature review of the qualitative and quantitative composition of commercial and non-commercial lovage oils of various origins and with data from the ISO standard (no chromatographic profile in the standard available) has been published in 2016 (3).

Table 6.42.1 Ten ingredients with the highest concentrations in commercial lovage oils (3)

Name	Concentration range	Name	Concentration range
(*Z*)-Ligustilide	4.9 - 85.2%	Linalool	trace - 4.4%
(*Z*)-Butylidenephthalide	1.1 - 28.6%	α-Pinene	0.2 - 3.1%
β-Phellandrene	0.07 - 15.5%	(*E*)-Butylidenephthalide	0.4 - 2.8%
β-Pinene	trace - 12.3%	(*E*)-Ligustilide	0.4 - 2.6%
Pentyl-1,5-cyclohexadiene	0.09 - 6.4%	β-Selinene	trace - 2.2%

CONTACT ALLERGY / ALLERGIC CONTACT DERMATITIS

Case reports and case series

A female patient became allergic to lovage oil from undiluted topical application; she reacted to the oil 5% in ethanol and to another essential oil product (mixture), to cananga oil, jasmine absolute (present in the essential oil mixture), eugenol and isoeugenol (1); lovage oil does not contain appreciable amounts of eugenol or isoeugenol (3). Lovage oil also sensitized a worker in the fragrance industry (2).

LITERATURE

1   Lapeere H, Boone B, Verhaeghe E, Ongenae K, Lambert J. Contact dermatitis caused by lovage (Levisticum officinalis) essential oil. Contact Dermatitis 2013;69:181-182

2   Calnan CD. Lovage sensitivity. Contact Dermatitis Newsletter 1969;5:99

3   De Groot AC, Schmidt E. Essential oils: contact allergy and chemical composition. Boca Raton, Fl., USA: CRC Press, Taylor and Francis Group, 2016 (ISBN 9781482246407)

Chapter 6.43   MANDARIN OIL

IDENTIFICATION

Description/definition	: Mandarin oil (essential oil of mandarin, Italian type) is the essential oil obtained from the pericarp (peel) of the mandarin (mandarin orange), *Citrus reticulata* Blanco (synonym: *Citrus nobilis* Andrews)
INCI name(s) EU	: Citrus nobilis peel oil (expressed)
INCI name(s) USA	: Citrus nobilis (mandarin orange) peel oil
CAS registry number(s)	: 8008-31-9; 84929-38-4
EC number(s)	: 284-521-0
CIR review(s)	: Final report 09/09/2014 (access: www.cir-safety.org/ingredients)
RIFM monograph(s)	: Food Chem Toxicol 1992;30:S69 (special issue VIII)
SCCS opinion(s)	: SCCNFP/0389/00, final (7)
ISO standard	: ISO 3528 Essential oil of mandarin, Italian type, 2012; Geneva, Switzerland, www.iso.org
Function(s) in cosmetics	: EU: masking; perfuming; skin condition; tonic. USA: fragrance ingredients; skin-conditioning agents - miscellaneous
Patch testing	: 2% pet.; test also limonene (see Chapter 3.95 Limonene)

GENERAL

Citrus reticulata Blanco, the mandarin orange (synonyms: mandarine, mandarin) is an evergreen thorny *Citrus* tree growing to 4.5-6 meter, which gives fruits resembling oranges. The mandarin orange has probably originated from Asia and is widely cultivated in the tropics and subtropics. The main producing countries are China (>50% of the world's production), Spain and Brazil, followed by Japan, Turkey, Italy, Egypt, South Korea, USA and Pakistan (8).

The essential oil expressed from the peel is employed commercially in flavoring hard candy, gelatins, ice cream, chewing gum, bakery goods, beverages and liqueurs. Mandarin essential oil is valued in perfume-manufacturing, particularly in the formulation of floral compounds and colognes, where the low volatile essential oil components play an important role as head notes. In pharmaceutical industries they are employed as flavoring agents to mask unpleasant tastes of drugs (2,3). Mandarin oils are also used in aromatherapy (4,5).

The history, global distribution, and nutritional importance of *Citrus* fruits have been reviewed in ref. 1.

CHEMICAL COMPOSITION

Mandarin oil is a clear mobile liquid with a light green to dark green, light yellow to dark orange or reddish to dark red color with blue influences, depending on the harvest time. In mandarin oils from various origins, over 255 chemicals have been identified. The ten chemicals that had the highest maximum concentrations in 98 commercial mandarin essential oil samples are shown in table 6.43.1 (Erich Schmidt, analytical data presented in ref. 8).

A full literature review of the qualitative and quantitative composition of commercial and non-commercial mandarin oils of various origins with data from the ISO standard has been published in 2016 (8).

Table 6.43.1 Ten ingredients with the highest concentrations in commercial mandarin oils (8)

Name	Concentration range	Name	Concentration range
Limonene	64.0 - 76.4%	*p*-Cymene	0.3 - 1.2%
γ-Terpinene	10.4 - 21.1%	Methyl *n*-methyl anthra-nilate	0.08 - 1.1%
Terpinolene	0.06 - 4.2%		
α-Pinene	1.2 - 3.1%	*trans*-Sabinene hydrate	0.01 - 1.1%
Myrcene	0.08 - 2.2%	α-Terpineol	0.07 - 1.1%
β-Pinene	0.5 - 2.2%		

CONTACT ALLERGY / ALLERGIC CONTACT DERMATITIS

General

Contact allergy to and possible allergic contact dermatitis from mandarin oil has been reported in one publication only (6). A false-positive patch test reaction due to the excited skin syndrome cannot be excluded.

Case reports and case series

An aromatherapist had occupational contact dermatitis with allergies to multiple essential oils used at work, including mandarin oil; the patient also reacted to geraniol, linalool, linalyl acetate, α-pinene, the fragrance mix and various other fragrance materials; α-pinene was demonstrated by GC-MS in the mandarin oil; limonene was not tested (6). α-Pinene may be present in commercial mandarin oils in concentrations up to 3% (8).

LITERATURE

1   Liu YQ, Heying E, Tanumihardjo SA. History, global distribution, and nutritional importance of *Citrus* fruits. Compreh Rev Food Sci Food Saf 2012;11:530–545

2   Dugo P, Bonaccorsi I, Ragonese C, Russo M, Donato P, Santi L, Mondello L. Analytical characterization of mandarin (*Citrus deliciosa* Ten.) essential oil. Flavour Fragr J 2011;26:34-46

3   Bourgou S, Rahali FZ, Ourghemmi I, Tounsi MS. Changes of peel essential oil composition of four Tunisian *Citrus* during fruit maturation. The Scientific World Journal 2012, Article ID 528593, 10 pages

4   Rhind JP. Essential oils. A handbook for aromatherapy practice, 2nd Edition. London: Singing Dragon, 2012

5   Lawless J. The encyclopedia of essential oils, 2nd Edition. London: Harper Thorsons, 2014

6   Dharmagunawardena B, Takwale A, Sanders KJ, Cannan S, Roger A, Ilchyshyn A. Gas chromatography: an investigative tool in multiple allergies to essential oils. Contact Dermatitis 2002;47:288-292

7   Opinion of the Scientific Committee on Cosmetic Products and Non-Food Products Intended for Consumers concerning 'The 1st update of the inventory of ingredients employed in cosmetic products. Section II: Perfume and aromatic raw materials', 24 October 2000, SCCNFP/0389/00, final. Available at: http://ec.europa.eu/health/ph_risk/committees/sccp/documents/out131_en.pdf

8   De Groot AC, Schmidt E. Essential oils: contact allergy and chemical composition. Boca Raton, Fl., USA: CRC Press, Taylor and Francis Group, 2016 (ISBN 9781482246407)

Chapter 6.44   MARJORAM OIL (SWEET)

IDENTIFICATION

Description/definition   : Sweet marjoram oil is the essential oil obtained from the flowering tops of the sweet marjoram, *Origanum majorana* L. (synonym: *Majorana hortensis* Moench)

INCI name(s) EU & USA   : Origanum majorana flower oil

CAS registry number(s)   : 8015-01-8; 82082-58-6

EC number(s)   : 282-004-4

RIFM monograph(s)   : Food Cosmet Toxicol 1976;14:469 (binder, page 517)

Merck Index monograph : 8164

Function(s) in cosmetics : EU: masking; refreshing. USA: fragrance ingredients

Patch testing   : 2% pet.; based on RIFM data, 6% pet. is probably not irritant (11)

GENERAL

Origanum majorana L., popularly known as sweet marjoram, is a herb or undershrub, which can grow to 40-60 cm. The plant is native to Cyprus and Turkey and sometimes naturalized, especially in the Mediterranean region. The sweet marjoram is one of the most important culinary herbs of the western world, widely cultivated in Europe, Africa, southern Asia and the Americas (10). The flowering tops of marjoram are steam-distilled to produce the essential oil of sweet marjoram, which is used in commercial food flavoring (e.g. baked goods, processed vegetables, condiments, soups, snack foods and gravies [3,4]), liqueurs, perfumes, cosmetics, pharmaceuticals and industrial products such as fungicides or insecticides (1,2,4).

Marjoram oil possesses antimicrobial properties against food borne bacteria and mycotoxigenic fungi and strong antioxidant activity (5), mainly because of its high content of phenolic acids and flavonoids, which is useful in health supplements and food preservation. Medicinal uses include external application for sprains and bruises; marjoram oils are also employed in aromatherapy (6,7),

The ethnopharmacology, phytochemistry, and biological activities of the sweet marjoram have been reviewed in 2017 (12).

CHEMICAL COMPOSITION

Sweet marjoram oil is a yellowish to yellow-green, clear mobile liquid which has an aromatic, herbaceous and spicy odor. In sweet marjoram oils from various origins, over 240 chemicals have been identified. About 55 per cent of these were found in a single reviewed publication only. The ten chemicals that had the highest maximum concentrations in 49 commercial marjoram essential oil samples are shown in table 6.44.1 (Erich Schmidt, analytical data presented in ref. 10).

A full literature review of the qualitative and quantitative composition of commercial and non-commercial sweet marjoram oils of various origins has been published in 2016 (10).

Table 6.44.1 Ten ingredients with the highest concentrations in commercial marjoram oils (10)

Name	Concentration range	Name	Concentration range
β-Phellandrene	1.1 - 50.2%	*trans*-Sabinene hydrate	0.06 - 15.5%
Terpinen-4-ol	0.5 - 29.7%	acetate	
trans-Sabinene hydrate	0.6 - 24.0%	α-Terpinene	0.07 - 10.3%
Linalool	0.2 - 23.5%	Sabinene	1.0 - 9.4%
γ-Terpinene	0.2 - 16.7%	*cis*-Sabinene hydrate	0.01 - 6.8%
		Terpinolene	0.2 - 6.8%

CONTACT ALLERGY / ALLERGIC CONTACT DERMATITIS

General

Allergic contact dermatitis from marjoram oil has been reported in two publications only, both of which concerned occupational contact dermatitis in aromatherapists (8,9). Linalool and possibly α-pinene and caryophyllene may have been allergens in one study (9). False-positive reactions due to the excited skin syndrome cannot be excluded in either study.

Case reports and case series

An aromatherapist had chronic hand dermatitis and was patch test positive to 17 of 20 oils used at her work (tested 1% and 5% in petrolatum), including marjoram oil (8). Two other aromatherapists had contact dermatitis (one occupational) with allergies to multiple essential oils used at their work, including marjoram oil. Both patients also reacted to geraniol, α-pinene, the fragrance mix and various other fragrance materials. In addition, one proved to be allergic to linalool and linalyl acetate, the other to caryophyllene. α-Pinene, linalool, geraniol and caryophyllene were demonstrated by GC-MS in both marjoram oils used by the patients (9). Linalool has been found in concentrations of up to 23.5% in commercial marjoram oils, α-pinene and caryophyllene in concentrations over 3% (table 6.44.1).

LITERATURE

1   Ramos S, Rojas LB, Lucena ME, Meccia G, Usubillaga A. Chemical composition and antibacterial activity of *Origanum majorana* L. essential oil from the Venezuelan Andes. J Essent Oil Res 2011;23:45-49

2   Schmidt E, Bail S, Buchbauer G, Stoilova I, Krastanov A, Stoyanova A, Jirovetz L. Chemical composition, olfactory evaluation and antioxidant effects of the essential oil of *Origanum majorana* L. from Albania, Nat Prod Commun 2008;3:1051-1056. Data also presented in ref. 58

3   Novak J, Lukas L, Franz CM. The essential oil composition of wild growing sweet marjoram (*Origanum majorana* L., Lamiaceae) from Cyprus—three chemotypes. J Essent Oil Res 2008;20:339-341

4   Sellami IH, Maamouri E, Chahed T, Wannes WA, Kchouk ME, Marzouk B. Effect of growth stage on the content and composition of the essential oil and phenolic fraction of sweet marjoram (Origanum majorana L.), Ind Crop Prod 2009;30:395-402

5   Baranauskiene R, Venskutonis PR, Demyttenaere JCR. Sensory and instrumental evaluation of sweet marjoram (*Origanum majorana* L.) aroma. Flavour Fragr J 2005;20:492-500

6   Rhind JP. Essential oils. A handbook for aromatherapy practice, 2nd Edition. London: Singing Dragon, 2012

7   Lawless J. The encyclopedia of essential oils, 2nd Edition. London: Harper Thorsons, 2014

8   Selvaag E, Holm J, Thune P. Allergic contact dermatitis in an aromatherapist with multiple sensitizations to essential oils. Contact Dermatitis 1995;33:354-355

9   Dharmagunawardena B, Takwale A, Sanders KJ, Cannan S, Roger A, Ilchyshyn A. Gas chromatography: an investigative tool in multiple allergies to essential oils. Contact Dermatitis 2002;47:288-292

10 De Groot AC, Schmidt E. Essential oils: contact allergy and chemical composition. Boca Raton, Fl., USA: CRC Press, Taylor and Francis Group, 2016 (ISBN 9781482246407)

11 De Groot AC. Patch Testing, 4th Edition. Wapserveen, The Netherlands: acdegroot publishing, 2018 (ISBN 978-90-813233-4-5)

12 Bina F, Rahimi R. Sweet Marjoram: A Review of ethnopharmacology, phytochemistry, and biological activities. J Evid Based Complementary Altern Med 2017;22:175-185

Chapter 6.45   MELISSA OIL (LEMON BALM OIL)

IDENTIFICATION

Description/definition   : Melissa oil (lemon balm oil) is the essential oil obtained from the aerial parts of the
                              melissa (lemon balm), *Melissa officinalis* L.
INCI name(s) EU & USA   : Melissa officinalis leaf oil
CAS registry number(s)   : 8014-71-9; 84082-61-1
EC number(s)   : 282-007-0
IFRA standard   : Restricted (www.ifraorg.org/en-us/standards-library) (table 6.45.1)
Function(s) in cosmetics   : EU: masking; perfuming; tonic. USA: fragrance ingredients
Patch testing   : 2% pet. (12)

Table 6.45.1 IFRA restrictions for melissa oil

Category [a]	Limits [b]	Category [a]	Limits [b]	Category [a]	Limits [b]
1	0.04%	5	0.33%	9	5.0%
2	0.05%	6	1.01%	10	2.5%
3	0.21%	7	0.11%	11	not restricted
4	0.63%	8	1.40%		

[a] For explanation of categories see pages 6-8
[b] Limits in the finished products

GENERAL

Melissa officinalis L. (lemon balm) is a perennial herb which can grow to a height of 70-150 cm and which has leaves with a gentle lemon scent. The lemon balm is native to the Madeira and Canary Islands, Morocco, Tunisia, temperate regions of Asia, Pakistan, and various countries in South and East Europe. The plant is cultivated for the herb as a spice, and as a medicinal, aromatic, ornamental and bee plant in Europe (Italy, Hungary), north-western Africa (Morocco, Algeria), Egypt, north, central and south America (Brazil, Peru), temperate Asia (Turkey, China, Korea, Russia), and Australia. It has escaped cultivation and established itself in England, continental Europe, North America and northern Iran (11).

The herb, the essential oil and extracts have many medicinal applications (2,3,4,5,6) and melissa is listed in a number of European Pharmacopoeias (3). The essential oil, which is obtained from the (often flowering) aerial parts of *M. officinalis*, is employed in liqueurs (Benedictine, Chartreuse), ice-cream, perfumes, cosmetics and furniture polishes (1). It is also used by the food industry to inhibit the spoilage yeast growth (1). The oil is very popular in aromatherapy (7,8) against nervous tension and may be used as a home remedy for headaches and toothaches (5).

The yield of essential oil of lemon balm is very low, so the production cost and price of the oil are very high. As a consequence, lemon balm oil is sometimes adulterated with other oils, e.g. from *Cymbopogon* spp. or *Citrus* peel oil (6).

CHEMICAL COMPOSITION

Melissa oil is a slightly yellowish to light brownish, clear mobile liquid which has a fresh, herbal, citrusy odor which can sometimes be recognized as lemon odor. In melissa oils from various origins, over 310 chemicals have been identified. About half of these were found in a single reviewed publication only. The ten chemicals that had the highest maximum concentrations in 53 commercial melissa essential oil samples are shown in table 6.45.2 (Erich Schmidt, analytical data presented in ref. 11).

A full literature review of the qualitative and quantitative composition of commercial and non-commercial melissa oils of various origins and their chemotypes has been published in 2016 (11).

Table 6.45.2 Ten ingredients with the highest concentrations in commercial melissa oils (11)

Name	Concentration range	Name	Concentration range
Geranial	0.2 - 41.7%	Geraniol	0.2 - 22.2%
Neral	0.5 - 31.0%	Methyl citronellate	0.03 - 19.2%
β-Caryophyllene	0.7 - 29.4%	Nerol	0.1 - 16.2%
α-Citronellal	0.5 - 29.2%	Citronellol	0.05 - 13.1%
Germacrene D	0.2 - 24.0%	(*E*)-β-Ocimene	0.05 - 9.3%

CONTACT ALLERGY / ALLERGIC CONTACT DERMATITIS

General
Only two case reports of allergic contact dermatitis from melissa oils have been found (9,10). In neither, false-positive patch tests due to the excited skin syndrome can be excluded. In one case, geraniol and caryophyllene may have been allergens in melissa oil (9).

Case reports and case series
An aromatherapist had non-occupational contact dermatitis with allergies to multiple essential oils used at work, including 'melissa blend'. The patient also reacted to geraniol, linalool, linalyl acetate, α-pinene, the fragrance mix and various other fragrance materials. Linalool, geraniol and caryophyllene were demonstrated by GC-MS in the melissa blend (9). High concentrations of geraniol (up to 22.2%) and caryophyllene (up to 29.4%) have been found in commercial melissa oils (table 6.45.2).

A female 'complementary therapist' developed occupational contact dermatitis from a multitude of essential oils used at work, including melissa oil (10).

LITERATURE

1   Khalid KA, Hu W, Cai W, Hussien MS. Influence of cutting and harvest day time on the essential oils of lemon balm (*Melissa officinalis* L.). J Essent Oil Bear Plants 2009;12:348-357
2   Khalid KA, Cai W, Ahmed AMA. Effect of harvesting treatments and distillation methods on the essential oil of lemon balm and apple geranium plants. J Essent Oil Bear Plants 2009;12:120-130
3   Rehman S-U, Latief R, Bhat KA, Khuroo MA, Shawl AS, Chandra S. Comparative analysis of the aroma chemicals of Melissa officinalis using hydrodistillation and HS-SPME techniques. Arab J Chem (2013). Available at: http://dx.doi.org/10.1016/j.arabjc.2013.09.015
4   Mimica-Dukic N, Bozin B, Sokovic M, Simin N. Antimicrobial and antioxidant activities of *Melissa officinalis* L. (Lamiaceae) essential oil. J Agric Food Chem 2004;52:2485-2489
5   Lemon balm. In: Charles DJ. Antioxidant properties of spices, herbs and other sources. New York Heidelberg: Springer, 2013:371-376
6   Sarý AO, Ceylan A. Yield characteristics and essential oil composition of lemon balm (*Melissa officinalis* L.) grown in the Aegean Region of Turkey. Turk J Agric Forest 2002;22:217-224
7   Rhind JP. Essential oils. A handbook for aromatherapy practice, 2nd Edition. London: Singing Dragon, 2012
8   Lawless J. The encyclopedia of essential oils, 2nd Edition. London: Harper Thorsons, 2014
9   Dharmagunawardena B, Takwale A, Sanders KJ, Cannan S, Roger A, Ilchyshyn A. Gas chromatography: an investigative tool in multiple allergies to essential oils. Contact Dermatitis 2002;47:288-292
10 Newsham J, Rai S, Williams JDL. Two cases of allergic contact dermatitis to neroli oil. Br J Dermatol 2011;165(suppl.1):76
11 De Groot AC, Schmidt E. Essential oils: contact allergy and chemical composition. Boca Raton, Fl., USA: CRC Press, Taylor and Francis Group, 2016 (ISBN 9781482246407)
12 De Groot AC. Patch Testing, 4th Edition. Wapserveen, The Netherlands: acdegroot publishing, 2018 (ISBN 978-90-813233-4-5)

Chapter 6.46 MYRRH OIL

IDENTIFICATION

Description/definition	: Myrrh oil is the essential oil obtained from the wood exudate of the (African) myrrh, *Commiphora myrrha* (Nees) Engl. and related species such as *Commiphora molmol* Engl. ex Tschirch (actually a synonym for *Commiphora myrrha* (Nees) Engl.), *Commiphora gileadensis* L. (Mecca myrrh, balm-of-Gilead), and *Commiphora abyssinica* (O. Berg) Engl. (preferred name: *Commiphora habessinica* (O. Berg) Engl.), also called Abyssinian myrrh or Yemen myrrh
INCI name(s) EU	: Commiphora myrrha gum oil; Commiphora abyssinica gum oil (both perfuming names, not INCI names proper)
INCI name(s) USA	: Not in the Personal Care Products Council Ingredient database
CAS registry number(s)	: 8016-37-3; 84929-26-0; 9000-45-7
EC number(s)	: 284-510-0; 232-543-6
RIFM monograph(s)	: Food Cosmet Toxicol 1976;14:621 (binder, page 581)
Merck Index monograph	: 7693
Function(s) in cosmetics	: EU: perfuming
Patch testing	: 2% pet.; based on RIFM data, 8% pet. is probably not irritant (10)

GENERAL

The *Commiphora* genus contains up to 200 species of often thorny shrubs or small- to medium-sized dioecious trees with a peeling, papery bark growing in sandy and rocky areas distributed across Africa (especially northern Africa: Somalia, Sudan, Ethiopia, Eritrea) and the Arabian peninsula (Yemen, Oman, Saudi Arabia), with four species also found in India (2,8). Myrrh is the dried gum oleoresin principally obtained from the schizogenous gum-oleoresin cavities in the stem or branches of the small tree *Commiphora myrrha* (Nees) Engl. (which produces true myrrh, also called Somalia myrrh, heerabol myrrh) or other *Commiphora* species such as *C. abyssinica* (*habessinica*) (Berg.) Engl., *Commiphora gileadensis* L. (produces Mecca balsam, also called mecca myrrh, opobalsam, balsam of Gilead), *Commiphora schimperi* (O. Berg) Engl. (CAS 89997-88-6; EC 289-725-3) and *Commiphora wildii* (CAS 1082996-27-7).

The myrrh balsam (oleoresin, gum) is obtained from these trees by incisions in the bark and is a yellowish exudate. On exposure to the air this exudate darkens, hardens and dries to rounded irregular tears, brownish-yellow to reddish-yellow in color. Myrrh comprises 30-60 per cent water-soluble gum, 25-40% alcohol-soluble resin and 3-8% essential oil and is used for perfume, medicinal purposes and as incense (4,8).

Myrrh oil is the essential oil obtained by hydro- or steam-distillation of myrrh wood exudate (resin). The oil is used in aromatherapy, perfumery, to flavor cosmetics such as toothpaste and mouthwash and is a flavor in alcoholic drinks, soft drinks, and food (1,3).

CHEMICAL COMPOSITION

Myrrh oil is a yellowish-brown to brownish clear viscous liquid, which has a warm-balsamic, sweet and spicy aromatic odor. In myrrh oils from various origins, over 110 chemicals have been identified. About 69 per cent of these were found in a single reviewed publication only. The ten chemicals that had the highest maximum concentrations in 46 commercial myrrh essential oil samples are shown in table 6.46.1 (Erich Schmidt, analytical data presented in ref. 8).

A review of the chemistry of myrrh is provided in ref. 9. A full literature review of the qualitative and quantitative composition of commercial and non-commercial myrrh oils of various origins has been published in 2016 (8).

Table 6.46.1 Ten ingredients with the highest concentrations in commercial myrrh oils (8)

Name	Concentration range	Name	Concentration range
Furanoeudesma-1,3-diene	5.9 - 36.2%	Lindestrene	2.7 - 9.6%
Curzerene	8.5 - 34.2%	α-Humulene	0.3 - 8.8%
Furanodiene	4.3 - 17.0%	β-Elemene	0.5 - 8.7%
α-Pinene	0.3 - 15.8%	2-Methoxyfuranodiene	1.7 - 7.4%
Curzerenone	1.2 - 12.0%	α-Copaene	0.1 - 5.5%

CONTACT ALLERGY / ALLERGIC CONTACT DERMATITIS

General
There are only three publications on contact allergy to myrrh oil. In two, aromatherapists reacted to the oil they used at work, but in neither of them can a false-positive patch test reaction from the excited skin syndrome be excluded.

Case reports and case series
An aromatherapist had chronic hand dermatitis and was patch test positive to 17 of 20 oils used at her work (tested 1% and 5% in petrolatum), including myrrh oil (6). One positive patch test to myrrh oil was seen in an aromatherapist with occupational contact dermatitis from (multiple) essential oils; however, this oil had not been used by the patient (5).

Another aromatherapist had occupational contact dermatitis with allergies to multiple essential oils used at work, including myrrh oil. The patient also reacted to geraniol, α-pinene, caryophyllene, the fragrance mix and various other fragrance materials; these chemicals could not be identified by GC-MS in the myrrh oil (7).

LITERATURE

1 Wanner J, Schmidt E, Bail S, Jirovetz L, Buchbauer G, Gochevd V, et al. Chemical composition and antibacterial activity of selected essential oils and some of their main compounds. Nat Prod Comm 2010;5:1359-1364
2 Shen T, Li G-H, Wang X-N, Lou H-X. The genus *Commiphora*: A review of its traditional uses, phytochemistry and pharmacology. J Ethnopharmacol 2012;142:319-330
3 Marongiu B, Piras A, Porcedda S, Scorciapino A. Chemical composition of the essential oil and supercritical CO2 extract of *Commiphora myrrha* (Nees) Engl. and of *Acorus calamus* L. J Agric Food Chem 2005;53:7939-7943
4 Lawrence BM. Progress in essential oils. Perfum Flavor 2004;29(October):88-? (last page unknown)
5 Bleasel N, Tate B, Rademaker M. Allergic contact dermatitis following exposure to essential oils. Australas J Dermatol 2002;43:211-213
6 Selvaag E, Holm J, Thune P. Allergic contact dermatitis in an aromatherapist with multiple sensitizations to essential oils. Contact Dermatitis 1995;33:354-355
7 Dharmagunawardena B, Takwale A, Sanders KJ, Cannan S, Roger A, Ilchyshyn A. Gas chromatography: an investigative tool in multiple allergies to essential oils. Contact Dermatitis 2002;47:288-292
8 De Groot AC, Schmidt E. Essential oils: contact allergy and chemical composition. Boca Raton, Fl., USA: CRC Press, Taylor and Francis Group, 2016 (ISBN 9781482246407)
9 Hanuš LO, Řezanka T, Dembitsky VM, Moussaieff A. Myrrh - Commiphora Chemistry. Biomedical Papers 2005;149:3-28
10 De Groot AC. Patch Testing, 4th Edition. Wapserveen, The Netherlands: acdegroot publishing, 2018 (ISBN 978-90-813233-4-5)

Chapter 6.47   NEEM OIL

IDENTIFICATION

Description/definition	: Neem oil (margosa oil) is the essential oil obtained from the seed of the neem (neem tree, Indian lilac, margosa tree), *Azadirachta indica* A. Juss. (synonym: *Melia azadirachta* L.)
INCI name(s) EU & USA	: Azadirachta indica seed extract; Melia azadirachta seed extract
Other names	: Margosa extract
CAS registry number(s)	: 84696-25-3; 90063-92-6
EC number(s)	: 283-644-7; 290-052-2
Function(s) in cosmetics	: EU: skin conditioning. USA: skin-conditioning agents - miscellaneous
Patch testing	: Pure

GENERAL

Azadirachta indica A. Juss. is a fast-growing evergreen tree from the mahogany family Meliaceae that can reach a height of 15-20 metres. The tree is indigenous to the dry forests of south and south-east Asia and is widely distributed in India, Nepal, Pakistan, Bangladesh, Sri Lanka, Myanmar, Thailand, Malaysia, Indonesia and Iran and cultivated in many countries. The neem tree is the holy tree of the Hindus and is considered a major component in Ayurvedic and Unani medicine (10).

Neem essential oil (margosa oil) is obtained by hydrodistillation of the seeds (3,4). There is very little information in literature on neem essential oils; virtually all studies on 'neem oils' pertain to the fixed (vegetable) oil of the seeds, which may be obtained by either cold-pressing or extraction with various solvents, or to essential oils from the leaves or flowers of the neem tree. The essential oil is apparently not used in aromatherapy (5).

Neem *essential* oil should not be confused with the INCI entry Melia azadirachta seed oil (CAS 8002-65-1), which is the fixed oil expressed or extracted from the seeds of the neem tree. It is uncertain whether the INCI nomenclature mentioned in the section 'Identification' above pertains to essential oils or solvent-extracted neem products. The fact that the functions are given as skin conditioning and not a fragrance ingredient, argues against it being an essential oil.

Biological, pharmacological and medicinal aspects of the (various parts of the) neem tree and its seed oil have been reviewed (1,2).

CHEMICAL COMPOSITION

Neem oil is a light brownish to brownish clear mobile liquid which has an oily, woody and dusty, slightly animalistic odor. In two neem oils obtained by hydrodistillation, over 65 chemicals have been identified. The 10 major compounds found in neem essential oil (one quantitative publication only [3]) are shown in table 6.47.1. Over 80% of the oil is composed of fatty acids (>60%) and alkanes (3).

A full literature review of the qualitative and quantitative composition of commercial and non-commercial neem oils of various origins has been published in 2016 (10).

Table 6.47.1 Ten ingredients with the highest concentrations in one neem essential oil sample (3)

Name	Concentration range	Name	Concentration range
Hexadecanoic acid (palmitic acid)	34.0%	Pentacosane	4.9%
		Methyl oleate	3.8%
Oleic acid	15.7%	Octadecanoic acid (stearic acid)	2.9%
5,6-Dihydro-2,4,6-tri-ethyl-(4*H*)-1,3,5-dithiazine	11.7%		
		Eudesm-7(11)-en-4-ol	2.7%
Tricosane	10.5%	Linoleic acid	2.4%
Tetradecanoic acid	6.8%		

CONTACT ALLERGY / ALLERGIC CONTACT DERMATITIS

General

There are six publications on contact allergy to neem oil. Five patients became sensitized from therapeutic use of the oil the 6th from the use of an antipsoriatic herbal preparation containing neem oil. The literature has been reviewed in 2017 (12).

Case reports and case series

One patient developed allergic contact dermatitis from neem oil in a poultice containing neem oil and tea tree oil for treatment of a furuncle; a patch test with pure neem oil was positive (6,8). Another patient became sensitized to neem oil which was used to treat alopecia areata (7). The antipsoriatic herbal preparation Psorigon® caused allergic contact dermatitis in one patient, who showed positive patch tests to the product and to 'Azadirachta indica' 1%, 2%, 5% and 10%. It is not certain that the ingredient was an essential oil (9).

A woman developed acute allergic contact dermatitis of the neck and in the retroauricular and laterocervical areas from treating her scalp psoriasis with pure neem oil with tocopherol. A patch test with the product was positive and to tocopherol negative, implicating neem oil as the offending agent (11).

A male patient presented himself with an itchy dermatitis on the forearms, backs of the hands, and legs. His job was to repair agricultural engines. By doing this, he had developed irritant contact dermatitis of the hands from contact with oil, frequent washing, and mechanical stress to the skin. For 2 months, the patient had been using neem oil on his hands, arms, and legs to treat his dry skin. Within 2 weeks, an itchy rash appeared at the sites of application. Patch tests revealed positive reactions to sodium metabisulfite, ketoconazole cream (which contains sodium sulfite), and neem oil. The product contained 99.9% neem oil and 0.1% tocopherol. Later, the patient was tested with tocopherol 10% and 30% in arachis oil and retested with the neem oil, which again gave a positive reaction to the oil; there were no reactions to tocopherol. Twenty-three controls were tested with the neem oil product with negative results. The reactions to sodium metabisulfite and ketoconazole cream were of past relevance (12).

Another case of allergic contact dermatitis caused by neem oil was reported from Spain; details are unknown (article not read) (13).

LITERATURE

1   Brahmachari G. Neem– an omnipotent plant: A retrospection. Chem Bio Chem 2004;5:408-421
2   Atawodi SE, Atawodi JC. *Azadirachta indica* (neem): a plant of multiple biological and pharmacological activities. Phytochem Rev 2009;8:601-620
3   Kurose K, Yatagai M. Components of the essential oils of *Azadirachta indica* A. Juss, *Azadirachta siamensis* Velton, and *Azadirachta excelsa* (Jack) Jacobs and their comparison. J Wood Sci 2005;51:185-188
4   Manzoor F, Naz N, Malik S, Siddiqui BS, Syed A, Perwaiz S. Chemical analysis and comparison of antitermitic activity of essential oils of Neem (*Azadirachta indica*), Vetiver (*Vetiveria zizanioides*) and Mint (*Mentha arvensis*) against *Heterotermes indicola* (Wasmann) from Pakistan. Asian J Chem 2012;24:2069-2072
5   Rhind JP. Essential oils. A handbook for aromatherapy practice, 2nd Edition. London: Singing Dragon, 2012
6   Greenblatt DT, Banerjee P, White JML. Allergic contact dermatitis to neem oil. Brit J Derm 2011;165(suppl. 1):74-75
7   Reutemann P, Ehrlich A. Neem oil: an herbal therapy for alopecia areata causes dermatitis. Dermatitis 2008;19:E12-E15
8   Greenblatt DT, Banerjee P, White JML. Allergic contact dermatitis caused by neem oil. Contact Dermatitis 2012;67:242-243
9   Ahmed I, Charles-Holmes R. Contact allergy to Psorigon®. Contact Dermatitis 2000;42:276
10 De Groot AC, Schmidt E. Essential oils: contact allergy and chemical composition. Boca Raton, Fl., USA: CRC Press, Taylor and Francis Group, 2016 (ISBN 9781482246407)
11 Lauriola MM, Corazza M. Allergic contact dermatitis caused by argan oil, neem oil, and Mimosa tenuiflora. Contact Dermatitis 2016;75:388-390
12 De Groot AC, Jagtman BA, Woutersen M. Contact allergy to neem oil. Dermatitis 2017;28:360-362
13 Sánchez-Gilo A, Nuño González A, Gutiérrez Pascual M, Vicente Martín FJ. Airborne allergic contact dermatitis caused by neem oil. Actas Dermosifiliogr 2018;109:449-450

Chapter 6.48   NEROLI OIL

IDENTIFICATION

Description/definition	: Neroli oil (essential oil of neroli) is the essential oil obtained from the flowers of the bitter orange, *Citrus aurantium* L. (synonyms: *Citrus aurantium* subsp. *amara* (Link) Engl., *Citrus amara* Link, *Citrus bigaradia* Loisel, *Citrus vulgaris* Risso)
INCI name(s) EU	: Citrus aurantium amara flower oil
INCI name(s) USA	: Citrus aurantium amara (bitter orange) flower oil
Other name(s)	: Oil of orange flowers
CAS registry number(s)	: 8016-38-4; 72968-50-4; 68916-04-1
EC number(s)	: 277-143-2
CIR review(s)	: Final report 12/06/2016 (access: www.cir-safety.org/ingredients)
RIFM monograph(s)	: Food Cosmet Toxicol 1976;14:813 (special issue III)
SCCS opinion(s)	: SCCS/1459/11 (21)
ISO standard	: ISO 3517 Essential oil of neroli, 2013; Geneva, Switzerland, www.iso.org
Merck Index monograph	: 8168
Function(s) in cosmetics	: EU: masking; skin conditioning. USA: fragrance ingredients; skin-conditioning agents – miscellaneous; solvents
Patch testing	: 2% and 5% pet. (SPCanada)

GENERAL

Citrus aurantium L. is an evergreen shrub or tree, 2-3 to 7-8 meter tall, with short and sharp spines, which produces ovoid or rounded greenish-yellow fruits with bitter acidic pulp. It probably has a multiple hybrid origin in China and elsewhere, and is widely cultivated in the tropics and subtropics. The countries producing the bitter orange trees and their essential oils include Spain, Italy, France, Egypt, Tunisia, Morocco, Uganda, Ivory Coast, Paraguay, Brazil, Argentina, and China (23).

The neroli essential oil, obtained from the flowers by steam- or hydrodistillation is used in the perfume (mainly fine fragrances) and soap industry. The volatile oil contains a sensual fragrance and forms the heart of one the world's most enduring perfumes, 'Eau de Cologne'. It also has limited use in flavoring candy, soft-drinks and liqueurs, ice cream, baked goods and chewing gum. In addition, neroli oil has applications in aromatherapy (2,3,23).

Citrus aurantium L. is not only used for the production of neroli oil, but is also the source for obtaining bitter orange oil from cold-pressing of the fruit peels (Chapter 6.52) and petitgrain bigarade oil from steam-distillation of the leaves, twigs and unripe fruit (Chapter 6.57).

CHEMICAL COMPOSITION

Neroli oil is a clear mobile liquid with pale yellow to light amber color, sometimes with slight blue influences and which has a flowery, sometimes harsh but fresh odor, reminding of natural orange blossoms. In neroli oils from various origins, over 190 chemicals have been identified. About 50 per cent of these were found in a single reviewed publication only. The ten chemicals that had the highest maximum concentrations in 79 commercial neroli essential oil samples are shown in table 6.48.1 (Erich Schmidt, analytical data presented in ref. 23).

A full literature review of the qualitative and quantitative composition of commercial and non-commercial neroli oils of various origins and with data from the ISO standard, has been published in 2016 (23). A slightly older but useful review of the chemical composition of neroli oils is provided in reference 1.

Table 6.48.1 Ten ingredients with the highest concentrations in commercial neroli oils (23)

Name	Concentration range	Name	Concentration range
Linalool	31.9-57.7%	α-Terpineol	3.2-7.6%
Limonene	10.1-20.3%	(*E*)-Nerolidol	1.7-4.9%
β-Pinene	3.8-16.9%	Geranyl acetate	1.7-3.7%
Linalyl acetate	1.4-15.1%	Geraniol	2.0-3.6%
(*E*)-β-Ocimene	3.5-7.9%	(*E,E*)-Farnesol	0.3-3.5%

CONTACT ALLERGY / ALLERGIC CONTACT DERMATITIS

General

The SCCS (Scientific Committee on Consumer Safety), in a 2012 Opinion on Fragrance allergens in cosmetic products, has marked neroli oil as 'established contact allergen in humans' (21,22).

Contact allergy to / allergic contact dermatitis from neroli oil has been reported in over 15 publications. In routine testing (one study), a prevalence rate of only 0.3% positive patch test reactions was observed. There have been several case reports of allergic contact dermatitis from neroli oil, mostly from its presence in topical pharmaceutical preparations and some from cosmetics. Also, several cases of occupational contact dermatitis from neroli oil have been documented, both in people who use the oils for massage (including aromatherapists) and patients sensitized from their work as bottle fillers in a perfume factory. In one case, geraniol may have been an allergen in neroli oil.

Testing in groups of patients

The results of patch tests with neroli oil in routine testing (consecutive patients suspected of contact dermatitis) and in groups of selected patients are shown in table 6.48.2. In routine testing, the rate of positive reactions was 0.3% (only one study performed), whereas between 0.7% and 20% of patients in selected groups had positive patch tests. The high positivity rate of 20% was seen in a very small group of 10 patients with fragrance contact allergy (6).

Table 6.48.2 Patch testing in groups of patients

Years and Country	Test conc. & vehicle	Number of patients tested | positive (%)		Selection of patients (S); Relevance (R); Comments (C)	Ref.
Routine testing					
2000-2007 USA	2% pet.	324	1 (0.3%)	R: 100%; C: weak study: a. high rate of macular erythema and weak reactions, b. relevance figures include 'questionable' and 'past' relevance	5
Testing in groups of selected patients					
2008-2014 UK	2% pet.	471	3 (0.6%)	S: patients tested with a fragrance series; R: not stated	24
2001-2010 Australia	2% pet.	477	20 (4.2%)	S: not specified; R: 65%	20
2000-2008 IVDK	2% pet.	6220	44 (0.7%)	S: patients with dermatitis suspected of causal exposure to fragrances; R: not stated	17
1989-1999 Portugal	2% pet.	67	4 (6.6%)	S: patients who had a positive patch test to the fragrance mix; R: not stated	19
1996-1997 UK	2% pet.	10	2 (20%)	S: patients suspected of cosmetic dermatitis and reacting to the fragrance mix; R: not stated	6

IVDK Information Network of Departments of Dermatology, Germany, Switzerland, Austria (www.ivdk.org); pet.: petrolatum

Case reports and case series

Occupational allergic contact dermatitis

Occupational allergic contact dermatitis developed in an aromatherapist who worked with many essential oils diluted to 5%; she reacted to neroli oil and lavender oil (9). A female 'complementary therapist' developed occupational contact dermatitis from a multitude of essential oils used at work, including neroli oil (11). One masseuse / reflexologist was seen with occupational dermatitis from contact allergy to neroli oil and other essential oils (10).

Three people working in a perfume factory as bottle fillers developed occupational allergic contact dermatitis from neroli oil they worked with and from various other essential oils; there was also one positive patch test reaction among 20 workers without dermatitis (12).

Non-occupational allergic contact dermatitis

Two positive patch test reactions to neroli oil, which was present in cosmetics that had given a positive patch test or had been positive in a usage test, were seen in a 9-year period in one clinic in Belgium (16). One case of allergic contact dermatitis from a facial moisturizer was due to its ingredient neroli oil (11). Fourteen cases of contact sensitization to neroli oil present in topical pharmaceutical preparations have been observed (4).

Five cases of contact allergy to 'oil of orange flowers' in topical pharmaceutical preparations were reported (7). Two positive patch test reactions to neroli oil (of which one was photoaggravated) were due to its presence in a topical NSAID preparation used by patients suspected to be allergic to the NSAID (18). There may be some overlap in these three reports from Belgium.

Miscellaneous

In a number of publications, positive patch tests to neroli oil have been reported with unknown, uncertain or unstated relevance. These include (literature screened up to 2014 [23]) the following. One positive patch test to neroli oil in an aromatherapist with occupational contact dermatitis from (multiple) essential oils; this oil had not been used by the patient (8). A patient suffering from airborne contact dermatitis caused by (other) essential oils had a positive patch test to 'pomerance flower oil' (14). An aromatherapist had chronic hand dermatitis and was patch test positive to 17 of 20 oils used at her work (tested 1% and 5% in petrolatum) and to neroli oil, with which she had no contact (13). One positive patch test to neroli oil occurred in a case of occupational hand dermatitis in a cook / entration rangegrower from contact allergy to lemon (oil), who also reacted to lemongrass oil and geraniol. The patient was patch tested with 'essences' (no concentration mentioned), but from the text it seems that this would indicate essential oils (15); geraniol may be present in commercial neroli oils in concentrations up to 3.6% (table 6.48.1).

Photosensitivity

Photosensitivity from neroli oil has been cited in ref. 25.

REFERENCES

1 Dugo G, Peyron L, Bonaccorsi I. Extracts from the bitter orange flowers (*Citrus aurantium* L.): Composition and adulteration. In: G Dugo and L Mondello, Eds. Citrus oils. Composition, advanced analytical techniques, contaminants, and biological activity. Boca Raton, USA: CRC Press, 2010:333-348

2 Rhind JP. Essential oils. A handbook for aromatherapy practice, 2nd Edition. London: Singing Dragon, 2012

3 Lawless J. The encyclopedia of essential oils, 2nd Edition. London: Harper Thorsons, 2014

4 Nardelli A, D'Hooge E, Drieghe J, Dooms M, Goossens A. Allergic contact dermatitis from fragrance components in specific topical pharmaceutical products in Belgium. Contact Dermatitis 2009;60:303-313

5 Wetter DA, Yiannias JA, Prakash AV, Davis MD, Farmer SA, el-Azhary RA, et al. Results of patch testing to personal care product allergens in a standard series and a supplemental cosmetic series: an analysis of 945 patients from the Mayo Clinic Contact Dermatitis Group, 2000-2007. J Am Acad Dermatol 2010;63:789-798

6 Thomson KF, Wilkinson SM. Allergic contact dermatitis to plant extracts in patients with cosmetic dermatitis. Br J Dermatol 2000;142:84-88

7 Devleeschouwer V, Roelandts R, Garmyn M, Goossens A. Allergic and photoallergic contact dermatitis from ketoprofen: results of (photo) patch testing and follow-up of 42 patients. Contact Dermatitis 2008;58:159-166

8 Bleasel N, Tate B, Rademaker M. Allergic contact dermatitis following exposure to essential oils. Australas J Dermatol 2002;43:211-213

9 Keane FM, Smith HR, White IR, Rycroft RJG. Occupational allergic contact dermatitis in two aromatherapists. Contact Dermatitis 2000;43:49-51

10 Trattner A, David M, Lazarov A. Occupational contact dermatitis due to essential oils. Contact Dermatitis 2008;58:282-284

11 Newsham J, Rai S, Williams JDL. Two cases of allergic contact dermatitis to neroli oil. Br J Dermatol 2011;165(suppl.1):76

12 Schubert HJ. Skin diseases in workers at a perfume factory. Contact Dermatitis 2006;55:81-83

13 Selvaag E, Holm J, Thune P. Allergic contact dermatitis in an aromatherapist with multiple sensitizations to essential oils. Contact Dermatitis 1995;33:354-355

14 Schaller M, Korting HC. Allergic airborne contact dermatitis from essential oils used in aromatherapy. Clin Exp Dermatol 1995;20:143-145

15 Audicana M, Bernaola G. Occupational contact dermatitis from citrus fruits: Lemon essential oils. Contact Dermatitis 1994;31:183-185

16 Nardelli A, Drieghe J, Claes L, Boey L, Goossens A. Fragrance allergens in 'specific' cosmetic products. Contact Dermatitis 2011;64:212-219

17 Uter W, Schmidt E, Geier J, Lessmann H, Schnuch A, Frosch P. Contact allergy to essential oils: current patch test results (2000–2008) from the Information Network of Departments of Dermatology (IVDK). Contact Dermatitis 2010;63:277-283

18 Matthieu L, Meuleman L, van Hecke E, Blondeel A, Dezfoulian B, Constandt L, Goossens A. Contact and photocontact allergy to ketoprofen. The Belgian experience. Contact Dermatitis 2004;50:238-241

19 Manuel Brites M, Goncalo M, Figueiredo A. Contact allergy to fragrance mix - a 10-year study. Contact Dermatitis 2000;43:181-182

20 Toholka R, Wang Y-S, Tate B, Tam M, Cahill J, Palmer A, Nixon R. The first Australian Baseline Series: Recommendations for patch testing in suspected contact dermatitis. Australas J Dermatol 2015;56:107-115

21 SCCS (Scientific Committee on Consumer Safety). Opinion on Fragrance allergens in cosmetic products, 26-27 June 2012, SCCS/1459/11. Available at:
    https://ec.europa.eu/health/sites/health/files/scientific_committees/consumer_safety/docs/sccs_o_102.pdf

22 Uter W, Johansen JD, Börje A, Karlberg A-T, Lidén C, Rastogi S, Roberts D, White IR. Categorization of fragrance contact allergens for prioritization of preventive measures: clinical and experimental data and consideration of structure–activity relationships. Contact Dermatitis 2013;69:196-230

23 De Groot AC, Schmidt E. Essential oils: contact allergy and chemical composition. Boca Raton, Fl., USA: CRC Press, Taylor and Francis Group, 2016 (ISBN 9781482246407)

24 Sabroe RA, Holden CR, Gawkrodger DJ. Contact allergy to essential oils cannot always be predicted from allergy to fragrance markers in the baseline series. Contact Dermatitis 2016;74:236-241

25 De Groot AC. Patch Testing, 4th Edition. Wapserveen, The Netherlands: acdegroot publishing, 2018 (ISBN 978-90-813233-4-5)

Chapter 6.49   NIAOULI OIL

IDENTIFICATION

Description/definition	: Niaouli oil is the essential oil obtained from the leaves and twigs of the broad-leaved paperbark (paper bark tea tree, niaouli), *Melaleuca quinquenervia* (Cav.) S.T. Blake
INCI name(s) EU	: Melaleuca quinquenervia oil (perfuming name, not an INCI name proper)
INCI name(s) USA	: Not in the Personal Care Products Council Ingredient Database
CAS registry number(s)	: 8014-68-4
EC number(s)	: No EC number found
Function(s) in cosmetics	: EU: perfuming
Patch testing	: 1% alc. (14)

GENERAL

Melaleuca quinquenervia (Cav.) S.T. Blake, also called niaouli (3), is a small to medium-sized evergreen tree, which grows as a spreading tree up to 20 m high, with the trunk covered by a white, beige and grey thick papery bark and grey-green ovate (egg-shaped) leaves. It is native to Papua New Guinea, the coastal areas of North and East Australia, Indonesia and New Caledonia (where it is one of the most widespread trees [3]). The niaouli tree is naturalized in southern Africa, India, Malaysia, the Philippines, USA (Florida, Hawaii, where it is an invasive weed [2,4]), the Caribbean (West Indies) and it is cultivated in Madagascar (4,5,6,11).

The essential oil of the leaves and twigs of *Melaleuca quinquenervia* is called niaouli oil, which is used in a variety of cosmetic products, especially in Australia. The oil is reported to be used in herbalism and natural medicine (1). It has also been used in aromatherapy for a long time (1,3). Oils having high concentrations of (*E*)-nerolidol and linalool are used in fragrances (4).

CHEMICAL COMPOSITION

Niaouli oil of the 1,8-cineole type is a clear, colorless mobile liquid which has a fresh, herbal odor reminding of soft eucalyptus oil. In niaouli oils from various origins, over 150 chemicals have been identified. About 46 per cent of these were found in a single reviewed publication only. The ten chemicals that had the highest maximum concentrations in 39 commercial niaouli essential oil samples are shown in table 6.49.1. (Erich Schmidt, analytical data presented in ref. 11). There are several chemotypes and the composition of niaouli oils may vary extremely.

A full literature review of the qualitative and quantitative composition of commercial and non-commercial niaouli oils of various origins and their chemotypes has been published in 2016 (11).

Table 6.49.1 Ten ingredients with the highest concentrations in commercial niaouli oils (11)

Name	Concentration range	Name	Concentration range
(*E*)-Nerolidol	0.3 - 80.3%	α-Terpineol	2.1 - 9.2%
1,8-Cineole	45.3 - 61.2%	γ-Terpinene	0.02 - 5.2%
Viridiflorol	1.0 - 22.6%	Ledol	0.6 - 4.8%
α-Pinene	4.7 - 15.0%	β-Caryophyllene	0.5 - 4.1%
Limonene	0.8 - 9.9%	β-Myrcene	0.3 - 3.8%

CONTACT ALLERGY / ALLERGIC CONTACT DERMATITIS

General

There have been six publications on allergic contact dermatitis from niaouli oil. In one case, α-pinene may have been an allergen in niaouli oil (8).

Case reports and case series

In a clinic in Belgium, in the period 1990-2016, two cases of dermatitis caused by contact allergy to niaouli oil from its presence as active principle in 'topical botanical medicines' have been observed (13). In Strasbourg, France, in the period 1967-1972, 276 patients with plant allergy were seen. 'Niaouli and thyme oils' (test concentration unknown) reacted in 12 (4.3%) (12).

An aromatherapist had non-occupational contact dermatitis with allergies to multiple essential oils used at work, including niaouli oil. The patient also reacted to geraniol, linalool, linalyl acetate, α-pinene, the fragrance mix and various other fragrance materials. α-Pinene was demonstrated by GC-MS in niaouli oil (8). In commercial oils, α-pinene has been found in a maximum concentration of 15.0% (table 6.49.1).

A positive patch test reaction to niaouli oil, which was present in a cosmetic that had given a positive patch test or had been positive in a usage test in patients, was seen in a 9-year period in one clinic in Belgium (9). Two positive patch tests to niaouli oil, probably from its presence in a topical pharmaceutical preparation, have been observed (7). There may be overlap between refs. 7,9 and 13.

Additional information on contact allergy to niaouli oil may be found in ref. 10 (article not read).

LITERATURE

1 Barbosa LCA, Silva CJ, Teixeira RR, Meira RMSA, Pinheiro AL. Chemistry and biological activities of essential oils from *Melaleuca* L. species. Agriculturae Conspectus Scientificus 2013;78:11-23

2 Wheeler GS, Pratt PD, Giblin-Davis RM, Ordung KM. Intraspecific variation of *Melaleuca quinquenervia* leaf oils in its naturalized range in Florida, the Caribbean, and Hawaii. Biochem Syst Ecol 2007;35:489-500

3 Trilles BL, Bombarda I, Bouraïma-Madjebi S, Raharivelomanana P, Bianchini J-P, Gaydou EM. Occurrence of various chemotypes in niaouli [*Melaleuca quinquenervia* (Cav.) S.T. Blake] essential oil from New Caledonia. Flavour Fragr J 2006;21:677-682

4 Ireland BF, Hibbert DB, Goldsack RJ, Doran JC, Brophy JJ. Chemical variation in the leaf oil of *Melaleuca quinquenervia* (Cav.) S.T. Blake. Biochem Syst Ecol 2002;30:457-470

5 Ramanoelina PAR, Viano J, Bianchini J-P, Gaydou EM. Occurrence of various chemotypes in niaouli (*Melaleuca quinquenervia*) essential oils from Madagascar using multivariate statistical analysis. J Agric Food Chem 1994;42:1177-1182

6 Lawrence BM. Progress in essential oils. Perfum Flavor 2013;38(5):44-48

7 Nardelli A, D'Hooge E, Drieghe J, Dooms M, Goossens A. Allergic contact dermatitis from fragrance components in specific topical pharmaceutical products in Belgium. Contact Dermatitis 2009;60:303-313

8 Dharmagunawardena B, Takwale A, Sanders KJ, Cannan S, Roger A, Ilchyshyn A. Gas chromatography: an investigative tool in multiple allergies to essential oils. Contact Dermatitis 2002;47:288-292

9 Nardelli A, Drieghe J, Claes L, Boey L, Goossens A. Fragrance allergens in 'specific' cosmetic products. Contact Dermatitis 2011;64:212-219

10 Escande JP, Foussereau J, Lantz JP, Basset A. Le problème des fausses sensibilisations croisées dans les allergies de groupe aux allergènes vegetaux. Rev Fr Allergol 1973;13:70-75 (article in French)

11 De Groot AC, Schmidt E. Essential oils: contact allergy and chemical composition. Boca Raton, Fl., USA: CRC Press, Taylor and Francis Group, 2016 (ISBN 9781482246407)

12 Fousserau J, Meller JC, Benezra C. Contact allergy to Frullania and Laurus nobilis: cross-sensitization and chemical structure of the allergens. Contact Dermatitis 1975;1:223-230

13 Gilissen L, Huygens S, Goossens A. Allergic contact dermatitis caused by topical herbal remedies: importance of patch testing with the patients' own products. Contact Dermatitis 2018;78:177-184

14 De Groot AC. Patch Testing, 4th Edition. Wapserveen, The Netherlands: acdegroot publishing, 2018 (ISBN 978-90-813233-4-5)

Chapter 6.50   NUTMEG OIL

IDENTIFICATION

Description/definition	: Nutmeg oil (essential oil of nutmeg) is the essential oil obtained from the seed of the nutmeg, *Myristica fragrans* Houtt.
INCI name(s) EU	: Myristica fragrans kernel oil
INCI name(s) USA	: Myristica fragrans (nutmeg) kernel oil
Other names	: Myristica oil; mace oil
CAS registry number(s)	: 8008-45-5; 84082-68-8
EC number(s)	: 282-013-3
RIFM monograph(s)	: Food Cosmet Toxicol 1976;14:631 (binder, page 596)
ISO standard	: ISO 3215 Essential oil of nutmeg, Indonesian type, 1998; Geneva, Switzerland, www.iso.org
Merck Index monograph	: 8088 (Nutmeg)
Function(s) in cosmetics	: EU: masking; skin conditioning. USA: flavoring agents; fragrance ingredients; skin-conditioning agents - miscellaneous
Patch testing	: 2% pet.; based on RIFM data, 8% pet. is probably not irritant (9)

GENERAL

Myristica fragrans Houtt. is a spreading, medium- to large-sized, aromatic evergreen tree usually growing to around 5-13 meter high, occasionally 20 meter. The origin of the nutmeg is uncertain but may include the Indonesian Molucca Islands (the 'spice islands'). The tree is cultivated in India, Sri Lanka, Indonesia, Malaysia, the Caribbean (Grenada) and to a lesser extent elsewhere, mainly for its nutmegs, the hard kernels of its seed (3,4,7). The export of nutmeg is dominated by Indonesia and Grenada, and broadly speaking both nutmeg and its derivatives are classified as East Indian (Indonesia, Malaysia, Sri Lanka) or West Indian (Carribean, Grenada) (2,3). The East Indian nutmeg is superior in flavor to the West Indian (3,4,7). Nutmeg is the hard kernel of the seed of *M. fragrans*; dried crimson aril (bright red cover of the seed) is the spice mace.

The essential oil of nutmeg is obtained by steam-distillation of ground nutmeg. Nutmeg oil is used in the flavoring of meat products, pastry, liqueurs, in ketchups and soft drinks, and in the pharmaceutical, perfumery and cosmetics (mainly for men) industry and to flavor tobacco (1,2). The oil is used both externally and internally for medical conditions (8) and its use through aromatherapy is gaining in importance (4,5).

Mace oil (the essential oil obtained from the aril [i.e., the bright red cover of the seed]) has a composition which is similar to nutmeg oil and therefore is a direct substitute for nutmeg oil (4).

Nutmeg essential oil should not be confused with the fixed oil (vegetable oil) of the nutmeg, also called nutmeg butter.

CHEMICAL COMPOSITION

Nutmeg oil is a nearly colorless to pale yellow clear mobile liquid which has a spicy, aromatic, slight peppery sweet odor. In nutmeg oils from various origins, over 120 chemicals have been identified. The ten chemicals that had the highest maximum concentrations in 51 commercial nutmeg essential oil samples are shown in table 6.50.1 (Erich Schmidt, analytical data presented in ref. 7).

A full literature review of the qualitative and quantitative composition of commercial and non-commercial nutmeg oils of various origins and with data from the ISO standard has been published in 2016 (7).

Table 6.50.1 Ten ingredients with the highest concentrations in commercial nutmeg oils (7)

Name	Concentration range	Name	Concentration range
Sabinene	16.5 - 36.7%	Terpinen-4-ol	0.2 - 8.4%
α-Pinene	12.6 - 25.3%	γ-Terpinene	3.6 - 7.4%
β-Pinene	2.6 - 16.5%	α-Terpinene	2.4 - 4.6%
Myrcene	2.3 - 10.5%	Limonene	3.8 - 4.5%
Myristicin	1.7 - 9.9%	β-Phellandrene	1.9 - 3.2%

CONTACT ALLERGY / ALLERGIC CONTACT DERMATITIS

General
There has been only one publication on contact allergy to / allergic contact dermatitis from nutmeg oil.

Case reports and case series
Four positive patch test reactions to nutmeg oil were observed in a group of 14 patients (29%) with oral lichen planus and contact allergy to spearmint oil (6). The high percentage of co-reactivity may possibly be explained by their common ingredients limonene (highest concentrations in commercial spearmint and nutmeg oils 23.7% resp. 4.5%) and myrcene (highest concentration in commercial spearmint and nutmeg oils 2.6% resp. 10.5%) (7).

LITERATURE

1   Dupuy N, Molinet J, Mehl F, Nanlohy F, Le Dréau Y, Kister J. Chemometric analysis of mid infrared and gas chromatography data of Indonesian nutmeg essential oils. Ind Crops Prod 2013;43:596- 601
2   Ehlers D, Kirchhoff J, Gerard D, Quirin K-W. High-performance liquid chromatography analysis of nutmeg and mace oils produced by supercritical CO2 extraction – comparison with steam-distilled oils – comparison of East Indian, West Indian and Papuan oils. Int J Food Sci Technol 1998;33:215-223
3   Charles DJ. Nutmeg. In: Antioxidant Properties of Spices, Herbs and Other Sources. New York: Springer Science + Business Media, 2013: 427-433
4   Rema J, Rishnamoorthy B. Nutmeg and Mace. In: Peter KV, Ed. Handbook of herbs and spices, 2nd Ed, Vol. 1. Oxford-Cambridge-Philadelhia-New Delhi: Woodhead Publishing Ltd, 2012:399-416
5   Lawless J. The encyclopedia of essential oils, 2nd Edition. London: Harper Thorsons, 2014
6   Gunatheesan S, Tam MM, Tate B, Tversky J, Nixon R. Retrospective study of oral lichen planus and allergy to spearmint oil. Australas J Dermatol 2012;53:224-228
7   De Groot AC, Schmidt E. Essential oils: contact allergy and chemical composition. Boca Raton, Fl., USA: CRC Press, Taylor and Francis Group, 2016 (ISBN 9781482246407)
8   Ogunwande IA, Olawore NO, Adeleke KA, Ekundayo O. Chemical composition of essential oil of *Myristica fragrans* Houtt (nutmeg) from Nigeria. J Essent Oil Bear Plants 2003;6:21-26
9   De Groot AC. Patch Testing, 4th Edition. Wapserveen, The Netherlands: acdegroot publishing, 2018 (ISBN 978-90-813233-4-5)

Chapter 6.51   OLIBANUM OIL (FRANKINCENSE OIL)

IDENTIFICATION

Description/definition   : Olibanum oil (frankincense oil) is the essential oil obtained from the wood exudate of
                            the olibanum tree (frankincense), *Boswellia sacra* Flueck. (synonym: *Boswellia carteri*
                            Birdw.) and other *Boswellia* species
INCI name(s) EU   : Boswellia carterii oil; Boswellia carterii gum oil (perfuming name, not an INCI name
                            proper)
INCI name(s) USA   : Boswellia carterii oil
Other names   : Frankincense oil
CAS registry number(s)   : 8016-36-2; 89957-98-2
EC number(s)   : 289-620-2
RIFM monograph(s)   : Food Cosmet Toxicol 1978;16:835 (special issue IV) (olibanum absolute); Food
                            Cosmet Toxicol 1978;837 (special issue IV) (olibanum gum)
Merck Index monograph : 8196 (Olibanum)
Function(s) in cosmetics : EU: masking; perfuming; tonic. USA: fragrance ingredients
Patch testing   : 2% pet.

GENERAL

Boswellia sacra Flueck. is a small deciduous tree, which reaches a height of 2 to 8 meters, with one or more trunks. Its bark has the texture of paper and can be removed easily. It is native to Somalia, Ethiopia, Oman and Yemen and is cultivated in Somalia and Oman (4) for the production of a gum oleoresin. The resin, which is called olibanum or frankincense, is harvested by making a small, shallow incision on the trunk or branches of the tree or by removing a portion of the crust of it. This allows a milky substance to seep from the wounds. This material is left on the tree to dry in the sun for a few days, after which the so called 'resin tears' can be scraped off and the olibanum is collected by hand. The color of the material varies from light yellow to dark brown (2,3,11). Olibanum consist of 60% resin (of which 50% are boswellic acids), 20% rubber, 6-8% bassorine (an α-D-galacturonic acid polysaccharide), 5-15% essential oils and 0.5% bitter and mucilage compounds (3).

Olibanum (either from *Boswellia sacra* Flueck. or other species of the genus *Boswellia*) has a long history of medicinal, religious (e.g. as incense in the Catholic Church and other religious ceremonies), social and other uses (4). The essential oil of olibanum is obtained by steam-distillation of the olibanum oleoresin and is one of the most commonly used oils in aromatherapy practice (1,6). In perfumery, frankincense oil is used as a fixative and for its fresh balsamic, dry, resinous, somewhat green note fragrance (4). It is also added as a fixative and fragrance to soaps, creams, lotions and detergents (6).

The chemistry and biology of essential oils of the genus *Boswellia* are described in ref. 12. Pharmacological and medical aspects of olibanum have been reviewed (5). The name *Boswellia carterii*, found not only in INCI but also in (most) other publications, is incorrect and should read *Boswellia carteri* (11).

CHEMICAL COMPOSITION

Olibanum oil is a mobile, colorless to yellowish, sometimes slightly green liquid which has a balsamic, slightly terpenic, spicy warm and tender sweet odor. In *B. sacra* olibanum oils from various origins, over 245 chemicals have been identified. About 58 per cent of these were found in a single reviewed publication only. The ten chemicals that had the highest maximum concentrations in 28 commercial olibanum (frankincense) essential oil samples are shown in table 6.51.1 (Erich Schmidt, analytical data presented in ref. 11).

A full literature review of the qualitative and quantitative composition of commercial and non-commercial olibanum oils of various origins has been published in 2016 (11).

Table 6.51.1 Ten ingredients with the highest concentrations in commercial olibanum oils (11)

Name	Concentration range	Name	Concentration range
α-Pinene	14.8 - 46.5%	Sabinene	0.5 - 7.2%
α-Thujene	1.6 - 25.8%	Terpinen-4-ol	0.2 - 5.8%
Limonene	5.5 - 18.5%	*p*-Cymene	2.7 - 4.9%
Myrcene	1.8 - 10.4%	β-Caryophyllene	1.1 - 4.7%
Octyl acetate	0.04 - 7.8%	(*Z*)-β-Ocimene	0.01 - 4.5%

CONTACT ALLERGY / ALLERGIC CONTACT DERMATITIS

General
There are only three publications on contact allergy to / allergic contact dermatitis from olibanum (frankincense) oil, all concerning occupational contact dermatitis in aromatherapists. In two and possibly all, a false-positive patch test reaction due to the excited skin syndrome cannot be excluded. In one report, α-pinene and possibly caryophyllene may have been allergens in the olibanum oil (9).

Case reports and case series
An aromatherapist had chronic hand dermatitis and was patch test positive to 17 of 20 oils used at her work (tested 1% and 5% in petrolatum), including olibanum oil (8). Another aromatherapist had occupational contact dermatitis with allergies to multiple essential oils used at work, including frankincense oil. The patient also reacted to geraniol, α-pinene, caryophyllene, the fragrance mix and various other fragrance materials. α-Pinene and caryophyllene were demonstrated by GC-MS in the olibanum oil (9). α-Pinene is the major ingredient in olibanum oil: concentrations in commercial olibanum oils were found to be 14.8-46.5%, whereas caryophyllene may be present in such oils in concentrations of up to 4.7% (table 6.51.1).

A positive patch test reaction to frankincense oil was observed in an aromatherapist with occupational contact dermatitis from multiple essential oils; apparently she had no previous contact with olibanum oil (7). Contact dermatitis from contact allergy to olibanum *extract* (from *Boswellia serrata*) present in a 'naturopathic cream' has been observed (10).

LITERATURE

1   Chen Y, Zhou C, Ge Z, Liu Z, Liu Y, Feng W, et al. Composition and potential anticancer activities of essential oils obtained from myrrh and frankincense. Oncol Lett 2013;6:1140-1146
2   Van Vuuren SF, Kamatou GPP, Viljoen AM. Volatile composition and antimicrobial activity of twenty commercial frankincense essential oil samples. S Afr J Bot 2010;76:686–691
3   Mertens M, Buettner A, Kirchhoff E. The volatile constituents of frankincense – a review. Flavour Fragr J 2009;24:279-300
4   Al-Saidi S, Rameshkumar KB, Hisham A, Sivakumar N, Al-Kindy S. Composition and antibacterial activity of the essential oils of four commercial grades of Omani Luban, the oleo-gum resin of *Boswellia sacra* Flueck. Chem Biodivers 2012;9:615-624
5   Moussaieff A, Mechoulam R. Boswellia resin: from religious ceremonies to medical uses; a review of *in-vitro, in-vivo* and clinical trials. J Pharm Pharmacol 2009;61:1281-1293
6   Camarda L, Dayton T, Di Stefano V, Pitonzo R, Schillaci D. Chemical composition and antimicrobial activity of some oleogum resin essential oils from *Boswellia* spp. Ann Chim 2007;97:837-844
7   Bleasel N, Tate B, Rademaker M. Allergic contact dermatitis following exposure to essential oils. Australas J Dermatol 2002;43:211-213
8   Selvaag E, Holm J, Thune P. Allergic contact dermatitis in an aromatherapist with multiple sensitizations to essential oils. Contact Dermatitis 1995;33:354-355
9   Dharmagunawardena B, Takwale A, Sanders KJ, Cannan S, Roger A, Ilchyshyn A. Gas chromatography: an investigative tool in multiple allergies to essential oils. Contact Dermatitis 2002;47:288-292
10 Acebo E, Raton JA, Sautua S, Eizaguirre X, Trébol I, Díaz Pérez JL. Allergic contact dermatitis from *Boswellia serrata* extract in a naturopathic cream. Contact Dermatitis 2004;51:91-92
11 De Groot AC, Schmidt E. Essential oils: contact allergy and chemical composition. Boca Raton, Fl., USA: CRC Press, Taylor and Francis Group, 2016 (ISBN 9781482246407)
12 Hussain H, Al-Harrasi A, Al-Rawahi Ahmed, Hussain Javid. Chemistry and biology of essential oils of genus Boswellia. Evidence-based Complementary & Alternative Medicine (eCAM) 2013:1-12

Chapter 6.52   ORANGE OIL

There are two types of 'orange oil': bitter orange oil produced from *Citrus aurantium* L. (the bitter orange) and sweet orange oil produced from *Citrus sinensis* (L.) Osbeck, both from cold pressing of the pericarp (cold-pressed peel oils). In non-botanical literature, including the literature on contact allergy / allergic contact dermatitis, usually the term 'orange oil' is used, without specifying its botanical source.

6.52.1 BITTER ORANGE OIL

IDENTIFICATION

Description/definition	: Bitter orange oil (essential oil of bitter orange) is the essential oil obtained from the pericarp (peel) of the bitter orange, *Citrus aurantium* L. (synonyms: *Citrus amara* Link, *Citrus bigaradia* Loisel, *Citrus vulgaris* Risso)
INCI name(s) EU	: Citrus aurantium amara peel oil
INCI name(s) USA	: Citrus aurantium amara (bitter orange) peel oil
Other names	: Bitter orange oil; oil of bitter orange
CAS registry number(s)	: 68916-04-1; 72968-50-4
EC number(s)	: 277-143-2
CIR review(s)	: Final report 09/09/2014 (access: www.cir-safety.org/ingredients)
RIFM monograph(s)	: Food Cosmet Toxicol 1974;12:735
SCCS opinion(s)	: SCCNFP/0392/00, final (17); SCCNFP/0389/00, final (18); SCCS/1459/11 (19)
IFRA standard	: Restricted (www.ifraorg.org/en-us/standards-library) (table 6.52.1.1)
ISO standard	: ISO 9844 Essential oil of bitter orange, 2006; Geneva, Switzerland, www.iso.org
Merck Index monograph	: 8149
Function(s) in cosmetics	: EU: skin conditioning. USA: fragrance ingredients; skin-conditioning agents – miscellaneous
Patch testing	: 2% pet. (SPEurope, SPCanada) (sweet orange oil); test also limonene (see Chapter 3.95 Limonene)

Table 6.52.1.1 IFRA restrictions for bitter orange peel oil expressed

Leave-on products:	0.4%
Rinse-off products:	no restriction
Non-skin contact products:	no restriction

The limit only applies to applications on skin exposed to sunshine, excluding rinse-off products. If combinations of phototoxic fragrance ingredients are used, the use levels have to be reduced accordingly. The sum of the concentrations of all phototoxic ingredients, expressed in % of their recommended maximum level in the consumer product shall not exceed 100

GENERAL

Citrus aurantium L., commonly named bigarade or bitter (sour) orange, is an evergreen shrub or tree, 2-3 to 7-8 meter tall, with short and sharp spines, which produces ovoid or rounded greenish-yellow fruit, 25-70 mm in diameter. It probably has a multiple hybrid origin in China and elsewhere, and is widely cultivated in the tropics and subtropics, important areas of cultivation being Paraguay, Morocco, and Spain (21).

The bitter orange oil, obtained from the peel by cold pressing, is used for flavoring baked goods, chewing gum, ice cream, soft drinks, liqueurs (Cointreau, Curaçao, Licor Beirão) and as a fragrance in perfumery and cosmetics. The role of essential oils and antioxidants derived from *Citrus* by-products in food protection and medicine has been reviewed (1). Besides these uses, undiluted essential oils are sold on the international market of aromatherapy.

The history, global distribution, and nutritional importance of *Citrus* fruits have been reviewed in ref. 22. *Citrus aurantium* L. is not only used for the production of bitter orange (peel) oil, but also for obtaining neroli oil from the flowers (Chapter 6.48 Neroli oil) and petitgrain bigarade oil from the leaves, twigs and unripe fruits (Chapter 6.57 Petitgrain bigarade oil).

CHEMICAL COMPOSITION

Bitter orange oil is a clear mobile liquid, which has a light, pale yellow to brownish green color and a fresh-citrusy note with characteristic odor of the scratched peel of the bitter orange. In bitter orange oils from various origins, over 215 chemicals have been identified. The ten chemicals that had the highest maximum concentrations in 72 commercial bitter orange essential oil samples are shown in table 6.52.1.2 (Erich Schmidt, analytical data presented in ref. 21).

A full literature review of the qualitative and quantitative composition of commercial and non-commercial bitter orange oils of various origins and with data from the ISO standard has been published in 2016 (21).

Table 6.52.1.2 Ten ingredients with the highest concentrations in commercial bitter orange oils (21)

Name	Concentration range	Name	Concentration range
Limonene	92.2 - 95.6%	β-Phellandrene	0.2 - 0.6%
Myrcene	1.5 - 2.5%	Linalyl acetate	0.05 - 0.4%
β-Pinene	0.2 - 0.8%	Decanal	0.02 - 0.3%
α-Pinene	0.4 - 0.7%	Linalool	0.1 - 0.3%
(E)-β-Ocimene	0.02 - 0.6%	n-Octanal	0.01 - 0.3%

6.52.2 SWEET ORANGE OIL

IDENTIFICATION

Description/definition	: Sweet orange oil (essential oil of sweet orange) is the essential oil obtained by expression from the pericarp (peel) of the (sweet) orange, *Citrus sinensis* (L.) Osbeck
INCI name(s) EU	: Citrus sinensis (Valencia) peel oil expressed (not officially an INCI name but perfuming name)
INCI name(s) USA	: Citrus aurantium dulcis (orange) peel oil (wrong name, also in INCI EU; *Citrus aurantium dulcis* is *not* a synonym for *Citrus sinensis* (L.) Osbeck.)
Other names	: Sweet orange oil; orange oil
CAS registry number(s)	: 97766-30-8; 8028-48-6; 8008-57-9
EC number(s)	: 307-891-8; 232-433-8
CIR review(s)	: Final report 09/09/2014 (access: www.cir-safety.org/ingredients)
RIFM monograph(s)	: Food Cosmet Toxicol 1974;12:733 (binder, page 607)
SCCS opinion(s)	: SCCNFP/0389/00, final (18); SCCS/1459/11 (19)
ISO standard	: ISO 3140 Essential oil of sweet orange, 2010: Geneva, Switzerland, www.iso.org
Merck Index monograph	: 8167
Function(s) in cosmetics	: EU: perfuming. USA: fragrance ingredients; skin-conditioning agents - miscellaneous
Patch testing	: 2% pet. (SPEurope, SPCanada); test also limonene (see Chapter 3.95 Limonene)

GENERAL

Citrus species may have originated in India 30 to 40 million years ago. *Citrus* fruits subsequently spread to East Asia and the Mediterranean region, where a great number of varieties were born by numerous mutations. The most popular citrus fruit is the sweet orange, *Citrus sinensis* (L.) Osbeck. This is a tree, up to 10 m tall, with few slender and flexible spines and aromatic leaves of 7.5-11 cm. China is the origin of sweet oranges: *sinensis* in its botanical name, *Citrus sinensis* (L.) Osbeck refers to China. Oranges are grown widely in the tropics and subtropics. Brazil produces the greatest volume of this species, followed by the United States, China, Mexico, Spain, India, Egypt and Morocco (21).

Orange peel oil is a by-product of orange juice production and obtained by cold pressing. These essential oils have wide commercial applications in food processing, pharmaceutical preparations, perfumery and cosmetics because of its flavor and fragrance (21). Sweet orange oils are also employed in aromatherapy practices.

CHEMICAL COMPOSITION

Sweet orange oil is a clear mobile, yellow to orange-brown liquid which has a fresh citrusy odor reminding of fresh scratched orange peel. In sweet orange oils from various origins, over 335 chemicals have been identified. The ten chemicals that had the highest maximum concentrations in 422 commercial sweet orange essential oil samples are shown in table 6.52.2.1 (Erich Schmidt, analytical data presented in ref. 21).

A full literature review of the qualitative and quantitative composition of commercial and non-commercial sweet orange oils of various origins and with data from the ISO standard, has been published in 2016 (21). The history, global distribution, and nutritional importance of *Citrus* fruits have been reviewed in ref. 22.

Table 6.52.2.1 Ten ingredients with the highest concentrations in commercial sweet orange oils (21)

Name	Concentration range	Name	Concentration range
Limonene	94.7 - 95.7%	Decanal	0.09 - 0.6%
Myrcene	1.4 - 3.5%	γ-Terpinene	0.01 - 0.6%
α-Pinene	0.2 - 1.0%	n-Octanal	0.07 - 0.5%
Sabinene	0.02 - 0.7%	β-Pinene	0.01 - 0.5%
β-Phellandrene	0.02 - 0.7%	Undecanal	0.01 - 0.4%

CONTACT ALLERGY / ALLERGIC CONTACT DERMATITIS

Orange oil (unspecified)

General

Contact allergy to / allergic contact dermatitis from orange oil (unspecified whether bitter or sweet orange oil) has been reported in over 10 publications. In groups of consecutive patients suspected of contact dermatitis, prevalence rates of up to 3.2% positive patch test reactions have been observed, but adequate relevance data are lacking. Most case reports concern occupational contact dermatitis in aromatherapists and other whose massage clients with oils and in patients working in a perfume factory.

Testing in groups of patients

The results of patch tests with orange oil in routine testing (consecutive patients suspected of contact dermatitis) and in groups of selected patients are shown in table 6.52.2.2. In routine testing, rates of positive reactions were 0.6% to 3.2% in two studies, whereas between 0.1% and 4.5% of patients in selected groups had positive patch tests. However, relevance data are lacking.

Table 6.52.2.2 Patch testing in groups of patients

Years and Country	Test conc. & vehicle	Number of patients tested | positive (%)		Selection of patients (S); Relevance (R); Comments (C)	Ref.
Routine testing					
2000-2007 USA	2% pet.	678	4 (0.6%)	R: 100%; C: weak study: a. high rate of macular erythema and weak reactions, b. relevance figures include 'questionable' and 'past' relevance	4
1967-1970 Italy	20% pet.	590	19 (3.2%)	R: not stated, but in the population tested (which included patients with dermatitis other than contact dermatitis) many had regular contact with oranges	9
Testing in groups of selected patients					
2000-2008 IVDK	2% pet.	6246	10 (0.2%)	S: patients with dermatitis suspected of causal exposure to fragrances; R: not stated; C: no frequent co-reactivity to limonene, the main component of all citrus oils	13
1997-2000 Austria	2% pet.	747	1 (0.1%)	S: patients suspected of fragrance allergy: R: not stated	5
1989-1999 Portugal	2% pet.	67	3 (4.5%)	S: patients who had a positive patch test to the fragrance mix; R: not stated	14

IVDK Information Network of Departments of Dermatology, Germany, Switzerland, Austria (www.ivdk.org); pet.: petrolatum

Case reports and case series

An aromatherapist had chronic hand dermatitis and was patch test positive to 17 of 20 oils used at her work (tested 1% and 5% in petrolatum), including orange oil (6). A physiotherapist had occupational contact dermatitis from orange oil and other essential oils (8). Two cases of occupational allergy to 'orange oil terpenenes' (tested 1% in olive oil) in bottle fillers in a perfume factory were seen; another two positive patch test reactions were observed among 20 workers in the same factory who did not have dermatitis (11).

Irritant contact dermatitis of the hands was diagnosed in a male masseur who worked with essential oils regularly; he had positive patch test reactions to orange oil and lemongrass oil but it was not mentioned whether he had used these oils (10). One positive patch test reaction to orange oil, which was present in a cosmetic that had given a positive patch test or had been positive in a usage test in patients, was seen in a 9-year period in a clinic in Belgium (12).

Additional information on allergy to orange oil can be found in refs. 7 and 25 (articles not read).

Orange oil bitter

General

The SCCS (Scientific Committee on Consumer Safety), in a 2012 Opinion on Fragrance allergens in cosmetic products, has marked bitter orange oil as 'established contact allergen in humans' (19,20).

Contact allergy to bitter orange oil has been reported in two publications only. In a group of consecutive patients suspected of contact dermatitis, the prevalence rate of positive patch test reactions was 1.5%, but relevance data are lacking.

Testing in groups of patients

Two hundred dermatitis patients from Poland were tested with bitter orange oil 2% in petrolatum and three (1.5%) reacted. The same authors also patch tested 51 patients allergic to Myroxylon pereirae resin (balsam of Peru) and/or turpentine and/or wood tar and/or colophony and three (5.9%) had a positive patch test; relevance data were not provided (16). A group of 86 patients from Poland previously reacting to the fragrance mix was tested with bitter orange oil and two (2.3%) had a positive patch test reaction; relevance data were not provided (15).

Orange oil sweet

General

The SCCS (Scientific Committee on Consumer Safety), in a 2012 Opinion on Fragrance allergens in cosmetic products, has marked Citrus sinensis peel oil expressed as 'established contact allergen in humans' (19,20).

Fresh sweet orange oil is probably little allergenic. However, during use, exposure to light and oxygen (2), and even during storage in the dark (27), strongly allergenic limonene hydroperoxides are formed, which may increase the risk of allergic reactions. See Chapter 3.95 Limonene for further details.

Contact allergy to / allergic contact dermatitis from sweet orange oil has been reported in a few publications only.   In a group of consecutive patients suspected of contact dermatitis (one study only), the prevalence rate of positive patch test reactions was 0.5%, but relevance data are lacking. In one patient, limonene may have been an allergen in (a positive patch test to) sweet orange oil (23).

Patch testing in groups of patients

Two hundred dermatitis patients from Poland were tested with sweet orange oil 2% in petrolatum and one (0.5%) reacted. The same authors also patch tested 51 patients allergic to Myroxylon pereirae resin (balsam of Peru) and/or turpentine and/or wood tar and/or colophony and two (3.9%) had a positive patch test; relevance data were not provided (16). A group of 86 patients from Poland previously reacting to the fragrance mix was tested with sweet orange oil and four (4.7%) had a positive patch test reaction; relevance data were not provided (15).

Case reports and case series

An aromatherapist had non-occupational allergic contact dermatitis with allergies to multiple essential oils used at work, including sweet orange oil. The patient also reacted to geraniol, linalool, linalyl acetate, α-pinene, the fragrance mix and various other fragrance materials; α-pinene was demonstrated by GC-MS in the orange oil, limonene was not tested (23). α-Pinene is not an important component of sweet orange oil.

A female patient developed allergic contact dermatitis from the perfume in an eye cream; she was patch tested with all 94 components of the perfume and reacted to 'orange sweet, terpeneless' (test concentration unknown) and eleven of the other chemicals in the perfume (24). One patient with allergic contact dermatitis from tea tree oil co-reacted to sweet orange oil and its main ingredient limonene (26); limonene may also be an allergen in tea tree oil.

Additional information on allergy to sweet orange oil can be found in refs. 7 and 25 (articles not read).

OTHER SIDE EFFECTS

Photosensitivity

Photosensitivity from both sweet and bitter orange oil has been cited in ref. 3.

LITERATURE

1   Hardin A, Crandall PG, Stankus T. Essential oils and antioxidants derived from Citrus by-products in food protection and medicine: An Introduction and review of recent literature. J Agric Food Inform 2010;11:99-122
2   Rudbäck J, Islam N, Nilsson U, Karlberg AT. A sensitive method for determination of allergenic fragrance terpene hydroperoxides using liquid chromatography coupled with tandem mass spectrometry. J Sep Sci 2013;36:1370-1378

3   De Groot AC. Patch Testing, 4th Edition. Wapserveen, The Netherlands: acdegroot publishing, 2018 (ISBN 978-90-813233-4-5)

4   Wetter DA, Yiannias JA, Prakash AV, Davis MD, Farmer SA, el-Azhary RA, et al. Results of patch testing to personal care product allergens in a standard series and a supplemental cosmetic series: an analysis of 945 patients from the Mayo Clinic Contact Dermatitis Group, 2000-2007. J Am Acad Dermatol 2010;63:789-798

5   Wöhrl S, Hemmer W, Focke M, Götz M, Jarisch R. The significance of fragrance mix, balsam of Peru, colophonium and propolis as screening tools in the detection of fragrance allergy. Br J Dermatol 2001;145:268-273

6   Selvaag E, Holm J, Thune P. Allergic contact dermatitis in an aromatherapist with multiple sensitizations to essential oils. Contact Dermatitis 1995;33:354-355

7   Rivasseau J. A propos des sensibilisations de groupe. Bull Soc Franç Derm Syph 1956;63:83-84 (article in French)

8   Trattner A, David M, Lazarov A. Occupational contact dermatitis due to essential oils. Contact Dermatitis 2008;58:282-284

9   Meneghini CL, Rantuccio F, Lomuto M. Additives, vehicles and active drugs of topical medicaments as causes of delayed-type allergic dermatitis. Dermatologica 1971;143:137-147

10   Jung P, Sesztak-Greinecker G, Wantke F, Götz M, Jarisch R, Hemmer W. Mechanical irritation triggering allergic contact dermatitis from essential oils in a masseur. Contact Dermatitis 2006;54:297-299

11   Schubert HJ. Skin diseases in workers at a perfume factory. Contact Dermatitis 2006;55:81-83

12   Nardelli A, Drieghe J, Claes L, Boey L, Goossens A. Fragrance allergens in 'specific' cosmetic products. Contact Dermatitis 2011;64:212-219

13   Uter W, Schmidt E, Geier J, Lessmann H, Schnuch A, Frosch P. Contact allergy to essential oils: current patch test results (2000–2008) from the Information Network of Departments of Dermatology (IVDK). Contact Dermatitis 2010;63:277-283

14   Manuel Brites M, Goncalo M, Figueiredo A. Contact allergy to fragrance mix - a 10-year study. Contact Dermatitis 2000;43:181-182

15   Rudzki E, Grzywa Z. Allergy to perfume mixture. Contact Dermatitis 1986;15:115-116

16   Rudzki E, Grzywa Z, Bruo WS. Sensitivity to 35 essential oils. Contact Dermatitis 1976;2:196-200

17   Opinion of the Scientific Committee on Cosmetic Products and Non-Food Products Intended for Consumers concerning 'An initial list of perfumery materials which must not form part of cosmetic products except subject to the Restrictions and Conditions laid down, 25 September 2001, SCCNFP/0392/00, final. Available at: http://ec.europa.eu/health/archive/ph_risk/committees/sccp/documents/out150_en.pdf

18   Opinion of the Scientific Committee on Cosmetic Products and Non-Food Products Intended for Consumers concerning 'The 1st update of the inventory of ingredients employed in cosmetic products. Section II: Perfume and aromatic raw materials', 24 October 2000, SCCNFP/0389/00, final. Available at: http://ec.europa.eu/health/ph_risk/committees/sccp/documents/out131_en.pdf

19   SCCS (Scientific Committee on Consumer Safety). Opinion on Fragrance allergens in cosmetic products, 26-27 June 2012, SCCS/1459/11. Available at: https://ec.europa.eu/health/sites/health/files/scientific_committees/consumer_safety/docs/sccs_o_102.pdf

20   Uter W, Johansen JD, Börje A, Karlberg A-T, Lidén C, Rastogi S, Roberts D, White IR. Categorization of fragrance contact allergens for prioritization of preventive measures: clinical and experimental data and consideration of structure–activity relationships. Contact Dermatitis 2013;69:196-230

21   De Groot AC, Schmidt E. Essential oils: contact allergy and chemical composition. Boca Raton, Fl., USA: CRC Press, Taylor and Francis Group, 2016 (ISBN 9781482246407)

22   Liu YQ, Heying E, Tanumihardjo SA. History, global distribution, and nutritional importance of Citrus fruits. Compreh Rev Food Sci Food Saf 2012;11:530-545

23   Dharmagunawardena B, Takwale A, Sanders KJ, Cannan S, Roger A, Ilchyshyn A. Gas chromatography: an investigative tool in multiple allergies to essential oils. Contact Dermatitis 2002;47:288-292

24   Larsen WG. Cosmetic dermatitis due to a perfume. Contact Dermatitis 1975;1:142-145

25   Michel PJ. Dermite des mains récidivante par contacts avec des oranges (intolerance à l'essence d'orange douce). Bull Soc Franç Derm Syph 1953;60:320 (article in French)

26   Kränke B. Allergisierende Potenz von Teebaumöl. Hautarzt 1997;48:203-204 (article in German)

27   Rudbäck J, Islam MN, Börje A, Nilsson U, Karlberg A-T.Essential oils can contain allergenic hydroperoxides at eliciting levels, regardless of handling and storage. Contact Dermatitis 2015;73:253-254

Chapter 6.53   OREGANO OIL

IDENTIFICATION

Description/definition : Oregano oil is the volatile oil distilled from the leaves and flowers of the wild marjoram, *Origanum vulgare* L., Labiatae
INCI name EU and USA : Origanum vulgare leaf oil; there is also an entry for flower *extract*, but not for flower *oil*
CAS registry number(s) : 84012-24-8
EC number(s) : 281-670-3
ISO standard : ISO 13171 Essential oil oregano, 2016; Geneva, Switzerland, www.iso.org
Merck Index monograph : 8169
Function(s) in cosmetics : EU: masking; refreshing. USA: flavoring agents
Patch testing : Commercial oregano essential oil, tested semi-open (1)

GENERAL

Origanum vulgare (European oregano, wild marjoram) is a hardy, bushy perennial herb up to 90 centimeter high with an erect hairy stem, dark-green ovate leaves and pinkish-purple flowers. It is a common garden plant with a strong aroma when the leaves are bruised. The wild marjoram is native to Europe and now cultivated all over the world. This is the 'true' oregano of the herb garden, which also has a very ancient medical reputation (2).

The essential is produced by steam-distillation of the dried flowering herb; they are mainly produced in the former USSR, Bulgaria and Italy. For commercial oregano oils, mostly *Origanum vulgare* L. subsp. *hirtum* (Link) letsw. is used. The oil is used as a fragrance component in soaps, colognes and perfumes, especially men's fragrances. It is also employed to some extent as a flavoring agent, mainly in meat products and pizzas. It has no applications in aromatherapy (2).

CHEMICAL COMPOSITION

At www.thegoodscentscompany.com, there is no description of the physical appearance, odor type and odor of Origanum vulgare leaf oil. The flower oil (from Albania) has been described as 'reddish in color and of a pourable viscosity. The aroma is herbal fresh, somewhat green, a tad woody and simply just like smelling a jar of oregano herbs' (www.thegoodscentscompany.com).

The ten chemicals that had the highest maximum concentrations in 24 commercial oregano essential oil samples obtained from the flowering tops of *Origanum vulgare* L. subsp. *hirtum* (Link) letsw. and analyzed between 2007 and 2017 are shown in table 6.53.1 (Erich Schmidt, personal communication, September 2018).

Table 6.53.1 Ten ingredients with the highest concentrations in commercial oregano oils

Name	Concentration range	Name	Concentration range
Carvacrol	28.4 - 75.0%	Linalool	1.2 - 4.2%
Thymol	0.4 - 29.2%	Caryophyllene	1.3 - 4.0%
p-Cymene	3.6 - 11.2%	Myrcene	0.7 - 2.6%
γ-Terpinene	1.9 - 9.3%	α-Terpinene	0.5 - 2.0%
α-Pinene	0.3 - 5.2%	Limonene	0.1 - 1.4%

CONTACT ALLERGY

General

There is only one case report of allergic contact dermatitis from oregano oil in literature.

Case reports and case series

A woman presented with a 1-year history of dermatitis that began on her right medial calf after a shave biopsy. She subsequently developed an infection at the biopsy site and began treatment with MelaGel, containing tea tree oil. She developed a peri-incisional red, indurated, weepy plaque, which subsequently spread to involve her lateral leg. The patient reported using other essential oils on her skin as well and in an aromatherapy diffuser. She had positive patch tests to oregano oil (commercial preparation, tested semi-open), MelaGel, tea tree oil, ylang-ylang oil and sandalwood oil, all of which she had used (1).

LITERATURE

1   Hagen SL, Grey KR, Warshaw EM. Patch testing to essential oils. Dermatitis 2016;27:382-384
2   Lawless J. The encyclopedia of essential oils, 2nd Edition. London: Harper Thorsons, 2014

Chapter 6.54   PALMAROSA OIL

IDENTIFICATION

Description/definition	: Palmarosa oil (essential oil of palmarosa) is the essential oil obtained from the aerial parts (leaves) of the motia grass (palmarosa), *Cymbopogon martini* (Roxb.) Will. Watson
INCI name(s) EU	: Cymbopogon martini motia herb oil (perfuming name, not an INCI name proper)
INCI name(s) EU	: Not in the Personal Care Products Council Ingredient Database
CAS registry number(s)	: 91722-54-2; 8014-19-5; 84649-81-0
EC number(s)	: 294-453-3; 283-461-2
RIFM monograph(s)	: Food Cosmet Toxicol 1974;12:947 (special issue I) (binder, page 614)
ISO standard	: ISO 4727 Essential oil of palmarosa, 1988: Geneva, Switzerland, www.iso.org; no chromatographic profile available
Function(s) in cosmetics	: EU: perfuming
Patch testing	: 2% pet.; based on RIFM data, 8% pet. is probably not irritant (11)

GENERAL

Cymbopogon martini (Roxb.) Will. Watson, commonly known as palmarosa, is a perennial, tufted, multi-harvest grass with numerous erect culms, 150-300 cm long, that arise from a short, stout and woody rhizome, and which has linear or lanceolate glaucous aromatic leaves, 25-50 cm long. It is native to India and Pakistan. The plant is naturalized in China, India, Indo-China, Malaysia, the western Indian Ocean, and Australia. The grass is cultivated in India, Indonesia, the Seychelles, Brazil and Madagascar (10).

The essential oil of palmarosa is obtained by steam-distillation of the leaves (ISO criterion) or the leaves plus inflorescences (flowering herbs) (5,7) of *Cymbopogon martini*, notably the variety *motia*. It is widely used as a perfumery raw material in soaps, floral, rose-like perfumes and cosmetics preparations. It is also used for flavoring tobacco products, foods, non-alcoholic beverages, for masking the odor of botanical pesticides (4) and in the preparation of mosquito repellent products. In medicine, the oil is used as a remedy for various diseases and symptoms and has also applications in aromatherapy (1,3,4,5,6).

The essential oil of palmarosa is highly valued in the perfumery industry as a source of high grade geraniol *ex* palmarosa, which is separated through fractional distillation (2,4); the olfactory note of this geraniol is considered superior to geraniol prepared from other sources (7).

In literature, the plant is often – incorrectly - termed *Cymbopogon martinii* (with double i).

CHEMICAL COMPOSITION

Palmarosa oil is a pale yellow to yellow, clear mobile liquid which has a sweet floral odor with aspects of geranium and rose. In palmarosa oils from various origins, over 155 chemicals have been identified. About half of these were found in a single reviewed publication only. The ten chemicals that had the highest maximum concentrations in 34 commercial palmarosa essential oil samples are shown in table 6.54.1 (Erich Schmidt, analytical data presented in ref. 10).

A full literature review of the qualitative and quantitative composition of commercial and non-commercial palmarosa oils of various origins with data from the ISO standard (no chromatographic profile available) has been published in 2016 (10).

Table 6.54.1 Ten ingredients with the highest concentrations in commercial palmarosa oils (10)

Name	Concentration range	Name	Concentration range
Geraniol	74.2 - 86.9%	(Z,E)-Farnesol	0.5 - 1.5%
Geranyl acetate	3.4 - 12.5%	Geranyl hexanoate	0.4 - 1.5%
Linalool	2.3 - 4.5%	Limonene	0.1 - 1.4%
β-Caryophyllene	1.7 - 2.5%	(Z)-β-Ocimene	0.3 - 0.7%
(E)-β-Ocimene	0.6 - 2.1%	Geranial	0.2 - 0.7%

CONTACT ALLERGY / ALLERGIC CONTACT DERMATITIS

General
Contact allergy to / allergic contact dermatitis from palmarosa oil has been reported in two publications only.

Case reports and case series
Contact allergy to palmarosa oil with cross-reactivity to citronella oil has been recorded (9, article not read). One positive patch test to palmarosa oil was observed in an aromatherapist with occupational contact dermatitis from multiple (other) essential oils; palmarosa oil itself had not been used by the patient. Geraniol, the major component of palmarosa oil, was negative (8).

LITERATURE
1   Rajeswara Rao BR, Rajput DK, Patel RP. Storage of essential oils: influence of presence of water for short periods on the composition of major constituents of the essential oils of four economically important aromatic crops. J Essent Oil Bear Plants 2011;14:673-678

2   Rajeswara Rao BR, Rajput DK, Patel RP. Essential oil profiles of different parts of palmarosa (*Cymbopogon martinii* (Roxb.) Wats. var. *motia* Burk.). J Essent Oil Res 2009;21:519-521

3   Fatima S, Abad Farooqi AH, Ansari SR, Sharma S. Effect of water stress on growth and essential oil metabolism in *Cymbopogon martinii* (palmarosa) cultivars. J Essent Oil Res 1999;11:491-496

4   Rajeswara Rao BR, Kaul PN, Syamasundar KV, Ramesh S. Chemical profiles of primary and secondary essential oils of palmarosa (*Cymbopogon martinii* (Roxb.) Wats. var. *motia* Burk.). Ind Crops Prod 2005;21:121-127

5   Rajeswara Rao BR. Biomass and essential oil yields of rainfed palmarosa (*Cymbopogon martinii* (Roxb.) Wats. var. *motia* Burk.) supplied with different levels of organic manure and fertilizer nitrogen in semi-arid tropical climate. Ind Crops Prod 2001;14:171-178

6   Dubey VS, Mallavarapu GR, Luthra R. Changes in the essential oil content and its composition during palmarosa (*Cymbopogon martinii* (Roxb.) Wats. var. *motia*) inflorescence development. Flavour Fragr J 2000;15:309-314

7   Mallavarapu GR, Rajeswara Rao BR, Kaul PN, Ramesh S, Bhattacharya AK. Volatile constituents of the essential oils of the seeds and the herb of palmarosa (*Cymbopogon martinii* (Roxb.) Wats. var. *motia* Burk.). Flavour Fragr J 1998;13:167-169

8   Bleasel N, Tate B, Rademaker M. Allergic contact dermatitis following exposure to essential oils. Australas J Dermatol 2002;43:211-213

9   Paschoud JM. Quelques cas d'eczema de contact avec sensibilisation de groupe. Dermatologica 1963;127:349

10 De Groot AC, Schmidt E. Essential oils: contact allergy and chemical composition. Boca Raton, Fl., USA: CRC Press, Taylor and Francis Group, 2016 (ISBN 9781482246407)

11 De Groot AC. Patch Testing, 4th Edition. Wapserveen, The Netherlands: acdegroot publishing, 2018 (ISBN 978-90-813233-4-5)

Chapter 6.55   PATCHOULI OIL

IDENTIFICATION

Description/definition	: Patchouli oil (essential oil of patchouli) is the essential oil obtained from the leaves of the patchouli plant, *Pogostemon cablin* (Blanco) Benth. (synonyms: *Mentha cablin* Blanco; *Pogostemon patchouli* Pellet)
INCI name(s) EU & USA	: Pogostemon cablin leaf oil
CAS registry number(s)	: 8014-09-3; 84238-39-1
EC number(s)	: 282-493-4
RIFM monograph(s)	: Food Cosmet Toxicol 1982;20:791 (special issue VI)
SCCS opinion(s)	: SCCS/1459/11 (15)
ISO standard	: ISO 3757 Essential oil of patchouli, 2002; Geneva, Switzerland, www.iso.org
Merck Index monograph	: 8170
Function(s) in cosmetics	: EU: masking. USA: fragrance ingredients
Patch testing	: 10% pet. (SPEurope, SPCanada)

GENERAL

Pogostemon cablin (Blanco) Benth. is a perennial aromatic herb or subshrub with erect stems, which can grow to a height of one meter. It is (possibly) native to the Philippines and is cultivated in the Western Indian Ocean Islands (Madagascar, Seychelles), China, Taiwan, India, Indonesia, Malaysia, Brazil and on a smaller scale in many other countries. The patchouli has occasionally escaped from cultivation and is now widely naturalized in south-east Asia, southern China, India, Sri Lanka, Mauritius, and Florida (17).

Patchouli essential oil is used in incense, and for flavoring tobacco, chewing gum, beverages, frozen dry desserts, candy, baked goods, gelatin, and meat and meat products. It is equally employed in scented industrial products such as paper towels, laundry detergents, and air fresheners. Patchouli oil is perceived to have many useful pharmacological and therapeutic properties. The oil is therefore used medicinally, notably in India, China and Japan and is also widely employed in aromatherapy practices (17).

A comprehensive review of the phytochemical constituents and pharmacological activities of *Pogostemon cablin* has been provided in 2015 (18).

CHEMICAL COMPOSITION

Patchouli oil is a mobile to highly viscous liquid, which has a woody, earthy, slightly camphoraceous and balsamic odor. In patchouli oils from various origins, over 210 chemicals have been identified. About 66 per cent of these were found in a single reviewed publication only. The ten chemicals that had the highest maximum concentrations in 52 commercial patchouli essential oil samples are shown in table 6.55.1 (Erich Schmidt, analytical data presented in ref. 17).

A full literature review of the qualitative and quantitative composition of commercial and non-commercial patchouli oils of various origins, their chemotypes and with data from the ISO standard, has been published in 2016 (17). Older literature is reviewed in refs. 1 and 2.

Table 6.55.1 Ten ingredients with the highest concentrations in commercial patchouli oils (17)

Name	Concentration range	Name	Concentration range
Patchouli alcohol (patchoulol)	22.3 - 33.9%	γ-Patchoulene	5.9 - 8.0%
		δ-Patchoulene	1.7 - 7.5%
α-Bulnesene	14.8 - 18.9%	β-Caryophyllene	3.0 - 4.7%
α-Guaiene	12.4 - 15.6%	Pogostol	1.6 - 4.5%
Seychellene	3.2 - 9.4%	β-Patchoulene	2.0 - 4.1%
α-Patchoulene	4.7 - 8.0%		

CONTACT ALLERGY / ALLERGIC CONTACT DERMATITIS

General

The SCCS (Scientific Committee on Consumer Safety), in a 2012 Opinion on Fragrance allergens in cosmetic products, has marked Pogostemon cablin extract as 'established contact allergen in humans' (15,16).

Contact allergy to / allergic contact dermatitis from patchouli oil has been reported in more than 10 publications. Pigmented cosmetic dermatitis from essential oils including patchouli oil used to be frequent in Japanese women. In groups of consecutive patients suspected of contact dermatitis, prevalence rates of up to 0.9% positive patch test reactions have been observed, but relevance data are lacking. Of four patients with allergic contact dermatitis from patchouli oil, three had used the oil occupationally.

Testing in groups of patients
The results of patch tests with patchouli oil in routine testing (consecutive patients suspected of contact dermatitis) and in groups of selected patients are shown in table 6.55.2. In routine testing, rates of positive reactions ranged from 0.6% to 0.9%, whereas between 0.4% and 14% of patients in selected groups had positive patch tests. The high percentage of 14 was in a small group of 21 patients with dermatitis caused by perfumes (13).

Table 6.55.2 Patch testing in groups of patients

Years and Country	Test conc. & vehicle	Number of patients tested | positive (%)		Selection of patients (S); Relevance (R); Comments (C)	Ref.
Routine testing					
2000-2008 IVDK	10% pet.	2446	14 (0.6%)	R: not stated	8
1999-2000 Denmark	10% pet.	318	3 (0.9%)	R: not specified; C: this study was part of the international study mentioned below (9)	14
1998-2000 six European countries	10% pet.	1606	13 (0.8%)	R: not specified for individual oils/chemicals	9
Testing in groups of selected patients					
2000-2008 IVDK	10% pet.	828	12 (1.4%)	S: patients with dermatitis suspected of causal exposure to fragrances; R: not stated	8
<1996 Japan, Ireland, USA, UK, Switzerland, Sweden	10% pet.	167	5 (3.0%)	S: patients known or suspected to be allergic to fragrances; R: not stated	3
<1986 France	3% pet.	21	3 (14%)	S: patients with dermatitis caused by perfumes; R: not stated	13
1971-1980 Japan	20% pet.	477	2 (0.4%)	S: patients with dermatoses other than pigmented cosmetic dermatitis and volunteers; R: not stated	6
<1974 Japan	?	183	11 (6.0%)	S: patients suspected of cosmetic dermatitis; R: unknown	10

IVDK Information Network of Departments of Dermatology, Germany, Switzerland, Austria (www.ivdk.org); pet.: petrolatum

Case reports and case series
A massage therapist had occupational contact dermatitis from allergies to various essential oils, including patchouli oil (4). Two patients, bottle fillers in a perfume factory, developed occupational contact allergy to patchouli oil and various other essential oils they worked with; in this study, there was also one positive patch test reaction to patchouli oil among 20 workers in the same factory who did not have dermatitis (5).

One patient developed allergic contact dermatitis from the application of pure patchouli oil to the skin behind the ears and in the axillae (12).

Pigmented cosmetic dermatitis
In Japan, in the 1960s and 1970s, many female patients developed facial pigmentation following dermatitis of the face (7). This so-called pigmented cosmetic dermatitis was shown to be caused by contact allergy to components of cosmetic products, notably essential oils, other fragrance materials, antimicrobials, preservatives and coloring materials (6,7). In a group of 620 Japanese patients with this condition investigated between 1970 and 1980, 1-3% had positive patch test reactions to patchouli oil 20% in petrolatum (6). The number of patients with pigmented cosmetic dermatitis decreased strongly after 1978, when major cosmetic companies began to eliminate strong contact sensitizers from their products (7).

LITERATURE

1   Lawrence BM. Progress in essential oils. Perfum Flavor 1990;15(2):75-79 (possibly 76-77)
2   Lawrence BM. Progress in essential oils. Perfum Flavor 1981;6(4):73-76(possibly 1981;6(5):73-76)
3   Larsen W, Nakayama H, Lindberg M, Fischer T, Elsner P, Burrows D, et al. Fragrance contact dermatitis: A worldwide multicenter investigation (Part 1). Am J Cont Derm 1996;7:77-83
4   Cockayne SE, Gawkrodger DJ. Occupational contact dermatitis in an aromatherapist. Contact Dermatitis 1997;37:306-307
5   Schubert HJ. Skin diseases in workers at a perfume factory. Contact Dermatitis 2006;55:81-83
6   Nakayama H, Matsuo S, Hayakawa K, Takhashi K, Shigematsu T, Ota S. Pigmented cosmetic dermatitis. Int J Dermatol 1984;23:299-305
7   Nakayama H, Harada R, Toda M. Pigmented cosmetic dermatitis. Int J Dermatol 1976;15:673-675

8   Uter W, Schmidt E, Geier J, Lessmann H, Schnuch A, Frosch P. Contact allergy to essential oils: current patch test results (2000–2008) from the Information Network of Departments of Dermatology (IVDK). Contact Dermatitis 2010;63:277-283

9   Frosch PJ, Johansen JD, Menné T, Pirker C, Rastogi SC, Andersen KE, et al. Further important sensitizers in patients sensitive to fragrances. II. Reactivity to essential oils. Contact Dermatitis 2002;47:279-287

10 Nakayama H, Hanaoka H, Ohshiro A. Allergen Controlled System (ACS). Tokyo, Japan: Kanehara Shuppan, 1974:42. Data cited in ref. 11

11 Mitchell JC. Contact hypersensitivity to some perfume materials. Contact Dermatitis 1975;1:196-199

12 Hausen BM, Kunze B. Kontaktallergie auf Patchouli-Öl. Akt Dermatol 1991;17:199-202

13 Meynadier JM, Meynadier J, Peyron JL, Peyron L. Formes cliniques des manifestations cutanées d'allergie aux parfums. Ann Dermatol Venereol 1986;113:31-39

14 Paulsen E, Andersen KE. Colophonium and Compositae mix as markers of fragrance allergy: Cross-reactivity between fragrance terpenes, colophonium and Compositae plant extracts. Contact Dermatitis 2005;53:285-291

15 SCCS (Scientific Committee on Consumer Safety). Opinion on Fragrance allergens in cosmetic products, 26-27 June 2012, SCCS/1459/11. Available at: https://ec.europa.eu/health/sites/health/files/scientific_committees/consumer_safety/docs/sccs_o_102.pdf

16 Uter W, Johansen JD, Börje A, Karlberg A-T, Lidén C, Rastogi S, Roberts D, White IR. Categorization of fragrance contact allergens for prioritization of preventive measures: clinical and experimental data and consideration of structure–activity relationships. Contact Dermatitis 2013;69:196-230

17 De Groot AC, Schmidt E. Essential oils: contact allergy and chemical composition. Boca Raton, Fl., USA: CRC Press, Taylor and Francis Group, 2016 (ISBN 9781482246407)

18 Swamy MK, Sinniah UR. A comprehensive review on the phytochemical constituents and pharmacological activities of *Pogostemon cablin* Benth.: An aromatic medicinal plant of industrial importance. Molecules 2015;20:8521-8547

Chapter 6.56 PEPPERMINT OIL

IDENTIFICATION

Description/definition	: Peppermint oil (essential oil of peppermint) is the essential oil obtained from the flowering aerial parts, leaves of the peppermint, *Mentha* x *piperita* L.
INCI name(s) EU	: Mentha piperita oil
INCI name(s) USA	: Mentha piperita (peppermint) oil
CAS registry number(s)	: 8006-90-4; 84082-70-2
EC number(s)	: 282-015-4
CIR review(s)	: Final report 03/06/2018; Int J Toxicol 2001;20(suppl.3):S61-S73 (access: www.cir-safety.org/ingredients)
SCCS opinion(s)	: SCCS/1459/11 (53)
ISO standard	: ISO 856 Essential oil of peppermint, 2006; Geneva, Switzerland, www.iso.org
Merck Index monograph	: 8528 (Peppermint)
Function(s) in cosmetics	: EU: masking; perfuming; refreshing; tonic. USA: fragrance ingredients; skin-conditioning agents - miscellaneous
Patch testing	: 10% pet. (Chemo, SPEurope, SPCanada)

GENERAL

Mentha x *piperita* L. is a herbaceous rhizomatous perennial plant growing to 30-90 cm tall. It is a sterile hybrid cross between *Mentha aquatica* and *Mentha spicata*. The peppermint is naturalized in the Azores, Siberia, Australia, New Zealand, all across Europe except the Scandinavian countries, Canada and the USA. The plant is cultivated in large parts of Europe, USA, Canada, Chile, Argentina, Australia, some African countries, Brazil and Japan and is widely used as medicinal plant and as flavoring agent in tea, ice cream, confectionery, chewing gum and toothpaste (55).

The essential oil of peppermint, obtained by steam-distillation of the leaves, has many pharmaceutical applications. The European Medicines Agency recently reviewed the pharmacological and clinical literature of peppermint oil and considered two indications as proven and well established: minor spasms of the gastrointestinal tract, flatulence and abdominal pain, especially in patients with irritable bowel syndrome (oral use) and mild tension type headache (cutaneous use) (3). Peppermint oil is also widely employed for flavoring chewing gum, cough drops, sweets, alcoholic drinks, toothpaste, mouth freshener and is also used for perfumes, other cosmetic products and in the tobacco industry. It is also a popular oil in aromatherapy (55).

Peppermint has been thoroughly reviewed in references 1 and 2. The biological properties of menthol, the main component of peppermint oil, are discussed in ref. 4.

CHEMICAL COMPOSITION

Peppermint oil is a colorless to pale greenish-yellow, clear mobile liquid which has a fresh, minty, cooling, green and sweetish odor, with variations depending on its origin. In peppermint oils from various origins, over 335 chemicals have been identified. About 59 per cent of these were found in a single reviewed publication only. The ten chemicals that had the highest maximum concentrations in 157 commercial peppermint essential oil samples are shown in table 6.56.1 (Erich Schmidt, analytical data presented in ref. 55).

A full literature review of the qualitative and quantitative composition of commercial and non-commercial peppermint oils of various origins, their chemotypes and with data from the ISO standard, has been published in 2016 (55).

Table 6.56.1 Ten ingredients with the highest concentrations in commercial peppermint oils (55)

Name	Concentration range	Name	Concentration range
Menthol	23.0 - 47.9%	α-Pinene	0.06 - 9.7%
Menthone	10.6 - 38.5%	Menthyl acetate	0.5 - 7.7%
Limonene	0.3 - 18.5%	Neomenthol	0.2 - 7.4%
Isomenthone	2.2 - 10.6%	Menthofuran	0.07 - 7.0%
1,8-Cineole	0.3 - 9.9%	β-Pinene	0.2 - 6.5%

CONTACT ALLERGY / ALLERGIC CONTACT DERMATITIS

General

The SCCS (Scientific Committee on Consumer Safety), in a 2012 Opinion on Fragrance allergens in cosmetic products, has marked Mentha piperita extract as 'established contact allergen in humans' (53,54).

Contact allergy to / allergic contact dermatitis from peppermint oil has been reported in over 50 publications. The oil (2% in petrolatum) has been included in the screening series of the North American Contact Dermatitis Group (NACDG) since 2009. In groups of consecutive patients suspected of contact dermatitis, prevalence rates of up to 1.8% positive patch test reactions have been observed. In most studies, no relevance data were provided, but in the NACDG investigations, 'definite' + 'probable' relevance was only 22-39%. There have been many case reports of allergic reactions to products with peppermint oil. Often, toothpastes, other oral products and peppermint in foods are causative products, which may induce oral discomfort, cheilitis, stomatitis, oral ulcers, burning mouth syndrome, lip swelling and lichenoid reactions of the oral mucosa. Some causative products were cosmetics. Occupational contact dermatitis does occur, but its share appears to be smaller than in some other essential oils.

A short review of contact allergy to peppermint oil has been provided in 2016 (67) and 2010 (21). Menthol, the main ingredient of peppermint oil, is said to have a low sensitizing potential (24). Older literature on contact allergy to peppermint oil can be found in ref. 31 (article not read).

Testing in groups of patients
The results of patch tests with peppermint oil in routine testing (consecutive patients suspected of contact dermatitis) are shown in table 6.56.2; those in groups of selected patients are shown in table 6.56.3. In routine testing, rates of positive reactions ranged from 0.3% to 1.8%, whereas between 0.1% and 19% of patients in selected groups had positive patch tests. The high positivity rate of 19% was seen in a small group of 16 patients known to be allergic to propolis and Myroxylon pereirae resin (48).

Table 6.56.2 Patch testing in groups of patients: Routine testing

Years and Country	Test conc. & vehicle	Number of patients tested | positive (%)		Selection of patients (S); Relevance (R); Comments (C)	Ref.
2015-2017 NACDG	2% pet.	5591	33 (0.6%)	R: definite + probable relevance: 27%	71
2013-14 USA, Canada	2% pet.	4859	27 (0.6%)	R: definite + probable relevance: 22%	68
2009-14 USA, Canada	2% pet.	13,398	71 (0.5%)	R: of 26 patients reacting, but negative to FM I, FM II and balsam of Peru, 23% had definite + probable relevance	66
2011-12 USA, Canada	2% pet.	4230	18 (0.4%)	R: definite + probable relevance: 39%	39
2009-10 USA, Canada	2% pet.	4303	26 (0.6%)	R: definite + probable relevance: 36%	22
2000-2007 USA	2% pet.	500	5 (1.0%)	R: 100%; C: weak study: a. high rate of macular erythema and weak reactions, b. relevance figures include 'questionable' and 'past' relevance	6
2002-2003 Korea	2% pet.	422	5 (1.2%)	R: not stated	19
1999-2000 Denmark	2% pet.	318	2 (0.6%)	R: not specified; C: this study was part of the international study mentioned below (ref. 40)	50
1998-2000 six European countries	2% pet.	1606	9 (0.6%)	R: not specified for individual oils/chemicals	40
1983-1984 Italy	2% pet.	1200	3 (0.3%)	R: not stated	51
<1977 Poland	2% pet.	400	7 (1.8%)	R: not stated	27
<1976 Poland	2% pet.	200	1 (0.5%)	R: not stated	13
<1973 Poland	2% pet.	200	2 (1.0%)	R: not stated	56
<1970 UK	?	1147	4 (0.3%)	data cited in ref. 18, no details known	19

Case reports and case series

Occupational allergic contact dermatitis
An aromatherapist had chronic hand dermatitis and was patch test positive to 17 of 20 oils used at her work (tested 1% and 5% in petrolatum), including peppermint oil (11). Another aromatherapist had occupational contact dermatitis with allergies to multiple essential oils used at work, including peppermint oil. The patient also reacted to geraniol, α-pinene, caryophyllene, the fragrance mix and various other fragrance materials; α-pinene and caryophyllene were demonstrated by GC-MS in the peppermint oil. Menthol, the main ingredient in peppermint oil, was not tested (12). α-Pinene has been found in commercial peppermint oils in a maximum concentration of 9.7% and caryophyllene in a maximum concentration of 5.2% (55).

Another aromatherapist had occupational contact dermatitis from contact allergy to various essential oils, including 'mint oil' (10). Occupational allergic contact dermatitis from peppermint oil also occurred in an unknown number of food handlers (49, article not read).

Cosmetics

Four patients developed allergic contact dermatitis of the lips (allergic contact cheilitis) and the perioral skin from peppermint oil in a lip balm (16). One positive patch test reaction to peppermint oil, which was present in a cosmetic that had given a positive patch test or had been positive in a usage test, was seen in a 9-year period in a clinic in Belgium (5). One patient developed allergic cosmetic dermatitis which proved to be caused by peppermint oil in a skin care product (52). In a group of 39 patients with cosmetic allergy, where the causative allergen was identified with certainty or high probability, peppermint oil was the allergen in one case (46). One case of allergic contact dermatitis caused by a depilatory product from its ingredient peppermint oil has been reported (47).

Table 6.56.3 Patch testing in groups of patients: Selected patient groups

Years and Country	Test conc. & vehicle	Number of patients tested	positive (%)	Selection of patients (S); Relevance (R); Comments (C)	Ref.
2008-2014 UK	2% pet.	471	3 (0.6%)	S: patients tested with a fragrance series; R: not stated	58
2011-2012 Italy	1% pet.	122	3 (2.5%)	S: patients who reported adverse cutaneous reactions to products (notably cosmetics) containing botanical ingredients in a questionnaire; they were tested with a 'botanical series'; R: all three reactions were relevant	36
2000-2008 IVDK	2% pet.	6546	39 (0.6%)	S: patients with dermatitis suspected of causal exposure to fragrances; R: not stated	37
<2005 USA	2% pet.	160	7 (4.4%)	S: patients using consumer products containing peppermint oil; R: 'at least possibly relevant'	32
1997-2000 Austria	2% pet.	747	1 (0.1%)	S: patients suspected of fragrance allergy; R: not stated	8
1997-1998 Italy	2% pet.	54	2 (3.7%)	S: patients with cheilitis suspected of toothpaste allergy; R: both reactions were relevant	41
1996-1997 UK	2% pet.	10	1 (10%)	S: patients suspected of cosmetic dermatitis and reacting to the fragrance mix; R: not stated	7
1994-1995 UK	2% pet.	40	2 (5%)	S: patients previously reacting to the fragrance mix; R: not stated; C: there was also one positive reaction in a patient negative to the fragrance mix	42
<1986 Poland	2% pet.	86	6 (7.0%)	S: patients previously reacting to the fragrance mix; R: not stated	26
<1983 Poland	2% pet.	16	3 (19%)	S: patients known to be allergic to propolis and Myroxylon pereirae; R: not stated	48
<1978 Denmark	5% pet.	38	2 (5.3%)	S: see text under Case reports	20
<1976 Poland	2% pet.	51	1 (2.0%)	S: patients allergic to Myroxylon pereirae resin (balsam of Peru) and/or turpentine and/or wood tar and/or colophony	13

IVDK Information Network of Departments of Dermatology, Germany, Switzerland, Austria (www.ivdk.org); pet.: petrolatum

Toothpastes and other oral products

Swelling of the tongue, lips and gingival mucosa was caused by contact allergy to peppermint oil in an antiseptic spray used in dentistry, a mouthwash and candies; the patient, who had been sensitized primarily by turpentine oil, also reacted to limonene and α-pinene (17). Limonene has been found in commercial peppermint oils in concentrations up to 18.5% and α-pinene in a maximum concentration of 9.7% (table 6.56.1). Six cases of allergic reactions to peppermint oil were found in patients with burning mouth syndrome (n=2), recurrent oral ulcers (n=2) or lichenoid mucosal reactions (n=2); five also reacted to menthol (main ingredient). The reactions to peppermint oil were considered to be relevant, but the causative products were not specified (18).

A patient with oral burning and discomfort and a lichenoid reaction of the oral mucosa had positive patch test reaction to peppermint oil and menthol; the symptoms improved after avoiding mint-flavored mouthwashes and food (25). Another individual had allergic contact cheilitis from peppermint oil in toothpaste (33). One patient developed stomatitis and lip dermatitis from contact allergy to peppermint oil and menthol present in toothpastes (43). Six cases of contact stomatitis and contact dermatitis from allergy to oil of peppermint, oil of spearmint, carvone and anethole in toothpastes have been described; it is unknown how many cases were caused by peppermint oil (45) (article not read).

A woman had cheilitis, erythema and burning of the oral mucosa from contact allergy to peppermint oil in toothpaste (57). One or more other individuals had stomatitis and perioral dermatitis from exposure to 'peppermint oil and/or menthol' in toothpastes (no details known, article not read) (64).

Other products

A patient developed allergic contact dermatitis from peppermint oil and its main component menthol in a transdermal therapeutic system (15). Three patients with allergic contact dermatitis from peppermint oil were seen in Japan (article not read); the allergens were menthol (the main component of peppermint oil), piperitone and pulegone (28). Both piperitone and pulegone have been found in a maximum concentration of 5.4% in commercial peppermint oils (55). One individual had orofacial granulomatosis, mainly of the lower lip; he was allergic to peppermint oil and menthol. An exclusion diet resulted in reduction of the swelling; upon re-exposure to menthol, further episodes of lip swelling occurred (30). One positive patch test reaction to peppermint oil was observed in a group of in 53 women with chronic anogenital dermatitis and was considered to be relevant (38).

A male individual presented with a 1-month history of dermatitis that began on his dorsal hands with subsequent widespread involvement of his arms, trunk, legs, feet, and face. The patient treated his rash with a lotion made by his wife, which included essential oils (not specified). Furthermore, the patient diffused patchouli, lavender, lemongrass, and peppermint oils at home. When patch tested, he had 22 positive patch test reactions, including to the homemade lotion, peppermint and lemongrass oil. Obviously, some of the many weak (+) reactions may have been false-positive from the excited skin syndrome (69).

Miscellaneous

In a number of publications, positive patch tests to peppermint oil have been reported with unknown, uncertain or unstated relevance. These include (literature screened up to 2014 [55]) the following. Two positive patch test reactions to peppermint oil were seen in a group of 32 patients with sore mouth, stomatitis and/or dermatitis around the mouth or dentist personnel. One also reacted to spearmint oil and its ingredient carvone. The causative products were supposed to be toothpastes (20). A positive patch test to peppermint oil was observed in an aromatherapist with occupational contact dermatitis from multiple essential oils; it was uncertain whether this oil had been used by the patient (9).

A positive patch test reaction to peppermint oil was seen in a patient who had airborne allergic contact dermatitis from tea tree oil and lavender oil (14). One positive patch test to peppermint oil was observed in a woman who drank large amounts of peppermint tea, which appeared to induce vulvar dermatitis (23). Four positive patch test reactions to peppermint oil occurred in 7 patients with allergic contact dermatitis from compound tincture of benzoin (27). Two patients with cheilitis, who both reacted to peppermint oil and to menthol have been presented; the causative products were not specified, but presumably toothpastes were implicated (29). One patient had prolonged lip swelling, apparently from contact allergy to peppermint oil and menthol (34). A positive patch test reaction to peppermint oil was seen in a patient allergic to ascaridole, an allergen in tea tree oil (35).

Ten patients allergic to peppermint oil (of who 4 co-reacted to spearmint oil) were patch tested with 24 ingredients. There were 4 positive reactions to menthol, one to menthyl acetate, 4 to piperitone, 3 to pulegone, 2 to tetrahydrodimethylbenzofuran (menthofuran), and one to dihydrocarveol (59); the latter is not an ingredient of peppermint oils (55). Further details are lacking (59, article in Japanese).

The allergens in peppermint oil

The main allergen is probably menthol, co-reacting with peppermint oil in at least 15 patients (15,18,25,28,29,30, 43,59,64). Other possible allergens, which have shown co-reactions with peppermint oil are α-pinene (12,17), limonene (17), caryophyllene (12), piperitone (28,59), pulegone (28,59), menthyl acetate (59) and menthofuran (59).

OTHER SIDE EFFECTS

Irritant contact dermatitis

Undiluted peppermint oil spilled on a previous skin graft on the dorsum of the hand of a pharmaceutical worker caused a chemical burn (60). In the mouth, 40 drops of undiluted peppermint oil taken orally for medicinal purposes caused chemical burns in the entire oral cavity and pharynx, producing edema of the upper and lower lips, the tongue, uvula, and soft palate (61). Oral intake or enteric-coated peppermint oil capsules may cause burning of the anal canal (62,63).

Immediate contact reactions

Immediate contact reactions (contact urticaria) from peppermint oil have been cited in ref. 70.

LITERATURE

1   Lawrence BM. The genus Mentha. Boca Raton, FL, USA: CRC Press, 2006
2   Lawrence BM. Peppermint oil. Carol Stream, IL, USA: Allured Publishing Corp, 2007

3   European Medicines Agency. Assessment report on *Mentha x piperita* L., aetheroleum. London, UK, Doc Ref EMEA/HMPC/349465/2006: 2008. Available at: http://www.ema.europa.eu

4   Kamatou GPP, Vermaak I, Viljoen AM, Lawrence BM. Menthol: A simple monoterpene with remarkable biological properties. Phytochem 2013;96:15-25

5   Nardelli A, Drieghe J, Claes L, Boey L, Goossens A. Fragrance allergens in 'specific' cosmetic products. Contact Dermatitis 2011;64:212-219

6   Wetter DA, Yiannias JA, Prakash AV, Davis MD, Farmer SA, el-Azhary RA, et al. Results of patch testing to personal care product allergens in a standard series and a supplemental cosmetic series: an analysis of 945 patients from the Mayo Clinic Contact Dermatitis Group, 2000-2007. J Am Acad Dermatol 2010;63:789-798

7   Thomson KF, Wilkinson SM. Allergic contact dermatitis to plant extracts in patients with cosmetic dermatitis. Br J Dermatol 2000;142:84-88

8   Wöhrl S, Hemmer W, Focke M, Götz M, Jarisch R. The significance of fragrance mix, balsam of Peru, colophonium and propolis as screening tools in the detection of fragrance allergy. Br J Dermatol 2001;145:268-273

9   Bleasel N, Tate B, Rademaker M. Allergic contact dermatitis following exposure to essential oils. Australas J Dermatol 2002;43:211-213

10   Boonchai W, Lamtharachai P, Sunthonpalin P. Occupational allergic contact dermatitis from essential oils in aromatherapists. Contact Dermatitis 2007;56:181-182

11   Selvaag E, Holm J, Thune P. Allergic contact dermatitis in an aromatherapist with multiple sensitizations to essential oils. Contact Dermatitis 1995;33:354-355

12   Dharmagunawardena B, Takwale A, Sanders KJ, Cannan S, Roger A, Ilchyshyn A. Gas chromatography: an investigative tool in multiple allergies to essential oils. Contact Dermatitis 2002;47:288-292

13   Rudzki E, Grzywa Z, Bruo WS. Sensitivity to 35 essential oils. Contact Dermatitis 1976;2:196-200

14   De Groot AC. Airborne allergic contact dermatitis from tea tree oil. Contact Dermatitis 1996;35:304-305

15   Foti C, Conserva A, Antelmi A, Lospalluti L, Angelini G. Contact dermatitis from peppermint and menthol in a local action transcutaneous patch. Contact Dermatitis 2003;49:312-313

16   Tran A, Pratt M, DeKoven J. Acute allergic contact dermatitis of the lips from peppermint oil in a lip balm. Dermatitis 2010;21:111-115

17   Dooms-Goossens A, Degreef H, Holvoet C, Maertens M. Turpentine-induced hypersensitivity to peppermint oil. Contact Dermatitis 1977;3:304-308

18   Morton CA, Garioch J, Todd P, Lamey PJ, Forsyth A. Contact sensitivity to menthol and peppermint in patients with intra-oral symptoms. Contact Dermatitis 1995;32:281-284

19   Calnan CD. Oil of cloves, laurel, lavender, peppermint. Contact Dermatitis Newsletter 1970;7:148

20   Andersen KE. Contact allergy to toothpaste flavors. Contact Dermatitis 1978;4:195-198

21   Herro E, Jacob SE. *Mentha piperita* (peppermint). Dermatitis 2010;21:327-329

22   Warshaw EM, Belsito DV, Taylor JS, Sasseville D, DeKoven JG, Zirwas MJ, et al. North American Contact Dermatitis Group patch test results: 2009 to 2010. Dermatitis 2013;24:50-59

23   Vermaat H, van Meurs T, Rustemeyer T, Bruynzeel DP, Kirtschig G. Vulval allergic contact dermatitis due to peppermint oil in herbal tea. Contact Dermatitis 2008;58:364-365

24   Ale SI, Hostynek JJ, Maibach HI. Menthol: a review of its sensitisation potential. Exog Dermatol 2002:1:74-80

25   Fleming CJ, Forsyth A. D5 patch test reactions to menthol and peppermint. Contact Dermatitis 1998;38:337

26   Rudzki E, Grzywa Z. Allergy to perfume mixture. Contact Dermatitis 1986;15:115-116

27   Fettig J, Taylor J, Sood A. Post-surgical allergic contact dermatitis to compound tincture of benzoin and association with reactions to fragrances and essential oils. Dermatitis 2014;25:211-212

28   Saito F, Oka K. Allergic contact dermatitis due to peppermint oil. Skin Res 1990;32:161-167 (article in Japanese)

29   Wilkinson SM, Beck MH. Allergic contact dermatitis from menthol in peppermint. Contact Dermatitis 1994;30:42-43

30   Lewis FM, Shah M, Gawkrodger DJ. Contact sensitivity to food additives can cause oral and perioral symptoms. Contact Dermatitis 1995;33:429-430

31   Smith IL. Acute allergic reaction following the use of toothpaste—a case report. Br Dent J 1968;125:304-305

32   Guin JD. Use of consumer product ingredients for patch testing. Dermatitis 2005;16:71-77

33   Freeman S, Stephens R. Cheilitis: Analysis of 75 cases referred to a contact dermatitis clinic. Am J Cont Derm 1999;10:198-200

34   Shah M, Lewis M, Gawkrodger DJ. Contact allergy in patients with oral symptoms: a study of 47 patients. Am J Cont Derm 1996;7:146-151

35   Christoffers WA, Blömeke B, Coenraads P-J, Schuttelaar M-LA. The optimal patch test concentration for ascaridole as a sensitizing component of tea tree oil. Contact Dermatitis 2014;71:129-137

36 Corazza M, Borghi A, Gallo R, Schena D, Pigatto P, Lauriola MM, et al. Topical botanically derived products: use, skin reactions, and usefulness of patch tests. A multicentre Italian study. Contact Dermatitis 2014;70:90-97

37 Uter W, Schmidt E, Geier J, Lessmann H, Schnuch A, Frosch P. Contact allergy to essential oils: current patch test results (2000–2008) from the Information Network of Departments of Dermatology (IVDK). Contact Dermatitis 2010;63:277-283

38 Vermaat H, Smienk F, Rustemeyer Th, Bruynzeel DP, Kirtschig G. Anogenital allergic contact dermatitis, the role of spices and flavour allergy. Contact Dermatitis 2008;59:233-237

39 Warshaw EM, Maibach HI, Taylor JS, Sasseville D, DeKoven JG, Zirwas MJ, et al. North American Contact Dermatitis Group patch test results: 2011-2012. Dermatitis 2015;26:49-59

40 Frosch PJ, Johansen JD, Menné T, Pirker C, Rastogi SC, Andersen KE, et al. Further important sensitizers in patients sensitive to fragrances. II. Reactivity to essential oils. Contact Dermatitis 2002;47:279-287

41 Francalanci S, Sertoli A, Giorgini S, Pigatto P, Santucci B, Valsecchi R. Multicentre study of allergic contact cheilitis from toothpastes. Contact Dermatitis 2000;43:216-222

42 Katsarma G, Gawkrodger DJ. Suspected fragrance allergy requires extended patch testing to individual fragrance allergens. Contact Dermatitis 1999;41:193-197

43 Downs AMR, Lear JT, Sansom JE. Contact sensitivity in patients with oral symptoms. Contact Dermatitis 1998; 39:258-259

44 Magnusson B, Wilkinson DS. Cinnamic aldehyde in toothpaste. 1. Clinical aspects and patch tests. Contact Dermatitis 1975;1:70-76

45 Hjorth N, Jervoe P. Allergisk Kontaktstomatitis og Kontaktdermatitis fremkaldt of smagsstoffer i tandpasta. Tandlaegebladet 1967;71:937-942. Data cited in ref. 44 (article in Danish)

46 De Groot AC. Contact allergy to cosmetics: causative ingredients. Contact Dermatitis 1987;17:26-34

47 Travassos AR, Claes L, Boey L, Drieghe J, Goossens A. Non-fragrance allergens in specific cosmetic products. Contact Dermatitis 2011;65:276-285

48 Rudzki E, Grzywa Z. Dermatitis from propolis. Contact Dermatitis 1983;9:40-45

49 Peltonen L, Wickstrom G, Vaahtoranta M. Occupational dermatoses in the food industry. Dermatosen 1985;33:166-169

50 Paulsen E, Andersen KE. Colophonium and Compositae mix as markers of fragrance allergy: Cross-reactivity between fragrance terpenes, colophonium and Compositae plant extracts. Contact Dermatitis 2005;53:285-291

51 Santucci B, Cristaudo A, Cannistraci C, Picardo M. Contact dermatitis to fragrances. Contact Dermatitis 1987;16:93-95

52 De Groot AC. Contact allergy to cosmetics: causative ingredients. Contact Dermatitis 1987;17:26-34

53 SCCS (Scientific Committee on Consumer Safety). Opinion on Fragrance allergens in cosmetic products, 26-27 June 2012, SCCS/1459/11. Available at: https://ec.europa.eu/health/sites/health/files/scientific_committees/consumer_safety/docs/sccs_o_102.pdf

54 Uter W, Johansen JD, Börje A, Karlberg A-T, Lidén C, Rastogi S, Roberts D, White IR. Categorization of fragrance contact allergens for prioritization of preventive measures: clinical and experimental data and consideration of structure–activity relationships. Contact Dermatitis 2013;69:196-230

55 De Groot AC, Schmidt E. Essential oils: contact allergy and chemical composition. Boca Raton, Fl., USA: CRC Press, Taylor and Francis Group, 2016 (ISBN 9781482246407)

56 Rudzki E, Kielak D. Sensitivity to some compounds related to Balsam of Peru. Contact Dermatitis Newsletter 1972;nr.13:335-336

57 Hausen BM. Toothpaste allergy. Dtsch Med Wochenschr 1984;109:300-302

58 Sabroe RA, Holden CR, Gawkrodger DJ. Contact allergy to essential oils cannot always be predicted from allergy to fragrance markers in the baseline series. Contact Dermatitis 2016;74:236-241

59 Saito F, Miyazaki T, Matsuoka Y. Peppermint oil contact allergy. Skin Res 1984;26:636-643 (article in Japanese).

60 Parys BT. Chemical burns resulting from contact with peppermint oil mar: a case report. Burns Incl Therm Inj 1983;9:374-375

61 Tamir S, Davidovich Z, Attal P, Eliashar R. Peppermint oil chemical burn. Otolaryngol Head Neck Surg 2005;133:801-802

62 Weston C F M. Anal burning and peppermint oil. Postgrad Med J 1987;63:717

63 Somerville KW, Richmond CR, Bell GD. Delayed release peppermint oil capsules (Colpermin) for the spastic colon syndrome: a pharmacokinetic study. Br J Clin Pharmacol 1984;18:638-640

64 Baer P N. Toothpaste allergies. J Clin Pediatr Dent 1992;16:230-231. Data cited in ref. 65

65 Calapai G, Minciullo PL, Miroddi M, Chinou I, Gangemi S, Schmidt RJ. Contact dermatitis as an adverse reaction to some topically used European herbal medicinal products - Part 3: *Mentha × piperita - Solanum dulcamara*. Contact Dermatitis 2016;74:131-144

66 Warshaw EM, Zug KA, Belsito DV, Fowler JF Jr, DeKoven JG, Sasseville D, et al. Positive patch-test reactions to essential oils in consecutive patients: Results from North America and Central Europe. Dermatitis 2017;28:246-252

67 De Groot AC, Schmidt E. Essential Oils, Part V: Peppermint oil, lavender oil, and lemongrass oil. Dermatitis 2016; 27:325-332

68 DeKoven JG, Warshaw EM, Belsito DV, Sasseville D, Maibach HI, Taylor JS, et al. North American Contact Dermatitis Group Patch Test Results: 2013-2014. Dermatitis 2017;28:33-46

69 Grey KR, Hagen SL, Warshaw EM. Essential oils: Emerging "medicaments". Dermatitis 2016;27:227-228

70 De Groot AC. Patch Testing, 4th Edition. Wapserveen, The Netherlands: acdegroot publishing, 2018 (ISBN 978-90-813233-4-5)

71 DeKoven JG, Warshaw EM, Zug KA, Maibach HI, Belsito DV, Sasseville D, et al. North American Contact Dermatitis Group patch test results: 2015-2016. Dermatitis 2018;29:297-309

Chapter 6.57   PETITGRAIN BIGARADE OIL

IDENTIFICATION

Description/definition	: Petitgrain bigarade oil (essential oil of bitter orange petitgrain, cultivated) is the essential oil obtained from the leaves and twigs with little green (unripe) fruits of the bitter orange, *Citrus aurantium* L. (synonyms: *Citrus amara* Link, *Citrus bigaradia* Loisel, *Citrus vulgaris* Risso)
INCI name(s) EU	: Citrus aurantium amara leaf/twig oil; Citrus aurantium leaf oil
INCI name(s) USA	: Citrus aurantium amara (bitter orange) leaf/twig oil
CAS registry number(s)	: 8014-17-3; 72968-50-4; 68916-04-1
EC number(s)	: 277-143-2
CIR review(s)	: Final report 12/06/2016 (access: www.cir-safety.org/ingredients)
RIFM monograph(s)	: Food Chem Toxicol 1992;30:S101 (special issue VIII); Food Chem Toxicol 1982;20:801 (special issue VI)
SCCS opinion(s)	: SCCS/1459/11 (10)
ISO standard	: ISO 8901 Essential oil of bitter orange petitgrain, cultivated, 2003; ISO 3064 Essential oil of petitgrain, Paraguayan type, 2015; Geneva, Switzerland, www.iso.org
Function(s) in cosmetics	: EU: flavouring; masking; perfuming. USA: flavoring agents; fragrance ingredients
Patch testing	: 5% pet. (SPEurope)

GENERAL

For a general introduction to the bitter orange tree *Citrus aurantium* L. see Chapter 6.52. Orange oil, bitter.

Petitgrain bigarade oil is obtained by steam-distillation of the leaves, or of the leaves, young branches and immature fruits of the bitter orange tree (1,3). It is widely used in perfumery for the sweet and fresh note it gives to colognes and lotions. The oils produced in the Mediterranean area are said to have better odor properties than those produced in Paraguay (2,3). Petitgrain bigarade oil is also employed in the fabrication of soaps because of its good resistance to an alkaline medium (1). In addition, bitter orange leaf oil may be added to foods and drinks as flavoring. The oil may also be employed in aromatherapy practices.

Citrus aurantium L. is not only used for the production of petitgrain bigarade oil, but is also the source for obtaining bitter orange oil from cold-pressing of the fruit peels (Chapter 6.52) and neroli oil from the flowers (Chapter 6.48).

CHEMICAL COMPOSITION

Petitgrain bigarade oil is a pale yellow to amber yellow clear mobile liquid with a slight blue fluorescence, which has a fresh ethereal, slightly orange and green odor. In petitgrain bigarade oils from various origins, over 157 chemicals have been identified. About 45 per cent of these were found in a single reviewed publication only. The ten chemicals that had the highest maximum concentrations in 47 commercial petitgrain bigarade essential oil samples are shown in table 6.57.1 (Erich Schmidt, analytical data presented in ref. 12).

A full literature review of the qualitative and quantitative composition of commercial and non-commercial petitgrain bigarade oils of various origins, their chemotypes and with data from the ISO standard, has been published in 2016 (12). Older reviews are presented in refs. 2 and 3.

Table 6.57.1 Ten ingredients with the highest concentrations in commercial petitgrain bigarade oils (12)

Name	Concentration range	Name	Concentration range
Linalyl acetate	41.3 - 54.0%	(E)-β-Ocimene	0.9 - 4.1%
linalool	19.8 - 34.0%	Myrcene	0.4 - 3.6%
α-Terpineol	4.6 - 7.5%	Neryl acetate	1.6 - 2.8%
Geranyl acetate	2.5 - 4.8%	Limonene	0.3 - 2.6%
Geraniol	0.9 - 4.4%	β-Pinene	0.09 - 1.9%

CONTACT ALLERGY / ALLERGIC CONTACT DERMATITIS

General

The SCCS (Scientific Committee on Consumer Safety), in a 2012 Opinion on Fragrance allergens in cosmetic products, has categorized Citrus aurantium amara leaf oil as 'possible fragrance contact allergen' (10,11). Fresh petitgrain bigarade oil is probably little allergenic. However, during use, exposure to light and oxygen (4) , and even during storage in the dark (13), strongly allergenic linalool and linalyl acetate hydroperoxides are formed, which may increase the risk of allergic reactions (see Chapter 3.96 Linalool and Chapter 3.97 Linalyl acetate for further details).

Contact allergy to / allergic contact dermatitis from petitgrain bigarade oil has been reported in four publications only. In a group of consecutive patients suspected of contact dermatitis, a prevalence rate of 0.5% positive patch test reactions has been observed; relevance data are lacking. Two published case reports both describe occupational contact dermatitis from petitgrain bigarade oil. In one case, linalool and possibly geraniol may have been allergens in the oil (6).

Testing in groups of patients

Two hundred dermatitis patients from Poland were tested with petitgrain bigarade oil 2% in petrolatum and one (0.5%) reacted. The same authors also patch tested 51 patients allergic to Myroxylon pereirae resin (balsam of Peru) and/or turpentine and/or wood tar and/or colophony and three (5.9%) had a positive patch test; relevance data were not provided (7).

A group of 86 patients from Poland previously reacting to the fragrance mix was tested with petitgrain bigarade oil and seven (8.1%) had a positive patch test reaction. Relevance data were not provided (9); there were also four reactions to 'petitgrain Paraguay oil' (9).

Case reports and case series

An aromatherapist had non-occupational contact dermatitis with allergies to multiple essential oils used at work, including petitgrain oil. The patient also reacted to geraniol, linalool, linalyl acetate, α-pinene, the fragrance mix and various other fragrance materials; α-pinene, linalool and geraniol were demonstrated by GC-MS in petitgrain oil (6). Linalool is an important chemical in petitgrain bigarade oils and has been found in commercial oils in concentrations of 20-34%; geraniol had a highest concentration of 4.4% (table 6.57.1).

Two bottle fillers in a perfume factory developed occupational allergic contact dermatitis from petitgrain bigarade oil and other essential oils they worked with; there was also one positive patch test reaction to petitgrain bigarade oil among twenty workers who did not have dermatitis (8).

OTHER SIDE EFFECTS

Photosensitivity Photosensitivity from petitgrain bigarade oil has been cited in ref. 5.

LITERATURE

1   Kirbaslar G, Kirbaslar SI. Composition of Turkish bitter orange and lemon leaf oils. J Essent Oil Res 2004;16:105-108

2   Mondello L, Dugo G, Dugo P, Bartle KD. Italian citrus petitgrain oils. Part I. Composition of bitter orange petitgrain oil. J Essent Oil Res 1996;8:597-609.

3   Dugo G, Cotroneo A, Bonaccorsi I. Composition of petitgrain oils In: G Dugo and L Mondello, Eds. Citrus oils: composition, advanced analytical techniques, contaminants, and biological activity. Boca Raton, USA: CRC Press, Taylor & Francis Group, 2011:253-330

4   Rudbäck J, Islam N, Nilsson U, Karlberg AT. A sensitive method for determination of allergenic fragrance terpene hydroperoxides using liquid chromatography coupled with tandem mass spectrometry. J Sep Sci 2013;36:1370-1378

5   De Groot AC. Patch Testing, 4th Edition. Wapserveen, The Netherlands: acdegroot publishing, 2018 (ISBN 978-90-813233-4-5)

6   Dharmagunawardena B, Takwale A, Sanders KJ, Cannan S, Roger A, Ilchyshyn A. Gas chromatography: an investigative tool in multiple allergies to essential oils. Contact Dermatitis 2002;47:288-292

7   Rudzki E, Grzywa Z, Bruo WS. Sensitivity to 35 essential oils. Contact Dermatitis 1976;2:196-200

8   Schubert HJ. Skin diseases in workers at a perfume factory. Contact Dermatitis 2006;55:81-83

9   Rudzki E, Grzywa Z. Allergy to perfume mixture. Contact Dermatitis 1986;15:115-116

10 SCCS (Scientific Committee on Consumer Safety). Opinion on Fragrance allergens in cosmetic products, 26-27 June 2012, SCCS/1459/11. Available at: https://ec.europa.eu/health/sites/health/files/scientific_committees/consumer_safety/docs/sccs_o_102.pdf

11 Uter W, Johansen JD, Börje A, Karlberg A-T, Lidén C, Rastogi S, Roberts D, White IR. Categorization of fragrance contact allergens for prioritization of preventive measures: clinical and experimental data and consideration of structure–activity relationships. Contact Dermatitis 2013;69:196-230

12 De Groot AC, Schmidt E. Essential oils: contact allergy and chemical composition. Boca Raton, Fl., USA: CRC Press, Taylor and Francis Group, 2016 (ISBN 9781482246407)

13 Rudbäck J, Islam MN, Börje A, Nilsson U, Karlberg A-T.Essential oils can contain allergenic hydroperoxides at eliciting levels, regardless of handling and storage. Contact Dermatitis 2015;73:253-254

Chapter 6.58   PINE NEEDLE OIL

IDENTIFICATION

Description/definition	: Pine needle oil is the essential oil obtained from the needles and twigs of the Scotch pine, *Pinus sylvestris* L.
INCI name(s) EU & USA	: Pinus sylvestris leaf oil
Other names	: Scots pine oil; pine scotch oil
CAS registry number(s)	: 8023-99-2; 84012-35-1
EC number(s)	: 281-679-2
RIFM monograph(s)	: Food Cosmet Toxicol 1976;14:845 (special issue III)
IFRA specification	: Essential oils and isolates derived from the Pinacea family, including *Pinus* and *Abies* genera, should only be used when the level of peroxides is kept to the lowest practicable level, for instance by adding antioxidants at the time of production; such products should have a peroxide value of less than 10 millimoles peroxide per liter, determined according to the FMA method (www.ifraorg.org/en-us/standards-library)
SCCS opinion(s)	: SCCNFP/0392/00, final (12); SCCNFP/0389/00, final (13)
Merck Index monograph	: 8172
Function(s) in cosmetics	: EU: masking. USA: fragrance ingredients
EU cosmetic restrictions	: Regulated in Annex III/110 of the Regulation (EC) No. 344/2013
Patch testing	: 2% pet.; based on RIFM data, 12% pet. is probably not irritant (17)

GENERAL

Pinus sylvestris L. (sometimes termed *Pinus silvestris* - botanically incorrect, but linguistically correct, sylvestris being derived from the Latin word silva, forest) is an evergreen coniferous tree that can grow up to 25-40 meter tall and 0.5-1.2 meter in diameter. It is native to the temperate regions of Asia and Europe, grows naturally from Scotland to the Pacific Ocean and from above the Arctic Circle to the Mediterranean. *P. sylvestris* has been widely planted in New Zealand and in the colder regions of North America and is listed as an invasive species in some areas there. It is the world's most widespread pine (14)

Pine needle essential oils are widely used as fragrances in perfumes and other cosmetics, in pharmaceuticals, as flavoring additives for food and beverages, as scenting agents in a variety of household products, and as intermediates in the synthesis of perfume chemicals. Scots pine oil is believed to possess a wide range of pharmacological properties and is used in various illnesses. Its insecticidal and deodorant properties are also well known. Pine needle oils are also applied in aromatherapy (14).

CHEMICAL COMPOSITION

Pine needle oil is a colorless clear mobile liquid, which has a harsh, fresh and coniferous terpeny and woody odor. In pine needle oils from various origins, over 255 chemicals have been identified. About 56 per cent of these were found in a single reviewed publication only. The ten chemicals that had the highest maximum concentrations in 112 commercial pine needle essential oil samples are shown in table 6.58.1 (Erich Schmidt, analytical data presented in ref. 14).

A full literature review of the qualitative and quantitative composition of commercial and non-commercial pine needle oils of various origins and their chemotypes has been published in 2016 (14).

Table 6.58.1 Ten ingredients with the highest concentrations in commercial pine needle oils (14)

Name	Concentration range	Name	Concentration range
Limonene	3.1 - 30.1%	δ3-Carene	1.4 - 13.0%
Bornyl acetate	8.4 - 29.9%	β-Pinene	0.9 - 7.1%
Camphene	4.2 - 27.4%	β-Phellandrene	0.1 - 6.0%
α-Pinene	13.3 - 20.4%	α-Phellandrene	0.04 - 5.3%
Myrcene	0.4 - 13.5%	γ-Cadinene	0 - 5.3%

CONTACT ALLERGY / ALLERGIC CONTACT DERMATITIS

General

Contact allergy to / allergic contact dermatitis from pine needle oil has been reported in 12 publications. In groups of consecutive patients suspected of contact dermatitis, prevalence rates of up to 2.0% positive patch test reactions have been observed, but relevance data are lacking. In one case report, α-pinene may have been an allergen in the oil (4).

Testing in groups of patients

Routine testing
Between 1973 and 1977, 3500 patients were tested in Spain with 'pine oil' and fifteen (0.4%) had a positive patch test (7). Four positive patch test reactions to pine needle oil were seen in 200 (2.0%) consecutive patients with dermatitis (5). Relevance data were not provided in either study.

Testing in groups of selected patients
In a group of 51 patients allergic to Myroxylon pereirae resin (balsam of Peru) and/or turpentine and/or wood tar and/or colophony, there were 15 (29.4%) positive reactions to pine needle oil (5). The high percentage is likely related to the fact that all these products are obtained from trees, three of them (pine needle oil, turpentine and colophony) from *Pinus* species.

In another study from these authors, a group of 86 patients from Poland previously reacting to the fragrance mix was tested with pine needle oil and three (3.4%) had a positive patch test reaction (6). Relevance data were not provided in either study (5,6). In a group of 21 patients with dermatitis caused by perfumes and tested with a series of essential oils, three (14%) reacted to pine (*Pinus sylvestris*) oil; relevance data were not provided (8).

Case reports and case series
In a clinic in Belgium, in the period 1990-2016, one case of dermatitis caused by contact allergy to pine oil from its presence as active principle in 'topical botanical medicines' has been observed (16).

An aromatherapist had non-occupational contact dermatitis with allergies to multiple essential oils used at work, including pine oil. The patient also reacted to geraniol, linalool, linalyl acetate, α-pinene, the fragrance mix and various other fragrance materials; α-pinene was demonstrated by GC-MS in the pine oil (4). α-Pinene is an important component of pine needle oil and may be found in concentrations of 13.3-20.4% in commercial needle oils (table 6.58.1).

Four cases (1) and two (2) of contact sensitization to pine needle oil in topical pharmaceutical preparations have been reported; there may be overlap between these studies. One patient working as painter and car mechanic developed occupational contact dermatitis from a wax polish. He reacted to the wax polish and its ingredients pine oil (5% and 10% in olive oil) and dipentene (*d,l*-limonene) and co-reacted to turpentine oil, which also contains limonene and is obtained from *Pinus* species, just as pine oil (11).

A car mechanic had occupational contact dermatitis of the hands and forearms for 3 years. Patch testing gave positive reactions to dipentene (*D,L*-limonene) and pine oil 5% pet. The patient usually washed his hands with a homemade hand-washing paste, prepared by the owner of the garage, at the end of the working day. This paste was obtained by mixing dish soap powder and fine sawdust from Swedish pine wood. On day 4, the patient showed a positive patch test reaction to the hand-washing paste (5% in water). Patch tests with this paste in 10 healthy volunteers gave negative results. The reaction was ascribed to pine oil and limonene present in the pine wood (18).

In a number of publications, positive patch tests to pine needle oil have been reported with unknown, uncertain or unstated relevance. These include (literature screened up to 2014 [14]) the following. One positive patch test was obtained to pine needle oil and dwarf pine needle oil in a patient allergic to Melaleuca alternifolia (tea tree) oil (3). One case of allergic contact dermatitis from a 'natural' deodorant containing lichen acids has been reported; the patient reacted to the deodorant, lichen acid mix, usnic acid and some essential oils including pine oil (9). In Poland, 30% of patients allergic to turpentine oil also react to pine needle oil; α-pinene is the major ingredient of turpentine oil and also an important component of pine needle oil (10).

OTHER SIDE EFFECTS

Immediate contact reactions
Immediate contact reactions (contact urticaria) from pine oil have been cited in ref. 17.

Systemic side effects
A 12-month-old healthy girl may have developed systemic toxicity with irregular breathing, cyanosis and seizures from five prolonged baths containing an unknown quantity of essential oils of eucalyptus, pine, and thyme over a 4-day period for a benign and afebrile upper respiratory tract infection (15).

LITERATURE

1   Nardelli A, D'Hooge E, Drieghe J, Dooms M, Goossens A. Allergic contact dermatitis from fragrance components in specific topical pharmaceutical products in Belgium. Contact Dermatitis 2009;60:303-313

2   Devleeschouwer V, Roelandts R, Garmyn M, Goossens A. Allergic and photoallergic contact dermatitis from ketoprofen: results of (photo) patch testing and follow-up of 42 patients. Contact Dermatitis 2008;58:159-166

3   Hausen BM, Reichling J, Harkenthal M. Degradation products of monoterpenes are the sensitizing agents in tea tree oil. Am J Contact Dermat 1999;10:68-77

4   Dharmagunawardena B, Takwale A, Sanders KJ, Cannan S, Roger A, Ilchyshyn A. Gas chromatography: an investigative tool in multiple allergies to essential oils. Contact Dermatitis 2002;47:288-292

5   Rudzki E, Grzywa Z, Bruo WS. Sensitivity to 35 essential oils. Contact Dermatitis 1976;2:196-200

6   Rudzki E, Grzywa Z. Allergy to perfume mixture. Contact Dermatitis 1986;15:115-116

7   Romaguera C, Grimalt F. Statistical and comparative study of 4600 patients tested in Barcelona (1973–1977). Contact Dermatitis 1980;6:309-315

8   Meynadier JM, Meynadier J, Peyron JL, Peyron L. Formes cliniques des manifestations cutanées d'allergie aux parfums. Ann Dermatol Venereol 1986;113:31-39

9   Sheu M, Simpson EL, Law SV, Storrs FJ. Allergic contact dermatitis from a natural deodorant: A report of 4 cases associated with lichen acid mix allergy. J Am Acad Dermatol 2006;55:332-337

10 Rudzki E, Berova N, Czernielewski A, Grzywa Z, Hegyi E, Jirásek J, et al. Contact allergy to oil of turpentine: a 10-year retrospective view. Contact Dermatitis 1991;24:317-318

11 Martins C, Gonçalo M, Gonçalo S. Allergic contact dermatitis from dipentene in wax polish. Contact Dermatitis 1995;33:126-127

12 Opinion of the Scientific Committee on Cosmetic Products and Non-Food Products Intended for Consumers concerning 'An initial list of perfumery materials which must not form part of cosmetic products except subject to the Restrictions and Conditions laid down, 25 September 2001, SCCNFP/0392/00, final. Available at: http://ec.europa.eu/health/archive/ph_risk/committees/sccp/documents/out150_en.pdf

13 Opinion of the Scientific Committee on Cosmetic Products and Non-Food Products Intended for Consumers concerning 'The 1st update of the inventory of ingredients employed in cosmetic products. Section II: Perfume and aromatic raw materials', 24 October 2000, SCCNFP/0389/00, final. Available at: http://ec.europa.eu/health/ph_risk/committees/sccp/documents/out131_en.pdf

14 De Groot AC, Schmidt E. Essential oils: contact allergy and chemical composition. Boca Raton, Fl., USA: CRC Press, Taylor and Francis Group, 2016 (ISBN 9781482246407)

15 Burkhard PR, Burkhardt K, Haenggeli CA, Landis T. Plant-induced seizures: Reappearance of an old problem. J Neurol 1999;246:667-670

16 Gilissen L, Huygens S, Goossens A. Allergic contact dermatitis caused by topical herbal remedies: importance of patch testing with the patients' own products. Contact Dermatitis 2018;78:177-184

17 De Groot AC. Patch Testing, 4th Edition. Wapserveen, The Netherlands: acdegroot publishing, 2018 (ISBN 978-90-813233-4-5)

18 D'Erme AM, Francalanci S, Milanesi N, Ricci L, Gola M. Contact dermatitis due to dipentene and pine oil in an automobile mechanic. Occup Environ Med 2012;69:452

Chapter 6.59   RAVENSARA OIL

IDENTIFICATION

Description/definition : Ravensara oil is the essential oil obtained from the twigs with leaves of the ravensara, *Ravensara aromatica* Sonn. (synonym: *Cryptocarya agathophylla* van der Werff)

INCI name(s) EU : Ravensara aromatica leaf oil; Ravensara aromatica twig oil (perfuming name, not an INCI name proper)

INCI name(s) USA : Ravensara aromatica leaf oil

CAS registry number(s) : 91770-56-8

EC number(s) : 294-842-8

Function(s) in cosmetics : EU: masking; perfuming. USA: fragrance ingredients

Patch testing : 2% pet. (11)

GENERAL

Ravensara aromatica Sonnerat is an evergreen aromatic tree which can grow up to 20 meter and has a deep rich reddish brown bark. It is native to the wet forests of east Madagascar and is cultivated in Mauritius (1,2,4,10). The whole tree is strongly aromatic. Both the leaves and bark of *Ravensara aromatica* are rich in essential oils. These oils are commercialized in Madagascar and in Northern hemisphere countries under the name of 'Ravensara' or 'Ravensare' (2), mainly (in Europe and the USA) for aromatherapy (1,6,7,10).

Ravensara oil should not be confused – but often is - with ravintsara oil, the essential oil obtained from the species *Cinnamomum camphora*. Many commercial oils sold as 'ravensara' are in fact ravintsara oils. These oils usually contain high concentrations of 1,8-cineole (eucalyptol) or camphor, chemicals mostly not present or in low concentrations in oils obtained from *R. aromatica* (3,5,10).

CHEMICAL COMPOSITION

Ravensara oil is a yellowish to greenish yellow easily mobile liquid, which has an aromatic, phenolic to spicy anise odor. In ravensara oils from various origins, over 95 chemicals have been identified. About 39 per cent of these were found in a single reviewed publication only. The ten chemicals that had the highest maximum concentrations in 41 commercial ravensara essential oil samples are shown in table 6.59.1 (Erich Schmidt, analytical data published in ref. 10).

A full literature review of the qualitative and quantitative composition of commercial and non-commercial ravensara oils of various origins, their chemotypes and with data from the ISO standard, has been published in 2016 (10).

Table 6.59.1 Ten ingredients with the highest concentrations in commercial ravensara oils (10)

Name	Concentration range	Name	Concentration range
1,8-Cineole [a]	0.1 - 68.0%	β-Pinene	0.1 - 15.7%
Sabinene	0.1 - 25.5%	α-Terpineol	0.2 - 14.7%
Methyl eugenol	trace - 21.4%	Linalool	0.05 - 12.4%
Methyl chavicol	0.04 - 19.9%	α-Phellandrene	0.04 - 11.8%
Limonene	0.08 - 19.4%	α-Pinene	0.3 - 8.3%

[a] the high concentrations of 1,8-cineole indicate that some commercial ravensara oils were in fact ravintsara oils obtained from *Cinnamomum camphora*

CONTACT ALLERGY / ALLERGIC CONTACT DERMATITIS

General

There have been two case reports of allergic contact dermatitis from ravensara oils only, both in an occupational setting, in an aromatherapist and a complementary therapist. In one, α-pinene and possibly linalool may have been allergens in the ravensara oils (8).

Case reports and case series

An aromatherapist had occupational contact dermatitis with allergies to multiple essential oils used at work, including ravensara oil. The patient also reacted to geraniol, linalool, linalyl acetate, α-pinene, the fragrance mix and various other fragrance materials; α-pinene was demonstrated by GC-MS in the ravensara oil (8). This chemical has been found in commercial ravensara oils in concentrations of up to 8.3% and linalool in a maximum concentration of 12.4% (table 6.59.1).

A female 'complementary therapist' developed occupational contact dermatitis from a multitude of essential oils used at work, including ravensara oil (9).

LITERATURE

1   Andrianoelisoa HS, Menut C, Ramanoelina P, Raobelison F, Collas de Chatelperron P, Danthu P. Chemical composition of essential oils from bark and leaves of individual trees of *Ravensara aromatica* Sonnerat. J Essent Oil Res 2010;22:66-70

2   Andrianoelisoa HS, Menut C, Collas de Chatelperron P, Saracco J, Ramanoelina P, Danthu P. Intraspecific chemical variability and highlighting of chemotypes of leaf essential oils from *Ravensara aromatica* Sonnerat, a tree endemic to Madagascar. Flavour Fragr J 2006;21:833-838

3   Andrianoelisoa H, Menut C, Danthu P. *Ravensara aromatica* ou *Ravintsara*: une confusion qui perdure parmi les distributeurs d'huiles essentielles en Europe et en Amérique du Nord. phytothérapie 2012;10:161-169

4   Holm Y, Hiltunen R. Chemical composition of a commercial oil of *Ravensara aromatica* Sonn. used in aromatherapy. J Essent Oil Res 1999;11:677-678

5   Juliani HR, Kapteyn J, Jones D, Koroch AR, Wang M, Charles D, Simon JE. Application of near-infrared spectroscopy in quality control and determination of adulteration of African essential oils. Phytochem Anal 2006;17:121-128

6   Rhind JP. Essential oils. A handbook for aromatherapy practice, 2nd Edition. London: Singing Dragon, 2012

7   Lawless J. The encyclopedia of essential oils, 2nd Edition. London: Harper Thorsons, 2014

8   Dharmagunawardena B, Takwale A, Sanders KJ, Cannan S, Roger A, Ilchyshyn A. Gas chromatography: an investigative tool in multiple allergies to essential oils. Contact Dermatitis 2002;47:288-292

9   Newsham J, Rai S, Williams JDL. Two cases of allergic contact dermatitis to neroli oil. Br J Dermatol 2011;165(suppl.1):76

10 De Groot AC, Schmidt E. Essential oils: contact allergy and chemical composition. Boca Raton, Fl., USA: CRC Press, Taylor and Francis Group, 2016 (ISBN 9781482246407)

11 De Groot AC. Patch Testing, 4th Edition. Wapserveen, The Netherlands: acdegroot publishing, 2018 (ISBN 978-90-813233-4-5)

Chapter 6.60   ROSE OIL

IDENTIFICATION

Description/definition : Rose oil (essential oil of rose) is the essential oil obtained from the flowers of the
damask rose, *Rosa* x *damascena* Mill.

INCI name(s) EU & USA : Rosa damascena flower oil

CAS registry number(s) : 8007-01-0; 90106-38-0

EC number(s) : 290-260-3

RIFM monograph(s) : Food Cosmet Toxicol 1974;12:979,981 (special issue I); Food Cosmet Toxicol
1975;13:913

SCCS opinion(s) : SCCS/1459/11 (28)

ISO standard : ISO 9842 Essential oil of rose, 2003; Geneva, Switzerland, www.iso.org

Merck Index monograph : 8173

Function(s) in cosmetics : EU: masking; skin conditioning. USA: fragrance ingredients; skin-conditioning agents –
miscellaneous

Patch testing : 2% pet. (Chemo, absolute); 0.5% pet. (SPCanada)

GENERAL

Rosa x *damascena* Mill. is a deciduous shrub growing to 2.2 meters tall, the stems densely armed with stout, curved prickles and stiff bristles. It is commonly called the damask rose, as the plant was originally brought to Europe from Damascus, Syria. The damask rose is cultivated in Bulgaria, Turkey, India, Iran, southern France, southern Italy, Morocco, Ukraine, Caucasus, Syria, and China. The whole rose oil industry in Bulgaria and Turkey, which are the main producers of rose essential oil, is based on a single genotype which has been vegetatively propagated for centuries (30).

Rose essential oil is obtained from the fresh flowers of *R. damascena* by hydro- or steam-distillation. Because of the labor-intensive production process and the low content of oil in rose blooms (about 3,500 to 4,000 kilograms of rose flowers are necessary to produce one kilogram of rose oil), rose oil is very expensive and is often called 'liquid gold'. Rose oil is primarily used as a fragrance ingredient in the perfumery and cosmetics industry and is included in a large number of fine fragrances, creams, soaps, lotions and other cosmetic products.

However, rose oil also has pharmacological applications, and it is claimed to have many biological properties. Traditionally, rose oil is used as a remedy for anxiety, depression and for the treatment of stress-related conditions, but the oil has also been used in many other diseases and in aromatherapy (26,27,30). Its therapeutic efficacy has been reviewed in 2018 (32).

CHEMICAL COMPOSITION

Rose oil is a light yellow, crystallized or mobile liquid (depending on the temperature), which has a strong floral odor with subtle fruity or green, sweet honey-like background notes. In rose oils from various origins, over 440 chemicals have been identified. About 56 per cent of these were found in a single reviewed publication only. The ten chemicals that had the highest maximum concentrations in 51 commercial rose essential oil samples are shown in table 6.60.1 (Erich Schmidt, analytical data presented in ref. 30).

A full literature review of the qualitative and quantitative composition of commercial and non-commercial rose oils of various origins and with data from the ISO standard has been published in 2016 (30).

Table 6.60.1 Ten ingredients with the highest concentrations in commercial rose oils (30)

Name	Concentration range	Name	Concentration range
Citronellol	0.5 - 44.8%	α-Terpineol	0.06 - 7.5%
Geraniol	4.9 - 23.8%	Linalool	0.02 - 6.4%
Heneicosane	0.8 - 21.0%	Ethanol	0.03 - 4.9%
Nonadecane	6.3 - 15.9%	Methyl eugenol	0.06 - 4.3%
Nerol	0.6 - 11.0%	Eicosane (*n*-)	0.1 - 4.0%

CONTACT ALLERGY / ALLERGIC CONTACT DERMATITIS

General

The SCCS (Scientific Committee on Consumer Safety), in a 2012 Opinion on Fragrance allergens in cosmetic products, has marked *Rosa* species as 'established contact allergen in humans' (28,29).

Contact allergy to / allergic contact dermatitis from rose oils has been reported in over 25 publications. In groups of consecutive patients suspected of contact dermatitis, prevalence rates of 1.2% and 1.6% positive patch test reactions have been observed, but reliable relevance data are lacking. There have been several case reports on allergic contact dermatitis from rose oil, mostly from its presence in perfumes or other cosmetics. Geraniol may have been an allergen in rose oil in several cases, citronellol (the main ingredient) and linalool each in one rose oil-allergic individual. In addition, there are many descriptions of positive patch test reactions to rose oil (which is often tested in a fragrance series), where the relevance was uncertain. Most of these occurred in aromatherapists and others working occupationally with (other) essential oils. Many also reacted to geraniol, which may have been the primary sensitizer in these patients; the positive patch test reaction to rose oil then was the result of the presence of geraniol in the patch test material.

Testing in groups of patients
The results of patch tests with rose oil in routine testing (consecutive patients suspected of contact dermatitis) and in groups of selected patients are shown in table 6.60.2. In routine testing, the rates of positive reactions were 1.2% and 1.6% in 2 studies, whereas between 0.4% and 30% of patients in selected groups had positive patch tests. The high positivity rate of 30% was found in a very small group of 10 patients strongly suspected of fragrance allergy and reacting to the fragrance mix (4).

Table 6.60.2 Patch testing in groups of patients

Years and Country	Test conc. & vehicle	Number of patients tested	positive (%)	Selection of patients (S); Relevance (R); Comments (C)	Ref.
Routine testing					
2000-2007 USA	2% pet.	679	11 (1.6%)	R: 100%; C: weak study: a. high rate of macular erythema and weak reactions, b. relevance figures include 'questionable' and 'past' relevance	2
2002-2003 Korea	2% pet.	422	5 (1.2%)	R: not stated	17
Testing in groups of selected patients					
2011-2015 Spain	2% pet.	607	24 (3.9%)	S: patients previously reacting to FM I, FM II, Myroxylon pereirae resin or hydroxyisohexyl 3-cyclohexene carboxaldehyde in the baseline series and subsequently tested with a fragrance series; R: not stated; C: the test material was an *extract*	33
2008-2014 UK	2% pet.	471	3 (0.6%)	S: patients tested with a fragrance series; R: not stated	31
2004-2008 Spain	2% pet.	86	6 (7.0%)	S: patients previously reacting to the fragrance mix I or Myroxylon pereirae (n=54) or suspected of fragrance contact allergy (n=32); R: not stated; C: almost all patients also reacted to geraniol, one of its major components	13
<2004 Israel	2% pet.	91	2 (2.2%)	S: patients who had shown a doubtful or positive reaction to the fragrance mix I and/or Myroxylon pereirae resin and/or one or two commercial fine fragrances; R: not stated	18
1989-1999 Portugal	2% pet.	67	3 (4.5%)	S: patients who had a positive patch test to the fragrance mix; R: not stated	20
1990-1998 Japan	5% pet.	1483	6 (0.4%)	S: patients suspected of cosmetic contact dermatitis, virtually all were women; range of annual frequency of sensitization: 0-0.9%; R: not stated; C: tested was 'rose oil Bulgarian'	5
1996-1997 UK	2% pet.	10	3 (30%)	S: patients strongly suspected of fragrance allergy and reacting to the fragrance mix; R: not stated; C: tested was 'rose oil, Bulgarian'	4
<1994 Japan	?	?	? (3.9%)	S and R: unknown. Possibly routine testing	21
<1974 Japan	?	137	4 (2.9%)	S: patients suspected of cosmetic dermatitis; R: unknown	23

Case reports and case series
Two aromatherapists developed occupational contact dermatitis from contact allergy to multiple essential oils; they both reacted to rose oil Bulgarian in the fragrance series, which reactions were considered to be relevant (7). A massage therapist had occupational contact dermatitis from allergies to many essential oils; she reacted to rose oil, Bulgarian, in the fragrance series, which reaction was judged to be clinically relevant (9). A patient with hand dermatitis reacted to rose oil, geraniol and several other fragrances and essential oils; she used a 'fragrance-free' hand soap containing rose oil (11); commercial rose oils contain up to 23.8% geraniol (table 6.60.1).

One individual developed allergic cosmetic dermatitis from rose oil in a face cream (19). Two positive patch test reactions to rose oil, which was present in cosmetics that had given a positive patch test or had been positive in a usage test in patients, were seen in a 9-year period in one clinic in Belgium (12). One patient had allergic contact dermatitis from 'Rose Absolute' perfume and a body lotion containing *Rosa centifolia*; she reacted to her own products, *Rosa centifolia*, rose oil Bulgarian, several indicators of fragrance allergy, two other essential oils and various individual fragrance chemicals including linalool and citral (the combination of geranial and neral) (14); linalool has been found in commercial rose oils in concentrations up to 6.4%; geranial has been found in a lower concentration (max. 1.8%), but neral is not an important constituent of rose oils (30).

A patient developed contact allergy to a perfume; she reacted to the fragrance mix, Bulgarian rose oil and geraniol; chromatographic analysis of the perfume showed it to contain 33% citronellol and 20% geraniol, but the perfume, quite curiously, was not analyzed (22). Five cases of contact sensitization to rose oil present in topical pharmaceutical preparations have been reported from Belgium (1).

Miscellaneous

In a number of publications, positive patch tests to rose oil have been reported with unknown, uncertain or unstated relevance. These include (literature screened up to 2014 [30]) the following. In a group of 819 patients suspected of contact dermatitis, there were four positive patch test reactions to Bulgarian rose oil (3). Four positive patch tests to rose oil Bulgarian oil were observed in four massage therapists / aromatherapists with occupational contact dermatitis from (multiple) essential oils; one had not used this oil, in the other three this was uncertain (6).

Two aromatherapists with occupational contact dermatitis from other essential oils co-reacted to rose oil Bulgarian in the fragrance series (7). A naturopathic therapist and a masseuse with occupational contact dermatitis to various essential oils also reacted to Bulgarian rose oil in the fragrance series (8). Two positive patch tests to Bulgarian rose oil were seen in two aromatherapists allergic to multiple essential oils; they did not use rose oils themselves, but were allergic to geraniol, which is after citronellol the most important component of rose oils (10).

A patient with allergic contact cheilitis from geraniol in ice cream, candy and gum had a positive patch test to rose oil and the fragrance mix I, both of which contain geraniol (15). One patient with allergic contact cheilitis from lime reacted to lime, rose oil, geranium oil Bulgarian and their important component geraniol (16). Another patient developed disseminated allergic contact dermatitis from geraniol and lavender essence in a cream; the patient also reacted to Bulgarian rose oil and geranium oil Bourbon, both of which contain high concentrations of geraniol (25).

LITERATURE

1   Nardelli A, D'Hooge E, Drieghe J, Dooms M, Goossens A. Allergic contact dermatitis from fragrance components in specific topical pharmaceutical products in Belgium. Contact Dermatitis 2009;60:303-313
2   Wetter DA, Yiannias JA, Prakash AV, Davis MD, Farmer SA, el-Azhary RA, et al. Results of patch testing to personal care product allergens in a standard series and a supplemental cosmetic series: an analysis of 945 patients from the Mayo Clinic Contact Dermatitis Group, 2000-2007. J Am Acad Dermatol 2010;63:789-798
3   Kohl L, Blondeel A, Song M. Allergic contact dermatitis from cosmetics: retrospective analysis of 819 patch-tested patients. Dermatology 2002;204:334-337
4   Thomson KF, Wilkinson SM. Allergic contact dermatitis to plant extracts in patients with cosmetic dermatitis. Br J Dermatol 2000;142:84-88
5   Sugiura M, Hayakawa R, Kato Y, Sugiura K, Hashimoto R. Results of patch testing with lavender oil in Japan. Contact Dermatitis 2000;43:157-160
6   Bleasel N, Tate B, Rademaker M. Allergic contact dermatitis following exposure to essential oils. Australas J Dermatol 2002;43:211-213
7   Boonchai W, Lamtharachai P, Sunthonpalin P. Occupational allergic contact dermatitis from essential oils in aromatherapists. Contact Dermatitis 2007;56:181-182
8   Trattner A, David M, Lazarov A. Occupational contact dermatitis due to essential oils. Contact Dermatitis 2008;58:282-284
9   Cockayne SE, Gawkrodger DJ. Occupational contact dermatitis in an aromatherapist. Contact Dermatitis 1997;37:306-307
10 Dharmagunawardena B, Takwale A, Sanders KJ, Cannan S, Roger A, Ilchyshyn A. Gas chromatography: an investigative tool in multiple allergies to essential oils. Contact Dermatitis 2002;47:288-292
11 Scheinman PL. Is it really fragrance free? Am J Cont Derm 1997;8:239-242
12 Nardelli A, Drieghe J, Claes L, Boey L, Goossens A. Fragrance allergens in 'specific' cosmetic products. Contact Dermatitis 2011;64:212-219
13 Cuesta L, Silvestre JF, Toledo F, Lucas A, Pérez-Crespo M, Ballester I. Fragrance contact allergy: a 4-year retrospective study. Contact Dermatitis 2010;63:77-84
14 Nardelli A, Thijs L, Janssen K, Goossens A. *Rosa centifolia* in a 'non-scented' moisturizing body lotion as a cause of allergic contact dermatitis. Contact Dermatitis 2009;61:306-309
15 Tamagawa-Mineoka R, Katoh N, Kishimoto S. Allergic contact cheilitis due to geraniol in food. Contact Dermatitis 2007;56:242-243

16 Thomson MA, Preston PW, Prais L, Foulds IS. Lime dermatitis from gin and tonic with a twist of lime. Contact Dermatitis 2007;56:114-115

17 An S, Lee AY, Lee CH, Kim D-W, Hahm JH, Kim K-J, et al. Fragrance contact dermatitis in Korea: a joint study. Contact Dermatitis 2005;53:320-323

18 Trattner A, David M. Patch testing with fine fragrances: comparison with fragrance mix, balsam of Peru and a fragrance series. Contact Dermatitis 2004;49:287-289

19 Penchalaiah K, Handa S, Lakshmi SB, Sharma VK, Kumar B. Sensitizers commonly causing allergic contact dermatitis from cosmetics. Contact Dermatitis 2000;43:311-313

20 Manuel Brites M, Goncalo M, Figueiredo A. Contact allergy to fragrance mix - a 10-year study. Contact Dermatitis 2000;43:181-182

21 Sugai T. Group study IV – farnesol and lily aldehyde. Environ Dermatol 1994;1:213-214

22 Vilaplana J, Romaguera C, Grimalt F. Contact dermatitis from geraniol in Bulgarian rose oil. Contact Dermatitis 1991;24:301

23 Nakayama H, Hanaoka H, Ohshiro A. Allergen Controlled System (ACS). Tokyo, Japan: Kanehara Shuppan, 1974:42. Data cited in ref. 24

24 Mitchell JC. Contact hypersensitivity to some perfume materials. Contact Dermatitis 1975;1:196-199

25 Juarez A, Goiriz R, Sanchez-Perez J, Garcia-Diez A. Disseminated allergic contact dermatitis after exposure to a topical medication containing geraniol. Dermatitis 2008;19:163

26 Rhind JP. Essential oils. A handbook for aromatherapy practice, 2nd Edition. London: Singing Dragon, 2012

27 Lawless J. The encyclopedia of essential oils, 2nd Edition. London: Harper Thorsons, 2014

28 SCCS (Scientific Committee on Consumer Safety). Opinion on Fragrance allergens in cosmetic products, 26-27 June 2012, SCCS/1459/11. Available at: https://ec.europa.eu/health/sites/health/files/scientific_committees/consumer_safety/docs/sccs_o_102.pdf

29 Uter W, Johansen JD, Börje A, Karlberg A-T, Lidén C, Rastogi S, Roberts D, White IR. Categorization of fragrance contact allergens for prioritization of preventive measures: clinical and experimental data and consideration of structure–activity relationships. Contact Dermatitis 2013;69:196-230

30 De Groot AC, Schmidt E. Essential oils: contact allergy and chemical composition. Boca Raton, Fl., USA: CRC Press, Taylor and Francis Group, 2016 (ISBN 9781482246407)

31 Sabroe RA, Holden CR, Gawkrodger DJ. Contact allergy to essential oils cannot always be predicted from allergy to fragrance markers in the baseline series. Contact Dermatitis 2016;74:236-241

32 Mohebitabar S, Shirazi M, Bioos S, Rahimi R, Malekshahi F, Nejatbakhsh F. Therapeutic efficacy of rose oil: A comprehensive review of clinical evidence. Avicenna J Phytomed 2017;7:206-213

33 Silvestre JF, Mercader P, González-Pérez R, Hervella-Garcés M, Sanz-Sánchez T, Córdoba S, et al. Sensitization to fragrances in Spain: A 5-year multicentre study (2011-2015). Contact Dermatitis. 2018 Nov 14. doi: 10.1111/cod.13152. [Epub ahead of print]

Chapter 6.61   ROSEMARY OIL

IDENTIFICATION

Description/definition	: Rosemary oil (essential oil of rosemary) is the essential oil obtained from the leaves and flowering tops of the rosemary, *Rosmarinus officinalis* L.
INCI name(s) EU	: Rosmarinus officinalis leaf oil
INCI name(s) USA	: Rosmarinus officinalis (rosemary) leaf oil
CAS registry number(s)	: 8000-25-7; 84604-14-8
EC number(s)	: 283-291-9
CIR review(s)	: Final report 06/10/2014 (access: www.cir-safety.org/ingredients)
RIFM monograph(s)	: Food Cosmet Toxicol 1974;12:977 (special issue I) (binder, page 665)
ISO standard	: ISO 1342 Essential oil of rosemary, 2012; Geneva, Switzerland, www.iso.org
Merck Index monograph	: 9665 (Rosemary)
Function(s) in cosmetics	: EU: masking; skin conditioning. USA: fragrance ingredients; skin-conditioning agents – miscellaneous
Patch testing	: 0.5% pet. (SPCanada); based on RIFM data, 10% pet. is probably not irritant (15)

GENERAL

Rosmarinus officinalis L. is a woody evergreen perennial herb, up to 1.5 meter tall, which has strongly aromatic, needle-like evergreen leaves. Rosemary is native to the Madeira Islands, the Canary Islands, northern Africa, the Mediterranean European countries, Cyprus, Turkey, and the Caucasus (GRIN Taxonomy for Plants). The plant is widely cultivated for medicinal, culinary, cosmetic and ornamental purposes. Rosemary is one of the most prized culinary herbs, especially in Mediterranean cuisine (6). *R. officinalis* has also been extensively used in traditional folk medicine.

The essential oil of rosemary, which is obtained by steam-distillation from the leaves and flowering tops of the plant, is widely used as an ingredient in rubefacients, liniments, inhalants, perfumes, soaps, deodorants, bath essences, hair lotions, shampoos and other cosmetics, room sprays, detergents, softeners, disinfectants and insecticides (1,2,4,5,6,7). Rosemary oil is also utilized as a seasoning for foodstuffs such as meat dishes, salami and sauces and for flavoring liquors (3,4). The oil has many applications in traditional medicine (2,3) and is also used in aromatherapy (6,8).

The phytochemistry and biological activities of *R. officinalis* have been reviewed in 2018 (16).

CHEMICAL COMPOSITION

Rosemary oil is a colorless to pale yellow clear mobile liquid, sometimes with a greenish touch, which has a herbal, fresh green, terpeny and somewhat aromatic-spicy odor. In rosemary oils from various origins, over 505 chemicals have been identified. About 53 per cent of these were found in a single reviewed publication only. The ten chemicals that had the highest maximum concentrations in 108 commercial rosemary essential oil samples are shown in table 6.61.1 (Erich Schmidt, analytical data presented in ref. 13).

A full literature review of the qualitative and quantitative composition of commercial and non-commercial rosemary oils of various origins, their chemotypes and with data from the ISO standard, has been published in 2016 (13).

Table 6.61.1 Ten ingredients with the highest concentrations in commercial rosemary oils (13)

Name	Concentration range	Name	Concentration range
1,8-Cineole	7.6 - 59.8%	Camphene	0.06 - 12.0%
Myrcene	0.2 - 46.0%	β-Pinene	0.3 - 10.3%
α-Pinene	1.9 - 46.0%	Limonene	0.7 - 6.7%
Camphor	2.9 - 24.2%	Borneol	0.4 - 6.3%
Bornyl acetate	0.2 - 13.1%	β-Caryophyllene	0.7 - 6.2%

CONTACT ALLERGY / ALLERGIC CONTACT DERMATITIS

General

Contact allergy to / allergic contact dermatitis from rosemary oil has been reported in a few publications only. Routine testing has apparently not been performed. Three case reports of allergic contact dermatitis from rosemary oil were from occupational exposure in an aromatherapist, a masseuse and a physiotherapist. In one patient, α-pinene and possibly linalool may have been allergens in rosemary oil (9).

Testing in groups of patients

A group of 86 patients from Poland previously reacting to the fragrance mix was tested with rosemary oil and three (3.4%) had a positive patch test reaction; relevance data were not provided (11).

Case reports and case series

An aromatherapist had occupational contact dermatitis with allergies to multiple essential oils used at work, including rosemary oil; the patient also reacted to geraniol, linalool, linalyl acetate, α-pinene, the fragrance mix and various other fragrance materials; α-pinene and linalool were detected in the rosemary oil by GC-MS (9). α-Pinene has been found in commercial rosemary oils in a maximum concentration of 5.0%, linalool in lower concentrations up to 2.1% (table 6.61.1).

Two masseuses and one physiotherapist had occupational allergic contact dermatitis from rosemary oil and other essential oils (10). One positive patch test reaction has been observed to rosemary oil 0.5% petrolatum; its relevance was not stated (cited in ref. 12).

OTHER SIDE EFFECTS

In France, two children aged 2 years and 3 months who received a cosmetic baby balm on the skin of their thorax containing eucalyptus, rosemary and lavender essential oils, developed convulsions. As there was no other explanation for this and the 'neurologic toxicity of terpene derivatives is well known' (referring to studies on camphor toxicity), the cosmetic was suspected to be the culprit product. Although no specific terpene ingredient was blamed, the authors discussed the possible role of camphor, menthol and eucalyptol (1,8-cineole). On the basis of these 2 hardly convincing cases, the product was withdrawn from the market (14).

LITERATURE

1   Apostolides NA, El Beyrouthy M, Dhifi W, Najm S, Cazier F, Najem W, Labaki M, Aboukaïs A. Chemical composition of aerial parts of *Rosmarinus officinalis* L. essential oil growing wild in Lebanon. J Essent Oil Bear Plants 2013;16:274-282
2   Akrout A, Hajlaoui H, Mighri H, Najjaa H, El Jani H, Zaidi S, Neffati M. Chemical and biological characteristics of essential oil of Rosmarinus officinalis cultivated in Djerba. J Essent Oil Bear Plants 2010;13:398-411
3   Mikre W, Rohloff J, Hymete A. Volatile constituents and antioxidant activity of essential oils obtained from important aromatic plants of Ethiopia. J Essent Oil Bear Plants 2007;10:465-474
4   Guazzi E, Maccioni S, Monti G, Flamini G, Cioni PL, Morelli I. *Rosmarinus officinalis* L. in the gravine of Palagianello (Taranto, South Italy). J Essent Oil Res 2001;13:231-233
5   Arnold N, Valentini G, Bellomaria B, Hocine L. Comparative study of the essential oils from *Rosmarinus eriocalyx* Jordan & Fourr. from Algeria and *R. officinalis* L. from other countries. J Essent Oil Res 1997;9:167-175
6   Kabouche Z, Boutaghane N, Laggoune S, Kabouche A, Ait-Kaki Z, Benlabed Z. Comparative antibacterial activity of five Lamiaceae essential oils from Algeria. Int J Aromather 2005;15:129-133.
7   Flamini G, Cioni PL, Morelli I, Macchia M, Ceccarini L. Main agronomic-productive characteristics of two ecotypes of *Rosmarinus officinalis* L. and chemical composition of their essential oils. J Agric Food Chem 2002;50:3512-3517
8   Tigrine-Kordjani N, Meklati BY, Chemat F, Guezil FZ. kinetic investigation of rosemary essential oil by two methods: solvent-free microwave extraction and hydrodistillation. Food Anal Methods 2012;5:596-603
9   Dharmagunawardena B, Takwale A, Sanders KJ, Cannan S, Roger A, Ilchyshyn A. Gas chromatography: an investigative tool in multiple allergies to essential oils. Contact Dermatitis 2002;47:288-292
10   Trattner A, David M, Lazarov A. Occupational contact dermatitis due to essential oils. Contact Dermatitis 2008;58:282-284
11   Rudzki E, Grzywa Z. Allergy to perfume mixture. Contact Dermatitis 1986;15:115-116
12   Hjorther AB, Christophersen C, Hausen BM, Menné T. Occupational allergic contact dermatitis from carnosol, a naturally-occurring compound present in rosemary. Contact Dermatitis 1997;37:99-100
13   De Groot AC, Schmidt E. Essential oils: contact allergy and chemical composition. Boca Raton, Fl., USA: CRC Press, Taylor and Francis Group, 2016 (ISBN 9781482246407)
14   Laribière A, Miremont-Salamé G, Bertrand S, François C, Haramburu F. Terpènes dans les cosmétiques: 2 cas d'épilepsie. Thérapie 2005;60: 607-609
15   De Groot AC. Patch Testing, 4th Edition. Wapserveen, The Netherlands: acdegroot publishing, 2018 (ISBN 978-90-813233-4-5)
16   Andrade JM, Faustino C, Garcia C, Ladeiras D, Reis CP, Rijo P. *Rosmarinus officinalis* L.: an update review of its phytochemistry and biological activity. Future Sci OA 2018;4(4):FSO283. doi: 10.4155/fsoa-2017-0124

Chapter 6.62   ROSEWOOD OIL

IDENTIFICATION

Description/definition	: Rosewood oil (essential oil of rosewood, Brazilian type) is the essential oil obtained from the wood of the rosewood, *Aniba rosaeodora* Ducke (and possibly from other *Aniba* species such as *Aniba parviflora* (Meisn.) Mez.)
INCI name(s) EU	: Aniba rosaeodora wood oil
INCI name(s) USA	: Aniba rosaeodora (rosewood) wood oil
Other names	: Bois de rose oil
CAS registry number(s)	: 8015-77-8; 83863-32-5
EC number(s)	: 281-093-7
RIFM monograph(s)	: Food Cosmet Toxicol 1978;16:653 (special issue IV)
ISO standard	: ISO 3761 Essential oil of rosewood, 2005; Geneva, Switzerland, www.iso.org
Function(s) in cosmetics	: EU: astringent; masking; perfuming; skin conditioning; tonic. USA: fragrance ingredients; skin-conditioning agents - miscellaneous
Patch testing	: 5% pet. (8); test also linalool (see Chapter 3.96 Linalool)

GENERAL

Aniba rosaeodora Ducke (synonyms: *Aniba rosaeodora* var. *amazonica* Ducke, *Aniba duckei* Kostermans) is a massive, evergreen fragrant tree, up to 30 meters in height and two meters in diameter. It is native to French Guyana, Columbia, Ecuador, Suriname, Venezuela, Brazil and Peru (1,4). Because of overuse of the trees in the past (notably for production of essential oil), *A. rosaeodora* is now an endangered species (4).

Rosewood oil is obtained by felling wild *Aniba rosaeodora* Ducke trees ('bois de rose' or 'bois de rose fenelle' in French; 'pau-rosa' in Brazilian) and possibly other species of *Aniba* such as *Aniba parviflora* (3) and steam-distilling the comminuted trunk wood. The oil possesses a characteristic aroma and is a long-established ingredient in the more expensive perfumes and a perfume fixative (1,2,4). It is cited to be used in food production also (1). The oil is used in aromatherapy formulations, but has become less attractive as environmental concerns have grown over the destructive nature of rosewood oil production in Brazil (1).

CHEMICAL COMPOSITION

Rosewood oil is a colorless to pale yellow clear mobile liquid which has a fresh, floral and tender woody odor. In rosewood oils from various origins, over 60 chemicals have been identified (only few analytical studies found). About 42 per cent of these were found in a single reviewed publication only. The ten chemicals that had the highest maximum concentrations in 36 commercial rosewood essential oil samples are shown in table 6.62.1 (Erich Schmidt, analytical data presented in ref. 7).

A full literature review of the qualitative and quantitative composition of commercial and non-commercial rosewood oils of various origins and with data from the ISO standard has been published in 2016 (7).

Table 6.62.1 Ten ingredients with the highest concentrations in commercial rosewood oils (7)

Name	Concentration range	Name	Concentration range
Linalool	73.0 - 88.4%	α-Copaene	0.2 - 2.1%
α-Terpineol	1.9 - 8.8%	*cis*-Linalool oxide, furanoid	0.03 - 2%
trans-Sabinene hydrate	0.01 - 3.3%	*trans*-Linalool oxide	0.9 - 2.0%
Geraniol	0.7 - 2.3%	*trans*-Linalool oxide,	0.06 - 1.7%
α-Pinene	0.2 - 2.2%	furanoid	
cis-Linalool oxide	0.9 - 2.1%		

CONTACT ALLERGY / ALLERGIC CONTACT DERMATITIS

General

Contact allergy to / allergic contact dermatitis from rosewood oil has been reported in two case reports only. In one, linalool may have been an allergen in rosewood oil (5).

Case reports and case series

One patient had airborne contact dermatitis from contact allergy to rosewood oil and two other essential oils in aromatherapy lamps, whereby the water vapour produced distributes the essential oils as an aerosol in the air; the patient also reacted to linalool, which is an important constituent of all three oils (5). In commercial rosewood oils, linalool is the dominant ingredient with concentrations of 73-88% (table 6.62.1).

An aromatherapist had occupational contact dermatitis from multiple essential oil sensitizations, including rosewood (6).

LITERATURE

1   Coppen JJW. Rosewood oil. In: Non-wood forest products. Flavours and fragrances of plant origin. Rome: Food and Agriculture Organization of the United Nations, 1995:29-36
2   Chantraine J-M, Dhénin J-M, Moretti C. Chemical variability of rosewood (*Aniba rosaeodora* Ducke) essential oil in French Guiana. J Essent Oil Res 2009;21:486-495
3   Santana A, Ohashi S, de Rosa L, Green CL. Brazilian rosewood oil: The prospect for sustainable production and oil quality management. Int J Aromather 1997;8:16-20
4   Convention on International Trade in Endangered Species of Wild Fauna and Flora. Fifteenth meeting of the Conference of the Parties, Doha (Qatar), 13-25 March 2010. Available at: http://www.cites.org/eng/cop/15/prop/E-15-Prop-29.pdf
5   Schaller M, Korting HC. Allergic airborne contact dermatitis from essential oils used in aromatherapy. Clin Exp Dermatol 1995;20:143-145
6   Selvaag E, Holm J, Thune P. Allergic contact dermatitis in an aromatherapist with multiple sensitizations to essential oils. Contact Dermatitis 1995;33:354-355
7   De Groot AC, Schmidt E. Essential oils: contact allergy and chemical composition. Boca Raton, Fl., USA: CRC Press, Taylor and Francis Group, 2016 (ISBN 9781482246407)
8   De Groot AC. Patch Testing, 4th Edition. Wapserveen, The Netherlands: acdegroot publishing, 2018 (ISBN 978-90-813233-4-5)

Chapter 6.63   SAGE OIL

There are two major commercial sage oils: Sage oil Dalmatian, obtained from *Salvia officinalis* L. and sage oil Spanish, which is obtained from *Salvia lavandulifolia* Vahl.

6.63.1 SAGE OIL DALMATIAN

IDENTIFICATION

Description/definition	: Dalmatian sage oil (essential oil of Dalmatian sage) is the essential oil obtained from the flowering tops of the sage, *Salvia officinalis* L.
INCI name(s) EU	: Salvia officinalis oil
INCI name(s) USA	: Salvia officinalis (sage) oil
CAS registry number(s)	: 8022-56-8; 84082-79-1
EC number(s)	: 282-025-9
RIFM monograph(s)	: Food Cosmet Toxicol 1974;12:987 (special issue I) (binder, page 672)
SCCS opinion(s)	: SCCS/1459/11 (11)
ISO standard	: ISO 9909 Essential oil of Dalmatian sage, 1997; Geneva, Switzerland, www.iso.org
Merck Index monograph	: 9750 (Salvia)
Function(s) in cosmetics	: EU: masking; tonic. USA: fragrance ingredients
Patch testing	: 2% pet.; based on RIFM data, 8% pet. is probably not irritant (18)

GENERAL

Salvia officinalis L. is a perennial, evergreen subshrub, up to 60 cm tall, with a woody base, soft gray-green oval leaves and a mass of blue or violet inflorescences (2). The name Salvia comes from the Latin salvere, which means 'to be well, to be in good health', indicating the (perceived) medical value of the plant (3). The Dalmatian sage is native to south-eastern Europe (Albania, former Yugoslavia, Greece, Italy) and is now widely cultivated in many (warm)-temperate regions of the world, mainly to obtain dried leaves to be used as a raw material in medicine, perfumery, and the food industry (1, 13).

The essential oil of sage, which is obtained by steam-distillation of the flowering tops or the leaves, is used in traditional medicine and by the pharmaceutical, perfumery, liqueur and food industry (3,5). It is also employed in incense and for aromatherapy, though it often considered too toxic for that practice because of the high thujone content (7,8,9). A variety of pharmacological activities has been ascribed to the essential oils of sage. However, the European Medicines Agency in 2009 assessed the safety and efficacy of their use in minor indications that do not require supervision of a medical practitioner, and concluded that the benefit-risk analysis of sage essential oil is negative, warning for the toxicity of thujone, usually the main ingredient of commercial sage oils (4).

CHEMICAL COMPOSITION

Dalmatian sage oil is a colorless to yellow clear mobile liquid, which has an herbaceous, aromatic-spicy green camphoraceous odor. In Dalmatian sage oils from various origins, over 310 chemicals have been identified. About 47 per cent of these were found in a single reviewed publication only. The ten chemicals that had the highest maximum concentrations in 55 commercial Dalmatian sage essential oil samples are shown in table 6.63.1.1 (Erich Schmidt, analytical data presented in ref. 13).

A full literature review of the qualitative and quantitative composition of commercial and non-commercial sage oils Dalmatian of various origins, their chemotypes and with data from the ISO standard, has been published in 2016 (13). Literature on sage oils from before 1997 has been reviewed in ref. 14.

Table 6.63.1.1 Ten ingredients with the highest concentrations in commercial Dalmatian sage oils (13)

Name	Concentration range	Name	Concentration range
α-Thujone	14.0 - 39.9%	β-Pinene	1.0 - 9.2%
Camphor	8.5 - 22.6%	Camphene	1.2 - 7.9%
α-Humulene	2.5 - 12.4%	β-Caryophyllene	1.9 - 7.7%
1,8-Cineole	2.1 - 12.1%	α-Pinene	1.1 - 6.5%
β-Thujone (*cis-*)	2.5 - 9.6%	Limonene	0.4 - 6.2%

6.63.2 SAGE OIL SPANISH

IDENTIFICATION

Description/definition	: Spanish sage oil (essential oil of sage, Spanish) is the essential oil obtained from the flowering tops of the Spanish sage, *Salvia lavandulifolia* Vahl.
INCI name(s) EU	: Salvia lavandulifolia leaf oil; Salvia lavandulifolia herb oil (perfuming name, not an INCI name proper)
INCI name(s) USA	: Salvia lavandulaefolia leaf oil (botanical name incorrect)
CAS registry number(s)	: 90106-49-3; 95371-15-6
EC number(s)	: 290-272-9
RIFM monograph(s)	: Food Cosmet Toxicol 1976;14:857 (special issue III)
SCCS opinion(s)	: SCCS/1459/11 (11)
ISO standard	: ISO 3526 Oil of sage, Spanish, 2005; Geneva, Switzerland, www.iso.org
Merck Index monograph	: 9750 (Salvia)
Function(s) in cosmetics	: EU: masking; perfuming. USA: fragrance ingredients
Patch testing	: 2% pet.; based on RIFM data, 8% pet. is probably not irritant (18)

GENERAL

Salvia lavandulifolia Vahl is a small woody and densely branched herbaceous perennial with wiry stems, growing 30-50 cm tall and up to 60 cm wide (16). The plant is native to northern Africa (Algeria, Morocco) and south-western Europe (France, Spain) and is endemic in Turkey (17). The Spanish sage grows in the wild and inhabits stony slopes, rock crevices, and oak and pine woodlands (15). It is cultivated on a small scale in Spain. The essential oil of Spanish sage, which is obtained mostly from wild plants in Spain (province of Granada) is used for cosmetics (soap, toothpaste), desserts, soft drinks, alcoholic beverages and as medicine, and in Spain also for cooking (13). In addition, it is employed in aromatherapy practices (7,8).

CHEMICAL COMPOSITION

Spanish type sage oil is a colorless to pale yellow liquid, which has a fresh herbaceous, camphoraceous odor, reminding of eucalyptus. In Spanish sage oils from various origins, over 120 chemicals have been identified. About 41 per cent of these were found in a single reviewed publication only. The ten chemicals that had the highest maximum concentrations in 42 commercial Spanish sage essential oil samples are shown in table 6.63.2.1 (Erich Schmidt, analytical data presented in ref. 13).

A full literature review of the qualitative and quantitative composition of commercial and non-commercial Spanish sage oils of various origins and with data from the ISO standard has been published in 2016 (13).

Table 6.63.2.1 Ten ingredients with the highest concentrations in commercial Spanish sage oils (13)

Name	Concentration range	Name	Concentration range
Camphor	11.0 - 36.0%	Borneol	1.0 - 7.0%
1,8-Cineole	10.0 - 30.0%	Limonene	2.0 - 6.0%
α-Pinene	4.0 - 11.0%	Linalyl acetate	0.1 - 5.0%
Sabinyl acetate	0.5 - 9.0%	Linalool	0.3 - 4.0%
Terpinyl acetate	0.5 - 9.0%	Sabinene	0.1 - 3.5%

CONTACT ALLERGY / ALLERGIC CONTACT DERMATITIS

Sage oil, unspecified

The SCCS (Scientific Committee on Consumer Safety), in a 2012 Opinion on Fragrance allergens in cosmetic products, has categorized as *Salvia* species as 'possible fragrance contact allergen' (11,12).

General

Contact allergy to and possible allergic contact dermatitis from sage oil has been reported in one publication only. A false-positive patch test reaction due to the excited skin syndrome cannot be excluded (10).

Case reports and case series
An aromatherapist had chronic hand dermatitis and was patch test positive to 17 of 20 oils used at her work (tested 1% and 5% in petrolatum), including sage oil (10).

<u>Sage oil Dalmatian</u>
No reports on contact allergy to sage oil, specifically mentioned to be obtained from *Salvia officinalis*, have been found. Allergy to sage oils (botanical source unspecified) is discussed above.

<u>Sage oil Spanish</u>
No reports on contact allergy to sage oil, specifically mentioned to be obtained from *Salvia lavandulifolia*, have been found. Allergy to sage oils (botanical source unspecified) is discussed above.

LITERATURE

1   Khalid KA. Evaluation of *Salvia officinalis* L. essential oil under selenium treatments. J Essent Oil Res 2011;23: 57-60

2   Awen BZ, Unnithan CR, Ravi S, Kermagy A, Prabhu V, Hemlal H. Chemical composition of *Salvia officinalis* essential oil of Libya. J Essent Oil Bear Plants 2011;14:89-94

3   Damjanovic-Vratnica B, Đakov T, Šukovic D, Damjanovic J. Chemical composition and antimicrobial activity of essential oil of wild-growing *Salvia officinalis* L. from Montenegro. J Essent Oil Bear Plants 2008;11:79-89

4   Tognolini M, Barocelli E, Ballabeni V, Bruni R, Bianchi A, Chiavarini M, Impicciatore M. Comparative screening of plant essential oils: Phenylpropanoid moiety as basic core for antiplatelet activity. Life Sciences 2006;78:1419-1432

5   Raal A, Orav A, Arak E. Composition of the essential oil of *Salvia officinalis* L. from various European countries. Nat Prod Res 2007;21:406-411

6   Committee on Herbal Medicinal Products. Public statement on *Salvia officinalis* L., Aetheroleum. London: European Medicines Agency, 2009
     http://www.ema.europa.eu/docs/en_GB/document_library/Public_statement/2010/02/WC500070841.pdf

7   Rhind JP. Essential oils. A handbook for aromatherapy practice, 2nd Edition. London: Singing Dragon, 2012

8   Lawless J. The encyclopedia of essential oils, 2nd Edition. London: Harper Thorsons, 2014

9   Davis P. Aromatherapy. An A-Z, 3rd Edition. London: Vermilion, 2005

10   Selvaag E, Holm J, Thune P. Allergic contact dermatitis in an aromatherapist with multiple sensitizations to essential oils. Contact Dermatitis 1995;33:354-355

11   SCCS (Scientific Committee on Consumer Safety). Opinion on Fragrance allergens in cosmetic products, 26-27 June 2012, SCCS/1459/11. Available at:
     https://ec.europa.eu/health/sites/health/files/scientific_committees/consumer_safety/docs/sccs_o_102.pdf

12   Uter W, Johansen JD, Börje A, Karlberg A-T, Lidén C, Rastogi S, Roberts D, White IR. Categorization of fragrance contact allergens for prioritization of preventive measures: clinical and experimental data and consideration of structure–activity relationships. Contact Dermatitis 2013;69:196-230

13   De Groot AC, Schmidt E. Essential oils: contact allergy and chemical composition. Boca Raton, Fl., USA: CRC Press, Taylor and Francis Group, 2016 (ISBN 9781482246407)

14   Boelens MH, Boelens H. Chemical and sensory evaluation of sage oils. Perfum Flavor 1997;22(2):19-40

15   Zrira S, Menut C, Bessière CM, Elamrani A, Benjilali B. A study of the essential oil of *Salvia lavandulifolia* Vahl from Morocco. J Essent Oil Bear Plants 2004;7:232-238

16   Usano-Alemany J, Palá-Paúl J, Herráiz-Peñalver D. Temperature stress causes different profiles of volatile compounds in two chemotypes of *Salvia lavandulifolia* Vahl. Biochem System Ecol 2014;54:166-171

17   Herraiz-Peñalver D, Usano-Alemany J, Cuadrado J, Jordán MJ, Lax V, Sotomayor JA, Palá-Paúl J. Essential oil composition of wild populations of *Salvia lavandulifolia* Vahl. from Castilla-La Mancha (Spain). Biochem Syst Ecol 2010;38:1224-1230

18   De Groot AC. Patch Testing, 4th Edition. Wapserveen, The Netherlands: acdegroot publishing, 2018 (ISBN 978-90-813233-4-5)

Chapter 6.64   SANDALWOOD OIL

There are three varieties of sandalwood oil: East Indian sandalwood oil obtained from the wood of *Santalum album* L., Australian sandalwood oil obtained from *Santalum spicatum* (R. Br.) A. DC., and New Caledonian sandalwood oil, prepared from the wood of *Santalum austrocaledonicum* Vieill. The East Indian variety has not commercially been available since 2008, as *Santalum album* is on the endangered species list of the International Union for the Conservation of Nature (IUCN) and Indian law prohibits the export of sandalwood oil.

In non-botanical literature, including reports of contact allergy, almost always the general term 'sandalwood oil' is used, without specifying its botanical source.

6.64.1   SANDALWOOD OIL EAST INDIA

IDENTIFICATION

Description/definition	: Sandalwood oil East India (essential oil of sandalwood) is the essential oil obtained from the wood of the East Indian sandalwood, *Santalum album* L.
INCI name(s) EU	: Santalum album oil
INCI name(s) USA	: Santalum album (sandalwood) oil
Other names	: Oil of santal
CAS registry number(s)	: 8006-87-9; 84787-70-2
EC number(s)	: 284-211-1
RIFM monograph(s)	: Food Cosmet Toxicol 1974;12:989 (special issue I) (binder, page 675)
SCCS opinion(s)	: SCCS/1459/11 (44)
ISO standard	: ISO 3518 Essential oil of sandalwood, 2002; Geneva, Switzerland, www.iso.org
Merck Index monograph	: 9760 (Sandalwood)
Function(s) in cosmetics	: EU: masking. USA: fragrance ingredients; solvents
Patch testing	: 2% pet. (Chemo); 10% pet. (SPEurope, SPCanada)

GENERAL

Santalum album L. is a small evergreen tree, which can grow to a height of 20 meter with a girth of up to 2.4 meter. The plant is found distributed in India, Indonesia, New Caledonia, Philippine Islands, Malaysia and Sri Lanka. India used to account for virtually all of the world's production of sandalwood and its oil (2). *Santalum album* is a partial parasite that attaches to the roots of other trees; it needs 'nurse' species in the area of planting out. About 500 potential host plants are known; for sandalwood cultivation, *Cassia siamea* has been favored in general (2,46).

Distillation of the powdered heartwood yields the East Indian sandalwood oil (Oleum santali) (the sapwood contains little, if any, detectable oils) (1). Its main use is in the creation of perfumes. *S. album* produces excellent fragrant material, and is one of the oldest and most expensive perfumery raw materials. The oil is highly rated for its fixative properties and for its persistent, heavy, sweet, woody odor (2,3). The oil is also used extensively in the cosmetics industry in the manufacture of soaps, face creams, toilet powders and air fresheners (2).

In addition, sandalwood oil has applications in many food products, alcoholic and non-alcoholic beverages, for flavoring chewing tobacco and is a very popular oil in aromatherapy and in Ayurveda and other medicinal systems (2,4,5). East Indian sandalwood oil is also said to show promise as treatment of acne, psoriasis, eczema, common warts, and mollusca contagiosa because of anti-inflammatory, anti-microbial, and anti-proliferative effects of the oil (32).

Since 2008, *Santalum album* is on the International Union for the Conservation of Nature (IUCN) list of endangered species. As a consequence, the governments of the two sandalwood production areas of India, Madras and Mysore, decided to stop the production of the oil and any export. However, small quantities are illegally being sold and are subsequently adulterated (46).

CHEMICAL COMPOSITION

Sandalwood oil is a clear, slightly viscous, and colorless to pale yellow liquid, which has a soft, sweet and woody note with long lasting powdery odor. In sandalwood oils from various origins, over 125 chemicals have been identified. About 69 per cent of these were found in a single reviewed publication only. The ten chemicals that had the highest maximum concentrations in 39 commercial East Indian sandalwood essential oil samples are shown in table 6.64.1.1 (Erich Schmidt, analytical data presented in ref. 46).

A full literature review of the qualitative and quantitative composition of commercial and non-commercial East Indian sandalwood oils of various origins and with data from the ISO standard, has been published in 2016 (46). A comprehensive review on the constituents of the heartwood from fragrant sandalwood species including *S. album* obtained by hydrodistillation and solvent extraction is presented in ref. 7 (essential oil composition not separated from solvent extracts).

Table 6.64.1.1 Ten ingredients with the highest concentrations in commercial East Indian sandalwood oils (46)

Name	Concentration range	Name	Concentration range
(Z)-α-Santalol	43.4 - 53.3%	(Z)-Lanceol	0.7 - 3.3%
(Z)-β-Santalol	15.6 - 23.6%	(E)-Nuciferol	0.3 - 2.9%
(Z)-trans-α-Bergamotol	4.5 - 8.6%	(E)-α-Santalal	1.0 - 2.8%
epi-β-Santalol	3.2 - 6.6%	epi-β-Santalene	0.3 - 2.3%
β-Santalene	0.5 - 3.6%	(E)-β-Santalol	0.5 - 2.0%

6.64.2 SANDALWOOD OIL AUSTRALIA

IDENTIFICATION

Description/definition	: Sandalwood oil Australia (essential oil of Australian sandalwood) is the essential oil obtained from the wood of the Australian sandalwood, *Santalum spicatum* (R. Br.) A. DC.
INCI name(s) EU	: Santalum spicata wood oil (perfuming name, not an INCI name proper)
INCI name(s) USA	: Not in the Personal Care Products Council Ingredient Database
CAS registry number(s)	: 8024-35-9; 92875-02-0; 1175539-50-0
EC number(s)	: 296-618-5
ISO standard	: ISO 22769 Essential oil of Australian sandalwood, 2009; Geneva, Switzerland, www.iso.org
Merck Index monograph	: 9760 (Sandalwood)
Function(s) in cosmetics	: EU: perfuming
Patch testing	: 2% pet. (Chemo); 10% pet. (SPEurope, SPCanada) (ex *Santalum album*)

GENERAL

The West Australian sandalwood *Santalum spicatum* (R. Br.) A. DC. (synonyms: *Eucarya spicata* (R. Br.) Sprague & Summerh.; *Fusanus spicatus* R. Br.) is an evergreen tree that grows from three up to eight meters tall. It is native to West Australia. *Santalum spicatum* is used for the production of furniture but mainly for producing an essential oil. Distillation of the stem wood, butt wood and roots yields the Australian sandalwood oil. This oil is employed for the production of cosmetics such as soaps, powder and creams (2) as well as for medicinal purposes (6). Sandalwood oils are widely used in aromatherapy; their presumed properties and medicinal applications have been reviewed (5).

CHEMICAL COMPOSITION

Australian sandalwood oil a clear, slightly viscous, colorless to brownish liquid which has a soft, woody and sweet note with long lasting dry powdery odor. In Australian sandalwood oils from various origins, over 90 chemicals have been identified. About 70 per cent of these were found in a single reviewed publication only. The ten chemicals that had the highest maximum concentrations in 23 commercial Australian sandalwood essential oil samples are shown in table 6.64.2.1 (Erich Schmidt, analytical data presented in ref. 46).

A full literature review of the qualitative and quantitative composition of commercial and non-commercial Australian sandalwood oils of various origins with data from the ISO standard has been published in 2016 (46). A comprehensive review on the constituents of the heartwood from fragrant sandalwood species including *S. spicatum* obtained by hydrodistillation and solvent extraction is presented in ref. 7 (essential oil composition not separated from solvent extracts).

Table 6.64.2.1 Ten ingredients with the highest concentrations in commercial Australian sandalwood oils (46)

Name	Concentration range	Name	Concentration range
(Z)-α-Santalol	17.0 - 42.9%	(Z)-Nuciferol	0.6 - 10.7%
(E,E)-Farnesol	1.4 - 18.4%	(E)-Nuciferol	3.9 - 9.1%
(Z)-β-Santalol	6.4 - 17.7%	(Z)-trans-α-Bergamotol	1.0 - 8.9%
epi-α-Bisabolol	0.4 - 12.8%	α-Santalene	0.4 - 4.9%
(Z)-Lanceol	0.8 - 10.8%	epi-β-Santalene	0.3 - 4.8%

6.64.3   SANDALWOOD OIL NEW CALEDONIA

IDENTIFICATION

Description/definition   : Sandalwood oil New Caledonia is the essential oil obtained from the wood of the New
                            Caledonian sandalwood, *Santalum austrocaledonicum* Vieill.
INCI name(s) EU & USA   : Santalum austrocaledonicum wood oil
Other names   : Oil of santal
CAS registry number(s)   : 91845-48-6
EC number(s)   : 295-223-5
Merck Index monograph   : 9760 (Sandalwood)
Function(s) in cosmetics : EU: flavouring; masking; perfuming. USA: flavoring agents; fragrance ingredients
Patch testing   : 2% pet. (Chemo); 10% pet. (SPEurope, SPCanada) (ex *Santalum album*)

GENERAL

Santalum austrocaledonicum Vieill. is an evergreen tree that grows from three up to eight meters tall. It is native to the islands of Vanuatu and Nouméa (New Caledonia). It is a partial parasite that attaches to the roots of other trees; it needs 'nurse' species in the area of planting out. In the forest, 'false guaiac' (*Acacia spirobis)* is observed as symbiosis plant, but also other plants can be linked with it. The new Caledonian sandalwood is used for the production of furniture, but mainly for producing essential oil. Distillation of the stem wood, butt wood and roots yields the New Caledonian sandalwood oil. This oil is employed in the production of cosmetics such as soaps, powder and creams (2). Sandalwood oils are widely used in aromatherapy; their presumed properties and medicinal applications have been reviewed (5).

CHEMICAL COMPOSITION

Sandalwood oil New Caledonia is a clear, slightly viscous, colorless to pale yellow liquid which has a soft, woody sweet and note with long lasting powdery odor. In New Caledonian sandalwood oils from various origins, over 90 chemicals have been identified. The ten chemicals that had the highest maximum concentrations in 39 commercial New Caledonian sandalwood essential oil samples are shown in table 6.64.3.1 (Erich Schmidt, analytical data presented in ref. 46).

A full literature review of the qualitative and quantitative composition of commercial and non-commercial New Caledonian sandalwood oils of various origins has been published in 2016 (46). A comprehensive review on the constituents of the heartwood from fragrant sandalwood species including *S. austrocaledonicum* obtained by hydrodistillation and solvent extraction is presented in ref. 7 (essential oil composition not separated from solvent extracts).

Table 6.64.3.1 Ten ingredients with the highest concentrations in commercial New Caledonian sandalwood oils (46)

Name	Concentration range	Name	Concentration range
(*Z*)-α-Santalol	38.6 - 46.6%	epi-β-Santalol	2.2 - 4.4%
(*Z*)-β-Santalol	13.2 - 19.2%	α-Bisabolol	0.6 - 2.9%
(*Z*)-Lanceol	5.0 - 15.2%	epi-β-Santalene	0.5 - 2.8%
(*Z*)-*trans*-α-Bergamotol	5.0 - 8.6%	(*E*)-Nuciferol	0.6 - 2.6%
α-Santalene	0.2 - 6.5%	Santene	0.1 - 2.3%

CONTACT ALLERGY / ALLERGIC CONTACT DERMATITIS

General

The SCCS (Scientific Committee on Consumer Safety), in a 2012 Opinion on Fragrance allergens in cosmetic products, has marked Santalum album extract as 'established contact allergen in humans' (44,45). Sandalwood oil has been added to the German baseline series in 2010 (49).

Contact allergy to / allergic contact dermatitis from sandalwood oil (botanical source rarely stated) has been reported in over 35 publications. Pigmented cosmetic dermatitis from sandalwood oil used to be frequent in Japanese women. In groups of consecutive patients suspected of contact dermatitis, prevalence rates of up to 2.4% positive patch test reactions have been observed, but reliable relevance data are lacking. There are only a few case reports of allergic contact dermatitis from sandalwood oil. In one of these, santalol may have been an allergen in the oil.

A short review of contact allergy to sandalwood oil has been provided in 2016 (51).

Testing in groups of patients

The results of patch tests with sandalwood oil in routine testing (consecutive patients suspected of contact dermatitis) are shown in table 6.64.3.2; those in groups of selected patients are shown in table 6.64.3.3. In routine testing, rates of positive reactions ranged from 0.1% to 2.4%, whereas between 0.6% and 20% of patients in selected groups had positive patch tests. The high positivity rate of 20% was seen in a very small group of 10 patients strongly suspected of fragrance allergy and reacting to the fragrance mix (15).

Table 6.64.3.2 Patch testing in groups of patients: Routine testing

Years and Country	Test conc. & vehicle	Number of patients tested	positive (%)	Selection of patients (S); Relevance (R); Comments (C)	Ref.
2010-2014 IVDK	10% pet.	48,956	676 (1.4%)	R: not stated	50
2010-2012, Germany, Austria, Switzerland	10% pet.	9598	(1.6%)	R: not stated; C: range per country: 1.3-2.9%	49
2000-2008 IVDK	10% pet.	3671	46 (1.3%)	R: not stated	28
2000-2007 USA	2% pet.	870	17 (2.0%)	R: 82%; C: weak study: a. high rate of macular erythema and weak reactions, b. relevance figures include 'questionable' and 'past' relevance	14
2002-2003 Korea	2% pet.	422	10 (2.4%)	R: not stated	29
1999-2000 Denmark	2% pet.	318	4 (1.3%)	R: not specified; C: this study was part of the international study mentioned below (ref. 30)	41
	10% pet.	318	5 (1.6%)		
1998-2000 six European countries	10% pet.	1606	15 (0.9%)	R: not specified for individual oils/chemicals; the test substance was prepared from East Indian sandalwood oil	30
	2% pet.	1606	7 (0.4%)		
1979-1990 Japan	2% pet.	3152	44 (1.4%)	R: not stated	33
1983-1984 Italy	2% pet.	1200	1 (0.1%)	R: not stated	34

Case reports and case series

Sandalwood oil was responsible for 3 out of 399 cases of cosmetic (photo)allergy where the causal allergen was identified in a study of the NACDG, USA, 1977-1983 (11). A patient suspected to be allergic to incense had positive patch tests to two brands of incense, sandalwood oil, musk ambrette and santalol; gas chromatography of pentane:ether extracts of the incense showed 9% and 34% musk ambrette and 8% santalol in both incenses. The sandalwood oil extract contained 73% santalol, which is the dominant component of sandalwood oil (43).

A bottle filler in a perfume factory developed occupational allergy to East Indian sandalwood oil and some other essential oils he had contact with at work (22). Four positive patch tests to sandalwood and three photopatch tests were seen in an investigation in New York, 1986-1993; some (number not specified) of these were considered to be relevant (10).

A woman presented with a 1-year history of dermatitis that began on her right medial calf after a shave biopsy. She subsequently developed an infection at the biopsy site and began treatment with MelaGel, containing tea tree oil. She developed a peri-incisional red, indurated, weepy plaque, which subsequently spread to involve her lateral leg. The patient reported using other essential oils on her skin as well in an aromatherapy diffuser. She had positive patch tests to sandalwood oil, MelaGel, tea tree oil, ylang-ylang oil and oregano oil, all of which she had used (52).

Miscellaneous

In a number of publications, positive patch tests to sandalwood oil have been reported with unknown, uncertain or unstated relevance. These include (literature screened up to 2014 [46]) the following. Three positive patch tests to sandalwood oil occurred in massage therapists / aromatherapists with occupational contact dermatitis from multiple essential oils; it is uncertain whether sandalwood oil had been used by the patients (20). Of seven patients allergic to the fragrance farnesol, 4 (57%) co-reacted to sandalwood oil (and various other fragrances) (39). One positive patch test reaction to 'sandal oil' was seen in a group of 460 patients with positive patch tests related to cosmetics (35).

Additional information on contact allergy to sandalwood oil can be found in ref. 42 (article not read).

Pigmented cosmetic dermatitis

In Japan, in the 1960s and 1970s, many female patients developed pigmentation following dermatitis of the face (24). This so-called pigmented cosmetic dermatitis was shown to be caused by contact allergy to components of cosmetic products, notably essential oils, other fragrance materials, antimicrobials, preservatives and coloring materials (23,24). In a group of 620 Japanese patients with this condition investigated between 1970 and 1980, 3-5% had positive patch test reactions to sandalwood oil 10% in petrolatum (23). The number of patients with pigmented cosmetic dermatitis decreased strongly after 1978, when major cosmetic companies began to eliminate strong contact sensitizers from their products (23).

Table 6.64.3.3 Patch testing in groups of patients: Selected patient groups

Years and Country	Test conc. & vehicle	Number of patients tested | positive (%)		Selection of patients (S); Relevance (R); Comments (C)	Ref.
2011-2015 Spain	2% pet.	607	19 (3.1%)	S: patients previously reacting to FM I, FM II, Myroxylon pereirae resin or hydroxyisohexyl 3-cyclohexene carboxaldehyde in the baseline series and subsequently tested with a fragrance series; R: not stated	53
2008-2014 UK	2% pet.	471	4 (0.8%)	S: patients tested with a fragrance series; R: not stated; the test material was from *Santalum album*	48
2003-2014 IVDK	10% pet.	5202	(3.1%)	S: patients with stasis dermatitis / chronic leg ulcers; R: not stated; C: percentage of reactions significantly higher than in a control group of routine testing	47
2006-2010 USA	2% pet.	100	4 (4%)	S: patients with eyelid dermatitis; R: not stated	17
2001-2010 Australia	2% pet.	986	51 (5.2%)	S: not specified; R: 28%	38
2001-2010 Canada	not stated	160	20 (12.5%)	S: patients with suspected photosensitivity and patients who developed pruritus or a rash after sunscreen application; R: not stated; C: weak study: inadequate reading of test results, erythema only was considered to represent a positive patch test reaction	19
2000-2008 IVDK	10% pet.	1002	18 (1.8%)	S: patients with dermatitis suspected of causal exposure to fragrances; R: not stated	28
2004-2008 Spain	2% pet.	86	2 (2.3%)	S: patients previously reacting to the fragrance mix I or Myroxylon pereirae (n=54) or suspected of fragrance contact allergy (n=32); R: not stated	27
1993-2006 USA	2% pet.	76	1 (1.3%)	S: not stated; R: not specified	13
2000-2005 USA	2% pet.	182	2 (1.1%)	S: patients with suspected photodermatoses and/or with suspected allergic reactions to sunscreen products; R: one reaction was relevant; C: there were also three patients with *photo*allergic reactions to sandalwood oil	26
1989-1999 Portugal	2% pet.	67	4 (6.0%)	S: patients who had a positive patch test to the fragrance mix; R: not stated	31
1996-1997 UK	2% pet.	10	2 (20%)	S: patients suspected of cosmetic dermatitis and reacting to the fragrance mix; R: not stated	15
1990-1998 Japan	2% pet.	1483	12 (0.8%)	S: patients suspected of cosmetic contact dermatitis, virtually all were women; range of annual frequency of sensitization: 0-1.9%; R: not stated	18
<1996 Japan, Ireland, USA, UK, Switzerland, Sweden	10% pet.	167	11 (6.6%)	S: patients known or suspected to be allergic to fragrances; R: not stated	16
1985-1990 USA	undiluted	176	1 (0.6%)	S: patients with history of photosensitivity; R: not stated	9
<1986 Poland	2% pet.	86	2 (2.3%)	S: patients previously reacting to the fragrance mix; R: not stated	25
<1986 France	2% pet.	21	4 (19%)	S: patients with dermatitis caused by perfumes; R: not stated	40
<1976 France	2% pet.	51	2 (3.9%)	S: patients allergic to Myroxylon pereirae resin (balsam of Peru) and/or turpentine and/or wood tar and/or colophony; R: not stated	21
<1974 Japan	?	137	14 (10.2%)	S: patients suspected of cosmetic dermatitis; R: unknown	36

IVDK Information Network of Departments of Dermatology, Germany, Switzerland, Austria (www.ivdk.org); pet.: petrolatum

OTHER SIDE EFFECTS

Sandalwood oil has also been responsible for a number of cases of *photo*contact allergy (8,9,10,11,12,13,19). It concerned positive photopatch tests in serial photopatch testing, virtually always of unknown relevance.

LITERATURE

1   Jones CG, Plummer JA, Barbour EL. Non-destructive sampling of Indian sandalwood (*Santalum album* L.) for oil content and composition. J Essent Oil Res 2007;19:157-164
2   Venkatesha Gowda VS, Patil KB, Ashwath DS. Manufacturing of sandalwood oil, market potential demand and use. J Essent Oil Bear Plants 2004;7:293-297
3   Braun NA, Meier M, Pickenhagen W. Isolation and chiral GC analysis of β-bisabolols—trace constituents from the essential oil of *Santalum album* L. (Santalaceae). J Essent Oil Res 2003;15: 63-65
4   Kuriakose S, Joe IH. Feasibility of using near infrared spectroscopy to detect and quantify an adulterant in high quality sandalwood oil. Spectrochim Acta Part A: Mol Biomol Spectrosc 2013;115:568-573

5   Erligmann A. Sandalwood oils. Int J Aromather 2001;11:186-192

6   Brophy JJ, Fookes CJR, Lassak EV. Constituents of *Santalum spicatum* (R. Br.) A. DC. wood oil. J Essent Oil Res 1991;3:381-385

7   Baldovini N, Delasalle C, Joulain D. Phytochemistry of the heartwood from fragrant *Santalum* species: a review. Flavour Fragr J 2011;26:7-26

8   Pigatto PD, Legori A, Bigardi AS, Guarrera M, Tosti A, Santucci B, et al. Gruppo Italiano recerca dermatiti da contatto ed ambientali Italian multicenter study of allergic contact photodermatitis: epidemiological aspects. Am J Cont Derm 1996;7:158-163

9   DeLeo VA, Suarez SM, Maso MJ. Photoallergic contact dermatitis. Results of photopatch testing in New York, 1985 to 1990. Arch Dermatol 1992;128:1513-1518

10   Fotiades J, Soter NA, Lim HW. Results of evaluation of 203 patients for photosensitivity in a 7.3 year period. J Am Acad Dermatol 1995;33:597-602

11   Adams RM, Maibach HI. A five-year study of cosmetic reactions. J Am Acad Dermatol 1985;13:1062-1069

12   Starke JC. Photoallergy to sandalwood oil. Arch Dermatol 1967;96:62-63

13   Victor FC, Cohen DE, Soter NA. A 20-year analysis of previous and emerging allergens that elicit photoallergic contact dermatitis. J Am Acad Dermatol 2010;62:605-610

14   Wetter DA, Yiannias JA, Prakash AV, Davis MD, Farmer SA, el-Azhary RA, et al. Results of patch testing to personal care product allergens in a standard series and a supplemental cosmetic series: an analysis of 945 patients from the Mayo Clinic Contact Dermatitis Group, 2000-2007. J Am Acad Dermatol 2010;63:789-798

15   Thomson KF, Wilkinson SM. Allergic contact dermatitis to plant extracts in patients with cosmetic dermatitis. Br J Dermatol 2000;142:84-88

16   Larsen W, Nakayama H, Lindberg M, Fischer T, Elsner P, Burrows D, et al. Fragrance contact dermatitis: A worldwide multicenter investigation (Part 1). Am J Cont Derm 1996;7:77-83

17   Wenk KS, Ehrlich AE. Fragrance series testing in eyelid dermatitis. Dermatitis 2012;23:22-26

18   Sugiura M, Hayakawa R, Kato Y, Sugiura K, Hashimoto R. Results of patch testing with lavender oil in Japan. Contact Dermatitis 2000;43:157-160

19   Greenspoon J, Ahluwalia R, Juma N, Rosen CF. Allergic and photoallergic contact dermatitis: A 10-year experience. Dermatitis 2013;24:29-32

20   Bleasel N, Tate B, Rademaker M. Allergic contact dermatitis following exposure to essential oils. Australas J Dermatol 2002;43:211-213

21   Rudzki E, Grzywa Z, Bruo WS. Sensitivity to 35 essential oils. Contact Dermatitis 1976;2:196-200

22   Schubert HJ. Skin diseases in workers at a perfume factory. Contact Dermatitis 2006;55:81-83

23   Nakayama H, Matsuo S, Hayakawa K, Takhashi K, Shigematsu T, Ota S. Pigmented cosmetic dermatitis. Int J Dermatol 1984;23:299-305

24   Nakayama H, Harada R, Toda M. Pigmented cosmetic dermatitis. Int J Dermatol 1976;15:673-675

25   Rudzki E, Grzywa Z. Allergy to perfume mixture. Contact Dermatitis 1986;15:115-116

26   Scalf LA, Davis MDP, Rohlinger AL, Connolly SM. Photopatch testing of 182 patients: a 6-year experience at the Mayo Clinic. Dermatitis 2009;20:44-52

27   Cuesta L, Silvestre JF, Toledo F, Lucas A, Pérez-Crespo M, Ballester I. Fragrance contact allergy: a 4-year retrospective study. Contact Dermatitis 2010;63:77-84

28   Uter W, Schmidt E, Geier J, Lessmann H, Schnuch A, Frosch P. Contact allergy to essential oils: current patch test results (2000–2008) from the Information Network of Departments of Dermatology (IVDK). Contact Dermatitis 2010;63:277-283

29   An S, Lee AY, Lee CH, Kim D-W, Hahm JH, Kim K-J, et al. Fragrance contact dermatitis in Korea: a joint study. Contact Dermatitis 2005;53:320-323

30   Frosch PJ, Johansen JD, Menné T, Pirker C, Rastogi SC, Andersen KE, et al. Further important sensitizers in patients sensitive to fragrances. II. Reactivity to essential oils. Contact Dermatitis 2002;47:279-287

31   Manuel Brites M, Goncalo M, Figueiredo A. Contact allergy to fragrance mix - a 10-year study. Contact Dermatitis 2000;43:181-182

32   Moy RL, Levenson C. Sandalwood album oil as a botanical therapeutic in dermatology. J Clin Aesthet Dermatol 2017;10:34-39

33   Utsumi M, Sugai T, Shoji A, Watanabe K, Asoh S, Hashimoto Y. Incidence of positive reactions to sandalwood oil and its related fragrance materials in patch tests and a case of contact allergy to natural and synthetic sandalwood oil in a museum worker. Skin Res 1992;34(suppl.14):209-213 (article in Japanese)

34   Santucci B, Cristaudo A, Cannistraci C, Picardo M. Contact dermatitis to fragrances. Contact Dermatitis 1987;16:93-95

35   Romaguera C, Camarasa JMG, Alomar A, Grimalt F. Patch tests with allergens related to cosmetics. Contact Dermatitis 1983;9:167-168

36 Nakayama H, Hanaoka H, Ohshiro A. Allergen Controlled System (ACS). Tokyo, Japan: Kanehara Shuppan, 1974:42. Data cited in ref. 37

37 Mitchell JC. Contact hypersensitivity to some perfume materials. Contact Dermatitis 1975;1:196-199

38 Toholka R, Wang Y-S, Tate B, Tam M, Cahill J, Palmer A, Nixon R. The first Australian Baseline Series: Recommendations for patch testing in suspected contact dermatitis. Australas J Dermatol 2015;56:107-115

39 Goossens A, Merckx L. Allergic contact dermatitis from farnesol in a deodorant. Contact Dermatitis 1997;37:179-180

40 Meynadier JM, Meynadier J, Peyron JL, Peyron L. Formes cliniques des manifestations cutanées d'allergie aux parfums. Ann Dermatol Venereol 1986;113:31-39 (article in French)

41 Paulsen E, Andersen KE. Colophonium and Compositae mix as markers of fragrance allergy: Cross-reactivity between fragrance terpenes, colophonium and Compositae plant extracts. Contact Dermatitis 2005;53:285-291

42 Sugai T. Historical data of the JSCD Group study III – Fragrance materials. Environ Dermatol 1994;1:209-212 (article in Japanese)

43 Hayakawa R, Matsunaga K, Arima Y. Depigmented contact dermatitis due to incense. Contact Dermatitis 1987;16:272-274

44 SCCS (Scientific Committee on Consumer Safety). Opinion on Fragrance allergens in cosmetic products, 26-27 June 2012, SCCS/1459/11. Available at: https://ec.europa.eu/health/sites/health/files/scientific_committees/consumer_safety/docs/sccs_o_102.pdf

45 Uter W, Johansen JD, Börje A, Karlberg A-T, Lidén C, Rastogi S, Roberts D, White IR. Categorization of fragrance contact allergens for prioritization of preventive measures: clinical and experimental data and consideration of structure–activity relationships. Contact Dermatitis 2013;69:196-230

46 De Groot AC, Schmidt E. Essential oils: contact allergy and chemical composition. Boca Raton, Fl., USA: CRC Press, Taylor and Francis Group, 2016 (ISBN 9781482246407)

47 Erfurt-Berge C, Geier J, Mahler V. The current spectrum of contact sensitization in patients with chronic leg ulcers or stasis dermatitis - new data from the Information Network of Departments of Dermatology (IVDK). Contact Dermatitis 2017;77:151-158

48 Sabroe RA, Holden CR, Gawkrodger DJ. Contact allergy to essential oils cannot always be predicted from allergy to fragrance markers in the baseline series. Contact Dermatitis 2016;74:236-241

49 Frosch PJ, Johansen JD, Schuttelaar M-LA, Silvestre JF, Sánchez-Pérez J, Weisshaar E, et al. (on behalf of the ESSCA network). Patch test results with fragrance markers of the baseline series – analysis of the European Surveillance System on Contact Allergies (ESSCA) network 2009–2012. Contact Dermatitis 2015;73:163-171

50 Warshaw EM, Zug KA, Belsito DV, Fowler JF Jr, DeKoven JG, Sasseville D, et al. Positive patch-test reactions to essential oils in consecutive patients: Results from North America and Central Europe. Dermatitis 2017;28:246-252

51 De Groot AC, Schmidt E. Essential oils, Part VI: Sandalwood oil, ylang-ylang oil, and jasmine absolute. Dermatitis 2017;28:14-21

52 Hagen SL, Grey KR, Warshaw EM. Patch testing to essential oils. Dermatitis 2016;27:382-384

53 Silvestre JF, Mercader P, González-Pérez R, Hervella-Garcés M, Sanz-Sánchez T, Córdoba S, et al. Sensitization to fragrances in Spain: A 5-year multicentre study (2011-2015). Contact Dermatitis. 2018 Nov 14. doi: 10.1111/cod.13152. [Epub ahead of print]

Chapter 6.65   SILVER FIR OIL

IDENTIFICATION

Description/definition	: Silver fir oil is the essential oil obtained from the needles of the (European) silver fir, *Abies alba* Mill.
INCI name(s) EU & USA	: Abies alba leaf oil
Other names	: Fir needle oil; Abies alba needle oil
CAS registry number(s)	: 8021-27-0; 90028-76-5
EC number(s)	: 289-870-2
RIFM monograph(s)	: Food Cosmet Toxicol 1974;12:811 (special issue I) (binder, page 17)
IFRA specification	: Essential oils and isolates derived from the Pinacea family, including *Pinus* and *Abies* genera, should only be used when the level of peroxides is kept to the lowest practicable level, for instance by adding antioxidants at the time of production; such products should have a peroxide value of less than 10 millimoles peroxide per liter, determined according to the FMA method (www.ifraorg.org/en-us/standards-library)
SCCS opinion(s)	: SCCNFP/0392/00, final (6); SCCNFP/0389/00, final (7)
Merck Index monograph	: 8154 (Oil of fir); 8155 (Oils of Fir – Siberian)
Function(s) in cosmetics	: EU: masking; perfuming; tonic. USA: fragrance ingredients
EU cosmetic restrictions	: Regulated in Annex III/103 of the Regulation (EC) No. 344/2013
Patch testing	: 2% pet.; based on RIFM data, 20% pet. is probably not irritant (9)

GENERAL

The common silver fir *Abies alba* Mill., also known as the Christmas tree, is an evergreen tree up to 45-55 meter tall and a diameter of 200-260 cm. It is native to middle and south European countries, Ukraine and Belarus. The tree is found at altitudes of 300-1,700 meter on mountains with a rainfall of over 1,000 mm. The silver fir is widely cultivated (1,8).

In Europe, the essential oil obtained from the needles is said to be used in perfumes, room sprays, deodorants and bath preparations (we doubt whether this oil is used in fragrances and cosmetics). Silver for oil is also employed in inhalants for the treatment of colds, and in medicinal preparations against rheumatism and similar ailments and is said to have soothing qualities (8). It is also employed in aromatherapy practices (2,3).

CHEMICAL COMPOSITION

Silver fir oil is a colorless mobile liquid which has a fresh coniferous, slightly camphoraceous odor. In silver fir oils from various origins, over 110 chemicals have been identified. About 42 per cent of these were found in a single reviewed publication only. The ten chemicals that had the highest maximum concentrations in 16 commercial silver fir essential oil samples are shown in table 6.65.1 (Erich Schmidt, analytical data presented in ref. 8).

A full literature review of the qualitative and quantitative composition of commercial and non-commercial silver fir oils of various origins and their chemotypes has been published in 2016 (8).

Table 6.65.1 Ten ingredients with the highest concentrations in commercial silver fir oils (8)

Name	Concentration range	Name	Concentration range
Limonene	6.1 - 54.7%	β-Phellandrene	0.01 - 4.9%
α-Pinene	0.5 - 32.8%	β-Caryophyllene	0.1 - 4.2%
β-Pinene	7.4 - 31.7%	Tricyclene	0.5 - 2.6%
Camphene	5.8 - 17.3%	Myrcene	0.7 - 2.5%
Bornyl acetate	0.4 - 14.2%	α-Terpineol	0.07 - 2.3%

CONTACT ALLERGY / ALLERGIC CONTACT DERMATITIS

General

Contact allergy to silver fir oil has been reported in two publications, but no cases of allergic contact dermatitis from the oil have been identified.

Testing in groups of patients

Two hundred dermatitis patients from Poland were tested with silver fir oil 2% in petrolatum and two (1%) reacted. The same authors also patch tested 51 patients allergic to Myroxylon pereirae resin (balsam of Peru) and/or turpentine and/or wood tar and/or colophony and nine (17.6%) had a positive patch test; relevance data were not provided (4). This high percentage can likely be explained by the fact that all materials tested originate from trees.

A group of 86 patients from Poland previously reacting to the fragrance mix was tested with silver fir oil and two (2.3%) had a positive patch test reaction; relevance data were not provided (5).

LITERATURE

1   Roussis V, Couladis M, Tzakou O, Loukis A, Petrakis PV, Dukic NM, et al. A comparative study on the needle volatile constituents of three *Abies* species grown in south Balkans. J Essent Oil Res 2000;12:41-46
2   Rhind JP. Essential oils. A handbook for aromatherapy practice, 2nd Edition. London: Singing Dragon, 2012
3   Lawless J. The encyclopedia of essential oils, 2nd Edition. London: Harper Thorsons, 2014
4   Rudzki E, Grzywa Z, Bruo WS. Sensitivity to 35 essential oils. Contact Dermatitis 1976;2:196-200
5   Rudzki E, Grzywa Z. Allergy to perfume mixture. Contact Dermatitis 1986;15:115-116
6   Opinion of the Scientific Committee on Cosmetic Products and Non-Food Products Intended for Consumers concerning 'An initial list of perfumery materials which must not form part of cosmetic products except subject to the Restrictions and Conditions laid down, 25 September 2001, SCCNFP/0392/00, final. Available at: http://ec.europa.eu/health/archive/ph_risk/committees/sccp/documents/out150_en.pdf
7   Opinion of the Scientific Committee on Cosmetic Products and Non-Food Products Intended for Consumers concerning 'The 1st update of the inventory of ingredients employed in cosmetic products. Section II: Perfume and aromatic raw materials', 24 October 2000, SCCNFP/0389/00, final. Available at: http://ec.europa.eu/health/ph_risk/committees/sccp/documents/out131_en.pdf
8   De Groot AC, Schmidt E. Essential oils: contact allergy and chemical composition. Boca Raton, Fl., USA: CRC Press, Taylor and Francis Group, 2016 (ISBN 9781482246407)
9   De Groot AC. Patch Testing, 4th Edition. Wapserveen, The Netherlands: acdegroot publishing, 2018 (ISBN 978-90-813233-4-5)

Chapter 6.66   SPEARMINT OIL

IDENTIFICATION

Description/definition	: Spearmint oil (essential oil of spearmint) is the essential oil obtained from the flowering aerial parts and leaves of the spearmint, *Mentha spicata* L. (synonyms: *Mentha viridis, Mentha spicata* ssp. *spicata)* and *Mentha crispa* L.)
INCI name(s) EU	: Mentha viridis leaf oil; Mentha spicata herb oil (perfuming name, not officially an INCI name)
INCI name(s) USA	: Mentha viridis (spearmint) leaf oil
CAS registry number(s)	: 84696-51-5; 8008-79-5
EC number(s)	: 283-656-2
RIFM monograph(s)	: Food Cosmet Toxicol 1978;16:871 (special issue IV)
SCCS opinion(s)	: SCCS/1459/11 (27)
ISO standard	: ISO 3033 Parts 1-4 Essential oil of spearmint, 2005; Geneva, Switzerland, www.iso.org
Merck Index monograph	: 10135 (Spearmint)
Function(s) in cosmetics	: EU: astringent; masking; skin conditioning; perfuming. USA: cosmetic astringents; flavoring agents; fragrance ingredients; skin-conditioning agents - miscellaneous
Patch testing	: 2% pet.; based on RIFM data, 4% pet. is probably not irritant (3); test also carvone (see Chapter 3.30 Carvone)

GENERAL

Mentha spicata L. is an herbaceous creeping rhizomatous perennial plant growing 30-100 cm tall with a strong aromatic odor. Its leaves have serrated margins and pointed tips, which explains the 'spear' in the name spearmint. The plant is native to western Asia (Cyprus, Lebanon, Syria, Turkey) and south-eastern Europe (Albania, Bulgaria, former Yugoslavia, Greece, Italy). It is naturalized widely and found in many places around the world as garden escapes. The spearmint is cultivated in Africa, Asia (Turkey, China, Japan, India, Pakistan), Australia, New Zealand, Europe, Canada, USA and the Caribbean (2).

Spearmint essential oil, obtained by distillation of aerial flowering parts and the leaves of *Mentha spicata* L., is rich in carvone and presents a characteristic spearmint odor (1). This oil (as well as other mint oils) and carvone are used in perfumery, cosmetics, pharmaceuticals and in the food industries. As flavor or fragrance, spearmint oils are widely added to products such as toothpastes, mouth-washes, cigarettes, chewing gum and alcoholic drinks. They are also employed in aromatherapy practices (2).

CHEMICAL COMPOSITION

Spearmint oil is a colorless to pale yellow clear mobile liquid, which has a fresh herbal, minty soft aromatic odor. In spearmint oils from various origins, over 250 chemicals have been identified. About 45 per cent of these were found in a single reviewed publication only. The ten chemicals that had the highest maximum concentrations in 71 commercial spearmint essential oil samples are shown in table 6.66.1 (Erich Schmidt, analytical data presented in ref. 2).

A full literature review of the qualitative and quantitative composition of commercial and non-commercial spearmint oils of various origins, their chemotypes and with data from the ISO standard, has been published in 2016 (2).

Table 6.66.1 Ten ingredients with the highest concentrations in commercial spearmint oils (2)

Name	Concentration range	Name	Concentration range
Carvone	60.6 - 82.3%	*cis*-Dihydrocarvone	0.3 - 3.3%
Limonene	0.4 - 23.7%	β-Caryophyllene	0.09 - 3.0%
Dihydrocarveol	0.05 - 5.1%	Myrcene	0.01 - 2.6%
1,8-Cineole	0.01 - 4.4%	3-Octanol	0.01 - 2.2%
trans-Dihydrocarvyl acetate	0.1 - 3.7%	Menthol	0.2 - 2.2%

CONTACT ALLERGY / ALLERGIC CONTACT DERMATITIS

General

The SCCS (Scientific Committee on Consumer Safety), in a 2012 Opinion on Fragrance allergens in cosmetic products, has marked spearmint oil as 'established contact allergen in humans' (10,27).

Contact allergy to / allergic contact dermatitis from spearmint oil has been reported in over 20 publications. In groups of consecutive patients suspected of contact dermatitis, prevalence rates of up to 1.6% positive patch test reactions have been observed, but relevance data are lacking. At least ten case reports of contact allergic reactions to spearmint oil have been reported. Nearly all were from its presence in toothpastes, causing stomatitis, cheilitis, perioral dermatitis, sore mouth and possibly oral lichenoid reactions (table 6.66.2). In about half the cases where carvone, the dominant (60-80%) ingredient of spearmint oils, was also tested, co-reactivity occurred, and this is likely the main allergen.

Testing in groups of patients

The results of patch tests with spearmint oil in routine testing (consecutive patients suspected of contact dermatitis) and in groups of selected patients are shown in table 6.66.2. In routine testing, rates of positive reactions ranged from 0.8% to 1.6%, whereas between 0.1% and 10% of patients in selected groups had positive patch tests.

Table 6.66.2 Patch testing in groups of patients

Years and Country	Test conc. & vehicle	Number of patients tested	positive (%)	Selection of patients (S); Relevance (R); Comments (C)	Ref.
Routine testing					
2000-2007 USA	2% pet.	500	5 (1.0%)	R: 100%; C: weak study: a. high rate of macular erythema and weak reactions, b. relevance figures include 'questionable' and 'past' relevance	4
1999-2000 Denmark	2% pet.	318	5 (1.6%)	R: not specified; C: this study was part of the international study mentioned below (12)	26
1998-2000 six European countries	2% pet.	1606	13 (0.8%)	R: not specified for individual oils/chemicals	12
Testing in groups of selected patients					
1999-2011 Australia	5% pet.	1467	73 (5.0%)	S: patients tested with the 'toothpaste, essential oils and fragrance (rare) series'; R: 19/73 (26%) relevant; 14/19 had biopsy-proven oral lichen planus (OLP); in ten of these, the OLP improved >80% after avoidance of spearmint; C: 50% had a positive patch test to carvone and 8/14 (57%) to 'sassafras'; the latter reactions were considered cross-reactions to spearmint oil	24, 25
2001-2010 Australia	5% pet.	1383	68 (4.9%)	S: not specified; R: 31%	23
<2005 USA	2% pet.	111	4 (3.6%)	S: patients using consumer products containing spearmint oil; R: 'at least possibly relevant'	7
2000 USA, Japan and 4 European countries	5% pet.	178	9 (5.1%)	S: patients previously shown to be allergic to fragrances; R: not stated	14
1997-2000 Austria	2% pet.	747	1 (0.1%)	S: patients suspected of fragrance allergy; R: not stated	8
1997-1998 Italy	2% pet.	54	4 (7.4%)	S: patients with cheilitis suspected of toothpaste allergy; R: all reactions were relevant	15
1996-1997 UK	2% pet.	10	1 (10%)	S: patients suspected of cosmetic dermatitis and reacting to the fragrance mix; R: not stated	??
<1978 Denmark	5% pet.	40	4 (10%)	S: see text under case reports	6

pet.: petrolatum

Case reports and case series

An aromatherapist had occupational contact dermatitis with allergies to multiple essential oils used at work, including spearmint oil; carvone was not tested (5). A case of occupational contact allergy to spearmint oil in a chewing gum finisher has been reported (11). Four positive patch test reactions to spearmint oil were seen in a group of 40 patients with sore mouth, stomatitis and/or dermatitis around the mouth or who were dentist personnel. Two also reacted to anethole (not an important component), two to carvone (the main ingredient of spearmint oil, 60-80% of the total oil) and one to peppermint oil. The causative products were supposed to be toothpastes (6).

One patient with oral lichen planus developed allergic contact stomatitis from spearmint oil in mouth rinse and chewing gum (9). In another patient, contact allergy to spearmint oil in toothpaste caused sore mouth, fissuring of the lips and dermatitis of the surrounding skin; a patch test with anethole 5% in petrolatum was negative (16). One individual had erosive cheilitis from contact allergy to spearmint oil and its main component carvone in toothpaste (17). Four patients developed stomatitis and dermatitis from contact allergy to spearmint oil in toothpastes (22).

Some additional cases of contact allergy to spearmint oil in toothpastes have been reported (19,20). One positive patch test reaction to spearmint oil (and peppermint oil) was seen in a patient with contact dermatitis from compresses with an infusion of fresh leaves of *Mentha spicata* (13). One patient had a positive patch test reaction to spearmint oil 0.1% in petrolatum, considered to be clinically relevant, in a group of 146 patients referred for cheilitis to a UK hospital between 1982 and 2001 (8).

LITERATURE

1   Chauhan RS, Nautiyal MC, Tava A. Essential oil composition from aerial parts of *Mentha spicata* L. J Essent Oil Bear Plants 2010;13:353-356

2   De Groot AC, Schmidt E. Essential oils: contact allergy and chemical composition. Boca Raton, Fl., USA: CRC Press, Taylor and Francis Group, 2016 (ISBN 9781482246407)\

3   De Groot AC. Patch Testing, 4th Edition. Wapserveen, The Netherlands: acdegroot publishing, 2018 (ISBN 978-90-813233-4-5)

4   Wetter DA, Yiannias JA, Prakash AV, Davis MD, Farmer SA, el-Azhary RA, et al. Results of patch testing to personal care product allergens in a standard series and a supplemental cosmetic series: an analysis of 945 patients from the Mayo Clinic Contact Dermatitis Group, 2000-2007. J Am Acad Dermatol 2010;63:789-798

5   Dharmagunawardena B, Takwale A, Sanders KJ, Cannan S, Roger A, Ilchyshyn A. Gas chromatography: an investigative tool in multiple allergies to essential oils. Contact Dermatitis 2002;47:288-292

6   Andersen KE. Contact allergy to toothpaste flavors. Contact Dermatitis 1978;4:195-198

7   Guin JD. Use of consumer product ingredients for patch testing. Dermatitis 2005;16:71-77

8   Strauss RM, Orton DI. Allergic contact cheilitis in the United Kingdom: a retrospective study. Dermatitis 2003;14:75-77

9   Clayton R, Orton D. Contact allergy to spearmint oil in a patient with oral lichen planus. Contact Dermatitis 2004;51:314-315

10 Uter W, Johansen JD, Börje A, Karlberg A-T, Lidén C, Rastogi S, Roberts D, White IR. Categorization of fragrance contact allergens for prioritization of preventive measures: clinical and experimental data and consideration of structure–activity relationships. Contact Dermatitis 2013;69:196-230

11 Morris GE. Dermatoses among food handlers. Ind Med Surg 1954;23:343.

12 Frosch PJ, Johansen JD, Menné T, Pirker C, Rastogi SC, Andersen KE, et al. Further important sensitizers in patients sensitive to fragrances. II. Reactivity to essential oils. Contact Dermatitis 2002;47:279-287

13 Bonamonte D, Mundo L, Daddabbo M, Foti C. Allergic contact dermatitis from *Mentha spicata* (spearmint). Contact Dermatitis 2001;45:298

14 Larsen W, Nakayama H, Fischer T, Elsner P, Frosch P, Burrows D, et al. Fragrance contact dermatitis: a worldwide multicenter investigation (Part II). Contact Dermatitis 2001;44:344-346

15 Francalanci S, Sertoli A, Giorgini S, Pigatto P, Santucci B, Valsecchi R. Multicentre study of allergic contact cheilitis from toothpastes. Contact Dermatitis 2000;43:216-222

16 Skrebova N, Brocks K, Karlsmark T. Allergic contact cheilitis from spearmint oil. Contact Dermatitis 1998;39:35-36

17 Worm M, Jeep S, Sterry W, Zuberbier T. Perioral contact dermatitis caused by L-carvone in toothpaste. Contact Dermatitis 1998;38:338

18 Sainio E-L, Kanerva L. Contact allergens in toothpastes and a review of their hypersensitivity. Contact Dermatitis 1995;33:100-105

19 Grattan CEH, Peachy RD. Contact sensitization to toothpaste flavouring. J Royal Coll Gen Pract 1985;35:498. Data cited in ref. 18

20 Baer ON. Toothpaste allergies. J Clin Pediatr Dent 1992;16:230-231. Data cited in ref. 18

21 Magnusson B, Wilkinson DS. Cinnamic aldehyde in toothpaste. 1. Clinical aspects and patch tests. Contact Dermatitis 1975;1:70-76

22 Hjorth N, Jervoe P. Allergisk Kontaktstomatitis og Kontaktdermatitis fremkaldt of smagsstoffer i tandpasta. Tandlaegebladet 1967;71:937-942. Data cited in ref. 21

23 Toholka R, Wang Y-S, Tate B, Tam M, Cahill J, Palmer A, Nixon R. The first Australian Baseline Series: Recommendations for patch testing in suspected contact dermatitis. Australas J Dermatol 2015;56:107-115

24 Gunatheesan S, Tam MM, Tate B, Tversky J, Nixon R. Retrospective study of oral lichen planus and allergy to spearmint oil. Australas J Dermatol 2012;53:224-228

25 Cahill J, Gunatheesan S, Tam M, Tate B, Nixon R. Oral lichen planus and allergy to spearmint oil. Contact Dermatitis 2012;66 (Suppl. 2):38 (FC1.03)

26 Paulsen E, Andersen KE. Colophonium and Compositae mix as markers of fragrance allergy: Cross-reactivity between fragrance terpenes, colophonium and Compositae plant extracts. Contact Dermatitis 2005;53:285-291

27 SCCS (Scientific Committee on Consumer Safety). Opinion on Fragrance allergens in cosmetic products, 26-27 June 2012, SCCS/1459/11. Available at: https://ec.europa.eu/health/sites/health/files/scientific_committees/consumer_safety/docs/sccs_o_102.pdf

Chapter 6.67   SPIKE LAVENDER OIL

IDENTIFICATION

Description/definition	: Spike lavender oil (essential oil of spike lavender, Spanish type) is the essential oil obtained from the flowering top of the spike lavender, *Lavandula latifolia* Medik. (synonym: *Lavandula spica* L.).
INCI name(s) EU	: Lavandula spica flower oil; Lavandula latifolia herb oil (perfuming name, not an INCI name proper)
INCI name(s) USA	: Lavandula spica (lavender) flower oil
CAS registry number(s)	: 8016-78-2; 84837-04-7; 97722-12-8
EC number(s)	: 307-762-6; 284-290-6
RIFM monograph(s)	: Food Cosmet Toxicol 1976;14:453 (binder, page 488)
SCCS opinion(s)	: SCCS/1459/11 (8)
ISO standard	: ISO 4719 Essential oil of spike lavender, Spanish type, 2012; Geneva, Switzerland, www.iso.org
Merck Index monograph	: 6715 (Lavender)
Function(s) in cosmetics	: EU: masking; perfuming. USA: fragrance ingredients
Patch testing	: 2% pet.; based on RIFM data, 8% pet. is probably not irritant (11)

GENERAL

Lavandula latifolia Medik., commonly known as spike lavender, is a strongly aromatic evergreen shrub growing to 30-80 cm tall. It is native to Italy, France and Spain and is naturalized in other Mediterranean countries (1). The plant is cultivated as an essential oil plant, for scent, ornament, and as a bee plant (3,10). In Spain, the culture of spike lavender is said to have been largely replaced in the last years by the more productive species lavandin (*Lavandula x intermedia* Emeric ex Loisel; *Lavandula hybrida*) (1).

The essential oil of spike lavender is obtained by steam-distillation of the flowering tops of both cultivated and wild *L. latifolia* populations, but often, stems and leaves are also distilled together with the inflorescences (4). Spike lavender oils are used in perfumery, cosmetics, as flavor in food products, in technical preparations such as room sprays and disinfectants, and in veterinary medicine (liniments) (1,2). Spike lavender oil is believed to have many pharmacological activities and is widely used in aromatherapy (1,2,3).

The most important ingredients of the oil are linalool, 1,8-cineole and camphor, together accounting for more than 80% of the oil (3). The relative concentration of camphor and linalool determines the quality and prize of the product. The most appreciated oils for the perfume and cosmetic industries are those with high content in linalool and low content in camphor, while those richer in camphor are mainly used in aromatherapy and phytotherapy (1).

CHEMICAL COMPOSITION

Spike lavender oil is a light yellow to orange-yellow liquid which has a fresh and floral but also camphoraceous-minty odor. In spike lavender oils from various origins, over 395 chemicals have been identified, of which 225 only before 1986 (when analytical apparatus were less reliable). The ten chemicals that had the highest maximum concentrations in 24 commercial spike lavender essential oil samples are shown in table 6.67.1 (Erich Schmidt, analytical data presented in ref. 10).

A full literature review of the qualitative and quantitative composition of commercial and non-commercial spike lavender oils of various origins with data from the ISO standard has been published in 2016 (10). A review of various aspects of lavenders (lavender, lavandin, spike lavender), written from the industry's perspective, can be found (on-line) in a dissertation from the International Centre for Aroma Trades Studies, Plymouth, UK (5).

Table 6.67.1 Ten ingredients with the highest concentrations in commercial spike lavender oils (10)

Name	Concentration range	Name	Concentration range
Linalool	0.6 - 42.3%	Limonene	0.2 - 3.0%
Camphor	8.0 - 35.1%	1-Octen-3-ol	0.04 - 2.6%
1,8-Cineole	3.2 - 31.2%	β-Pinene	0.4 - 2.6%
(*E*)-β-Farnesene	0.2 - 4.3%	β-Caryophyllene	0.03 - 1.9%
α-Pinene	0.6 - 3.6%	Caryophyllene oxide	trace - 1.7%

CONTACT ALLERGY / ALLERGIC CONTACT DERMATITIS

General

The SCCS (Scientific Committee on Consumer Safety), in a 2012 Opinion on Fragrance allergens in cosmetic products, has categorized Lavandula spica extract as 'possible fragrance contact allergen' (8,9).

Contact allergy to spike lavender oil has been reported in two publications, but no cases of allergic contact dermatitis from the oil have been identified.

Testing in groups of patients

Two hundred dermatitis patients from Poland were tested with spike lavender oil 2% in petrolatum and one (0.5%) reacted. The same authors also patch tested 51 patients allergic to Myroxylon pereirae resin (balsam of Peru) and/or turpentine and/or wood tar and/or colophony and one (2.0%) had a positive patch test; relevance data were not provided (6).

A group of 86 patients from Poland previously reacting to the fragrance mix was tested with spike lavender oil and eight (9.3%) had a positive patch test reaction; relevance data were not provided (7).

LITERATURE

1   Herraiz-Peñalver D, Ángeles Cases M, Varela F, Navarrete P, Sánchez-Vioque R, Usano-Alemany J. Chemical characterization of Lavandula latifolia Medik. essential oil from Spanish wild populations. Biochem System Ecol 2013;46:59-68

2   Eikani MH, Golmohammad F, Shokrollahzadeh S, Mirza M, Rowshanzamir S. Superheated water extraction of Lavandula latifolia Medik volatiles: Comparison with conventional techniques. J Essent Oil Res 2008;20:482-487

3   Munoz-Bertomeu J, Arrillaga I, Segura J. Essential oil variation within and among natural populations of Lavandula latifolia and its relation to their ecological areas. Biochem System Ecol 2007;35:479-488

4   Boelens MH. The essential oil of spike lavender Lavandula latifolia Vill. (L. spica D.C.). Perfum Flavor 1986;11(5):43-63

5   Bosilcov A. Lavender: A key perfumery material. Dissertation. International Centre for Aroma Trades Studies, Plymouth University, Plymouth, UK, 2010

6   Rudzki E, Grzywa Z, Bruo WS. Sensitivity to 35 essential oils. Contact Dermatitis 1976;2:196-200

7   Rudzki E, Grzywa Z. Allergy to perfume mixture. Contact Dermatitis 1986;15:115-116

8   SCCS (Scientific Committee on Consumer Safety). Opinion on Fragrance allergens in cosmetic products, 26-27 June 2012, SCCS/1459/11. Available at: https://ec.europa.eu/health/sites/health/files/scientific_committees/consumer_safety/docs/sccs_o_102.pdf

9   Uter W, Johansen JD, Börje A, Karlberg A-T, Lidén C, Rastogi S, Roberts D, White IR. Categorization of fragrance contact allergens for prioritization of preventive measures: clinical and experimental data and consideration of structure–activity relationships. Contact Dermatitis 2013;69:196-230

10 De Groot AC, Schmidt E. Essential oils: contact allergy and chemical composition. Boca Raton, Fl., USA: CRC Press, Taylor and Francis Group, 2016 (ISBN 9781482246407)

11 De Groot AC. Patch Testing, 4th Edition. Wapserveen, The Netherlands: acdegroot publishing, 2018 (ISBN 978-90-813233-4-5)

Chapter 6.68   SPRUCE OIL

IDENTIFICATION
There are several spruce species from which essential oils can be obtained, including the Hemlock or Eastern spruce *Tsuga canadensis*, Norway or common spruce *Picea abies*, white spruce *Picea glauca* and black spruce *Picea mariana*. As the botanical origin of the spruce oil in the article discussed below was not mentioned, no further data can be provided.

CONTACT ALLERGY

Case reports and case series
An inhalant ointment, consisting entirely of eucalyptus oil and spruce oil, that helps to relieve nasal congestion due to upper respiratory tract infections, was applied to the collar of the pajamas of a female child and caused dermatitis in the neck and on the upper chest. Patch tests were positive to eucalyptus oil (probably tested 2% pet.) and spruce oil 5% pet. Three controls were negative (1).

LITERATURE
1   Kartal D, Kartal L, Çinar S, Borlu M. Allergic contact dermatitis caused by both eucalyptus oil and spruce oil. Int J Med Pharm Case Rep 2016;7:1-3

Chapter 6.69   STAR ANISE OIL

IDENTIFICATION

Description/definition	: Star anise oil (essential oil of star anise, Chinese type) is the essential oil obtained from the fruit of the (Chinese) star anise, *Illicium verum* Hook. f.
INCI name(s) EU	: Illicium verum fruit/seed oil
INCI name(s) USA	: Illicium verum (anise) fruit/seed oil
CAS registry number(s)	: 8007-70-3; 84650-59-9; 68952-43-2
EC number(s)	: 283-518-1
RIFM monograph(s)	: Food Cosmet Toxicol 1975;13:715 (special issue II) (binder, page 99)
SCCS opinion(s)	: SCCS/1459/11 (14)
ISO standard	: ISO 11016 Essential oil of star anise, 1999; Geneva, Switzerland, www.iso.org
Merck Index monograph	: 1927 (Anise)
Function(s) in cosmetics	: EU: masking; oral care; tonic. USA: flavoring agents; fragrance ingredients
Patch testing	: 0.5% pet.; test also Anethole (see Chapter 3.11 Anethole) (16)

GENERAL

Illicium verum Hook. f. is an aromatic evergreen tree that grows up to 15 meter tall. It is native to southern China and Vietnam and is cultivated mainly in these countries. The tree can also be found in Jamaica, Laos, Philippines, Korea, Japan, and Taiwan (10). Star anise, the star-shaped dried composite fruit of *Illicium verum*, is widely used in Chinese (as an ingredient of the traditional five-spice powder of Chinese cooking), Indian, Malaysian and Indonesian cuisines and also in the production of alcoholic beverages such as sambuca, pastis and some types of absinthe (1,2,3,4,5,8, 9,10). Star anise is also very important in Chinese traditional medicine (1,2,4,7). Furthermore, star anise is the industrial source of shikimic acid, a primary ingredient used to create the antiviral drug, oseltamivir phosphate which is regarded as a remedy for the bird flu H5N1 strain of virus (1,2).

The essential oil of star anise, obtained by steam-distillation of the dried fruits, is located in the meso- and pericarp and has a hot, sweet and aniseed-like taste (6). Chinese star anise essential oils have a wide range of commercial applications in the production of perfumes, cosmetics (including toothpastes), soaps, food and beverage flavorings and pharmaceutical preparations such as cough lozenges (6,7,10). The oil of star anise is considered to have beneficial pharmacological properties and may be used for medicinal purposes. It is employed in aromatherapy practices, but aromatherapy experts caution for the risk of toxicity due to the high anethole content (11,12).

Star anise oil should not be confused with aniseed oil, obtained from *Pimpinella anisum* L. (see Chapter 6.2 Aniseed oil).

CHEMICAL COMPOSITION

Star anise oil is a clear, mobile liquid, which will become a solid crystalline mass when cold (below 15°C), and which has an intense typical anise and fennel seed odor. In star anise oils from various origins, over 160 chemicals have been identified. About 54 per cent of these were found in a single reviewed publication only. The ten chemicals that had the highest maximum concentrations in 41 commercial star anise essential oil samples are shown in table 6.69.1 (Erich Schmidt, analytical data presented in ref. 16).

A full literature review of the qualitative and quantitative composition of commercial and non-commercial star anise oils of various origins with data from the ISO standard has been published in 2016 (16).

Table 6.69.1 Ten ingredients with the highest concentrations in commercial star anise oils (16)

Name	Concentration range	Name	Concentration range
(*E*)-Anethole	84.3 - 90.1%	Linalool	0.2 - 1.3%
Methyl chavicol	0.2 - 5.9%	*p*-Anisaldehyde	0.2 - 0.9%
Limonene	0.2 - 3.3%	β-Caryophyllene	0.2 - 0.8%
α-Pinene	0.3 - 1.8%	δ3-Carene	0.03 - 0.7%
(*E*)-Foeniculin	0.09 - 1.7%	α-Phellandrene	0.2 - 0.6%

CONTACT ALLERGY / ALLERGIC CONTACT DERMATITIS

General

The SCCS (Scientific Committee on Consumer Safety), in a 2012 Opinion on Fragrance allergens in cosmetic products, has categorized Illicium verum fruit oil as 'possible fragrance contact allergen' (14,15).

Contact allergy to star anise oil has been reported in one publication only. No clinical records of allergic contact dermatitis from star anise oils have been found. The main compound, anethole (84-90% of the entire oil) is also the principal allergen; possible other allergens are methyl chavicol and limonene.

Testing in groups of patients

One hundred consecutive patients with dermatitis were tested with star anise oil 0.5%, 1% and 2% in petrolatum; over 1/3 had positive reactions to the 1% and the 2% concentration, indicating that these concentrations are irritant. In five, patch test sensitization occurred, with flare-up of the 1% and 2% concentrations. Three were tested with anethole 1% in petrolatum (the main ingredient of star anise oil, present in concentrations of 84-90% in commercial oils; table 6.69.1), and all reacted. Another of these actively sensitized patients was tested with 9 components of star anise oil and reacted to anethole, α-pinene (maximum concentration in commercial star anise essential oils 1.8%), safrole and methyl chavicol (maximum concentration in commercial star anise essential oils 5.9%, table 6.69.1), all tested 1% in petrolatum (13).

Fifteen patients positive to 1% star anise oil, negative to 0.5% but positive to one or more 'balsams' (Myroxylon pereirae resin, turpentine, wood tars, colophony) were also tested with these 9 components with the following results: 5 reactions to anethole, 8 to α-pinene (who all co-reacted to turpentine, α-pinene is an important allergen in turpentine oil), 3 to limonene and one to safrole (limonene was found in commercial star anise oils in a maximum concentration of 3.3%, table 6.69.1). A concentration of 0.5% star anise oil may not be irritant, but detected only one sensitization out of the 5 actively sensitized patients. There was no cross- or pseudo-cross-reactivity to other essential oils. No mention was made of any clinical relevance of the reactions, which presumably there was not (13).

LITERATURE

1   Huang B, Liang J, Wang G, Qin L. Comparison of the volatile components of *Illicium verum* and *I. lanceolatum* from East China. J Essent Oil Bear Plants 2012;15:467-475
2   Wang G-W, Hu W-T, Huang BK, Qin L-P. *Illicium verum*: A review on its botany, traditional use, chemistry and Pharmacology. J Ethnopharmacol 2011;136:10-20
3   Howes M-JR, Kite GC, Simmonds MSJ. Distinguishing Chinese star anise from Japanese star anise using thermal desorption-gas chromatography-mass Spectrometry. J Agric Food Chem 2009;57:5783-5789
4   Cai M, Guo X, Liang H, Sun P. Microwave-assisted extraction and antioxidant activity of star anise oil from *Illicium verum* Hook.f. Int J Food Sci Technol 2013;48:2324-2330
5   Singh G, Maurya S, de Lampasona MP, Catalan C. Chemical constituents, antimicrobial investigations and antioxidative potential of volatile oil and acetone extract of star anise fruits. J Sci Food Agric 2006;86:111-121
6   Bernard T, Perineau F, Delmas M, Gaset A. Extraction of essential oils by refining plant materials. II. Processing of products in the dry state: *Illicium verum* Hooker (fruit) and *Cinnamomum zeylanicum* Nees (bark). Flavour Fragr J 1989;4:85-90
7   Li G, Sun Z, Xia L, Shi J, Liu Y, Suoa Y, et al. Supercritical CO2 oil extraction from Chinese star anise seed and simultaneous compositional analysis using HPLC by fluorescence detection and online atmospheric CI-MS identification. J Sci Food Agric 2010;90:1905-1913
8   Tonutti I, Liddle P. Aromatic plants in alcoholic beverages. A review. Flavour Fragr J 2010;25:341-350
9   Wang Q, Jiang L, Wen Q. Effect of three extraction methods on the volatile component of *Illicium verum* Hook. f. analyzed by GC–MS. Wuhan Univ J Nat Sci 2007;12: 529-534
10 Orwa C, Mutua A, Kindt R, Jamnadass R, Simons A. Agroforestree Database: a tree reference and selection guide version 4.0 (2009). Available at http://www.worldagroforestry.org/treedb2/AFTPDFS/Illicium_verum.pdf
11 Rhind JP. Essential oils. A handbook for aromatherapy practice, 2nd Edition. London: Singing Dragon, 2012
12 Lawless J. The encyclopedia of essential oils, 2nd Edition. London: Harper Thorsons, 2014
13 Rudzki E, Grzywa Z. Sensitizing and irritating properties of star anise oil. Contact Dermatitis 1976;2:305-306
14 SCCS (Scientific Committee on Consumer Safety). Opinion on Fragrance allergens in cosmetic products, 26-27 June 2012, SCCS/1459/11. Available at:
    https://ec.europa.eu/health/sites/health/files/scientific_committees/consumer_safety/docs/sccs_o_102.pdf
15 Uter W, Johansen JD, Börje A, Karlberg A-T, Lidén C, Rastogi S, Roberts D, White IR. Categorization of fragrance contact allergens for prioritization of preventive measures: clinical and experimental data and consideration of structure–activity relationships. Contact Dermatitis 2013;69:196-230
16 De Groot AC, Schmidt E. Essential oils: contact allergy and chemical composition. Boca Raton, Fl., USA: CRC Press, Taylor and Francis Group, 2016 (ISBN 9781482246407)

Chapter 6.70   TANGERINE OIL

IDENTIFICATION

Description/definition	: Tangerine oil is the essential oil obtained from the pericarp (peel) of the tangerine, *Citrus tangerina* Hort. Ex Tan. (synonym: *Citrus tangerina* Tanaka).
INCI name(s) EU	: Citrus tangerina peel oil
INCI name(s) USA	: Citrus tangerina (tangerine) peel oil
CAS registry number(s)	: 223748-44-5
CIR review(s)	: Final report 09/09/2014 (access: www.cir-safety.org/ingredients)
RIFM monograph(s)	: Food Chem Toxicol 1982;20:831 (special Issue VI)
SCCS opinion(s)	: SCCS/1459/11 (6)
Function(s) in cosmetics	: EU: masking; skin conditioning. USA: fragrance ingredients; skin-conditioning agents – miscellaneous
Patch testing	: 2% and 10% pet. (5); test also limonene (see Chapter 3.95 Limonene)

GENERAL

Citrus tangerina Hort. Ex Tan. (tangerine) is an orange-colored citrus fruit. It originates presumably from China, where it can also be found in wild state. The tangerine is cultivated in China, Japan and the USA (8). Varieties are the cultivar Dancy (formerly the most popular form) and the hybrids Sunburst, Robinson and Murcott. The name 'Tangerine' comes from Tangiers, a city in Morocco, where the first shipment of tangerines was allegedly sent to mainland Europe around 1845 (1).

Tangerines are most commonly peeled and eaten out of hand. The fresh fruit is also used in salads, desserts and main dishes. The peel is dried and used in Sichuan cuisine. The fruit is popular throughout the world and highly revered; the tangerine is a symbol of luck in China and regarded as a remedy for indigestion in France (1). In botanical terms, the tangerine is a type of mandarin orange, closely related to *Citrus reticulata* Blanco. However, in the flavor and fragrance industry, differences are said to exist between the varieties both in terms of juice and essential oil (1). Tangerine oil, which is obtained by cold-pressing the pericarp (peel) of the tangerines, is employed in aromatherapy practices (3,4).

The history, global distribution, and nutritional importance of *Citrus* fruits have been reviewed in ref. 2.

CHEMICAL COMPOSITION

Tangerine oil is a yellowish orange to deep orange, clear mobile liquid which has a fresh juicy, citrusy peel note odor. In tangerine oils from various origins, over 125 chemicals have been identified. About 46 per cent of these were found in a single reviewed publication only. The ten chemicals that had the highest maximum concentrations in 28 commercial tangerine essential oil samples are shown in table 6.70.1 (Erich Schmidt, analytical data presented in ref. 8).

A full literature review of the qualitative and quantitative composition of commercial and non-commercial tangerine oils of various origins has been published in 2016 (8).

Table 6.70.1 Ten ingredients with the highest concentrations in commercial tangerine oils (8)

Name	Concentration range	Name	Concentration range
Limonene	81.8 - 97.8%	*p*-Cymene	0.4 - 1.1%
γ-Terpinene	0.1 - 5.6%	α-Thujene	0.08 - 1.2%
Terpinolene	0.2 - 2.9%	β-Pinene	trace - 0.9%
Myrcene	0.1 - 2.2%	Sabinene	0.1 - 0.6%
α-Pinene	0.08 - 1.9%	Decanal	0.1 - 0.5%

CONTACT ALLERGY / ALLERGIC CONTACT DERMATITIS

General

The SCCS (Scientific Committee on Consumer Safety), in a 2012 Opinion on Fragrance allergens in cosmetic products, has categorized Citrus tangerina extract as 'possible fragrance contact allergen' (6,7).

Allergic contact dermatitis from tangerine oil has been reported in one publication only.

Case reports and case series

One individual developed allergic contact dermatitis from a perfume; all (coded) ingredients were tested, and there were strongly positive patch test reactions to tangerine oil 2% and 10% in petrolatum only (5).

LITERATURE

1   Reeve D, Arthur D. Riding the citrus trail: When is a mandarin a tangerine? Perfum Flavor 2002;27(July/August): 20-22

2   Liu YQ, Heying E, Tanumihardjo SA. History, global distribution, and nutritional importance of Citrus fruits. Compreh Rev Food Sci Food Saf 2012;11:530–545

3   Rhind JP. Essential oils. A handbook for aromatherapy practice, 2nd Edition. London: Singing Dragon, 2012

4   Lawless J. The encyclopedia of essential oils, 2nd Edition. London: Harper Thorsons, 2014

5   Vilaplana J, Romaguera C. Contact dermatitis from the essential oil of tangerine in fragrance. Contact Dermatitis 2002;46:108

6   SCCS (Scientific Committee on Consumer Safety). Opinion on Fragrance allergens in cosmetic products, 26-27 June 2012, SCCS/1459/11. Available at: https://ec.europa.eu/health/sites/health/files/scientific_committees/consumer_safety/docs/sccs_o_102.pdf

7   Uter W, Johansen JD, Börje A, Karlberg A-T, Lidén C, Rastogi S, Roberts D, White IR. Categorization of fragrance contact allergens for prioritization of preventive measures: clinical and experimental data and consideration of structure–activity relationships. Contact Dermatitis 2013;69:196-230

8   De Groot AC, Schmidt E. Essential oils: contact allergy and chemical composition. Boca Raton, Fl., USA: CRC Press, Taylor and Francis Group, 2016 (ISBN 9781482246407)

Chapter 6.71   TEA TREE OIL

IDENTIFICATION

Description/definition : Tea tree oil (essential oil of Melaleuca, terpinen-4-ol type) is the volatile oil obtained from the leaves and terminal branchlets of either the narrow-leaf tea-tree *Melaleuca alternifolia* (Maiden et Betche) Cheel, the flax-leaf (narrow-leaf) tea-tree *Melaleuca linariifolia* Smith, or the creek tea-tree *Melaleuca dissitiflora* F. Muell.

INCI name(s) EU : Melaleuca alternifolia leaf oil

INCI name(s) USA : Melaleuca alternifolia (tea tree) leaf oil

CAS registry number(s) : 68647-73-4; 85085-48-9

EC number(s) : 285-377-1

RIFM monograph(s) : Food Chem Toxicol 1988;26:407 (special issue VII)

SCCS opinion(s) : SCCP/08438/04 (91); SCCP/1155/08 (92)

ISO standard : ISO 4730 Essential oil of Melaleuca, terpinen-4-ol type (Tea Tree oil), 2017 and 2004; Geneva, Switzerland, www.iso.org

Merck Index monograph : 10496

Function(s) in cosmetics : EU: antioxidant; perfuming. USA: antioxidants; fragrance ingredients

Patch testing : 5% pet., oxidized (Chemo, SPCanada)

GENERAL

Melaleuca alternifolia is a tall shrub or small tree up to 15 meters high with a bushy crown and papery bark. This tree is native to Australia. Tea tree oil, which is obtained from the leaves (and terminal branchlets) by steam-distillation, has been reported to have multiple biological activities. It is marketed as a 'natural' topical antimicrobial. The product is present in many different formulations including pure oil (also for aromatherapy [20,25,26]), ointments, wart-paint (2), acne treatments (3,96) and household products such as fabric softeners, detergents and cleansers (4,20,22). In a monograph by the European Medicines Agency (16), tea tree oil was considered to be suitable for the treatment of small superficial wounds and insect bites, small boils (furuncles and mild acne), itching and irritation in cases of mild athlete's foot, and minor inflammation of oral mucosa (16). The oil is also used in many types of cosmetic products (5,20,22).

Useful reviews on various aspects of tea tree oil are provided in references 1,4,5,8,9,10,11,15,16,17,19,20,66. The author has published a full review of contact allergy to tea tree oil in 2016 (94) and of its constituents in the same year (93).

CHEMICAL COMPOSITION

Tea tree oil is a colorless to pale yellow, clear mobile liquid which has a terpeny, coniferous and minty-camphoraceus odor. In tea tree oils from various origins, over 220 chemicals have been identified. About 55 per cent of these were found in a single reviewed publication only. The ten chemicals that had the highest maximum concentrations in 97 commercial tea tree essential oil samples are shown in table 6.71.1 (Erich Schmidt, analytical data presented in ref. 93).

A full literature review of the qualitative and quantitative composition of commercial and non-commercial tea tree oils of various origins, their chemotypes and with data from the ISO standard, has been published in 2016 (93).

CONTACT ALLERGY / ALLERGIC CONTACT DERMATITIS

General

Of all essential oils, tea tree oil has caused most allergic reactions since the first case reports were published in 1991 from Australia, where tea tree oil is produced. The oil has been extensively investigated. Neat tea tree oil is a moderate sensitizer in humans (38,40,45,66,67,71). Undiluted oils and formulations containing 5% tea tree oil can also induce irritation of the skin / irritant contact dermatitis (40,65,66,71). Contact allergy to / allergic contact dermatitis from tea tree oil has been reported frequently. There are many reports of routine testing; tea tree oil 5% (oxidized) was added to the screening series of the North American Contact Dermatitis Group (NACDG) in 2003.

In groups of consecutive patients suspected of contact dermatitis, prevalence rates of up to 2.5% positive patch test reactions have been observed. In two well-documented studies, current relevance was found in 41% and 56% of the positive patch tests (35,42). In the NACDG studies, 'definite' + 'probable' relevance ranged from 20% to 56%. Many case reports of allergic contact dermatitis have been documented. Nearly 70% were caused by the application of pure tea tree oil on damaged skin, followed by cosmetics (16%) and topical pharmaceutical preparations (10%); there were also 6 cases of occupational allergic contact dermatitis in two aromatherapists, a complementary therapist, two pedicures and a beautician.

Table 6.71.1 Ten ingredients with the highest concentrations in commercial tea tree oils (93)

Name	Concentration range	Name	Concentration range
Terpinolene	0.04 - 45.7%	1,8-Cineole	0.5 - 18.3%
Terpinen-4-ol	6.2 - 44.9%	α-Terpinene	2.3 - 11.7%
γ-Terpinene	3.1 - 23.0%	α-Pinene	1.8 - 9.2%
cis-Sabinene hydrate	trace - 19.4%	β-Phellandrene	trace - 5.2%
p-Cymene	0.3 - 19.4%	α-Terpineol	1.9 - 4.2%

Testing in groups of patients

The results of patch tests with tea tree oil in routine testing (consecutive patients suspected of contact dermatitis) are shown in table 6.71.2, those of testing in groups of selected patients are shown in table 6.71.3. In routine testing, rates of positive reactions ranged from 0.1% to 2.5%, whereas between 0.5% and 41% of patients in selected groups had positive patch tests. The very high positivity rate of 41% was seen in a small group of 17 patients suspected of cosmetic dermatitis and tested with the undiluted oil, which may give rise to irritant reactions (although 6/7 reactions were considered to be relevant) (31). In two well-documented studies, current relevance was found in 41% and 56% of the positive patch tests (35,42). In the NACDG studies, 'definite' + 'probable' relevance ranged from 20% to 56%.

Table 6.71.2 Results of testing groups of patients: Routine testing

Years and Country	Test conc. & vehicle	Number of patients tested | positive (%)		Selection of patients (S); Relevance (R); Comments (C)	Ref.
2015-2017 NACDG	5% pet. ox.	5593	66 (1.2%)	R: definite + probable relevance: 24%	107
2011-2015 USA	5% pet. ox.	1687	22 (1.3%)	R: not stated	108
2013-14 USA, Canada	5% pet., ox.	4859	44 (0.9%)	R: definite + probable relevance: 55%	105
2009-14 USA, Canada	5% pet., oxidized	13,398	123 (0.9%)	R: of 63 patients reacting, but negative to FM I, FM II and balsam of Peru, 52% had definite + probable relevance	104
2011-2013 The Netherlands	5% pet.	221	2 (0.9%)	R: not relevant; C: both patients also reacted to ascaridole	81
2011-12 USA, Canada	5% pet., oxidized	4231	36 (0.9%)	R: definite + probable relevance: 56%	86
2009-10 USA, Canada	5% pet.	4299	43 (1.0%)	R: definite + probable relevance: 50%; the test material was oxidized	33
2001-2010 Australia	10% pet.	5087	129 (2.5%)	R: 33%	89
<2010 Australia	5% pet.	794	28 (3.5%)	R: 43%; not absolutely certain that there was no selection	89
2007-8 USA, Canada	5% pet.	5078	71 (1.4%)	R: definite + probable relevance: 37%	50
2000-2007 USA	5% pet.	869	18 (2.1%)	R: 100%; C: weak study: a. high rate of macular erythema and weak reactions, b. relevance figures include 'questionable' and 'past' relevance	29
<2006 USA, Canada	5% pet.	1603	5 (0.3%)	R: definite + probable relevance: 20%	80
2005-6 USA, Canada	5% pet.	4435	62 (1.4%)	R: definite + probable relevance: 36%	49
2003-4 USA, Canada	5% pet.	5137	45 (0.9%)	R: not stated	51
2000-2004 Australia	10% and 5% pet.	2320	41 (1.8%)	R: 17/41 (41%); only 4 patients had used cosmetic products containing tea tree oil (soap, hand cream, face cream, deodorant and hand lotion, one product each); 66% of the 41 patients recalled prior use of tea tree oil and 20% specified application of neat (100%) tea tree oil	35
<2004 USA	5% pet.	1603	5 (0.3%)	C: no details known	52
2002-2003 Denmark	10% pet.	377	1 (0.3%)	R: probably relevant	65
1999-2003 Germany	5% DEP, oxidized	2284	21 (0.9%)	R: percentage not specified; some patients had used (self-made) cosmetics containing tea tree oil, others had used the neat oil for eczema, acne, fleabites, muscle pain, and for evaporation in the sauna or indoors to banish wasps	69
2001 United Kingdom	pure, oxidized	550	13 (2.4%)	R: 4 relevant, 5 possibly relevant, 4 relevance unknown; C: 2 cases of occupational allergy in a beauty therapist and a complementary therapist; other exposures included the use of a shaving gel and children's shampoo; 38% irritant patch test reactions to pure oxidized tea tree oil	73
< 2000 Italy	5%, 1% and 0.1%, pet., undiluted	725	1 (0.1%)	C: details not known; irritant reactions to undiluted tea tree oil	41
1999-2000 Germany, Austria	5% DEP, oxidized	3375	36 (1.1%)	R: current relevance 56%; range of positive patch tests per centre: 0%-2.3%; co-reactivity to oil of turpentine: 39%	42

Table 6.71.2 Results of testing groups of patients: Routine testing (continued)

Years and Country	Test conc. & vehicle	Number of patients tested	positive (%)		Selection of patients (S); Relevance (R); Comments (C)	Ref.
1999 Australia	?	477	12	(2.5%)	R: not stated; C: in a group of 45 patients reacting to compound tincture of benzoin, there were 15 (33%) reactions to tea tree oil	85
1997 France	5-10-50% in arachis oil and pure	1216	7	(0.6%)	R: the patients used pure oils, creams and hair products containing tea tree oil	47

Table 6.71.3 Results of testing groups of patients: Selected patient groups

Years and Country	Test conc. & vehicle	Number of patients tested	positive (%)		Selection of patients (S); Relevance (R); Comments (C)	Ref.
2014-2016 USA	5% pet.	103	2	(2%)	S: patients tested with a screening fragrance series; R: not stated	109
2014 The Netherlands	5% pet., oxidized	29	4	(13.8%)	S: patients with dermatitis who had previously been tested with ascaridole and had a (doubtful) positive or irritant reaction to ascaridole at that time; R: no relevance found	81
2008-2014 UK	5% pet.	2104	11	(0.5%)	S: patients tested with a cosmetics series; R: not stated	98
2011-2012 Italy	5% pet.	122	2	(1.6%)	S: patients who reported adverse cutaneous reactions to products (notably cosmetics) containing botanical ingredients in a questionnaire; they were tested with a 'botanical series'; R: both reactions were relevant	83
2001-2010 Australia	5% pet.	794	28	(3.5%)	S: not specified; R: 43%	89
2001-2002 Sweden	5% alc.	1075	29	(2.7%)	S: patients referred for routine testing willing to participate in a study on cosmetic use and adverse reactions; R: not stated	30
1998-1999 Australia	pure and 10% pet.	216	6	(2.8%)	S: healthy adult volunteers; R: not stated; C: the patients were patch tested with ten different samples. when 'indistinguishable' reactions were counted, the percentage of positive reactions rose to 4.8%; in the subgroup of patients (63%) who had previously come into contact with tea tree oil, the percentages were 4.6% (without 'indistinguishable' reactions) and 7.6% (with such reactions); probably an overestimation	39
1996-1997 UK	pure	17	7	(41%)	S: patients suspected of cosmetic dermatitis; R: 6/7 relevant	31

DEP: diethyl phthalate; pet.: petrolatum

Case reports and case series

Details of published case reports of allergic contact dermatitis to tea tree oil are summarized in table 6.71.4. Over 100 patients with allergic contact dermatitis from tea tree oil have been reported. Of the cases where the products responsible for the allergic reactions were specified, nearly 70% related to pure tea tree oil applied for therapeutic purposes on a variety of skin conditions including acne, eczema, sunburn, wounds (of any cause), warts, herpes and fungal infections. This category was followed by cosmetics (16%) and topical pharmaceutical preparations (10%); there were also 6 cases of occupational allergic contact dermatitis in two aromatherapists, a complementary therapist, two pedicures and a beautician. See table 6.71.4 and also data from refs. 35 and 69 in table 6.71.2).

Table 6.71.4 Case reports of allergic contact dermatitis from tea tree oil

Years and country	Nr. of patients allergic to tea tree oil	Causative products, clinical data and comments	Ref.
2016 USA	1	Gel for wound treatment	106
1990-2016 Belgium	12	Six pure oils, 6 topical pharmaceuticals; widespread dermatitis in 2 patients from application of the undiluted oil	103
2016 Ireland	1	Hydrogel and dressing for the treatment of burn injuries	102
2015 Australia	1	Pure oil; the dermatitis was pustular, as was the patch test reaction to tea tree oil; the relevance was 'past'	101
2015 Spain	5	Pure oils	95
2013 The Netherlands	2	Soap and cream containing tea tree oil in one patient, shaving oil in the second patient who had the clinical picture of folliculitis barbae; both patients also reacted to ascaridole	84

Table 6.71.4 Case reports of allergic contact dermatitis from tea tree oil (continued)

Years and country	Nr. of patients allergic to tea tree oil	Causative products, clinical data and comments	Ref.
2011 UK	1	Essential oil used by a 'complementary therapist' with contact allergy to many other oils	79
2000-2010 Belgium	5	Skin care products; this represented 0.5% of 959 cases of cosmetic allergy where the causal allergen was found	28
2000-2009 Belgium	1	Skin care product	88
1978-2008 Belgium	2	Topical pharmaceutical preparations	27
2007 USA	1	Pure oil used for aromatherapy	77
2007 Australia	1	The patient was sensitized by pure oil used for acne, and later developed allergic contact dermatitis of the eyelids from using a tea tree oil-containing shampoo	55
2004 Canada	1	Pure oil for aromatherapy	76
2004 Germany	1	Pure oil on the face of a 12-year-old boy for a 'minimal skin affection'	68
2003 United Kingdom	1	Pure oil on a piercing wound; contact allergy may have precipitated linear IgA disease	46
2002 United Kingdom	1	Pure tea tree oil; the patient was a professional aroma-therapist, who also reacted to many other essential oils	75
2000 United Kingdom	1	'Tea tree oil products' used for vulvovaginitis	62
2000 Germany	1	No details known	74
2000 USA	1	Erythema multiforme-like contact dermatitis ('id-') from application of pure oil to a wound	63
1999 Germany	8	Pure oil in seven patients for treatment of eczema, plantar warts and sunburn	43
<1999 Germany	16	Ten patients had used pure oil for skin disorders such as eczema, warts, sunburn and herpes (n=9) and for 'hygiene and cosmetic purposes (n=1); one patient developed dermatitis from shampoo to which pure oil had been added; no data for the other 5 cases	36
1998 Germany	1	Pure oil on psoriasis	59
1997 United Kingdom	1	Wart paint with tea tree oil	54
1997 France	7	Pure oils and cosmetics containing tea tree oil	47
1997 Sweden	1	Pure oil on skin irritation	60
1997 Germany	2	Pure oil, in one patient used on basal cell carcinoma; one also reacted to limonene and sweet orange oil	61
1996 USA	12	Details not known	56
1996 The Netherlands	1	Airborne allergic contact dermatitis from inhalation of aqueous solution of tea tree oil; source of primary sensitization not mentioned	64
1995 Norway	1	Hand dermatitis in an aromatherapist, primarily sensiti-zed to lemongrass oil; positive patch test reaction to tea tree oil used at her work. Cajeput was mentioned as synonym, so possibly it was not the oil from *Melaleuca alternifolia*	57
1994 Germany	7	Pure oil on skin disorders such as fungal infection, dog scratches, insect bites, and hand rashes	44
1994 Netherlands	3	Pure oil; occupational contact dermatitis in two pedicures and a beautician	48
1994 Norway	1	Pure oil for treatment of acne	87
1992 Netherlands	1	Pure oil for treatment of dermatitis; systemic contact dermatitis after oral administration; the patient co-reacted to 1,8-cineole, an ingredient of the oil	34
1992 Australia	2	Undiluted oil; first two cases of contact allergy reported	37

Products with low concentrations (<2%) of tea tree oil will infrequently induce contact allergy or elicit allergic reactions. Thus, of twenty-seven cases of contact dermatitis to products with tea tree oil that were reported to the Swedish MPA (Medicinal Products Agency), all had a tea tree oil concentration of 2% or higher (70).

The allergens in tea tree oil

Melaleuca oil is a moderate sensitizer in animal and human experiments (40,45,66,67,71); skin sensitization may be enhanced by irritancy (66). The composition of tea tree oil changes particularly in the presence of atmospheric oxygen but also when the oil is exposed to light, humidity and higher temperatures. Under these conditions, the antioxidants α-terpinene, γ-terpinene and terpinolene oxidize to p-cymene. Consequently, the levels of α-terpinene, γ-terpinene and terpinolene decrease whereas the level of p-cymene increases up to tenfold (14,23). Hence, the concentration of p-cymene is a good measure of the oxidative degradation of tea tree oil (24). Oxidation processes further lead to the formation of peroxides, endoperoxides and epoxides such as ascaridole (12) and 1,2,4-trihydroxymenthane (13,14,23), which are strong sensitizers (18,36,53). Air exposure leads to a 3-fold increase in the sensitization potency for tea tree oil (36). Auto-oxidation of α-terpinene to allylic epoxides and other oxidation products may be contributory (78).

In 1994 and 1999, the main sensitizers were identified (32,36). Since then, especially German investigators have tested a considerable number of patients allergic to tea tree oil with one ingredient or a battery of its constituents to identify the main sensitizers. The results are shown in table 6.71.5.

Table 6.71.5 Testing with ingredients in patients with positive patch test reactions to tea tree oil

Years and country	Nr. tested allergic to tea tree oil (test conc./veh.)	Ingredients tested, test concentration and vehicle, numbers positive, percentage positive (in brackets) and comments	Ref.
2011-2013 Netherlands	6 (5% pet.)	All reacted to ascaridole 1% and/or 2% and/or 5% in petrolatum	81
2009-2013 Spain	4 (5% pet. and pure)	All reacted to oxidized d-limonene (concentration/vehicle unknown)	82
1999-2003 Germany	20 (5% DEP)	Terpinolene 5% DEP: n=17 (85%); Ascaridole 5% DEP: n=15 (75%); α-Terpinene 5% DEP: n=16 (80%); 1,2,4-Trihydroxymenthane 5% pet.: n=13 (65%); α-Phellandrene 5% DEP: n=7 (35%); d-Limonene 5% DEP: n=11 (55%); Myrcene 5% DEP: n=7 (35%); Viridiflorene 5% DEP: n=1 (5%); d-Carvone 5% DEP: n=4 (20%); l-Carvone 5% DEP: n=4 (20%); Aromadendrene 5% DEP: n=1 (5%); Sabinene 5% DEP: n=2 (10%); Terpinen-4-ol 5% DEP: n=1 (5%)	69
2000 Germany	8 (20% olive oil)	Terpinolene 10% aqua: n=7 (88%); Ascaridole (5% aqua): n=7 (88%); α-Terpinene 5% aqua: n=6 (75%); α-Phellandrene 5% aqua: n= 5 (63%); 1,2,4-Trihydroxymenthane 5% pet.: n=2 (25%); d-Carvone (5% aqua): n=1 (13%); Terpinen-4-ol 10% aqua: n=1 (13%)	43
2000 Germany	15 (test conc./veh. not specified)	All were tested with 1,2,4-dihydroxymenthane and 11 (73%) reacted positively	53
1999-2000 Germany, Austria	10 (5% DEP)	Terpinolene 10% DEP: n= 10 (100%); Ascaridole 5% DEP: n=10 (100%); α-Terpinene 5% DEP: n= 10 (100%); 1,2,4-Trihydroxymenthane 5% DEP: n=9 (90%); α-Phellandrene 5% DEP: n=6 (60%); d-Limonene 5% DEP: n=4 (40%); Myrcene 5% DEP: n=1 (10%); Viridiflorene 5% DEP: n= 1 (10%)	42
1999 Germany	16 (test vehicle not mentioned)*	Terpinolene 10%: n=16 (100%); Ascaridole 5%: n=12 (75%); α-Terpinene 5%: n=11 (69%); 1,2,4-Trihydroxymenthane 5%: n=8 (50%); α-Phellandrene 5%: n= 5 (31%); Myrcene 5%: n=2 (13%); d-Limonene 5%: n=1 (6%); Viridiflorene 5%: n=1 (6%)	36
1998 Germany	1 (conc./veh. ?)	1 reaction to ascaridole; article not read	58
1997 Australia	3 (varying test concentrations)	α-Terpinene: n=1; 3 patients reacted to a sesquiterpenoid hydrocarbon fraction and sesquiterpenoid mixed with paraffin to obtain a concentration as in 25% tea tree oil	40, 45
1994 Germany	7 (1% solution)	Limonene 1% alc.: n= 6 (86%); α-Terpinene 1% alc.: n= 5 (71%); Aromadendrene 1% alc.: n=5 (71%); Terpinen-4-ol 1% and 5% alc.: n=2 (29%); p-Cymene 1% alc.: n=1 (14%); α-Phellandrene 1% alc.: n=1 (14%)	44
1992 Netherlands	1 (pure)	1,8 Cineole (eucalyptol)	34

conc.: concentration; DEP: diethyl phthalate; Nr.: number; veh.: vehicle

* Test concentrations were probably 5% DEP for all allergens except 1,2,4-trihydroxymenthane, which was tested in petrolatum (118)

The most important sensitizers in tea tree oil appear to be terpinolene, ascaridole, α-terpinene (and its oxidation products, [78]), 1,2,4-trihydroxymenthane, α-phellandrene, d-limonene and myrcene. Other chemicals which may be responsible for tea tree oil allergy, albeit less frequently, include aromadendrene, d-carvone, l-carvone, terpinen-4-

ol, viridiflorene, sabinene, *p*-cymene and possibly 1,8-cineole (34,36,42,43,44,69,81,82,84,90). Most of these have been found in low concentrations or not at all in commercial tea tree oils, which can be explained by the fact that these were fresh oil samples.

Conversely, of 14 patients with occupational contact dermatitis from *d*-limonene and patch tested with tea tree oil 5% in petrolatum, 5 (36%) had a positive (n=4) or doubtful positive (n=1) reaction to tea tree oil. This indicates that previous contact allergy to limonene may result in a positive patch test to tea tree oil (90).

OTHER SIDE EFFECTS

Immediate-type reactions
A man experienced immediate flushing, pruritus, throat constriction, and lightheadedness after topical application of tea tree oil. The patient had placed a drop of tea tree oil on his finger and had applied this to psoriatic lesions on his leg. Skin-prick and intradermal testing was performed, as well as enzyme-linked immunosorbent assays for specific IgG and IgE against tea tree oil. The patient had a positive wheal and flare reaction on intradermal testing with tea tree oil. All five patient controls were negative on skin testing. No specific IgG or IgE was detected (97).

Systemic side effects
Repeated topical exposure to products containing lavender and tea tree oil was suggested to be the cause of prepubertal gynecomastia in three prepubertal boys. The explanation was that these oils may have estrogenic and antiandrogenic activity (99). The article received many critical reactions, but in a review article on side effects of essential oils in aromatherapy, the causality was classified as 'likely' (100). Although there has been another case report of (unilateral) gynecomastia in a young male alledgedly caused by tea tree oil (6, no details available, article in Spanish only), currently the postulation that tea tree oil can effect puberty lacks solid evidence (72).

LITERATURE

1   Pazyar N, Yaghoobi R, Bagherani N, Kazerouni A. A review of applications of tea tree oil in dermatology. Int J Dermatol 2013;52:784-790

2   Bhushan M, Beck MH. Allergic contact dermatitis from tea tree oil in a wart paint. Contact Dermatitis 1997;36:117-118

3   Enshaieh S, Jooya A, Siadat AH, Iraji F. The efficacy of 5% topical tea tree oil gel in mild to moderate acne vulgaris: a randomized, double-blind placebo-controlled study. Indian J Dermatol Venereol Leprol 2007;73:22-25

4   Crawford GH, Sciacca JR, James WD. Tea tree oil: cutaneous effects of the extracted oil of *Melaleuca alternifolia*. Dermatitis 2004;15:59-66

5   Scientific Committee on Consumer products (SCCP). Opinion on tea Tree Oil. Adopted by the SCCP during the 18th plenary meeting of 16 December 2008. SCCP Report 1155/08. Available at: http://ec.europa.eu/health/ph_risk/committees/04_sccp/docs/sccp_o_160.pdf

6   Lopez-Rodriguez JA, Duelo Marcos M. Unilateral gynecomastia in young male due to tea tree oil. An Pediatr (Barc) 2014;81:e18-19 (article in Spanish)

7   Carson CF, Hammer KA, Riley TV. Compilation and review of published and unpublished tea tree oil literature. A report for the Rural Industries Research and Development Corporation. Barton, Austra: RIRDC Publication No 05/151, 2005, ISBN 1 74151 214 X. Available at https://rirdc.infoservices.com.au/downloads/05-151

8   Carson CF, Riley TV. Safety, efficacy and provenance of tea tree (*Melaleuca alternifolia*) oil. Contact Dermatitis 2001;45:65-67

9   Southwell IA. Tea tree oil stability and evaporation rate. An addendum to *p*-cymene and peroxides, indicators of oxidation in tea tree oil. A report for the Rural Industries Research and Development Corporation by Ian Southwell, September 2006, RIRDC Publication No 06/112, RIRDC Project No ISO-2A., Annex 9 of the dossier

10   Hausen BM. "Wundermittel" mit Tücken: Teebaumöl. Ärzt Prax Dermatol 1999;9-10

11   Beckmann B, Ippen H. Teebaum-Öl. Dermatosen 1998;46:120-124

12   Hausen BM. Kontaktallergie auf Teebaumöl und Ascaridol. Akt Derm 1998;24:60-62

13   Harkenthal M, Reichling J, Geiss HK, Saller R. Oxidationsprodukte als mögliche Ursache von Kontaktdermatitiden. Pharmazeut Z 1998;47:4092

14   Harkenthal M, Hausen BM, Reichling J. 1,2,4-Trihydroxy menthane, a contact allergen from oxidized Australian tea tree oil. Pharmazie 2000;55:153-154

15   Brophy JJ, Craven LA, Doran JC. Melaleucas: their botany, essential oils and uses. ACIAR Monograph No. 156. Canberra: Australian Centre for International Agricultural Research, 2013. Available at: http://aciar.gov.au/publication/mn156

16 European Medicines Agency. Assessment report on *Melaleuca alternifolia* (Maiden and Betch) Cheel, *M. linariifolia* Smith, *M. dissitiflora* F. Mueller and/or other species of *Melaleuca*, aetheroleum. Committee on Herbal Medicinal Products (HMPC) 2013, EMA/HMPC/320932/2012

17 Almeida Barbosa LC, Silva CJ, Teixeira RR, Strozi Alves Meira RM, Lelis Pinheiro A. Chemistry and biological activities of essential oils from *Melaleuca* L. species. Agriculturae Conspectus Scientificus 2013;78:11-23

18 Sciarrone D, Ragonese C, Carnovale C, Piperno A, Dugo P, Dugo G, Mondello L. Evaluation of tea tree oil quality and ascaridole: A deep study by means of chiral and multi heart-cuts multidimensional gas chromatography system coupled to mass spectrometry detection. J Chromatogr A 2010;1217:6422-6427

19 Carson CF, Hammer KA, RileyTV. *Melaleuca alternifolia* (tea tree) oil: a review of antimicrobial and other medicinal properties. Clin Microbiol Rev 2006;19:50-62

20 Hartford O, Zug KA. Tea tree oil. Cutis 2005;76:178-180

21 Shellie R, Marriott P, Zappia G, Mondello L, Dugo G. Interactive use of linear retention indices on polar and apolar columns with an MS-library for reliable characterization of Australian tea tree and other *Melaleuca* sp. oils, J Essent Oil Res 2003;15:305-312

22 Cox SD, Mann CM, Markham JL. Interactions between components of the essential oil of *Melaleuca alternifolia*. J Appl Microbiol 2001;91:492-497

23 Brophy JJ, Davies NW, Southwell IA. Gas chromatographic quality control for oil of *Melaleuca* terpinen-4-ol type (Australian tea tree). J Agric Food Chem 1989;37:1330-1335

24 Southwell I. *p*-Cymene and organic peroxides as indicators of oxidation in tea tree oil. A report for the Rural Industries Research and Development Corporation. Australian Government, Rural Industries Research and Development Corporation, 2006. RIRDC Publication No 06/112, RIRDC Project No ISO-2A. Available at: https://rirdc.infoservices.com.au/downloads/06-112

25 Rhind JP. Essential oils. A handbook for aromatherapy practice, 2nd Edition. London: Singing Dragon, 2012

26 Lawless J. The encyclopedia of essential oils, 2nd Edition. London: Harper Thorsons, 2014

27 Nardelli A, D'Hooge E, Drieghe J, Dooms M, Goossens A. Allergic contact dermatitis from fragrance components in specific topical pharmaceutical products in Belgium. Contact Dermatitis 2009;60:303-313

28 Travassos AR, Claes L, Boey L, Drieghe J, Goossens A. Non-fragrance allergens in specific cosmetic products. Contact Dermatitis 2011;65:276-285

29 Wetter DA, Yiannias JA, Prakash AV, Davis MD, Farmer SA, el-Azhary RA, et al. Results of patch testing to personal care product allergens in a standard series and a supplemental cosmetic series: an analysis of 945 patients from the Mayo Clinic Contact Dermatitis Group, 2000-2007. J Am Acad Dermatol 2010;63:789-798

30 Lindberg M, Tammela M, Bostrom A, Fischer T, Inerot A, Sundberg K, Berne B. Are adverse skin reactions to cosmetics underestimated in the clinical assessment of contact dermatitis? A prospective study among 1075 patients attending Swedish patch test clinics. Acta Derm Venereol 2004;84:291-295

31 Thomson KF, Wilkinson SM. Allergic contact dermatitis to plant extracts in patients with cosmetic dermatitis. Br J Dermatol 2000;142:84-88

32 Knight TE, Hausen BM. Melaleuca oil (tea-tree oil) dermatitis. J Am Acad Dermatol 1994;30:423-427

33 Warshaw EM, Belsito DV, Taylor JS, Sasseville D, DeKoven JG, Zirwas MJ, et al. North American Contact Dermatitis Group patch test results: 2009 to 2010. Dermatitis 2013;24:50-59

34 De Groot AC, Weijland JW. Systemic contact dermatitis from tea tree oil. Contact Dermatitis 1992;27:279-280

35 Rutherford T, Nixon R, Tam M, Tate B. Allergy to tea tree oil: retrospective review of 41 cases with positive patch tests over 4.5 years. Australas J Dermatol 2007;48:83-87

36 Hausen BM, Reichling J, Harkenthal M. Degradation products of monoterpenes are the sensitizing agents in tea tree oil. Am J Cont Derm 1999;10:68-77

37 Apted JH. Contact dermatitis associated with the use of tea-tree oil. Australas J Dermatol 1991;32:177

38 Satchell AC, Saurajen A, Bell C, Barnetson RS. Treatment of interdigital tinea pedis with 25% and 50% tea tree oil solution: a randomized, placebo-controlled, blinded study. Australas J Dermatol 2002;43:175-178

39 Greig JE, Carson CF, Stuckey MS, Riley TV. Skin sensitivity testing for tea tree oil – A Report for the Rural Industries Research and Development Corporation. Rural Industries Research and Development Corporation, Barton Act Australia Report no. 99. 1999. Available at: https://rirdc.infoservices.com.au/items/99-102

40 Southwell I, Freeman S, Rubel DM. Skin irritancy of tea tree oil. J Essent Oil Res 1997;9:47-52

41 Lisi P, Meligeni L, Pigatto P, et al. The prevalence of sensitivity to melaleuca essential oil. It Ann Clin Exp Allergol Dermat 2000;54:141-144

42 Pirker C, Hausen BM, Uter W, Hillen U, Brasch J, Bayerl C, et al. Sensitization to tea tree oil in Germany and Austria. A multicenter study of the German Contact Dermatitis group. J Dtsch Dermatol Ges 2003;1:629-634

43 Lippert U, Walter A, Hausen BM, Fuchs Th. Increasing incidence of contact dermatitis to tea tree oil. J Allergy Clin Immunol 2000;105;S43 (abstract 127)

44 Knight TE, Hausen BM. Melaleuca oil (tea tree oil) dermatitis. J Am Acad Dermatol 1994;30:423-427

45 Rubel DM, Freeman S, Southwell I. Tea tree oil allergy: what is the offending agent? Report of three cases of tea tree oil allergy and review of the literature. Australas J Dermatol 1998;39:244-247

46 Perrett CM, Evans AV, Russell-Jones R. Tea tree oil dermatitis associated with linear IgA disease. Clin Exp Dermatol 2003;28:167-170

47 Fritz TM, Burg G, Krasovec M. Allergic contact dermatitis to cosmetics containing Melaleuca alternifolia (tea tree) oil. Ann Dermatol Venereol 2001;128:123-126

48 Van der Valk PG, de Groot AC, Bruynzeel DP, Coenraads PJ, Weijland JW. Allergic contact eczema due to tea tree oil. Ned Tijdschr Geneeskd 1994;138:823-825 (in Dutch)

49 Zug KA, Warshaw EM, Fowler JF Jr, Maibach HI, Belsito DL, Pratt MD, et al. Patch-test results of the North American Contact Dermatitis Group 2005-2006. Dermatitis 2009;20:149-160

50 Fransway AF, Zug KA, Belsito DV, DeLeo VA, Fowler JF Jr, Maibach HI, et al. North American Contact Dermatitis Group patch test results for 2007-2008. Dermatitis 2013;24:10-21

51 Warshaw EM, Belsito DV, DeLeo VA, Fowler JF Jr, Maibach HI, Marks JG, et al. North American Contact Dermatitis Group patch-test results, 2003-2004 study period. Dermatitis 2008;19:129-136

52 Crawford GH, Sciacca JR, James WD. Tea tree oil: cutaneous effects of the extracted oil of Melaleuca alternifolia. Dermatitis 2004;15:59-66

53 Harkenthal M, Hausen BM, Reichling J. 1,2,4-Trihydroxymenthane, a contact allergen from oxidized Australian tea tree oil. Pharmazie 2000;55:153-154

54 Bhushan M, Beck MH. Allergic contact dermatitis from tea tree oil in a wart paint. Contact Dermatitis 1997;36:117-118

55 Williams JD, Nixon RL, Lee A. Recurrent allergic contact dermatitis due to allergen transfer by sunglasses. Contact Dermatitis 2007;57:120-121

56 Fransway A. Allergy to oil of Melaleuca: Report of 12 cases. American Contact Dermatitis Society Meeting. 9.02.1996, Washington DC, USA (abstract)

57 Selvaag E, Holm J, Thune P. Allergic contact dermatitis in an aromatherapist with multiple sensitizations to essential oils. Contact Dermatitis 1995;33:354-355

58 Hausen BM. Kontaktallergie auf Teebaumöl und Ascaridol. Akt Derm 1998;24:60-62

59 Fritz TM, Elmer P. Allergisches Kontaktekzem auf Teebaumöl bei einer Patientin mit Psoriasis. Akt Derm 1998;24:7-10

60 Hackzell-Bradley M, Bradley T, Fischer T. Kontaktallergi av 'tea tree-oil'. Lakartidningen 1997:94:4359-4361

61 Kränke B. Allergisierende Potenz von Teebaumöl. Hautarzt 1997;48:203-204

62 Varma S, Blackford S, Statham BN, Blackwell A. Combined contact allergy to tea tree oil and lavender oil complicating chronic vulvovaginitis. Contact Dermatitis 2000;42:309-310

63 Khanna M, Qasem K, Sasseville D. Allergic contact dermatitis to tea tree oil with erythema multiforme-like Id reaction. Dermatitis 2000;11:238-242

64 De Groot AC. Airborne allergic contact dermatitis from tea tree oil. Contact Dermatitis 1996;35:304-305

65 Veien NK, Rosner K, Skovgaard GL. Is tea tree oil an important contact allergen? Contact Dermatitis 2004;50:378-379

66 Scientific Committee on Consumer products (SCCP). Opinion on tea Tree Oil. Adopted by the SCCP during the 18th plenary meeting of 16 December 2008. SCCP Report 1155/08. Available at: http://ec.europa.eu/health/ph_risk/committees/04_sccp/docs/sccp_o_160.pdf

67 Anonymous. Human studies Draize method, study no. DT-029. Skin & Cancer Foundation, Australia, 1997

68 Kütting B, Brehler R, Traupe H. Allergic contact dermatitis in children – strategies of prevention and risk management. Eur J Dermatol 2004;14:80-85

69 Hausen BM. Evaluation of the main contact allergens in oxidized tea tree oil. Dermatitis 2004;15:213-214

70 Anonymous. Tea Tree Oil (TTO) Monograph on active ingredient being used in cosmetic products, prepared by the Norwegian delegation to the Council of Europe Committee of experts on cosmetic products, 2001, RD 4-3/35.

71 Aspres N, Freeman S. Predictive testing for irritancy and allergenicity of tea tree oil in normal human subjects. Exogen Dermatol 2003;2:258-261

72 Carson CF, Tisserand R, Larkman T. Lack of evidence that essential oils affect puberty. Reprod Toxicol 2014;44:50-51

73 Coutts I, Shaw S, Orton D. Patch testing with pure tea tree oil - 12 months experience. Br J Dermatol 2002;147(Suppl. 62):70

74 Reindl H, Gall H, Hausen BM, Peter U. Akutes Kontaktekzem nach Anwendung von Teebaumöl. Allergo J 2000;9:100-103

75 Dharmagunawardena B, Takwale A, Sanders KJ, Cannan S, Roger A, Ilchyshyn A. Gas chromatography: an investigative tool in multiple allergies to essential oils. Contact Dermatitis 2002;47:288-292

76 Monthrope Y, Shaw J. A 'natural' dermatitis: Contact allergy to tea tree oil. Univ Toronto Med J 2004;82:59-60

77 Stonehouse A, Studdiford J. Allergic contact dermatitis from tea tree oil. Department of Family & Community Medicine Faculty Papers. Paper 12:2007 (not further specified, cited by Posadzki P, Alotaibi A, Ernst E. Adverse effects of aromatherapy: A systematic review of case reports and case series. Int J Risk Saf Med 2012;24:147-161)

78 Rudbäck J, Andresen Bergström M, Börje A, Nilsson U, Karlberg AT. α-Terpinene, an antioxidant in tea tree oil, autoxidizes rapidly to skin allergens on air exposure. Chem Res Toxicol 2012;25:713-721

79 Newsham J, Rai S, Williams JDL. Two cases of allergic contact dermatitis to neroli oil. Br J Dermatol 2011;165(suppl.1):76

80 Belsito DV, Fowler JF Jr, Sasseville D, Marks JG Jr, De Leo VA, Storrs FJ. Delayed-type hypersensitivity to fragrance materials in a select North American population. Dermatitis 2006;17:23-28

81 Christoffers WA, Blömeke B, Coenraads P-J, Schuttelaar M-LA. The optimal patch test concentration for ascaridole as a sensitizing component of tea tree oil. Contact Dermatitis 2014;71:129-137

82 Santesteban R, Loidi L, Agulló A, Hervella M, Larrea M, Yanguas I. Allergic contact dermatitis to tea tree oil. Contact Dermatitis 2014;70 (suppl.1):102

83 Corazza M, Borghi A, Gallo R, Schena D, Pigatto P, Lauriola MM, et al. Topical botanically derived products: use, skin reactions, and usefulness of patch tests. A multicentre Italian study. Contact Dermatitis 2014;70:90-97

84 Christoffers WA, Blömeke B, Coenraads P-J, Schuttelaar M-LA. Co-sensitization to ascaridole and tea tree oil. Contact Dermatitis 2013;69:187-189

85 Scardamaglia L, Nixon R, Fewings J. Compound tincture of benzoin: a common contact allergen? Australas J Dermatol 2005;44:180-184

86 Warshaw EM, Maibach HI, Taylor JS, Sasseville D, DeKoven JG, Zirwas MJ, et al. North American Contact Dermatitis Group patch test results: 2011-2012. Dermatitis 2015;26:49-59

87 Selvaag E, Eriksen B, Thune P. Contact allergy due to tea tree oil and cross-sensitization to colophony. Contact Dermatitis 1994;31:124-125

88 Nardelli A, Drieghe J, Claes L, Boey L, Goossens A. Fragrance allergens in 'specific' cosmetic products. Contact Dermatitis 2011;64:212-219

89 Toholka R, Wang Y-S, Tate B, Tam M, Cahill J, Palmer A, Nixon R. The first Australian Baseline Series: Recommendations for patch testing in suspected contact dermatitis. Australas J Dermatol 2015;56:107-115

90 Pesonen M, Suomela S, Kuuliala O, Henriks-Eckerman M-L, Aalto-Korte K. Occupational contact dermatitis caused by D-limonene. Contact Dermatitis 2014;71:273-279

91 SCCP (Scientific Committee on Consumer Products). Opinion on tea tree oil, 7 December 2004, SCCP/08438/04. Available at: http://ec.europa.eu/health/ph_risk/committees/04_sccp/docs/sccp_o_00c.pdf

92 SCCP (Scientific Committee on Consumer Products). Opinion on tea tree oil, 16 December 2008, SCCP/1155/08. Available at: http://ec.europa.eu/health/ph_risk/committees/04_sccp/docs/sccp_o_160.pdf

93 De Groot AC, Schmidt E. Essential oils: contact allergy and chemical composition. Boca Raton, Fl., USA: CRC Press, Taylor and Francis Group, 2016 (ISBN 9781482246407)

94 De Groot AC, Schmidt E. Tea tree oil: contact allergy and chemical composition. Contact Dermatitis 2016;75:129-143

95 Santesteban Muruzábal R, Hervella Garcés M, Larrea García M, Loidi Pascual L, Agulló Pérez A, Yanguas Bayona I. Secondary effects of topical application of an essential oil. Allergic contact dermatitis due to tea tree oil. An Sist Sanit Navar 2015;38:163-167 (article in Spanish).

96 Hammer KA. Treatment of acne with tea tree oil (melaleuca) products: a review of efficacy, tolerability and potential modes of action. Int J Antimicrob Agents 2015;45:106-110

97 Mozelsio NB, Harris KE, McGrath KG, Grammer LC. Immediate systemic hypersensitivity reaction associated with topical application of Australian tee tree oil. Allergy Asthma 2003;24:73-75

98 Sabroe RA, Holden CR, Gawkrodger DJ. Contact allergy to essential oils cannot always be predicted from allergy to fragrance markers in the baseline series. Contact Dermatitis 2016;74:236-241

99 Henley DV, Lipson N, Korach KS, Bloch CA. Brief report - Prepubertal gynecomastia linked to lavender and tea tree oils. N Engl J Med 2007;356:479-485

100 Posadzki P, Alotaibi A, Ernst E. Adverse effects of aromatherapy: a systematic review of case reports and case series. Int J Risk Saf Med 2012;24:147-161

101 Verma A, Tancharoen C, Tam MM, Nixon R. Pustular allergic contact dermatitis caused by fragrances. Contact Dermatitis 2015;72:245-248

102 Storan ER, Nolan U, Kirby B. Allergic contact dermatitis caused by the tea tree oil-containing hydrogel Burnshield®. Contact Dermatitis 2016;74:309-310

103 Gilissen L, Huygens S, Goossens A. Allergic contact dermatitis caused by topical herbal remedies: importance of patch testing with the patients' own products. Contact Dermatitis 2018;78:177-184

104 Warshaw EM, Zug KA, Belsito DV, Fowler JF Jr, DeKoven JG, Sasseville D, et al. Positive patch-test reactions to essential oils in consecutive patients: Results from North America and Central Europe. Dermatitis 2017;28:246-252

105 DeKoven JG, Warshaw EM, Belsito DV, Sasseville D, Maibach HI, Taylor JS, et al. North American Contact Dermatitis Group Patch Test Results: 2013-2014. Dermatitis 2017;28:33-46

106 Hagen SL, Grey KR, Warshaw EM. Patch testing to essential oils. Dermatitis 2016;27:382-384

107 DeKoven JG, Warshaw EM, Zug KA, Maibach HI, Belsito DV, Sasseville D, et al. North American Contact Dermatitis Group patch test results: 2015-2016. Dermatitis 2018;29:297-309

108 Veverka KK, Hall MR, Yiannias JA, Drage LA, El-Azhary RA, Killian JM, et al. Trends in patch testing with the Mayo Clinic standard series, 2011-2015. Dermatitis 2018;29:310-315

109 Nath NS, Liu B, Green C, Atwater AR. Contact allergy to hydroperoxides of linalool and *d*-limonene in a US population. Dermatitis 2017;28:313-316

Chapter 6.72 THUJA OIL

IDENTIFICATION

Description/definition	: Thuja oil is the essential oil obtained from the twigs with leaves of the (northern) white cedar, *Thuja occidentalis* L. and from other *Thuja* species, including *Thuja plicata*
INCI name(s) EU & USA	: Thuja occidentalis leaf oil
Other names	: Cedar leaf oil
CAS registry number(s)	: 90131-58-1; 8007-20-3
EC number(s)	: 290-370-1
RIFM monograph(s)	: Food Cosmet Toxicol 1974;12:843 (special issue I) (binder, 197)
SCCS opinion(s)	: SCCNFP/0392/00 (10); SCCNFP/0389/00 (11)
Merck Index monograph	: 10813 (Thuja)
Function(s) in cosmetics	: EU: masking; perfuming; tonic. USA: fragrance ingredients
EU cosmetic restrictions	: Regulated in Annex III/119 of the Regulation (EC) No. 344/2013
Patch testing	: 2% pet.; based on RIFM data, 4% pet. is probably not irritant (13)

GENERAL

Thuja occidentalis L. is an evergreen coniferous tree which grows up to 25 meter tall and one meter in diameter. It is native to Canada and the USA and is cultivated in China, Korea, Russia (European part), and Europe, often for ornamental purposes (2,12). One of its common names is 'Arborvitae', which is particularly used in the horticultural trade in the United States and is Latin for 'tree of life' - due to the supposed medicinal properties of the sap, bark and twigs. In folk medicine, *Thuja occidentalis* has been used to treat various diseases (2). It has a myriad of applications in Western herbal medicine, traditional Chinese medicine, homeopathy and aromatherapy. The pharmaceutical, pharmacological and clinical properties of *Thuja occidentalis* (products) have been reviewed (3,4).

Cedar leaf essential oil, made from the twigs with leaves of *Thuja occidentalis* L. by steam-distillation or hydrodistillation, has been used for perfumes, cleansers, disinfectants, hair preparations, room sprays, deodorants and soft soaps (2). It is also approved for use in food in the USA and the EU (5). It is still used in some mainstream over-the-counter preparations to relieve congestion in the upper respiratory tract, the best-known of which is Vicks VapoRub™. Thuja leaf oil is also added to pest repellant sprays and paints to protect against mites, moths, and rodents (4). The major constituent of the oil of *T. occidentalis* foliage, thujone, is used pharmacologically as active ingredient in the production of nasal decongestants and cough suppressants, perfumes, shoe polishes and soaps (1,2). Thuja oil is, however, considered too toxic (due to the high thujone content) for aromatherapy practices (6,7,8).

CHEMICAL COMPOSITION

Thuja oil is a clear, colorless to slightly greenish mobile liquid, which has a strong, fresh camphoraceous and greenish odor. In thuja oils from various origins, over 120 chemicals have been identified. About 42 per cent of these were found in a single reviewed publication only. The ten chemicals that had the highest maximum concentrations in 44 commercial thuja essential oil samples are shown in table 6.72.1 (Erich Schmidt, analytical data presented in ref. 12).

A full literature review of the qualitative and quantitative composition of commercial and non-commercial thuja oils of various origins has been published in 2016 (12).

Table 6.72.1 Ten ingredients with the highest concentrations in commercial thuja oils (12)

Name	Concentration range	Name	Concentration range
α-Thujone	47.8 - 66.3%	α-Pinene	1.4 - 3.6%
Fenchone	12.4 - 15.7%	Terpinen-4-ol	1.5 - 3.4%
β-Thujone (*cis*-thujone)	6.8 - 10.8%	(Z)-3-Hexenol	0.07 - 3.0%
δ3-Carene	0.7 - 8.2%	Limonene	1.1 - 2.7%
Sabinene	1.7 - 4.4%	Bornyl acetate	0.9 - 2.5%

CONTACT ALLERGY / ALLERGIC CONTACT DERMATITIS

General
Allergic contact dermatitis from thuja oil has been reported in one publication only.

Case reports and case series
One individual developed erythema multiforme-like contact dermatitis from the application of thuja essential oil on hemorrhoids. He reacted to thuja oil (pure and 1% in petrolatum), the fragrance mix, colophony, juniper tar and pine tar, which are, with the exception of the fragrance mix, all tree products (9).

OTHER SIDE EFFECTS

Photosensitivity
Photosensitivity from thuja oil has been cited in ref. 13.

LITERATURE

1   Kamdem PD, Hanover JW, Gage DA. Contribution to the study of the essential oil of *Thuja occidentalis* L. J Essent Oil Res 1993;5:117-122
2   Tsiri D, Graikou K, Poblocka-Olech L, Krauze-Baranowska M, Spyropoulos C, Chinou I. Chemosystematic value of the essential oil composition of *Thuja* species cultivated in Poland - antimicrobial activity. Molecules 2009;14:4707-4715
3   Naser B, Bodinet C, Tegtmeier M, Lindequist U. *Thuja occidentalis* (Arbor vitae): A review of its pharmaceutical, pharmacological and clinical properties. eCAM 2005;2:69-78
4   Brijesh K, Ruchi R, Sanjita D, Saumya D. Phytoconstituents and therapeutic potential of *Thuja occidentalis*. Res J Pharm Biol Chem Sci 2012;3:354-362
5   Jirovetz L, Buchbauer G, Denkova Z, Slavchev A, Stoyanova A, Schmidt E. Chemical composition, antimicrobial activities and odor descriptions of various *Salvia* sp. and *Thuja* sp. essential oils. Ernährung/Nutrition 2006;30:152-159
6   Rhind JP. Essential oils. A handbook for aromatherapy practice, 2nd Edition. London: Singing Dragon, 2012
7   Lawless J. The encyclopedia of essential oils, 2nd Edition. London: Harper Thorsons, 2014
8   Davis P. Aromatherapy. An A-Z, 3rd Edition. London: Vermilion, 2005
9   Puig L, Alomar A, Randazzo L, Cuatrecasas M. Erythema multiformlike reaction caused by topical application of thuja essential oil. Am J Cont Derm 1994;5:94-97
10 Opinion of the Scientific Committee on Cosmetic Products and Non-Food Products Intended for Consumers concerning 'An initial list of perfumery materials which must not form part of cosmetic products except subject to the Restrictions and Conditions laid down, 25 September 2001, SCCNFP/0392/00, final. Available at: http://ec.europa.eu/health/archive/ph_risk/committees/sccp/documents/out150_en.pdf
11 Opinion of the Scientific Committee on Cosmetic Products and Non-Food Products Intended for Consumers concerning 'The 1st update of the inventory of ingredients employed in cosmetic products. Section II: Perfume and aromatic raw materials', 24 October 2000, SCCNFP/0389/00, final. Available at: http://ec.europa.eu/health/ph_risk/committees/sccp/documents/out131_en.pdf
12 De Groot AC, Schmidt E. Essential oils: contact allergy and chemical composition. Boca Raton, Fl., USA: CRC Press, Taylor and Francis Group, 2016 (ISBN 9781482246407)
13 De Groot AC. Patch Testing, 4th Edition. Wapserveen, The Netherlands: acdegroot publishing, 2018 (ISBN 978-90-813233-4-5)

Chapter 6.73   THYME OIL

There are two major thyme oils: thyme oil obtained from *Thymus vulgaris* L. and oil of thyme containing thymol, Spanish type, obtained from *Thymus zygis* L. In botanical literature, including reports on contact allergy, nearly always the name 'thyme oil' is used, without specifying the botanical source.

6.73.1 THYME OIL (ex Thymus vulgaris L.)

IDENTIFICATION

Description/definition	: Thyme oil is the essential oil obtained from the flowering tops of the (English, common, garden) thyme, *Thymus vulgaris* L.
INCI name(s) EU	: Thymus vulgaris flower/leaf oil
INCI name(s) USA	: Thymus vulgaris (thyme) flower/leaf oil
CAS registry number(s)	: 8007-46-3; 84929-51-5
EC number(s)	: 284-535-7
RIFM monograph(s)	: Food Cosmet Toxicol 1974;12:1003 (special issue I) (binder, page 704) (thyme oil red)
ISO standard	: ISO 19817 Essential oil of thyme (*Thymus vulgaris* L. and *Thymus zygis* L.), thymol type, 2017; Geneva, Switzerland, www.iso.org
SCCS opinion(s)	: SCCS/1459/11 (14)
Merck Index monograph	: 8177 (Thyme)
Function(s) in cosmetics	: EU: masking; skin conditioning; tonic. USA: fragrance ingredients; skin-conditioning agents - miscellaneous
Patch testing	: 2% pet.; 5% alc. (25)

GENERAL

Thymus vulgaris L. (common thyme, garden thyme or just 'thyme') is a bushy, woody-based evergreen subshrub with small, highly aromatic, grey-green leaves growing to 15-30 centimeter tall by 40 centimeter wide. It is native to Italy, France, Spain and Morocco. The thyme is widely cultivated as a spice and medicinal plant in the Mediterranean area, Europe and many other countries (1,2,6). In Europe and North America the plant sometimes escaped from cultivation and became naturalized (16).

Thyme oil is obtained by steam-distillation of fresh or dried leaves and flowering tops of the plant (2). Most commercial oils are of the thymol chemotype and generally contain 35-55% thymol. This oil is considered to have various pharmacological activities. It is used in foods (not only to flavor, but also to preserve meat and fats) (3), cosmetics, perfumery (to create spicy, leathery notes) and pharmaceuticals such as oral hygiene products (3,4,5,6). In addition, It is extensively used in phytotherapy and aromatherapy, though usually in low concentrations in the case of high carvacrol content (8,16).

Health aspects and potential uses of *Thymus vulgaris* and its ingredient thymol have been reviewed in 2018 (26).

CHEMICAL COMPOSITION

Thyme oil is a colorless to dark red, clear mobile liquid which has a characteristic odor, ranging from aromatic, spicy and medicinal-phenolic, over citrusy fresh and aromatic, to natural floral, woody and herbaceous, depending on the chemotype. In thyme oils from various origins, over 325 chemicals have been identified. About 50 per cent of these were found in a single reviewed publication only. The ten chemicals that had the highest maximum concentrations in 25 commercial thyme essential oil samples are shown in table 6.73.1.1 (Erich Schmidt, analytical data presented in ref. 16).

A full literature review of the qualitative and quantitative composition of commercial and non-commercial thyme oils of various origins and their chemotypes has been published in 2016 (16).

Table 6.73.1.1 Ten ingredients with the highest concentrations in commercial thyme oils (16)

Name	Concentration range	Name	Concentration range
Carvacrol	trace - 77.8%	Geraniol	0 - 26.0%
Linalool	0.03 - 68.5%	α-Thujene	0.2 - 25.9%
Thymol	0.2 - 47.8%	*p*-Cymene	0.5 - 25.7%
1,8-Cineole	0.2 - 36.5%	Geranyl acetate	0 - 21.8%
cis-Sabinene hydrate	0.07 - 32.7%	γ-Terpinene	0.2 - 21.2%

6.73.2   THYME OIL SPANISH

IDENTIFICATION

Description/definition   : Thyme oil containing thymol, Spanish type (essential oil of thyme containing thymol,
                             Spanish type) is the essential oil obtained from the flowering tops of the Spanish thyme,
                             Thymus zygis L.
INCI name(s) EU and USA : Thymus zygis flower oil
Other names   : Red thyme oil
CAS registry number(s)   : 85085-75-2
EC number(s)   : 285-397-0
RIFM monograph(s)   : Food Cosmet Toxicol 1974;12:1003 (special issue I) (binder, page 704) (thyme oil red)
SCCS opinion(s)   : SCCS/1459/11 (14)
ISO standard   : ISO 19817 Essential oil of thyme (*Thymus vulgaris* L. and *Thymus zygis* L.), thymol type,
                             2017; ISO 14715 Essential oil of thyme containing thymol, Spanish type, 2008; Geneva,
                             Switzerland, www.iso.org
Merck Index monograph : 8177 (Thyme)
Function(s) in cosmetics : EU: masking. USA: fragrance ingredients
Patch testing   : 2% pet.; based on RIFM data, 8% pet. is probably not irritant (25)

GENERAL

Thymus zygis L. (Spanish thyme, sauce thyme, red thyme) is an evergreen shrub growing to 0.3 meter high. It is native to Morocco, Portugal and Spain (8). The Spanish thyme, notably the *gracilis* subspecies, is sometimes cultivated but is also collected on a large scale in the wild, for the production of leaves and essential oil (3,5). Spain is responsible for some 85% of the world's production of *Thymus zygis* products (2).

The flowering herb is employed in the production of Spanish (red) thyme essential oil, which is used as aroma in the food industry, utilized in the cosmetics and fragrances industries and also employed for pharmaceutical purposes (4). The oils with high thymol content are highly valued. Thyme oils are also employed in aromatherapy practices, but usually in low concentrations in case of high thymol content (6,7).

CHEMICAL COMPOSITION

Thyme oil containing thymol, Spanish type, is a yellowish to red clear mobile liquid, which has an intense aromatic – phenolic, spicy and slightly woody odor. In Spanish thyme oils from various origins, over 170 chemicals have been identified. About 47 per cent of these were found in a single reviewed publication only. The ten chemicals that had the highest maximum concentrations in 38 commercial Spanish thyme essential oil samples are shown in table 6.73.2.1 (Erich Schmidt, analytical data presented in ref. 16).

A full literature review of the qualitative and quantitative composition of commercial and non-commercial Spanish thyme oils of various origins, their chemotypes and with data from the ISO standard, has been published in 2016 (16). A 1960-1989 literature review on *Thymus zygis* L. and other *Thymus* species is provided in ref. 17.

Table 6.73.2.1 Ten ingredients with the highest concentrations in commercial Spanish thyme oils (16)

Name	Concentration range	Name	Concentration range
Thymol	39.2 - 56.2%	Camphene	0.3 - 4.2%
p-Cymene	12.8 - 25.4%	α-Terpinene	0.7 - 3.3%
γ-Terpinene	3.4 - 9.8%	Limonene	1.8 - 2.3%
Carvacrol	0.2 - 5.3%	β-Caryophyllene	0.6 - 2.2%
Linalool	3.2 - 5.2%	Borneol	0.3 - 2.1%

CONTACT ALLERGY / ALLERGIC CONTACT DERMATITIS

Thyme oil (unspecified)

General

The SCCS (Scientific Committee on Consumer Safety), in a 2012 Opinion on Fragrance allergens in cosmetic products, has categorized *Thymus* species as 'possible fragrance contact allergen' (14,15).

Contact allergy to thyme oil (botanical origin not specified) been reported in 6 publications. Routine testing has not been performed; there are some studies in which groups of selected patients were tested, but without data on relevance.

Patch testing in groups of patients

One positive patch test reaction to thyme oil was observed in a group of 51 patients (2%) allergic to Myroxylon pereirae resin (balsam of Peru) and/or turpentine and/or wood tar and/or colophony, tested with thyme oil 2% in petrolatum (10). Another group of 86 patients from Poland previously reacting to the fragrance mix was tested with thyme oil and four (4.6%) had a positive patch test reaction (11). In neither of these studies were data on relevance provided. In a group of 100 patients with ulcus cruris and tested with a special series including thyme oil, five (5%) had a positive patch test reaction; relevance is unknown (article not read) (13).

In Strasbourg, France, in the period 1967-1972, 276 patients with plant allergy were investigated. 'Thyme and niaouli oils' (test concentration unknown) reacted in 12 (4.3%) of the patients (22).

Case reports and case seriess

In one clinic in Belgium, in the period 1990-2016, three cases of dermatitis caused by contact allergy to thyme oil from its presence as active principle in 'topical botanical medicines' have been observed (24).

Additional information on contact allergy to thyme oil may be found in ref. 12 (article not read).

Thyme oil ex *Thymus vulgaris*

General

Allergic contact dermatitis from thyme oil obtained from *Thymus vulgaris* has been reported in one publication only. The patient reacted to 'sweet thyme oil', which probably is the oil from *Thymus vulgaris* of the linalool chemotype. Linalool and possibly α-pinene may have been allergens in the oil in this case report (9).

Case reports and case series

An aromatherapist had non-occupational contact dermatitis with allergies to multiple essential oils used at work, including sweet thyme oil. The patient also reacted to geraniol, linalool, linalyl acetate, α-pinene, the fragrance mix and various other fragrance materials; α-pinene and linalool were demonstrated by GC-MS in the thyme oil (9). Sweet thyme oil is presumably the essential oil obtained from the linalool chemotype of *Thymus vulgaris.* In commercial thyme oils, linalool concentrations of up to 68.5% have been found and α-pinene had a maximum concentration of 5.1% (16).

Spanish thyme oil

No reports on contact allergy to thyme oil, specifically mentioned to be obtained from *Thymus zygis*, have been found.

OTHER SIDE EFFECTS

Systemic side effects

A 12-month-old healthy girl may have developed systemic toxicity with irregular breathing, cyanosis and seizures from five prolonged baths containing an unknown quantity of essential oils of eucalyptus, pine, and thyme over a 4-day period for a benign and afebrile upper respiratory tract infection (23).

LITERATURE

1   Edris AE, Shalaby AS, Fadel HM. Effect of organic agriculture practices on the volatile flavor components of some essential oil plants growing in Egypt: III. *Thymus vulgaris* L. essential oil. J Essent Oil Bear Plants 2009;12:319-326
2   Arraiza MP, Andrés MP, Arrabal C, López JV. Seasonal variation of essential oil yield and composition of thyme (*Thymus vulgaris* L.) grown in Castilla—La Mancha (central Spain). J Essent Oil Res 2009;21:360-362
3   Omidbaigi R, Kazemi Sh, Daneshfar E. Harvest time effecting on the essential oil content and compositions of *Thymus vulgaris*. J Essent Oil Bear Plants 2008;11:162-167
4   Atti-Santos AC, Pansera MR, Paroul N, Atti-Serafini L, Moyna P. Seasonal variation of essential oil yield and composition of *Thymus vulgaris* L. (Lamiaceae) from south Brazil. J Essent Oil Res 2004;16:294-295
5   Baranauskiene R, Venskutonis PR, Viskelis P, Dambrauskiene E. Influence of nitrogen fertilizers on the yield and composition of thyme (*Thymus vulgaris*). J Agric Food Chem 2003;51:7751-7758
6   Echeverrigaray G, Agostini G, Tai-Serfeni L, Paroul N, Pauletti GF, Atti dos Santos AC. Correlation between the chemical and genetic relationships among commercial thyme cultivars. J Agric Food Chem 2001;49:4220-4223
7   Rhind JP. Essential oils. A handbook for aromatherapy practice, 2nd Edition. London: Singing Dragon, 2012
8   Lawless J. The encyclopedia of essential oils, 2nd Edition. London: Harper Thorsons, 2014
9   Dharmagunawardena B, Takwale A, Sanders KJ, Cannan S, Roger A, Ilchyshyn A. Gas chromatography: an investigative tool in multiple allergies to essential oils. Contact Dermatitis 2002;47:288-292

10   Rudzki E, Grzywa Z, Bruo WS. Sensitivity to 35 essential oils. Contact Dermatitis 1976;2:196-200

11   Rudzki E, Grzywa Z. Allergy to perfume mixture. Contact Dermatitis 1986;15:115-116

12   Escande JP, Foussereau J, Lantz JP, Basset A. Le problème des fausses sensibilisations croisées dans les allergies de groupe aux allergènes vegetaux. Rev Fr Allergol 1973;13:70-75

13   Le Roy R, Grosshans E, Foussereau J. Recherche d'allergie de contact dans 100 cas d'ulcère de jambe. Dermatosen in Beruf und Umwelt 1981;29(6):168-170

14   SCCS (Scientific Committee on Consumer Safety). Opinion on Fragrance allergens in cosmetic products, 26-27 June 2012, SCCS/1459/11. Available at: https://ec.europa.eu/health/sites/health/files/scientific_committees/consumer_safety/docs/sccs_o_102.pdf

15   Uter W, Johansen JD, Börje A, Karlberg A-T, Lidén C, Rastogi S, Roberts D, White IR. Categorization of fragrance contact allergens for prioritization of preventive measures: clinical and experimental data and consideration of structure–activity relationships. Contact Dermatitis 2013;69:196-230

16   De Groot AC, Schmidt E. Essential oils: contact allergy and chemical composition. Boca Raton, Fl., USA: CRC Press, Taylor and Francis Group, 2016 (ISBN 9781482246407)

17   Stahl-Biskup E. The chemical composition of thymus oils: A review of the literature 1960–1989. J Essent Oil Res 1991;3:61-82

18   Pérez-Sánchez R, Ubera JL, Lafont F, Gálvez C. Composition and variability of the essential oil in *Thymus zygis* from Southern Spain. J Essent Oil Res 2008;20:192-200

19   Sotomayor JA, Martínez RM, García, AJ, Jordán MJ. Thymus *zygis* subsp. *gracilis*: watering level effect on phytomass production and essential oil quality. J Agric Food Chem 2004;52:5418–5424

20   Amarti F, El Ajjouri M, Ghanmi M, Satrani B, Aafi A, Farah A, et al. Composition chimique, activité antimicrobiennne et antioxydante de l'huile essentielle de *Thymus zygis* du Maroc. Phytothérapie 2011;9:149-157

21   Lawrence BM. Progress in essential oils. Perfum Flavor 2008;(May):58-? (last page unknown)

22   Fousserau J, Meller JC, Benezra C. Contact allergy to Frullania and Laurus nobilis: cross-sensitization and chemical structure of the allergens. Contact Dermatitis 1975;1:223-230

23   Burkhard PR, Burkhardt K, Haenggeli CA, Landis T. Plant-induced seizures: Reappearance of an old problem. J Neurol 1999;246:667-670

24   Gilissen L, Huygens S, Goossens A. Allergic contact dermatitis caused by topical herbal remedies: importance of patch testing with the patients' own products. Contact Dermatitis 2018;78:177-184

25   De Groot AC. Patch Testing, 4th Edition. Wapserveen, The Netherlands: acdegroot publishing, 2018 (ISBN 978-90-813233-4-5)

26   Salehi B, Mishra AP, Shukla I, Sharifi-Rad M, Contreras MDM, Segura-Carretero A, et al. Thymol, thyme, and other plant sources: Health and potential uses. Phytother Res 2018;32:1688-1706

Chapter 6.74   TURMERIC OIL

IDENTIFICATION

Description/definition	: Turmeric oil is the oil obtained by steam-distillation from the dried root of the turmeric, *Curcuma longa* L., Zingiberaceae
INCI name USA	: Curcuma longa root oil
INCI name USA	: Curcuma longa (turmeric) root oil
CAS registry number(s)	: 84775-52-0; 8024-37-1
EC number(s)	: 283-882-1
RIFM monograph(s)	: Food Chem Toxicol 1983;21:839
Merck Index monograph	: 11275 (Turmeric)
Function(s) in cosmetics	: EU: perfuming; skin conditioning. USA: skin-conditioning agents - miscellaneous
Patch testing	: unknown; suggested: 2% and 5% pet.

GENERAL

Turmeric is a perennial tropical herb up to 1 meter high, with thick rhizome roots, which are deep orange inside. The plant is native to south-eastern Asia and extensively cultivated in India, China, Indonesia, Jamaica and Haiti. The main active ingredients of turmeric are curcuminoids and chemicals in the essential oil which are synthesized in the leaves and stored in the rhizome (3). Traditionally, turmeric has been used as a spice, in cosmetics, as coloring material and as flavor in the food industries (3). The root is used extensively in Chinese herbalism and as a local home medicine.

Turmeric essential oil is obtained by steam-distillation from the 'cured' rhizome – boiled, cleaned and sun-dried. It is employed in perfumery work for oriental and fantasy-type fragrances and also in aromatherapy (2).

CHEMICAL COMPOSITION

There is no description of the physical appearance, odor type and odor of turmeric essential oil available at www.thegoodscentscompany.com. It has been described as a yellowish-orange liquid with a faint blue fluorescence and a fresh spicy woody odor (2). The composition of turmeric essential oil is extremely variable. The main ingredients generally are ar-turmerone (up to 60%), α- and β-turmerone (together up to 49%, mostly α- > β-), ar-curcumene (up to 34%) and zingiberene (up to 17%) (4).

CONTACT ALLERGY

Case reports and case series

A male patient presented with a 2-week history of an itchy rash on both knees that subsequently spread to the neck, trunk, and arms. He had applied turmeric oil for approximately 14 days to his right knee for osteoarthritis pain. The patient had no preceding illness, herpes labialis, or change in medications. On examination, he was generally uncomfortable with a low-grade fever. The right knee had a sharply demarcated violaceous plaque with overlying scale and desquamation, at the primary site of turmeric application. At sites where the oil had not been applied, including the posterior neck, chest, abdomen, back, penile shaft, bilateral arms, and legs, there were erythematous targetoid papules and plaques.

Biopsies were obtained from both arms and pathology showed orthokeratosis, spongiosis, interface dermatitis, and Civatte bodies with perivascular and interstitial eosinophils. Thus, the clinical and histopathologic findings were consistent with erythema multiforme-like allergic contact dermatitis to turmeric oil. Patch testing to turmeric oil was offered for confirmation of the diagnosis but declined by the patient (1).

LITERATURE

1   Huber J, deShazo R, Powell D, Duffy K, Hull C. Erythema multiforme-like allergic contact dermatitis to turmeric essential oil. Dermatitis 2016;27:385-386
2   Lawless J. The encyclopedia of essential oils, 2nd Edition. London: Harper Thorsons, 2014
3   Mostajeran A, Gholaminejad A, Asghari G. Salinity alters curcumin, essential oil and chlorophyll of turmeric (*Curcuma longa* L.). Res Pharm Sci 2014;9:49-57
4   Lawrence BM. Progress in essential oils. Turmeric oil. Perfumer and Flavorist 2000;25:32-37

Chapter 6.75   TURPENTINE OIL

IDENTIFICATION

Description/definition	: Turpentine oil (essential oil of turpentine) is the essential oil obtained by steam-distillation of the gum resin of *Pinus massoniana* Lamb. (Chinese turpentine oil), *Pinus pinaster* Aiton (Iberian turpentine oil), and other *Pinus* species
INCI name(s) EU	: Turpentine, steam distilled (*Pinus* spp.)
INCI name(s) USA	: Turpentine (defined as: Turpentine is a mixture of terpene hydrocarbons obtained from various species of *Pinus*)
CAS registry number(s)	: 8006-64-2
EC number(s)	: 232-350-7
IFRA specification	: Essential oils and isolates derived from the Pinacea family, including *Pinus* and *Abies* genera, should only be used when the level of peroxides is kept to the lowest practicable level, for instance by adding antioxidants at the time of production; such products should have a peroxide value of less than 10 millimoles peroxide per liter, determined according to the FMA method (www.ifraorg.org/en-us/standards-library)
SCCS opinion(s)	: SCCNFP/0392/00, final (48); SCCNFP/0389/00, final (49); SCCS/1459/11 (50)
ISO standard	: ISO/DIS 21389 Essential oil of gum turpentine, Chinese type, 2003; ISO 11020 Essential oil of turpentine, Iberian type, 1998; Geneva, Switzerland, www.iso.org
Merck Index monograph	: 11277 (Turpentine)
Function(s) in cosmetics	: EU: perfuming. USA: external analgesics; fragrance ingredients; viscosity decreasing agents
EU cosmetic restrictions	: Regulated in Annex III/126 of the Regulation (EC) No. 344/2013
Patch testing	: 0.4% pet. (Chemo, hydroperoxides); 10% pet. (SPEurope, SPCanada); test also α-pinene (see Chapter 3.139 α-Pinene)

GENERAL

Turpentine oil (often simply called 'turpentine') is obtained by steam-distillation of the oleoresin of *Pinus pinaster* Aiton (Iberian turpentine oil), *Pinus massoniana* Lamb. (Chinese turpentine oil) and other *Pinus* species. What is left after distillation (the non-volatile residue) is called rosin (colophony, colophonium). Oil of turpentine formerly was widely used as paint-thinner and for cleaning paints brushes, but this application has largely been abandoned and has been replaced with other solvents. Turpentine oil is an ingredient in many liniments, cold remedies, and veterinary medications. It may also be used in topical NSAID pharmaceutical preparations.

Other commonly used products traditionally containing turpentine include varnishes, sealing wax, dry cleaning materials, shoe and floor polishes, printers' ink, and various adhesives, including adhesive tape (2,9,10,45). The oil is not applied *per se* in perfumes and cosmetics, but is used for the production of α- and β- pinene and limonene. Despite its strong terpeny odor and known risk of sensitization, turpentine oils may also be employed in aroma-therapy practices (47). In earlier days it was utilized for cutting pine needle oils and other oils with high concentrations of pinenes (adulteration).

CHEMICAL COMPOSITION

Chinese turpentine oil

Turpentine oil, Chinese type, is a colorless, clear mobile liquid, which has a strong terpeny and resinous odor. The ten chemicals that had the highest maximum concentrations in 52 commercial Chinese turpentine essential oil samples are shown in table 6.75.1 (Erich Schmidt, analytical data presented in ref. 52).

Table 6.75.1 Ten ingredients with the highest concentrations in commercial Chinese turpentine oils (52)

Name	Concentration range	Name	Concentration range
α-Pinene	57.1 - 74.4%	β-Myrcene	0.6 - 1.2%
β-Pinene	11.4 - 20.8%	Camphene	0.7 - 1.1%
Limonene	1.3 - 13.6%	β-Phellandrene	0.4 - 1.1%
β-Caryophyllene	0.9 - 4.1%	α-Terpineol	0.2 - 1.0%
Longifolene	0.1 - 2.1%	α-Terpinolene	0.05 - 0.9%

Iberian turpentine oil

Turpentine oil, Iberian type, is a colorless, clear mobile liquid, which has a strong terpeny, mildly coniferous, resinous odor. The ten chemicals that had the highest maximum concentrations in 47 commercial Iberian turpentine essential oil samples are shown in table 6.75.2 (Erich Schmidt, analytical data presented in ref. 52).

Table 6.75.2 Ten ingredients with the highest concentrations in commercial Iberian turpentine oils (52)

Name	Concentration range	Name	Concentration range
α-Pinene	68.2 - 81.9%	Camphene	0.04 - 1.9%
β-Pinene	4.8 - 17.3%	p-Cymene	trace - 1.7%
β-Caryophyllene	0.3 - 4.4%	α-Terpineol	trace - 1.2%
Limonene	0.5 - 3.9%	β-Myrcene	0.01 - 1.1%
Longifolene	0.1 - 2.4%	Pinocarveol	0.05 - 1.0%

As can be seen from tables 6.75.1 and 6.75.2, turpentine oils consist mainly of α-pinene, with variable amounts of β-pinene, limonene, β-caryophyllene, camphene, p-cymene, longifolene and myrcene. The relative proportions of these chemicals vary with the country of origin and the *Pinus* species from which the gum is obtained (5). An important variable is the amount of δ3-carene (should be low, as oxidized δ3-carene causes allergic reactions), which is high in turpentines from Scandinavia, the East-European countries, Russia and Indonesia (46) and low in turpentine oils from the south of France, Spain, Portugal and China (21).

CONTACT ALLERGY / ALLERGIC CONTACT DERMATITIS

General

The SCCS (Scientific Committee on Consumer Safety), in a 2012 Opinion on Fragrance allergens in cosmetic products, has marked turpentine (oil) as 'established contact allergen in humans' (50,51).

Turpentine oil is often loosely referred to as 'turpentine'. However, 'turpentine' does not always indicate the *essential oil of turpentine*, which is obtained by steam-distillation of the gum resin of *Pinus* species and which is also known as gum turpentine or balsam oil. Turpentine can also be a byproduct of the sulfate extraction process in which pine wood is converted into paper pulp. This oil (*not* essential) of turpentine is known as sulfate oil or sulfate turpentine (27). In literature on contact allergy to / allergic contact dermatitis from turpentine oil presented here (which is largely restricted to the period after 1975), a distinction between these two turpentine products can usually not be made.

Turpentine oil is both an irritant and a sensitizer. Old, oxidized turpentine is more irritating and sensitizing than is the freshly made product. When turpentine oil is allowed to stand, especially with exposure to light, oxidation results in the formation of formic acid and aldehydes, which may be irritating to the skin. Oxidation products of turpentine may also cause allergic contact sensitization (2,10). Indeed, up to the mid-1970s, occupational dermatitis from turpentine oil was well known in painters and home decorators, workers in the pottery industries (8), mechanics using impregnated soaps and shoe repairers (5,6,10). The main allergens were considered to be oxidation products of δ3-carene, δ3-carene hydroperoxides (also sometimes called turpentine peroxides), notably in oils from Sweden and Finland, which contained high concentrations of this component (7,8,10,28). However, other components were also allergens in turpentine oil, including α-pinene, dipentene (*dl*-limonene) and β-pinene (see below: The allergens in turpentine oil).

When turpentine oils rich in δ3-carene (from Sweden, Finland, Indonesia, Hungary, Poland, Russia) (21) were gradually replaced with oils with low concentrations of δ3-carene (Spain, Portugal, China) (4,21) and turpentine oil was also widely replaced with cheaper substitutes such as petroleum-based white spirit and other organic solvents, the incidence of allergic contact dermatitis to turpentine oil subsequently dropped (27,29,38). In 1979, turpentine peroxides (tested since 1972 instead of turpentine oil to avoid irritant reactions) were removed from the European standard series by the ICDRG (International Contact Dermatitis Research group) because of low rates of positive reactions (in 1975 and 1976 0.7% in 11,798 patients patch tested in 5 European countries and the USA) (27).

However, turpentine oil continued to be used in the pottery industry and Indonesian turpentine oil caused a cluster of cases of occupational contact dermatitis in 1996 in the UK (5). From 1996 to 1998, a sudden increase of rates of sensitization to turpentine oil was observed in Germany, Austria and Switzerland to 4.4% in 1998 (10). It was assumed that the oil of turpentine patch test was a surrogate marker for terpenes present in alternative cosmetic and medical products recovered from plants, e.g., tea tree oil, which showed frequent concomitant reactions with oil of turpentine (12). However, thereafter, the prevalence rates decreased again from 4.4% in 1998 to 1.6% in 2002 (11) and 1.95% in the period 1999 to 2012 (53).

Testing in groups of patients

General population
In the general German adult population, 2.5% of 1141 test subjects reacted to oil of turpentine, 4.3% of the women and 0.7% of the men (13). The estimated 10-year prevalence rate of sensitization to turpentine oil in the general German population in the period 1992-2002 varied from 0.3% (medium case scenario) to 0.8% (worst case scenario) (41).

Patch testing in groups of patients
The results of patch tests with turpentine oil in routine testing (consecutive patients suspected of contact dermatitis) are shown in table 6.75.3; those in groups of selected patients are shown in table 6.75.4. In routine testing, rates of positive reactions ranged from 1.2-4.2%, whereas between 0.8% and 58% (aimed testing in pottery workers with dermatitis) of patients in selected groups had positive patch tests.

Table 6.75.3 Patch testing in groups of patients: Routine testing

Years and Country	Test conc. & vehicle	Number of patients tested | positive		Selection of patients (S); Relevance (R); Comments (C)	Ref.
1996-2015 IVDK	10% pet.	143966	2952 (1.9%)	R: not stated	57
2009-2012, Germany, Austria, Switzerland, Finland	10% pet.	14,071	(2.2%)	R: not stated; C: range per country: 1.3-3.3%	55
1999-2012 IVDK	10% pet.	131,595	2568 (2.0%)	R: not stated	53
2007-2008 five European countries	10% pet.	6647	102 (1.5%)	R: not stated	3
2005-2008 IVDK	10% pet.	37,163	669 (1.8%)	R: not stated	15
2004-2008 Iran	10% pet.	469	7 (1.5%)	R: not stated	44
2002-2003 some European countries	10% pet.	3767	60 (1.6%)	R: not stated; rates ranged from 0.4% to 4.3% in various centers (both in Germany)	14
1996-2002 IVDK	10% pet.	60,737	1595 (2.6%)	R: not stated; annual prevalence was highest in 1998 (4.4%) and thereafter declined to 1.95% in 1999-2012 (53)	11
1992-1997 IVDK	10% pet.	45,005	560 (1.2%)	R: not specified; C: the prevalence rates were low from 1992-1995 (0.3-0.6%), but rose to 1.8% in 1996 and 3.2% in 1997; the cause of this increase was unknown	10
1984-1988 five East-European countries	10% o.o.	48,020	887 (1.8%)	R: not specified; 30% of the patients from Poland co-reacted to pine needle oil, which also contains high concentrations of α-pinene	21
<1986, Spain	?	1610	67 (4.2%)	R: not specified, but occupations were mentioned, including 7 painters; Scandinavian turpentine was used for patch testing; there were 36 co-reactions to α-pinene, 25 to β-pinene, 16 to δ3-carene, 7 to l-limonene and 5 to d-limonene in patients allergic to turpentine	22
1979-1983 five East-European countries	10% o.o.	36,431	596 (1.6%)	R: not specified	21
1979-1983 Portugal	10% pet.	4316	99 (2.3%)	R: not stated; C: the prevalence of sensitization declined steadily from 3.6% in 1979 to 1.3% in 1983; turpentine oil from Portugal is made from P. pinaster and P. pinea, both of which do not contain δ3-carene; 22 patients allergic to turpentine oils were tested with a number of its ingredients and δ3-carene; there were 17 reactions to α-pinene, 15 to dipentene (dl-limonene), 4 to δ3-carene, 3 to α-terpineol and 2 to β-pinene	4
1973-1977 Denmark	?	3225	45 (1.4%)	R: not stated	26
1973-1977 Spain	10% lanette wax	4600	35 (0.8%)	R: not stated	25
1972-1976 Canada	1% o.o.	1075	28 (2.6%)	R: not stated	24

Table 6.75.4 Patch testing in groups of patients: Selected patient groups

Years and Country	Test conc. & vehicle	Number of patients tested	positive	Selection of patients (S); Relevance (R); Comments (C)	Ref.
2003-2014 IVDK	10% pet.	5202	(3.1%)	S: patients with stasis dermatitis / chronic leg ulcers; R: not stated; C: percentage of reactions significantly higher than in a control group of routine testing	54
2003-2012 IVDK	10% pet.	2046	36 (1.8%)	S: nurses with occupational contact dermatitis; R: not stated; C: the prevalence did not differ significantly from the group of nurses without occupational contact dermatitis	39
1996-2009 IVDK	10% pet.	744	17 (2.3%)	S: the group consisted of female cleaners; R: not stated; the rate of positive reactions was not higher than in control groups of females (without cleaners) with occupational contact dermatitis and females without occupational contact dermatitis	17
1993-2003 IVDK	10% pet.	1224	15 (1.2%)	S: patients with scalp dermatitis; R: not specified	42
1998-2002 IVDK	10% pet.	304	18 (5.9%)	S: patients with a positive patch test to skin care creams; R: not stated; C: this percentage was significantly higher than in the group of patients who did *not* react to skin creams (2.9%)	18
1998-2002 IVDK	10% pet.	70	6 (8.6%)	S: patients with a positive patch test to bath and shower products; R: not stated; C: the percentage was higher than in patients without positive reactions to bath and shower products (3.5%), but the difference was not significant	18
1995-1999 IVDK	10% pet.	969	21 (2.2%)	S: patients with periorbital allergic contact dermatitis; R: not stated; C: the percentage positives was about the same as in patients with dermatitis other than periorbital	1
<1996 UK	10% pet.	24	14 (58%)	S: patients with occupational hand dermatitis working in the pottery industry and exposed to Indonesian turpentine oil; 7 co-reacted to α-pinene, 4 to δ3-carene	5
1975-1980 Denmark	?	?	36 (?)	S: not specified for this particular allergen; R: 39%, of which 36% was occupational (occupations not specified)	16

IVDK Information Network of Departments of Dermatology, Germany, Switzerland, Austria (www.ivdk.org); o.o.: olive oil; pet.: petrolatum

Case reports and case series

Occupational allergic contact dermatitis

An artist painter developed occupational hand dermatitis from contact allergy to turpentine oil he used to dilute paints and clean brushes (2). A porcelain painter had occupational allergic contact dermatitis due to oil of turpentine, oil of aniseed and lavender oil, that were mixed with pigments for painting (19). In a group of 37 painters, varnishers and lacquerers seen between 1970 and 1993 in a clinic and Portugal and suspected of occupational contact dermatitis, 8 (22%) reacted to turpentine, which reactions were probably (but not implicitly) being considered relevant (20).

Occupational contact dermatitis of the hands developed in a patient working in a laboratory and handling the oil at work; later, he developed stomatitis from pharmaceutical products containing peppermint oil; he reacted to turpentine peroxides, peppermint oil, limonene (*d*- and *l*-) and α-pinene, chemicals which are present in both peppermint and turpentine oils (32). An oil painter had contact allergy to turpentine and developed dermatitis from its use at work; he also reacted to epoxy resin in a spray varnish (36).

Non-occupational allergic contact dermatitis

A woman developed hand dermatitis from washing the clothes of her husband, which were impregnated with an NSAID-solution, that he used daily as sports trainer; the patient reacted to the topical pharmaceutical product and its ingredient oil of turpentine (9). Two patients had allergic contact dermatitis from turpentine in topical pharmaceutical products (30). Hand dermatitis from contact allergy to Portuguese turpentine oil in a paint brush cleaner developed in a patient who painted his own house (31).

A patient developed allergic contact dermatitis from the scalp, trunk and hands from turpentine present in a hair piece adhesive (34). Two out of three patients known to be sensitive to turpentine developed perianal dermatitis when suppositories containing turpentine were inserted (35). One case of airborne allergic contact dermatitis from turpentine in a patient who had previously worked as a painter has been described (43). A hobby painter developed allergic contact dermatitis from turpentine oil used to dilute paints and clean brushes (45).

Miscellaneous

In a number of publications, positive patch tests to turpentine oil have been reported with unknown, uncertain or unstated relevance. These include (literature screened up to 2014 [52]) the following. In a group of 460 patients who were considered to have positive patch tests related to cosmetics, 37 (8%) had positive tests to turpentine (23). One positive patch test to turpentine oil occurred in a car mechanic and painter, who had allergic contact dermatitis from wax polish; the patient reacted to its ingredients pine oil and dipentene (d,l-limonene); turpentine oil also contains limonene and is obtained from Pinus species, just as pine oil (40).

The allergens in turpentine oil

Traditionally, δ3-carene hydroperoxides are considered to be the main allergens in turpentine oil, at least in Scandinavian turpentine oil (7). There can be no doubt, however, that there are also other sensitizers, some of which are important. Already in 1957 it was shown that oxidized limonene could elicit positive reactions in patients sensitized to turpentine (37). In Spain, where mainly Scandinavian turpentine was used, 67 patients allergic to turpentine oil were tested with a battery of its ingredients. There were 36 reactions to α-pinene (15% in olive oil), 25 to β-pinene (15% in olive oil), 16 to δ3-carene (15% in olive oil), 7 to l-limonene (1% in alcohol) and 5 to d-limonene (1% in alcohol) (22). In Portugal, of 22 turpentine-allergic patients, 17 reacted to α-pinene, 15 to dipentene (dl-limonene), 3 to α-terpineol, 2 to β-pinene and 4 to δ3-carene. Portugal was an important producer of turpentine oil with low or no δ3-carene content, obtained from P. pinaster and P. pinea (4).

In 14 pottery workers with occupational contact dermatitis after contact with Indonesian (high δ3-carene concentration) turpentine oil, 7 co-reacted to α-pinene and 4 to δ3-carene (5). Of 40 Polish patients allergic to turpentine oil and tested with both Polish turpentine (high carene content) and Chinese turpentine oil (no carenes), 19 reacted to both (probably pinenes and limonene as allergens) and 17 only to Polish turpentine (presumably δ3-carene as the allergen) (21). Thus, it appears that α-pinene may be equally important if not more important than δ3-carene as contact allergen in turpentine oils. In Bulgarian turpentine oil, α-phellandrene was shown to be a sensitizer (33).

OTHER SIDE EFFECTS

Immediate contact reactions

Immediate contact reactions (contact urticaria) from 'turpentine' have been cited in ref. 56.

LITERATURE

1   Herbst RA, Uter W, Pirker C, Geier J, Frosch PJ. Allergic and non-allergic periorbital dermatitis: patch test results of the Information Network of the Departments of Dermatology during a 5-year period. Contact Dermatitis 2004;51:13-19

2   Laube S, Tan BB. Contact dermatitis from turpentine in a painter. Contact Dermatitis 2004;51:41-42

3   Uter W, Aberer W, Armario-Hita JC, Fernandez-Vozmediano JM, Ayala F, Balato A, et al. Current patch test results with the European baseline series and extensions to it from the 'European Surveillance System on Contact Allergy' network, 2007–2008. Contact Dermatitis 2012;67:9-19

4   Cachao P, Menezes Brandao F, Carmo M, Frazao S, Silva M. Allergy to oil of turpentine in Portugal. Contact Dermatitis 1986;14:205-208

5   Lear JT, Heagerty AH, Tan BB, Smith AG, English JS. Transient re-emergence of oil of turpentine allergy in the pottery industry. Contact Dermatitis 1996;35:169-172

6   Pirilä V, Pirilä L. Terpentinallergie. Berufsdermatosen 1964;12:163-167

7   Pirilä V, Kilpio O, Olkknen A, Pirilä L, Siltanen E. On the chemical nature of the eczematogens in oil of turpentine. V. Dermatologica 1969;139:183-194

8   Benezra C, Fousserea J, Maleville J. L'identification chimique des allergènes vegetaux et son interêt dans la prévention de nombreux eczémas allergiques professionels. Maladies Professionelles de Médecine du Travail et de Sécurite Sociale 1970;31:539-543 (data cited in ref. 5)

9   Borrego L, Hernandez N, Martel R, Almeida P. Turpentine sensitization in a nonsteroidal anti-inflammatory solution user. Dermatitis 2012;23:182-183

10 Treudler R, Richter G, Geier J, Schnuch A, Orfanos CE, Tebbe B. Increase in sensitization to oil of turpentine: recent data from a multicenter study on 45,005 patients from the German-Austrian information network of departments of dermatology (IVDK). Contact Dermatitis 2000;42:68-73

11 Schnuch A, Lessmann H, Geier J, Frosch PJ, Uter W. Contact allergy to fragrances: frequencies of sensitization from 1996 to 2002. Results of the IVDK. Contact Dermatitis 2004;50:65-76

12 Pirker C, Hausen BM, Uter W, Hillen U, Brasch J, Bayerl C, et al. Sensitization to tea tree oil in Germany and Austria. A multicenter study of the German Contact Dermatitis Group. J Dtsch Dermatol Ges 2003;1:629-634

13 Schäfer T, Böhler E, Ruhdorfer S, Weigl L, Wessner D, Filipiak B, et al. Epidemiology of contact allergy in adults. Allergy 2001;56:1192-1196

14 Uter W, Hegewald J, Aberer W, Ayala F, Bircher AJ, Brasch J, et al. The European standard series in 9 European countries, 2002/2003 – first results of the European Surveillance System on Contact Allergies. Contact Dermatitis 2005;53:136-145

15 Uter W, Geier J, Frosch PJ, Schnuch A. Contact allergy to fragrances: current patch test results (2005 to 2008) from the IVDK network. Contact Dermatitis 2010; 63:254-261

16 Veien NK, Hattel T, Justesen O, Norholm A. Patch testing with substances not included in the standard series. Contact Dermatitis 1983;9:304-308

17 Liskowsky J, Geier J, Bauer A. Contact allergy in the cleaning industry: analysis of contact allergy surveillance data of the Information Network of Departments of Dermatology. Contact Dermatitis 2011;65:159-166

18 Uter W, Balzer C, Geier J, Frosch PJ, Schnuch A. Patch testing with patients' own cosmetics and toiletries – results of the IVDK, 1998–2002. Contact Dermatitis 2005;53:226-233

19 Vente C, Fuchs T. Contact dermatitis due to oil of turpentine in a porcelain painter. Contact Dermatitis 1997;37:187

20 Moura C, Dias M, Vale T. Contact dermatitis in painters, polishers and varnishers. Contact Dermatitis 1994;31:51-53

21 Rudzki E, Berova N, Czernielewski A, Grzywa Z, Hegyi E, Jirásek J, et al. Contact allergy to oil of turpentine: a 10-year retrospective view. Contact Dermatitis 1991;24:317-318

22 Romaguera C, Alomar A, Conde-Salazar L, Camarasa JMG, Grimalt F, Martin Pascual A, et al. Turpentine sensitization. Contact Dermatitis 1986;14:197

23 Romaguera C, Camarasa JMG, Alomar A, Grimalt F. Patch tests with allergens related to cosmetics. Contact Dermatitis 1983;9:167-168

24 Lynde CW, Warshawski L, Mitchell JC. Screening patch tests in 4190 eczema patients 1972-81. Contact Dermatitis 1982;8:417-421

25 Romaguera C, Grimalt F. Statistical and comparative study of 4600 patients tested in Barcelona (1973-1977). Contact Dermatitis 1980;6:309-315

26 Hammershøy O. Standard patch test results in 3225 consecutive Danish patients from 1973 to 1977. Contact Dermatitis 1980;6:263-268

27 Cronin E. Oil of turpentine – a disappearing allergen. Contact Dermatitis 1979;5:308-311

28 Pirilä V, Siltanen E. On the chemical nature of the eczematogenic agent in oil of turpentine. III. Dermatologica 1958;117:1-8

29 Foussereau J. Allergy to turpentine, lanolin and nickel in Strasbourg. Contact Dermatitis 1978;4:300

30 Nardelli A, D'Hooge E, Drieghe J, Dooms M, Goossens A. Allergic contact dermatitis from fragrance components in specific topical pharmaceutical products in Belgium. Contact Dermatitis 2009;60:303-313

31 Calnan CD. Turpentine in paint brush cleaner. Contact Dermatitis 1978;4:57-58

32 Dooms-Goossens A, Degreef H, Holvoet C, Maertens M. Turpentine-induced hypersensitivity to peppermint oil. Contact Dermatitis 1977;3:304-308

33 Michailov P, Berowa N, Zuzulowa A. Klinische und biochemische Untersuchungen über die berufsbedingten allergischen und toxischen Erscheinungen durch Terpentin. Allergie und Asthma 1970;16:201-205

34 Kanof NB. Eczematous contact dermatitis to turpentine signaled by a reaction to a hair piece adhesive. Contact Dermatitis 1977;3:108

35 Klaschka F. Allergy to turpentine: Examination of systemic trigger action. Contact Dermatitis 1975;1:319-320

36 Conde-Salazar L, Romero L, Guimaraens D, Harto A. Contact dermatitis in an oil painter. Contact Dermatitis 1982;8:209-210

37 Hellerström S, Thyresson N, Widmark G. Chemical aspects on turpentine eczema. Dermatologica 1957;115:277-286

38 Gollhausen R, Enders F, Przybilla B, Burg G, Ring J. Trends in allergic contact sensitization. Contact Dermatitis 1988;18:147-154

39 Molin S, Bauer A, Schnuch A, Geier J. Occupational contact allergy in nurses: results from the Information Network of Departments of Dermatology 2003–2012. Contact Dermatitis 2015;72:164-171

40 Martins C, Gonçalo M, Gonçalo S. Allergic contact dermatitis from dipentene in wax polish. Contact Dermatitis 1995;33:126-127

41 Thyssen JP, Uter W, Schnuch A, Linneberg A, Johansen JD. 10-year prevalence of contact allergy in the general population in Denmark estimated through the CE-DUR method. Contact Dermatitis 2007;57:265-272

42 Hillen U, Grabbe S, Uter W. Patch test results in patients with scalp dermatitis: analysis of data of the Information Network of Departments of Dermatology. Contact Dermatitis 2007;56:87-93

43 Dooms-Goossens AE, Debusschere KM, Gevers DM, Dupré KM, Degreef HJ, et al. Contact dermatitis caused by airborne agents: A review and case reports. J Am Acad Dermatol 1986;15:1-10

44 Firooz A, Nassiri-Kashani M, Khatami A, Gorouhi F, Babakoohi S, Montaser-Kouhsari L, et al. Fragrance contact allergy in Iran. J Eur Acad Dermatol Venereol 2010;24:1437-1441

45 Barchino-Ortiz L, Cabeza-Martínez R, Leis-Dosil VM, Suárez-Fernández RM, Lázaro-Ochaita P. Allergic contact hobby dermatitis from turpentine. Allergol Immunopathol (Madr) 2008;36:117-119

46 Sukarno A, Hardiyanto EB, Marsoem SN, Na'iem M. Oleoresin production, turpentine yield and components of *Pinus merkusii* from various Indonesian provenances. J Trop Forest Sci 2015;27:136-141

47 Lawless J. The encyclopedia of essential oils, 2nd Edition. London: Harper Thorsons, 2014

48 Opinion of the Scientific Committee on Cosmetic Products and Non-Food Products Intended for Consumers concerning 'An initial list of perfumery materials which must not form part of cosmetic products except subject to the Restrictions and Conditions laid down, 25 September 2001, SCCNFP/0392/00, final. Available at: http://ec.europa.eu/health/archive/ph_risk/committees/sccp/documents/out150_en.pdf

49 Opinion of the Scientific Committee on Cosmetic Products and Non-Food Products Intended for Consumers concerning 'The 1st update of the inventory of ingredients employed in cosmetic products. Section II: Perfume and aromatic raw materials', 24 October 2000, SCCNFP/0389/00, final. Available at: http://ec.europa.eu/health/ph_risk/committees/sccp/documents/out131_en.pdf

50 SCCS (Scientific Committee on Consumer Safety). Opinion on Fragrance allergens in cosmetic products, 26-27 June 2012, SCCS/1459/11. Available at: https://ec.europa.eu/health/sites/health/files/scientific_committees/consumer_safety/docs/sccs_o_102.pdf

51 Uter W, Johansen JD, Börje A, Karlberg A-T, Lidén C, Rastogi S, Roberts D, White IR. Categorization of fragrance contact allergens for prioritization of preventive measures: clinical and experimental data and consideration of structure–activity relationships. Contact Dermatitis 2013;69:196-230

52 De Groot AC, Schmidt E. Essential oils: contact allergy and chemical composition. Boca Raton, Fl., USA: CRC Press, Taylor and Francis Group, 2016 (ISBN 9781482246407)

53 Geier J, Uter W, Lessmann H, Schnuch A. Fragrance mix I and II: results of breakdown tests. Flavour Fragr J 2015;30:264-274

54 Erfurt-Berge C, Geier J, Mahler V. The current spectrum of contact sensitization in patients with chronic leg ulcers or stasis dermatitis - new data from the Information Network of Departments of Dermatology (IVDK). Contact Dermatitis 2017;77:151-158

55 Frosch PJ, Johansen JD, Schuttelaar M-LA, Silvestre JF, Sánchez-Pérez J, Weisshaar E, et al. (on behalf of the ESSCA network). Patch test results with fragrance markers of the baseline series – analysis of the European Surveillance System on Contact Allergies (ESSCA) network 2009–2012. Contact Dermatitis 2015;73:163-171

56 De Groot AC. Patch Testing, 4th Edition. Wapserveen, The Netherlands: acdegroot publishing, 2018 (ISBN 978-90-813233-4-5)

57 Claßen A, Buhl T, Schubert S, Worm M, Bauer A, Geier J, Molin S; Information Network of Departments of Dermatology (IVDK) study group. The frequency of specific contact allergies is reduced in patients with psoriasis. Br J Dermatol. 2018 Aug 12. doi: 10.1111/bjd.17080. [Epub ahead of print]

Chapter 6.76   VALERIAN OIL

IDENTIFICATION

Description/definition   : Valeriana officinalis root oil is the volatile oil obtained from the root of the valerian,
Valeriana officinalis, Valerianaceae (Caprifoliaceae)
INCI name(s) EU & USA   : Valeriana officinalis root oil
CAS registry number(s)   : 8008-88-6
EC number(s)   : 308-322-6
Merck Index monograph   : 11359 (Valerian)
Function(s) in cosmetics   : EU: masking; perfuming. USA: fragrance ingredients
Patch testing   : 2% pet. (10)

GENERAL

Valeriana officinalis L. (the common valerian) is a hardy perennial flowering plant, which reaches a height of 0.6-1.2 meter. It is native to western Asia (Iran, Turkey), the Caucasus, Siberia, China, Japan, Korea, Taiwan, and all across Europe; the valerian is naturalized elsewhere. Cultivars selected for high contents of pharmacologically active substances are cultivated in temperate Europe, Korea, Japan, as well as Africa and USA (9). The valerians are highly respected medicinal plants listed in many Pharmacopoeias (7). Their underground parts, the rhizomes and roots, contain pharmacologically active substances, notably the ester iridoids (also named valepotriates) valerenic acid, its derivatives and an essential oil (i.e. substances which can be obtained as an essential oil by hydrodistillation).

Valerian roots (*Valerianae radix*) and their isolates (including essential oils) are employed in folk medicine, modern phytotherapy and aromatherapy, but also as official drugs (2,5,6,7). They are widely used in western Europe and many other countries in the world, mainly for their sedative, calming and hypnotic effects (2,3,4,5). Valerian roots and its products may also be used for food flavoring, e.g., in ice cream, baked goods and condiments (3,7,9), rarely for perfumery (low concentrations, traces) and in cosmetic products (1,2,5,6), as poison antidotes and deodorants (4), as natural repellents of insects, pests, and some rodents (5,6) and in veterinary practice (2,5,6,7).

CHEMICAL COMPOSITION

Valerian oil is a yellowish-green to brownish yellow, clear mobile liquid when fresh, which turns into a dark-brown and viscous liquid when aging; it has a slightly aromatic, tobacco-amber and woody odor when fresh, but acidic sharp, cheesy and disgusting odor when older. In valerian oils from various origins, over 330 chemicals have been identified. About 50 per cent of these were found in a single reviewed publication only. The ten chemicals that had the highest maximum concentrations in 11 commercial valerian essential oil samples are shown in table 6.76.1 (Erich Schmidt, analytical data reported in ref. 9).

A full literature review of the qualitative and quantitative composition of commercial and non-commercial valerian oils of various origins has been published in 2016 (9).

Table 6.76.1 Ten ingredients with the highest concentrations in commercial valerian oils (9)

Name	Concentration range	Name	Concentration range
Kessanyl acetate	1.3 - 29.5%	Kessane	2.3 - 6.7%
Camphene	0.6 - 24.1%	Myrtenyl acetate	0.9 - 6.1%
Bornyl acetate	9.8 - 21.4%	β-Pinene	0.3 - 4.9%
Valerianol (kusunol)	6.3 - 19.8%	Borneol	0.06 - 4.3%
Valerenal	0.6 - 8.6%	β-Eudesmol	1.3 - 4.3%

CONTACT ALLERGY / ALLERGIC CONTACT DERMATITIS

General
Contact allergy to and possible allergic contact dermatitis from valerian oil has been reported in one publication only. A false-positive patch test reaction due to the excited skin syndrome cannot be excluded (8).

Case reports and case series
An aromatherapist had occupational contact dermatitis with allergies to multiple essential oils used at work, including valerian oil. The patient also reacted to geraniol, α-pinene, caryophyllene, the fragrance mix and various other fragrance materials. None of these were identified with GC-MS in the valerian oil sample (8).

REFERENCES

1 Huynh L, Pacher T, Tran H, Novak J. Comparative analysis of the essential oils of *Valeriana hardwickii* Wall. from Vietnam and *Valeriana officinalis* L. from Austria. J Essent Oil Res 2013;25:409-414

2 Seidler-Lozykowska K, Mielcarek S, Baraniak M. Content of essential oil and valerenic acids in valerian (*Valeriana offcinalis* L.) roots at the selected developmental phases. J Essent Oil Res 2009;21:413-416

3 Raal A, Arak E, Orav A, Kailas T, Müürisepp M. Variation in the composition of the essential oil of commercial *Valeriana officinalis* L. roots from different countries. J Essent Oil Res 2008;20:524-529

4 Pavlovic M, Kovacevic N, Tzakou O, Couladis M. The essential oil of *Valeriana officinalis* L. *s.l.* growing wild in western Serbia. J Essent Oil Res 2004;16:397-399

5 Safaralie A, Fatemi S, Sefidkon F. Essential oil composition of *Valeriana officinalis* L. roots cultivated in Iran. Comparative analysis between supercritical CO2 extraction and hydrodistillation. J Chromat A 2008;1180:159-164

6 Letchamo W, Ward W, Heard B, Heard D. Essential oil of *Valeriana officinalis* L. cultivars and their antimicrobial activity as influenced by harvesting time under commercial organic cultivation. J Agric Food Chem 2004;52:3915-3919

7 Asadollahi-Baboli M. Comprehensive analysis of *Valeriana officinalis* L. essential oil using GC-MS coupled with integrated chemometric resolution techniques. Int J Food Prop 2015;18:597-607

8 Dharmagunawardena B, Takwale A, Sanders KJ, Cannan S, Roger A, Ilchyshyn A. Gas chromatography: an investigative tool in multiple allergies to essential oils. Contact Dermatitis 2002;47:288-292

9 De Groot AC, Schmidt E. Essential oils: contact allergy and chemical composition. Boca Raton, Fl., USA: CRC Press, Taylor and Francis Group, 2016 (ISBN 9781482246407)

10 De Groot AC. Patch Testing, 4th Edition. Wapserveen, The Netherlands: acdegroot publishing, 2018 (ISBN 978-90-813233-4-5)

Chapter 6.77   VETIVER OIL

IDENTIFICATION

Description/definition : Vetiver oil (essential oil of vetiver) is the essential oil obtained from the roots of the vetiver, *Chrysopogon zizanioides* (L.) Roberty (synonym: *Vetiveria zizanioides* (L.) Nash)

INCI name(s) EU & USA : Vetiveria zizanoides root oil

Other names : Khas khas oil; khus oil; cus cus oil

CAS registry number(s) : 8016-96-4; 84238-29-9

EC number(s) : 282-490-8

RIFM monograph(s) : Food Cosmet Toxicol 1974;12:1013 (special issue 1) (binder, page 728)

SCCS opinion(s) : SCCNFP/0389/00, final (15); SCCS/1459/11 (23)

ISO standard : ISO 4716 Essential oil of vetiver, 2013; Geneva, Switzerland, www.iso.org

Merck Index monograph : 8178

Function(s) in cosmetics : EU: masking; perfuming; tonic. USA: fragrance ingredients

Patch testing : 5% pet. (11)

GENERAL

Chrysopogon zizanioides (L.) (synonym: *Vetiveria zizanioides* (L)), commonly known as vetiver, is a perennial grass of the Poaceae family, native to India. In western and northern India, it is popularly known as khus. Vetiver can grow up to 1.5 meters high and form clumps as wide. Unlike most grasses, which form horizontally spreading, mat-like root systems, vetiver's roots grow downward, two to four meter in depth. It can be found, either wild or cultivated, in a wide range of areas from highlands to lowlands widely spread in subtropical and tropical regions of Asia, Africa, Oceania, and Central and South America (18).

Steam-distillation of the roots produces vetiver essential oil. The oil is used as perfumery source, as an aroma in food and as flavor agent in some beverages (1-5,8,9,10). Essential oil of vetiver is one of the most viscous oils with an extremely slow rate of volatility, which makes it very persistent and one of the finest fixatives known. The oil and its constituents are used extensively for blending oriental type of perfumes and floral compounds and are a main ingredient in about one-third of all western quality perfumes and 20% of all men's fragrances (6). Vetiver essential oil is also very popular in aromatherapy. It has many claimed biological properties and may be used in the treatment of a wide variety of diseases (7,8).

CHEMICAL COMPOSITION

Vetiver oil is a yellowish to reddish brown viscous liquid, which has a woody, earthy, slightly dusty and balsamic odor. In vetiver oils from various origins, over 445 chemicals have been identified. About 55 per cent of these were found in a single reviewed publication only. The ten chemicals that had the highest maximum concentrations in 51 commercial vetiver essential oil samples are shown in table 6.77.1 (Erich Schmidt, analytical data presented in ref. 18).

A full literature review of the qualitative and quantitative composition of commercial and non-commercial vetiver oils of various origins and with data from the ISO standard has been published in 2016 (18).

Table 6.77.1 Ten ingredients with the highest concentrations in commercial vetiver oils (18)

Name	Concentration range	Name	Concentration range
Khusimol	4.8 - 18.8%	β-Vetispirene	0.8 - 5.2%
(*E*)-Isovalencenol	1.0 - 17.7%	Vetiselinol	1.5 - 4.9%
β-Vetivene	0.3 - 10.4%	γ-Vetivenene	0.2 - 4.8%
α-Vetivone (isonootkatone)	1.8 - 6.1%	Zizanoic acid (khusenic acid)	0 - 4.3%
β-Vetivone	1.9 - 5.7%	α-Cadinol	0 - 3.5%

CONTACT ALLERGY / ALLERGIC CONTACT DERMATITIS

General

The SCCS (Scientific Committee on Consumer Safety), in a 2012 Opinion on Fragrance allergens in cosmetic products, has categorized 'Vetiveria zizanoides extract' as 'possible fragrance contact allergen' (16,17).

Contact allergy to vetiver oil has been reported in two publications, and two possible cases of allergic contact dermatitis from the oil have been identified (in both of which false-positive patch test reactions due to the excited skin syndrome cannot be excluded) (11,12).

Testing in groups of patients

Two hundred dermatitis patients from Poland were tested with vetiver oil 2% in petrolatum and one (0.5%) reacted. The same authors also patch tested 51 patients allergic to Myroxylon pereirae resin (balsam of Peru) and/or turpentine and/or wood tar and/or colophony and two (3.9%) had a positive patch test; relevance data were not provided (13).

A group of 86 patients from Poland previously reacting to the fragrance mix was tested with vetiver oil and nine (10.4%) had a positive patch test reaction; relevance data were not provided (14).

Case reports and case seriess

An aromatherapist had chronic hand dermatitis and was patch test positive to 17 of 20 oils used at her work (tested 1% and 5% in petrolatum), including vetiver oil (11).

Another aromatherapist had occupational contact dermatitis with allergies to multiple essential oils used at work, including vetiver oil. The patient also reacted to geraniol, α-pinene, caryophyllene, the fragrance mix and various other fragrance materials, but none of these chemicals was identified by GC-MS in the vetiver oil sample (12).

LITERATURE

1 Mallavarapu GR, Syamasundar KV, Ramesh S, Rao BR. Constituents of south Indian vetiver oils. Nat Prod Commun 2012;7:223-225
2 Lavinia UC. Other uses, and utilization of vetiver: Vetiver Oil. Proceedings of the Third International Conference on Vetiver and Exhibition, Guangzhou, China, 6-9 October 2003. Beijing: China Agricultural Press, 2003:486-491. Available at: http://www.vetiver.com/ICV3-Proceedings/IND_vetoil.pdf
3 Martinez J, Rosa PTV, Menut C. Valorization of Brazilian vetiver (Vetiveria zizanoides (L.) Nash ex Small) oil. J Agric Food Chem 2004;52:6578-6584
4 Filippi J-J, Belhassena E, Baldovinia N, Brevard H, Meierhenrich UJ. Qualitative and quantitative analysis of vetiver essential oils by comprehensive two-dimensional gas chromatography and comprehensive two-dimensional gas chromatography/mass spectrometry. J Chromatogr A 2013;1288:127-148
5 Lawrence BM. Essential oils 2008-2011. Carol Stream IL: Alluredbooks, 2012:57-72
6 Schmidt E. Vetiveröl – Duft und Analytik. Forum 2008;32:41-43
7 Bharat B, Sharma SK, Singh T, Singh L, Arya H. Vetiveria zizanoides (Linn.) Nash: a pharmacological overview. Int Res J Pharm 2013;4:18-20
8 Balasankar D, Vanilarasu K, Preetha PS, Umadevi SRM, Bhowmik D. Traditional and medicinal uses of vetiver. J Med Plants Studies 2013;1:191-200
9 Gupta S, Dwivedi GR, Darokar MP, Srivastava SK. Antimycobacterial activity of fractions and isolated compounds from Vetiveria zizanioides. Med Chem Res 2012;21:1283-1289
10 Chou S-T, Lai C-P, Lin C-C, Shih Y. Study of the chemical composition, antioxidant activity and anti-inflammatory activity of essential oil from Vetiveria zizanioides. Food Chem 2012;134:262-268
11 Selvaag E, Holm J, Thune P. Allergic contact dermatitis in an aromatherapist with multiple sensitizations to essential oils. Contact Dermatitis 1995;33:354-355
12 Dharmagunawardena B, Takwale A, Sanders KJ, Cannan S, Roger A, Ilchyshyn A. Gas chromatography: an investigative tool in multiple allergies to essential oils. Contact Dermatitis 2002;47:288-292
13 Rudzki E, Grzywa Z, Bruo WS. Sensitivity to 35 essential oils. Contact Dermatitis 1976;2:196-200
14 Rudzki E, Grzywa Z. Allergy to perfume mixture. Contact Dermatitis 1986;15:115-116
15 Opinion of the Scientific Committee on Cosmetic Products and Non-Food Products Intended for Consumers concerning 'The 1st update of the inventory of ingredients employed in cosmetic products. Section II: Perfume and aromatic raw materials', 24 October 2000, SCCNFP/0389/00, final. Available at: http://ec.europa.eu/health/ph_risk/committees/sccp/documents/out131_en.pdf
16 SCCS (Scientific Committee on Consumer Safety). Opinion on Fragrance allergens in cosmetic products, 26-27 June 2012, SCCS/1459/11. Available at: https://ec.europa.eu/health/sites/health/files/scientific_committees/consumer_safety/docs/sccs_o_102.pdf
17 Uter W, Johansen JD, Börje A, Karlberg A-T, Lidén C, Rastogi S, Roberts D, White IR. Categorization of fragrance contact allergens for prioritization of preventive measures: clinical and experimental data and consideration of structure–activity relationships. Contact Dermatitis 2013;69:196-230
18 De Groot AC, Schmidt E. Essential oils: contact allergy and chemical composition. Boca Raton, Fl., USA: CRC Press, Taylor and Francis Group, 2016 (ISBN 9781482246407)

Chapter 6.78 YLANG-YLANG OIL

IDENTIFICATION

Description/definition	: Ylang-ylang oil (essential oil of ylang-ylang) is the essential oil obtained from the flowers of the ylang-ylang tree, *Cananga odorata* (Lam.) Hook f. et Thomson, forma *genuina*
INCI name(s) EU & USA	: Cananga odorata flower oil
CAS registry number(s)	: 8006-81-3; 83863-30-3
EC number(s)	: 281-092-1
RIFM monograph(s)	: Food Cosmet Toxicol 1974;12:1015 (special issue I) (binder, page 731)
IFRA standard	: Restricted (www.ifraorg.org/en-us/standards-library) (table 6.78.1)
SCCS opinion(s)	: SCCS/1459/11 (57)
ISO standard	: ISO 3063 Essential oil of ylang-ylang 'extra'; 'first'; 'second'; 'third', 2004; Geneva, Switzerland, www.iso.org
Merck Index monograph	: 11568 (ylang-ylang)
Function(s) in cosmetics	: EU: masking; perfuming. USA: fragrance ingredients
Patch testing	: 2% pet. (Chemo, SPCanada); 10% pet. (SPEurope)

Table 6.78.1 IFRA restrictions for ylang-ylang extracts

Category [a]	Limits [b]	Category [a]	Limits [b]	Category [a]	Limits [b]
1	0.05%	5	0.40%	9	5.00%
2	0.06%	6	1.30%	10	2.50%
3	0.27%	7	0.10%	11	not restricted
4	0.80%	8	1.80%		

[a] For explanation of categories see pages 6-8
[b] Limits in the finished products

GENERAL

Cananga odorata Hook. fil. et Thomson, commonly known as kenanga (Indonesia), ylang-ylang (Philippines), canang odorant (French) and cananga (English), is an evergreen medium-sized tree growing 10-30 meter in height. Its flowers blossom throughout the year and are very fragrant. The cananga is native to Malaysia and Indonesia, but is now naturalized to most of the larger Pacific Island groups, northern Australia, Thailand, and Vietnam. The tree has long been cultivated on a large scale in South East Asia and some islands of the Indian Ocean, mainly Madagascar and the Comoro Islands, for the production of essential oil from the flowers (59).

There are two forms of *Cananga odorata*: the forma *genuina* and the forma *macrophylla*. From both species essential oils are produced, mostly by steam-distillation of fresh mature flowers: cananga oil from the *macrophylla* form and the more precious ylang-ylang essential oil from *C. odorata* forma *genuina*. The applications of both oils, which were formerly considered to be identical and are still often used – incorrectly – as synonyms, are broadly the same. However, the ylang-ylang oil is generally preferred, notably in the fragrance industry.

Ylang-ylang oil is mainly used for fine (floral) fragrances, but also for other cosmetics including soaps and skin lotions and detergents. The oil may also be utilized as flavoring agent for beverages, ice cream, candies, chewing gums and baked goods. In folk medicine and aromatherapy, ylang-ylang oil is claimed to be useful for various diseases (59).

Traditional uses, phytochemistry, and bioactivities of ylang-ylang oil have been reviewed in 2015 (67).

Grades (fractions) of ylang-ylang oil

Ylang-ylang essential oil production has the particularity of relying on a fractionation based on distillation times, resulting in four to five grades (fractions) of oil that have different commercial applications: 'extra super', 'extra' (30 minutes distillation time), 'first' (2-5 hours), 'second' (6-10 hours), and 'third' (up to 12 hours). The commercial grades differ considerably in their chemical composition; the first fractions are the most valuable for the production of fine fragrances. There are also commercial 'complete' ylang-ylang oils, which result from 24 hours distillation of the flowers without removal of earlier fractions. Most of the oils on the market are mixtures of various fractions, but are sold as one particular fraction (59).

The various grades (fractions, qualities) of ylang-ylang oils have different compositions and there are different ISO norms for each grade. It should be realized, that there are no absolute boundaries between the various qualities and that overlap of a quality in some studies with different grades in other investigations may be considerable.

A full literature review of the qualitative and quantitative composition of commercial and non-commercial ylang-ylang oils of various origins with data from the ISO standards has been published in 2016 (59). Older reviews of ylang-ylang oils include refs. 1-5. It should be appreciated that there is a real possibility that, especially in older scientific literature, ylang-ylang and cananga oils have been mixed up.

CHEMICAL COMPOSITION

YLANG-YLANG OIL 'EXTRA'
Ylang-ylang oil 'extra' is the first (and most valuable) fraction of the essential oil obtained with 30 minutes distillation time. Ylang-ylang oil 'extra' is a clear mobile liquid with pale yellowish to darker yellow color, which has an intense exotic, somewhat jasmine-like, floral odor with an aromatic woody note in the background. In ylang-ylang oils 'extra' from various origins, over 190 chemicals have been identified. About 56 per cent of these were found in a single reviewed publication only. The ten chemicals that had the highest maximum concentrations in 51 commercial ylang-ylang 'extra' essential oil samples are shown in table 6.78.2 (Erich Schmidt, analytical data presented in ref. 59).

Table 6.78.2 Ten ingredients with the highest concentrations in commercial ylang-ylang 'extra' oils (59)

Name	Concentration range	Name	Concentration range
Germacrene D	11.7 - 21.3%	β-Caryophyllene	3.6 - 10.1%
Benzyl acetate	3.8 - 16.9%	Geranyl acetate	2.9 - 9.4%
Linalool	5.8 - 13.5%	Benzyl benzoate	2.7 - 9.3%
p-Cresyl methyl ether	3.5 - 11.4%	Methyl benzoate	2.1 - 6.0%
(E,E)-α-Farnesene	5.6 - 10.3%	(E)-Cinnamyl acetate	1.3 - 5.6%

YLANG-YLANG OIL 'FIRST'
Ylang-ylang oil 'first' is the second fraction of the essential oil obtained with 2-5 hours distillation time. Ylang-ylang oil 'first' is a clear mobile liquid with pale yellowish to darker yellow color, which has a strong exotic, somewhat jasmine-like, floral odor with an aromatic woody note in the background. In ylang-ylang oils 'first' from various origins, over 145 chemicals have been identified. About 55 per cent of these were found in a single reviewed publication only. The ten chemicals that had the highest maximum concentrations in 12 commercial ylang-ylang 'first' essential oil samples are shown in table 6.78.3 (Erich Schmidt, analytical data presented in ref. 59).

Table 6.78.3 Ten ingredients with the highest concentrations in commercial ylang-ylang 'first' oils (59)

Name	Concentration range	Name	Concentration range
Germacrene D	13.6 - 15.8%	Methyl benzoate	4.5 - 5.6%
Benzyl acetate	12.0 - 15.1%	Geranyl acetate	4.4 - 5.5%
Linalool	9.8 - 11.3%	(E)-Cinnamyl acetate	3.9 - 4.6%
p-Cresyl methyl ether	8.0 - 10.7%	Benzyl benzoate	4.0 - 4.5%
(E,E)-α-Farnesene	8.1 - 10.2%	β-Caryophyllene	3.7 - 4.2%

YLANG-YLANG OIL 'SECOND'
Ylang-ylang oil 'second' is the third fraction of the essential oil obtained with 6-10 hours distillation time. Ylang-ylang oil 'second' is a clear mobile liquid with yellowish to darker yellow color, which has a typical exotic floral, somewhat jasmine-like, and woody odor. In ylang-ylang oils 'second' from various origins, over 120 chemicals have been identified. About 52 per cent of these were found in a single reviewed publication only. The ten chemicals that had the highest maximum concentrations in 42 commercial ylang-ylang 'second' essential oil samples are shown in table 6.78.4 (Erich Schmidt, analytical data presented in ref. 59).

Table 6.78.4 Ten ingredients with the highest concentrations in commercial ylang-ylang 'second' oils (59)

Name	Concentration range	Name	Concentration range
Germacrene D	12.2 - 26.4%	p-Cresyl methyl ether	3.5 - 11.4%
(E,E)-α-Farnesene	5.2 - 19.7%	Benzyl benzoate	4.3 - 11.0%
β-Caryophyllene	4.9 - 18.8%	Benzyl acetate	0.3 - 8.4%
Linalool	0.1 - 13.2%	Methyl benzoate	0.8 - 5.4%
Geranyl acetate	3.0 - 11.8%	(E,E)-Farnesyl acetate	1.2 - 4.9%

YLANG-YLANG OIL 'THIRD'
Ylang-ylang oil 'third' is the fourth fraction of the essential oil obtained with distillation times up to 12 hours. Ylang-ylang oil 'third' is a clear mobile liquid with yellow to yellow brownish color, which has a typical exotic floral, somewhat jasmine-like, and woody odor. In ylang-ylang oils 'third' from various origins, over 170 chemicals have

been identified. About 58 per cent of these were found in a single reviewed publication only. The ten chemicals that had the highest maximum concentrations in 22 commercial ylang-ylang 'third' essential oil samples are shown in table 6.78.5 (Erich Schmidt, analytical data presented in ref. 59).

Table 6.78.5 Ten ingredients with the highest concentrations in commercial ylang-ylang 'third' oils (59)

Name	Concentration range	Name	Concentration range
(*E,E*)-α-Farnesene	6.3 - 28.9%	Benzyl acetate	0.3 - 6.3%
Germacrene D	11.7 - 25.8%	Geranyl acetate	0.8 - 6.2%
β-Caryophyllene	5.2 - 16.3%	δ-Cadinene	2.2 - 5.6%
Benzyl benzoate	3.5 - 14.0%	(*E,E*)-Farnesyl acetate	1.3 - 5.5%
Linalool	0.5 - 6.7%	α-Humulene	1.6 - 4.6%

DIFFERENCES IN COMPOSITION OF THE VARIOUS QUALITIES (FRACTIONS) OF YLANG-YLANG OILS

The four fractions (qualities) of ylang-ylang essential oils differ mainly in the quantities of their main ingredients. This is readily shown in the ISO values for the four qualities: 'extra', 'first', 'second' and 'third'. The main constituents of the 'extra' quality ylang-ylang oils (upper ISO limits given) are linalool (24%), germacrene D (20%), benzyl acetate (17.5%), *p*-cresyl methyl ether (16.0%), (*E,E*)-α-farnesene (15.0%), and geranyl acetate (14.0%). For some of these chemicals, there is a steady decrease of their concentrations towards the quality 'third': linalool (from 24.0 to 4.0%), benzyl acetate (from 17.5% to 3.0%), *p*-cresyl methyl ether (from 16.0% to 1.4%), geranyl acetate (from 14.0 to 6.6%) and methyl benzoate (from 9.0% to 0.9%). Conversely, other chemicals increase in concentration from the 'extra' to the 'third' quality: germacrene D (from 20.0 to 35.0%), (*E,E*)-α-farnesene (from 15.0 to 29.0%), and β-caryophyllene (from 8.5% to 19.0%). Thus, the third quality is dominated by these three compounds: germacrene D, (*E,E*)-α-farnesene and β-caryophyllene. The other ingredients mentioned in ISO remain more or less stable in all fractions and/or are quantitatively less important.

CONTACT ALLERGY / ALLERGIC CONTACT DERMATITIS

General

The SCCS (Scientific Committee on Consumer Safety), in a 2012 Opinion on Fragrance allergens in cosmetic products, has marked ylang-ylang oil as 'established contact allergen in humans' (57,58).

Contact allergy to / allergic contact dermatitis from ylang-ylang oil has been reported in at least 60 publications. Ylang-ylang oil used to be a frequent sensitizer in Japan, causing many cases of pigmented cosmetic dermatitis. In the 1990s, the frequency of allergy to this oil decreased, presumably from the elimination of its main sensitizer, dihydro-isoeugenol (20,21). The oil (2% in petrolatum) has been included in the screening series of the North American Contact Dermatitis Group (NACDG) since 2001 and in 2010 (10% pet.) to the German baseline series (61).

In groups of consecutive patients suspected of contact dermatitis, prevalence rates of up to 2.5% positive patch test reactions have been observed, but percentages of 'definite' relevance and even 'probable' relevance are low. There have been 15 descriptions in case reports of allergic contact dermatitis from ylang-ylang oil; in 11, the cause was occupational exposure to the oil (8 in aromatherapists / massagists, 2 in workers in the cosmetic industry and one in a beautician). In one patient each, linalool and caryophyllene may have been an allergen in ylang-ylang oil.

A short review of contact allergy to ylang-ylang oil has been provided in 2016 (64).

Testing in groups of patients

The results of patch tests with ylang-ylang oil in routine testing (consecutive patients suspected of contact dermatitis) are shown in table 6.78.6 and those of testing in groups of selected patients in table 6.78.7. In routine testing, rates of positive reactions ranged from 0.7-2.6%, whereas between 0.8% and 38% of patients in selected groups had positive patch tests. The very high positivity rate of 38% was seen in a group of 21 patients with dermatitis caused by fragrances (54).

Table 6.78.6 Patch testing in groups of patients: Routine testing

Years and Country	Test conc. & vehicle	Number of patients tested | positive (%)	Selection of patients (S); Relevance (R); Comments (C)	Ref.
2015-2017 NACDG	2% pet.	5594 71 (1.3%)	R: definite + probable relevance: 18%	71
2013-14 USA, Canada	2% pet.	4859 59 (1.2%)	R: definite + probable relevance: 12%	65
2010-2014 IVDK	10% pet.	48,956 1175 (2.4%)	R: not stated	63
2009-14 USA, Canada	2% pet.	13,398 146 (1.1%)	R: of 35 patients reacting, but negative to FM I, FM II and balsam of Peru, 14% had definite + probable relevance	63
2011-12 USA, Canada	2% pet.	4230 30 (0.7%)	R: definite + probable relevance: 27%	42

Table 6.78.6 Patch testing in groups of patients: Routine testing (continued)

Years and Country	Test conc. & vehicle	Number of patients tested | positive (%)		Selection of patients (S); Relevance (R); Comments (C)	Ref.
2010-2012, Germany, Austria, Switzerland	10% pet.	9596	(2.8%)	R: not stated; C: range per country: 2.43-4.5%	61
2009-10 USA, Canada	2% pet.	4303	56 (1.3%)	R: definite + probable relevance: 27%	19
2000-2008 IVDK	10% pet.	3175	80 (2.5%)	R: not stated	41
2007-8 USA, Canada	2% pet.	5080	71 (1.4%)	R: definite + probable relevance: 17%	12
2000-2007 USA	2% pet.	870	8 (0.9%)	R: 100%; C: weak study: a. high rate of macular erythema and weak reactions, b. relevance figures include 'questionable' and 'past' relevance	6
2005-6 USA, Canada	2% pet.	4434	67 (1.5%)	R: definite + probable relevance: 15%	11
<2006 USA, Canada	2% pet.	1603	11 (0.7%)	R: definite + probable relevance: 0%	36
2003-4 USA, Canada	2% pet.	5137	64 (1.2%)	R: not stated	13
2001-2 USA, Canada	2% pet.	4893	49 (1.0%)	R: definite + probable relevance: 22%	37
1999-2000 Denmark	10% pet. (I)	318	5 (1.6%)	R: not specified; C: this study was part of the international study mentioned below (ref. 44)	55
	10% pet. (II)	318	6 (1.9%)		
1998-2000 six European countries	10% pet. (I)	1606	42 (2.6%)	R: not specified for individual oils/chemicals	44
	10% pet. (II)	1606	41 (2.6%)		
1998-9 Netherlands	4% pet.	1825	18 (1.0%)	R: not stated; C: 15/18 also reacted to the fragrance mix	46
<1976 Poland	2% pet.	200	4 (2.0%)	R: not stated	27

Case reports and case series

Occupational allergic contact dermatitis

Three massage therapists / aromatherapists with occupational contact dermatitis from (multiple) essential oils had positive patch tests to ylang-ylang oil; one patient had used the oil, in the other two it was uncertain (16). An aromatherapist developed occupational contact dermatitis from contact allergy to multiple essential oils; she reacted to both ylang-ylang and cananga oil in the fragrance series, which reactions were considered to be relevant (17).

Another aromatherapist developed occupational contact dermatitis from ylang-ylang oil; she also reacted to angelica oil and geraniol (24), which is not an important component of ylang-ylang oil. Yet another two aromatherapists had contact dermatitis (one occupational) with allergies to multiple essential oils used at work, including ylang-ylang oil; both patients also reacted to geraniol, α-pinene, the fragrance mix and various other fragrance materials. In addition, one proved to be allergic to linalool and linalyl acetate, the other to caryophyllene; α-pinene, linalool, and caryophyllene were demonstrated by GC-MS in many essential oils (25). Caryophyllene is an important component of ylang-ylang oil, which has been present in certain grades of commercial ylang-ylang oils in a concentration of 18.8%; linalool may reach concentrations >13%.

A massage therapist had occupational contact dermatitis from allergies to many essential oils including ylang-ylang oil, while cananga oil reacted in the fragrance series (28). A patient working in a cosmetic factory had occupational dermatitis from contact allergy to ylang-ylang oil in a fragrance mixture he was handling daily; he also reacted to aniseed oil, with which he had no contact (33).

A woman packing cosmetics developed occupational allergic contact dermatitis oil from ylang-ylang oil; she also reacted to other fragrance materials (22). A beautician developed occupational contact dermatitis from contact allergy to ylang-ylang oil in a massage lotion (29). An aromatherapist had chronic hand dermatitis and was patch test positive to 17 of 20 oils used at her work (tested 1% and 5% in petrolatum), including ylang-ylang oil (23).

Non-occupational allergic contact dermatitis

A patient developed allergic contact dermatitis from the perfume in an eye cream; she was patch tested with all 94 components of the perfume and reacted to ylang-ylang oil (test concentration unknown) and eleven of the other chemicals in the perfume (50). Two positive patch tests to ylang-ylang oil, possibly from its presence in topical pharmaceutical preparations, have been observed (56).

A woman presented with a 1-year history of dermatitis that began on her right medial calf after a shave biopsy. She subsequently developed an infection at the biopsy site and began treatment with MelaGel, containing tea tree oil. She developed a peri-incisional red, indurated, weepy plaque, which subsequently spread to involve her lateral leg. The patient reported using other essential oils on her skin as well in an aromatherapy diffuser. She had positive patch tests to ylang-ylang oil, MelaGel, tea tree oil, sandalwood oil and oregano oil, all of which she had used (66).

Another female patient presented with a 1-year history of dermatitis that began on the anterior shins and was treated with a variety of essential oils in coconut and sweet almond carrier oils. Her dermatitis initially improved but then flared again after a vacation during which she used essential oils. The patient also developed bilateral eyelid swelling and pruritus, which spread to involve her right ear and drained clear fluid. She used an aromatherapy diffuser at home and applied essential oils to herself and family members. The patient had positive patch tests to various fragrances, ylang-ylang oil, and a body lotion and ointment, both containing ylang-ylang oil (66).

Table 6.78.7 Patch testing in groups of patients: Selected patient groups

Years and Country	Test conc. & vehicle	Number of patients tested	positive (%)		Selection of patients (S); Relevance (R); Comments (C)	Ref.
2014-2016 USA	2% pet.	103	2	(2%)	S: patients tested with a screening fragrance series; R: not stated	72
2011-2015 Spain	2% pet.	607	29	(4.8%)	S: patients previously reacting to FM I, FM II, Myroxylon pereirae resin or hydroxyisohexyl 3-cyclohexene carboxaldehyde in the baseline series and subsequently tested with a fragrance series; R: not stated	70
2008-2014 UK	2% pet.	475	5	(1.1%)	S: patients tested with a fragrance series; R: not stated	68
2003-2014 IVDK	10% pet.	5202		(3.8%)	S: patients with stasis dermatitis / chronic leg ulcers; R: not stated	60
2003-2012 IVDK		917	23	(2.5%)	S: nurses with occupational contact dermatitis; R: not stated	62
2007-2011 IVDK	10% pet.	99	6	(6.1%)	S: physical therapists; R: not stated	69
2001-2010 Australia	2% pet.	1020	64	(6.3%)	S: not specified; R: 30%	52
2006-2010 USA	2% pet.	100	6	(6.0%)	S: patients with eyelid dermatitis; R: not stated	14
2004-2008 Spain	2% pet.	86	12	(13.9%)	S: patients previously reacting to the fragrance mix I or Myroxylon pereirae (n=54) or suspected of fragrance contact allergy (n=32); R: not stated	40
2000-2008 IVDK	10% pet.	2155	85	(3.9%)	S: patients with dermatitis suspected of causal exposure to fragrances; R: not stated	41
<2004 Israel	2% pet.	91	2	(2.2%)	S: patients who had shown a doubtful or positive reaction to the fragrance mix I and/or Myroxylon pereirae resin and/or one or two commercial fine fragrances; R: not stated	43
2001-2004 USA	2% pet.	611	17	(2.8%)	S: men with presumed cosmetic allergy; R: not specified	7
1989-1999 Portugal	2% pet.	67	9	(13.4%)	S: patients who had a positive patch test to the fragrance mix; R: not stated	45
1990-1998 Japan	5% pet.	1483	33	(2.2%)	S: patients suspected of cosmetic contact dermatitis, virtually all were women; range of annual frequency of sensitization: 0-4.3%; R: not stated	15
1989-1998 India	2% pet.	10	2	(20%)	S: patients previously reacting to the fragrance mix and/ or Myroxylon pereirae resin; R: not stated	47
1996-1997 UK	2% pet.	10	3	(30%)	S: patients strongly suspected of fragrance allergy; all also reacted to the fragrance mix; R: not stated	9
<1996 Japan, Ireland, USA, UK, Switzerland, Sweden	10% pet.	167	29	(17.4%)	S: patients known or suspected to be allergic to fragrances; R: not stated	10
<1986 Poland	2% pet.	86	8	(9.3%)	S: patients previously reacting to the fragrance mix; R: not stated	32
<1986 France	2.5% pet.	21	8	(38%)	S: patients with dermatitis caused by perfumes; R: not stated	54
1971-1980 Japan	5% pet.	477	4	(0.8%)	S: patients with dermatoses other than pigmented cosmetic dermatitis and volunteers; R: not stated	30
<1976 Poland	2% pet.	51	3	(5.9%)	S: patients allergic to Myroxylon pereirae resin (balsam of Peru) and/or turpentine and/or wood tar and/or colophony	27
<1974 Japan	?	183	25	(13.7%)	S: patients suspected of cosmetic dermatitis; R: unknown; in many, there was co-reactivity with benzyl salicylate, which may be present in commercial ylang-ylang oils in concentrations of up to 4.7% and to geraniol, which may reach concentrations of up to 2.0% in such oils	48

IVDK Information Network of Departments of Dermatology, Germany, Switzerland, Austria (www.ivdk.org); pet.: petrolatum

Miscellaneous

In a number of publications, positive patch tests to ylang-ylang oil have been reported with unknown, uncertain or unstated relevance. These include (literature screened up to 2014 [59]) the following. In a group of 819 patients suspected of contact dermatitis, four had positive patch test reactions to ylang-ylang oil (8). A naturopathic therapist and a masseuse with occupational contact dermatitis from various (other) essential oils reacted to ylang-ylang oil in the fragrance series (26). Positive patch test reactions to ylang-ylang oil were seen in three patients with allergic contact dermatitis of the lips (cheilitis) and the perioral skin from peppermint oil in lip balm (31).

A patient had hand dermatitis from contact allergy to geraniol and rose oil in a 'fragrance-free' hand soap; she also reacted to ylang-ylang oil and several other fragrances and essential oils (34). Four positive patch test reactions to ylang-ylang oil were observed in 7 patients with allergic contact dermatitis from compound tincture of benzoin (35). A beautician with occupational allergic hand dermatitis from products containing citral and certain essential oils co-reacted to ylang-ylang oil (38); citral (neral + geranial) is not an important component of ylang-ylang oil. Three positive reactions were seen to ylang-ylang oil, which was tested in seven patients out of a group of 63 who were patch test positive to their own shaving product/eau de toilette/perfume (39).

Two positive reactions were observed to ylang-ylang oil, which was tested in 43 patients out of a group of 819 who were patch test *negative* to their own shaving product/eau de toilette/perfume (39). Five female patients from India, two with facial hyperpigmentation, three with erythema of the face, reacted to ylang-ylang oil and other fragrances; two used aromatic oils on the face for headaches. In one a Repeated Open Application Test (ROAT) was positive. It was uncertain whether these products contained ylang-ylang oil (51). Of seven patients allergic to the fragrance farnesol, 3 (43%) co-reacted to ylang-ylang oil (and various other fragrances) (53).

Co-reactivity to cananga oil
Co-reactivity between ylang-ylang oil and cananga oil and vice versa is discussed in Chapter 6.11 Cananga oil.

Pigmented cosmetic dermatitis
In Japan, in the 1960s and 1970s, many female patients developed facial pigmentation following dermatitis of the face (18). This so-called pigmented cosmetic dermatitis was shown to be caused by contact allergy to components of cosmetic products, notably essential oils, other fragrance materials, antimicrobials, preservatives and coloring materials (18,30). In a group of 620 Japanese patients with this condition investigated between 1970 and 1980, 6-14% had positive patch test reactions to ylang-ylang oil 5% in petrolatum (30). In a group of 222 patients with pigmented cosmetic dermatitis investigated in the period 1975-1977, the rate of positive reactions was even 20% (20).

The number of patients decreased strongly after 1978, when major cosmetic companies began to eliminate strong contact sensitizers from their products, including dihydro-isoeugenol from ylang-ylang oil (20,21,30). Yet, even today cases of (presumed) pigmented cosmetic dermatitis from ylang-ylang oil are being reported (51).

LITERATURE
1   Fournier G, Leboeuf M, Cavé A. Annonaceae essential oils: A review. J Essent Oil Res 1999;11:131-142
2   Lawrence BM. Progress in essential oils. Perfum Flavor 1986;11:111-125
3   Lawrence BM. Progress in essential oils. Perfum Flavor 1989;14:71-80
4   Lawrence BM. Progress in essential oils. Perfum Flavor 1995;20:49-58
5   Ekundayo O. A review of the volatiles of the Annonaceae. J Essent Oil Res 1989;1:223-245
6   Wetter DA, Yiannias JA, Prakash AV, Davis MD, Farmer SA, el-Azhary RA, et al. Results of patch testing to personal care product allergens in a standard series and a supplemental cosmetic series: an analysis of 945 patients from the Mayo Clinic Contact Dermatitis Group, 2000-2007. J Am Acad Dermatol 2010;63:789-798
7   Warshaw EM, Buchholz HJ, Belsito DV, Maibach HI, Folwer JF Jr, Rietschel RL, et al. Allergic patch test reactions associated with cosmetics: Retrospective analysis of cross-sectional data from the North American Contact Dermatitis Group, 2001-2004. J Am Acad Dermatol 2009;60:23-38
8   Kohl L, Blondeel A, Song M. Allergic contact dermatitis from cosmetics: retrospective analysis of 819 patch-tested patients. Dermatology 2002;204:334-337
9   Thomson KF, Wilkinson SM. Allergic contact dermatitis to plant extracts in patients with cosmetic dermatitis. Br J Dermatol 2000;142:84-88
10 Larsen W, Nakayama H, Lindberg M, Fischer T, Elsner P, Burrows D, et al. Fragrance contact dermatitis: A worldwide multicenter investigation (Part 1). Am J Cont Derm 1996;7:77-83
11 Zug KA, Warshaw EM, Fowler JF Jr, Maibach HI, Belsito DL, Pratt MD, et al. Patch-test results of the North American Contact Dermatitis Group 2005-2006. Dermatitis 2009;20:149-160
12 Fransway AF, Zug KA, Belsito DV, DeLeo VA, Fowler JF Jr, Maibach HI, et al. North American Contact Dermatitis Group patch test results for 2007-2008. Dermatitis 2013;24:10-21
13 Warshaw EM, Belsito DV, DeLeo VA, Fowler JF Jr, Maibach HI, Marks JG, et al. North American Contact Dermatitis Group patch-test results, 2003-2004 study period. Dermatitis 2008;19:129-136
14 Wenk KS, Ehrlich AE. Fragrance series testing in eyelid dermatitis. Dermatitis 2012;23:22-26
15 Sugiura M, Hayakawa R, Kato Y, Sigiura K, Hashimoto R. Results of patch testing with lavender oil in Japan. Contact Dermatitis 2000;43:157-160
16 Bleasel N, Tate B, Rademaker M. Allergic contact dermatitis following exposure to essential oils. Australas J Dermatol 2002;43:211-213

17 Boonchai W, Lamtharachai P, Sunthonpalin P. Occupational allergic contact dermatitis from essential oils in aromatherapists. Contact Dermatitis 2007;56:181-182

18 Nakayama H, Harada R, Toda M. Pigmented cosmetic dermatitis. Int J Dermatol 1976;15:673-675

19 Warshaw EM, Belsito DV, Taylor JS, Sasseville D, DeKoven JG, Zirwas MJ, et al. North American Contact Dermatitis Group patch test results: 2009 to 2010. Dermatitis 2013;24:50-59

20 Sugawara M, Nakayama H, Watanabe S. Contact hypersensitivity to ylang-ylang oil. Contact Dermatitis 1990;23:248-249

21 Toyoda T, Watanabe S, Kawasaki M, et al. Dihydro-isoeugenol found in ylang-ylang oil. Skin Res 1989;31 (suppl.7):35-43 (in Japanese)

22 Kanerva L, Estlander T, Jolanki R. Occupational allergic contact dermatitis caused by ylang-ylang oil. Contact Dermatitis 1995;33:198-199

23 Selvaag E, Holm J, Thune P. Allergic contact dermatitis in an aromatherapist with multiple sensitizations to essential oils. Contact Dermatitis 1995;33:354-355

24 Keane FM, Smith HR, White IR, Rycroft RJG. Occupational allergic contact dermatitis in two aromatherapists. Contact Dermatitis 2000;43:49-51

25 Dharmagunawardena B, Takwale A, Sanders KJ, Cannan S, Roger A, Ilchyshyn A. Gas chromatography: an investigative tool in multiple allergies to essential oils. Contact Dermatitis 2002;47:288-292

26 Trattner A, David M, Lazarov A. Occupational contact dermatitis due to essential oils. Contact Dermatitis 2008;58:282-284

27 Rudzki E, Grzywa Z, Bruo WS. Sensitivity to 35 essential oils. Contact Dermatitis 1976;2:196-200

28 Cockayne SE, Gawkrodger DJ. Occupational contact dermatitis in an aromatherapist. Contact Dermatitis 1997;37:306-307

29 Romaguera C, Vilaplana J. Occupational contact dermatitis from ylang-ylang oil. Contact Dermatitis 2000;43:251

30 Nakayama H, Matsuo S, Hayakawa K, Takhashi K, Shigematsu T, Ota S. Pigmented cosmetic dermatitis. Int J Dermatol 1984;23:299-305

31 Tran A, Pratt M, DeKoven J. Acute allergic contact dermatitis of the lips from peppermint oil in a lip balm. Dermatitis 2010;21:111-115

32 Rudzki E, Grzywa Z. Allergy to perfume mixture. Contact Dermatitis 1986;15:115-116

33 Rudzki E, Rebandel P, Grzywa Z. Occupational dermatitis from cosmetic creams. Contact Dermatitis 1993;29:210

34 Scheinman PL. Is it really fragrance free? Am J Contact Dermatitis 1997;8:239-242

35 Fettig J, Taylor J, Sood A. Post-surgical allergic contact dermatitis to compound tincture of benzoin and association with reactions to fragrances and essential oils. Dermatisis 2014;25:211-212

36 Belsito DV, Fowler JF Jr, Sasseville D, Marks JG Jr, De Leo VA, Storrs FJ. Delayed-type hypersensitivity to fragrance materials in a select North American population. Dermatitis 2006;17:23-28

37 Pratt MD, Belsito DV, DeLeo VA, Fowler JF Jr, Fransway AF, Maibach HI, et al. North American Contact Dermatitis Group patch-test results, 2001-2002 study period. Dermatitis 2004;15:176-183

38 De Mozzi P, Johnston GA. An outbreak of allergic contact dermatitis caused by citral in beauticians working in a health spa. Contact Dermatitis 2014;70:377-379

39 Uter W, Geier J, Schnuch A, Frosch PJ. Patch test results with patients' own perfumes, deodorants and shaving lotions: results of the IVDK 1998–2002. J Eur Acad Dermatol Venereol 2007;21:374-379

40 Cuesta L, Silvestre JF, Toledo F, Lucas A, Pérez-Crespo M, Ballester I. Fragrance contact allergy: a 4-year retrospective study. Contact Dermatitis 2010;63:77-84

41 Uter W, Schmidt E, Geier J, Lessmann H, Schnuch A, Frosch P. Contact allergy to essential oils: current patch test results (2000–2008) from the Information Network of Departments of Dermatology (IVDK). Contact Dermatitis 2010;63:277-283

42 Warshaw EM, Maibach HI, Taylor JS, Sasseville D, DeKoven JG, Zirwas MJ, et al. North American Contact Dermatitis Group patch test results: 2011-2012. Dermatitis 2015;26:49-59

43 Trattner A, David M. Patch testing with fine fragrances: comparison with fragrance mix, balsam of Peru and a fragrance series. Contact Dermatitis 2004;49:287-289

44 Frosch PJ, Johansen JD, Menné T, Pirker C, Rastogi SC, Andersen KE, et al. Further important sensitizers in patients sensitive to fragrances. II. Reactivity to essential oils. Contact Dermatitis 2002;47:279-287

45 Manuel Brites M, Goncalo M, Figueiredo A. Contact allergy to fragrance mix - a 10-year study. Contact Dermatitis 2000;43:181-182

46 De Groot AC, Coenraads PJ, Bruynzeel DP, Jagtman BA, van Ginkel CJW, Noz K, van der Valk PGM, et al. Routine patch testing with fragrance chemicals in The Netherlands. Contact Dermatitis 2000;42:184-185

47 Gupta N, Shenoi SD, Balachandran C. Fragrance sensitivity in allergic contact dermatitis. Contact Dermatitis 1999;40:53-54

48 Nakayama H, Hanaoka H, Ohshiro A. Allergen Controlled System (ACS). Tokyo, Japan: Kanehara Shuppan, 1974:42. Data cited in ref. 49

49 Mitchell JC. Contact hypersensitivity to some perfume materials. Contact Dermatitis 1975;1:196-199

50 Larsen WG. Cosmetic dermatitis due to a perfume. Contact Dermatitis 1975;1:142-145

51 Srivastava PK, Bajaj AK. Ylang-ylang oil not an uncommon sensitizer in India. Indian J Dermatol 2014;59:200-201

52 Toholka R, Wang Y-S, Tate B, Tam M, Cahill J, Palmer A, Nixon R. The first Australian Baseline Series: Recommendations for patch testing in suspected contact dermatitis. Australas J Dermatol 2015;56:107-115

53 Goossens A, Merckx L. Allergic contact dermatitis from farnesol in a deodorant. Contact Dermatitis 1997;37:179-180

54 Meynadier JM, Meynadier J, Peyron JL, Peyron L. Formes cliniques des manifestations cutanées d'allergie aux parfums. Ann Dermatol Venereol 1986;113:31-39

55 Paulsen E, Andersen KE. Colophonium and Compositae mix as markers of fragrance allergy: Cross-reactivity between fragrance terpenes, colophonium and Compositae plant extracts. Contact Dermatitis 2005;53:285-291

56 Nardelli A, D'Hooge E, Drieghe J, Dooms M, Goossens A. Allergic contact dermatitis from fragrance components in specific topical pharmaceutical products in Belgium. Contact Dermatitis 2009;60:303-313

57 SCCS (Scientific Committee on Consumer Safety). Opinion on Fragrance allergens in cosmetic products, 26-27 June 2012, SCCS/1459/11. Available at: https://ec.europa.eu/health/sites/health/files/scientific_committees/consumer_safety/docs/sccs_o_102.pdf

58 Uter W, Johansen JD, Börje A, Karlberg A-T, Lidén C, Rastogi S, Roberts D, White IR. Categorization of fragrance contact allergens for prioritization of preventive measures: clinical and experimental data and consideration of structure–activity relationships. Contact Dermatitis 2013;69:196-230

59 De Groot AC, Schmidt E. Essential oils: contact allergy and chemical composition. Boca Raton, Fl., USA: CRC Press, Taylor and Francis Group, 2016 (ISBN 9781482246407)

60 Erfurt-Berge C, Geier J, Mahler V. The current spectrum of contact sensitization in patients with chronic legulcers or stasis dermatitis - new data from the Information Network of Departments of Dermatology (IVDK). Contact Dermatitis 2017;77:151-158

61 Frosch PJ, Johansen JD, Schuttelaar M-LA, Silvestre JF, Sánchez-Pérez J, Weisshaar E, et al. (on behalf of the ESSCA network). Patch test results with fragrance markers of the baseline series – analysis of the European Surveillance System on Contact Allergies (ESSCA) network 2009–2012. Contact Dermatitis 2015;73:163-171

62 Molin S, Bauer A, Schnuch A, Geier J. Occupational contact allergy in nurses: results from the Information Network of Departments of Dermatology 2003–2012. Contact Dermatitis 2015;72:164-171

63 Warshaw EM, Zug KA, Belsito DV, Fowler JF Jr, DeKoven JG, Sasseville D, et al. Positive patch-test reactions to essential oils in consecutive patients: Results from North America and Central Europe. Dermatitis 2017;28:246-252

64 De Groot AC, Schmidt E. Essential oils, Part VI: Sandalwood oil, ylang-ylang oil, and jasmine absolute. Dermatitis 2017;28:14-21

65 DeKoven JG, Warshaw EM, Belsito DV, Sasseville D, Maibach HI, Taylor JS, et al. North American Contact Dermatitis Group Patch Test Results: 2013-2014. Dermatitis 2017;28:33-46

66 Hagen SL, Grey KR, Warshaw EM. Patch testing to essential oils. Dermatitis 2016;27:382-384

67 Tan LT, Lee LH, Yin WF, Chan CK, Abdul Kadir H, Chan KG, Goh BH. Traditional uses, phytochemistry, and bioactivities of Cananga odorata (Ylang-ylang). Evid Based Complement Alternat Med 2015;2015:896314. doi: 10.1155/2015/896314

68 Sabroe RA, Holden CR, Gawkrodger DJ. Contact allergy to essential oils cannot always be predicted from allergy to fragrance markers in the baseline series. Contact Dermatitis 2016;74:236-241

69 Girbig M, Hegewald J, Seidler A, Bauer A, Uter W, Schmitt J. Type IV sensitizations in physical therapists: patch test results of the Information Network of Departments of Dermatology (IVDK) 2007-2011. J Dtsch Dermatol Ges 2013;11:1185-1192

70 Silvestre JF, Mercader P, González-Pérez R, Hervella-Garcés M, Sanz-Sánchez T, Córdoba S, et al. Sensitization to fragrances in Spain: A 5-year multicentre study (2011-2015). Contact Dermatitis. 2018 Nov 14. doi: 10.1111/cod.13152. [Epub ahead of print]

71 DeKoven JG, Warshaw EM, Zug KA, Maibach HI, Belsito DV, Sasseville D, et al. North American Contact Dermatitis Group patch test results: 2015-2016. Dermatitis 2018;29:297-309

72 Nath NS, Liu B, Green C, Atwater AR. Contact allergy to hydroperoxides of linalool and d-limonene in a US population. Dermatitis 2017;28:313-316

Chapter 6.79   ZDRAVETZ OIL

IDENTIFICATION

Description/definition	: Zdravetz oil is the essential oil obtained from the aerial parts (above ground plant) of the bigroot (Bulgarian) geranium (zdravetz) *Geranium macrorrhizum* L.
INCI name(s) EU	: Geranium macrorrhizum herb oil (perfuming name, not officially an INCI name)
INCI name(s) USA	: Not in the Personal Care Products Council Ingredient Database
CAS registry number(s)	: 92347-05-2; 68991-32-2
EC number(s)	: 296-192-0
Function(s) in cosmetics	: EU: perfuming
Patch testing	: 2% pet. (8)

GENERAL

Geranium macrorrhizum L. (zdravetz) is a hardy, flowering, perennial plant that grows to a height of 30-50 cm and has a thick, succulent rhizome (underground stem, hence the name 'macrorrhizum', big root) and soft aromatic leaves. It is native to middle Europe (Austria), south-eastern Europe (Albania, Bulgaria, Croatia, Greece, Italy, Romania, Serbia, Slovenia) and south-western Europe (France) and naturalized elsewhere. In Bulgaria, *G. macrorrhizum* is widely grown as a cultural symbol associated with health and good luck and for its aromatic properties (2,7). 'Zdrave' is the Bulgarian word for 'health' (3); the common name of the plant in Serbian is 'zdravats', which could be translated as 'health' or 'to be healthy' (1).

Steam-distillation of the aerial parts of *Geranium macrorrhizum* yields the essential oil which is called zdravetz oil (sometimes spelled zdravets). The oil is used in traditional medicine, is also used in limited quantities in cigarette flavorings and is (rarely) employed in aromatherapy practices (4). The commercial oil, produced solely in Bulgaria, is mainly obtained from wild-growing plants and the total annual amount exported from Bulgaria may be very limited (possibly only several hundred kilograms) (2,3).

CHEMICAL COMPOSITION

Zdravetz oil at a temperature of over 20°C is a light to dark green clear liquid, which has a floral herbaceous, soft earthy odor. At lower temperatures, over half of the oil volume is taken up by large colorless prismatic crystals with no odor, formed by the ingredient germacrone. The liquid portion called 'eleoptene' contains all odorous components (2,3). Very little research on the composition of zdravetz oil has been performed. In fact, only one analytical study investigating the essential oil (one lab-hydrodistilled oil sample) of *G. macrorrhizum* has been published in the last 10 years (2).

In zdravetz oils from various origins, over 275 chemicals have been identified. About 79 per cent of these (notably chemicals found in traces in ref. 2, one lab-hydrodistilled oil from plants growing wild in Serbia) were found in a single reviewed publication only. The high percentage is strongly influenced by the paucity of recently reported studies on *G. macrorrhizum* essential oil. The ten chemicals that had the highest maximum concentrations in 8 commercial zdrawetz essential oil samples are shown in table 6.79.1 (Erich Schmidt, analytical data presented in ref. 7).

A full literature review of the qualitative and quantitative composition of commercial and non-commercial zdravetz oils of various origins has been published in 2016 (7).

Table 6.79.1 Ten ingredients with the highest concentrations in commercial zdravetz oils (7)

Name	Concentration range	Name	Concentration range
(*E,E*)-Germacrone	45.5 - 66.6%	γ-Eudesmol	0.4 - 2.5%
Germacrene B	4.5 - 11.2%	γ-Curcumene	1.0 - 2.4%
trans-β-Elemenone	1.4 - 5.9%	α-Pinene	0.05 - 2.1%
α-Eudesmol	0 - 5.3%	β-Eudesmol	0.4 - 2.1%
α-Bisabolol	0.06 - 2.8%	(*Z*)-β-Ocimene	0.8 - 1.6%

CONTACT ALLERGY / ALLERGIC CONTACT DERMATITIS

General

Contact allergy to zdravetz oil has been reported in two publications, but no cases of allergic contact dermatitis from the oil have been identified.

Patch testing in groups of patients

Two hundred dermatitis patients from Poland were tested with zdravetz oil 2% in petrolatum and one (0.5%) reacted. The same authors also patch tested 51 patients allergic to Myroxylon pereirae resin (balsam of Peru) and/or turpentine and/or wood tar and/or colophony and one (2.0%) had a positive patch test; relevance data were not provided (5). A group of 86 patients from Poland previously reacting to the fragrance mix was tested with zdravetz oil and four (4.6%) had a positive patch test reaction; relevance data were not provided (6).

LITERATURE

1   Chalchat J-C, Petrovic SD, Maksimovic ZA, Gorunovic MS. A comparative study on essential oils of *Geranium macrorrhizum* L. and *Geranium phaeum* L., Geraniaceae from Serbia. J Essent Oil Res 2002;14:333-335
2   Radulović NS, Dekić MS, Stojanović-Radić ZZ, Zoranić SK. *Geranium macrorrhizum* L. (Geraniaceae) essential oil: A potent agent against *Bacillus subtilis*. Chem Biodivers 2010;7:2783-2800
3   Ognyanov I. Bulgarian zdravets oil. Perfum Flavor 1985;10(Oct/Nov):39-44
4   Rhind JP. Essential oils. A handbook for aromatherapy practice, 2nd Edition. London: Singing Dragon, 2012
5   Rudzki E, Grzywa Z, Bruo WS. Sensitivity to 35 essential oils. Contact Dermatitis 1976;2:196-200
6   Rudzki E, Grzywa Z. Allergy to perfume mixture. Contact Dermatitis 1986;15:115-116
7   De Groot AC, Schmidt E. Essential oils: contact allergy and chemical composition. Boca Raton, Fl., USA: CRC Press, Taylor and Francis Group, 2016 (ISBN 9781482246407)
8   De Groot AC. Patch Testing, 4th Edition. Wapserveen, The Netherlands: acdegroot publishing, 2018 (ISBN 978-90-813233-4-5)

Monographs in Contact Allergy, Volume 2
Fragrances and Essential oils

SECTION 4

LISTS OF SYNONYMS AND INDEX

CHAPTER 7 LIST OF SYNONYMS OF FRAGRANCES

In this chapter, all synonyms of chemicals (including IUPAC names), used in this book by their INCI names, are listed alphabetically in the left column of table 7.1. In the right column, their corresponding INCI names are given (or Monograph names where no INCI names are available). These are all discussed in separate Monographs/Chapters. The page numbers of these Chapters (where the corresponding synonyms can be found) are listed in the Index and the Contents section.

Table 7.1 List of synonyms: Conversion of synonyms to INCI names or Chapter names

Synonym	INCI name / Chapter name
A	
Acetivenol ®	Vetiveryl acetate
5-Acetyl-1,1,2,3,3,6-hexamethylindan	Acetyl hexamethyl indan
6-Acetyl-1,1,2,4,4,7-hexamethyltetralin	Acetyl hexamethyl tetralin
Acetyl isoeugenol	Isoeugenyl acetate
4-(Acetyloxymethyl)-10-formyl-3,9-dihydroxy-1,7-dimethyl-6-oxobenzo[b][1,4]benzodioxepine-2-carboxylic acid	Physodalic acid
Alcohol C-8	Caprylic alcohol
Alcohol C-9	Nonyl alcohol
Aldehyde C-7	Heptanal
Aldehyde C-9	Nonanal
5-Allyl-1,3-benzodioxole	Safrole
Allyl cyclohexanepropionate	Allyl cyclohexylpropionate
1-Allyl-4-methoxybenzene	Allylanisole
4-Allylveratrole	Methyl eugenol
Ambretone ®	5-Cyclohexadecenone
α-Amylcinnamaldehyde	Amyl cinnamal
α-Amylcinnamic alcohol	Amylcinnamyl alcohol
α-Amyl cinnamic aldehyde	Amyl cinnamal
Anise camphor	Anethole
Anisic alcohol	Anise alcohol
Anisyl alcohol	Anise alcohol
Artificial almond oil	Benzaldehyde
Atranoric acid	Atranorin
B	
Balsam fir oleoresin (*Abies balsamea* (L.) Mill.)	Myroxylon pereirae resin
Balsam Peru	Myroxylon pereirae resin
Benzenecarbaldehyde	Benzaldehyde
Benzene carboxaldehyde	Benzaldehyde
Benzeneethanol	Phenethyl alcohol
Benzeneethanol, α,α-dimethyl-, acetate	Dimethylbenzyl carbinyl acetate
Benzenepropanol	Phenylpropanol
1,3-Benzodioxole-5-carbaldehyde	Heliotropine
3-(1,3-Benzodioxol-5-yl)-2-methylpropanal	Methylenedioxyphenyl methylpropanal
Benzoic acid, 2-hydroxy-, hexyl ester	Hexyl salicylate
2*H*-1-Benzopyran-2-one	Coumarin
Benzyl 2-hydroxybenzoate	Benzyl salicylate
Benzyl (*E* or *Z*)-3-(3-hydroxy-4-methoxyphenyl)prop-2-enoate	Benzyl isoferulate
2-Benzylideneheptanal	Amyl cinnamal
2-Benzylideneheptan-1-ol	Amylcinnamyl alcohol
2-Benzylideneoctanal	Hexyl cinnamal
Benzyl 3-phenylprop-2-enoate	Benzyl cinnamate
Benzyl propanoate	Benzyl propionate
Bergamol	Linalyl acetate

Table 7.1 List of synonyms: Conversion of synonyms to INCI names or Chapter names (continued)

Synonym	INCI name / Chapter name
2-(4-*tert*-Butylbenzyl)propionaldehyde	Butylphenyl methylpropional
1-(4-*tert*-Butyl-2,6-dimethyl-3,5-dinitrophenyl)ethenone	Musk ketone
1-*tert*-Butyl-3,5-dimethyl-2,4,6-trinitrobenzene	Musk xylene
1-*tert*-Butyl-2-methoxy-4-methyl-3,5-dinitrobenzene	Musk ambrette
p-tert-Butyl-α-methylhydrocinnamic aldehyde	Butylphenyl methylpropional
3-(4-*tert*-Butylphenyl)-2-methylpropanal	Butylphenyl methylpropional
1-*tert*-Butyl-3,4,5-trimethyl-2,6-dinitrobenzene	Musk tibetene
5-*tert*-Butyl-1,2,3-trimethyl-4,6-dinitrobenzene	Musk tibetene

C

Cajeputene	*D,L*-Limonene
Cajeputol	Eucalyptol
Camphogen	*p*-Cymene
(+)-Camphor	*D*-Camphor
(-)-Camphor	*L*-Camphor
(*R*)-Camphor	*D*-Camphor
(*S*)-Camphor	*L*-Camphor
Capryl alcohol	Caprylic alcohol
4-[[(*E*)-3-Carboxyprop-2-enoyl]oxymethyl]-10-formyl-3,9-dihydroxy-1,7-dimethyl-6-oxobenzo[b][1,4]benzodioxepine-2-carboxylic acid	Fumarprotocetraric acid
delta-3- / δ-3- / *S*-3-Carene	3-Carene
4-Carvomenthenol	4-Terpineol
3-Carvomenthenone	Piperitone
Caryophyllene	beta-Caryophyllene
trans-Caryophyllene	beta-Caryophyllene
Cashmeran ®	Dihydro pentamethylindanone
Cedramber	Cedrol methyl ether
Cephrol	β-Citronellol
3-Chloro-2,6-Dihydroxy-4-methylbenzaldehyde	Chloroatranol
Chromen-2-one	Coumarin
1,8-Cineole	Eucalyptol
Cinnamaldehyde	Cinnamal
Cinnamein	Benzyl cinnamate
Cinnamic acid, methyl ester	Methyl cinnamate
Cinnamic alcohol	Cinnamyl alcohol
Cinnamic aldehyde	Cinnamal
cis-Citral	Neral
trans-Citral	Geranial
α-Citral	Geranial
β-Citral	Neral
Citral A	Geranial
Citral B	Neral
α-Citronellol	Rhodinol
DL-Citronellol	β-Citronellol
Coniferol	Coniferyl alcohol
Cyclacet ®	Verdyl acetate
Cyclohexadec-5-en-1-one	5-Cyclohexadecenone
Cyclohexanol, 5-methyl-2-(1-methylethyl)-, acetate	Menthyl acetate
Cyclopentaneacetic acid, 3-oxo-2-pentyl-, methyl ester	Methyldihydrojasmonate
Cycloverdyl acetate	Verdyl acetate
p-Cymen-3-ol	Thymol
p-Cymol	*p*-Cymene

Table 7.1 List of synonyms: Conversion of synonyms to INCI names or Chapter names (continued)

Synonym	INCI name / Chapter name
D	
Damascenone	Rose ketone-4
2,6-Diacetyl-7,9-dihydroxy-8,9b-dimethyldibenzofuran-1,3-dione	Usnic acid
1,1-Diethoxy-3,7-dimethylocta-2,6-diene	Citral diethyl acetal
Diethyl (Z)-but-2-enedioate	Diethyl maleate
Dihydroambrettolide	Hexadecanolactone
3,4-Dihydro-2H-1-benzopyran-2-one	Dihydrocoumarin
3,4-Dihydrochromen-2-one	Dihydrocoumarin
2,3-Dihydrocitral	Citronellal
Dihydro-p-cymene	alpha-Phellandrene
6,7-Dihydro-1,1,2,3,3-pentamethyl-4(5H)-indanone	Dihydro pentamethylindanone
2,6-Dihydroxy-4-methylbenzaldehyde	Atranol
3,9-Dihydroxy-6-oxo-7-(2-oxoheptyl)-1-pentylbenzo[b][1,4]-benzodioxepine-2-carboxylic acid	Physodic acid
Diisoeugenol, dehydro-	Dehydrodiisoeugenol
1,2-Dimethoxy-4-prop-1-enylbenzene	Methyl isoeugenol
1,2-Dimethoxy-4-prop-2-enylbenzene	Methyl eugenol
3,4-Dimethoxypropenylbenzene	Methyl isoeugenol
2-(6,6-Dimethyl-4-bicyclo[3.1.1]hept-3-enyl)ethyl acetate	Nopyl acetate
2,4-Dimethylcyclohex-3-ene-1-carbaldehyde	2,4-Dimethyl-3-cyclohexene carboxaldehyde
2,4(or 3,5)-Dimethyl-3-cyclohexene-1-carboxaldehyde	Dimethyltetrahydro benzaldehyde
1-(1,1-Dimethylethyl)-3,5-dimethyl-2,4,6-trinitrobenzene	Musk xylene
3,7-Dimethyl-7-methoxyoctan-2-ol	Methoxytrimethylheptanol
Dimethyl-2-methylbut-2-enedioate	Dimethyl citraconate
6,6-Dimethyl-4-methylidenebicyclo[3.1.1]heptane	beta-Pinene
(4R)-3,3-Dimethyl-2-methylidenebicyclo[2.2.1]heptane; 2-methoxyphenol	2-Methoxyphenol/2,2-dimethyl-3-methyl-idenebicycloheptane hydrogenated
Dimethyl methyl maleate	Dimethyl citraconate
2,2-Dimethyl-3-(3-methylphenyl)propan-1-ol	Trimethylbenzenepropanol
3,7-Dimethyl-2,6-octadienal	Citral
(2E)-3,7-Dimethyl-2,6-octadienal	Geranial
(2Z)-3,7-Dimethylocta-2,6-dienal	Neral
3,7-Dimethyl-2,6-octadienal diethyl acetal	Citral diethyl acetal
3,7-Dimethylocta-1,6-dien-3-ol	Linalool
(2E)-3,7-Dimethylocta-2,6-dien-1-ol	Geraniol
(2Z)-3,7-Dimethylocta-2,6-dien-1-ol	Nerol
trans-3,7-Dimethyl-2,6-octadien-1-ol	Geraniol
3,7-Dimethylocta-1,6-dien-3-yl acetate	Linalyl acetate
[(2E)-3,7-Dimethylocta-2,6-dienyl] acetate	Geranyl acetate
3,7-Dimethyloctane-1,7-diol	Hydroxycitronellol
Dimethyl octanol	Dihydrocitronellol
3,7-Dimethyl-1-octanol	Dihydrocitronellol
3,7-Dimethyloct-6-enal	Citronellal
3,7-Dimethyloct-6-en-1-ol	β-Citronellol
(3S)-3,7-Dimethyloct-7-en-1-ol	Rhodinol
α,α-Dimethylphenethyl acetate	Dimethylbenzyl carbinyl acetate
1,1-Dimethyl-2-phenylethyl acetate	Dimethylbenzyl carbinyl acetate
(4,8-Dimethyl-2-propan-2-ylidene-3,3a,4,5,6,8a-hexahydro-1H-azulen-6-yl) acetate	Vetiveryl acetate
3,6-Dimethyl-4,5,6,7-tetrahydro-1-benzofuran	Tetrahydro-dimethylbenzofuran
5-(2,3-Dimethyl-4,5,6,7-tetrahydro-1H-tricyclo[2.2.1.0^{2,6}]heptan-3-yl)-2-methylpent-2-en-1-ol	α-Santalol
2,2-Dimethyl-3-(3-tolyl)propan-1-ol	Trimethylbenzenepropanol
1,4-Dioxacyclohexadecane-5,16-dione	Ethylene dodecanedioate

Table 7.1 List of synonyms: Conversion of synonyms to INCI names or Chapter names (continued)

Synonym	INCI name / Chapter name
Dipentene	*D,L*-Limonene

E

Ebanol ®	3-Methyl-5-(2,2,3-trimethyl-3-cyclo-pentenyl)pent-4-en-2-ol
Elenol	β-Citronellol
Estragole	Allylanisole
Ethenol, 2-phenyl-, 1-acetate	Styryl acetate
3-Ethoxy-4-hydroxybenzaldehyde	Ethyl vanillin
Ethyl 4-methoxybenzoate	Ethyl anisate
Ethyl *p*-methoxybenzoate	Ethyl anisate
Eugenyl methyl ether	Methyl eugenol

F

Farnesyl alcohol	Farnesol
Fixolide	Acetyl hexamethyl tetralin
Fixolide ®	Acetyl hexamethyl indan
Floropal ®	2,4,6-Trimethyl-4-phenyl-1,3-dioxane
4-Formyl-1,3-dimethylcyclohex-1-ene	2,4-Dimethyl-3-cyclohexene carboxaldehyde

G

Galaxolide ®	Hexamethylindanopyran
Galbanum resin / gum	Ferula galbaniflua gum
Gardenia acetal	2,4,6-Trimethyl-4-phenyl-1,3-dioxane
Geranial diethyl acetal	Citral diethyl acetal
(*Z*)-Geraniol	Nerol
Geraniol acetate	Geranyl acetate
Geranyl alcohol	Geraniol
Greenyl acetate	Verdyl acetate

H

Hedione ®	Methyldihydrojasmonate
Helional ®	Methylenedioxyphenyl methylpropanal
Heptaldehyde	Heptanal
Hesperetic acid	Isoferulic acid
Hexadecanolide	Hexadecanolactone
Ω-6-Hexadecenlactone	Ambrettolide
6-Hexadecen-16-olide	Ambrettolide
1,3,4,6,7,8-Hexahydro-4,6,6,7,8,8-hexamethylindeno(5,6-c)pyran	Hexamethylindanopyran
3a,4,5,6,7,7a-Hexahydro-4,7-methanoinden-6-yl acetate	Verdyl acetate
(3*R*-(3α,3αβ,7b,8aα))-1-(2,3,4,7,8,8a-Hexahydro-3,6,8,8-tetramethyl-1*H*-3a,7-methanoazulen-5-yl)ethan-1-one	Acetylcedrene
1-(3,5,5,6,8,8-Hexamethyl-6,7-dihydronaphthalen-2-yl)ethanone	Acetyl hexamethyl tetralin
1,1,2,3,3,6-Hexamethylindan-5-yl methyl ketone	Acetyl hexamethyl indan
1-(1,1,2,3,3,6-Hexamethyl-2*H*-inden-5-yl)ethenone	Acetyl hexamethyl indan
4,6,6,7,8,8-Hexamethyl-1,3,4,7-tetrahydrocyclopenta[g]isochromene	Hexamethylindanopyran
[(*Z*)-Hex-3-enyl] 2-hydroxybenzoate	*cis*-3-Hexenyl salicylate
α-Hexylcinnamaldehyde	Hexyl cinnamal
Hexyl cinnamic aldehyde	Hexyl cinnamal
Hexyl 2-hydroxybenzoate	Hexyl salicylate
HICC	Hydroxyisohexyl 3-cyclohexene carboxaldehyde

Table 7.1 List of synonyms: Conversion of synonyms to INCI names or Chapter names (continued)

Synonym	INCI name / Chapter name
Hivertal ®	Dimethyltetrahydro benzaldehyde
Hyacinthin	Phenylacetaldehyde
Hydrocinnamic alcohol	Phenylpropanol
Hydrocinnamyl alcohol	Phenylpropanol
2-Hydroxybenzaldehyde	Salicylaldehyde
2-Hydroxy-*p*-cymene	Carvacrol
7-Hydroxy-3,7-dimethyloctanal	Hydroxycitronellal
2-Hydroxy-4-(2-hydroxy-4-methoxy-6-methylbenzoyl)oxy-6-methylbenzoic acid	Evernic acid
γ-Hydroxyisoeugenol	Coniferyl alcohol
4-Hydroxy-3-methoxybenzaldehyde	Vanillin
(3-Hydroxy-4-methoxycarbonyl-2,5-dimethylphenyl) 3-formyl-	Atranorin
3-Hydroxy-4-methoxycinnamic acid	Isoferulic acid
4-Hydroxy-3-methoxycinnamyl alcohol	Coniferyl alcohol
(*E*)-3-(3-Hydroxy-4-methoxyphenyl)prop-2-enoic acid	Isoferulic acid
3-(4-Hydroxy-3-methoxyphenyl)-2-propen-1-ol	Coniferyl alcohol
3-(4-Hydroxy-3-methoxyphenyl)prop-2-enyl benzoate	Coniferyl benzoate
3 and 4-(4-Hydroxy-4-methylpentyl)cyclohex-3-ene-1-carbaldehyde	Hydroxyisohexyl 3-cyclohexene carboxaldehyde
3-Hydroxy-2-methylpyran-4-one	Maltol
4-(3-Hydroxyprop-1-enyl)-2-methoxyphenol	Coniferyl alcohol

I

Synonym	INCI name / Chapter name
α-Irone	5-Methyl-alpha-ionone
Isoanethole	Allylanisole
Isobornyl cyclohexanol	Camphylcyclohexanol
Isobornyl cyclohexanol	5,5,6-Trimethylbicyclohept-2-ylcyclohexanol
Isocamphyl cyclohexanol (mixed isomers)	5,5,6-Trimethylbicyclohept-2-ylcyclohexanol
Isocyclemone E	Tetramethyl acetyloctahydronaphthalene
Isodiprene	3-Carene
Isoestragole	Anethole
Iso E super ®	Tetramethyl acetyloctahydronaphthalene
Isoeugenol benzyl ether	Benzyl isoeugenol
Isoeugenol, dehydrodi-	Dehydrodiisoeugenol
Isoeugenyl methyl ether	Methyl isoeugenol
Isoeugenyl α-toluate	Isoeugenyl phenylacetate
Isolongifolene ketone	Isolongifolanone
Isomethyleugenol	Methyl isoeugenol
α-Isomethyl ionone	Methyl ionones
β-Isomethyl ionone	Methyl ionones
Isopentyl 2-hydroxybenzoate	Isoamyl salicylate
4-Isopropylbenzaldehyde	Cuminaldehyde
Isopropyl-*m*-cresol	Thymol
5-Isopropyl-*o*-cresol	Carvacrol
4-Isopropylidene-1-methylcyclohexene	Terpinolene
4-Isopropyl-1-methylcyclohexane-1,2,4-triol	1,2,4-Trihydroxymenthane
1-Isopropyl-4-methylenebicyclo[3.1.0]hexane	Sabinene
4-Isopropyltoluene	*p*-Cymene
Isoterpinene	Terpinolene
Isothymol	Carvacrol
2,4-Ivy carbaldehyde	2,4-Dimethyl-3-cyclohexene carboxaldehyde

J

Synonym	INCI name / Chapter name
Juniperolactone	Hexadecanolactone

Table 7.1 List of synonyms: Conversion of synonyms to INCI names or Chapter names (continued)

Synonym	INCI name / Chapter name

L

Larixinic acid	Maltol
Lignyl acetate	Nopyl acetate
Ligustral ®	2,4-Dimethyl-3-cyclohexene carboxaldehyde
Lilial ®	Butylphenyl methylpropional
Lily propanol	Trimethylbenzenepropanol
(+)-Limonene	*D*-Limonene
(-)-limonene	*L*-Limonene
α-Limonene	*D*-Limonene
β-Limonene	*L*-Limonene
(*R*)-Limonene	*D*-Limonene
(*S*)-Limonene	*L*-Limonene
Linalyl alcohol	Linalool
Lyral ®	Hydroxyisohexyl 3-cyclohexene carboxaldehyde

M

Majantol ®	Trimethylbenzenepropanol
Melaleucol	Nerolidol
Melilotin	Dihydrocoumarin
p-Mentha-1,3-diene	alpha-Terpinene
p-Mentha-1,4(8)-diene	Terpinolene
p-Mentha-1,5-diene	alpha-Phellandrene
p-Mentha-1,8-diene	*D,L*-Limonene
(*R*)-*p*-Mentha-1,8-diene	*D*-Limonene
(*S*)-*p*-Mentha-1,8-diene	*L*-Limonene
1,8(9)-*p*-Menthadiene	*D,L*-Limonene
1-*p*-Menthen-4-ol	4-Terpineol
p-Menth-1-en-8-ol	alpha-Terpineol
p-Menth-8-en-2-ol	Dihydrocarveol
p-Menth-8-en-3-ol	Isopulegol
p-Menth-1-en-3-one	Piperitone
(1*R*)-(+)-*p*-Menth-4(8)-en-3-one	*D*-Pulegone
p-Menth-1-en-8-yl acetate	α-Terpinyl acetate
Menthofuran	Tetrahydro-dimethylbenzofuran
(+)-Menthol	*D*-Menthol
(-)-Menthol	*L*-Menthol
2-(*o*-) or 4-(*p*)-Methoxycinnamaldehyde	Methoxycinnamal
o- or *p*-Methoxycinnamic aldehyde	Methoxycinnamal
7-Methoxy-3,7-dimethyloctanal	Methoxycitronellal
7-Methoxy-3,7-dimethyloctan-2-ol	Methoxytrimethylheptanol
2-Methoxy-4-[7-methoxy-3-methyl-5-[(*E*)-prop-1-enyl]-2,3-dihydro-1-benzofuran-2-yl]phenol	Dehydrodiisoeugenol
4-(4-Methoxyphenyl)-3-buten-2-one	Anisylidene acetone
(4-Methoxyphenyl)methanol	Anise alcohol
2-Methoxy-1-phenylmethoxy-4-prop-1-enylbenzene	Benzyl isoeugenol
3-(2-Methoxyphenyl)prop-2-enal	Methoxycinnamal
1-Methoxy-4-(1-propenyl)benzene	Anethole
1-Methoxy-4-prop-2-enylbenzene	Allylanisole
2-Methoxy-4-(prop-1-enyl)phenol	Isoeugenol
2-Methoxy-4-prop-2-enylphenol	Eugenol
(2-Methoxy-4-prop-1-enylphenyl) acetate	Isoeugenyl acetate
(2-Methoxy-4-prop-1-enylphenyl) benzoate	Isoeugenyl benzoate
2-Methoxy-4-prop-1-enylphenyl phenylacetate	Isoeugenyl phenylacetate
Methyl 2-aminobenzoate	Methyl anthranilate

Table 7.1 List of synonyms: Conversion of synonyms to INCI names or Chapter names (continued)

Synonym	INCI name / Chapter name
Methyl 4-anisate	Methyl *p*-anisate
α-Methyl-1,3-benzodioxole-5-propionaldehyde	Methylenedioxyphenyl methylpropanal
3-Methylbutyl 2-hydroxybenzoate	Isoamyl salicylate
Methyl cedryl ketone	Acetylcedrene
Methyl chavicol	Allylanisole
6-Methylchromen-2-one	6-Methyl coumarin
Methyl coumarin	6-Methyl coumarin
2-(4-Methylcyclohex-3-en-1-yl)propan-2-ol	alpha-Terpineol
2-(4-Methylcyclohex-3-en-1-yl)propan-2-yl acetate	Terpineol acetate
Methyl heptine carbonate	Methyl 2-octynoate
Methyl 2-hydroxybenzoate	Methyl salicylate
2-Methyl-3-hydroxypyrone	Maltol
4-Methylidene-1-propan-2-ylbicyclo[3.1.0]hexane	Sabinene
Methyl-γ-ionone	alpha-Isomethyl ionone
α-Methyl ionone	Methyl ionones
β-Methyl ionone	Methyl ionones
γ-Methylionone	alpha-Isomethyl ionone
6-Methylionone	5-Methyl-alpha-ionone
6-Methyl-α-ionone	5-Methyl-alpha-ionone
1-Methyl-4-isopropenyl-1-cyclohexene	*D,L*-Limonene
1-Methyl-4-isopropyl-1,3-cyclohexadiene	alpha-Terpinene
Methyl 4-methoxybenzoate	Methyl *p*-anisate
1-Methyl-1-(4-methylcyclohex-3-enyl)ethyl ethanoate	α-Terpinyl acetate
(4*R*)-1-Methyl-4-(1-methylethenyl)cyclohexene	*D*-Limonene
1-Methyl-4-(1-methylethyl)benzene	*p*-Cymene
4-Methyl-1-(1-methylethyl)-3-cyclohexen-1-ol	4-Terpineol
2-Methyl-5-(1-methylethyl)phenol	Carvacrol
5-Methyl-2-(1-methylethyl)phenol	Thymol
7-Methyl-3-methylideneocta-1,6-diene	Myrcene
2-Methyl-5-(3-methyl-2-methylidene-3-bicyclo[2.2.1]hepta-nyl)pent-2-en-1-ol	β-Santalol
2-Methyl-5-(1-methylvinyl)cyclohexanol	Dihydrocarveol
Methyl non-2-ynoate	Methyl octine carbonate
Methyl 2-nonynoate	Methyl octine carbonate
Methyl oct-2-ynoate	Methyl 2-octynoate
Methyl 2-(3-oxo-2-pentylcyclopentyl)acetate	Methyldihydrojasmonate
Methyl pentylacetylenecarboxylate	Methyl 2-octynoate
Methyl phenylacetate	Benzyl acetate
Methyl 3-phenylacrylate	Methyl cinnamate
(2-Methyl-1-phenylpropan-2-yl) acetate	Dimethylbenzyl carbinyl acetate
Methyl 3-phenylprop-2-enoate	Methyl cinnamate
1-Methyl-4-propan-2-ylbenzene	*p*-Cymene
1-Methyl-4-propan-2-ylcyclohexa-1,3-diene	alpha-Terpinene
2-Methyl-5-propan-2-ylcyclohexa-1,3-diene	alpha-Phellandrene
1-Methyl-4-propan-2-ylcyclohexane-1,2,4-triol	1,2,4-Trihydroxymenthane
5-Methyl-2-propan-2-ylcyclohexan-1-ol	*DL*-Menthol
(1*R*,2*S*,5*R*)-5-Methyl-2-propan-2-ylcyclohexan-1-ol	*L*-Menthol
(1*S*,2*R*,5*S*)-5-Methyl-2-propan-2-ylcyclohexan-1-ol	*D*-Menthol
4-Methyl-1-propan-2-ylcyclohex-3-en-1-ol	4-Terpineol
3-Methyl-6-propan-2-ylcyclohex-2-en-1-one	Piperitone
(5-Methyl-2-propan-2-ylcyclohexyl) acetate	Menthyl acetate
1-Methyl-4-propan-2-yl-2,3-dioxabicyclo[2.2.2]oct-5-ene	Ascaridole
(5*R*)-5-Methyl-2-propan-2-ylidenecyclohexan-1-one	*D*-Pulegone
1-Methyl-4-propan-2-ylidenecyclohexene	Terpinolene
2-Methyl-5-propan-2-ylphenol	Carvacrol
5-Methyl-2-propan-2-ylphenol	Thymol

Table 7.1 List of synonyms: Conversion of synonyms to INCI names or Chapter names (continued)

Synonym	INCI name / Chapter name
2-Methyl-5-prop-1-en-2-ylcyclohexan-1-ol	Dihydrocarveol
5-Methyl-2-prop-1-en-2-ylcyclohexan-1-ol	Isopulegol
1-Methyl-4-prop-1-en-2-ylcyclohexene	*D,L*-Limonene
(4*R*)-1-Methyl-4-prop-1-en-2-ylcyclohexene	*D*-Limonene
(4*S*)-1-Methyl-4-prop-1-en-2-ylcyclohexene	*L*-Limonene
(5*R* or 5*S*)-2-Methyl-5-prop-1-en-2-ylcyclohex-2-en-1-one	Carvone
Methyl α-toluate	Benzyl acetate
3-Methyl-4-(2,6,6-trimethylcyclohex-1-en-1-yl)but-3-en-2-one	Methyl ionones
3-Methyl-4-(2,6,6-trimethylcyclohex-2-en-1-yl)but-3-en-2-one	alpha-Isomethyl ionone
3-Methyl-4-(2,6,6-trimethylcyclohex-2-en-1-yl)but-3-en-2-one	Methyl ionones
3-Methyl-5-(2,2,3-trimethylcyclopent-3-en-1-yl)pentan-2-ol	Pentamethylcyclopent-3-ene-butanol
3-Methyl-5-(2,2,3-trimethylcyclopent-3-en-1-yl)pent-4-en-2-ol	3-Methyl-5-(2,2,3-trimethyl-3-cyclopentenyl)pent-4-en-2-ol
Moschus moschiferus L.	Musk
Moschus moschiferus L. pod grain absolute	Musk
Moskene	Musk moskene
Musk amberol	5-Cyclohexadecenone
Musk indane	Acetyl hexamethyl indan
Musk indanone	Dihydro pentamethylindanone
Muskonate	Ethylene dodecanedioate
Musk tetralin	Acetyl hexamethyl tetralin
Musk tonquin	Musk
Musk tonquin absolute	Musk
Musk xylol	Musk xylene
β-Myrcene	Myrcene

N

Narcissus absolute	Narcissus poeticus flower extract
Neomenthyl acetate	Menthyl acetate
Neroli oil, artificial	Methyl anthranilate
Neryl alcohol	Nerol
Nonan-1-ol	Nonyl alcohol
1-Nonanol	Nonyl alcohol
Nopinene	beta-Pinene
Nopol acetate	Nopyl acetate
Normuscone	Cyclopentadecanone

O

Oakmoss absolute	Evernia prunastri extract
Oakmoss extract	Evernia prunastri extract
(3*R*-(3α,3aβ,6β,7β,8aα))-Octahydro-6-methoxy-3,6,8,8-tetramethyl-1*H*-3a,7-methanoazulene	Cedrol methyl ether
1-(1,2,3,4,5,6,7,8-Octahydro-2,3,8,8-tetramethyl-2-naphthyl)ethan-1-one	Tetramethyl acetyloctahydronaphthalene
Octanol	Caprylic alcohol
Octan-1-ol	Caprylic alcohol
Octyl alcohol	Caprylic alcohol
Osyrol	Methoxytrimethylheptanol
Oxacycloheptadecan-2-one	Hexadecanolactone
Oxacycloheptadec-7-en-2-one	Ambrettolide

P

Parmelin	Atranorin
Parmelin acid	Atranorin

Table 7.1 List of synonyms: Conversion of synonyms to INCI names or Chapter names (continued)

Synonym	INCI name / Chapter name
Patchouli ethenone	Tetramethyl acetyloctahydronaphthalene
Pelargol	Dihydrocitronellol
Pelargonaldehyde	Nonanal
α,β,2,2,3-Pentamethylcyclopent-3-ene-1-butanol	Pentamethylcyclopent-3-ene-butanol
1,1,3,3,5-Pentamethyl-4,6-dinitro-2*H*-indene	Musk moskene
1,1,2,3,3-Pentamethyl-2,5,6,7-tetrahydroinden-4-one	Dihydro pentamethylindanone
Pentyl cinnamate	Amyl cinnamate
2-Pentylcinnamic alcohol	Amylcinnamyl alcohol
Pentyl 2-hydroxybenzoate	Amyl salicylate
Pentyl 3-phenyl-2-propenoate	Amyl cinnamate
2-Pentyl-3-phenylprop-2-en-1-ol	Amylcinnamyl alcohol
Pentyl salicylate	Amyl salicylate
1,4-Peroxido-*p*-menthene-2	Ascaridole
Peruviol	Nerolidol
Phantolide ®	Acetyl hexamethyl indan
Phenethyl carbinol	Phenylpropanol
Phenol, 4-(3-(benzoyloxy)-1-propenyl)-2-methoxy-	Coniferyl benzoate
Phenol, 2-methoxy-4-(1-propenyl)-, benzoate	Isoeugenyl benzoate
2-Phenylacetaldehyde	Phenylacetaldehyde
3-Phenylacrylic acid	Cinnamic acid
3-Phenylallyl benzoate	Cinnamyl benzoate
4-Phenylbut-3-en-2-one	Benzylidene acetone
2-Phenylethanol	Phenethyl alcohol
2-Phenylethenyl acetate	Styryl acetate
Phenylethyl alcohol	Phenethyl alcohol
Phenylmethanol	Benzyl alcohol
Phenylmethyl propionate	Benzyl propionate
3-Phenylpropan-1-ol	Phenylpropanol
3-Phenylprop-2-enal	Cinnamal
3-Phenylprop-2-enoic acid	Cinnamic acid
3-Phenylprop-2-en-1-ol	Cinnamyl alcohol
3-Phenyl-2-propenyl benzoate	Cinnamyl benzoate
3-Phenylprop-2-enyl 3-phenylprop-2-enoate	Cinnamyl cinnamate
Physodalin	Physodic acid
2-Pinene	alpha-Pinene
Piperonal	Heliotropine
Propanoic acid, phenylmethyl ester	Benzyl propionate
4-Propan-2-ylbenzaldehyde	Cuminaldehyde
5-Prop-2-enyl-1,3-benzodioxole	Safrole
5-[(*E* or *Z*)-Prop-1-enyl]-1,3-benzodioxole	Isosafrole
Prop-2-enyl 3-cyclohexylpropanoate	Allyl cyclohexylpropionate
2-Propenyl 3-cyclohexylpropanoate	Allyl cyclohexylpropionate
Propenylguaiacol benzoate	Isoeugenyl benzoate
Propenylguaiacol phenylacetate	Isoeugenyl phenylacetate
3-Propylidene-2-benzofuran-1-one	Propylidene phthalide
Pseudopinene	beta-Pinene
(+)-Pulegone	*D*-Pulegone
(*R*)-Pulegone	*D*-Pulegone

R

Rhodinol	β-Citronellol
Rose dihydroketone	beta-Damascone
Rose ketone-2 (*cis*- and *trans*-)	beta-Damascone

Table 7.1 List of synonyms: Conversion of synonyms to INCI names or Chapter names (continued)

Synonym	INCI name / Chapter name
S	
Sandal hexanol	5,5,6-Trimethylbicyclohept-2-ylcyclohexanol
Sandal octanol	Methoxytrimethylheptanol
Sandalore ®	Pentamethylcyclopent-3-ene-butanol
Sandal pentanol	Pentamethylcyclopent-3-ene-butanol
Sandal pentenol	3-Methyl-5-(2,2,3-trimethyl-3-cyclopentenyl)pent-4-en-2-ol
Santalex T ®	Camphylcyclohexanol
Santall	Camphylcyclohexanol
Shikimole	Safrole
Styracin	Cinnamyl cinnamate
Synthetic sweet birch oil	Methyl salicylate
Synthetic wintergreen oil	Methyl salicylate
T	
Terpenol	alpha-Terpineol
Terpen-4-ol	4-Terpineol
Terpinen-4-ol	4-Terpineol
4-Terpinenol	4-Terpineol
4,5,6,7-Tetrahydro-3,6-dimethylbenzofuran	Tetrahydro-dimethylbenzofuran
Tetrahydrogeraniol	Dihydrocitronellol
1-(5,6,7,8-Tetrahydro-3,5,5,6,8,8-hexamethyl-2-naphthyl)ethan-1-one	Acetyl hexamethyl tetralin
4-(2,5,6,6-Tetramethylcyclohex-2-en-1-yl)but-3-en-2-one	5-Methyl-alpha-ionone
1,1,4,7-Tetramethyl-1a,2,3,5,6,7,7a,7b-octahydrocyclopropa[e]azulene	Ledene
2,2,8,8-Tetramethyl-octahydro-1H-2,4a-methanonapthalene-10-one	Isolongifolanone
1-(2,3,8,8-Tetramethyl-1,2,3,4,5,6,7,8-octahydronaphthalen-2-yl)ethanone	Tetramethyl acetyloctahydronaphthalene
2,2,7,7-Tetramethyltricyclo[6.2.1.0^{1,6}]undecan-5-one	Isolongifolanone
3,3,7,11-Tetramethyltricyclo[6.3.0.02.4]undec-7-ene	Ledene
4(10)-Thujene	Sabinene
α-Tolualdehyde	Phenylacetaldehyde
Tonalide ®	Acetyl hexamethyl tetralin
Treemoss absolute	Evernia furfuracea extract
Treemoss extract	Evernia furfuracea extract
Tricyclo decenyl acetate	Verdyl acetate
Tricyclo(5.2.1.02,6)dec-4-en-8-yl acetate	Verdyl acetate
β,β,3-Trimethylbenzenepropanol	Trimethylbenzenepropanol
4,7,7-Trimethylbicyclo[2.2.1]heptan-3-one	*DL*-Camphor
(1*R*,4*R*)-4,7,7-Trimethylbicyclo[2.2.1]heptan-3-one	*D*-Camphor
(1*S*,4*S*)-4,7,7-Trimethylbicyclo[2.2.1]heptan-3-one	*L*-Camphor
1-(1,7,7-Trimethylbicyclo[2.2.1]heptan-2-yl)cyclohexan-1-ol	Camphylcyclohexanol
1-(4,7,7-Trimethyl-3-bicyclo[2.2.1]heptanyl)cyclohexan-1-ol	Camphylcyclohexanol
3-(2,2,3-Trimethyl-5-bicyclo[2.2.1]heptanyl)cyclohexan-1-ol	5,5,6-Trimethylbicyclohept-2-ylcyclohexanol
3-(5,5,6-Trimethylbicyclo[2.2.1]heptan-2-yl)cyclohexanol	5,5,6-Trimethylbicyclohept-2-ylcyclohexanol
3,7,7-Trimethylbicyclo[4.1.0]hept-3-ene	3-Carene
4,6,6-Trimethylbicyclo[3.1.1]hept-3-ene	alpha-Pinene
1-(2,6,6-Trimethyl-1,3-cyclohexadien-1yl)-2-buten-1-one	Rose ketone-4
1-(2,6,6-Trimethyl-2-cyclohexen-1-yl)-2-buten-1-one	alpha-Damascone
1-(2,6,6-Trimethylcyclohexen-1-yl)but-2-en-1-one (*E*- or *Z*-)	beta-Damascone
(*E*)-4-(2,6,6-Trimethyl-1-cyclohexen-1-yl)but-3-en-2-one	beta-Ionone

Table 7.1 List of synonyms: Conversion of synonyms to INCI names or Chapter names (continued)

Synonym	INCI name / Chapter name
(*E*)-4-(2,6,6-Trimethyl-2-cyclohexen-1-yl)but-3-en-2-one	alpha-Ionone
1-(2,6,6-Trimethylcyclohex-1-en-1-yl)pent-1-en-3-one	Methyl ionones
1-(2,6,6-Trimethylcyclohex-2-en-1-yl)pent-1-en-3-one	Methyl ionones
3,7,11-Trimethyldodeca-1,6,10-trien-3-ol	Nerolidol
3,7,11-Trimethyldodeca-2,6,10-trien-1-ol	Farnesol
1,1,7-Trimethyl-4-methylene-2,3,4a,5,6,7,7a,7b-octahydro-1a*H*-cyclopropa[e]azulene	Aromadendrene
(1*R*-(1*R**,4*R**,6*R**,10*S**))-4,12,12-Trimethyl-9-methylene-5-oxatricyclo[8.2.0.04,6]dodecane	Caryophyllene oxide
(1*R*,4*E*,9*S*)-4,11,11-Trimethyl-8-methylidenbicyclo[7.2.0]undec-4-ene	beta-Caryophyllene
1,2,3-Trimethyl-5-(2-methyl-2-propanyl)-4,6-dinitrobenzene	Musk tibetene
2,2,4-Trimethyl-3-oxabicyclo[2.2.2]octane	Eucalyptol
Triplal ®	2,4-Dimethyl-3-cyclohexene carboxaldehyde
Tropional	Methylenedioxyphenyl methylpropanal

U

Usmarin	Atranorin
Usmarin acid	Atranorin

V

Vanillaldehyde	Vanillin
Vanillic aldehyde	Vanillin
Vertofix ®	Acetylcedrene
Vetiver acetate	Vetiveryl acetate
Vetiverol acetate	Vetiveryl acetate
Violet leaves absolute	Viola odorata leaf extract
Viridiflorene / Viridiflorine / Viridoflorene	Ledene

Chapter 8   LIST OF SYNONYMS OF ESSENTIAL OILS

For convenience sake, for the monograph titles of essential oils, their 'common' names are used instead of their (more difficult and less well known) INCI names. In table 8.1, all synonyms of these essential oils, including their INCI names, are listed alphabetically in the left column. In the right column, their corresponding Monograph (Chapter) names are shown. The page numbers of these Chapters (where the corresponding synonyms can be found) are listed in the Index and the Contents section.

Table 8.1 List of synonyms: Conversion of synonyms and INCI names to Chapter names

Synonym or INCI name	Chapter name
A	
Abies alba leaf / needle oil	Silver fir oil
Acorus calamus root oil	Calamus oil
Angelica archangelica seed / root oil	Angelica oil (fruit, root)
Aniba rosaeodora (rosewood) wood oil	Rosewood oil
Anthemis nobilis flower oil	Chamomile oil (Roman)
Azadirachta indica seed extract	Neem oil
B	
Bay leaf oil	Bay oil
Bay oil, sweet	Laurel leaf oil
Bergamot orange oil	Bergamot oil
Boswellia carterii oil / gum oil	Olibanum oil
Bulnesia sarmientoi wood oil	Guaiacwood oil
C	
Cajuput oil	Cajeput oil
Cananga odorata flower oil	Ylang-ylang oil
Cananga odorata macrophylla flower extract	Cananga oil
Canarium luzonicum gum oil	Elemi oil
Cedar leaf oil	Thuja oil
Cedrus atlantica wood oil	Cedarwood oil (Atlas)
Cedrus deodara wood oil	Cedarwood oil (Himalaya)
Chamomile oil Hungarian	Chamomile oil (German)
Chamomilla recutita flower oil	Chamomile oil (German)
Chamomilla recutita (matricaria) flower oil	Chamomile oil (German)
Chinese cinnamon oil	Cassia bark oil
Cinnamomum cassia leaf oil	Cassia leaf oil
Cinnamomum cassia oil	Cassia bark oil
Cinnamomum zeylanicum bark / leaf oil	Cinnamon oil (bark, leaf)
Citrus aurantium amara (bitter orange) flower oil	Neroli oil
Citrus aurantium amara (bitter orange) leaf / twig oil	Petitgrain bigarade oil
Citrus aurantium amara (bitter orange) peel oil	Orange oil (bitter)
Citrus aurantium bergamia (bergamot) fruit / peel oil	Bergamot oil
Citrus aurantium dulcis (orange) peel oil	Orange oil (sweet)
Citrus aurantium leaf oil	Petitgrain bigarade oil
Citrus limon (lemon) peel oil	Lemon oil
Citrus nobilis (mandarin orange) peel oil	Mandarin oil
Citrus paradisi (grapefruit) peel oil	Grapefruit oil
Citrus sinensis (Valencia) peel oil expressed	Orange oil (sweet)
Citrus tangerina (tangerine) peel oil	Tangerine oil
Commiphora myrrha / abyssinica gum oil	Myrrh oil
Coriandrum sativum (coriander) fruit oil	Coriander fruit oil
Cupressus funebris wood oil	Cedarwood oil (China)
Cupressus sempervirens (leaf) oil	Cypress oil

Table 8.1 List of synonyms: Conversion of synonyms and INCI names to Chapter names (continued)

Synonym or INCI name	Chapter name
Cus cus oil	Vetiver oil
Cymbopogon citratus leaf oil	Lemongrass oil (West Indian)
Cymbopogon flexuosus oil	Lemongrass oil (East Indian)
Cymbopogon martini motia herb oil	Palmarosa oil
Cymbopogon nardus (citronella) oil	Citronella oil (Sri Lanka)
Cymbopogon winterianus herb oil	Citronella oil (Java)

D

Daucus carota fruit oil	Carrot seed oil

E

Elettaria cardamomum seed oil	Cardamom oil
English chamomile oil	Chamomile oil (Roman)
Eucalyptus citriodora oil	Eucalyptus oil (citriodora)
Eucalyptus globulus leaf / twig oil	Eucalyptus oil (globulus)
Eugenia caryophyllus (clove) bud / leaf / stem oil	Clove oil (bud, leaf, stem)

F

Ferula galbaniflua (galbanum) resin oil	Galbanum resin oil
Fir needle oil	Silver fir oil
Frankincense oil	Olibanum oil

G

Geranium macrorrhizum herb oil	Zdravetz oil

H

Hyssopus officinalis leaf oil	Hyssop oil

I

Illicium verum (anise) fruit / seed oil	Star anise oil

J

Jasminum grandiflorum / sambac (jasmine) flower extract	Jasmine absolute (grandiflorum, sambac)
Juniperus communis fruit oil	Juniper berry oil
Juniperus mexicana (wood) oil	Cedarwood oil (Texas)
Juniperus virginiana (wood) oil	Cedarwood oil (Virginia)

K

Khas khas oil	Vetiver oil
Khus oil	Vetiver oil

L

Laurus nobilis leaf oil	Laurel leaf oil
Lavandula angustifolia (lavender) oil	Lavender oil
Lavandula hybrida abrial / grosso herb oil	Lavandin oil (Abrial, Grosso))
Lavandula hybrida (herb) oil	Lavandin oil
Lavandula intermedia oil	Lavandin oil
Lavandula latifolia herb oil	Spike lavender oil
Lavandula officinalis flower oil	Lavender oil

Table 8.1 List of synonyms: Conversion of synonyms and INCI names to Chapter names (continued)

Synonym or INCI name	Chapter name
Lavandula spica (spike lavender) flower oil	Spike lavender oil
Levisticum officinale oil	Lovage oil

M

Margosa oil / extract	Neem oil
Matricaria oil	Chamomile oil (German)
Matricaria recutita flower oil	Chamomile oil (German)
Melaleuca alternifolia (tea tree) leaf oil	Tea tree oil
Melaleuca leucadendron cajaput / cajuputi leaf oil	Cajeput oil
Melaleuca quinquenervia oil	Niaouli oil
Melia azadirachta seed extract	Neem oil
Mentha piperita (peppermint) oil	Peppermint oil
Mentha spicata herb oil	Spearmint oil
Mentha viridis (spearmint) leaf oil	Spearmint oil
Myristica fragrans (nutmeg) kernel oil	Nutmeg oil

N

Nigella sativa seed extract	Black cumin oil

O

Ocimum basilicum (basil) flower/leaf extract	Basil oil
Ocimum basilicum herb oil	Basil oil
Oil of santal	Sandalwood oil (East India)
Origanum majorana flower oil	Marjoram oil

P

Pelargonium graveolens oil	Geranium oil
Pimenta acris (bay) leaf oil	Bay oil
Pimpinella anisum (anise) fruit oil	Aniseed oil
Pine scotch oil	Pine needle oil
Pinus mugo leaf oil	Dwarf pine oil
Pinus pumilio branch / leaf oil	Dwarf pine oil
Pinus sylvestris leaf oil	Pine needle oil
Piper nigrum (pepper) fruit oil	Black pepper oil
Pogostemon cablin leaf oil	Patchouli oil

R

Ravensara aromatica leaf / twig oil	Ravensara oil
Roman chamomile oil	Chamomile oil (Roman)
Rosa damascena flower oil	Rose oil
Rosmarinus officinalis (rosemary) leaf oil	Rosemary oil

S

Salvia lavandulifolia leaf / herb oil	Sage oil (Spanish)
Salvia officinalis (sage) oil	Sage oil (Dalmatian)
Salvia sclarea (flower) oil	Clary sage oil
Santalum album (sandalwood) oil	Sandalwood oil (East India)
Santalum austrocaledonicum wood oil	Sandalwood oil (New Caledonia)
Santalum spicata wood oil	Sandalwood oil (Australia)
Scots pine oil	Pine needle oil
Sweet bay oil	Laurel leaf oil

Table 8.1 List of synonyms: Conversion of synonyms and INCI names to Chapter names (continued)

Synonym or INCI name	Chapter name
T	
Thuja occidentalis leaf oil	Thuja oil
Thymus vulgaris (thyme) flower / leaf oil	Thyme oil
Thymus zygis flower oil	Thyme oil (Spanish)
V	
Valeriana officinalis root oil	Valerian oil
Vetiveria zizanoides root oil	Vetiver oil
Z	
Zingiber officinale (ginger) root oil	Ginger oil

Index

SYNONYMS AND THEIR LOCATIONS IN THE BOOK CAN BE FOUND IN CHAPTERS 7 and 8

SYNONYMS AND THEIR LOCATIONS IN THE BOOK CAN BE FOUND IN CHAPTERS 7 and 8

M (continued)

Methyl anthranilate, 474
Methyl benzoate, 529
alpha-Methylbenzyl alcohol, 529
Methyl cinnamate, 476
6-Methyl coumarin, 478
Methyldihydrojasmonate, 482
Methylenedioxyphenyl methylpropanal, 484
Methyl eugenol, 485
3'-Methylevernic acid, 274
2'-O-Methylevernic acid, 274
2,2'-di-O-Methylgyrophoric acid, 274
2'',4-di-O-Methylgyrophoric acid, 274
Methyl haematommate, 268
Methyl ionones, 487
5-Methyl-alpha-ionone, 489
Methyl isoeugenol, 491
Methyl 3'-methyllecanorate, 274
Methyl octine carbonate, 493
Methyl 2-octynoate, 495
Methyl beta-orcinolcarboxylate, 268

Methyl orsellinate, 268
2'-O-Methylphysodic acid, 268
2'-O-Methylphysodone, 268
Methyl salicylate, 500
3-Methyl-5-(2,2,3-trimethyl-3-cyclopen-
tenyl)pent-4-en-2-ol, 504
Methyl vanillyl ketone, 529
Microphyllinic acid, 268
Monoaryl compounds, 268
Musk, 506
Musk ambrette, 507
Musk ketone, 516
Musk moskene, 519
Musk tibetene, 521
Musk xylene, 523
alpha-Muurolene, 529
Myrcene, 525
Myristic acid, 529
Myroxylon pereirae resin, 527
Myrrh oil, 816

N

Naphthalene, 529
Narcissus poeticus flower extract, 553
Neem oil, 818
Neral, 555
Nerol, 557
Nerolidol, 559

Neroli oil, 820
Niaouli oil, 824
Nonanal, 561
Nonyl alcohol, 562
Nopyl acetate, 563
Nutmeg oil, 826

O

Ocimene, 529
1-Octacosanol, 529
Octadecanoic acid, 529
Olibanum oil (frankincense oil), 828
Olivetolcarboxylic acid, 268
Olivetonide, 268

Olivetoric acid, 268
Orange oil, 830
beta-Orcinol, 268
beta-Orcinolcarboxylic acid, 268
Orcinol monomethylether, 268
Oregano oil, 835

P

Palmarosa oil, 836
Palmitic acid, 529
Patchoulene, 529
Patchouli oil, 838
Pentamethylcyclopent-3-ene-butanol, 565
5-Pentylresorcinol, 268
Peppermint oil, 841
Perlatolic acid, 268
Petitgrain bigarade oil, 848
alpha-Phellandrene, 566
Phenethyl alcohol, 568
Phenylacetaldehyde, 570
1-Phenylethanol, 529

Phenylpropanol, 573
3-Phenylpropanol, 529
Physodalic acid, 658
Physodic acid, 659
Physodone, 268
alpha-Pinene, 574
Pine needle oil, 850
beta-Pinenes, 578
Piperitone, 581
Propylidene phthalide, 583
Prunastric acid, 274
Prunastrin, 274
D-Pulegone, 585